# Stroke Rehabilitation

## A Function-Based Approach

# Stroke Rehabilitation

## A Function-Based Approach

**GLEN GILLEN, EdD, OTR/L, BCN, FAOTA**

Assistant Professor in Clinical Occupational Therapy
Programs in Occupational Therapy
College of Physicians and Surgeons
Columbia University
New York, New York

**ANN BURKHARDT, OTD, OTR/L, BCN, FAOTA**

Director of Occupational Therapy
New York-Presbyterian Hospital
Columbia University Medical Center
Associate Clinical Instructor
Programs in Occupational Therapy
Columbia University
New York, New York

**SECOND EDITION**

*With **31** contributing authors*
*With **469** illustrations*

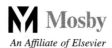

Mosby
*An Affiliate of Elsevier*

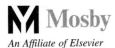 Mosby

*An Affiliate of Elsevier*

11830 Westline Industrial Drive
St. Louis, Missouri 63146

STROKE REHABILITATION: A FUNCTION-BASED APPROACH,
2ND EDITION

---

### NOTICE

Occupational therapy is an ever-changing field. Standard safety precautions must be followed, but as new research and clinical experience broaden our knowledge, changes in treatment and drug therapy may become necessary or appropriate. Readers are advised to check the most current product information provided by the manufacturer of each drug to be administered to verify the recommended dose, the method and duration of administration, and contraindications. It is the responsibility of the licensed health care provider, relying on experience and knowledge of the patient, to determine dosages and the best treatment for each individual patient. Neither the publisher nor the editors assume any liability for any injury and/or damage to persons or property arising from this publication.

---

Previous edition copyrighted 1998

**Library of Congress Cataloging-in-Publication Data**

Stroke rehabilitation: a function-based approach / [edited by] Glen Gillen, EdD, OTR/L, BCN, FAOTA, Assistant Professor in Clinical Occupational Therapy, Ann Burkhardt, OTD, OTR/L, BCN, FAOTA; with 37 contributing authors.–2nd ed.
    p. cm.
Includes bibliographical references and index.
  ISBN-13: 978-0-323-02431-0     ISBN-10: 0-323-02431-9
   1. Cerebrovascular disease–Patients–Rehabilitation. I. Gillen, Glen. II. Burkhardt, Ann.
  RC388.5.S85625 2004
  616.8'106–dc22

                                                 2004042561

*Publishing Director:* Linda Duncan
*Managing Editor:* Kathy Falk
*Associate Developmental Editor:* Melissa Kuster Deutsch
*Publishing Services Manager:* Patricia Tannian
*Senior Project Manager:* Anne Altepeter
*Book Design Manager:* Gail Morey Hudson

ISBN-13: 978-0-323-02431-0
ISBN-10: 0-323-02431-9

Printed in the United States of America

Last digit is the print number:  9  8  7  6  5  4  3

# Contributors

**Lorraine Aloisio, OT/L**
Private Practitioner and Consultant
Long Island, New York

**Guðrún Árnadóttir, MA, BOT**
Private Practitioner, Associate Professor
Division of Occupational Therapy, Faculty of Health
University of Akureyri, Iceland
Coordinator of Occupational Therapy Research and
  Development Projects, Occupational Therapy
Grensás, Landspítali, University Hospital
Reykjavík, Iceland

**Wendy Avery-Smith, MS, OTR/L**
Occupational Therapist
Whittier Rehabilitation Hospital
Haverhill, Massachusetts
Professional Associate
Department of Rehabilitation Medicine
New York-Presbyterian Hospital
New York Weill Cornell Center
New York, New York

**Beverly K. Bain, EdD, OTR, FAOTA**
Consultant to Occupational Therapy and Rehabilitation
  Departments
Matheny School and Hospital
Peapack, New Jersey

**Matthew N. Bartels, MD, MPH**
Assistant Professor of Clinical Rehabilitation Medicine
Columbia University
New York, New York

**Carolyn M. Baum, PhD, OTR, FAOTA**
Associate Professor of Occupational Therapy and Neurology
Washington University School of Medicine
St. Louis, Missouri

**Karen A. Buckley, MA, OT/L**
Clinical Assistant Professor
Department of Occupational Therapy, New York University
New York, New York

**Ann Burkhardt, MA, OTR/L, BCN, FAOTA**
Director of Occupational Therapy
New York-Presbyterian Hospital
Columbia University Medical Center
Associate Clinical Instructor, Columbia University
Programs in Occupational Therapy
New York, New York

**Helen S. Cohen, EdD, OTR, FAOTA**
Associate Professor
Bobby R. Alford Department of Otorhinolaryngology and
  Communicative Sciences
Baylor College of Medicine
Houston, Texas

**Catherine A. Duffy, OTR/L, BCN**
Advanced Clinician, Occupational Therapy Department
New York-Presbyterian Hospital
Columbia University Medical Center
Instructor in Clinical Occupational Therapy, Programs in
  Occupational Therapy
Columbia University
New York, New York

**Janet Falk-Kessler, EdD, OTR, FAOTA**
Associate Professor in Clinical Occupational Therapy
Director, Programs in Occupational Therapy
Columbia University
New York, New York

**Jessica Farman, MS, OTR/L**
Occupational Therapist
Hebrew Rehabilitation Center for the Aged
Boston, Massachusetts

**Judith Dicker Friedman, MA, OTR/L, BCN**
Adjunct Assistant Professor
Occupational Therapy Department, New York University
New York, New York

**Salvatore DiMauro, MD**
Lucy G. Moses Professor of Neurology
College of Physicians and Surgeons
Columbia University
New York, New York

**Glen Gillen, MPA, OTR/L, BCN**
Associate in Clinical Occupational Therapy, Programs in
  Occupational Therapy
College of Physicians and Surgeons, Columbia University
New York, New York

**Michele G. Hahn, MSOT, OTR/L**
Clinical Laboratory Supervisor
Program in Occupational Therapy
Washington University
St. Louis, Missouri

**Sheila M. Hayes, BSN, MS, PT**
Senior Physical Therapist
Helen Hayes Hospital
West Haverstraw, New York

**Leslie A. Kane, MA, OTR/L**
Therapy Manager, Brain Injury Program
Mount Sinai Medical Center
New York, New York

**Virgil Mathiowetz, PhD, OTR, FAOTA**
Associate Professor
Program in Occupational Therapy
University of Minnesota
Minneapolis, Minnesota

**Stephanie M. Milazzo, MA, OTR, CHT**
Director of Rehabilitation
Rehab Resources Unlimited
Ossining, New York

**Barbara E. Neuhaus, EdD, OTR**
Adjunct Associate Professor (Retired)
Programs in Occupational Therapy
Columbia University
New York, New York

**Steve Park, MS, OTR/L**
Associate Professor
School of Occupational Therapy
Pacific University
Forest Grove, Oregon

**Susan L. Pierce, OTR, CDRS**
Certified Driver Rehabilitation Specialist
Adaptive Mobility Services, Inc.
Orlando, Florida

**Ashwini K. Rao, EdD, OTR/L**
Assistant Professor of Clinical Physical Therapy
Physical Therapy Program, Department of Rehabilitation
  Medicine
Columbia University
New York, New York

**Kerry Brockmann Rubio, MHS, OTR/L, BCN**
Lead Occupational Therapist
Maria Parham Hospital
Henderson, North Carolina

**Patricia A. Ryan, MA, OTR/L**
Senior Occupational Therapist
Department of Occupational Therapy
New York-Presbyterian Hospital
Columbia University Medical Center
Instructor in Clinical Occupational Therapy, Programs in
  Occupational Therapy
Columbia University
New York, New York

**Joyce Shapero Sabari, PhD, OTR, BCN, FAOTA**
Associate Professor and Chair
Occupational Therapy Program
State University of New York—Downstate Medical Center
Brooklyn, New York

**Mary Shea, MA, OTR, ATP**
Occupational Therapist
Clinical Specialist
Mount Sinai Medical Center
New York, New York

**Jennie W. Sullivan, OTR/L**
Occupational Therapist
East Tennessee Children's Hospital
Knoxville, Tennessee

**Jeffrey L. Tomlinson, OTR, CSW**
Senior Occupational Therapist
New York State Psychiatric Institute
New York, New York

**Carolyn A. Unsworth, PhD, BAppSc (OccTher),
  AccOT, OTR**
Associate Professor
School of Occupational Therapy, La Trobe University
Bundoora, Victoria, Australia

# Contributors
to the Previous Edition

Susan M. Donato

Lauren Joachim

Christine M. Johann

Karen Halliday Pulaski

Denise A. Supon

Nancy C. Whyte

*For*
**Michael**
GLEN GILLEN

*To*
**Ken, Betty, Hattie,** and **Elva,**
who always told me I could
ANN BURKHARDT

# Foreword
## from the First Edition

In an era of scientific breakthroughs the reality that 550,000 men and women are affected by strokes each year serves as a strong motivator to search for the most effective ways of providing services to this special population. Equally, the fact that a majority of employed occupational therapists treat stroke patients gives rise to the imperative underlying the publication of *Stroke Rehabilitation: A Function-Based Approach*, the first comprehensive text on stroke written primarily by and for occupational therapists and other neurorehabilitation specialists. This book is long overdue—a text that provides professionals an exhaustive resource in a single volume. Editors Glen Gillen and Ann Burkhardt are to be commended for taking on the immense task of conceptualizing and organizing the book. Both have considerable experience as clinicians and educators and know the needs of learners at all levels. They have succeeded in selecting a group of authors with extensive knowledge in particular aspects of stroke rehabilitation.

The overall plan for the book reflects the global nature of a full rehabilitation program that takes the patient from acute care through all aspects of therapy to reentry into community living. The 32 chapters cover direct intervention with patients, approaches that address environmental changes for facilitating function, and approaches that focus on aspects of the total system in which the rehabilitation takes place. This structure allows for presentation of issues such as psychosocial aspects of coping with stroke; working with families; the partnership between the occupational therapist and the certified occupational therapy assistant; total quality assurance; and topics such as sexuality, leisure, and driving that are particularly relevant for patients nearing the end of their rehabilitation.

Each author introduces new information through a thorough review of literature on the chapter topic. The writing also keeps the focus on function in its broadest sense. The content is directed toward remediation, as well as attaining function through adaptation. This function-based approach to stroke rehabilitation not only acknowledges the complexity of patient needs, but also the economic realities of providing health care in an environment of managed care and reimbursement restrictions. The sound, practical focus of the book's content provides a solid foundation for students who are learning about stroke rehabilitation for the first time, as well as for occupational therapy practitioners who need to enrich their clinical base with new knowledge. Each chapter provides useful learning tools such as objectives, key terms, and review questions to develop the reasoning skills of the learners. The case studies that accompany the chapters furnish readers with helpful examples of ways to apply theoretical information. An extensive list of references on each topic directs the reader to additional resources. The numerous illustrations throughout the text and the detailed information regarding several standardized assessment tools are particularly valuable.

*Stroke Rehabilitation: A Function-Based Approach* fills a vital need for current clinical information and will be a valuable addition to rehabilitation literature.

**Barbara E. Neuhaus, EdD, OTR, FAOTA***

*Adjunct Associate Professor*
*Programs in Occupational Therapy*
*Columbia University*
*New York, New York*

---

*Shortly after the first edition of this text was published, Dr. Neuhaus survived a stroke. She shares her experiences in Chapter 30 of this edition.

# Preface

Since publication of the first edition of *Stroke Rehabiliation: A Function-Based Approach*, understanding has increased among members of the community of those who provide services to stroke survivors of the need to document the effectiveness of various interventions—in other words, further blending of the art and science of stroke rehabilitation.

The current text combines aspects of background medical information, a comprehensive review of standardized and nonstandardized evaluation procedures and assessments, treatment techniques, and evidence-based interventions. It contains the most up-to-date research on stroke rehabilitation from a variety of rehabilitation settings and professions without losing its holistic perspective on the overall care of the people whose lives we as clinicians touch.

This text has overarching themes. First and foremost, clinicians are provided with specific suggestions to maintain a client-centered approach when working with stroke survivors. Furthermore, clinicians are challenged to use the most up-to-date treatment approaches (including both remediation and adaptation approaches) to decrease impairments, prevent secondary complications, improve the client's ability to perform meaningful activities, and, most important, to decrease participation restrictions and improve quality of life.

Although this book is written primarily by occupational therapists, it is an appropriate reference for a variety of rehabilitation professionals, including physiatrists, physical therapists, speech and language pathologists, rehabilitation nurses, social workers, vocational counselors, and therapeutic recreation specialists. The immense value of an interdisciplinary team approach when working with the stroke survivor population cannot be overestimated. This text may also be beneficial to therapists who practice virtually alone in the community or as a case manager because its research on the specific topic of stroke rehabilitation is comprehensive. The terms *patient* and *client* have been used interchangeably; it is recognized that stroke rehabilitation can take place in multiple settings.

Educators and students can use this text in the classroom setting. Key terms, chapter objectives, review questions, and case studies have been provided as learning tools. A text that can appeal to the basic learner and the specialist alike, this book is a good investment for any clinician who plans to work with neurologically impaired persons—specifically, adults who have had a stroke. This text spans the continuum of care—from acute to long-term management—in a variety of roles and settings.

The first five chapters provide the necessary medical and therapeutic foundations that should be the basis of any treatment plan. The information in Chapter 2, Psychological Aspects of Stroke Rehabilitation, as well as in Chapter 3, Improving Participation and Quality of Life Through Occupation, should be implicit in any therapeutic interaction with this population. Chapters 4, Task-Oriented Approach to Stroke Rehabilitation, and 5, Activity-Based Intervention in Stroke Rehabilitation, provide readers with an overall view of current therapeutic approaches and should be understood before the chapters on specialized topics are read.

Chapters 6 through 15 focus on the motor control aspects of stroke rehabilitation. Chapter 6, Approaches to Motor Control Dysfunction: An Evidence-Based Review, provides the reader with critical information to critique traditional and current practice approaches. Specific topics related to motor control that are covered include trunk control (Chapter 7), balance (Chapter 8) and vestibular dysfunction (Chapter 9), comprehensive approaches to upper extremity function and management (Chapter 10), edema control (Chapter 11), splinting (Chapter 12), casting (Chapter 13), functional mobility (Chapter 14), and gait (Chapter 15).

The following four chapters provide readers with insight into managing simple and complex visual, perceptual, and cognitive impairments. Chapters focus on assessment and interventions related to primary visual skills (Chapter 16), clinical reasoning during assessment and treatment planning (Chapter 17), standardized assessment of the impact of cognitive-perceptual impairments on meaningful tasks (Chapter 18), and evidence-based approaches to management (Chapter 19).

This text contains comprehensive chapters on specific aspects of daily living after a stroke, such as driving, sexuality, leisure, instrumental activities of daily living, mobility, and self-care. Specific interventions highlighted include dysphagia management, home adaptation, wheeled mobility and seating prescription, working with families, and the integration of assistive technology for the stroke population. Finally, two stroke survivors who share their thoughts, frustrations, and experiences provide readers with invaluable insights to the stroke recovery process.

It is my hope that this text will challenge practicing clinicians to consider their present approaches to stroke rehabilitation and serve as a foundation on which students can build their philosophies for intervention with the stroke population.

**Glen Gillen**

# Acknowledgments

We are grateful to all of the professionals from our own community, across the country, and internationally for their contributions to this book. They accepted our challenge to put their knowledge and skill base into words. Their dedication to this project will inspire future generations of clinicians. In addition, Jeanne Robertson's artistic talent continues to amaze!

We appreciate the dedication and persistence of the staff at Elsevier, specifically Kathy Falk, Melissa Kuster, and Anne Altepeter. Their encouragement and support throughout this project were invaluable.

# Contents

matthew n. bartels

**chapter 1**

# Pathophysiology and Medical Management of Stroke

**key terms**

hemorrhagic stroke

stroke diagnosis

stroke prevention

ischemic stroke

stroke management

**chapter objectives**

After completing this chapter, the reader will be able to accomplish the following:

1. Describe the pathophysiology of stroke.
2. Explain the diagnostic workup of stroke survivors.
3. Understand the medical management of various stroke syndromes.
4. Describe interventions to prevent the recurrence of stroke and its complications.

## PREVALENCE AND IMPACT OF STROKE

Stroke is the third leading cause of mortality in the United States after cardiovascular disease and cancer, accounting for 10% to 12% of all deaths.[12] An estimated 550,000 strokes occur each year, resulting in 150,000 deaths and more than 300,000 individuals with significant disability.[96] The United States has an estimated 3 million stroke survivors today, which is double the number of survivors 25 years ago.[45] The economic impact of stroke in 1993 was estimated at $30 billion, of which $17 billion were direct medical costs and $13 billion were indirect costs from lost productivity.[96] Fortunately, modern medical interventions (mostly risk factor modifications) have decreased stroke mortality by approximately 7% per year in industrialized nations since 1970.[12]

## EPIDEMIOLOGY OF STROKE

Stroke is essentially a preventable disease with known, manageable risk factors.[13] The established risk factors for stroke include hypertension, cigarette smoking, obesity, elevated serum fibrinogen levels, diabetes, a sedentary lifestyle, and the use of contraceptives with high doses of estrogen.[81] The most important and easily treated of these risk factors is systolic hypertension. In the Multiple Risk Factor Intervention Trial, 40% of strokes were attributed to systolic blood pressures greater than 140 mm Hg.[105] Stroke incidence also increases exponentially with aging, with an increase in stroke from 3 in 100,000 individuals per year in the third and fourth decades of age to 300 in 100,000 individuals per year in the eighth and ninth decades of life.[13] Eighty-eight percent of stroke

**Table 1-1**

**Modifiable and Nonmodifiable Risks**

| TYPE OF RISK | RELATIVE RISK (PER 1000 PERSONS) |
|---|---|
| **Modifiable Risks** | |
| Hypertension | 4.0-5.0 |
| Cardiac disease | 2.0-4.0 |
| Atrial fibrillation | 5.6-17.6 |
| Diabetes mellitus | 1.5-3.0 |
| Cigarette smoking | 1.5-2.9 |
| Alcohol abuse | 1.0-4.0 |
| Hyperlipidemia | 1.0-2.0 |
| **Nonmodifiable Risks** | |
| Age | 1-2/1000 at age 45-54 to 20/1000 at age 75-84 |
| Gender | 1.2-2.1 |
| Race (black or Hispanic) | 2.0 |
| Heredity | |

deaths occur among persons aged 65 or older[12] (Table 1-1 outlines modifiable and nonmodifiable risks).

Stroke prevention interventions have reduced mortality in industrialized nations primarily through treating hypertension in the elderly. Another cause of decreased mortality has been the establishment of dedicated stroke units that can prevent acute death and later development of life-threatening complications.

## PATHOGENESIS AND PATHOLOGY OF STROKE

### Definition and Description of Stroke Syndromes

*Stroke.* Stroke is essentially a disease of the cerebral vasculature in which a failure to supply oxygen to brain cells, which are the most susceptible to ischemic damage, leads to their death. The syndromes that lead to stroke compose two broad categories: ischemic and hemorrhagic stroke. Ischemic strokes account for approximately 80% of strokes, whereas hemorrhagic strokes account for the remaining 20%.[104]

*Transient Ischemic Attack.* Symptoms of a transient ischemic attack (TIA) include the focal deficits of an ischemic stroke and a clearly vascular distribution, but TIAs are reversible defects because no cerebral infarction ensues. The causes of TIAs can be thrombotic and embolic and also could result from a cerebral vasospasm. By definition, the effects of TIAs must resolve in less than 24 hours. A patient who has had a TIA should have a complete evaluation for cerebrovascular disease and sources of embolism because 35% of patients who have had TIAs have a stroke within 5 years.[132] The treatment

of TIAs depends on the source of the emboli or thrombi and can include anticoagulation therapy and/or surgery.

### Ischemic Stroke

An ischemic stroke is the most common form of stroke, and its cause varies. The one common factor among all the different subtypes of ischemic strokes is that the cause of injury is tissue anoxia caused by cessation of cerebral blood flow.

*Embolic Stroke.* Cerebral embolic strokes are the most common ischemic stroke subtype. Embolic strokes usually are characterized by an abrupt onset, although they also can be associated with stuttering symptoms. Usually no heralding events occur, such as TIAs or previous small strokes evolving into larger strokes.[66] Microemboli that cause smaller events are uncommon, and the usual clue to a possible embolic source is a completed stroke.[104] The source of approximately 40% of embolic strokes is unknown, even after the common sources have been evaluated extensively. Most embolic strokes of known cause occur after emboli that are cardiac in origin.[21] The second most common sources of emboli are atherothrombotic lesions that result in artery-to-artery embolisms. These lesions can be in the aorta, the carotid and vertebrobasilar systems, and, less frequently, smaller arteries.

### Sources of Emboli

*Cardiac Sources.* Cardiac emboli can develop from numerous areas in the heart. Cardiac arrhythmias, structural anomalies, and acute infarctions can be sources of emboli. Classically, the most common source is the left atrium in patients with atrial fibrillation. Atrial fibrillation causes thrombi through clot formation in the left atrial appendage, which then breaks off and embolizes through the arterial system. Patients older than age 60 are particularly prone to this type of embolization.

The most common cardiac structural cause of a cerebral embolism is a result of a myocardial infarction.[66] In patients with left ventricular infarcts, particularly anterior wall and apical infarctions, the endocardial damage associated with a subendocardial or transmural infarction is an excellent nidus (a focal point where bacteria or other infectious agents thrive) for thrombus formation. The emboli most often develop during the first several weeks after the infarction, although the risk for developing them can persist for much longer.

Valvular heart disease also can result in thrombi, but they more frequently develop after valve replacement rather than result directly from the native valve. More commonly the native valvular heart disease causes the patient to be in atrial fibrillation and then to develop an embolus. Mechanical heart valves (e.g., St. Jude valves) are much more likely to cause emboli than porcine valves, so patients with the mechanical type always continue to receive anticoagulation therapy.

Much less common sources of cardiac emboli are the vegetations resulting from bacterial endocarditis. These emboli cause small septic infarcts called *mycotic aneurysms*, which are at high risk of conversion to hemorrhagic infarcts. Other rare causes of cardiac emboli are atrial myxomas, which are tumors of the heart endocardium. In addition, embolic infarctions also may result from cardiac and thoracic surgery.[66]

Cardiac emboli usually (80% of the time) occlude the middle cerebral artery, 10% of cardiac emboli occlude the posterior cerebral artery, and the rest occlude the vertebral artery or its branches.[66] Anterior cerebral artery embolization from the heart is rare. The severity of the clinical syndrome is related to the size of the embolus. An embolus of 3 to 4 mm can cause a large stroke by occluding the larger brain arteries. Blood clots undergo lysis over a few days with the establishment of recanalization through the clot. Because clots naturally lyse, a stroke can convert from ischemic to hemorrhagic when reperfusion distal to the occlusion is present because the blood vessels in the ischemic distribution may no longer be intact. This can lead to leakage from these damaged arteries, arterioles, and capillaries, leading to a phenomenon called *hemorrhagic conversion*. The possibility of hemorrhagic conversion contraindicates the use of anticoagulation therapy as initial treatment for large embolic strokes.

*Vascular Sources.* Strokes that are vascular in origin are far less common than cardiac strokes but are still one major type of embolic stroke. The sources of vascular emboli are usually atheromatous plaques in the walls of the aorta, carotid arteries, or smaller vessels in the cerebral circulation. Platelet activation and the formation of a fibrin clot can occur rapidly. The most common areas affected by the emboli of the vascular system are the same as those affected by cardiac sources of emboli. The most common areas for ulcerated plaques in the cerebral blood supply are the aorta and the proximal internal carotid artery. The plaques in the carotid artery can be visualized by Doppler sonography of the carotid artery system.[104]

*Paradoxical Sources.* Congenital atrial septal defects can create the opportunity for emboli to cross from the right-sided (venous) circulation to the left-sided (arterial) circulation, a rare source of cerebral emboli. A common source of paradoxical embolic material is deep venous thrombosis (DVT). The modern techniques of transesophageal echocardiography with a "bubble study" help identify patients at risk for this condition. One performs a bubble study by injecting a small bolus of air into the venous circulation while the echocardiographer observes the heart. If the air bolus, which is seen easily, has no portion cross over to the left-sided circulation, then no shunt is present. If the bubbles cross into the left-sided circulation, then a shunt is possible. One of the most common

atrial shunting abnormalities is a patent foramen ovale. In young patients or patients who have had TIAs or strokes, the treatment of choice is surgical repair of the lesion.

*Unknown Sources.* Thrombi of unknown source often occur in patients with known hypercoagulability syndromes. These syndromes can result from acquired diseases (e.g., lupus anticoagulant and metastatic tumors) or inborn errors of the coagulation system (e.g., protein S and C deficiencies). Surgery or medication therapies such as estrogen replacement can induce iatrogenic causes of hypercoagulable states. Even when the patient is known to be in a hypercoagulable state, the source of the emboli may remain unknown. In many patients the entire workup is unrevealing.

### Thrombotic Stroke

A thrombotic stroke can result from a variety of causes, but most causes are related to the development of abnormalities in the arterial vessel wall. Atherosclerosis, arteritis, dissections, and external compression of the vessels are causes. In addition, some patients with hematologic disorders develop thrombosis. The spectrum of disease includes stroke and TIA, and often the difference between a thrombotic and an embolic stroke may be difficult to determine. Thrombosis and embolism are often both present, especially in patients with atherosclerotic disease. The exact mechanism of infarction from thrombosis still is being debated, but atherosclerosis does play a significant role. Hypertension with associated microtrauma of the arterial intima is thought to play a role, as is hypercholesterolemia.[84,104] Transient ischemic attacks may result from the formation of microthrombi and their embolization. Large vessel thrombosis also can occur in extracranial vessels, such as the vertebral and carotid arteries, leading to devastating strokes.[94]

*Pathophysiology.* Atherosclerotic plaque formation is greatest at the branching points of major vessels and also forms in areas of turbulent flow. Chronic hypertension is a common precursor, and damage to the intimal wall may be followed by lymphocyte infiltration. Foam cells then develop, and the first stage of atherosclerosis is formed. Calcification and narrowing with resultant turbulent flow follow. In this setting of turbulent flow, plaque ulceration can become a site for thrombus formation. If the thrombus forms and is degraded rapidly, a transient ischemic phenomenon can occur, which is the setting of a TIA. Classically, the symptoms of internal carotid disease include amaurosis fugax and monocular blindness. If the clot does not break up or lyse, a cerebral infarction can occur. The size and severity of the infarction depends on available collateral circulation and the size of the occluded vessel. In patients with extensive atherosclerotic disease, however, a limited amount of collateral circulation is available, and the sparing from collateral circulation may be limited.

***Atherothrombotic Disease.*** The most common site for the development of atherosclerosis and the subsequent development of atherothrombosis that leads to TIAs and stroke in the anterior circulation is the origin of the carotid artery and in the posterior circulation is the top of the basilar artery. Other sites of atherosclerosis include the carotid siphon and the stems (bases) of the middle cerebral artery, anterior cerebral artery, and origin of the basilar artery.[42] The atheromatous plaques are sources of emboli that can cause distal symptoms in a TIA or stroke.

These embolic events are similar events from other embolic sources (Table 1-2 lists common stroke syndromes and Figures 1-1 to 1-3 explain the anatomy of these strokes). Atherosclerotic disease is screened most readily by carotid Doppler ultrasonography and transcranial Doppler imaging. Magnetic resonance angiography and carotid and cerebral angiography can further elucidate lesions, which can be treated surgically or medically.

***Lacunar Syndrome.*** A lacunar stroke occurs in one of the perforating branches of the circle of Willis, the middle cerebral artery stem, or the vertebral or basilar arteries. The occlusion of these vessels results from the

**Table 1-2**

## Common Stroke Syndromes

| ANATOMIC DISTRIBUTION | STROKE SYNDROME |
|---|---|
| **Common Carotid Artery** | Often resembles middle cerebral artery (MCA) but can be asymptomatic if circle of Willis is competent |
| **Internal Carotid Artery** | Often resembles MCA but can be asymptomatic if circle of Willis is competent |
| **Middle Cerebral Artery** | |
| Main stem | Contralateral hemiplegia |
| | Contralateral hemianopia |
| | Contralateral hemianesthesia |
| | Head/eye turning toward the lesion |
| | Dysphagia |
| | Uninhibited neurogenic bladder |
| | Dominant hemisphere |
| |    Global aphasia |
| |    Apraxia |
| | Nondominant hemisphere |
| |    Aprosody and affective agnosia |
| |    Visuospatial deficit |
| |    Neglect syndrome |
| Upper division | Contralateral hemiplegia; leg more spared |
| | Contralateral hemianopia |
| | Contralateral hemianesthesia |
| | Head/eye turning toward the lesion |
| | Dysphagia |
| | Uninhibited neurogenic bladder |
| | Dominant hemisphere |
| |    Broca's (motor) aphasia |
| |    Apraxia |
| | Nondominant hemisphere |
| |    Aprosody and affective agnosia |
| |    Visuospatial deficit |
| |    Neglect syndrome |
| Lower division | Contralateral hemianopia |
| | Dominant hemisphere |
| |    Wernicke's aphasia |
| | Nondominant hemisphere |
| |    Affective agnosia |

**Table 1-2**

## Common Stroke Syndromes—cont'd

| ANATOMIC DISTRIBUTION | STROKE SYNDROME |
|---|---|
| **Anterior Cerebral Artery (ACA)** | |
| Proximal (precommunal) segment (A1) | Can be asymptomatic if circle of Willis is competent, but if both ACAs arise from the same stem, then: |
| |     Profound abulia (akinetic mutism) |
| |     Bilateral pyramidal signs |
| |     Paraplegia |
| Postcommunal segment (A2) | Contralateral hemiplegia; arm more spared |
| | Contralateral hemianesthesia |
| | Head/eye turning toward the lesion |
| | Grasp reflex, sucking reflex, gegenhalten |
| | Disconnection apraxia |
| | Abulia |
| | Gait apraxia |
| | Urinary incontinence |
| Anterior choroidal artery | Contralateral hemiplegia |
| | Hemianesthesia |
| | Homonymous hemianopsia |
| **Posterior Cerebral Artery** | |
| Proximal (precommunal) segment (P1) | Thalamic syndrome: |
| |     Choreoathetosis |
| |     Spontaneous pain and dysesthesias |
| |     Sensory loss (all modalities) |
| |     Intention tremor |
| |     Mild hemiparesis |
| | Thalamoperforate syndrome: |
| |     Crossed cerebellar ataxia |
| |     Ipsilateral third nerve palsy |
| | Weber's syndrome: |
| |     Contralateral hemiplegia |
| |     Ipsilateral third nerve palsy |
| | Contralateral hemiplegia |
| | Paralysis of vertical eye movement |
| | Contralateral action tremor |
| Postcommunal segment (P2) | Homonymous hemianopsia |
| | Cortical blindness |
| | Visual agnosia |
| | Prosopagnosia |
| | Dyschromatopsia |
| | Alexia without agraphia |
| | Memory deficits |
| | Complex hallucinations |
| **Vertebrobasilar Syndromes** | |
| Superior cerebellar artery | Ipsilateral cerebellar ataxia |
| | Nausea/vomiting |
| | Dysarthria |
| | Contralateral loss of pain and temperature sensation |
| | Partial deafness |
| | Horner' syndrome |
| | Ipsilateral ataxic tremor |

*Continued*

**Table 1-2**

**Common Stroke Syndromes—cont'd**

| ANATOMIC DISTRIBUTION | STROKE SYNDROME |
|---|---|
| Anterior inferior cerebellar artery | Ipsilateral deafness |
| | Ipsilateral facial weakness |
| | Nausea/vomiting |
| | Vertigo |
| | Nystagmus |
| | Tinnitus |
| | Cerebellar ataxia |
| | Paresis of conjugate lateral gaze |
| | Contralateral loss of pain and temperature sensation |
| Medial basal midbrain (Weber's syndrome) | Contralateral hemiplegia |
| | Ipsilateral third nerve palsy |
| Tegmentum of midbrain (Benedikt's syndrome) | Ipsilateral third nerve palsy |
| | Contralateral loss of pain and temperature sensation |
| | Contralateral loss of joint position sensation |
| | Contralateral ataxia |
| | Contralateral chorea |
| Bilateral basal pons (locked-in syndrome) | Bilateral hemiplegia |
| | Bilateral cranial nerve palsy (upward gaze spared) |
| Lateral pons (Millard-Gubler syndrome) | Ipsilateral sixth nerve palsy |
| | Ipsilateral facial weakness |
| | Contralateral hemiplegia |
| Lateral medulla (Wallenberg's syndrome) | Ipsilateral hemiataxia |
| | Ipsilateral loss of facial pain and sensation |
| | Contralateral loss of body pain and temperature sensation |
| | Nystagmus |
| | Ipsilateral Horner's syndrome |
| | Dysphagia and dysphonia |

atherothrombotic or lipohyalinotic blockage of one of these arteries. The development of disease in these arteries correlates closely with the presence of chronic hypertension and diabetic microvascular disease.[87,104] These are small vessels, 100 to 300 µm in diameter, that branch off the main artery and penetrate into the deep gray or white matter of the cerebrum.[87] The resulting infarcts are from 2 mm to 3 cm in size and account for roughly 20% of all strokes. These types of strokes usually evolve over a few hours and sometimes can be heralded by transient symptoms in lacunar TIAs. Lacunar strokes can cause recognizable syndromes (Table 1-3). The basic lacunar syndromes are (1) pure motor hemiparesis from an infarct in the posterior limb of the interior capsule or pons, (2) pure sensory stroke from an infarct in the ventrolateral thalamus, (3) ataxic hemiparesis from an infarct in the base of the pons or the genu of the internal capsule, and (4) pure motor hemiparesis with motor apraxia resulting from an infarct in the genu of the anterior limb of the internal capsule and the adjacent white matter in the corona radiata. Recovery from a lacunar stroke often can be dramatic, and in some individuals, near complete or complete resolution of deficits can occur in several weeks or months. In patients who have had multiple lacunar infarcts, a syndrome characterized by emotional instability, slow abulia (impairment in or loss of volition), and bilateral pyramidal signs known as *pseudobulbar palsy* will develop. This diagnosis is based on the symptoms and the use of computerized tomography (CT) or magnetic resonance imaging (MRI). Magnetic resonance imaging is especially useful in this situation for detecting small lesions in the deep brain structures or brainstem; the ability of CT to see lesions clearly in these areas is limited.[22]

*Hemorrhagic Conversion.* As a sequela of an embolic or ischemic infarction, a purely ischemic infarct may convert into a hemorrhagic lesion. Thrombi can migrate, lyse, and reperfuse into an ischemic area, leading to small hemorrhages (petechial hemorrhages) because the damaged capillaries and small blood vessels no longer maintain their integrity. These damaged areas then can coalesce (combine) and form a hemorrhage into ischemia.[66] These conversions are more common in large infarcts, such as an occluded middle cerebral artery, or in a large infarction in the distribution of a lenticulostriate artery. In patients who have large infarcts with possibility of hemorrhage, anticoagulation therapy is not used because of the risk of hemorrhagic conversion. These types of hemorrhages have characteristics in common with hemorrhagic strokes.

### Hemorrhagic Stroke

Hemorrhagic strokes have numerous causes. The four most common types are deep hypertensive intracerebral hemorrhages, ruptured saccular aneurysms, bleeding from an arteriovenous malformation (AVM), and spontaneous lobar hemorrhages.[66]

*Hypertensive Bleed.* Hypertensive cerebral hemorrhages usually occur in four sites: the putamen and internal capsule, the pons, the thalamus, and the cerebellum. Usually these hemorrhages develop from small penetrating arteries in the deep brain that have had damage from hypertension. The pathologic features of hypertension include lipohyalinosis (fat infiltration of pathologically degenerated tissue) and Charcot-Bouchard aneurysms.[41] The usual hypertensive intracerebral hemorrhage (ICH) develops over the span of a few minutes but occasionally can take as long as 60 minutes. Unlike ischemic infarcts, hemorrhagic bleeds do not follow the anatomic distribution of blood vessels but dissect through tissue planes spherically. This commonly leads to severe damage and

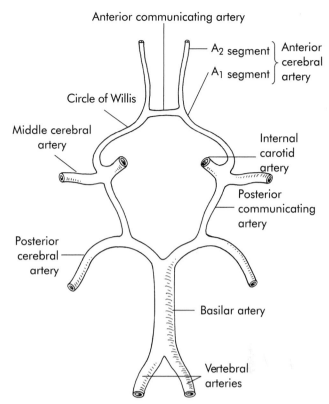

**Figure 1-1**   Circle of Willis and cerebral circulation.

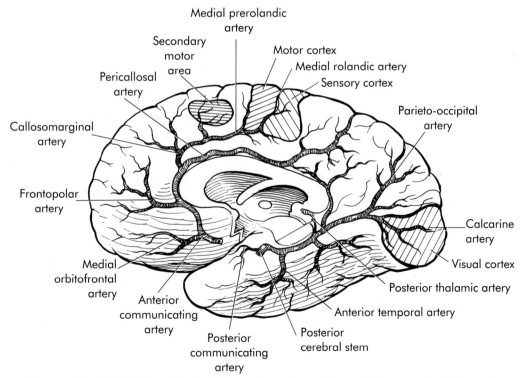

**Figure 1-2**   Medial view of brain with anterior and posterior cerebral artery circulation and areas of cortical function.

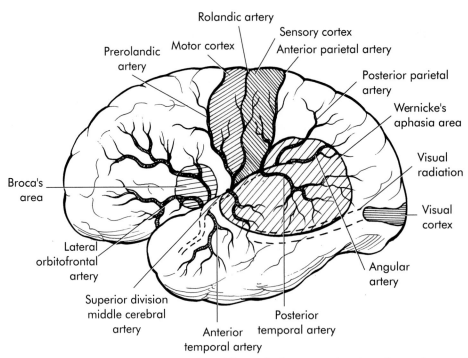

**Figure 1-3**   Lateral view of brain with middle cerebral artery and its branches and areas of cortical function.

**Table 1-3**

**Lacunar Stroke Syndromes and Their Anatomic Sites**

| LACUNAR SYNDROME | ANATOMIC SITES |
|---|---|
| Pure motor | Posterior limb of internal capsule |
|  | Basis pontis |
|  | Pyramids |
| Pure sensory | Ventrolateral thalamus |
|  | Thalamocortical projections |
| Ataxic hemiparesis | Pons |
|  | Genu of internal capsule |
|  | Corona radiata |
|  | Cerebellum |
| Motor hemiparesis with apraxia | Genu of the anterior limb of the internal capsule |
|  | Corona radiata |
| Hemiballismus | Head of caudate |
|  | Thalamus |
|  | Subthalamic nucleus |
| Dysarthria/clumsy hand | Base of pons |
|  | Genu of anterior limb of the internal capsule |
| Sensory/motor | Junction of the internal capsule and thalamus |
| Anarthric psuedobulbar | Bilateral internal capsule |

complications such as hydrocephalus and mass shift (movement of brain tissues to one side to accommodate the volume of the hemorrhage).[66,104] Within 48 hours of the hemorrhage, macrophages begin to phagocytize the hemorrhage at its outer margins. Patients with a cerebral hemorrhage often experience a rapid recovery within the first 2 to 3 months after the hemorrhage. Intracerebral hemorrhages usually occur while patients are awake and often while they are under emotional stress. Vomiting and headache are associated commonly with ICH and are unique features that differentiate ICHs from ischemic strokes. (Table 1-4 outlines the four major hypertensive ICH syndromes.)

***Lobar Intracerebral Bleed.***   Lobar hemorrhages are ICHs that occur outside the basal ganglia and thalamus in the white matter of the cerebral cortex. These types of hemorrhages and hypertension are not correlated clearly; the most common underlying condition in patients with this type of ICH is the presence of AVMs.[66] Other associated conditions include bleeding diatheses, tumors (e.g., melanoma or glioma), aneurysms in the circle of Willis, and a large number of idiopathic cases.[40] Patients with lobar ICH initially have acute onset of symptoms, and most lobar ICHs are small enough to cause discrete clinical syndromes that may resemble focal ischemic events. Because lobar bleeds occur far from the thalamus and the brainstem, coma and stupor are much less common than they are in patients with

**Table 1-4**

**The Four Major Hypertension Intracerebral Hemorrhage Syndromes**

| TYPE | STRUCTURES INVOLVED | CLINICAL SYNDROME | COMMENTS |
|---|---|---|---|
| Putamenal | Internal capsule<br>Basal ganglia | Contralateral hemiplegia<br>Coma in large infarcts<br>Eyes deviate away from lesion<br>Can have stupor/coma with brainstem compression<br>Decerebrate rigidity | Most common |
| Thalamic | Thalamus<br>Internal capsule | Contralateral hemiplegia<br>Prominent contralateral sensory deficit for all modalities<br>Aphasia if dominant (left) thalamus involved<br>Homonymous visual field defect<br>Gaze palsies<br>Horner's syndrome<br>Eyes deviate downward | |
| Pontine | Pons<br>Brainstem<br>Midbrain | Coma<br>Quadriparesis<br>Decerebrate rigidity<br>Severe acute hypertension<br>Death | Can lead to a locked-in syndrome |
| Cerebellar | Cerebellum | Nausea and vomiting<br>Ataxia<br>Vertigo/dizziness<br>Occipital headache<br>Gaze toward the lesion<br>Occasional dysarthria and dysphagia | Nystagmus and limb ataxia are rare |

hypertensive ICHs. Headaches are also common and can help differentiate lobar bleeds from ischemic strokes, which they can resemble so closely.[103] Detection of a hemorrhage on a CT scan or MRI is the best way to distinguish these two entities.

***Saccular Aneurysm and Subarachnoid Bleed.*** A saccular aneurysm rupture is the most common cause of a subarachnoid hemorrhage (SAH).[120] Saccular aneurysms occur at the bifurcation (branching) points of the large arteries in the brain and most commonly are found in the anterior portion of the circle of Willis.[66] An estimated 0.5% to 1% of normal individuals harbor saccular aneurysms.[126] Despite the high number, bleeding from them is rare (6 to 16 per 100,000). Unlike other stroke syndromes, however, the incidence of SAH has not declined since 1970.[82] The rupture risk correlates best with the size of the aneurysm. Aneurysms smaller than 3 mm have little chance of hemorrhage, whereas aneurysms 10 mm or larger have the greatest chance of rupture.[77] Subaracnoid hemorrhage usually is characterized by acute, abrupt onset of a severe headache of atypical quality.[82] These headaches are often the most severe that patients have ever experienced. A brief loss of consciousness, nausea

and vomiting, focal neurologic deficits, and a stiff neck at the onset of symptoms also may occur. The diagnosis is based on clinical suspicion, subarachnoid blood found on the CT scan, or blood found in the cerebrospinal fluid from a spinal tap. One determines the definitive location of the aneurysm by cerebral angiography.

The development of further delayed neurologic deficits result from three major events: rerupture, hydrocephalus, and cerebral vasospasm. Rerupture occurs in 20% to 30% of cases within 1 month if treatment is not aggressive, and rebleeding has an associated mortality rate of up to 70%.[82] Hydrocephalus occurs in up to 20% of cases, and aggressive management often is required. Chronic hydrocephalus is also common and often requires permanent cerebrospinal fluid drainage (shunting). Vasospasm also is a common problem after SAHs, occurring in approximately 30% of cases.[82] The normal time course for vasospasm is an onset in 3 to 5 days, peak narrowing in 5 to 14 days, and resolution in 2 to 4 weeks. In one half of cases, the vasospasm is severe enough to cause a cerebral infarction with resulting stroke or death. Even with modern management, 15% to 20% of patients who develop vasospasms still suffer strokes or die.[78] A permanent ischemic deficit develops in approximately 50% of patients with symptomatic vasospasms after SAHs.[55] Vasospasm therefore must be treated rapidly and as aggressively as possible to prevent permanent ischemic damage.

*Arteriovenous Malformation.* Arteriovenous malformations are found throughout the body and can occur in any part of the brain. They are usually congenital and consist of an abnormal tangle of blood vessels between the arterial and venous systems. They range from a few millimeters in size to large masses that can increase cardiac output because of the amount of their blood flow. The larger AVMs in the brain tend to be found in the posterior portions of the cerebral hemispheres.[41] Arteriovenous malformations occur more frequently in men, and if found in one family member, they have a tendency to be found in other members. Arteriovenous malformations are present from birth, but bleeding most often occurs in the second and third decades of life. Headaches and seizures are common symptoms, as is hemiplegia. Half of AVMs initially occur as intracerebral hemorrhages. Although rebleeding in the first month is rare, rebleeding is common in larger lesions as more time passes. Contrast CT, magnetic resonance angiography, and MRI are useful noninvasive tests, whereas cerebral angiography is the best test for delineating the nature of the lesion. The management of these lesions is accomplished best by a team approach, a combination of surgical treatment and interventional angiography for definitive management. Treatment of hydrocephalus and increased intracranial pressure is the same as treatment for SAH and ICH.

*Posttraumatic Hemorrhagic Stroke.* A traumatic brain injury commonly results in hemorrhagic damage to the brain in addition to ischemic and other injuries. The four major types of injury caused by traumatic brain injury include SAH and ICH, diffuse axonal injury, contusions, and anoxic injury from hypoperfusion (decreased flow in the vessels) and hypoxemia (decreased oxygen level). This combination of injuries leads to a constellation of findings that mixes the features of a number of individual ischemic and hemorrhagic injuries.

### Other Causes of Stroke and Strokelike Syndromes

*Arterial and Medical Disease.* Numerous medical conditions can result in arterial system diseases and lead to thrombosis and thromboembolism. Some conditions may cause disease in the cerebral vasculature (Table 1-5).

*Strokelike Syndromes.* A number of conditions in addition to TIAs and cerebral infarctions can cause transient paralysis. These conditions generally resolve spontaneously with no long-term sequelae. The most common cause of transient hemiparesis is Todd's paralysis, which develops postictally (after a seizure). Todd's

paralysis results from neurotransmitter depletion and neuronal fatigue in focal areas of the brain caused by the extremely high neuronal firing rate during a seizure.[29] Patients usually regain function within 24 hours. Another common cause of focal neurologic deficits is migraine headaches. These headaches actually are thought to result from cerebral vasospasms, but an actual ischemic infarct rarely if ever occurs. The deficits resolve with the resolution of the migraine and are not permanent.

*Cerebral Neoplasm.* Obviously, cerebral neoplasms (whether primary or metastatic) can lead to focal neurologic deficits that resemble a stroke. The treatment of the sequelae and the long-term management of the deficits are the same as they are in stroke patients. Treating the primary lesions is the focus of the acute care. Often the initial symptoms are seizures and ICHs.

## STROKE DIAGNOSIS

The diagnosis of stroke and differentiation of stroke from strokelike syndromes is based on the clinical presentation and physical examination of the patient. The examiner needs to differentiate a true stroke from syndromes that can mimic a stroke, such as Todd's paralysis, seizures, multiple sclerosis, tumors, and metabolic syndromes. Most often, the patient's symptoms in the emergency room include an acute onset of weakness or other neurologic deficits. The patient history can help identify the risk factors for stroke and the nature of the lesion. The physical examination includes a general medical examination and a neurologic examination. Only after a diagnosis of stroke based on the clinical history and examination can a further diagnostic evaluation be performed. Modern technology has improved the tools available for the accurate diagnosis of stroke and includes an armamentarium of imaging studies to diagnose the exact nature of the lesions that may cause neurologic deficits. Each imaging study available has benefits and limitations that are useful to know for assessing a patient who has had a stroke. The stroke evaluation also should include an evaluation for the cause of the stroke.

### Cerebrovascular Imaging

The main tool used in stroke diagnostic evaluations is cerebral imaging, which historically included pneumoencephalography and other studies that are no longer performed. Computed tomography is probably the most common and the best known of the studies. Magnetic resonance imaging is becoming more common and has some advantages over CT, but availability and cost are still prohibitive. Positron emission tomography scans and single-photon emission computerized tomography scans are just being introduced and may have a role in stroke diagnosis.

**Table 1-5**

## Medical Conditions That Cause Arterial System Disease

| CONDITION | FEATURES* | TREATMENT |
|---|---|---|
| **Vasculitic/Inflammatory** | | |
| Systemic lupus erythematosus | Most commonly associated vasculitis with stroke<br>Vasculitic, thrombotic, and embolic events occur<br>Greater than 50% recurrence rate<br>Antiphospholipid antibody may play a role | Treat lupus<br>Anticoagulation with warfarin |
| Binswanger's disease | Rare condition<br>Diffuse subcortical infarction<br>Diffuse lipohyalinosis of small arteries | No clear treatment<br>Anticoagulation |
| Scleroderma | Stroke in 6% of patients<br>Antiphospholipid antibody may play a role | No clear treatment<br>Anticoagulation |
| Periarteritis nodosa | Can cause a CNS vasculitis<br>Can cause embolic stroke | Treat underlying condition |
| Temporal arteritis | Can cause a CNS vasculitis<br>Can cause embolic stroke | Treat underlying condition |
| Wegener's granulomatosis | Can cause a CNS necrotizing vasculitis<br>Can cause thrombotic stroke | Treat underlying condition |
| Takayasu's arteritis | Can cause embolic stroke | Treat underlying condition<br>Anticoagulation |
| Isolated angiitis of the CNS | Rare primary CNS vasculitis<br>Headache, multiinfarct dementia, lethargy | Treat underlying condition |
| Fibromuscular dysplasia | Mostly in young women<br>Often asymptotic<br>Can be associated with TIA and stroke | Anticoagulation<br>Surgical dilation of the carotid arteries (if necessary) |
| Moyamoya disease | Vasooclusive disease of the large intracranial arteries<br>Mainly in Asian population<br>Cause of strokes in children and young adults | Role of anticoagulation controversial because of risk of hemorrhage<br>Role of surgery controversial |
| **Hypercoagulable State** | | |
| Antiphospholipid antibodies | Associated with recurrent thrombosis<br>Embolic and thrombotic strokes occur | Anticoagulation with warfarin |
| Oral contraceptive agents | Relative risk increased 4 times over controls<br>Thought to be caused by hypercoagulability | Stop oral contraceptives |
| Sickle cell disease | Microvascular occlusion caused by sickled cells<br>Seen in 5%-17% of patients with sickle cell disease | No good treatments exist |
| Polycythemia | Vascular occlusion caused by increased viscosity and hypercoagulability | Treat underlying cause (if known) |
| Inherited thrombotic tendencies | Include many familial clotting abnormalities | Treat abnormality (if possible)<br>Anticoagulation |
| **Others** | | |
| Venous thrombosis | Seen in meningitis, hypercoagulable states, and after trauma<br>Increased intracranial pressure, headache, seizures<br>Focal neurologic signs, especially in legs more than arms<br>Diagnosed with angiography | Anticoagulation<br>May need surgical decompression |
| Arterial dissection | More common in children and young adults<br>May present with TIA<br>Often preceded by trauma, mild to severe | Surgical treatment as needed<br>Anticoagulation after acute state |

*CNS, Central nervous system; TIA, transient ischemic attack.

## Computerized Axial Tomography

Computed tomography is a readily available and useful technique that has become the standard for the evaluation of a patient experiencing an acute onset of stroke. The most important functions of CT scanning in an acute patient are ruling out other conditions (e.g., tumor or abscess) and helping identify whether evidence exists of hemorrhage into the infarction. In the acute phase of stroke, most CT scans are actually negative with no clear evidence of abnormalities. A negative immediate CT scan with an acute neurologic deficit determined by physical examination actually can verify the impression of stroke because it rules out tumors, hemorrhages, and other brain lesions. The few changes seen in an acute stroke by CT are subtle and can include loss of distinction between gray and white matter and sulcal effacement. Acute bleeding, however, is visible on CT scanning and can be present in as many as 39% to 43% of patients.[22] By definition, hemorrhagic infarction occurs within 24 hours of infarction, and hemorrhagic transformation occurs after 24 hours of infarction. The cause of the hemorrhagic change is thought to result from reperfusion into areas of damaged capillary endothelium and is common in large infarcts with extensive injury. Hemorrhagic transformation occurs equally in all distributions of infarcts[90] and is not associated necessarily with hypertension or older age.[21] Hemorrhagic transformation can be detected in the acute phase by CT; in this case, one should not use anticoagulants because they may increase in the severity of the cerebral hemorrhage.

In the subacute phase the findings from CT clearly show the development of cerebral edema within 3 days, which then fades over the next 2 to 3 weeks; then a decrease in the signal intensity occurs over the infarction. This decrease corresponds with the change from the positive mass effect (swelling) of the acute phase to the negative mass effect (shrinkage) of the chronic phase. The infarct actually may be difficult to see again in 2 to 3 weeks but is clearly visible with the addition of contrast material. Long-term parenchymal enhancement develops, which is consistent with the scar formation that becomes the permanent CT finding. The loss of tissue volume (negative mass effect) and the permanent scar tissue are the characteristic features of a chronic infarct (Figures 1-4 to 1-8).

## Magnetic Resonance Imaging

Magnetic resonance imaging is now as commonly used in acute patients as CT, because cost and availability have improved. The MRI also has the advantage of allowing earlier detection of infarcts and, as more acute interventions have become common, allows for better evaluation of the course of acute treatment. Newer techniques such as diffusion-weighted averaging have been used to help in

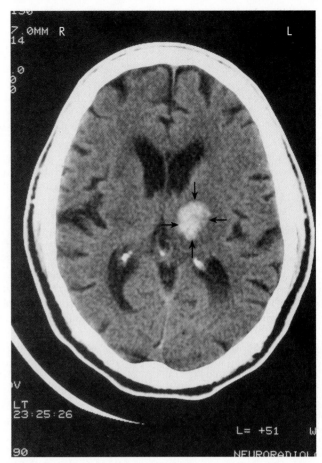

**Figure 1-4**   Magnetic resonance image of brain without gadolinium demonstrates an acute large left basal ganglia infarct. An acute infarct on the image appears white and is indicated by arrows.

the identification of early infarcts.[46,112] Magnetic resonance imaging also can rule out other conditions and screen for acute bleeding. In addition, MRI can be more sensitive for detecting cerebral infarctions in acute patients. Magnetic resonance images are created by mapping out the relaxation of protons after the imposition of a strong magnetic field. These images then are taken in two ways: T1- and T2-weighted images. In T1 images, fat and tissues with similar proton densities are enhanced (bright). In T2 images, water and tissues that are rich in water are enhanced. As in CT scans, sulcal effacement can be seen, but hyperintensity is also evident in affected areas on the T1-weighted images. Magnetic resonance images can show meningeal enhancement over the dura, which occurs in 35% of acute stroke cases.[35] Magnetic resonance imaging also can detect hemorrhage in much the same way as CT does.

The subacute changes of edema and mass effect can be seen with MRI, and use of contrast may be necessary to elucidate an infarct in the 2- to 3-week window. Magnetic resonance imaging has an advantage in determining a

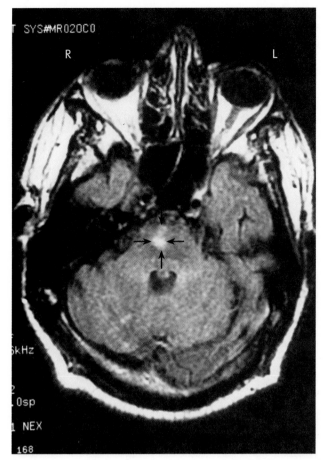

**Figure 1-5**  Magnetic resonance image of the brainstem and cerebellum without gadolinium demonstrates an acute right pontine infarct. The infarct appears white and is indicated by arrows.

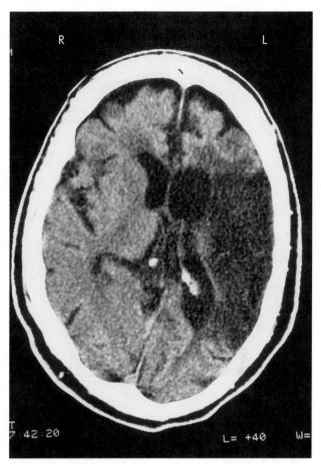

**Figure 1-6**  Computed tomography scan of the brain without contrast demonstrates a large, previous, left middle cerebral artery distribution infarction. Loss of mass of brain tissue has occurred with dilated ventricles. Bleeding or acute infarction is not evident.

hemorrhage in a late stage because it can detect the degradation products of hemoglobin (*hemosiderin deposits*) and show hemorrhage areas well after CT can no longer detect a bleed. The changes on MRI in a chronic infarction are similar to those on a CT scan.

### Positron Emission Tomography and Single-Photon Emission Computerized Tomography Scanning

Positron emission tomography and single-photon emission computerized tomography scanning are new techniques that are only available at selected centers. They have no clear role in the acute-stage evaluation of stroke.[2] In the subacute and chronic stages of stroke, these techniques help to distinguish between infarcted and noninfarcted tissue and can help delineate areas of dysfunctional but potentially salvageable brain tissue. These studies also can be used to try to assess brain function in the chronic setting. However, because of cost, limited availability, and an unclear definition of their use, they are essentially only research tools and do not have a role in the routine management of stroke patients.

## WORKUP FOR CAUSE OF STROKE

The workup for the diagnosis of stroke is aimed at answering three main questions:
1. Is the stroke thrombotic or embolic?
2. Does an underlying cause require treatment?
3. Do any risk factors require modification?

### Transcranial and Carotid Doppler

Transcranial and carotid Doppler studies allow for noninvasive visualization of the cerebral vessels. The advantages are that they provide useful therapeutic information on the state of the cerebral vessels and the blood flow to the brain. Approximately one third of patients who have had ischemic strokes that are cardiac in origin have significant cerebrovascular disease.[20] Patients with symptoms or evidence of posterior circulation disease are tested best with a transcranial Doppler study including examination of the vertebrobasilar system. The cost is low compared with other tests such as magnetic resonance angiography or

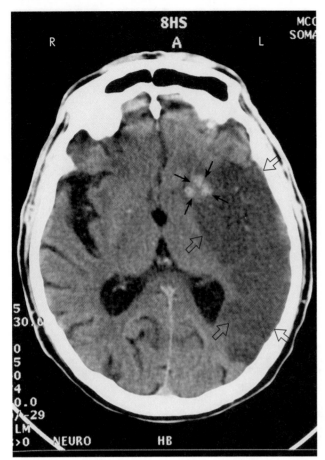

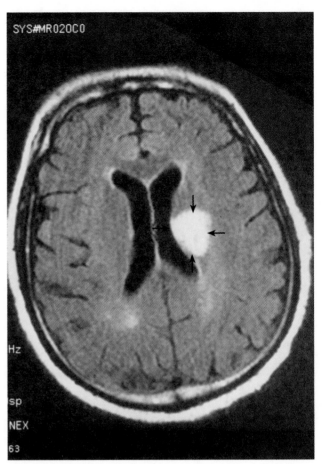

**Figure 1-7**    Computed tomography scan of the brain without contrast demonstrates a large subacute left middle cerebral artery distribution infarction, indicated by the hollow arrows. No loss of brain tissue mass has occurred compared with Figure 1-6. Evidence of acute bleeding is in the basal ganglia on the left, which is white on the scan and indicated with solid arrows.

**Figure 1-8**    Computed tomography scan of the brain without contrast demonstrates a large, acute left thalamic hemorrhage. The acute bleeding in the thalamus on the left is white on the scan and is indicated with arrows.

cerebral angiography, which has significant associated morbidity and mortality. The evidence of carotid disease can help shape the patient's treatment plan and encourage pursuit of definitive treatments such as carotid endarterectomy.

### Electrocardiography

Electrocardiography is used to evaluate patients with stroke symptoms to detect arrhythmias (which may be a source of embolic material) or myocardial infarction or other acute cardiac events that may be related to an acute stroke.

### Echocardiography

In patients with a history of cardiac disease and stroke, echocardiography usually is warranted. The types of cardiac disease that usually cause emboli and should be investigated with an echocardiograph include congestive heart failure, valvular heart disease, arrhythmias, and a

recent myocardial infarction. In some individuals, a patent foramen ovale (the fetal opening between the right and left sides of the heart) persists into adulthood and can be the source of a paradoxical embolus from the venous circulation that crosses from the right atrium into the left atrium. A transesophageal echocardiogram then can be useful in combination with a bubble study to assess for a right-to-left shunt. This specialized study also can visualize parts of the heart better in the search for emboli in areas such as the left atrial appendage when the standard transthoracic echocardiogram is inconclusive.

### Blood Work

The standard acute evaluation of the stroke patient includes a complete screening set of blood analyses, including hematologic studies, serum electrolyte levels (ionizing substances such as sodium and potassium), and renal (e.g., serum creatinine) and hepatic chemical analyses (liver function tests). The typical hematologic evaluation has a complete blood count, platelet count, prothrombin time, and partial thromboplastin time.

These studies help to rule out other causes of strokelike symptoms, diagnose complications, and allow for a baseline analysis before the initiation of therapies such as anticoagulation. The blood chemistry analyses allow metabolic abnormalities to be ruled out, as do the renal and hepatic chemistry analyses. The latter part of the stroke evaluation can involve numerous specialized tests that are chosen according to the clinical symptoms and development of the differential diagnosis as the evaluation progresses (Figure 1-9). (Table 1-6 provides a sample of some of these studies and their associated conditions.)

## MEDICAL STROKE MANAGEMENT

### Principal Goals

As in the medical management of all patients, the care of stroke management requires good general patient care. All phases include caring for the conditions the patient may have and preventing medical complications and anticipating needs that will arise as the patient progresses through the acute phase into the convalescent, rehabilitative, and long-term maintenance phases after stroke. Care for acute patients is provided best in a specialized stroke unit that commonly deals with the issues and concerns unique to these patients.[2,82] Outcome studies have demonstrated the benefit of these units in the care of stroke patients.[73] Medical rehabilitation units also have been shown to be beneficial in the improvements of outcomes in the subacute and convalescent phases.

### Acute Stroke Management

In management of acute stroke patients, basic medical needs have to be addressed and include essentials such as airway protection, maintenance of adequate circulation, and the treatment of fractures or other injuries and conditions that are present at the time of admission. The neurologic management of the acute stroke problems focus on identifying the cause of the stroke, preventing progression of the lesion, and treating acute neurologic complications. Some specific approaches apply to treatment of each of the different types of stroke.

### General Principles

The general principles of acute stroke management include attempting to stop progression of the lesion to

**Table 1-6**

## Medical Studies Used to Clarify Differential Diagnoses in Stroke Evaluation

| SPECIALIZED STUDIES TO EVALUATE STROKE | ASSOCIATED CONDITIONS |
| --- | --- |
| Proteins S and C | Hypercoagulable state |
| Anticardiolipin antibodies (lupus anticoagulant) | Lupus erythematosis, hypercoagulable state |
| Erythrocyte sedimentation rate | Collagen vascular disease |
| Rheumatoid factor | Lupus erythematosis, collagen vascular disease |
| Antinuclear antibody | Lupus erythematosis, collagen vascular disease |
| Hemoglobin | Polycythemia |
| Sickle cell preparation | Sickle cell disease |
| Hemoglobin electrophoresis | Sickle cell disease |
| Blood and tissue cultures | Infectious emboli |

limit deficits, reducing cerebral edema, decreasing the risk of hydrocephalus, treating seizures, and preventing complications such as DVT or aspiration that may lead to severe illness. (See the previous sections for a discussion of the studies used in acute patients to diagnose stroke.) Once the type of lesion has been defined, specific treatment can be instituted. Although numerous studies have been performed and are underway on the reduction of stroke mortality or disability,[110] no routine medical or surgical treatment has been shown to be effective. Currently, more aggressive methods such as angioplasty and thrombolysis are being studied, and the results of these trials are expected to lead to treatments that actually will improve the outcomes for individuals who have had strokes.

The basic principles in the approach to the treatment of acute stroke include an attempt to achieve improvement in cerebral perfusion by reestablishing blood flow, decreasing neuronal damage at the site of ischemia by modifying the pathophysiologic process, and decreasing edema in the area of damaged tissue (which often can lead to secondary damage to nonischemic brain tissue). Many pharmacologic and surgical treatments have been targeted toward at least one of these areas. Depending on

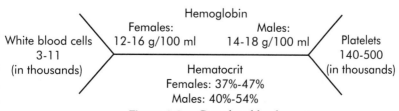

**Figure 1-9**   Complete blood count.

the stroke mechanism, the agents and techniques of choice are used.

## Ischemic Stroke

In patients who have had ischemic strokes, the restoration of blood flow and the control of neuronal damage at the area of ischemia are of the highest priority. In large strokes, edema can play a significant role, and mass shift can even lead to hydrocephalus. The pharmacologic therapies are divided broadly into antithrombotic, thrombolytic, neuroprotective, and antiedema therapies. The surgical therapies include endarterectomy, extracranial-intracranial bypass, and balloon angioplasty.

### Pharmacologic Therapies

*Antithrombotic Therapy (Antiplatelet and Anticoagulation).* The principal rationale behind the use of antiplatelet and anticoagulation agents is that rapid recanalization and reperfusion of occluded vessels reduces the infarction area. The theoretical benefit also exists of preventing clot propagation and recurring vascular thrombosis. The risks associated with the use of these treatments includes hemorrhagic conversion, hemorrhage, and increased cerebral edema, all of which are associated with worse outcomes.[72] Current research has not established a clear advantage to the use of aspirin or heparin in acute stroke patients, but these agents still are used commonly in the hope that they may decrease injury from acute stroke. Aspirin, an irreversible antiplatelet agent, is administered when symptoms appear. Heparin is administered intravenously in a continuous infusion.[57] Both of these agents are started only after determination by CT or MRI that no hemorrhage is associated with the stroke. Ticlopidine, another antiplatelet agent, has been even less well studied, and its role, if any, in acute stroke treatment is unclear. A recent meta-analysis of the trials of heparin and oral anticoagulation therapy in acute stroke treatment showed a marginal benefit from treatments with anticoagulation compared with no treatment at all.[109] Currently, numerous large, multicentric studies in the United States and Europe are examining the best approach to the antithrombotic treatment of stroke that should provide better guidance as their results become known in the next few years.

*Thrombolytic Therapy.* Thrombolytic therapy is attractive as a therapy for acute stroke, because it opens up occluded cerebral vessels and immediately restores blood flow to ischemic areas. However, a problem in using these agents in stroke treatment is that the treatment must start in 6 hours from onset of symptoms to be therapeutic. Most patients are symptomatic at a much later stage, and even if they have symptoms early enough, a rapid workup to rule out a cerebral bleed must be performed before initiation of therapy. The successful use of these agents—primarily urokinase, streptokinase, and tissue plasminogen activator—in the treatment of myocardial ischemia has aroused interest in similar use of these agents for acute stroke treatment. The mechanism of action of these agents is to cause fibrin breakdown in the clots that have been formed and thus lead to lysis of the occlusions in the blood vessels. Reviews of thrombolytic therapy for stroke treatment have shown some reduction in mortality, but no definitive answer is available to date concerning efficacy.[128] Currently, streptokinase is out of favor because of increased mortality and morbidity from intracranial hemorrhage,[100,124] but tissue plasminogen activator, a more specific thrombolytic agent, has been able to achieve favorable results. The National Institute of Neurological Disorders and Stroke trial was the cornerstone trial in approval of treatment of acute ischemic stroke with thrombolytics.[3,5,83,125] The trial was a double-blind, placebo-controlled trial that revealed an improvement in early outcomes in 24 hours of treatment and demonstrated an increase in symptom-free survival from 38% (placebo) to 50% (treatment) at 3 months. The strict use of a 3-hour window from the onset of symptoms and the rigid blood pressure guidelines of the National Institute of Neurological Disorders and Stroke trial are probably contributors to the excellent outcomes; the exact treatment protocols still are being defined. On reexamination at 1 year, the treated patients continued to show a benefit, and this has encouraged the use of this agent in selected groups.[70] Other thrombolytic agents such as alteplase also have shown benefit and are being used routinely. The results are at the same level of effectiveness as tissue plasminogen activator.[4] Unfortunately, the 3-hour window of efficacy limits the number of individuals who can receive benefit, and studies to expand the window of intervention to 6 hours or more have not shown clear benefits.[23,51] In the patient with stroke beyond 3 hours, the currently recommended interventions are mostly limited to the use of anticoagulants and antiplatelet agents to prevent further events.[83] Further active investigation continues to search for effective treatments in this large group of individuals with late presentation of stroke.

*Other Treatments for Altering Cerebral Perfusion.* A number of different treatments aimed at lowering blood viscosity or cerebral perfusion have been used, including hemodilution with agents such as dextran, albumin, and hetastarch. None of the 12 studies reviewed by Asplund demonstrated any clear benefit.[7] Similarly, studies of prostacyclins and several different types of cerebral vasodilators also have shown no clear evidence of increased survival rates or improvement in outcomes after treatment.[72] Research continues to be active in these areas, but so far none of these alternative treatments for increasing cerebral perfusion has yielded a favorable outcome.

*Neuroprotective Agents.* Neuroprotective agents are medications that can alter the course of metabolic events after the onset of ischemia and therefore have the potential to reduce stroke damage. No agent has shown clear benefits among this group of treatments. These agents include calcium channel blockers, naloxone, gangliosides, glutamate antagonists, and free-radical scavengers. Each of these agents has had promise in the theoretical or laboratory realm, but none have proved to be clinically efficacious.

The use of naloxone, a narcotic antagonist, is based on the in vitro observation that naloxone has neuroprotective effects. Unfortunately, the clinical trials to date have not demonstrated any benefit.[26] The therapeutic rationale of using calcium channel blockers is that they prevent injury to ischemic neurons by preventing calcium influx, which decreases metabolic activity in the neuron.[72] Initial hope was that the treatment results for SAH, in which nimodipine decreases secondary ischemia, would be similar for stroke. Unfortunately, the results of several studies have not shown any clear benefits from treatment with these agents,[88] and none of them currently are used routinely for stroke treatment.

In animal experiments, glutamate antagonists decrease the size of infarction area in stroke.[72] However, the few studies done in human beings have been inconclusive and have shown serious neuropsychiatric side effects.[26]

Gangliosides may reduce ischemic damage by counteracting toxic amino acids in ischemic tissue. Despite the many studies that have been performed, no clearly demonstrated benefits have resulted from use of these agents.[26]

The free-radical scavengers include 21-amino steroids (lazaroids), ascorbic acid (vitamin C), and tocopherol (vitamin E). They have not been well evaluated, and some studies to establish their clinical use are being undertaken.[72] However, vitamin E has been demonstrated clinically to reduce the risk of heart disease, so secondarily its use may decrease the risk of stroke.

*Agents for Cerebral Edema.* Agents that reduce cerebral edema include corticosteroids, mannitol, glycerol, vinca alkaloids, and piracetam. All the studies done on persons receiving steroids[99] after an acute stroke demonstrated no clear benefits, and steroid use creates a risk of diabetes and deep vein thrombosis.[49] Use of the other agents also has no clear benefit in the treatment of acute stroke and also are not used routinely.

### Surgical Therapies

*Endarterectomy.* A carotid endarterectomy is the surgical opening of the carotid arteries to remove plaque. This therapy has been shown to be useful in preventing recurrent strokes or development of stroke in individuals with TIAs, but it has not been used to treat acute stroke. In theory, the opening of the carotids could subject ischemic areas and their blood vessels to excessive pressure from restored blood flow and lead to hemorrhage.[32] Concerns about using major anesthesia in a patient with a new stroke makes this surgery too risky to treat acute stroke.

*Extracranial-Intracranial Bypass.* Despite the initial attraction of bringing extracranial blood flow into the intracranial vessels through the use of bypass procedures, the large trial done in the 1980s demonstrated no improvement in patient outcomes, and the procedure has been largely abandoned.[38]

*Balloon Angioplasty.* Despite its efficacy in opening blocked coronary arteries in patients with heart disease and its successful treatment of acute myocardial infarction, the use of balloon angioplasty in acute stroke has not been studied. Clinical centers are actively investigating its possible uses.

### Hemorrhagic Stroke

In patients who have had a hemorrhagic stroke, the size and location of the lesion determines the overall prognosis; supratentorial lesions greater than 5 cm have a poor prognosis, and brainstem lesions of 3 cm are usually fatal.[40] In these cases the control of edema is important, and the techniques described previously can be used. In patients with SAH, the treatment regimen is usually more aggressive and focuses on several issues, which include the control of intracranial pressure, prevention of rebleeding, maintenance of cerebral perfusion, and control of vasospasm.

*Prevention of Rebleeding.* Before 1980, 6 weeks of bed rest were prescribed routinely for the care of patients with acute SAH to prevent rebleeding. In 1981 a study demonstrated that bed rest was inferior to surgical treatment, lowering of blood pressure, and carotid ligation.[126] Antihypertensive medications for the prevention of rebleeding are still controversial, and no consensus exists as to their use. Carotid ligation used to be popular, but more recent reevaluations of the benefits of the technique have not been as conclusive, and because of its surgical risks, direct repair of the aneurysm is a better choice. Antifibrinolytic agents have been studied as well and also have been beneficial for low-risk patients in whom surgery must be delayed, but they seem to increase the risk of ischemic events. The placement of intraluminal coils, balloons, and polymers has shown some benefit in the short-term prevention of rebleeding, but the long-term efficacy is still unclear and the techniques remain experimental.[82] Because the risk of rebleeding is also very high in post-SAH seizures even though the incidence of seizure is low, the recommendation is that patients receive antiseizure medications for prophylaxis.

*Control of Vasospasm.* The treatment of vasospasm is important for the reasons previously outlined. The current treatments include the use of orally administered nimodipine, a calcium channel blocker that has been shown to improve outcomes of patients who have had an SAH with vasospasm. The results of using other calcium channel antagonists are unclear. The use of hypertension/hypervolemia/hemodilution has been recommended by some studies. Creating more volume than normal results in hypertension. The stretch caused by the volume stimulates the smooth muscle pressure receptors that line the vessels. These receptors inhibit muscle action by a protective response, and the blood vessel dilates to accommodate the increased volume. Hypertension/hypervolemia/hemodilution is most effective in preventing vasospasm after surgically clipping the aneurysm. Significant cardiac and hemodynamic risks are associated with this therapy, so intensive care unit monitoring is required.[82]

## PREVENTION OF STROKE RECURRENCE

### Ischemic Stroke

In general, the strategies to prevent recurrence of ischemic stroke can be divided into two areas: risk factor modification (which also applies to primary prevention) and secondary prevention to treat the underlying cause of stroke in individuals with a history of stroke. Following is a discussion of the secondary interventions that can be used to prevent recurrence of stroke.

*Hypertension.* Although the treatment of hypertension is an important primary preventive measure in the management of stroke, whether blood pressure reduction after stroke is beneficial has not been proved definitively. The transient rise in blood pressure after stroke usually settles without intervention.[129] Because of the uncertainty about whether overaggressive treatment of acute elevated blood pressure is harmful, definitive antihypertensive therapy probably should be delayed for 2 weeks.[72] At that time, one should follow the usual recommendations regarding adequate control of hypertension because some evidence indicates that it is beneficial. This seems especially appropriate in patients who have had a lacunar stroke because the development of multiple lacunae is related to uncontrolled blood pressure.

*Antiplatelet Medications.* In patients who have had a TIA or stroke, long-term use of aspirin has been shown to decrease the incidence of death, myocardial infarction, and recurrent events by up to 23%.[6] The doses of aspirin in numerous studies have ranged from 30 mg to 600 mg; all doses resulted in a 14% to 18% reduction in recurrent cerebral events, but gastrointestinal complications increased with the higher doses.[1,39,122] In general, a standard dosage of one regular adult aspirin (325 mg a day) is the usual treatment for recurrent ischemic stroke. Studies are under way that compare the efficacy of warfarin versus aspirin in treating ischemic stroke; the results of these studies are not yet available. Ticlopidine is another antiplatelet medication that has been effective in reducing the incidence of recurrent stroke.[65] Ticlopidine is most efficacious in women, patients who are not helped by aspirin therapy, and patients with vertebrobasilar symptoms, hypertension, diabetes, and no severe carotid disease.[49]

*Anticoagulation.* The incidence of recurrent stroke and TIA in patients with atrial fibrillation is approximately 7% per year. For patients who have atrial fibrillation with cardiac sources of emboli, warfarin is the clear treatment of choice; this is true for primary and secondary prevention. Although aspirin has some preventive effects, it is not *as* efficacious. In the presence of structural cardiac disease or atrial fibrillation, aspirin should be used only to treat patients in whom warfarin anticoagulation is contraindicated.[72]

The odds ratio for recurrence is approximately 0.36 in those treated with warfarin versus control and 0.84 for those treated with aspirin versus control.[36] However, problems exist with warfarin anticoagulation in the elderly. Cognitive and compliance difficulties can lead to an increase in complications. Unclear issues in anticoagulation use include when to start anticoagulants after stroke, the safety of anticoagulants in clinical practice, and the optimum anticoagulant blood level. Several studies currently are examining these questions.

*Treatment of Arrhythmias or Underlying Disease.* Obviously, primary and secondary prevention should treat the underlying cause of the ischemic stroke. Prevention can include cardioversion to normal sinus rhythm and treatment with antiarrhythmic medications, as well as treatment of underlying medical conditions if they can be found. Unfortunately, only a small proportion of patients who have had TIAs and strokes can benefit from these specific treatments.

*Carotid Endarterectomy.* The surgical treatment of carotid artery stenosis has been shown to be beneficial in recent studies of stroke recurrence in patients with severely (>70%) stenosed carotid arteries.[10,37] The data on the intermediate group of patients (stenosis from 30% to 70%) are being collected. For patients with high-grade stenosis, carotid endarterectomy reduces the range of stroke risk from 22% to 26% down to 8% to 12%.

### Hemorrhagic Stroke

The mainstay of ICH prevention is controlling systolic and diastolic hypertension. No clear benefit exists for one group of treatment agents versus another as long as adequate hypertension control is maintained. In patients in whom the ICH follows vasculitis or the use of anticoagulants, the treatment for preventing recurrence includes treating the vasculitis or terminating anticoagulant use.[104]

The secondary prevention of recurrent stroke and SAH of AVMs and/or aneurysms includes surgical management of the lesions (the treatment of choice). Clipping or microsurgical dissection of the lesions is performed whenever possible and as soon as the patient is able safely to undergo the procedure.[82,119] In surgically unresectable lesions, alternatives include sclerotherapy, coating, trapping, and proximal arterial occlusion.[82]

## PREVENTION OF COMPLICATIONS AND LONG-TERM SEQUELAE

### General Principles

To prevent complications and long-term sequelae after a stroke, maximizing function, decreasing morbidity, and preventing rehospitalization from a complication are important. Prevention of these complications begins on the day the patient arrives at the hospital with symptoms of acute stroke. Many complications are associated with bed rest in general, but some are specific to stroke.

### Musculoskeletal Complications

*Contractures.* Contractures are periarticular motion impairments that result from loss of elasticity in the periarticular tissues, which include muscles, tendons, and ligaments. Contractures can occur in any immobilized joint but are particularly prevalent in the paretic limbs after a stroke. In fact, only 10% of stroke patients recover limb strength and mobility rapidly enough to avoid developing contractures.[50] Shoulder pain, contractures, and muscle pain occur in 70% to 80% of patients who have had a hemiplegic stroke.[104] Chapter 10 addresses the management and related issues of the hemiplegic shoulder. Contractures also occur in other areas and begin to be problematic within a few days of onset or several days after the stroke when symptoms of immobility and spasticity may begin to develop. Usually contractures occur in a pattern of flexion, adduction, and internal rotation; muscles that span two joints are more susceptible to contracture formation.[52] To prevent shortening of the connective tissue in muscles and joints, an active range of motion (ROM) program must be initiated. Because certain muscles span two joints, joints must be positioned to allow full physiologic stretch of the muscles involved. Once a contracture is present, the mainstay of treatment is gradual, prolonged stretch. The minimal treatment is a sustained stretch greater than 30 minutes.[67] Other treatments include serial casting and splinting, deep-heating modalities,[18] and possible surgical release for long-standing, tight contractures.[52] (For a more detailed overview of these treatments, see Chapters 12 and 13.)

*Osteoporosis.* Bone is a metabolically active tissue that is normally in a state of equilibrium between active bone resorption and deposition. The ratio of bone formation to bone resorption is influenced by the stressors to which the bone is subjected, a relationship that is known as *Wolff's law.*[18] The lack of weight bearing and normal stress on long bones on the hemiplegic side of a stroke patient leads to a predominance of bone resorption. This loss of bone mass can start as early as 30 hours after the beginning of immobility[123] and with bed rest can be as high as 25% to 45% in 30 to 36 weeks.[31] In patients who have had a stroke, osteoporosis is often worse and the rate of hip fracture is far higher on the side of the hemiplegia.[53]

Osteoporosis prevention is accomplished best with measures that include active weight-bearing exercise and active muscle contraction (see Chapters 8 and 15). Medical therapies for individuals at risk for osteoporosis should be initiated. Therapies include bone-forming agents, calcium and vitamin D supplementation, hormone replacement, and other measures as needed. (Box 1-1 shows some of the medical treatments available for osteoporosis.)

*Heterotopic Ossification.* Heterotopic ossification is the deposition of calcium in the form of mature bone in the soft tissues. The condition is not particularly common after stroke but occurs with increased incidence after traumatic brain injury. The incidence ranges from 11% to 76% in various studies.[14] Spasticity is associated with the development of heterotopic ossification as are long-bone fractures and a prolonged coma. Symptoms of heterotopic ossification usually develop 1 to 3 months after injury with pain and limited ROM.[19] The diagnosis is based on clinical examination, elevated alkaline phosphatase levels in the serum, and a positive bone scan.

Treatment for heterotopic ossification includes active ROM; no studies indicate that the condition is caused or worsened by active ROM exercises.[14] Pharmacologic treatment options include the use of etidronate disodium and nonsteroidal antiinflammatory drugs.[19] Other treatments include radiation therapy and, for refractory cases after the lesion has matured, surgical excision of the

**Box 1-1**

**Treatments for Osteoporosis**

Bone forming agents (etidronate and others)
Estrogen replacement
Calcitonin
Calcium supplementation
Vitamin D supplementation
Fluoride supplementation
Weight-bearing exercises

heterotopic ossification. Performance of ROM exercises after surgery is particularly important. Low-dose radiation or etidronate disodium also can be used to prevent recurrence.[27]

***Falls.*** Falls are of particular concern in survivors of stroke. These patients are at increased risk of hip fracture because of developed osteoporosis, and the acuity of their balance, visual perceptions, and spatial perceptions is decreased. The increased risk of falls has been documented in several studies and is greater in patients who have had a right hemispheric stroke.[28,86,95] Fall prevention should emphasize balance and cognitive training, removing environmental hazards, and using adaptive devices. (These measures are reviewed in Chapters 8, 19, 25, and 27.)

### Neurologic Complications

***Seizures.*** Seizures after strokes have been documented since the nineteenth century. The incidence of late-onset seizures (epilepsy) in the individuals who have had strokes ranges from 6% to 18%,[54,127] whereas the incidence of early seizures is approximately 10%, with reports ranging from 3% to 38%.[11,133] The risk for seizures is highest right after stroke; 57% of seizures occur in the first week, and 88% of all seizures after strokes occur in the first year.[11] Seizures are more common in patients who have had an SAH; 85% of these seizures are early seizures.[118] The timing of seizures that occur after stroke varies according to the mechanism of injury. The timing of seizures after thrombotic and embolic strokes seems to be about equal. Patients with SAH have more seizures soon after the stroke, whereas patients with ICH are more similar to patients with ischemic stroke and may have more late-onset seizures.[133]

The treatment and management of seizures associated with stroke are usually straightforward, and monotherapy often produces adequate results. If the patient only has acute-onset seizures in the setting of their stroke, the patient often does not require long-term antiseizure medication. A single, brief seizure or a nongeneralizing local seizure also often can be managed conservatively. If seizures do require treatment, a single agent usually suffices and is beneficial because the drug interactions are fewer and the compliance is better with monotherapy. Carbamazepine and phenytoin are the preferred agents for treating epilepsy after stroke. Management of the medication requires close follow-up to ensure that the desired outcome is achieved: an asymptomatic, seizure-free patient. Excessive medication can lead to a number of symptoms (Box 1-2). Inadequate control of the condition leads to additional seizures. For situations in which seizures become refractory to treatment, one must remember several factors.[133] Intercurrent illness or metabolic disarray that lowers the seizure threshold may make the seizures more frequent and difficult to treat. Patient

---

**Box 1-2**

**Signs of Excessive Antiseizure Medication**

Lethargy
Drowsiness
Depression
Nystagmus
Ataxia
Irritability
Distractibility
Poor cognition
Poor memory

---

compliance may be a problem, especially if the stroke created cognitive and behavioral deficits. Progressive lesions or new infarcts are also causes of increasing seizure frequency. Finally, a stroke that occurs in highly epileptogenic areas—such as the hippocampus, the parietooccipital cortex surrounding the rolandic fissure, and calcarine cortex—may engender refractory epilepsy and require combination therapy. (Table 1-7 lists the common seizure medications and their side effects.)

***Hydrocephalus.*** Hydrocephalus can occur acutely, especially in patients with SAH and ICH as discussed previously, or it can develop symptoms insidiously later. Hydrocephalus usually is heralded by the gradual onset of a triad of symptoms, including lethargy with decreased mental function, ataxia, and urinary incontinence. Once hydrocephalus is suspected, one should perform a CT scan promptly because the increasing size of the ventricles are readily visible. Once diagnosed, one should surgically place a ventricular shunt. The procedure is well tolerated and can lead to resolution of all the symptoms of hydrocephalus if performed promptly. Patients with an occluded shunt have symptoms that mimic the initial symptoms of hydrocephalus.

***Spasticity.*** *Spasticity* is defined as a motor disorder characterized by a velocity-dependent increase in tonic stretch reflexes with exaggerated tendon jerks. Spasticity results from hyperexcitability of the stretch reflex (which is one component of the upper motor neuron syndrome).[71] In a normal recovery after a flaccid stroke, an initial period occurs with little resistance to passive motion of the muscles and joints. Approximately 48 hours after the stroke, tendon reflexes and muscle resistance to passive motion begin to return.[52] Spasticity is most pronounced in the flexor muscles and occurs throughout the hemiplegic side. The lower extremity later develops a component of extensor spasticity that can assist with function, whereas the upper extremity spasticity is usually in a flexor pattern.[8]

The management of spasticity includes encouraging voluntary movement, ROM exercises, and a func-

**Table 1-7**

**Medical Management of Seizures: Drug Therapy**

| MEDICATION | SIDE EFFECTS | PRINCIPLE USES |
|---|---|---|
| Phenytoin | Ataxia<br>Incoordination<br>Confusion<br>Rash<br>Gum hyperplasia<br>Hirsutism<br>Osteomalacia | Tonic-clonic (grand mal)<br>Partial |
| Carbamazepine | Ataxia<br>Dizziness<br>Diplopia<br>Vertigo<br>Bone marrow suppression<br>Hepatotoxicity | Tonic-clonic (grand mal)<br>Partial |
| Phenobarbital | Sedation<br>Ataxia<br>Confusion<br>Dizziness<br>Depression<br>Decreased libido<br>Rash | Tonic-clonic (grand mal)<br>Partial |
| Primidone | Same as phenobarbital | Tonic-clonic (grand mal)<br>Partial |
| Valproic acid | Ataxia<br>Sedation<br>Tremor<br>Bone marrow suppression<br>Hepatotoxicity<br>Weight gain<br>Transient alopecia | Absence (petit mal)<br>Atypical absence<br>Myoclonic<br>Tonic-clonic (grand mal) |
| Clonazepam | Ataxia<br>Sedation<br>Lethargy<br>Anorexia | Absence (petit mal)<br>Atypical absence<br>Myoclonic |
| Ethosuximide | Ataxia<br>Lethargy<br>Rash<br>Bone marrow suppression | Absence (petit mal) |

tional rehabilitative approach.[52] The research data on the different neurorehabilitative treatment approaches do not define clearly which approach is most effective, so an individualized approach to treating each patient is the best course. Pharmacologic treatments for spasticity are numerous, and they need to be tailored to each patient to find the best balance of side effects and efficacy. The most commonly used agents are baclofen, dantrolene sodium, and diazepam. These medications and a representative sample of the other medications used to treat patients who have had a stroke are presented in the table of medications and their side effects on the inside cover of the book. Other treatments for severe spasticity that are more invasive include phenol blocks and neurolysis,

botulinum toxin (Botox) injections, and implantable baclofen pumps. Botox injections and baclofen pumps are still experimental approaches, and ongoing studies will elucidate their future roles (see Chapter 10).

**Other Complications**

***Deconditioning.*** Physiologic deconditioning in patients after a stroke results from the acute medical illness and the associated bed rest and immobility that may result. (Box 1-3 lists some of the effects of deconditioning.) All of these factors can alter the ability of the patient to recover. Therefore, to get the patient out of bed and to increase activity as early and aggressively as possible is important.

**Box 1-3**

**Deconditioning Effects of Stroke**

**MUSCULOSKELETAL**

Atrophy
↓ Strength of tendons, ligaments, bones, and muscles
Depression
Anxiety
Sleep disturbance

**CARDIOVASCULAR**

↓ Stroke volume
↑ Heart rate
↓ VO$_2$max
↑ Respiratory rate
↓ Lean body mass
↑ Body fat
Orthostatic hypotension

**NEUROLOGIC/EMOTIONAL**

Sensory deprivation
↓ Balance
↓ Coordination
Fatigue

**GENITOURINARY**

Diuresis
Difficulty voiding

**ENDOCRINE**

Impaired glucose tolerance
Altered regulation of hormones

**BODY COMPOSITION AND METABOLISM**

Nitrogen loss
Calcium loss
Potassium loss
Phosphorus loss
Sulfur loss

*Psychological Complications.* Stroke is a major life event and is associated with significant alterations in the individual's well-being and independence. Negative emotional reactions are common in patients following a stroke[121] and can have a significant effect on the patient's eventual outcome. After a stroke, patients may go through the four stages of bereavement described by Worden.[137] These include accepting the loss, experiencing the pain of the loss, adjusting to a new environment in which previous abilities are missing, and investing in new activities. Not all patients become depressed, and this lack of depression does not necessarily mean the patient is in denial.[138] Denial is a normal defense mechanism, and as long as it does not interfere with the rehabilitative process, it is not a concern.[121] The indifference reaction, a persistent denial reaction, is more common in

patients who have had a right-sided stroke than a left-sided stroke.[44]

Another common consequence of stroke is emotional lability, which is rapidly shifting from one extreme emotion to another. Approximately 20% of patients have emotional lability 6 months after a stroke, and up to 10% have lability for 1 year. Emotional lability is more common in patients with pseudobulbar palsy and right hemispheric strokes, particularly if the patient is depressed.[60]

Anxiety is also common after stroke and is more frequent in patients with left hemispheric strokes[76] and cortical lesions.[115] Many sources of anxiety exist, including financial affairs, family issues, and a fear of dying or recurrent stroke. Reassurance and constant positive feedback during rehabilitation can help, and in severe cases, treatment with anxiolytics and psychological support may be needed.

Fortunately, outbursts and aggressive behavior are rare after a stroke, but when they occur, they are more common in patients with left-sided infarcts who are more aware of their deficits. The approach to management of these outbursts should not include restraints and threats but should be based on avoiding excessive frustration in the patient by removing emotional triggers and alternating easy and difficult tasks.[121]

Depression is common after stroke, developing in 20% to 50% of stroke survivors, with 30% being the most commonly accepted figure.[121] The depression can be a reaction to the stroke or a neuropsychological sequela of the stroke. The consequences of depression after stroke are numerous: hospital stays are longer,[33] cognitive impairment is greater,[102] and motivation decreases.[111] Depression is more common in patients with left cortical lesions[116] and lesions close to the frontal poles and is shorter in patients with subcortical and brainstem lesions. Depression after stroke often is treated best with antidepressant medications.[121] In patients who are unable to tolerate antidepressants, are unresponsive to therapy, or have active suicidal ideation, electroconvulsive therapy can be a last resort.[89] (See Chapter 2 for more information about the psychological effects of stroke.)

*Urinary Tract Dysfunction.* Urinary incontinence is common after stroke, affecting 51% to 60% of patients,[16] and can cause difficulties with rehabilitation, influence eventual discharge location, and place stress on caregivers.[34] One month and 6 months after stroke, 29% and 14% of patients, respectively, still have urinary incontinence.[9] The usual pathophysiology of incontinence is detrusor hyperreflexia, which is common in patients with cortical lesions. The incontinence assessment includes a thorough history of the urinary symptoms and can include urodynamic studies to help define the problem. Incontinence treatment includes timed voiding and use of pharmacologic agents and intermittent catheterization. If these treatments do not work, incontinence may need to be treated by indwelling catheterization. This is performed on patients who cannot independently self-catheterize and do not have caretakers who can provide this care or in patients who have physical barriers such as urethral strictures that prevent regular catheterizations. Unfortunately, indwelling catheters have a high incidence of associated urinary tract infections. Male patients also may use external condom catheters, which can provide socially acceptable continence when the individual is traveling or physically active. Patients with continuous dribbling also benefit from condom catheters. The goal of all of these therapies is to maintain continence and prevent urinary tract infections and other complications such as skin breakdown from skin maceration.

***Skin Breakdown and Decubitus Ulcers.*** Pressure ulcer formation is a serious health problem in debilitated and immobilized patients. After a stroke, patients are at particular risk for pressure ulcers because they have numerous factors contributing to skin breakdown. Abnormal sensation, contracture, malnutrition, immobility, and muscle and soft-tissue atrophy often develop and may be complicated by advanced age. Prevention of pressure ulcers, rather than treatment of developing ulcers, should be the focus of care. Preventive measures include frequent repositioning, keeping skin clean and dry, maintaining an adequate level of nutrition, and, in especially high-risk patients, using pressure-relief mattresses.[106] Once pressure ulcers have formed, in addition to strictly observing the preventive and pressure relieving measures previously noted, treatments include meticulous wound care with a variety of agents and possibly surgical reconstruction.

***Dysphagia.*** Swallowing disorders are common after a stroke. Dysphagia is more common in the elderly, with an incidence of 25% to 45%.[47,48] Aspiration can lead to pneumonia, and a decreased eating ability can lead to dehydration and malnutrition. Chapter 22 covers the details of the pathology of aspiration and the methods of its treatment.

***Aspiration.*** Aspiration causes chemical pneumonitis that can lead to a secondary bacterial infection. Because numerous anaerobic organisms are in the mouth, aspiration pneumonia can develop into an anaerobic abscess.[74] Such abscesses occur less frequently in edentulous individuals because they have less oral flora and can occur in up to a third of cases in hospitalized patients.[79] The treatment of choice is to reduce the risk of aspiration and administer antibiotics. Examining a radiographic film for evidence of abscess cavities and the sputum for organisms can help one develop a specific medical treatment. Sputum culture growth often requires up to 3 or 4 days,

so initial treatment is often empiric and should be the administration of a wide-spectrum antibiotic that is effective against hospital-acquired organisms (which are often resistant to certain antibiotics) and anaerobic bacteria.[74] The usual course of antibiotics is 7 to 10 day, but cavitary pneumonia may require far longer treatment for eradication of the organism.[75] Determination of which specific antibacterial agents to use depends on the resistance patterns in the institution in which the aspiration takes place; the infectious disease team at that institution should make the decision about which antibiotics to use.

***Deep Venous Thrombosis.*** Deep venous thrombosis is a common problem after stroke and has an incidence of 23% to 75% depending on the severity of the stroke. Most of the morbidity and mortality associated with DVT results from venous thromboembolism (VTE). Pulmonary embolism after stroke has an incidence of 10% to 29% and a mortality rate of 10%.[15] The formation of DVT is caused by the triad of risk factors outlined by Virchow's postulates: altered blood flow, damage to the blood vessel wall, and altered blood coagulability. Box 1-4 lists the common risk factors for DVT. Of the risk factors for DVT, stasis is one of the most important. After a stroke, DVT is 10 times more common in the paretic leg.[130] Deep venous thrombosis usually begins in the calf, and although the emboli from calf thrombi are not dangerous, these thrombi propagate in about 20% of cases, and about 50% of the proximal deep venous thrombi embolize. About 20% of symptomatic pulmonary emboli are fatal.[108] After a stroke, ambulation in itself is not preventive in the subacute setting: pulmonary embolism occurred in 57% of ambulatory patients in the rehabilitation setting.[117] Lower extremity and pelvic DVT are the most common, but proximal upper extremity DVT also can occur, although it is rare. All of the diagnostic and management issues discussed in the section on VTE that follows applies to this condition as well.

The diagnosis of DVT in the clinical setting is unreliable,[15] and many patients with life-threatening embolism

**Box 1-4**

**Risk Factors for Deep Venous Thrombosis**

Immobilization
Postoperative state
Age >40
Cardiac disease
Limb trauma
Coagulation disorders
Obesity
Advanced neoplasm
Pregnancy

and thrombosis have no clinical symptoms of DVT. Other patients with swelling and tenderness may not have DVT at all and may have any of a number of other diagnoses. The differential diagnosis of lower extremity pain and swelling includes trauma, fracture, gout, cellulitis, and superficial phlebitis. The usual clinical signs of DVT include pain and tenderness, swelling, the presence of Homan's sign, superficial venous distention, a palpable cord, and fever. Some of these signs, such as Homan's, are unreliable indicators. Homan's sign is present in less than one third of patients with DVT and is present in half of patients without DVT.[59] Objective testing for DVT has venography as the gold standard, but this procedure is associated with significant risks, including anaphylaxis and causing DVT. More commonly used, risk-free procedures are impedance plethysmography, which is a noninvasive test that measures volume changes in the leg with circumferential calf electrodes,[61] and Doppler ultrasound, which is also a noninvasive test that uses a handheld probe to detect blood flow in deep leg veins.[131] Doppler ultrasound and impedance plethysmography have similar sensitivities and specificities for DVT detection, but Doppler ultrasound is not as portable and has a higher cost than impedance plethysmography.[15]

The clinical diagnosis of pulmonary embolism is also unreliable, and only 30% of patients with pulmonary embolism have clinical DVT, even though 70% have venographic evidence of DVT.[15] The symptoms of submassive pulmonary embolism overlap with the symptoms of many other pulmonary conditions, including tachypnea, tachycardia, rales, hemoptysis, pleuritic chest pain, pleural effusion, general malaise, bronchospasm, and fever. In patients with massive pulmonary embolism with greater than 60% of the pulmonary circulation obstructed, patients are critically ill and develop heart failure, circulatory collapse, hypotension, and coma and can die suddenly.[117] The gold standard for testing for pulmonary embolism is the pulmonary angiogram, but its use is associated with significant morbidity and mortality. The preferred noninvasive test is the ventilation/perfusion scan.[85]

The best approach to VTE is to prevent DVT. The National Institutes of Health Consensus Conference on the Prevention of Venous Thrombosis and Pulmonary Embolism recommends using low doses of subcutaneously administered heparin in all stroke patients with no hemorrhagic components.[98] In all other patients, external pneumatic calf compression is recommended. More recently, low-molecular-weight heparin has been introduced and actually may be more effective than standard heparin for DVT prophylaxis.[58] Low doses of warfarin for DVT prophylaxis in stroke patients has not been well studied, but its use in other conditions has proved its effectiveness in DVT reduction. Dextran, aspirin, and static compression stockings are not effective for preventing DVT.[15] Physical treatments alone, such as ROM exercises, have not been studied. Ambulatory patients must be able to walk at least 50 feet to have a reduction in risk of DVT,[17] but as previously stated, the risk of pulmonary embolism in ambulatory patients is still significant.[117] The length of time prophylaxis should continue is still not definite, but evidence shows that continuing prophylaxis well into the subacute phase is warranted.[15]

The treatment of VTE (DVT and pulmonary embolism) is based on preventing pulmonary embolism, which can be fatal. A patient who is identified with acute VTE is started on intravenous heparin as long as no contraindications to anticoagulation exist.[56] The effectiveness of the heparin is determined by monitoring the partial thromboplastin time, and the heparin is adjusted to a dose between 1.5 and 2.5 times control. In a patient with only DVT, warfarin can be started on the first day, and the heparin can be discontinued when the warfarin dose is therapeutic as measured by the increase in the prothrombin time or international normalized ration. Targets are a prothrombin time of 1.25 to 1.5 times control or an international normalized ratio of 2 to 3.[15] In patients with pulmonary embolism, warfarin may be started a few days later, and after management of the acute stage, the patient keeps receiving it longer; patients with DVT receive warfarin for approximately 3 months, and patients with pulmonary embolism, for 6 months.[58] All patients who recently have been diagnosed with VTE are placed on bed rest initially and usually are allowed to become mobile 2 days after the partial thromboplastin time has become therapeutic.[62] The rehabilitation of patients with VTE who are beginning treatment should continue at the bedside, and in the case of patients with lower extremity DVT the rehabilitation program should include activity of daily living training, upper extremity programs, communication work, and dysphagia treatments.

## FUTURE TRENDS IN MEDICAL STROKE MANAGEMENT

### Improved Primary Stroke Prevention

Because the treatments for stroke are so limited and the deficits that can result are so devastating, the primary prevention of stroke has to be the essential strategy to decrease morbidity and mortality from stroke. With a good understanding of the risk factors for stroke, risk factor modification can be targeted at groups and individuals who are at risk. Table 1-1 lists the preventable and nonpreventable risk factors for stroke. Fortunately, many of the risk factors for stroke are the same as those for myocardial infarction and vascular disease leading to death, so the modification of stroke risk factors also decreases the risk of cardiac-related morbidity and mortality. As a result of greater awareness and risk factor modification and largely through the treatment of blood pressure, a decline of greater than 50% in the stroke mortality rate has occurred in the past 20 years.[134] Each of the modifiable risk factors are considered separately.

## Hypertension

Diastolic and systolic hypertension are each independently and strongly implicated in causing stroke. Hypertension increases the risk of stroke in all age groups of men and women.[134] In fact, no threshold level of blood pressure exists below which the risk curve plateaus.[80] For every 7.5 mm Hg increase in diastolic pressure is a 46% increase in stroke incidence and a 29% increase in coronary heart disease (CHD). Reducing blood pressure in hypertensive patients has been shown to decrease the risk of stroke significantly, with an average reduction of 5.8 mm Hg leading to a reduction in stroke incidence of 42% but only a 14% reduction in CHD incidence.[25] Because these trials only spanned 2 to 5 years, the reduction in stroke incidence is a direct result of decreased blood pressure and not an alteration in atherogenesis (production of plaque in the arteries), which would take longer to develop.[134] Systolic blood pressure is also a factor; the treatment of isolated systolic hypertension (>160 mm Hg) has been shown to reduce the incidence of stroke by 36% and CHD by 27% over 4.5 years.[97] Treating all forms of hypertension in the older age groups is therefore essential because they are at increased risk for stroke, and most strokes occur in this age group. Screening for hypertension and aggressively treating systolic and diastolic hypertension should be the cornerstone of any primary prevention program for stroke.

## Cigarette Smoking

The results of the Framingham Study and the Nurses' Health Study demonstrate that the cessation of cigarette smoking should lead to a prompt reduction in stroke mortality.[24,136] Risk of CHD decreases by 50% in 1 year and reaches the level of a nonsmoker's risk in 5 years. Smoking increases stroke risk by 40% in men and 60% in women (with no other risk factors being considered), and it seems to follow that smoking cessation leads to a reduction in stroke risk that is similar to the reduction in CHD incidence.

## Cardiac Arrhythmia and Myocardial Infarction

Coronary heart disease, atrial fibrillation, and congestive heart failure lead to an increased incidence of stroke.[134] Preventing these conditions by modifying their associated risk factors leads to a reduction in incidence of stroke. In addition, treating patients who have established arrhythmias and congestive heart failure with anticoagulants such as warfarin decreases the incidence of stroke (as explained previously).

## Blood Lipids

The development of carotid artery atherosclerotic disease has been shown to be related to the levels of serum lipids.[107] However, to relate accelerated atherosclerosis clearly to an increase in the incidence of stroke has been difficult because other pathologies related to serum lipids have been observed. Levels of total serum cholesterol less than 160 mg/dl seem to be associated with ICH and SAH, whereas higher levels of serum cholesterol are associated with atherothrombosis. No relationship has been demonstrated between cholesterol and lacunar strokes.[134] This unusual relationship of low serum lipids and higher hemorrhagic infarct has been demonstrated in Japan and also recently in the United States in the group of patients studied in the Multiple Risk Factor Intervention Trial.[63,101] Because of the ambiguity of these data, a clear statement of guidelines for the management of cholesterol to reduce incidence is difficult to make.

## Diabetes

The rate of atherosclerosis development in coronary, femoral, and cerebral vessels is increased in diabetics. Stroke is increased 2.5 to 4 times in diabetics compared with nondiabetics.[69] In the Framingham Study, glucose intolerance (a blood sugar greater than 150 mg/ml) is only a significant, independent contributor to stroke in older women and is greater for women than men at any age.[64] Because of the associated risk of stroke, careful management of diabetes in addition to all other risk factors is prudent.

## Oral Contraceptives

In female patients over the age of 35 who have other stroke risk factors, oral contraceptive use is associated with increased incidence of stroke.[113] The relative risk for oral contraceptive users is approximately 5 times greater if they are already in the high-risk group. With the use of lower estrogen formulation oral contraceptives, the risk has decreased substantially in recent years.[114] That the incidence of fatal SAH increased in oral contraceptive–using women with concomitant smoking is noteworthy; in the group over age 35 the incidence is 4 times higher.[43] Therefore the recommendation is that women over the age of 35 avoid using oral contraceptives, and younger women who smoke should be advised of the increased risks associated with concurrent oral contraceptive use.

## Alcohol

Heavy alcohol consumption is related to an increase in stroke and stroke deaths, whereas light to moderate alcohol consumption is associated with a reduced incidence of CHD.[30,68] Alcohol is clearly related to hemorrhagic stroke events, but the association with thromboembolic events is not definite. Regardless, patients at risk for stroke should avoid heavy alcohol consumption.

## Physical Activity

Despite the clear benefits of physical activity in the reduction of CHD morbidity and mortality, no clear association exists between physical activity and the incidence of stroke.[91,92]

## Public Education

The primary goal of primary and secondary prevention programs should be to educate individuals about risk factors and then to teach them the way to modify their risks. During routine visits, a physician should be able to identify at-risk patients through a combination of a history and physical. Routine blood pressure screening should be included in all evaluations, and patients who have hypertension should be treated. A stroke risk profile has been assembled from the Framingham Study data and can be used by physicians[135] (e.g., to help a physician decide which borderline hypertensive patients to treat). Education can start in the physician's office and be continued by all the other health professionals with whom the patient comes into contact. If the community at large is educated about the risk factors of stroke, those individuals who are at highest risk can seek out the attention they require. This model has been implemented and supported through research such as the Agency for Health Care Policy and Research *Smoking Cessation Clinical Practice Guidelines*.[93]

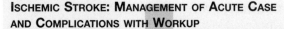

**Case Study 1**

### ISCHEMIC STROKE: MANAGEMENT OF ACUTE CASE AND COMPLICATIONS WITH WORKUP

G.H. is a 76-year-old woman who has a history of hypertension and diabetes mellitus and had a myocardial infarction 2 years ago. She arrives at her local emergency room 4 hours after an acute onset of weakness in her left arm and leg. She fell at home after trying to get up, and it was only after her neighbors heard her calls for help that the emergency services rescue team came to her aid. On admission to the emergency room, she has an elevated blood pressure of 200/100 and is alert and oriented. Her initial physical examination reveals left-sided weakness and sensory loss that is greater in her arm than her leg. The emergency room team has the impression that she has an acute stroke in evolution, so an emergency CT scan is ordered. The initial blood work and electrocardiogram are unremarkable. While she is in the CT scanner, the on-call resident is paged and asked to come see her because the radiology technician notes that she has become unable to move while in the machine. She now has a dense left hemiplegia. Because of fear of stroke progression, she is admitted to the intensive care unit.

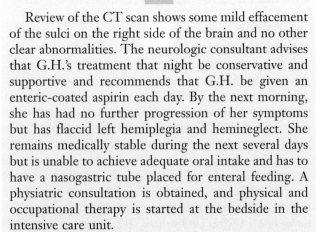

Review of the CT scan shows some mild effacement of the sulci on the right side of the brain and no other clear abnormalities. The neurologic consultant advises that G.H.'s treatment that night be conservative and supportive and recommends that G.H. be given an enteric-coated aspirin each day. By the next morning, she has had no further progression of her symptoms but has flaccid left hemiplegia and hemineglect. She remains medically stable during the next several days but is unable to achieve adequate oral intake and has to have a nasogastric tube placed for enteral feeding. A physiatric consultation is obtained, and physical and occupational therapy is started at the bedside in the intensive care unit.

Another CT scan is performed on the third hospital day, which reveals a clear, acute infarct in the right temporoparietal area with associated edema and no mass effect or hemorrhage, so the neurologist recommends an extended workup. Carotid Doppler images are normal, and the electrocardiogram indicates stability, but the echocardiogram reveals that G.H. has a decreased ejection fraction of 25% with a visible apical thrombus in the area of her previous myocardial infarction. The neurologist and cardiologist concur on anticoagulation with heparin followed by conversion to warfarin. Anticoagulant therapy is initiated, and the aspirin is no longer administered.

On the sixth hospital day, G.H. is started successfully on warfarin, her hemiparesis has improved, and she is able to move her leg against gravity and with gravity eliminated. However, she is still unable to swallow safely and still has a nasogastric tube. G.H. is accepted for inpatient rehabilitation and is transferred to the rehabilitation service on the eighth hospital day.

G.H.'s rehabilitation course is notable because of swelling and pain in her left leg, which is by duplex Doppler scanning found to result from a DVT. Because she developed the thrombosis while receiving adequate anticoagulation medication, she has an umbrella filter placed in her inferior vena cava to prevent development of a pulmonary embolus. G.H. becomes severely depressed and after consultation with the psychiatry service begins receiving antidepressant medication, which has good results. G.H. progresses in therapy, but her left shoulder becomes painful because of a shoulder-hand syndrome, which responds well to aggressive therapeutic intervention. She also develops a progressive increase in skeletal muscle activity, particularly in her left hand, which only can be kept under control with aggressive ROM exercises. At the time of her discharge, she is able to move short distances with a hemiwalker and needs assistance with dressing her lower extremities and setting up for her basic activities of daily living.

G.H.'s 1-year follow-up is notable for the continuing intractable painful spasticity in her left arm, so treatment with Botox is instituted and results in adequate pain relief. She remains stable until 5 years after her stroke, when she suffers a fall with a subsequent hip fracture. Evaluation of bone density shows accelerated osteoporosis in the left hip. She needs left hip hemiarthroplasty but is unable to regain her previous level of function despite aggressive therapy and finally has to be admitted to a nursing home when discharged from the hospital.

### Case Study 2

#### HEMORRHAGIC STROKE: MANAGEMENT OF ACUTE CASE WITH WORKUP

C.C. is a 25-year-old man who works as a sales manager in a local retail store. While dismissing a store clerk whom he caught stealing from the store safe, he suddenly complains of a severe headache, sinks to the chair in his office, and slumps over to the right. Within a few minutes he is unconscious, and the staff calls the ambulance. C.C. is admitted to the emergency room within 20 minutes, accompanied by the fired clerk who is proclaiming loudly that she has done nothing to him. In the emergency room, C.C. is in a deep coma, breathing deeply, and has dilated pupils and absent reflexes. He is intubated immediately for airway protection and is taken for an emergency CT scan. The study is not completed because C.C. has a seizure while in the CT scanner, but the partially completed study shows a great deal of blood in the ventricles. C.C. is diagnosed with a presumed SAH and treatment is started. Hyperventilation and treatment with mannitol begin. An intracranial pressure monitor is inserted, and C.C. is given phenytoin and nimodipine. C.C. is managed closely in the intensive care unit and after 3 days comes out of the coma. He remains intubated and has an MRI/magnetic resonance angiography performed that shows a probable berry aneurysm on the anterior communicating artery.

A cerebral angiogram is performed, and a 2 cm aneurysm is clearly visible. C.C. has a good response to the treatment and is extubated on the sixth hospital day. His neurologic examination reveals mild disorientation, dysarthria, and tetraparesis that is more pronounced on the right than the left.

The neurologic and neurosurgical team, patient, and family have a discussion and decide that surgical clipping of the aneurysm is the best approach to treating the lesion. C.C. is scheduled for operative intervention the next day. However, in the middle of the night, he suddenly loses consciousness and stops breathing. He has a cardiac arrest but is resuscitated successfully. An emergency CT scan reveals a large recurrent hemorrhage that extends into the cerebral cortex and a herniated brainstem. Aggressive treatments are instituted, but despite all measures the herniation progresses, and C.C. lapses into an irreversible coma. One week later C.C. is declared brain dead, and according to his family's wishes, his organs are donated for transplantation.

### REVIEW QUESTIONS

1. Which stroke risk factors are considered modifiable?
2. Which procedures are used to diagnose a stroke?
3. Which clinical signs indicate a patient is receiving excessive seizure medication?
4. What are the risk factors and recommended treatments for DVTs?
5. Other than neurologic, what are the common complications that follow a stroke?

### REFERENCES

1. A comparison of two doses of aspirin (30 mg versus 283 mg a day) in patients after a transient ischemic attack or minor ischemic stroke, the Dutch TIA Trial Study Group, *N Engl J Med* 325(18):1261-1266, 1991.
2. Adams HP Jr, Brott TG, Crowell RM, et al: Guidelines for the management of patients with acute ischemic stroke: a statement for healthcare professionals from a special writing group of the Stroke Council, American Heart Association, *Circulation* 90(3):1588-1601, 1994.
3. Adams HP Jr, Brott TG, Furlan AJ, et al: Guidelines for thrombolytic therapy for acute stroke: a supplement to the guidelines for the management of patients with acute ischemic stroke—a statement for healthcare professionals from a Special Writing Group of the Stroke Council, American Heart Association, *Circulation* 94(5):1167-1174, 1996.
4. Albers GW, Bates VE, Clark WM, et al: Intravenous tissue-type plasminogen activator for treatment of acute stroke: the standard

treatment with alteplase to reverse stroke (STARS) study, *JAMA* 283(9):1145-1150, 2000.

5. Alberts MJ: Diagnosis and treatment of ischemic stroke, *Am J Med* 106(2):211-221, 1999.

6. Antiplatelet Trialists' Collaboration: Collaborative overview of randomized trials of antiplatelet therapy. I. Prevention of death, myocardial infarction, and stroke by prolonged antiplatelet therapy in various categories of patients, *BMJ* 308(6921):81-106, 1994.

7. Asplund K: Hemodilution in acute stroke, *Cerebrovasc Dis* 1(suppl):129, 1991.

8. Bach-y-Rita P: Process of recovery from stroke. In Brandstser ME, Basmajian JV, editors: *Stroke rehabilitation*, Baltimore, 1987, Williams & Wilkins.

9. Barer DH: Continence after stroke: useful predictor or goal of therapy? *Age Ageing* 18(3):183-191, 1989.

10. Beneficial effect of carotid endarterectomy in symptomatic patients with high grade stenosis, North American Symptomatic Carotid Endarterectomy Trial Collaborators, *N Engl J Med* 325(7):445-453, 1991.

11. Black SE, Norris JW, Hachinski VC: Post stroke seizures, *Stroke* 14:134, 1983.

12. Bonita R: Epidemiology of stroke, *Lancet* 339(8789):342-344, 1992.

13. Bonita R, Beaglehole R, North JD: Event, incidence and case fatality rates of cerebrovascular disease in Auckland, New Zealand, *Am J Epidemiol* 120(2):236-243, 1984.

14. Bontke CF, Boake C: Principles of brain injury rehabilitation. In Braddom RL, editor: *Physical medicine and rehabilitation*, Philadelphia, 1996, WB Saunders.

15. Brandstater ME, Roth EJ, Siebens HC: Venous thromboembolism in stroke: literature review and implication for clinical practice, *Arch Phys Med Rehabil* 73(suppl 5):S379-S391, 1992.

16. Brockhurst JC, Andrews K, Richards B, et al: Incidence and correlates of incontinence in stroke patients, *J Am Geriatr Soc* 33(8):540-542, 1985.

17. Bromfield EB, Reding MJ: Relative risk of deep venous thrombosis or pulmonary embolism post-stroke based on ambulatory status, *J Neurol Rehab* 2:51, 1988.

18. Bushbacher RM: Deconditioning, conditioning, and the benefits of exercise. In Braddom RL, editor: *Physical medicine and rehabilitation*, Philadelphia, 1996, WB Saunders.

19. Bushbacher R: Heterotopic ossification: a review, *Crit Rev Phys Med Rehabil* 4:199, 1992.

20. Caplan LR: Diagnosis and treatment of ischemic stroke, *JAMA* 266(17):2413-2418, 1991.

21. Cerebral Embolism Study Group: Immediate anticoagulation of embolic stroke, Brain Hemorrhage and Cerebral Embolism Task Force: cardiogenic brain embolism—the second report of the Cerebral Embolism Task Force, *Arch Neurol* 46:727, 1989.

22. Cinnamon J, Viroslav AB, Dorey JH: CT and MRI diagnosis of cerebrovascular disease: going beyond the pixels, *Semin Ultrasound CT MRI* 16(3):212-236, 1995.

23. Clark WM, Wissman S, Albers GW, et al: Recombinant tissue-type plasminogen activator (alteplase) for ischemic stroke 3 to 5 hours after symptom onset. The ATLANTIS study: a randomized controlled trial. Alteplase thrombolysis for acute noninterventional therapy in ischemic stroke, *JAMA* 282(21):2019-2026, 1999.

24. Colditz GA, Bonita R, Stampfer MJ, et al: Cigarette smoking and risk for stroke in middle-aged women, *N Engl J Med* 318(15): 937-941, 1988.

25. Collins R, Peto R, MacMahon S, et al: Blood pressure, stroke, and coronary heart disease. II. Short-term reductions in blood pressure: overview of randomised drug trials in an epidemiological context, *Lancet* 335(8693):827-838, 1990.

26. Counsel C, Sandercock P: The management of patients with acute ischemic stroke, *Curr Med Lit Geriatr* 7:99, 1994.

27. Coventry MB, Scanlon PW: The use of radiation to discourage ectopic bone: a nine-year study in surgery about the hip, *J Bone Joint Surg Am* 63(2):201-208, 1981.

28. DeVincenzo DK, Watkins S: Accidental falls in a rehabilitation setting, *Rehabil Nurs* 12(5):248-252, 1987.

29. Dichter MA: The epilepsies and convulsive disorders. In Isselbacher KJ, Braunwald E, Wilson JD, et al, editors: *Harrison's principles of internal medicine*, New York, 1994, McGraw-Hill.

30. Donahue RP, Abbott RD, Reed DM, et al: Alcohol and hemorrhagic stroke: the Honolulu Heart Program, *JAMA* 255(17):2311-2314, 1986.

31. Donaldson CL, Hulley SB, Vogel JM, et al: Effect of prolonged bed rest on bone mineral, *Metabolism* 19(12):1071-1084, 1970.

32. Dyken ML: Trends in management and prognosis in stroke, *Ann Epidemiol* 3:535, 1993.

33. Ebrahim S: *Clinical epidemiology of stroke*, Oxford, England, 1995, Oxford University Press.

34. Ebrahim S, Nouri F: Caring for stroke patients at home, *Int Rehabil Med* 8(4):171-173, 1987.

35. Elster AD, Moody DM: Early cerebral infarction: gadopentetate dimeglumine enhancement, *Radiology* 177(3):627-632, 1990.

36. European Atrial Fibrillation Trial Study Group: Secondary prevention in nonrheumatic atrial fibrillation after transient ischemic attack or minor stroke, *Lancet* 342(8882):1255-1262, 1993.

37. European Carotid Surgery Trial Collaborative Group: Medical research council carotid surgery trial: interim results for patients with severe (70% to 90%) or with mild (0% to 30%) carotid stenosis, *Lancet* 334:175, 1989.

38. Failure of extracranial-intracranial arterial bypass to reduce the risk of ischemic stroke: results of an international randomized trial, the EC/IC Bypass Study Group, *N Engl J Med* 313(19):1191-200, 1985.

39. Farrell B, Godwin J, Richards S, et al: The United Kingdom transient ischemic attack (UK-TIA) aspirin trial: final results, *J Neurol Neurosurg Psychiatry* 54:1044, 1991.

40. Fisher CM: Clinical syndromes in cerebral thrombosis, hypertensive hemorrhage, and ruptured saccular aneurysm, *Clin Neurosurg* 22:117-147, 1975.

41. Fisher CM: Pathological observations in hypertensive cerebral hemorrhage, *J Neuropathol Exp Neurol* 30(3):536-550, 1971.

42. Fisher CM: Atherosclerosis of the carotid and vertebral arteries: extracranial and intracranial, *J Neuropathol Exp Neurol* 24:455, 1965.

43. Further analyses of mortality in oral contraceptive users, Royal College of General Practicioners' Oral Contraceptive Study, *Lancet* 1(8219):541-546, 1981.

44. Gainotti G: Emotional behavior and hemispheric side of the lesion, *Cortex* 8(1):41-55, 1972.

45. Garraway WM, Whisnant JP, Drury I: The changing pattern of survival after stroke, *Stroke* 14:699, 1983.

46. Gonzalez RG, Schaefer PW, Buonanno FS, et al: Diffusion weighted MR imaging: diagnostic accuracy in patients imaged within 6 hours of stroke symptom onset, *Radiology* 210(1):155-162, 1999.

47. Gordon C, Hewer RL, Wade DT: Dysphagia in acute stroke, *Br J Med* 295(6595):411-414, 1987.

48. Groher ME, Bukatman R: The prevalence of swallowing disorders in two teaching hospitals, *Dysphagia* 1:3, 1986.

49. Grotta JC, Norris JW, Kamm B: Prevention of stroke with ticlopidine: who benefits most? TASS Baseline and Angiographic Data Subgroup, *Neurology* 42(1):111-115, 1992.

50. Hachinski V, Norris JW: *The acute stroke*, Philadelphia, 1985, FA Davis.

51. Hacke W, Kaste M, Fieschi C, et al: Randomized double-blind placebo-controlled trial of thrombolytic therapy with intravenous alteplase in acute ischemic stroke (ECASS II), Second European-Australian Acute Stroke Study Investigators, *Lancet* 352(9136): 1245-1251, 1998.

52. Harburn KL, Potter PJ: Spasticity and contractures, *Phys Med Rehabil State Art Rev* 7:113, 1993.

53. Hassenfeld M: Increased incidence of hip fracture on the hemiplegic side of post stroke patients. Unpublished work presented at Columbia Presbyterian Medical Center, May 1993, New York.

54. Hauser WA, Ramirez-Lassepas M, Rosenstein R: Risk for seizures and epilepsy following cerebrovascular insults, *Epilepsia* 25:666, 1984.

55. Heros RC, Zervas NT, Varsos V: Cerebral vasospasm after subarachnoid hemorrhage: an update, *Ann Neurol* 14(6):599-608, 1983.

56. Hirsh J: Heparin, *N Engl J Med* 324(22):1565-1574, 1991.

57. Hirsh J: From unfractionated heparins to low molecular weight heparins, *Acta Chir Scand Suppl* 556:42-50, 1990.

58. Hirsh J, Genton E, Hull R: *Venous thromboembolism*, New York, 1981, Grune & Stratton.

59. Hirsh J, Hull R: Natural history and clinical features of venous thrombosis. In Coleman RW, Hirsh J, Marder V, et al, editors: *Haemostasis and thrombosis: basic principles and clinical practice*, Philadelphia, 1982, Lippincott.

60. House A, Dennis M, Molyneux A, et al: Emotionalism after stroke, *BMJ* 298(6679):991-994, 1989.

61. Hull R, Hirsh J: Diagnosis of venous thromboembolism. In Coleman RW, Hirsh J, Marder V, et al, editors: *Haemostasis and thrombosis: basic principles and clinical practice*, Philadelphia, 1982, Lippincott.

62. Hull RD, Raskob GE, Rosenbloom D, et al: Heparin for 5 days as compared with 10 days in the initial treatment of proximal venous thrombosis, *N Engl J Med* 322(18):1260-1264, 1990.

63. Iso H, Jacobs DR Jr, Wentworth D, et al: Serum cholesterol levels and six year mortality from stroke in 350,977 men screened for the multiple risk factor intervention trial, *N Engl J Med* 320(14):904-910, 1989.

64. Kannel WB, McGee DL: Diabetes and cardiovascular disease: the Framingham Study, *JAMA* 241(19):2035-2038, 1979.

65. Kanter MC, Sherman DG: Strategies for preventing stroke, *Curr Opin Neurol Neurosurg* 6(1):60-65, 1993.

66. Kistler JP, Ropper AH, Martin JB: Cerebrovascular disease. In Isselbacher KJ, Braunwald E, Wilson, JD, et al, editors: *Harrison's principles of internal medicine*, New York, 1994, McGraw-Hill.

67. Kottke FJ, Pauley DL, Ptak RA: The rationale for prolonged stretching for correction of shortening of connective tissue, *Arch Phys Med Rehabil* 47(6):345-352, 1966.

68. Kozararevic D, McGee D, Vojvodic N, et al: Frequency of alcohol consumption and morbidity and mortality: the Yugoslavia Cardiovascular Disease Study, *Lancet* 1(8169):613-616, 1980.

69. Kuller LH, Dorman JS, Wolf PA: Cerebrovascular disease and diabetes. In *Diabetes in America: diabetes data compiled for 1984*, National Diabetes Data Group, NIH Pub No 85-1468, Bethesda, Md, August 1985, Department of Health and Human Services.

70. Kwiatkowski TG, Libman RB, Frankel M, et al: Effects of tissue plasminogen activator for acute ischemic stroke at one year, National Institute of Neurological Disorders and Stroke Recombinant Tissue Plasminogen Activator Stroke Study Group, *N Engl J Med* 340(23):1781-1787, 1999.

71. Lance JW: Pathophysiology of spasticity and clinical experience with baclofen. In Eldman RG, Young RR, Koella P, editors: *Spasticity-disordered motor control*, Chicago, 1980, Yearbook.

72. Langhorne P, Stott DJ: Acute cerebral infarction: optimal management in older patients, *Drugs Aging* 6(6):445-455, 1995.

73. Langhorne P, Williams BO, Gilchrist W, et al: Do stroke units save lives? *Lancet* 342(8868):395-398, 1993.

74. Levison ME: Pneumonia, including necrotizing pulmonary infections (lung abscesses). In Isselbacher KJ, Braunwald E, Wilson JD, et al, editors: *Harrison's principles of internal medicine*, New York, 1994, McGraw-Hill.

75. Levison ME, Bush L: Pharmacodynamics of antimicrobial agents: bactericidal and postantibiotic effects, *Infect Dis Clin North Am* 3(3):415-421, 1989.

76. Lezak MD: *Neuropsychological assessment*, ed 2, New York, 1983, Oxford University Press.

77. Locksley HB: Natural history of subarachnoid hemorrhage, intracranial aneurysms, and arteriovenous malformations: based on 6368 cases in a cooperative study. In Sahs AL, Perret G, Locksley HB, et al, editors: *Intracranial aneurysms and subarachnoid hemorrhage: a cooperative study*, Philadelphia, 1969, Lippincott.

78. Longstreth WT Jr, Nelson LM, Koepsell TD, et al: Clinical course of spontaneous subarachnoid hemorrhage: a population based study in King County, Washington, *Neurology* 43(4):712-718, 1993.

79. Lorber B, Swenson RM: Bacteriology of aspiration pneumonia: a prospective study of community and hospital acquired cases, *Ann Intern Med* 81(3):329-331, 1974.

80. MacMahon S, Peto R, Cutler J, et al: Blood pressure, stroke, and coronary heart disease. I. Prolonged differences in blood pressure: prospective observational studies corrected for regression dilution bias, *Lancet* 335(8692):765-774, 1990.

81. Marmot MG, Poulter NR: Primary prevention of stroke, *Lancet* 339(8789):344-347, 1992.

82. Mayerberg MR, Batjer HH, Dacey R, et al: Guidelines for the management of aneurysmal subarachnoid hemorrhage: a statement for healthcare professionals from a special writing group of the Stroke Council, American Heart Association, *Stroke* 25(11):2315-2328, 1994.

83. McCullough LD, Beauchamp NB, Wityk R: Recent advances in the diagnosis and treatment of stroke, *Surv Ophthalmol* 45(4): 317-330, 2001.

84. McGill HC Jr: The pathogenesis of atherosclerosis, *Clin Chem* 34(8B):B33-B39, 1988.

85. McNeil BJ, Bettman MA: The diagnosis of pulmonary embolism. In Coleman RW, Hirsh J, Marder V, et al, editors: *Haemostasis and thrombosis: basic principles and clinical practice*, Philadelphia, 1982, Lippincott.

86. Mion LC, Gregor S, Buettner M, et al: Falls in the rehabilitation setting: incidence and characteristics, *Rehabil Nurs* 14(1):17-22, 1989.

87. Mohr JP: Lacunes, *Stroke* 13(1):3-11, 1982.

88. Mohr JP, Orgogozo JM, Harrison MJG, et al: Meta-analysis of nimodipine trials in acute ischemic stroke, *Cerebrovasc Dis* 4:197, 1994.

89. Murray GB, Shea V, Conn DK: Electroconvulsive therapy for post-stroke depression, *J Clin Psychiatry* 47:258, 1986.

90. Okada Y, Yamaguchi T, Minematsu K, et al: Hemorrhagic transformation in cerebral embolism, *Stroke* 20(5):598-603, 1989.

91. Paffenbarger RS Jr, Laughlin ME, Gima AS, et al: Work activity of longshoremen as related to death from coronary heart disease and stroke, *N Engl J Med* 282(20):1109-1114, 1970.

92. Paffenbarger RS, Wing AL, Hyde RT: Physical activity as an index of heart attack risk in college alumni, *Am J Epidemiol* 108(3): 161-175, 1978.

93. Perry RF: Clinical practice guidelines for smoking cessation, *JAMA* 276(6):448, 1996.

94. Pessin MS, Duncan GW, Mohr JP, et al: Clinical and angiographic features of carotid transient ischemic attacks, *N Engl J Med* 296(7):358-362, 1977.

95. Poplingher AR, Pillar T: Hip fracture in stroke patients: epidemiology and rehabilitation, *Acta Orthop Scand* 56(3):226-227, 1985.

96. PORT Study (funded by the Agency for Health Care Policy and Research), Durham, NC, 1994, Duke University Medical Center.

97. Prevention of stroke by antihypertensive drug treatment in older persons with isolated systolic hypertension: final results of the Systolic Hypertension in the Elderly Program (SHEP), SHEP Cooperative Research Group, *JAMA* 265(24):3255-3264, 1991.

98. Prevention of venous thrombosis and pulmonary embolism, NIH Consensus Development, *JAMA* 256(6):744-749, 1986.

99. Quizilbash N, Murphy M: Meta-analysis of trials of corticosteroids in acute stroke, *Age Ageing* 22(suppl):2, 1993.

100. Randomised controlled trial of streptokinase, aspirin, and combination of both in treatment of acute stroke, Multicenter Acute Stroke Trial: Italy (MAST-I) Group, *Lancet* 346(8989):1509-1514, 1995.

101. Reed DM: The paradox of high risk of stroke in populations with low risk of coronary heart disease, *Am J Epidemiol* 131(4):579-588, 1990.

102. Robinson RG, Bolla-Wilson K, Kaplan E, et al: Depression influenced intellectual impairment in stroke patients, *Br J Psychiatry* 148:541, 1986.

103. Ropper AH, Davis KR: Lobar cerebral hemorrhages: acute clinical syndromes in 26 patients, *Ann Neurol* 8(2):141-147, 1980.

104. Roth EJ, Harvey RL: Rehabilitation of stroke syndromes. In Braddom RL, editor: *Physical medicine and rehabilitation*, Philadelphia, 1996, WB Saunders.

105. Rutan GH, Kuller LH, Neaton JD, et al: Mortality associated with diastolic hypertension and isolated systolic hypertension among men screened for the Multiple Risk Factor Intervention Trial, *Circulation* 77(3):504-514, 1988.

106. Salcido R, Hart D, Smith AM: The prevention and management of pressure ulcers. In Braddom RL, editor: *Physical medicine and rehabilitation*, Philadelphia, 1996, WB Saunders.

107. Salonen R, Seppanen K, Rauramaa R, et al: Prevalence of carotid atherosclerosis and serum cholesterol levels in eastern Finland, *Atherosclerosis* 8(6):788-792, 1988.

108. Salzman EW, Hirsh J: Prevention of venous thromboembolism. In Coleman RW, Hirsh J, Marder V, et al, editors: *Haemostasis and thrombosis: basic principles and clinical practice*, Philadelphia, 1982, Lippincott.

109. Sandercock PA, van den Belt AG, Lindley RI, et al: Antithrombotic therapy in acute ischemic stroke: an overview of the randomized trials, *J Neurol Neurosurg Psychiatry* 56(1):17-25, 1993.

110. Sandercock PAG, Willems H: Medical treatment of acute ischemic stroke, *Lancet* 339(8792):537-539, 1992.

111. Sinyor D, Amato P, Kaloupek DG, et al: Post-stroke depression: relationships to functional impairment, coping strategies and rehabilitation outcome, *Stroke* 17(6):1102-1107, 1986.

112. Sorenson AG, Buonanno FS, Gonzalez RG, et al: Hyperacute stroke: evaluation with combined multisection diffusion-weighted and hemodynamically weighted echo-planar MR imaging, *Radiology* 199(2):391-401, 1996.

113. Stadel BV: Oral contraceptives and cardiovascular disease, *N Engl J Med* 288:672, 1981.

114. Stampfer MJ, Willett WC, Colditz GA, et al: A prospective study of the past use of oral contraceptive agents and the risk of cardiovascular diseases, *N Engl J Med* 319(20):1313-1317, 1988.

115. Starkstein SE, Cohen BS, Fedoroff P, et al: Relationship between anxiety disorders and depressive disorders in patients with cerebrovascular injury, *Arch Gen Psychiatry* 47(3):246-251, 1990.

116. Starkstein S, Robinson R, Price TR: Comparison of cortical and subcortical lesions in the production of post stroke mood disorders, *Brain* 110:1045, 1987.

117. Subbarao J, Smith J: Pulmonary embolism during stroke rehabilitation, *Ill Med J* 165(5):328-332, 1984.

118. Sundaram MB, Chow F: Seizures associated with spontaneous subarachnoid hemorrhage, *Can J Neurol Sci* 13(3):229-231, 1986.

119. Sundt TM Jr, Kobayashi S, Fode NC, et al: Results and complications of surgical management of 809 intracranial aneurysms in 722 cases: related and unrelated to grade of patient, type of aneurysm, and timing of surgery, *J Neurosurg* 56(6):753-765, 1982.

120. Sundt TM Jr, Whisnant JP: Subarachnoid hemorrhage from intracranial aneurysms, *N Engl J Med* 299(3):116-122, 1978.

121. Swartzman L, Teasell RW: Psychological consequences of stroke, *Phys Med Rehabil State Art Rev* 7:179, 1993.

122. Swedish Aspirin Low-Dose Trial (SALT) of 75 mg aspirin as secondary prophylaxis after cerebrovascular ischemic events, the SALT Collaborative Group, *Lancet* 338(8779):1345-1349, 1991.

123. Thompson DD, Rodan GA: Indomethacin inhibition of tenotomy induced bone resorbtion in rats, *J Bone Miner Res* 3:409, 1988.

124. Thrombolytic therapy with streptokinase in acute ischemic stroke: the Multicenter Acute Stroke Trial—Europe Study Group, *New Engl J Med* 335(3):145-150, 1996.

125. Tissue plasminogen activator for acute ischemic stroke, the National Institute of Neurological Disorders and Stroke rt-PA Stroke Study Group, *New Engl J Med* 333(24):1581-1587, 1995.

126. Torner JC, Nibbelink DW, Burmeister LF: Statistical comparisons of end results of a randomized treatment study. In Sahs AL, Nibbelink DW, Torner JC, editors: *Aneurysmal subarachnoid hemorrhage: report of the cooperative study*, Baltimore, 1981, Urban & Schwarzenberg.

127. Viitanen M, Eriksson S, Asplund K: Risk of recurrent stroke, myocardial infarction and epilepsy during long-term follow-up after stroke, *Eur Neurol* 28(4):227-231, 1988.

128. Wardlaw JM, Warlow CP: Thrombolysis in acute ischemic stroke: does it work? *Stroke* 23(12):1826-1839, 1992.

129. Warlow C: Disorders of the cerebral circulation. In Walton J, editor: *Brain's disease of the nervous system*, ed 10, Oxford, England, 1993, Oxford University Press.

130. Warlow C, Ogston D, Douglas AS: Deep venous thrombosis of the legs after strokes. I. Incidence and predisposing factors; II. Natural history, *BMJ* 1(6019):1178-1181, 1976.

131. Wheeler HB, Anderson FA Jr: Diagnostic approaches for deep vein thrombosis, *Chest* 89(suppl 5):407S-412S, 1986.

132. Whisnant JP, Matsumotoa N, Elveback LR: The effect of anticoagulant therapy on the prognosis of patients with transient cerebral ischemic attacks in a community: Rochester, Minnesota, 1955-1969, *Mayo Clinic Proc* 48(12):844-848, 1973.

133. Wiebe-Velasquez S, Blume WT: Seizures, *Phys Med Rehabil State Art Rev* 7:73, 1993.

134. Wolf PA, Belanger AJ, D'Agostino RB: Management of risk factors, *Neurol Clin* 10:177, 1992.

135. Wolf PA, D'Agostino RB, Belanger AJ, et al: Probability of stroke: a risk profile from the Framingham Study, *Stroke* 22(3):312-318, 1991.

136. Wolf PA, D'Agostino RB, Kannel WB, et al: Cigarette smoking as a risk factor for stroke: the Framingham Study, *JAMA* 259(7):1025-1029, 1988.

137. Worden JW: *Grief counseling and grief therapy*, New York, 1982, Springer.

138. Wortman CB, Silver RC: The myths of coping with loss, *J Consult Clin Psychol* 57(3):349-357, 1989.

janet falk-kessler

**chapter 2**

# Psychological Aspects of Stroke Rehabilitation

## key terms

| | | |
|---|---|---|
| anxiety | defense mechanisms | personality traits |
| coping | depression | self-efficacy |
| cultural factors | | |

## chapter objectives

After completing this chapter, the reader will be able to accomplish the following:

1. Understand how to assess psychological manifestations comprehensively after a stroke.
2. Understand how to modify treatment approaches based on personality traits.
3. Understand how a variety of psychological impairments affect the recovery process.

Understanding the relationship between psychological factors and stroke is a complex undertaking. Anxiety, depression, aggression, and emotional lability are commonly seen in persons who have sustained a stroke, as each takes its toll on adjustment and each affects functional outcome. Psychiatric conditions restrict recovery and restrain quality of life, making their assessment and treatment of paramount importance. Although much evidence is available on the psychological consequences of stroke, as much a function of physiologic changes as one's emotional reaction to this life-altering event, one's personality constructs and cultural background play a role in recovery and outcome. The purpose of this chapter is to examine the various elements that singly and in combination compose what should be a multifactorial understanding of the psychological implications for an individual who has sustained a stroke.

A well-documented fact is that more than half a million persons each year suffer a stroke, and more than 150,000

die.[11] Despite the fact that stroke is the third leading cause of death in the United States, more than 4 million stroke victims survive,[1] 25% of whom have sustained functional limitations including difficulty with activities of daily living.[11] Stroke is one of the leading causes of serious, long-term disability. These statistics are staggering but are further compounded by the significant psychological impact of stroke on the victims and their families.

The estimates for the psychological impact of stroke are equally astounding. Although most researchers agree that some form of psychiatric diagnosis is made in approximately 20% of those who have sustained a stroke,[77] as many as 30% to 50% of stroke victims have been estimated to have had some significant psychological disorder, most commonly depression.[74] Given the profound impact psychological disorders have on recovery, understanding the relationship, the range, and the effect these disorders have on individuals with stroke is paramount, for psychological factors may be antecedents, consequences, and/or reactions to the traumatic neurologic experience.

## THE HOSPITAL EXPERIENCE

For many individuals experiencing an acute, traumatic event, emergency hospitalization is coupled with a barrage of confusing and frightening thoughts and sensations. Although the overt concern expressed by the patient and the hospital staff alike may be focused on the illness that facilitated the hospitalization, the patient nonetheless is acutely aware of the physical changes that have occurred and are occurring and is surrounded by an environment that is foreign and controlling.[27] For many, this leads to increased fear and anxiety, a sense of powerlessness, and even psychological regression. It is not uncommon, for example, for independent adults to become completely passive participants in their health care and become dependent on hospital staff, who in fact are strangers, for even their most personal needs. The stressors that arise from simply being hospitalized affect one's psychological well-being. These stressors include a threat to one's integrity, dependence on strangers, separation from home and family, fear of loss of approval, fear of loss of control, fear of loss of body parts, and guilt. The initial loss of control (not knowing what is happening), integrity (wearing a hospital gown or using a bedpan), and freedom (given a schedule to follow, transported by others, told what to eat and when to eat) are values that are underscored by society and, when challenged, further add to stigma, shame, and a sense of isolation.[72,94] This experience of hospitalization contributes to a diminished sense of self.

Although many emergency hospitalizations require the patient to attend to an acute situation or illness, individuals who have sustained a stroke have to juggle the emotions that are evoked by an acute illness and by a chronic one. Reactions to acute illness include increased anxiety over the unknown, a reaction that numbs one's emotions, and a clinging to small improvements as though they represent great advances and excellent prognoses. During this period, defense mechanisms may appear. These may serve to protect the individual from the overwhelming emotions that may arise or may add to one's difficulty in coping with their illness and disability.[60,94,95] Defense mechanisms typically used include *denial*, which negates the reality of what is happening and has happened; *avoidance*, in which the individual is aware of what is happening and has happened but avoids the implications; *regression*, in which one exhibits increased emotion and/or increased dependent behavior not characteristic of one's developmental level; *compensation*, in which one becomes adept in an area to counter an inability of another area; *rationalization*, which provides reasons or excuses for not being able to accomplish tasks or goals; and *diversion of feelings*, in which unacceptable feelings are altered into socially appropriate behaviors.[22] How defenses are used also can give rise to how one is viewed by the treating therapist. The therapist may misinterpret behavior that is guided by maladaptive defense mechanisms and label the individual as a difficult patient.[60]

As time passes and the chronicity of the disability becomes apparent, the individual and that individual's social network must deal with the long-term effects of the stroke. Most immediate is the perceived change in oneself. Because role, lifestyle, and where one is in one's life cycle affect one's emotional reaction, trauma brings forth changes not only in what one can do but also in how one sees oneself. Sometimes referred to as first- and second-order development changes, learning new things and the change in one's perception of status brings forth its own unique stress.[98] Although time may enable one to develop the adaptive defenses necessary to deal with the anxiety surrounding illness, disability, and the unknown, one's psychological adaptation indeed may be undermined if the symptoms are not alleviated. The resultant reaction to stress is often a universal loss of self-esteem followed by depression. Maladaptive uses of defenses then may ensue.[94]

Stress of illness and disability affects not only the person but also one's family. A paranormative event such as unexpected and disabling illness is one in which all family members must cope and find new ways of relating to one another.[98] Previously established roles, authority relationships, family-based activities, and occupations may change,[44] resulting in a structural shift that puts the entire family at risk for significant distress within the family dynamics and the larger social network. As a result of the disability, the potential for increased alienation of the individual and of the family adds to the psychological distress already being experienced.[31]

Clearly, a complex relationship exists between psychological factors and medical conditions; biologic, psychological, and social variables play a part. Indeed, "Psychological Factors Affecting Medical Condition" now is recognized as a diagnostic category[2] and should be considered when one treats individuals with medical conditions. Undesirable psychological features may have an adverse effect on recovery and outcome or may place an individual at risk for an unwanted outcome. Specific psychological symptoms, such as anxiety or depression; specific personality traits or coping styles, such as aggressive personality traits[21,105]; maladaptive health behaviors, such as tobacco or alcohol abuse; and stress-related physiologic responses[100] have been linked to stroke.[46]

## PERSONALITY TRAITS AND THEIR CONTRIBUTION TO ILLNESS, RECOVERY, AND REHABILITATION

The relationship between psychosocial factors and sustaining a stroke is compounded by the role personality, as well as culture, has in how one copes with traumatic illness. Psychological adjustment to illness and disability depends on personality constructs; consequently, individuals who have had strokes need to be understood from the perspective of their character traits, their cultural background, and the psychological consequences that are reactionary and physiologically based. Some evidence exists that personality characteristics play a role in the development of stroke, in the recovery from stroke, and in how one participates in treatment.

Almost a half a century ago, it was suggested that personality constructs characterize how one copes with illness and engages in treatment, and that health care professionals should understand and adapt their interactive styles based on the patient's character.[32] Although the classification system suggested for understanding personalities included characteristics typical of those with personality disorders, such as the dependent and overdemanding personality, the controlling personality, or the dramatic personality, what is most significant is how individuals use those characteristics to cope with the stress and anxiety associated with illness.[60] Simply put, individuals who have sustained a significant physical illness or injury are struggling with emotional crises and revert to using those characteristics that have been used in past situations.[27] Understanding personality and its role in coping is critical for rehabilitation, for different styles promote functional adjustment and improved quality of life.[20]

## CULTURAL FACTORS AND ILLNESS

Culture is a major determinant of one's beliefs and attitudes, plays a major role in how one perceives illness and disability, and may influence how one interacts with health care providers. The meaning one ascribes to illness and how one behaves toward illness may be a function of personal and cultural health traditions. Assuming the sick role, which demands that one adjust to the role of patient and then relinquish that role to resume independence, may be determined culturally. For some, one's cultural background indeed may promote motivation toward rehabilitation and recovery; for others, it might obstruct progress. Culture dictates how one interacts in any social organization (a clinic or hospital is a social organization), how and when one communicates, how one deals with personal space, particularly as others intrude on it, and how one considers future goals.[88] Cultural habits may influence how one expresses oneself and, if one is reserved, may be misperceived as one being unmotivated, guarded, or disrespectful.[47] Like personality traits, one's cultural habits may be expressed as a means to deal with stressful situations.

It may seem logical for one who has suffered a stroke to be open with health care provider with feelings, goals, and concerns. In patient-centered practice, health care professionals expect to rely on patients to inform and instruct them as they evaluate and plan treatment for optimal occupational performance. However, some cultures prefer the health care provider to assume somewhat of an authoritarian role,[38] others may express respect through the avoidance of eye contact yet expect the health care provider to be solicitous in recognition of social worthiness,[26] and others may appear mistrustful and as a result appear uncommunicative.[47]

Having a disability that challenges one's independence is particularly difficult for those individuals for whom independence, control, and individuality are important values.[47] Indeed, these attributes eventually may motivate one in the rehabilitative process but initially make it more difficult to deal with a trauma that robs one of these values. In addition, culture often prescribes the roles one assumes in a social or family structure. For these individuals, coping with role change becomes even more challenging.

The psychological conditions that are so prevalent following stroke are particularly difficult for individuals to deal with if their cultural heritage is intolerant of psychological conditions. Although some cultural groups rely on verbal expression and take pride in expressing their feelings, others are embarrassed to discuss personal issues with outsiders,[47] feel guilty if they share feelings with strangers, view any mental condition as one that would bring shame on a family, and expect only will power and character to overcome psychological problems.[38] Indeed, psychological issues for some are viewed from a spiritual context, with the expectation of spiritual interventions.[26] For others, psychological issues are expressed in physical terms; headaches or backaches, for example, may be how one communicates depression.[37] For many individuals, the ability to accept treatment for a mental health condition happens only when all other interventions have failed.[38]

Cultural attitudes add to the emotional reaction one might have to the physical consequences of stroke and make one more resistant to understanding the psychological implications of stroke. One also must remember that not everyone from a particular cultural heritage shares the stereotypical cultural beliefs. The imperative, therefore, is that all health care providers understand what the meaning of illness and recovery is for individuals, from their particular personal and cultural perspectives.

## PSYCHOLOGICAL FACTORS AS PREDICTORS OF STROKE

Traditional psychoanalytic theory led some to believe that intrapsychic conflict resulted in physical illness. Although these notions gave rise to psychosomatic medical beliefs, the tenets associating unconscious conflicts as the primary catalyst for serious illness are no longer held.[93] Nonetheless, a growing body of evidence continues the tradition of recognizing the important interaction of psychological and emotional factors on medical outcomes.

The examination of psychological factors as predictors of stroke is receiving attention. This area of inquiry is difficult to investigate because the psychological variables typically identified are linked to lifestyle behaviors that are considered risk factors for coronary heart disease, such as tobacco and alcohol use, and decreased physical activity, as well as to physiologic risk factors (e.g., hypertension).[46,105] Even so, beginning evidence indicates that personality traits may be associated with increased risk for stroke, even when controlling for the confounding variables. In eastern Finland, where the incidence of coronary heart disease is high, a longitudinal study was conducted with more than 2000 men in which the relationship of anger to stroke was examined. Participants with a pattern of outward expression of anger were twice as likely to sustain a stroke compared with even-tempered individuals. Individuals with a pattern of inward expression, as well as those who were able to control their anger, were not at any higher risk for stroke.[21] The personality trait of anger was also the focus in a study of nearly 14,000 men and women from a biethnic American population.[105] In this study, anger was linked significantly to the incident of stroke, but only in the younger participants, suggesting that the influence of anger on stroke decreases as one ages. Anger is not the only variable being looked at as a predictor. A 14-year prospective study was conducted on 2200 healthy, middle-aged men to examine the role general psychological distress has on fatal, nonfatal, first ischemic stroke, and on transient ischemic attacks. When adjusting for those variables that many individuals with psychological distress also had (i.e., unhealthy lifestyle behaviors), researchers found a significant relationship between psychological distress and fatal stroke.[46]

Intense levels of perceived stress also have been linked with risk of stroke, specifically fatal stroke.[100] In a prospective study of almost 20,000 persons, those who reported high, frequent levels of stress were at greatest risk of dying from stroke. No relationship exists between reported stress levels and nonfatal stroke. The speculation is that individuals with better coping skills may be able to handle stressful situations and may have fewer associated lifestyle risk factors, thereby reducing their risk.

## PRESTROKE PSYCHOLOGICAL FACTORS AS PREDICTORS OF RECOVERY AND REHABILITATION

A series of studies have been done that examine prestroke personality and psychological variables on poststroke recovery and rehabilitation. In one study, a history of affective disorders or anxiety disorders was demonstrated to put one at increased risk for developing major depression. The severity of the depression symptoms also depends on a personal *or* family history of affective or anxiety disorders.[56] Personality traits, such as introversion and depression, may increase the mortality risk following a stroke.[57] An impaired social relationship with a significant other before a stroke also puts individuals at significant risk for depression during the acute phase following a stroke and during the long term after the stroke.[77]

Personality factors are associated with the ability to resume independence. As a character trait, one's self-esteem has been linked with recovery and independence.[12] Personality factors along with occupational status, educational level, workplace accommodation, and occupational choice play a significant role in being able to return to work.[48] One's ability to handle life events, classified into coping strategies, also affects one's ability to resume daily living function. Individuals with a preference for active coping styles or with an extrovert personality trait show greater improvements in activities of daily living function than those individuals with passive or avoidant coping styles. These individuals are speculated to be more highly motivated and have a more realistic appraisal of their potential, which results in improved activities of daily living function.[20]

## PERSONALITY CHANGE FOLLOWING STROKE

While it has been noted that a change in personality may follow a stroke, and this may be related to lesion location,[6,62] the change is generally grouped as disinhibition and is characterized by an instability of appropriate social behavior. Although some of the symptoms may appear to be consistent with the signs and symptoms of specific psychiatric conditions, they often emerge as negative emotions or behaviors that do not meet the criteria for particular diagnoses. These can range from euphoria to uncontrollable tears, from worry to agitation, from disinterest to hostility, or from paranoia and guarded behavior to excessive dependency. Despite the behavioral expression of these emotions, they tend not to reflect an underlying mood and may add to the embarrassment experienced by the patient.[6] Like those mental conditions that do emerge following stroke, disinhibition may resolve spontaneously, can and should be treated with medication, and may respond to psychological and social interventions.

## DEPRESSION

Among the most significant considerations in understanding the characteristics and consequences of stroke is the relationship of depression to onset, recovery, and rehabilitation of persons with stroke. As a result of the neurophysiologic changes and as a reaction to the consequences of stroke, depression has major implications for the course of recovery. Despite the causes of depression, assessment and treatment of depression affects psychological, functional, and medical health.

The relationship between cerebrovascular disease and depression was first noted in the early twentieth century.[49] For nearly three quarters of a century, the assumption held that depression following a stroke was related only to the functional and social consequences of the disability and not to the neurologic damage of the stroke itself. In a study that compared depression in individuals with stroke to individuals with orthopedic conditions, with both groups being matched for functional ability, the significant increase of depression in the group with stroke led the researchers to believe that depression was related to something more than a reaction to functional inability.[25] Depression in stroke has been distinguished from depression in other disorders as well. For example, patients with stroke, as compared with those with myocardial infarction or acute spinal cord injury, tend to have a different sequela to depression, which often is accompanied by generalized anxiety.[23] With the acknowledgment that depression in individuals with stroke is different from depression with other medical conditions, the understanding of why depression emerges following stroke has expanded with the recognition that depression is a complex result of a neurologic event.

Although studies have demonstrated that depression occurs in individuals without regard to location of lesion,[18,53,63] what generally is accepted is that an association exists between lesion location, particularly left anterior lesions, with onset of depression during the acute phase, and an increased severity of depression the closer the lesion is to the left frontal pole,[41,74] and right parietal lesions with depression during the subacute period.[77] Studies suggest the existence of neuroanatomic bases for depression, implicating lesion size and location*; neuroanatomic bases for recovery of depression following stroke[63]; and a pathophysiologic basis for depression, which may result from a chemical change following brain infarction.[77,78]

The distinction between major depression and minor depression is important to any discussion on depression and stroke. Both forms are prevalent and have implications for recovery and rehabilitation. Although it has been demonstrated that even major depression lasts less than 1 year,[4,13,41] depression that also is accompanied by cognitive impairment has a greater duration.[29] Any poststroke depression that does not remit leads to a poorer, long-term functional outcome.[14,15,51,69]

Fairly consistent criteria have been used to define and distinguish major depression and minor depression. Although researchers may have relied on the diagnostic criteria of different versions of the *Diagnostic and Statistical Manual of Mental Disorders* or have used assessments such as the Hamilton Depression Scale for Depression or Beck's Depression Inventory, the signs and symptoms for depression have remained fairly constant. Major depression typically is characterized by an unrelenting feeling of sadness or apathy, accompanied by four or more of the following: feelings of helplessness, worthlessness, and/or hopelessness; loss of pleasure or interest in all activities; change in appetite, weight, or sleep pattern; psychomotor retardation or agitation; loss of energy; loss of concentration; or suicidal ideation.[13] Indeed, suicidal ideation, although prevalent in individuals with a variety of acute medical conditions,[36] is also prevalent in medical conditions that become chronic. For individuals with stroke the prevalence of suicidal ideation in fact increases over time.[35]

In addition to the symptoms already described, major depression also may be characterized by isolative behavior and irritable, angry, or hostile expression. These symptoms can occur to a lesser extent and have a less debilitating effect. When the symptoms are less frequent and less severe, one may have a dysthymia disorder or minor depression.[2]

The distinction between the two categories in individuals who have sustained a stroke is important to make, because the more severe form of depression is associated with higher rates of mortality[52] and impairment in activities of daily living and is linked with more severe neurologic deficits.[33] However, evidence is increasing that any form of depression has an effect on functional status in individuals with stroke and that depressive symptoms, even in the absence of any depression diagnosis, affect functional status.[30] In fact, even an attitude of helplessness affects one's survival rate.[39]

Individuals who have major depression tend to have a personal history or a family history of affective disorders. Individuals who have minor depression may have sustained a previous stroke.[58] Although most major depression resolves within 1 year of the stroke,[13,41] many individuals continue to be depressed for 2 to 3 years. Although minor depression tends to last only 3 months,[13] evidence indicates that this too can last for 2 to 3 years.[4] In addition, individuals who perceive a lack of social support tend to have a more severe depressive disorder that lasts longer.[55]

Major and minor depressions can occur at any time following stroke, and the symptoms used to diagnose major or minor depression may vary depending on whether the depression onset is early or late.[66,97] Regardless of onset or symptom clusters, poststroke depression has been found to affect negatively the physical recovery from stroke[13] and independence in activities of daily living.[14,15]

---

*References 53, 63, 67, 82, 83, 90.

## OTHER CONDITIONS ASSOCIATED WITH LESION LOCATION

Although significant research has been conducted on poststroke depression, depression is not the only psychological diagnosis that may have an anatomic basis. Emotional lability, characterized by extreme expression of emotion such as crying or laughing, but without the underlying feelings of sadness or depression, occurs independent of depression and may be associated with lesions in the anterior regions of the cerebral hemispheres.[54,77] Other psychological diagnoses sometimes are confused with depression, can occur concomitantly, and have a prevalence rate of between 19% and 22%. These diagnoses include apathy (low motivation and/or energy), anxiety disorder (excessive worrying, restlessness, irritability, and/or tension), and catastrophic reactions (sudden onset of anxiety, hostility, or crying) (Table 2-1). Each of these also may be linked with lesion location, specifically the left posterior internal capsule, left cortex, and left anterior subcortex, respectively.[77] Although many

of these studies certainly suggest a cause for many of the psychiatric conditions seen in patients with stroke, anatomic location does not seem to have any relationship to quality of life on recovery.[18]

## ANXIETY DISORDERS

It is well documented that a significant comorbidity exists between poststroke depression and anxiety.[13] Anxiety disorders, most commonly generalized anxiety disorder, can emerge during any phase of recovery, from the acute phase to the rehabilitation phase. Like depression, its cause may vary. Although compelling evidence suggests anxiety is often a reaction to loss of anticipated or actual functional ability,[13] some evidence links anxiety to lesion location when it occurs during the acute poststroke phase,[10] and other evidence links early onset with a previous history of psychiatric conditions.[9] Regardless of its cause, the presence of anxiety impairs the prognosis for recovery of major depression, and if not resolved within 1 year of onset, the individual is at risk for a chronic anx-

## Table 2-1

### Psychiatric Conditions Associated with Stroke

| CONDITION | APPROXIMATE PREVALENCE RATE | FEATURES |
|---|---|---|
| Poststroke depression | 35%[13] | Features consistent with major or minor depression |
| Major depression | 20%[79] | Depressed mood; feelings of helplessness; diminished energy, concentration, and interest; change in appetite; suicidal ideation |
| Minor depression | 21%[79] | Depressed mood that may or may not be accompanied with other features but does not meet the criteria of major depression; dysthymia |
| Suicidal ideation | 7% during acute phase 11% within 2 years after stroke[35] | Thoughts of suicide |
| Apathy | 22% (half with no depression comorbidity)[91] | Low motivation and/or energy |
| Generalized anxiety disorder | 28% during acute phase[3,10] 22% 3 months after stroke[3] 13% with no depression comorbidity[3] | Excessive anxiety and worry |
| State of worry | 14%[10] | Expressed anxiety but not fulfilling generalized anxiety disorder criteria |
| Emotional lability | 18%[54] | Awareness of uncontrollable emotion (pathologic laughing or crying) that is inconsistent with mood |
| Catastrophic reaction | 19%[91] | Sudden onset of anxiety, hostility, or crying |
| Psychotic disorders or symptoms | | |
| Schizophreniform | Uncommon[73] | Delusions or hallucinations |
| Paranoia | Uncommon except in those with prestroke history of psychosis[6,79] | An acute or systematic delusion of being singled out in a negative way |
| Mania | Uncommon[40] | Elevated mood (euphoria or agitation), flight of ideas, diminished sleep |
| Bipolar disorder | Uncommon[13] | Depression and mania |

iety condition. Anxiety also occurs in the absence of depression, especially in individuals who lived alone when the stroke occurred.[3] Anxiety, without regard to when it emerges, is associated with dependence in activities of daily living, reduced functional ability, and a diminished social network.[3,9]

## OTHER PSYCHOLOGICAL CONDITIONS

Catastrophic reactions in which individuals experience sudden and extreme feelings of anxiety are related to anxiety disorders. Although these reactions typically occur after the acute poststroke phase, the responses may be in reaction to frustration and depression and have implications for rehabilitation.[13] Catastrophic reactions are distinguished from emotional lability in that an underlying emotion is associated with it. The affect expressed with emotional lability, that is, sudden outbursts of laughter or crying, is not associated with one's mood.[57,80]

Apathy is another common psychiatric condition. Although apathy is a symptom of depression, it can occur in the absence of a depressive disorder and is associated with cognitive impairment and with deficits in functional ability.[89] By its very nature, the impact of apathy on energy and motivation clearly effects engagement in the recovery and rehabilitative process.

Psychotic conditions are rare consequences of stroke, but they can occur. Some evidence suggests that a psychosis type of syndrome, in which an individual experiences hallucinations or delusions, may occur in individuals who have preexisting neuroanatomic risk factors for developing this disorder.[5,73] Symptoms of hallucinations or delusions tend to be uncommon overall but are associated with older age. The development of paranoia also can occur and with greater frequency than other psychotic features. Paranoia also may be associated with lesion location.[77] Manic episodes have been reported to occur, but they are rare.[40] Most psychotic conditions that emerge after stroke are believed to emerge in individuals with a history of psychotic conditions or in individuals predisposed to developing these conditions.[6]

Cognitive deficits are also common consequences of stroke.[106] Although cognitive deficits may be related directly to lesion, the effect between depression and cognition is interactive, and distinguishing one from the other is sometimes difficult. Some evidence suggests that depression indeed leads to cognitive impairment[59] that might be classified as a pseudodementia[6] and that these conditions can benefit from adequate treatment of depression.[34] Dementia, as an example of a specific cognitive deficit disorder, is less common in individuals who have had stroke, although the term *dementia* sometimes is used broadly to describe the disinhibitory symptoms discussed previously.[6]

Cognitive ability is linked with one's ability to live independently. Although the attentional aspect of cognition is a predictor of motor recovery,[76] the relationship of attention to one's ability to learn is what affects functional outcome. Not surprisingly, cognitive ability is a significant predictor of ability to live independently[43] (see Chapters 17, 18, and 19).

## EMOTIONAL REACTION TO STROKE

Research has shown that depression and other psychological conditions may be the result of the physiologic damage caused by stroke and an emotional consequence of the often resultant physically disabling condition and subsequent social disruption. One's reaction to illness and disability, to loss of function, to change in body image, and to role change and possible social alienation can give rise to reactions of grief, anger, guilt, and fear,[22] all of which contribute to a sense of social stigma[29] and produce a myriad of feelings that contribute to depression and anxiety. Indeed, stroke has been suggested to be "an overwhelming psychological event that triggers a depressive episode in predisposed individuals."[103] Given this, additional issues need to be considered that contribute to one's emotional reaction to stroke.

If an individual seeks treatment early enough in the development of a nonhemorrhagic stroke, medication is available that may halt the progression of the stroke and even reverse the damage to the brain. However, the medication available is not without potentially fatal consequences. Whether the individual or the individual's family makes the decision to be treated with the medication, when the outcome with or without medication is poor, the family may be left with feelings of anger and guilt in addition to feelings of grief. If the individual delayed seeking treatment and did not avail himself or herself of potential medication, family members may attribute blame to the patient for the condition with which they now must cope.[92]

Certainly physical recovery plays a major role in one's emotional reaction and in psychological adaptation. The actual experience of stroke, as it is happening, brings forth fear of the unknown and distress that this experience actually is occurring. Although the initial recovery phase may be marked by some improvement in one's physical status, a plateau period during which progress is slowed often follows and may lead to frustration and sadness. One's emotional recovery is marked by a mix of emotions, including uncertainty, hope, loss of control, anger, and frustration. Social recovery similarly is challenged, as one needs to adjust to changing roles, isolation, and the perceived dissonance between past and current/future life.[7]

Lack of control over one's body, fear and shock of the rapidity of the physical changes, and feelings of loss around three particular areas—activities, abilities, and independence—contribute to the emotional challenge of accepting that one's life is changed in significant ways.[29] To be able to make the transition toward recovery, the argument has been that individuals must assess the psychological meaning of loss as it relates to self-concept. In other words, how might the loss of ability as it affects activity engagement affect one's personal meaning of quality of life?[8] But to be able eventually to accept a changed self, one's self-concept goes through a process of transformation.

Issues of recovery have been framed in terms of stages and reflect the interplay between physical recovery, emotional recovery, and psychological adaptation. Although progress takes different forms for each individual, survivors tend to deal with common themes, and each has its impact on adaptation.

Buscherhof[8] presents a series of stages that, as a stroke survivor, enabled her to make the transition. These stages include *denial*, which can protect one from initial overwhelming emotion; *grieving* (as distinguished from depression), in which one mourns the loss of function; *role transition*, to include "care-receiver"; the *development of optimal independence*, which includes compensatory techniques and adjustment to a new body; *rebuilding a social support system;* and *reintegration into the community* via instrumental activities of daily living. These stages promote the acceptance of any remaining disability and the return to a satisfying quality of life.

Emotional reaction following stroke has significant implications for recovery. Feelings of helplessness or hopelessness affect survival rate,[39] apathy affects functional ability,[89] and depression and anxiety affect function and recovery.[3,9,13-15,30,33]

One's cultural background also may play a role in how one copes with illness, disability, and rehabilitation. As stated earlier, cultural values and attitudes may devalue any form of dependency. Consequently, a disability may add to feelings of alienation. From a cultural perspective, psychological conditions also may be viewed as a weakness of character. This further stigmatizes the individual and leads to the avoidance of acknowledging feelings and of being treated.[47]

Health professionals, without intending to do so, may become enablers of the loss of personal identity and dignity and contribute to a diminished self-esteem. The physician William Osler is credited with saying, "Ask not what disease the person has, but rather what person the disease has."[84] When an individual is referred to in terms of a disabling condition (i.e., "a right hemi"), one's dignity and sense of personal worth are challenged. This adds to what may be emerging as a damaged sense of self within the context of social stigma. Many individuals go to great lengths to conceal their disabilities from others to avoid being identified as a stroke.[71]

Although much has been written regarding the negative emotional reaction to stroke, the suggestion also has been made that for individuals whose lives ordinarily are characterized by crises, dealing with the consequences of stroke is not considered an extraordinary event but just another life change.[70] Although this challenges the general assumption that anyone who has experienced a stroke also will experience grief, loss, and distress,[74] considering the context of one's life in which stroke occurs is important.[44]

## BIOLOGIC INTERVENTION

Clearly, any number of factors are associated with the cause of psychological conditions following stroke. Social and psychological stressors play a major role in the development of these conditions, as do anatomic lesions. Despite the debate regarding the primary cause of psychological conditions, leading some to conclude that no evidence supports a single theory on the origin of psychological conditions in persons with stroke,[103] no debate exists regarding the importance of taking a bio-psycho-social approach in understanding and treating stroke, as psychological conditions take their toll on recovery and functional ability.

Although medication is not sufficient to counter the effect of stroke on daily function,[14] it is a critical weapon in the treatment of psychological conditions. Without regard to the cause of the conditions, a number of studies have been conducted to determine the use of psychopharmacologic agents in treating psychological conditions. Antidepressants have been used in individuals with depression or with pathologic affect, with promising results; benzodiazepines have been used for generalized anxiety disorder, with limited success because of side effects; and poststroke psychosis appears to respond to neuroleptic medication.[13] Although many of the studies conducted have been challenged because of the limitations of these studies (i.e., number of subjects, mixed diagnoses, and length of treatment),[103] it is well accepted that any psychological condition following stroke should be treated as soon as it is diagnosed because of the significant negative implications on recovery if the condition is not treated.

## RECOVERY

One of the most important contributors to any recovery process is motivation. Although psychological conditions, particularly depression, often are characterized by low motivation, personal traits influence one's determination toward recovery.

Four factors affect motivation: locus of control, self-efficacy, self-esteem, and social support.[19] *Locus of control* deals with where one places the influence of one's future.

If, for example, individuals believe they can influence their health by eating right, exercising, and so on, then those individuals are viewed as having an internal locus of control. Individuals with an internal locus of control are thought to be more self-motivated.

*Self-efficacy* relates to one's confidence in what one can do. A strong sense of self-efficacy motivates an individual toward accomplishing a goal. Too strong a sense of self-efficacy, however, may be reflected in misjudging one's capabilities, leading to frustration and anger.

Promoting individual control over lifestyle and by focusing on what one *can* do and work toward indeed may mediate the negative effects of disability and promote psychological adaptation.[74,96] This is consistent with the social cognition model of setting personal goals within the context of appropriate outcome expectations, a model that has been used successfully in rehabilitation.[75] A personal belief that one *can* cope with illness or disability without reliance on others leads to better outcomes.[104] Also important in the transition to recovery is an emphasis on health promotion. Because stroke survivors sometimes return to an unhealthy lifestyle,[75] fostering the psychological skills that can promote self-efficacy becomes even more important.

As previously noted, individuals with depression have difficulty with self-efficacy, and individuals with poststroke depression have more negative cognitions than do individuals without depression who have had a stroke. Although individuals with stroke tend to focus on what they can no longer do, not surprisingly, they may not recognize those qualities and abilities they *do* have.[74] Given the effectiveness of cognitive behavioral approaches in treating depression, cognitive behavioral approaches have been suggested to be efficacious with poststroke depression as well.[64]

*Self-esteem* deals with one's perception of one's own worth. An adequate sense of self leads to pride of accomplishment and active participation in the recovery process. Coping strategies focused on personal worth and control help diminish the stress related to illness. These strategies include taking positive action to regain control of one's life.[7] Use of adaptive coping strategies that have worked in the past[20,60,74] also promotes adaptation.

*Social support* has a major influence on motivation. By not feeling isolated or abandoned, one is more likely to consider the future and work toward goals. The importance of social support to the recovery process cannot be understated. Individuals are able to cope better with their changed self and show adequate self-esteem when their social environment is perceived as adequate. In fact, social support is considered essential in the initial recovery stage following stroke.[79] Psychological adaptation and improvement in function, even if affected by depression, is fostered when family is involved in rehabilitation efforts.[29]

Equally important, families are expected to cope with the immediate health needs and subsequent rehabilitation needs of the family member who has had the stroke, and sometimes they feel unsupported. Entire families undergo role and status change, and for family members to experience depression and anxiety is not unusual.[98] In fact, depression in the primary support person is on average three times higher than in the general population.[85] This is particularly true if the primary support person is a spouse, has lower financial income, or has an unsatisfying social network.[99] Families as a whole also perceive a decreased quality of life because their social and leisure activities are affected when a family member has had a stroke.[65] When the needs of the family also are addressed, an individual is better able to handle community reintegration. Family members need honest information, must have health professionals that are accessible, and must receive support for themselves.[101] Although social support for family members affects how satisfied they are with quality of life, being able to problem solve affects depressive behavior[28] (see Chapter 32).

One of the measures of quality of life is social participation.[42] Yet despite the return of or compensation for physical functioning, most patients who have sustained a stroke report a decreased involvement in social activities.[29,65] Although depression is thought to contribute to some of this finding, body image, the stigma of evident disability, and dependence on others for transportation also have been speculated to contribute to the isolation and frustration that results.[29] Although physical changes may set in motion the factors that can decrease social involvement, the resultant inability to resume previously held roles, inability to work, and diminished social interaction may have the greatest impact on quality of life.[7,65] Attention to social involvement after rehabilitation becomes especially important in the maintenance of function and in leading a meaningful and fulfilling life (see Chapter 3).

## OCCUPATIONAL THERAPY PRACTICE

Throughout this chapter, reference has been made to the effect of psychological conditions and psychiatric disorders on recovery and rehabilitation. Personality traits[57] and levels of stress[46,100] have been linked with mortality rates from stroke, as have severe forms of depression.[52] Personality traits related to self-esteem and coping style have been linked with ability to resume independence.[12,20]

Depression and anxiety have perhaps the greatest impact on recovery and rehabilitation. Depression has been linked in general with recovery from stroke, with deficits in physical function,[33,67] and with deficits in impairment in daily living.[14,15,51,69] Even depressive symptoms without a clear diagnosis are linked poorer functional status.[30] The presence of anxiety also reduces functional ability and diminishes social networks.[3,9]

Assessment and treatment of psychological conditions and psychiatric disorders is critical when working with individuals who have had a stroke and with their families. As reviewed elsewhere, studies have repeatedly demonstrated that medication is effective in the prevention[61] and treatment of these conditions[13] but should be coupled with psychological and social interventions.

In 2002, the American Occupational Therapy Association published its *Occupational Therapy Practice Framework*.[16] Critical to the framework, which delineates the focus of practice and links evaluation and intervention with occupation, is the interdependency of performance in areas of occupation, skills, and patterns with context, activity demands, and patient factors. Key to the practice of occupational therapy is the understanding of how illness or disability affect occupation and how engagement in occupation depends on the interaction of physical, psychological, emotional, and social conditions.

When using the framework as a guide, which reinforces the traditions of occupational therapy practice, one is compelled to evaluate all the patterns and skills necessary to engage in activity and occupation.[16] Ability to engage in everyday activities leads to participation in patient-selected contexts and results in satisfactory quality of life. Because quality of life is measured through physical, psychological, and social indicators,[42,102] the areas identified within this chapter require attention: personality traits; cultural attitudes and beliefs; psychological and cognitive consequences of stroke; emotional reactions to illness, disability, and recovery; and social context and support. This information has a direct bearing on the occupational profile that is developed and affects physical, psychological, and social functioning and the potential for independence.

The patient-centered focus of practice[16] is consistent with what should be the focus of evaluation and intervention. Patients measure success not by the therapist's standards but by their personal goals.[29] Indeed, the benchmarks that professionals use to determine functional ability is typically related to physical performance, whereas patients use quality of life measures.[7]

## The Therapeutic Relationship

Every interaction between the patient and therapist provides a context for assessment and intervention.[74] Hence the relationship that develops presents an ongoing opportunity to consider personal and social needs, to clarify and refine goals, and to address the ambient emotional conditions that are affecting progress.

The therapeutic relationship begins the moment the patient and therapist interact. This actually may precede face-to-face contact, as each may have preconceived notions of what to expect. These notions may impede the therapeutic process, if they lead to assumptions that are not accurate or realistic, or they may facilitate the process, if they promote the awareness of conditions and contexts that must be considered.

Fundamental to the relationship is respect, trust, concern for dignity, honesty, and the ability to be empathetic.[68,86] As the therapist and patient work to develop a collaborative effort that will result in optimal occupational performance, each needs to engage in the therapeutic process to provide meaning and value for the patient. Above all, this engagement is based on respecting the patient's individuality, making it possible for the patient to identify valued goals, and maintaining sensitivity for the fears, concerns, frustrations and disappointments that emerge. A significant communicative tool in this relationship is empathy: the ability to convey an understanding of another's condition. Not to be confused with sympathy, pity, or identification, each of which can interfere with the therapeutic relationship,[17] empathy advances the helpful nature of the relationship. Conveying empathy, along with informing patients of the processes and rationale behind treatment, anticipating possible difficulties or obstacles, and soliciting social support from family or friends improves cooperation and compliance in treatment.[87]

## Evaluation

Evaluating the psychological conditions in an individual with stroke should be part of every therapist's assessment procedures. In addition to using specific measurement tools that target psychological and cognitive functions, the therapist should seek to answer a series of questions via interview of the patient and family and through observation. This process may be a challenge, particularly if speech, language, or visual spatial impairments are evident.

Psychological conditions may present at any time and with varying degrees of intensity. A change when participating in treatment (i.e. sudden disinterest in activities or goals, decreased energy, difficulty concentrating, increased worrying or agitation, or change in interpersonal interactions) may be indicators of the onset of depression or anxiety.

The mental status examination provides the initial and the ongoing evaluation of mental states. In addition to the examination providing a beginning assessment of a patient's cognitive state (orientation, memory, and attention), it provides the therapist with an assessment of mood and affect, speech and perceptual disturbances, thought processes, concentration ability, abstract thinking, judgment and insight, and reliability.[45] Although one's mental state can change from day to day, it is an important indicator of psychological functioning and provides the therapist with an understanding of the patient factors and performance skills that must be considered when planning treatment.

Character style plays a role in how one approaches illness and recovery, and as a result, understanding a patient's style should affect how the therapist interacts with the patient. If, for example, the patient is excessively dependent, the patient in fact may be fearful of being left alone, abandoned, or unprotected and would benefit from the therapist's ability to set limits while conveying the intent to help. For those patients who require details and facts, the therapist should provide adequate information to calm any anxiety, while encouraging the patient to take charge of certain aspects of treatment.[27] Giving the patient a structured way of keeping track of progress outside of the treatment session would engage the patient in a productive way.

The following questions reflect the different personality styles that a patient may exhibit[27]:

1. Does the patient need/demand special attention or appear particularly dependent?
2. Does the patient seek out as many facts as possible about the illness or recovery?
3. Is the patient particularly personable, and does the patient use charm to form relationships with the therapist?
4. Does the patient dwell on difficulties and suffering and not react positively to good news?
5. Does the patient overreact to criticism or feedback?
6. Does the patient act in a superior manner or seem entitled to special status?
7. Is the patient aloof, uninvolved, or appear excessively calm?

Being able to cope with trauma and life-altering events is important in one's recovery. Coping may be focused on the meaning of an event or situation, the problems that need to be solved, or the emotions that are elicited.[50] Appraisal-focused, problem-focused, and emotion-focused coping are active processes that enable one to deal with stressors.[24] This is consistent with other studies in which clusters of coping behavior have been categorized as active, passive, emotional, and avoidant.[20] Effective coping bolsters a sense of self-worth, which adds to diminishing the stress of illness.[70]

In addition to identifying which coping strategies are useful, being able to identify who can and cannot cope may depend on a series of exhibited characteristics.[27] Box 2-1 lists the traits that reflect good and poor coping.

To assess the meaning of illness, from a personal perspective and from a cultural perspective, is important. The meaning of health and illness may be related to having the physical and emotional capacity to do what one wants to do, when one wants to do it, and brings forth behaviors that support one's attitudes and values.[88] Personality and mental conditions may influence this assessment; depression, for example, may lessen one's energy, interest, and commitment to engage in treatment or plan for the future. In addition, how one values and

---

**Box 2-1**

**Characteristics of Coping[27]**

**POSITIVE CHARACTERISTICS**

Focused on immediate problems
Flexible optimism
Resourceful in selecting strategies
Conscious of emotions that can impair judgment

**NEGATIVE CHARACTERISTICS**

Intolerant of others
Excessive use of defenses such as denial or rationalization
Impulsive judgments
Rigid or inflexible
Tendency toward preconceived notions
Passive

---

manages time and space, illness and loss, role and family, and work and leisure; how one interacts with others; and most importantly, how one defines self-worth may be determined culturally.[47,88] Part of this process, however, is the recognition that the therapist is using one's own culture and personality through which to consider the patient, to define illness and health, and to develop a therapeutic relationship. Just as understanding the patient's personal and cultural view of illness and health is important to maintain a truly objective patient-centered approach, the therapist has an obligation for self-reflection on these same areas to avoid imposing one's own values and attitudes on evaluation and treatment.

## SUMMARY

From the initial onset of a stroke through the process of recovery, one follows an unpredictable path. The individual is faced with a plethora of choices and challenges that are as unexpected as they are difficult. One is asked to relearn the activities one has always taken for granted, to assume new roles that may be unfamiliar or that challenge one's self-worth, and to rewrite the future. Although patients' aspire to return to their prestroke existence, their struggles are compounded by the emotional reactions to the loss of activities, abilities, and independence,[29] by the potential of social stigma,[71] and for some, by the real presence of psychiatric conditions.[13]

The psychological effects of stroke, whether directly related to the neurologic insult or related to the emotional reaction to a disabling condition, must be assessed and treated to ensure optimal functional performance. Because stroke survivors are concerned not only with what they can do, but also with how others perceive and accept them,[74] addressing the psychological, social, and physical concerns with equal value results in a satisfactory quality of life.

# REFERENCES

1. American Heart Association: *2001 heart and stroke statistical update*, Dallas, 2000, AHA.

2. American Psychiatric Association: *DSM-IV-TR: diagnostic and statistical manual of mental disorders*, ed 4, Washington, DC, 2000, APA.

3. Åström M: Generalized anxiety disorder in stroke patients: a 3-year longitudinal study, *Stroke* 27(2):270-275, 1996.

4. Berg A, Paolmäki H, Lehtihalmes M, et al: Poststroke depression: an 18-month follow-up, *Stroke* 34(1):138-143, 2003.

5. Berthier M, Starkstein S: Acute atypical psychosis following a right hemisphere stroke, *Acta Neurol Belg* 87(3):125-131, 1987.

6. Birkett DP: *The psychiatry of stroke*, Washington, DC, 1996, American Psychiatric Press.

7. Burton CR: Living with stroke: a phenomenological study, *J Adv Nurs* 32(2):301-309, 2000.

8. Buscherhof J: From abled to disabled: a life transition, *Top Stroke Rehabil* 5(2):19-29, 1998.

9. Castillo C, Schultz S, Robinson R: Clinical correlates of early-onset and late-onset poststroke generalized anxiety, *Am J Psychiatry* 152(8):1174-1179, 1995.

10. Castillo C, Starkstein S, Fedoroff J, et al: Generalized anxiety disorder after stroke, *J Nerv Ment Dis* 181(2):100-106, 1993.

11. Centers for Disease Control and Prevention: *Atlas of stroke mortality: racial, ethnic, and geographic disparities in the United States, 2002*. Retrieved April 6, 2003, from http://cdc.gov.

12. Chang A, Mackenzie A, Yip M, et al: The psychosocial impact of stroke, *J Clin Nurs* 8(4):477478, 1999.

13. Chemerinski E, Robinson RG: The neuropsychiatry of stroke, *Psychosomatics* 41(1):5-14, 2000.

14. Chemerinski E, Robinson RG, Arndt S, et al: The effect of remission of poststroke depression on activities of daily living in a double-blind randomized treatment study, *J Nerv Ment Dis* 189(7):421-425, 2001.

15. Chemerinski E, Robinson RG, Kosier JT: Improved recovery in activities of daily living associated with remission of poststroke depression, *Stroke* 32(1):113-117, 2001.

16. Commission on Practice: *Occupational therapy practice framework: domain and process*, Bethesda, Md, 2002, American Occupational Therapy Association.

17. Davis CM: *Patient practitioner interaction: an experiential manual for developing the art of health care*, ed 3, Thorofare, NJ, 1998, Slack.

18. de Haan R, Limburg M, Van der Meulen J, et al: Quality of life after stroke: impact of stroke type and lesion location, *Stroke* 26(3):402-408, 1995.

19. Drench ME, Noonan AC, Sharby N, et al: *Psychosocial aspects of health care*, Upper Saddle River, NJ, 2003, Prentice Hall.

20. Elmståhl S, Sommer M, Hagberg B: A 3-year follow-up of stroke patients: relationships between activities of daily living and personality characteristics, *Arch Gerontol Geriatr* 22:233-244, 1996.

21. Everson SA, Kaplan GA, Goldberg DE, et al: Anger expression and incident stroke: prospective evidence from the Kuopio ischemic heart disease study, *Stroke* 30(3):523-528, 1999.

22. Falvo DR: *Medical and psychosocial aspects for chronic illness and disability*, ed 2, Gaithersburg, Md, 1999, Aspen.

23. Fedoroff JP, Lipsey JR, Starkstein SE, et al: Phenomenological comparisons of major depression following stroke, myocardial infarction or spinal cord lesions, *J Affect Disord* 22(1-2):83-89, 1991.

24. Folkman S, Lazarus RS: Stress processes and depressive symptomatology, *J Abnorm Psychol* 95:107-113, 1986.

25. Folstein M, Maiberger R, McHugh P: Mood disorder as a specific complication of stroke, *J Neurol Neurosurg Psychiatry* 40(10):1018-1020, 1977.

26. Garcia-Preto N: Peurto Rican families. In McGoldrick M, Giordano J, Pearce J, editors: *Ethnicity and family therapy*, ed 2, New York, 1996, Guilford Press.

27. Gazzola L, Muskin P: The impact of stress and the objectives of psychosocial interventions. In Schein L, Bernard H, Spitz H, et al, editors: *Psychosocial treatment for medical conditions*, New York, 2003, Brunner-Routledge.

28. Grant JS, Elliott TR, Giger JN, et al: Social problem-solving abilities, social support, and adjustment among family caregivers of individuals with a stroke, *Rehabil Psychol* 46(1):44-57, 2001.

29. Hafsteinsdóttir T, BGrypdonck M: Being a stroke patient: a review of the literature, *J Adv Nurs* 26(3):580-588, 1997.

30. Herrmann N, Black S, Lawrence J, et al: The Sunnybrook Stroke Study: a prospective study of depressive symptoms and functional outcome, *Stroke* 29(3):618-624, 1998.

31. Imber-Black E: Creating meaningful rituals for new life cycle transitions. In Carter B, McGoldrick M, editors: *Expanded family life cycle*, ed 3, Boston, 1999, Allyn & Bacon.

32. Kahana R, Bibring G: Personality types in medical management. In Zinberg N: *Psychiatry and medical practice in a general hospital*, New York, 1964, International University Press.

33. Kauhanen M-L, Korpelainen JP, Brusin E, et al: Poststroke depression correlates with cognitive impairment and neurological deficits, *Stroke* 30(9):1875-1880, 1999.

34. Kimura M, Robinson RG, Kosier JT: Treatment of cognitive impairment after poststroke depression: a double-blind treatment trial, *Stroke* 31(7):1482-1486, 2000.

35. Kishi Y, Robinson RG, Kosier JT: Suicidal ideation among patients during the rehabilitation period after life-threatening physical illness, *J Nerv Ment Dis* 189(9):623-628, 2001.

36. Kishi Y, Robinson RG, Kosier JT: Suicidal ideation among patients with acute life-threatening physical illness: patients with stroke, traumatic brain injury, myocardial infarction, and spinal cord injury, *Psychosomatics* 42(5):382-390, 2001.

37. Lee E: Asian American families: an overview. In McGoldrick M, Giordano J, Pearce J, editors: *Ethnicity and family therapy*, ed 2, New York, 1996, Guildford Press.

38. Lee E: Chinese families. In McGoldrick M, Giordano J, Pearce J, editors: *Ethnicity and family therapy*, ed 2, New York, 1996, Guildford Press.

39. Lewis SC, Dennis MS, O'Rourke SJ, et al: Negative attitudes among short-term stroke survivors predict worse long-term survival, *Stroke* 32(7):1640-1645, 2001.

40. Liu CY, Wang SJ, Fuh JL, et al: Bipolar disorder following a stroke involving the left hemisphere, *Aust N Z J Psychiatry* 30(5):688-691, 1996.

41. Lyketsos C, Treisman G, Lipsey JR, et al: Does stroke cause depression? *J Neuropsychiatry* 10(1):103-107, 1998.

42. Mackenzie AE, Chang AM: Predictors of quality of life following stroke, *Disabil Rehabil* 24(5):259-265, 2002.

43. MacNeill SE, Lichtenberg PA, LaBuda J: Factors affecting return to living alone after medical rehabilitation: a cross-validation study, *Rehabil Psychol* 45(4):356-364, 2000.

44. Mattingly CE, Lawlor MC: Disability experience from a family perspective. In Crepeau EB, Cohn ES, Schell BAB, editors: *Willard & Spackman's occupational therapy*, ed 10, Philadelphia, 2003, Lippincott Williams & Wilkins.

45. Maxmen JS, Ward NG: *Essential psychopathology and its treatment*, ed 2, New York, 1995, WW Norton.

46. May M, McCarron P, Stansfeld S, et al: Does psychological distress predict the risk of ischemic stroke and transient ischemic attack? The Caerphilly Study, *Stroke* 33(1):7-12, 2002.

47. McGoldrick M: Overview: ethnicity and family therapy. In McGoldrick M, Giordano J, Pearce J, editors: *Ethnicity and family therapy*, ed 2, New York, 1996, Guilford Press.

48. McMahon R, Crown DS: Return to work factors following stroke, *Top Stroke Rehabil* 5(2):54-60, 1998.
49. McNamara ME: Neurological conditions: depression and stroke, multiple sclerosis, Parkinson's disease, and epilepsy. In Stoudemire A, editor: *Psychological factors affecting medical conditions*, Washington, DC, 1995, American Psychiatric Press.
50. Moos RH, Schaefer JA: Life transitions and crises: a conceptual overview. In Moos RH, editor: *Coping with life crises: an integrated approach*, New York, 1986, Plenum Press.
51. Morris PL, Raphael B, Robinson RG: Clinical depression is associated with impaired recovery from stroke, *Med J Aust* 157(4):239-242, 1992.
52. Morris PL, Robinson RG, Andrzejewski P, et al: Association of depression with 10-year poststroke mortality, *Am J Psychiatry* 150(1):124-129, 1993.
53. Morris PL, Robinson RG, de Carvalho ML, et al: Lesion characteristics and depressed mood in the stroke data bank study, *J Neuropsychiatry Clin Neurosci* 8(2):153-159, 1996.
54. Morris PL, Robinson RG, Raphael B: Emotional lability after stroke, *Aust N Z J Psychiatry* 27(4):601-605, 1993.
55. Morris PL, Robinson RG, Raphael B, et al: The relationship between the perception of social support and post-stroke depression in hospitalized patients, *Psychiatry* 54(3):306-316, 1991.
56. Morris PL, Robinson RG, Raphael B, et al: The relationship between risk factors for affective disorder and poststroke depression in hospitalised stroke patients, *Aust N Z J Psychiatry* 26(2):208-217, 1992.
57. Morris PL, Robinson RG, Samuels J: Depression, introversion and mortality following stroke, *Aust N Z J Psychiatry* 27(3):443-449, 1993.
58. Morris PL, Shields RB, Hopwood MJ, et al: Are there two depressive syndromes after stroke? *J Nerv Ment Dis* 182(4):230-234, 1994.
59. Murata Y, Kimura M, Robinson RG: Does cognitive impairment cause post-stroke depression? *Am J Geriatr Psychiatry* 8(4):310-317, 2000.
60. Muskin P, Haase E: Personality disorders. In Noble J, editor: *Textbook of primary care medicine*, ed 3, St Louis, 2001, Mosby.
61. Narushima K, Kosier JT, Robinson RG: Preventing poststroke depression: a 12-week double-blind randomized treatment trial and 21-month follow-up, *J Nerv Ment Dis* 190(5):296-303, 2002.
62. Nelson LD, Cicchetti D, Satz P, et al: Emotional sequelae of stroke, *Neuropsychology* 7(4):553-560, 1993.
63. Nelson LD, Cicchetti D, Satz P, et al: Emotional sequelae of stroke: a longitudinal perspective, *J Clin Exp Neuropsychol* 16(5):796-806, 1993.
64. Nicholl CR, Lincoln NB, Muncaster K, et al: Cognitions and post-stroke depression, *Br J Clin Psychol* 41(3):221-231, 2002.
65. O'Connell B, Hanna B, Penney W, et al: Recovery after stroke: a qualitative perspective, *J Qual Clin Pract* 21:120-125, 2001.
66. Paradiso S, Ohkubo T, Robinson RG: Vegetative and psychological symptoms associated with depressed mood over the first two years after stroke, *Int J Psychiatry Med* 27(2):137-157, 1997.
67. Parikh RM, Lipsey JR, Robinson RG, et al: A two-year longitudinal study of poststroke mood disorders: prognostic factors related to one and two year outcome, *Int J Psychiatry Med* 18(1):45-56, 1988.
68. Peloquin SM: The therapeutic relationship: manifestations and challenges in occupational therapy. In Crepeau EB, Cohn ES, Schell BAB, editors: *Willard & Spackman's occupational therapy*, ed 10, Philadelphia, 2003, Lippincott Williams & Wilkins.
69. Pohjasvaara T, Vataja R, Leppävuori A, et al: Depression is an independent predictor of poor long-term functional outcome post-stroke, *Eur J Neurol* 8:315-319, 2001.
70. Pound P, Gompertz P, Ebrahim S: Illness in the context of older age: the case of stroke, *Sociol Health Illn* 20(4):489-506, 1998.
71. Pound P, Gompertz P, Ebrahim S: Social and practical strategies described by people living at home with stroke, *Health Soc Care Community* 7(2):120, 1999.
72. Purtilo R, Haddad A: Challenges to patients. In Purtilo R, Haddad A, editors: *Health professional and patient interaction*, ed 6, Philadelphia, 2002, WB Saunders.
73. Rabins PV, Starkstein SE, Robinson RG: Risk factors for developing atypical (schizophreniform) psychosis following stroke, *J Neuropsychiatry Clin Neurosci* 3(1):6-9, 1991.
74. Remer-Osborn J: Psychological, behavioral and environmental influences on post-stroke recovery, *Top Stroke Rehabil* 5(2):45-53, 1998.
75. Rimmer JH, Hedman G: A health promotion program for stroke survivors, *Top Stroke Rehabil* 5(2):30-44, 1998.
76. Robertson IH, Ridgeway V, Greenfield E, et al: Motor recovery after stroke depends on intact sustained attention: a 2-year follow-up study, *Neuropsychology* 11(2):290-295, 1997.
77. Robinson RG: An 82-year-old woman with mood changes following a stroke, *JAMA* 283(12):1607-1614, 2000.
78. Robinson RG, Chemerinski E, Jorge R: Pathophysiology of secondary depressions in the elderly, *J Geriatr Psychiatry Neurol* 12(3):128-136, 1999.
79. Robinson R, Murata Y, Shimoda K: Dimensions of social impairment and their effect on depression and recovery following stroke, *Int Psychogeriatr* 11(4):375-384, 1999.
80. Robinson R, Parikh R, Lipsey J, et al: Pathological laughing and crying following stroke; validation of a measurement scale and a double-blind treatment study, *Am J Psychiatry* 150(2):286-293, 1993.
81. Reference deleted in proofs.
82. Robinson RG, Starr LB, Kubos KL, et al: A two-year longitudinal study of post-stroke mood disorders: findings during the initial evaluation, *Stroke* 14(5):736-741, 1983.
83. Robinson RG, Starr LB, Lipsey JR, et al: A two-year longitudinal study of poststroke mood disorders: in-hospital prognostic factors associated with six-month outcome, *J Nerv Ment Dis* 173(4):221-226, 1985.
84. Sacks OW: *An anthropologist on Mars: seven paradoxical tales*, New York, 1995, Knopf.
85. Schulz R, Tompkins CA, Rau MT: A longitudinal study of the psychosocial impact of stroke on primary support persons, *Psychol Aging* 3(2):131-141, 1988.
86. Schwartzberg S: *Interactive reasoning in the practice of occupational therapy*, Upper Saddle River, NJ, 2002, Prentice Hall.
87. Sheridan CL, Radmacher SA: Significance of psychological factors to health and disease. In Schein L, Bernard H, Spitz H, et al, editors: *Psychosocial treatment for medical conditions: principles and techniques*, New York, 2003, Brunner-Routledge.
88. Spector RE: *Cultural diversity in health and illness*, ed 4, Stamford, Conn, 1996, Appleton & Lange.
89. Starkstein SE, Bryer JB, Berthier ML, et al: Depression after stroke: the importance of cerebral hemisphere asymmetries, *J Neuropsychiatry Clin Neurosci* 3(3):276-285, 1991.
90. Starkstein S, Fedoroff J, Price T, et al: Apathy following cerebrovascular lesions, *Stroke* 24(11):1625-1630, 1993.
91. Starkstein SE, Fedoroff JP, Price TR, et al: Catastrophic reaction after cerebrovascular lesions: frequency, correlates, and validation of a scale, *J Neuropsychiatry Clin Neurosci* 5(2):189-194, 1993.
92. Stevens L, Schulman J: Neurological illness. In Schein L, Bernard H, Spitz H, et al, editors: *Psychosocial treatment for medical conditions: principles and techniques*, New York, 2003, Brunner-Routledge.
93. Stoudemire A: *Psychological factors affecting medical conditions*, Washington, DC, 1995, American Psychiatric Press.

94. Strain JJ, Grossman S: Psychologicalal reactions to medical illness and hospitalization. In Strain JJ, Grossman S, editors: *Psychological care of the medically ill*, New York, 1975, Appleton-Century-Croft.

95. Strauss DH, Spitzer RL, Muskin PR: Maladaptive denial of physical illness: a proposal for DSM-IV, *Am J Psychiatry* 147(9): 1168-1172, 1990.

96. Stuifbergen AK, Gordon D, Clark AP: Health promotion: a complementary strategy for stroke rehabilitation, *Top Stroke Rehabil* 5(2):11-18, 1998.

97. Tateno A, Kimura M, Robinson RG: Phenomenological characteristics of poststroke depression: early-versus late-onset, *Am J Geriatr Psychiatry* 10(5):575-582, 2002.

98. Terkelsen K: Toward a theory of the family life cycle. In Carter EA, McGoldrick M, editors: *The family life cycle: a framework for family therapy*, New York, 1980, Gardner Press.

99. Tompkins CA, Schulz R, Rau MT: Post-stroke depression in primary support persons: predicting those at risk, *J Consult Clin Psychol* 56(4):502-508, 1988.

100. Truelsen T, Nielsen N, Boysen G, et al: Self-reported stress and risk of stroke: the Copenhagen City Heart Study, *Stroke* 34(4):856-862, 2003.

101. van der Smagt-Duijnstee ME, Hamers JPH, Abu-Saad HH, et al: Relatives of hospitalized stroke patients: their needs for information, counseling and accessibility, *J Adv Nurs* 33(3): 307-315, 2001.

102. van Straten A, de Haan RJ, Limburg M, et al: Clinical meaning of the stroke-adapted sickness impact profile-30 and the sickness impact profile-136, *Stroke* 31(11):2610-2615, 2000.

103. Whyte EM, Mulsant BH: Post stroke depression: epidemiology, pathophysiology, and biological treatment, *Biol Psychiatry* 52: 253-264, 2002.

104. Wilcox VL, Kasl SV, Berkman LF: Social support and physical disability in older people after hospitalization: a prospective study, *Health Psychol* 13(2):170-179, 1994.

105. Williams J, Nieto J, Sanford C, et al: The association between trait anger and incident stroke risk: the Atherosclerosis Risk in Communities (ARIC) Study, *Stroke* 33(1):13-19, 2002.

106. Zelinski EM, Crimmins E, Reynolds S, et al: Do medical conditions affect cognition in older adults? *Health Psychol* 17(6):504-512, 1998.

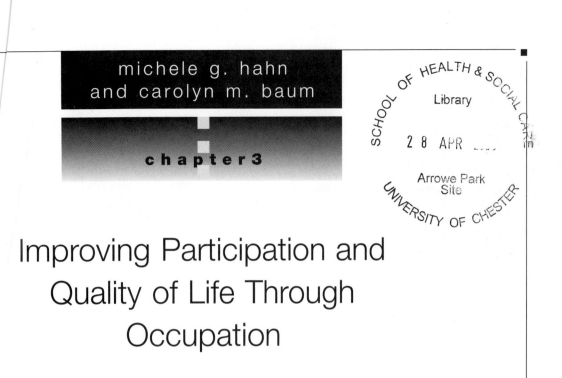

michele g. hahn
and carolyn m. baum

chapter 3

# Improving Participation and Quality of Life Through Occupation

**key terms**

| patient-centered care occupation | participation | quality of life |

**chapter objectives**

After completing this chapter, the reader will be able to accomplish the following:

1. Describe key concepts of participation, occupation, and quality of life.
2. Understand key measures to address participation, occupation, and quality of life in practice.
3. Address participation in the continuum of care from the acute episode to community life.
4. Describe barriers that threaten participation and quality of life.
5. Identify the key role that therapists have in fostering participation through occupation.

## CONCEPTS CENTRAL TO ENABLING PARTICIPATION

The term *participation* encompasses the concepts of personal independence and social and community integration.[54] Participation must be considered across the life span. A child plays with friends, engages in sports, goes to school, and is a member of a family; an adult participates in family, work, leisure, and community activities; an older adult may want to continue to work, travel, do volunteer work, and spend time with family. These activities reflect the individual's desire to participate fully in society, performing the occupations that are meaningful and important to them

Participation is easily taken for granted. Being able to do what one wants to do, go where one wants to go, and have freedom in the choice of activities at the time at which one wants do them is central to personal independence. Participation can be compromised after a stroke. Others obviously see that an individual's participation will be difficult if mobility problems impair balance or if the individual is using a wheelchair and faces stairs, narrow doorways, and steep inclines. What may not be so obvious are impairments that are not so visible, such as visual inattention, depression, and executive control.

Participation is supported or limited by the physiologic, psychological, cognitive, sensory, and motor capacities

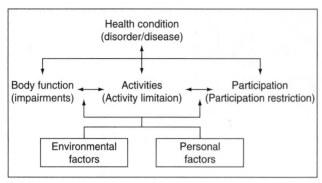

**Figure 3-1**    Interaction of concepts. (From World Health Organization: Introduction to the ICIDH-2: the International Classification of Function, Disability and Health, 2001. http://www3.who.int/ICF/ICFtemplate.cfm; retrieved Oct. 13, 2003.)

of the individual. Likewise, participation is supported or limited by environmental factors. Obvious environmental factors include the physical and social factors associated with accessibility and access to social support; others include governmental and organizational policies, especially as they affect employment.

In recent years, the concept of participation has become much more visible, for it is a central concept in the new International Classification of Functioning, Disability and Health approved as the new ICIDH-2.

Professionals from all of the health fields eventually will organize their services to support health, which, according to the International Classification of Functioning, Disability and Health, is the interaction of body function with engagement in activity and participation as influenced by environmental factors and personal choice (Figure 3-1). One must understand some key concepts to practice with participation as a central concept. These terms include *occupation, participation, patient-centered care,* and *quality of life.*

## OCCUPATION

To participate fully in a life that has meaning, independence, and choice, the individual engages in "occupations." *Occupation* has been defined as the "ordinary and familiar things that persons do every day."[15] Occupations have purpose, and perhaps most importantly, they have meaning for the person engaged in them. When individuals engage in occupations, they are engaged in activities that are directed by goals or are purposeful, are performed in situations or contexts that influence them, can be identified by the doer and others, and are meaningful.[14]

Occupations usually are classified into general categories, the most common classifications fall into the domains of work (or productivity), play or leisure, and self-maintenance (also referred to as *self-care* and *instrumental tasks*). These categories account for the cycle of

activities that constitutes the typical day, regardless of the culture being studied.[37]

### Work

Work is difficult to classify, for what is work to one may be play or leisure to another. Prineau[41] points out that some may derive relaxation and enjoyment in performing household chores, whereas others detest the experience. She asks readers to consider professional athletes who are paid well to exhibit their skills in tennis, golf, baseball, hockey, and other sports. These same occupations are pursued by amateurs as freely chosen recreational and leisure pastimes. The Canadian Association of Occupational Therapists has used the term *productivity* as a more useful alternative to *work*. *Productivity* is defined as "those activities and tasks which are done to enable the person to provide support to the self, family and society through the production of goods and services."[11]

### Play/Leisure

*Play* is a term used interchangeably with *leisure* to describe the nonwork activities of adults in addition to play as the chosen activities of children. Takata[43] asks one to consider that play is not defined by specific behaviors or activities but rather by attitudes and behavioral styles. Because of these characteristics, playfulness (or moments of play) can be experienced during (or enfolded within) work. Play and leisure must be considered central to the activities of individuals following stroke.

Leisure is thought to be a class of activities carried out in discretionary time.[21] Freedom of choice in participation without a particular goal other than enjoyment seems to be the defining characteristics of leisure activity.[24] No one can imagine lives devoid of play or leisure, and neither should a person who has had a stroke. That person's engagement in play and leisure should be enabled with tools, skills, and environments. (see Chapter 28).

### Self-Care: Maintaining Oneself in a Social World

Those activities that are necessary for maintenance of the self within the environment constitute another major classification of occupation. Often included in this category are activities related to personal care (eating, grooming, and hygiene), getting around (mobility), communicating, and performing basic tasks seen as fundamental to living in society; such activities include housecleaning, child care, banking, and shopping.

For a person to be self-reliant in any community, a level of competence is required that enables the accomplishment of tasks beyond those of basic self-care (which are referred to as physical self-maintenance). For this reason, Powell Lawton identified the use of the telephone, food preparation, housekeeping, laundry, shopping, money management, use of transportation, and medication management as important basic daily activities and proposed the term *instrumental activities of daily living* to describe them[33] (see Chapter 20).

Often when persons are hospitalized, the focus is on achieving independence in self-care. Christiansen[13] suggested that self-care tasks must be viewed as necessary from a societal point of view. Although eating and hygiene tasks are essential for survival and health, dressing and grooming are important to social interaction and participation. Some expect persons to care for themselves. Sometimes therapists go too far in expecting an individual to perform self-care; some individuals prefer to spend their time in other occupations and accept the help of others to do basic self-care. Therapists are familiar with the use of personal attendants with persons following spinal cord injuries; persons who have had a stroke benefit from a personal attendant so that they have choice in how they spend their time in occupations that are more important and meaningful to them.

A discussion of occupation cannot be complete without a discussion of self-efficacy and self-determination. Albert Bandura[2] used the term *self-efficacy* to describe the extent to which successes or failures influence expectations of future success or failure. The experience of success in doing things (occupations) contributes to a positive sense of oneself as effective or competent. In contrast, a negative view of self and one's ability to influence events can lead to perceptions of helplessness. Gage and Polatajko[20] observed that perceived self-efficacy has been shown to influence perseverance and well-being and that it can be modified through successful experiences.

According to self-determination theory,[42] intrinsic sources of motivation lead persons to encounter new challenges. An important (and logical) part of this theory is the claim that settings in which persons experience success helps them feel good about themselves. This enables persons to face their daily challenges more readily and in the process to develop an understanding of who they are and their place in the world.

Following stroke, many individuals are not able to engage in their occupations as they have in the past. Therapy must create the environment for learning that fosters a person's view of self so that successful experiences can be experienced and sustained. Opportunities for success must be fostered as well so that these persons are motivated to face their daily challenges.

Occupation is a concept that must be understood in terms of planning and describing the activities of an individual; it provides an important process that can and should be used in the rehabilitation program to improve a person's recovery. Box 3-1 highlights key statements that identify the importance of occupation; these can be translated directly into outcomes that practitioners can address today as they plan patient-centered care.

---

**Box 3-1**

**The Importance of Occupation**

- Occupation is the vehicle to acquire, maintain, or redevelop skills necessary to fulfill occupational roles and provide satisfaction.[19]
- The lack of occupation leads to a breakdown in habits and physiologic deterioration, which lead to loss of ability and competency to support daily life.[27]
- Individuals with cognitive loss who remain engaged in occupations retain higher levels of functional status and demonstrate fewer disturbing behaviors.[3]
- Engagement in individually motivating and ongoing occupations supplies sustenance for survival and safety and enhanced health.[49]
- Meaningful occupations provide individuals with exercise to maintain homeostasis and to keep body parts and neuronal physiology and mental capacities functioning at peak efficiency and enable maintenance and development of satisfying and stimulating social relationships.[49]

---

## PATIENT-CENTERED CARE

Patients who have had strokes need support to return to their lives as they lived them before the stroke. They require services that help them build endurance, increase movement and strength, increase awareness, obtain assistive devices such as wheelchairs and self-care tools, acquire accessible housing, and gain access to barrier-free workplaces and communities. These needs challenge rehabilitation professionals to extend their interventions beyond the patients' immediate impairments to focus on their long-term health needs by helping them develop healthy behaviors to improve their health and well-being and to minimize long-term health care costs associated with dysfunction.[6]

Rehabilitation traditionally has occurred in institutions and is a time-limited process aimed at helping a person with a stroke reach an optimum level of function. This approach labels the recipient of service as a patient, has led the patient to understand that the therapist would be fixing the problem, and has led the therapist to expect patients and their families to comply with his or her recommendations.[36] This approach does not reflect patient-centered care. To move from this traditional approach to a patient-centered approach, practitioners must shift from focusing on impairments to understanding why problems occur and what might be done about them.

A patient-centered approach requires a different orientation, one that engages the assistance and support of a therapist to facilitate the patient's problem solving and goal achievement.[36] In a patient-centered program, the practitioner and the patient bring important information to the partnership. For patients to understand why the practitioner is involved in their care and what they can expect to achieve through therapy is as important as for the therapist to understand the issues and needs of the patients. For patients to understand the scope of the therapist's knowledge also is important. The patient's knowledge of his or her condition and experience with the problem must become clear for the relationship to progress. If a person has a cognitive limitation, the person selected to be the guardian or caretaker must participate in treatment planning[6] to ensure protection of the patient's rights.

Early in the interaction, practitioners should obtain information from patients about their perception of the problem, needs, and goals. The implementation of a patient-centered approach requires the use of a top-down approach[35,45] in which patients identify what they perceive to be the important issues causing them difficulty in carrying out their daily activities in work, self-maintenance, leisure, and rest.[6]

A patient-centered approach requires practitioners to view patients in the contexts of their lives and help them not only to acquire the skills to handle the immediate issues that are influencing their health but also to learn strategies and link with community resources that promote, protect, and improve their health over the long term. This approach extends from the agency or institution into the community, requiring the practitioner to take an active role in advocating for healthy communities by removing attitudinal, economic, and physical barriers.[6]

## QUALITY OF LIFE

How do we think about the quality of our lives? In a recent discussion with students, not one student mentioned quality of life issues related to his or her health. Students' descriptions included being satisfied with their lives and doing what they want to do when and how they want to do it. In other words, they were expressing terms that relate to life satisfaction, well-being, and participation.

Rehabilitation professionals must think about their patients in terms of what will be the outcome of services as they affect the daily lives of the patients they serve, not merely the outcome achieved in a short-term goal. Quality is not achieved with strength, range, coordination, and balance. Quality is achieved by having meaningful relationships, having a job, being a good parent, and engaging in leisure interests, all which depend on having cognitive capacity, strength, endurance, and mobility, which may require new skills and new ways of doing things.

The concept of life satisfaction is subjective; what is satisfying to one is not necessarily satisfying to another. The concept reminds one of the importance of implementing a patient-centered plan to help the person do what he or she wants and needs to do. The concepts central to life satisfaction are happiness, having plans for the future, and engaging in interests and experiences that are meaningful.[39] All of these concepts are threatened when an individual's life changes abruptly with a stroke.

Well-being is one of the concepts that contributes to the individual's perception of quality of life. In addition to happiness, well-being includes the person's perception of confidence and self-esteem. Wilcock[49] encourages practitioners to consider relationships (including social friends, family, partnerships, neighbors, and strangers) and the availability of surroundings (including home, school, place of worship, peace, and weather and terrain) as central to the individual's perception of well-being. The World Health Organization Quality of Life Group[55] defines *quality of life* as an individuals' perceptions of their position in life in the context of the culture and value systems in which they live and in relation to their goals, expectations, standards, and concerns.

Being able to go where one wants to go and do what one wants to do is central to personal freedom. Participation should be the ultimate goal of medical and rehabilitative care and social services, for it describes the extent to which a person is engaged in life situations in a societal context.[54] Interventions must help patients participate in daily life, enabling them to develop the skills or build the adaptive strategies to do what is necessary for them to carry out their occupational roles. Practitioners carrying out their roles and doing what patients want and need them to do makes it possible for them to contribute to the patients' life satisfaction and sense of well-being. Such an approach makes a contribution to the health and well-being of patients, and collectively to society, for it enables quality in the lives of those served.

With the revisions to the World Health Organization International Classification of Functioning, Disability and Health, activity and participation have become issues central to care and must be included in treatment planning. Effective rehabilitation treatment begins with a sound assessment. In addition to determining the physical, cognitive, and psychological problems resulting from stroke, one must determine the patient's prior activities to establish the individual's identity so the person's interests are clear to all members of the team, for these interests serve to motivate the person during the rehabilitation.

### Assessment of Participation

A variety of measures are available to determine a patient's prior level of activity.[31] Traditionally, therapists have relied on activity checklists and open-ended interviews to obtain information regarding participation before stroke. Unfortunately, these interviews are limited by the patient's memory. Measures have been developed to provide therapists with a systematic and consistent method for evaluating participation. One such measure is the Activity Card Sort developed by Baum

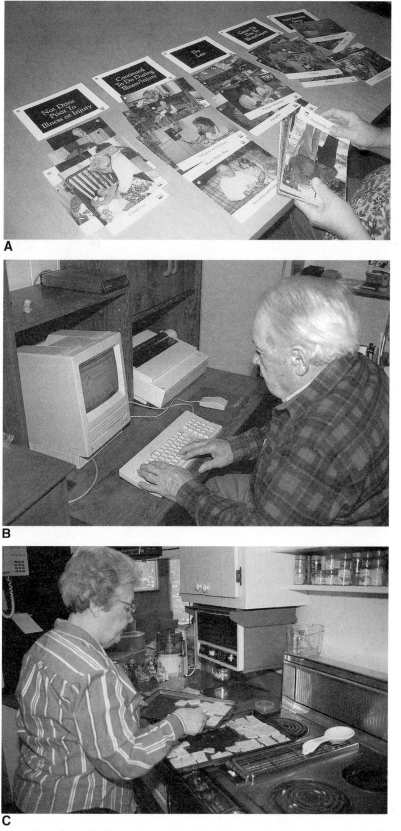

**Figure 3-2** Sample cards from the Activity Card Sort. **A,** Sorting the cards. **B,** Computer card. **C,** Cooking card.

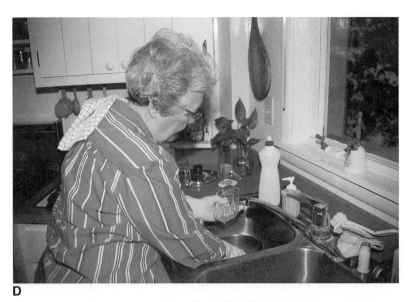

**Figure 3-2 cont'd    D,** Dish-washing card.

and Edwards[4] (Figure 3-2). The Activity Card Sort uses a Q-sort methodology to assess participation in 80 instrumental, social, and high- and low-demand physical leisure activities. Patients sort the cards into different piles to identify activities that were done before stroke, those activities they are doing less often, and those they have given up since their stroke. The Activity Card Sort uses cards with pictures of tasks that persons do every day.

These activities are documented in categories of instrumental, leisure, and social activities. Different versions of the card sort are available for the different contexts in which rehabilitation is occurring. The institutional version (for use in hospitals and nursing homes) sorts 80 cards into categories of activities done before illness and not done afterward. The recovering version identifies activities not done in the last 5 years, those given up because of illness, those one is beginning to do again, and those activities the patient is doing now. All versions allow one to determine a current activity level. The card sort takes approximately 30 minutes to administer and results in a score of percent of activities retained. The Activity Card Sort has been found to be a reliable and valid measure with individuals with cognitive loss[4] and stroke[26] and is available in several culture-specific formats. Adolescent and child versions are in development.

The Canadian Occupational Performance Measure, or COPM,[30,32] is an interview used to assess a patient's perception of recovery and goals. The COPM is based on a patient-centered practice framework. The COPM crosses all diagnoses and is not specific to any age group. The three primary areas identified are self-care, productivity, and leisure. The interview allows identification of problem areas. Satisfaction and importance of the problem areas are rated on a scale from 1 to 10. The COPM takes approximately 45 minutes to administer, but time can vary greatly with the interview. For this reason, the test may be difficult with individuals with cognitive deficits. Despite the length and cognitive difficulty, the assessment validity is good and the COPM is a patient-centered tool that facilitates development of treatment plans and therapeutic goals.

The Community Integration Questionnaire[51] originally was designed for individuals with traumatic brain injury and is particularly useful with younger stroke patients. The Community Integration Questionnaire measures handicap as a function of community integration.[34] The questionnaire has 15 items including questions such as "Who does the shopping in your household?" and "How many times a month do you leave the house to go shopping?" Four scores are calculated: home integration, community integration, productivity, and a total score. Each item has a possibility of three responses, with responses weighted numerically. A higher score indicates greater independence.

### Assessment of Quality of Life

The stroke outcome literature historically has reported survival from stroke. Medical advances may prolong life, but knowing how individuals feel regarding their lives after stroke is important.[37] Not until recently has the patient's perception of the quality of life been taken into account. A normal neurologic examination may not equate to good quality of life for the patient. Therefore, well-designed quality of life measures are essential.

The Reintegration to Normal Living[52,53] was developed to document reentry into everyday life following a sudden illness or event. The instrument is a functional status measure that quantitatively assesses the degree of reintegration to normal living achieved by patients after illness or trauma and is useful for individuals with physical or cognitive disabilities. The Reintegration to Normal Living assesses global function and the individual's satisfaction with basic self-care, in-home mobility, leisure activities, travel, and productive pursuits. The patient is provided with 11 statements. Some examples include "I am able to participate in recreational activities," "I assume a role in my family which meets my needs and those of the other family members," and "I am comfortable with how my self-care needs are met." The test can be completed using a pencil and paper format or an interview format. Reliability and validity have been established for persons with stroke.

The Medical Outcomes Study 36-item Short-Form Health Survey, or SF-36,[48] is the most commonly used life satisfaction scale. The SF-36 has been used extensively with many diagnoses, including stroke, and is quick and easy to administer. The SF-36 is a self-report measure of eight subcategories: physical functioning, physical role limitations, bodily pain, general health perceptions, energy/vitality, social functioning, emotional role limitations, and mental health.

Another quality of life scale is the Stroke Impact Scale (SIS). The SIS is a stroke-specific measure that incorporates function and quality of life into one measure.[29] The SIS III is a self-report measure including 59 items that form eight subgroups: strength, hand function, basic and instrumental activities of daily living, mobility, communication, emotion, memory and thinking, and participation. Duncan, Wallace, Lai, et al[18] have found the SIS to be valid, reliable, and sensitive to change in stroke populations. Furthermore, the SIS is reliable when responses are provided by proxy.[17]

The Stroke Adapted Sickness Impact Profile (SA-SIP)[47] is a shortened form of the more commonly know Sickness Impact Profile.[8] The SA-SIP has 30 true/false statements regarding a person's function and stroke-related symptoms. The statements are separated into seven categories: body care and movement, social interaction, mobility, emotional behavior, household management, alertness behavior, and ambulation. The SA-SIP has good reliability and validity (Table 3-1).

**Table 3-1**

**Summary of Tests and Availability**

| NAME OF TEST | REFERENCE | TIME TO ADMINISTER | SOURCE |
|---|---|---|---|
| **Participation Measures** | | | |
| Activity Card Sort | 5 | 30 minutes | Carolyn Baum, Program in Occupational Therapy, Box 8505, Washington University School of Medicine, 4444 Forest Park Ave., St. Louis, MO 63108 |
| Canadian Occupational Performance Measure | 12 | 30+ minutes | Law M, Baptiste S, Carswell A, et al: *Canadian occupational performance measure manual*, ed 3, Ottawa, 1998, CAOT Publications ACE. |
| Community Integration Questionnaire | 51 | 10 minutes | Willer B et al: Assessment of community integration following rehabilitation for traumatic brain injury, *J Head Trauma Rehabil* 8:75-87, 1993. |
| **Quality of Life Measures** | | | |
| Stroke Adapted Sickness Impact Profile) | 48 | 15 minutes | van Straten A, de Haan RJ, Limburg M, et al: A stroke-adapted 30-item version of the Sickness Impact Profile to assess quality of life (SAS-SIP30), *Stroke* 28:2155-2161, 1997. |
| Stroke Impact Scale | 18 | 30 minutes | User agreement and forms available at the following Web site: http://www2.kumc.edu/coa/SIS_Database/stroke-impact.htm |
| Reintegration to Normal Living | 54 | 10 minutes | Wood-Dauphinee SL, Opzoomer MA, Williams JI, et al: Assessment of global function: the Reintegration to Normal Living Index, *Arch Phys Med Rehabil* 69(8):583-590, 1988. |
| Medical Outcomes Study Short-Form Health Survey (SF-36) | 49 | 15 minutes | RAND Corporation, Santa Monica, California. |

## Barriers to Participation and Quality of Life

Once the practitioners identify problems with participation and quality of life, they must address barriers to resumption of activities. Such barriers can be divided into several subgroups including disability in basic and complex instrumental activities of daily living, decreased cognition, impaired motor function and balance, limited mobility, urinary incontinence, poor speech and language function, depression, decreased resource utilization, environmental inaccessibility, and diminishing social and community support. Each is discussed to highlight how rehabilitation can address the issues that may limit an individual's participation after stroke.

Persons who have had a stroke have impairments, that limit their ability to participate in activities outside the home. To go to the grocery store or to church, the individual must be dressed. Dinner with friends requires the motor ability to feed oneself, the cognitive capacity to carry on a conversation, and the judgment to select the appropriate diet. Difficulty with instrumental or more complex activities of daily living affects the person's ability to return to work, to drive, to manage finances, or to take the bus. See Chapters 20 and 21.

Even in the absence of motor impairment, a cognitive deficit can greatly impair the ability of an individual to return to tasks done before the stroke.[22] Cognitive deficits incorporate areas of attention, orientation, perception, praxis, visuomotor organization, memory, executive function, problem solving, planning, reasoning, and judgment.[28] Tatemichi, Desmond, Stern, et al[44] showed that cognitive dysfunction was a significant predictor for dependent living after discharge and found that quality of life is related to sequential aspects of behavior. Reading the newspaper, watching a movie, finding items on a grocery list, or knowing what to do if lost in the mall can be a challenge for some individuals following stroke.[25] Patients often report feeling overwhelmed with things that came automatically before the stroke. See Chapters 17, 18, and 19.

Impaired balance is cited in the literature as a key variable to independence in the community because of an increased risk of falls. For someone with impaired balance, a trip to the kitchen for a drink of water is a daunting task. Taking out the trash or resuming bowling may provoke enough fear to stop these activities. Addressing balance impairments in the hospital setting may not transfer to ability in the community. Testing of the individual's abilities outside of a sheltered rehabilitation clinic is essential. Decreased motor function and coordination contributes to poor participation in prior activities by limiting the ability to write, cut food, or resume playing tennis (see Chapters 8 and 9).

For individuals with limited mobility, home and community access is problematic. Difficulty with stairs or the inability to ambulate long distances limits the scope of activities for survivors of stroke. A home visit before discharge is recommended to resolve any immediate issues with inaccessibility. Commonly individuals receive equipment that does not fit in their homes. Obstacles including stairs, furniture, power cords, lighting, and noise affect ability to participate in activities inside and outside of the home. For working patients, job site evaluations are necessary for vocational success. For a full-time mother, this may include a comprehensive evaluation of the home and learning what tasks she performs to fulfill her roles (see Chapters 14 and 25).

Speech and language deficits occur in as many as 40% of individuals with strokes.[1] Poor speech and language functions deter patients from situations in which conversation is unavoidable. Persisting consequences adversely affect quality of life, ranging from loss of employment to feelings of isolation and depression. Therefore, addressing language barriers and educating patients and families in compensatory strategies alleviates some distress associated with speech and language deficits.

Depression is another common barrier to participation after stroke. The cause may be directly biologic depending on the location of the lesion in the brain or also may be a reaction to a sudden catastrophic event in the patient's life. Depression may affect participation and long-term outcome adversely.[1] Depression has been associated with longer hospital length of stay, poor performance in activities of daily living, and decreased socialization. Emotional issues such as fear and depression can lead to decreased reintegration into previous roles and occupations and to decreased quality of life. Following a life-altering event such as a stroke, a person may fear additional illness, injury, or another stroke. For this reason, patients may be hesitant to leave their homes and resume prior roles. In a study by Clarke, Marshall, Black, et al,[16] community-dwelling stroke survivors reported a lower sense of well-being than their healthy community-residing counterparts. Patients and their families should be educated regarding risk factors of stroke rehabilitation strategies and medical management following stroke. Additional education may decrease anxiety regarding a future stroke. Referral to a psychologist may be indicated for some individuals (see Chapter 2).

Urinary incontinence is a barrier to participation that frequently is overlooked by rehabilitation teams. Urinary incontinence generally is agreed to have a considerable effect on a person's quality of life and well-being. Between 9% and 40% of the individuals with stroke develop incontinence.[9,40] Incontinence has been identified as a predictor for nursing home placement and is associated with poor recovery from stroke.[9] Studies in the general population have shown that incontinence is associated with depression[46] and higher levels of anxiety.[7] Urinary incontinence often leads to a reduction in social activities and relationships, changes in physical activities, and elaborate planning and forethought before activities that previously could be done spontaneously.[23,38]

Although physical and cognitive impairments constrain the subjective well-being of stroke survivors living in the community, social resources can moderate the adverse effects of residual disabilities. Survivors who have adequate social support are less affected by functional dependence.[16] Social supports have been found to be associated with a higher quality of life in stroke survivors.[28] *Social participation* is defined as socially oriented sharing of resources[10] and is an essential component of quality of life. Therefore, poor resource use may be predictive of decreased quality of life following stroke. Individuals without family or close friends have difficulty reintegrating into prior roles after stroke. Many family members and friends must return to their prior roles several weeks after their loved one's stroke. This produces a gradual decrease in support over time. This decrease often occurs when home health staff have discharged the patient and additional resources such as transportation are required for outpatient therapy, grocery shopping, and medical appointments. This is a critical time for case management to secure the support of community organizations, transportation agencies, and outpatient therapy services. Too often, home health care is discontinued without further referral to a nearby outpatient facility. Although patients are no longer homebound following home care services, they are often in need of further rehabilitation to address the cognitive and emotional issues to help them return to activities, tasks, and roles in the family, work and the community.

## HOW TO FOSTER PARTICIPATION THROUGHOUT THE CONTINUUM OF CARE

No one method of treatment fosters participation in all avenues of rehabilitative care. The stroke team requires commitment and creativity to address the issue. The specific modality applied is not what enhances participation (and hopefully quality of life). Enhancement comes through the activities selected and the contexts in which they are performed. Only through the use of a patient-centered plan and the incorporation of meaningful activities in rehabilitation can the team foster participation to bring meaning to the individual in the rehabilitation program.

### Acute Care

In the acute care setting, acting as a triage team member is essential. This requires a thorough assessment battery. Identifying all the impairments that can improve performance in this setting allows for better discharge planning. Detailed evaluation improves the therapists' abilities to identify impairments from severe to subtle. Too often, assessments in the acute care setting are brief,

increasing the potential for error in discharge placement. Assessment in this phase of treatment should include not only basic measures of motor impairment, cognition, and language but also those of higher level functions, including balance, visual perception, and executive function. These elements are key to successful reentry into the community, participation in roles and activities done before the stroke, and maintenance of quality of life. Often the most problematic deficits are those that are not physically obvious. Patients and families are less likely to understand the impact of poor memory, impaired judgment, decreased language function, and limited balance. Translating these deficits to real-life tasks increases the tangibility for patients and their families and facilitates the transition through other avenues of care. Each level of rehabilitation encompasses increasingly complex tasks in varying contexts.

In some instances, patients do not move through acute care quickly. If treatment time is available, performance of basic tasks is critical. The most basic of self-care is required to go to church, to school, or work. The acute setting is ideal for beginning of basic activities of daily living including bathing, transfers, eating, and toileting as they are identified as meaningful for the patient. Some patients may chose to have an attendant help them with basic activities of daily living. In such cases, goals can evolve around other patient-centered tasks. For the person to do things that are important to them also is important, especially things such as talking on the phone or visiting with family. Emotional attachment to such activities is great. A loss or decrease in independence can produce an emotional response that increases disability.

### Inpatient Rehabilitation

According to the Agency for Healthcare Quality and Research, rehabilitation seeks to help the person with disabilities achieve the highest possible degree of performance. Rehabilitation is comparable to school in which the patient is provided an opportunity for instruction, support, protected practice, education, reassurance, direct assistance, and feedback. This is the "planned withdrawal" of support in which services are provided as needed and removed when no longer needed. The modalities of inpatient rehabilitation treatment are no different from acute care therapy or outpatient therapy; however, the tasks progress to be more difficult. Once the patient has mastered a task in a therapeutic context, the conditions are altered to more real-life situations. Inherent in this progression is that the patient is the leader. The therapist must recognize the need for preparing patients to go home beyond using basic activities of daily living performance as a discharge criteria, because this prepares patients to do well inside their homes but does not prepare patients to shop, go to work, or baby-sit a grandchild. The key to remember in the goal-setting process is the full range of tasks and roles to which the patient is returning. Furthermore, a prior level of function must be established and well documented. An occupational history makes it possible to integrate prior activities into the care plan. If the stroke is impairing prior function, the impairment is treatable and reimbursable. If the prior level of function is documented only in terms of basic self-care, patients will not have access to rehabilitation to return them to community life. By identifying what the person did before admission, one identifies goals to achieve after the prior level of function is achieved. The therapist has more time to achieve those goals once an independent level of self-care is achieved. Response to treatment is better if the patient is put in the context of something important to them. For example, a patient wants to work on writing. The practitioner provides handwriting exercises every day to complete as homework. However, the patient never completes the homework. The patient often is labeled unmotivated or uncooperative. The key question to ask is the type of writing the patient enjoys. Does the patient keep a journal? Does the patient enjoy crossword puzzles? These require different writing skills.

When a patient enters inpatient rehabilitation, an ongoing evaluation of capacities as well as patient goals is imperative. Through identification of higher-level tasks, patients can be challenged outside the walls of the rehabilitation hospital. For example, a patient walks down the hallway of the hospital. What is the response of the other therapists, nurses, and housekeepers in the hallway? What if 1 week after discharge that individual is negotiating a shopping mall. Will the persons in the mall have the same response as the hospital staff? A colleague of mine once referred to this concept as "rehab without walls," providing rehabilitation in the community rather than restricting it to the hospital setting is the best preparation for life after discharge.

## Home Health

The advantage to home health therapy is that the intervention takes place in the setting where the skills will be applied as they are being learned. One of the obvious goals of home health is to identify the physical barriers to the patient's success in the home environment. However, identification of the cognitive and perceptual barriers that limit performance in the home setting is key. In addition, patients may perform better in a familiar environment. As in inpatient rehabilitation, therapeutic activities should evolve around patient-centered goals and may include yard work, laundry, or cooking. The therapist has a dual role in home health therapy. In addition to helping remediate impairments from the stroke, the therapist modifies the environment to achieve maximum participation in goals. The environmental approach also involves educating those who are in the home to the person's

capabilities and how they can enable the person to be active to continue the recovery, as well as help the person gain self-management skills. Preparing the patient in the home environment is the first step in preparing the patient for community reentry. The downfall of home health therapy is the lack of peer support from other stroke patients and minimal patient-team interaction. Referral of the patient to outpatient therapy or a community support group once the patient is no longer restricted to the home setting is recommended.

## Outpatient Therapy

A good outpatient program involves a multidisciplinary team working with the patient to achieve maximum independence in all aspects of life the patient indicates as important. Outpatient therapy forces the patient to maintain a schedule of therapies, get ready in time for the appointment, arrange transportation to and from the appointment, and follow through with home programs that are jointly designed with the therapists. To get to therapy, the patient must have the physical endurance to participate in the preparation, the travel, and the therapy itself. The cognitive process involves initiation, planning, attention, organization, and sequencing. Before the patient reaches the door of the clinic, therapy already has begun.

A complete assessment includes an inventory of activities, responsibilities, and roles the patient likes to do and needs to do everyday. Patients can identify activities that are most important to them. Often outpatient therapy is difficult because of the broad spectrum of possibilities for patients in this setting. Generating a list of the patient's top five goals is recommended. From that point, additional goals can be formulated. In this setting, vocational issues can be addressed. Meeting with the patient's employer is important to address barriers in the workplace. Meeting with and educating the caregiver assists with the identification of barriers the patient may not see in the home. Addressing social support issues with family and friends also is important. An important strategy is to find activities that are enjoyable to the patient and the caregiver, so they can be involved in activities that they enjoy doing together.

## Case Study

### IMPROVING PARTICIPATION THROUGH OCCUPATION

Rosemary awoke one Saturday morning with slurred speech and difficulty walking. She decided to return to bed for additional rest. After sleeping for several more hours, she awoke with left-sided weakness and facial droop, worsening speech, and an inability to walk. She lived alone, was not married, and had no children. She promptly called 911. When paramedics reached her, the dysarthria was severe and she had complete left hemiplegia. She was oriented to her name and where she was but not to the date. In the emergency room, Rosemary was determined to have sustained a large right middle cerebral artery stroke. She was admitted immediately to the hospital and was referred to the stroke team for evaluation and treatment.

Rosemary's deficits included the following. She was unable to move her left arm or leg. She could roll in bed to her left side using the bed rail, but required maximum assistance to roll to the right. She was dependent with her transfers and basic activities of daily living. She had a left visual inattention and decreased sensation on the left side of her body. She was sleepy and was unable to work with a therapist for more than 30 minutes at a time.

Over her first few days in the hospital Rosemary began to improve. She was able to tolerate more time in therapy. Rosemary could support herself while sitting on the edge of the bed and began to play an active role in her activities of daily living. Rosemary was able to move from her bed to a chair with 75% assistance from the nursing and therapy staff. She was tolerating sitting up in bed and a chair for extended periods throughout the day. The team met to determine the course of Rosemary's rehabilitation. At the team meeting, Rosemary's living alone in a two-story home located in the city was revealed. Multiple steps were required to enter. She had two bathrooms in the house; however, the bathroom with a shower was located on the second floor. She had no family locally. Her home was located within walking distance of the doctor and a large grocery store.

Rosemary was a violinist in a local quartet and taught violin on the side. She had few friends other than those in the group with whom she worked. In addition, she was driving (and using public transportation), cooking, shopping, and managing her finances independently before her stroke. Because of these responsibilities and her lack of support at discharge, the team decided Rosemary would benefit from inpatient rehabilitation.

On admission to inpatient rehabilitation, Rosemary was evaluated by nursing, physical therapy, occupational therapy, and speech therapy staff members. She required moderate to maximum assistance with basic activities of daily living and transfers. She required 100% assistance to walk using a walker and an ankle/foot orthotic. She was able to move from her bed to a chair and back with 75% assistance. Her memory was good; however, she indicated that her attention was not, and she appeared easily distracted in the clinic. She was oriented to person, place, date, and situation. Her speech remained slurred, but her swallow was normal. Rosemary's endurance was improved greatly. She continued to show subtle signs of a left visual inattention. Her left arm continued to be weak throughout. Manual muscle test indicated strength at the shoulder and elbow was three fifths of normal. Strength in the wrist and hand was two fifths of normal. Sensation was normal to pin prick and temperature. She was diagnosed with depression and treated medically. The only interests stated in her chart included playing and teaching violin and playing bridge.

Following initial evaluation, the team met to discuss her goals and plans for discharge. Although she was improving daily, her ability to live alone was questionable because of her poor balance, limited attention, and decreased strength. Rosemary and the team set goals for her to be independent with basic activities of daily living and transfers from her bed, the bathtub, and the car. The team chose to address her ability to grocery shop and prepare a simple meal in the microwave. The case manager discussed these goals with Rosemary, and she agreed with the team's priorities.

At her second week of inpatient rehabilitation, Rosemary was able to dress herself independently using an adaptive strategy. She was walking with some assistance using an ankle/foot orthotic and a walker. She was able to prepare a bowl of cereal, a sandwich, and a microwave dinner. She was taken on trips to the gift shop and grocery store to evaluate her ability to follow a list, obtain objects on the list, and exchange money correctly. These trips were overstimulating to Rosemary, and her depression worsened. She missed her music and felt that her only love in life was the violin. She lived close to the hospital but did not have close friends or family to get her violin. Rosemary desperately wanted to do home visit and wanted to get her violin; however, the team thought it would increase her depression because her motor impairment would make it impossible for her to play. Despite the discouragement of the team, one of the therapists brought in a violin for Rosemary to play. The therapist went to a quiet treatment room with Rosemary.

## Case Study

### IMPROVING PARTICIPATION THROUGH OCCUPATION—cont'd

Although Rosemary was hesitant, she removed the violin from the case and asked the therapist to leave the room. She did not want anyone else to hear her attempts to play the violin for the first time. As the therapist closed the door, she could see the fear on Rosemary's face. The therapist returned to the room after 10 minutes. What she heard was amazing. When she opened the door, Rosemary was playing the violin. Her face beamed with pride as the team came in to hear her play. What they all felt was impossible was the key motivator for Rosemary. She began to practice several times a day.

At week 3 of her impatient rehabilitation, the team decided that Rosemary's progress had plateaued and that it was time to schedule discharge. Rosemary did not want to burden her small group of friends. She made the decision to transfer to a residential facility until her status improved. At discharge, she was independent with activities of daily living using some adaptive strategies and independent with transfers using adaptive equipment. Some assistance was required with walking using a quad cane and an ankle/foot orthotic, her speech remained slurred, and her facial droop persisted. Muscle strength throughout her arm was four fifths of normal, with poor coordination distally. She was able to balance a simulated checkbook, prepare simple meals independently (she was most comfortable with the microwave), and play her violin, but she could not drive. Rosemary had difficulty with higher-level tasks involving complex sequencing and organization. Performing multiple tasks at once was difficult for her.

Rosemary transferred to a residential facility for 2 months before returning home. At that time she was referred to outpatient therapy. Rosemary remained unable to drive but was proficient at using public transportation. She was independent with most basic and instrumental activities of daily living. A friend would pick her up weekly to take her to the grocery store. Her motor status was unchanged from her inpatient rehabilitation discharge. She continued to show four-fifths muscle strength proximally and improved coordination in her hand and fingers. Her speech was normal, and speech therapy was not required. Her higher-level executive functions were nearly normal. Her balance continued to be problematic, but she was walking with a straight cane and an ankle/foot orthotic. A comprehensive evaluation of her activities and quality of life revealed the following. Her Activity

Card Sort showed that she had retained only 35% of the activities she had done before the stroke, with the greatest loss in the areas of social activity and high-demand leisure activity. Rosemary's priorities indicated by the Activity Card Sort included the following (in order of importance): playing a musical instrument (her violin), driving, shopping, visiting with friends, and traveling. The Stroke Adapted Sickness Impact Profile (SA-SIP) revealed a score of 15 out of 30. Her score was in the midrange, indicating a decreased quality of life. Some of the problematic areas included "body care and movement," "mobility," and "ambulation." Rosemary received a score of 28 on the Reintegration to Normal Living Index. The scoring range of the index is from 11 to 55. A lower score indicates lower satisfaction. Rosemary's score was in the midrange, indicating some difficulty. Low scores included items regarding travel, spending days occupied with work that is important, getting around the community, and being comfortable in the company of others. The Community Integration Questionnaire indicated some severe difficulties in areas of home, social, and productivity. Rosemary's home integration score was a 3.6 out of 10 points, her social integration score was a 3 out of 12 points, her productivity score was a 1 out of 6 points, and her total score was 7.75 out of 28 points, indicating a poor level of independence. The team met with Rosemary to set her goals for outpatient therapy. Scores from her assessments were discussed. Rosemary identified that her primary barriers to satisfaction were her decreased ability to play her violin and her inability to drive. Because she was unable to drive, she had difficulty shopping, meeting friends, and traveling. Although she had friends to drive her to events or was able to use public transportation close to home, Rosemary felt a decrease in autonomy. This decrease in autonomy and an inability to continue her work added to her depression. Goals were set according to priorities outlined by Rosemary in her Activity Card Sort. The team set goals with Rosemary to improve her motor performance to improve her violin playing and walking independently while carrying a violin case. A driving evaluation was completed and indicated that she was able to return to driving. A trip to the grocery store and the mall allowed the therapists to determine her best method of negotiating the mall and for carrying bags to the car after shopping. Rosemary returned to therapy the second week with her violin. After an

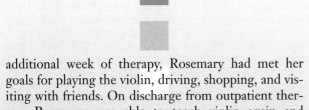

additional week of therapy, Rosemary had met her goals for playing the violin, driving, shopping, and visiting with friends. On discharge from outpatient therapy, Rosemary was able to teach violin again and hoped to return soon to concert performances. Her scores on the SA-SIP had increased to 3 out of 30. Her Community Integration Questionnaire scores returned to normal, and her activity level as measured by the Activity Card Sort returned to 85% of what it was before her stroke.

## REVIEW QUESTIONS

1. Describe the concepts encompassed in the word *participation* and the factors that affect participation.
2. What are three categories of occupation?
3. How may self-efficacy affect a client's recovery?
4. Define quality of life. What is the relationship between quality of life and activity and participation?
5. Describe some common assessments of participation and quality of life.
6. What are some common barriers limiting participation and quality of life?
7. How can therapists address participation through the continuum of care from acute care to the community?
8. What may have been done differently with Rosemary's care to facilitate her recovery? What did the therapists do well with Rosemary?

## REFERENCES

1. Agency for Health Care Policy and Research: *Post-stroke rehabilitation*, Rockville, Md, 1995, US Department of Health and Human Services, Public Health Service, Agency for Health Care Policy and Research.
2. Bandura A: *Social learning theory*, Englewood Cliffs, NJ, 1977, Prentice Hall.
3. Baum CM: The contribution of occupation to function in persons with Alzheimer's disease, *J Occup Sci Aust* 2(2):59-67, 1995.
4. Baum CM, Edwards D: *The Activity Card Sort: Form C*, Unpublished version, 2001.
5. Baum CM, Edwards DF, Morrow-Howell N: Identification and measurement of productive behaviors in senile dementia of the Alzheimer type, *Gerontologist* 33(3):403-408, 1993.
6. Baum CM, Law M: Occupational therapy practice: focusing on occupational performance, *Am J Occup Ther* 51(4):277-288, 1997.
7. Berglund AL, Eisemann M, Lalos O: Personality characteristics of stress incontinent women: a pilot study, *J Psychosom Obstet Gynaecol* 15(3):165-170, 1994.
8. Bergner M, Bobbitt RA, Carter WB, et al: The Sickness Impact Profile: development and final revision of a health status measure, *Med Care* 19(8):787-805, 1981.
9. Brittain KR, Peet SM, Castleden CM: Stroke and incontinence, *Stroke* 29(2):524-528, 1998.
10. Bukov A, Maas I, Lampert T: Social participation in very old age: cross sectional and longitudinal findings from BASE, *J Gerontol B Psychol Sci Soc Sci* 57(6):510-517, 2002.
11. Canadian Association of Occupational Therapists: *Guidelines for the client-centered practice of occupational therapy*, Toronto, 1995, The Association.
12. Chan C, Lee T: Validity of the Canadian occupational performance measure, *Occup Ther Int* 4:229-247, 1997.
13. Christiansen CH: A social-psychological approach to understanding self-care. In Christiansen CH, editor: *Ways of living: self-care strategies for special needs*, Bethesda, Md, 1994, American Occupational Therapy Association.
14. Christiansen CH, Baum C: *Occupational therapy: overcoming human performance deficits*, Thorofare, NJ, 1997, Slack.
15. Christiansen CH, Clark F, Kielhofner G, et al: Position paper: occupation, *Am J Occup Ther* 49(10):1015-1018, 1995.
16. Clarke P, Marshall V, Black SE, et al: Well-being after stroke in Canadian seniors: findings from the Canadian study of health and aging, *Stroke* 33(4):1016-1028, 2002.
17. Duncan PW, Lai SM, Tyler D, et al: Evaluation of proxy responses to the Stroke Impact Scale, *Stroke* 33(11):2593, 2002.
18. Duncan PW, Wallace D, Lai SM, et al: The Stroke Impact Scale version 2.0: evaluation of reliability, validity, and sensitivity to change, *Stroke* 30(10):2131-2140, 1999.
19. Fidler GS, Fidler JW: Doing and becoming: purposeful activity and self-actualization, *Am J Occup Ther* 32:305-310, 1978.
20. Gage M, Polatajko H: Enhancing occupational performance through an understanding of perceived self-efficacy, *Am J Occup Ther* 48(5):452-461, 1994.
21. Gunter BG, Stanley J: Theoretical issues in leisure study. In Gunter BG, Stanley J, St Clair R, editors: *Transitions to leisure: conceptual and human issues*, Lanham, Md, 1985, University Press of America.
22. Hochstenbach J, Anderson P, van Limbeek J, et al: Is there a relation between neuropsychologic variables and quality of life after stroke? *Arch Phys Med Rehabil* 82(10):1360-1366, 2001.
23. Hunskaar S, Vinsnes A: The quality of life in women with urinary incontinence as measured by the Sickness Impact Profile, *J Am Geriatr Soc* 39(4):378-382, 1991.
24. Iso-Ahola SE: Basic dimensions of definitions of leisure, *J Leisure Res* 1:28-39, 1979.
25. Katz N: *Cognitive rehabilitation: models for intervention in occupational therapy*, Stoneham, Mass, 1992, Butterworth-Heinemann.
26. Katz N, Karpin H, Lak A, et al: Participation and occupational performance: reliability and validity of the Activity Card Sort, *Occup Ther J Res* 23(1):10-17, 2003.
27. Kielhofner G: *Conceptual foundations of occupational therapy*, Philadelphia, 1992, FA Davis.
28. King RB: Quality of life after stroke, *Stroke* 27(9):1467-1472, 1996.
29. Lai S, Studenski S, Duncan P, et al: Persisting consequences of stroke measured by the stroke impact scale, *Stroke* 33(7):1840-1850, 2002.
30. Law M, Baptiste S, Mills J: Client-centred practice: what does it mean and does it make a difference? *Can J Occup Ther* 62:250-257, 1995.
31. Law M, Baum C, Dunn W: *Measuring occupational performance: supporting best practice in occupational therapy*, Thorofare, NJ, 2001, Slack.
32. Law M, Cooper BA, Strong S, et al: The person-environment-occupation model: a transactive approach to occupational performance, *Can J Occup Ther* 63:9-23, 1996.
33. Lawton MP: The functional assessment of elderly people, *J Am Geriatr Soc* 19(6):465-481, 1971.
34. Levine MN: Quality of life in stage II breast cancer: an instrument for clinical trials, *J Clin Oncol* 6:1798-1810, 1988.
35. Mathiowetz V, Bass-Haugen J: Motor behavior research: implications for therapeutic approaches to central nervous system dysfunction, *Am J Occup Ther* 48:733-745, 1994.

36. McColl MA, Gerein N, Valentine F: Meeting the challenges of disability: models for enabling function and well-being. In Christiansen C, Baum C, editors: *Occupational therapy: enabling function and well being*, ed 2, Thorofare, NJ, 1997, Slack.

37. Moore A: The band community: synchronizing human activity cycles for group cooperation. In Zemke R, Clark F, editors: *Occupational science: the evolving discipline*, Philadelphia, 1996, FA Davis.

38. Naughton M J, Wyman JF: Quality of life in geriatric patients with lower urinary tract dysfunction, *Am J Med Sci* 314(4):219-227, 1997.

39. Neugarten BL, Havinghurst RJ, Tobin SS: Measure of life satisfaction, *J Gerontol* 16:134-43, 1961.

40. Patel M, Coshall C, Lawrence E, et al: Recovery from poststroke urinary incontinence: associated factors and impact on outcome, *J Am Geriatr Soc* 49(9):1229-1233, 2001.

41. Primeau L: Work versus non-work: the case of household work. In Zemke R, Clark F, editors: *Occupational science: the evolving discipline*, Philadelphia, 1996, FA Davis.

42. Ryan RM, Deci EL: Self-determination theory and the facilitation of intrinsic motivation, social development, and well-being, *Am Psychol* 55(1):68-78, 2000.

43. Takata N: The play milieu: a preliminary appraisal, *Am J Occup Ther* 25:281-284, 1971.

44. Tatemichi T, Desmond D, Stern Y, et al: Cognitive impairment after stroke: frequency, patterns, and relationship to functional abilities, *J Neurol Neurosurg Psychiatry* 57:202-207, 1994.

45. Trombly CA: Occupation: purposefulness and meaningfulness as therapeutic mechanisms. The 1995 Eleanor Clarke Slagle Lecture, *Am J Occup Ther* 49:960-972, 1995.

46. Valvanne J, Juva K, Erkinjuntti T, et al: Major depression in the elderly: a population study in Helsinki, *Int Psychogeriatr* 8(3): 437-443, 1996.

47. van Straten A, de Haan RJ, Limburg M, et al: A stroke-adapted 30-item version of the Sickness Impact Profile to assess quality of life (SAS-SIP30), *Stroke* 28:2155-2161, 1997.

48. Ware JE, Sherbourne CD: The MOS 36-item Short-Form Health Survey (SF-36). I. Conceptual framework and item selection, *Med Care* 30(6):473-483, 1992.

49. Wilcock A: A theory of the human need for occupation, *Occup Sci Aust* 1(1):17-24, 1993.

50. Willer BS, Allen KM, Liss M, et al: Problems and coping strategies of individuals with traumatic brain injury and their spouses, *Arch Phys Med Rehabil* 72(7):460-464, 1991.

51. Willer B, Linn R, Allen K: Community integration and barriers to integration for individuals with brain injury. In Finlayson M, Garner S, editors: *Brain injury rehabilitation: clinical considerations*, Baltimore, 1993, Williams & Wilkins.

52. Wood-Dauphinee SL, Opzoomer MA, Williams JI, et al: Assessment of global function: The Reintegration to Normal Living Index, *Arch Phys Med Rehabil* 69(8):583-590, 1988.

53. Wood-Dauphinee SL, Williams J: Reintegration to normal living as a proxy to quality of life, *J Chronic Dis* 40(6):491-502, 1987.

54. World Health Organization: Introduction to the ICIDH-2: the International Classification of Function, Disability and Health, 2001. http://www3.who.int/ICF/ICFtemplate.cfm; retrieved Oct. 13, 2003.

55. World Health Organization Quality of Life Group: Development of the 3 WHO quality of life assessment, *Psychol Med* 28:551-558, 1998.

## SUGGESTED READINGS

American Occupational Therapy Association: Uniform terminology for occupational therapy (third edition), *Am J Occup Ther* 48(11):1047-1054, 1994.

Baum C, Christiansen C: The occupational therapy context: philosophy-principles-practice. In Christiansen C, Baum C, editors: *Occupational therapy: enabling function and well-being*, ed 2, Thorofare, NJ, 1997, Slack.

Buck D, Jacoby A, Massey A, et al: Evaluation of measures used to assess quality of life after stroke, *Stroke* 31(8):2004, 2000.

Edwards D: The effect of occupational therapy on function and well-being. In Christiansen C, Baum C, editors: *Occupational therapy: enabling function and well-being*, ed 2, Thorofare, NJ, 1997, Slack.

Meyer A: The philosophy of occupation therapy, *Arch Occup Ther* 1:10, 1922.

Ottenbacher KJ, Christiansen C: Occupational performance assessment. In Christiansen C, Baum C, editors: *Occupational therapy: enabling function and well-being*, ed 2, Thorofare, NJ, 1997, Slack.

Reed K: *Models of practice in occupational therapy*, Baltimore, 1984, Williams & Wilkins.

Rowland LP: *Merritt's textbook of neurology*, ed 9, Media, Penn, 1995, Williams & Wilkins.

Silverman M, McDowell BJ, Musa D, et al: To treat or not to treat: issues in decisions not to treat older persons with cognitive impairment, depression, and incontinence, *J Am Geriatr Soc* 45:1094-1101, 1997.

Steeman E, Defever M: Urinary incontinence among elderly persons who live at home: a literature review, *Geriatr Nurs* 22(3):441-455, 1998.

Wyman JF, Fantl JA, McClish DK, et al: Comparative efficacy of behavioral interventions in the management of female urinary incontinence, Continence Program for Women Research Group, *Am J Obstet Gynecol* 179(4):999-1007, 1998.

virgil mathiowetz

**chapter 4**

# Task-Oriented Approach to Stroke Rehabilitation

### key terms

model of motor behavior          motor development          occupational therapy task-
motor control          motor learning          oriented evaluation framework

### chapter objectives

After completing this chapter, the reader will be able to accomplish the following:

1. Describe the motor behavior (i.e., motor control, motor learning, and motor development) theories and model that support the occupational therapy task-oriented approach to persons after stroke.
2. Describe the evaluation framework for the occupational therapy task-oriented approach and identify specific assessments that are consistent with the approach.
3. Describe general treatment principles for the occupational therapy task-oriented approach and their application to persons after stroke.
4. Given a case study of a person after stroke, describe occupational therapy task-oriented approach evaluation and treatment strategies that you would use.

This chapter provides a theoretical foundation for the occupational therapy (OT) task-oriented approach or a function-based approach for persons after stroke. Mathiowetz and Bass-Haugen[53] proposed this approach in 1994 based on the motor behavior/motor control, motor development, and motor learning-theories and research of that time. Motor behavior, occupational therapy theories, and research have evolved since then, so the OT task-oriented approach has evolved as well.[5,51] This chapter represents the most recent thinking regarding this approach.

The theoretical assumptions of the neurophysiologic approaches, which include Rood's sensorimotor approach,[67] Knott and Voss's proprioceptive neuromuscular facilitation,[45] Brunnstrom's movement therapy,[11] and Bobath's neurodevelopmental treatment[8,9] were based on the empirical experience and research of their time. However, as the motor behavior theories changed in the 1980s and 1990s, the assumptions of the neurophysiologic approaches were challenged[32,73,74] and alternative approaches were proposed.[13,14,38,51-53] Recently the theoretical assumptions of the neurodevelopmental treatment approach were updated with current motor behavior theories.[39] However, many of the neurodevelopmental treatment techniques have changed little despite the changed theoretical assumptions. This may reflect the fact that neurodevelopmental treatment was developed empirically first, and then theoretical assumptions of the time were used to explain why it might work. In contrast, the OT task-oriented approach evaluation and interventions strategies emerged primarily from its theoretical assumptions (see Chapter 6).

## THEORETICAL ASSUMPTIONS AND MODEL UNDERLYING THE OCCUPATIONAL THERAPY TASK-ORIENTED APPROACH

### Systems Model of Motor Control

In the past 25 to 30 years, new models of motor control have evolved from the ecologic approach to perception and action[27,82] and from the study of complex, dynamical systems in mathematics and the sciences.[31] The new models emphasize the interaction between persons and their environments and suggest that motor behavior emerges from persons' multiple systems interacting with unique tasks and environmental contexts.[59] "Thus, the systems model of motor control is more interactive or heterarchical and emphasizes the role of the environment more than the earlier reflex-hierarchical models."[51]

In the systems model, the nervous system is viewed differently from earlier reflex-hierarchical models. Instead of being the primary system controlling movement, the nervous system now is considered only one system among many systems that affect motor behavior. "The nervous system itself is organized *heterarchically* such that higher centers interact with the lower centers but do not control them. Closed-loop and *open-loop systems* work cooperatively and both feedback and feedforward control are used to achieve task goals."[51] The central nervous system interacts with multiple personal and environmental systems as a person attempts to pursue a functional goal.

### Ecologic Approach to Perception and Action

The ecologic approach "emphasizes the study of interaction between the person and the environment during everyday, functional tasks and the close linkage between perception and action (i.e., purposeful movement)."[51] Gibson described the role of functional goals and the environment in the relationship between perception and action. He stated that direct perception involves the active search for affordances[28] or the functional utility of objects for a person with unique personal characteristics.[85] Therefore, Gibson's concept of affordances recognizes the close linkage between perception and action in terms of what the information available in the environment means to a specific person.[28]

Bernstein[7] also recognized the importance of the environment and personal factors other than the central nervous system in motor behavior. He explained the role that a particular muscle has in a movement is influenced by the context or circumstances. Bernstein[7] described three potential sources of variability in muscle function. Variability is due to anatomic factors. For example, from kinesiology one knows that in a standing position, the shoulder flexor muscles contract concentrically to bring the humerus to the 90-degree position. However, in the prone position with one's arm at one's side, shoulder extensor muscles contract eccentrically until reaching the 90-degree position. Thus, which muscles are activated depends on the initial position of the body. Another example relates to extending the shoulder from the 90-degree position when standing. If one wants to extend it quickly or against resistance, the shoulder extensor muscles contract. In contrast, if one extends the shoulder slowly against no resistance, the shoulder flexor muscles contract eccentrically and the shoulder extensor muscles do not need to contract at all. In both cases the role of the muscle is determined by the context in which it is used. A second source of variability is due to mechanical factors. Many nonmuscular forces, such as gravity and inertia, determine the degree to which a muscle needs to contract. For example, a muscle must exert much less force if contracting in a gravity-eliminated plane rather than against gravity. Likewise, the contraction of the elbow extensor muscles would be different if the shoulder were extending or flexing at the same time because of the effects of inertia. Again, the effect of a muscle contraction is related to the context. A third source of variability is the result of physiologic factors. "When higher centers send down a command for a muscle to contract, middle and lower centers have the opportunity to modify the command. Lower and middle centers receive peripheral sensory feedback. Thus, the impact of the command on the muscle will vary depending on the context and degree of influence of the middle and lower centers. As a result, the relationship between higher center or executive commands and muscle action is not a one-to-one."[51] Mathiowetz and Wade[54] also demonstrated the influence of context (informational support available in the environment) on movement. They reported that a natural informational support condition (e.g., eating applesauce with a spoon) elicited a smoother and more direct movement pattern than an impoverished informational support condition (e.g., pretending to eat applesauce with a spoon without any of the objects). Many have taken a dynamical systems view as a means to explain the complex person-environment interactions that occur in everyday life.

### Dynamical Systems Theory

The study of dynamical systems originated in the disciplines of mathematics, physics, biology, chemistry, psychology, and kinesiology and has been applied to the professions of occupational therapy, physical therapy, nursing, adapted physical education, and some areas of medicine.[12,50] Such study has influenced the development of a systems model of motor control as well. Dynamical systems theory proposes that behaviors emerge from the interaction of many systems and subsystems. Because the behavior is not specified but emergent, it is considered to be self-organizing.[43] Despite the many *degrees of freedom* or ways of performing a task available to persons, they tend to use relatively stable patterns of motor behavior.[79] For example, when one walks or brushes the teeth, one has many choices in how to perform the task, yet one tends to use preferred patterns. These relatively stable patterns of motor behavior, which are unique to each person, provide evidence of *self-organization.*

Behavior can shift between periods of stability and instability throughout life. For example, behaviors can change from being stable to being less stable as a result of a stroke or aging. In fact, "it is during unstable periods, characterized by a high variability of performance, that new types of behaviors may emerge either gradually or abruptly. These transitions in behavior, called *phase shifts*, are changes in preferred patterns of coordinated behavior to another."[51] A gradual phase shift occurs when an infant progresses from walking while holding on to a parent's hands to walking without a helping hand over several months. An abrupt phase shift in prehension pattern occurs when a person changes from picking up a small object such as a peanut to picking up a large object such as a large coffee mug. How can these phase shifts or changes in behavior be explained?

In the dynamical systems view, *control parameters* are variables that shift behavior from one form to another. They do not control the change but act as agents for reorganization of the behavior into a new form.[36] Control parameters are gradable in some way. In the infant example, the degree of parental support influenced the change or phase shift from walking with support to walking without support. As parental support decreases, infants need to rely more on their own ability to maintain balance and need to increase their strength to support and control their own body weight in an upright position. In the other example, increasing the size of the object to be grasped elicited the change in prehension pattern from tip prehension to cylindrical grasp. Consequently, object size also is considered a control parameter.

Explanations of changes in motor behavior in the systems model of motor control are different from earlier reflex-hierarchical models. Thelen[77] stated that an important characteristic of a system perspective is that the shift from one preferred movement pattern to another is marked by discrete, discontinuous transitions. These changes in only one or several personal or environmental systems (i.e., control parameters) can contribute to transitions in motor behavior.[17] In conclusion, no inherent ordering of systems exists in terms of their influence on motor behavior, and systems themselves are subject to change over time.

## SYSTEMS VIEW OF MOTOR DEVELOPMENT

A systems view of motor development suggests that changes over time are caused by multiple factors or systems such as maturation of the nervous system, biomechanical constraints and resources, and the impact of the physical and social environment.[36,51] For example, Thelen and Fisher[78] reported that the disappearance of the stepping reflex at 4 to 5 months of age is due to multiple factors internal and external to the child. Internal factors included the strength of the leg muscles, weight of the legs, and arousal level of the child. External factors included the varying effects of gravity in different environments. Thus, maturation of the nervous system alone cannot explain this change in developmental behavior. A systems view also suggests that normal development does not follow a rigid sequence, as the motor milestones would suggest. In fact, children follow variable developmental sequences because of their unique personal characteristics and environmental contexts. If the traditional developmental sequences are no longer sufficient as a guide for working with children, then they are certainly not appropriate as a guide for working with adults after stroke.[83]

In addition, the systems view suggests that behaviors observed after central nervous system damage result from patients' attempts to use their remaining resources to achieve functional goals. For example, the flexor pattern of spasticity often seen after stroke is due to various factors in addition to spasticity, such as weakness, inability to recruit appropriate muscles, biomechanical principles related to lever arms, and/or soft tissue tightness. Thus, when abnormal movement patterns are seen after stroke, therapists need to consider multiple factors as potential contributing variables (see Chapter 10).

## CONTEMPORARY VIEW OF MOTOR LEARNING

Schmidt[71] defined motor learning as "a set of processes associated with practice or experience leading to relatively permanent changes in the capabilities of responding." Thus, recent motor learning theories acknowledge that behavior changes observed during practice may be only temporary. As a result, contemporary motor learning research not only evaluates learning after the acquisition phase (i.e. immediate effects) but also after a retention phase (i.e., short-term or long-term effects) or a transfer test (i.e., ability to generalize to new task). As a consequence, new ways of thinking about motor learning have emerged. Motor learning research supports the idea that random practice (i.e., repetitive practice of several tasks in a varied sequence within a practice session) is better than blocked practice (i.e., repetitive practice of the same task within a practice session).[72]

Similarly, practicing variations of the same tasks in varied contexts is better than practicing the same task in the same context. In addition, practicing the whole task rather than parts of a task usually is better, especially if the parts are interdependent or relatively fast.[69]

McNevin, Wulf, and Carlson[55] summarized some additional principles. When persons are learning a new task such as golfing, they should focus on the movement effects (external focus on the golf club head) rather than on their own arm movements (internal focus). Self-controlled practice (i.e., a person being trained decides when and how feedback is given and whether assistive devices are used) is better than instructor-controlled practice. Finally, dyad training, in which a person is able to alternate observing and practicing a task, is beneficial to learning a new task.

Research on the role of feedback in learning demonstrates that physical and verbal guidance enhanced immediate performance but interfered with long-term learning.[69] Winstein and Schmidt[86] reported that 50% feedback (i.e., feedback after half of the trials) was better than 100% feedback. Faded or decreasing feedback was better than increasing feedback. Finally, summary feedback after multiple trials is better than immediate feedback after every trial.[70] In all cases, less feedback was better than more feedback.

Most research on motor learning has been performed on persons without disabilities using a brief, contrived task in laboratory environments. Therefore, therapists need to be cautious about applying these principles to persons with disabilities performing functional tasks in everyday, natural environments.

However, several studies have explored whether motor learning principles can be applied to persons after stroke. Hanlon[35] provided some evidence that random practice was better than blocked practice. Merians, Winstein, Sullivan, et al[56] reported that practice in a condition with reduced augmented feedback was beneficial for performance consistency but not for accuracy for persons with and without stroke. Dean and Shepherd[18] reported that task-related training using variable practice and varied contexts improved balance ability during seated reaching activities. Finally, Fasoli, Trombly, Tickle-Degnen, et al[20] reported that externally focused (task-related) instructions resulted in faster and more forceful movements than internally focused (movement-related) instructions for persons with and without stroke. Chapter 5 provides additional discussion of the application of motor learning principles to stroke rehabilitation.

## SYSTEMS MODEL OF MOTOR BEHAVIOR

The model in Figure 4-1 has been updated to include terminology from the Occupational Therapy Practice Framework.[1] The figure depicts the theoretical basis of

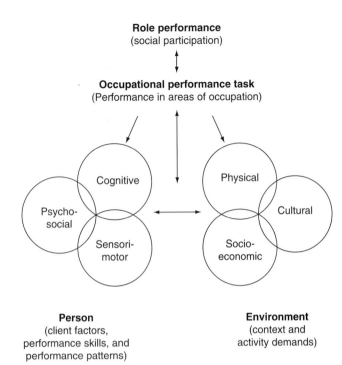

**Figure 4-1**    The systems model of motor behavior, which supports the occupational therapy task-oriented approach, emphasizes that occupational performance tasks and role performance emerge from an interaction of the person and their environment. In addition, any occupational performance task affects the person and environment. A continuous interaction occurs between role performance and occupational performance tasks. These interactions are ongoing across time. (Adapted from Mathiowetz V, Bass-Haugen: Assessing abilities and capacities: motor behavior. In Trombly CA, Radomski MV, editors: *Occupational therapy for physical dysfunction*, ed 5, Philadelphia, 2002, Lippincott Williams & Wilkins.)

the OT task-oriented approach. The model illustrates the interaction between the person (patient factors, performance skills, and performance patterns) and their environment (context and activity demands). Occupational performance tasks (i.e., activities of daily living, instrumental activities of daily living, work, education, and play/leisure) and role performance (social participation) emerge from the interaction between the systems of the person (cognitive, psychosocial, and sensorimotor) and the systems of the environment (physical, socioeconomic, and cultural). Changes in any one of these systems or subsystems can affect occupational performance tasks and/or role performance. "In some cases, only one primary factor might determine occupational performance. In most cases, occupational performance tasks emerge from the interaction of many systems. The on-going interactions between all components of the model reflect its heterarchical nature."[51]

In addition, any occupational performance task affects the environment in which it occurs and the person acting.

For example, if a patient with hemiplegia becomes independent in driving by using assistive technology and adaptive strategies, the patient's ability to drive would free family members from needing to provide transportation for appointments and social events. The patient would be able to resume a role of driver and the task of driving, which were likely meaningful to the patient's life. Thus the occupational performance task of driving affects persons and objects in the environment (i.e., assistive technology added to the car). The task also affects the person and the associated components. The ability to be less dependent on the family may affect the patient's self-esteem positively (i.e., psychosocial subsystem). The process of driving "provides the patient the opportunity to solve problems and to discover optimal strategies for performing tasks. This influences a client's cognitive and sensorimotor subsystems and the ability to perform other functional tasks."[51]

The specific components (subsystems) of the systems, which influence occupational performance tasks, may be framed in occupational therapy terminology.[1,2] Components of the cognitive system include orientation, attention span, memory, problem-solving calculations, learning, and generalization ability. Components of the psychosocial system include a person's values, interests, coping skills, self-concept, interpersonal skills, self-expression, time management, emotional functions, and self-control skills that could affect occupational performance tasks. Strength, endurance, range of motion, sensory functions and pain, perceptual function, and postural control are components associated with the sensorimotor system. The environment includes physical, socioeconomic, and cultural characteristics of the task itself and the broader environment. Components of the physical environment system include objects, tools, devices, furniture, plants, animals, and the natural and built environments, which could limit or enhance task performance. The social supports provided by the family, friends, caregivers, social groups, and community and financial resources are components of the socioeconomic system, which could influence choice in activities. Finally, components of the cultural system include customs, beliefs, activity patterns, behavioral standards, and societal expectations, which also could affect occupational performance tasks.

The inclusion of role performance in this systems model reflects an occupational therapy, not a motor behavior perspective. "Occupational therapists believe the roles that persons want and need to fulfill determine the occupational performance (i.e., the tasks and activities) they need to do. Conversely, the tasks and activities persons are able to do determine what roles they are able to fulfill."[51] Box 4-1 summarizes the assumptions of the OT task-oriented approach.

---

**Box 4-1**

### Assumptions of the Occupational Therapy Task-Oriented Approach Based on a Systems Model of Motor Behavior

- Personal and environmental systems, including the central nervous system, are heterarchically organized.
- Functional tasks help organize behavior.
- Occupational performance emerges from the interaction of persons and their environment.
- Experimentation with various strategies leads to optimal solutions to motor problems.
- Recovery is variable because patient factors and environmental contexts are unique.
- Behavioral changes reflect attempts to compensate and to achieve task performance.

Adapted from Mathiowetz V, Bass-Haugen J: Assessing abilities and capacities: motor behavior. In Trombly CA, Radomski MV, editors: *Occupational therapy for physical dysfunction*, ed 5, Philadelphia, 2002, Lippincott Williams & Wilkins.

---

## EVALUATION FRAMEWORK USING THE OCCUPATIONAL THERAPY TASK-ORIENTED APPROACH

The therapist conducts the evaluation using a top-down approach as suggested by Trombly.[81] Box 4-2 gives a framework for evaluation. Evaluation efforts focus initially on role performance and occupational performance tasks because they are the goals of motor behavior. A thorough understanding of the roles that a patient wants, needs, or is expected to perform and of the tasks needed to fulfill those roles enables therapists to plan meaningful and motivating treatment programs. After a patient has identified the most important role and occupational performance limitations, therapists use task analysis to identify which subsystem of the person or environment is limiting functional performance. This process may indicate the need for evaluation of selected subsystems of the person or environment.[23] The emphasis on role and occupational performance in the OT task-oriented approach is consistent with the idea that occupational therapy evaluation should be primarily at the participation and activities level rather than the impairment level, using World Health Organization[87] terminology. The therapist needs to use qualitative and quantitative measures during the evaluation process.[84] "Therefore, therapists use interviews, skilled observations, and standardized assessments to evaluate their clients. Although the client is the primary source of information, other sources including the client's records, caregivers, family members, and the physical environment contribute as well."[51] The evaluation framework is described in more detail subsequently.

**Box 4-2**

## Evaluation Framework for the Occupational Therapy Task-Oriented Approach Based on a Systems Model of Motor Behavior

1. Role Performance
   (Social participation)
   Identify past roles and whether they can be maintained or need to be changed.
   Determine how future roles will be balanced.
   Worker, student, volunteer, home maintainer, hobbyist/amateur, participant in organizations, friend, family member, caregiver, religious participant, other?

2. Occupational Performance Tasks
   (Performance in areas of occupation)
   **Activities of daily living:** bathing, feeding, bowel and bladder management, dressing, functional mobility, and personal hygiene and grooming
   **Instrumental activities of daily living:** home management, cooking, care of others, community mobility, shopping, financial management, and safety procedures
   **Work and/or education:** employment; volunteer and retirement activities
   **Play/leisure:** exploration and participation

3. Task Selection and Analysis
   What patient factors, performance skills and patterns, and/or contexts and activity demands limit or enhance occupational performance?

4. Person
   (Patient factors; performance skills and patterns)
   **Cognitive:** orientation, attention span, memory, problem solving, calculations, learning, and generalization
   **Psychosocial:** values, interests, coping skills, self-concept, interpersonal skills, self-expression, time management, and emotional functions and self-control
   **Sensorimotor:** strength, endurance, range of motion, sensory functions and pain, perceptual function, and postural control

5. Environment
   (Context and activity demands)
   **Physical:** objects, tools, devices, furniture, plants, animals, and built and natural environment
   **Socioeconomic:** social supports: family, friends, caregivers, social groups, and community and financial resources
   **Cultural:** customs, beliefs, activity patterns, behavior standards, and societal expectations

Adapted from Mathiowetz V, Bass-Haugen J: Assessing abilities and capacities: motor behavior. In Trombly CA, Radomski MV, editors: *Occupational therapy for physical dysfunction*, ed 5, Philadelphia, 2002, Lippincott Williams & Wilkins.

The first step in the evaluation process is to assess role performance. "Therapists must determine which roles clients had prior to the onset of disability, and which roles they can and cannot do at this time."[51] A discussion of roles that patients want or must do in the future helps determine which roles are most important to them. In addition, therapists need to explore ways that role changes have affected or will affect patients and their families, especially the primary caregivers. Jongbloed, Stanton, and Fousek[42] recommended that therapists ask questions such as "How have roles changed since the disability?" "How have family members reacted to these changes?" "Is there role flexibility when needed?" and "How competently do members perform roles?" The therapist may need to adjust these questions to the patient's level of understanding. The patient and significant others must participate in the evaluation of role performance whenever possible.

The therapist may assess role performance using a nonstandardized, semistructured interview. However, a standardized assessment tool such as the Role Checklist[4,60] is suggested. The Role Checklist is a self-report, written inventory designed for adolescent, adult, or geriatric populations. In Part One, patients check the 10 roles (Box 4-2) that they have performed in the past, are performing in the present, and plan to perform in the future. In Part Two, patients rate the value of each role to them on a scale from "not at all valuable," "somewhat valuable," to "very valuable." The Role Checklist takes 10 to 15 minutes to complete and has evidence of reliability and validity.

The therapist may use other assessment tools to gather information on role performance. For example, the Occupational Performance History Interview-II (OPHI-II)[44] is a broad, semistructured assessment of occupational life history including work, leisure, and daily life activities. One part of it explores life roles, whereas other parts explore interests, values, organization of daily routines, goals, perceptions of ability, and environmental influences. The complete OPHI-II takes about 50 minutes and has evidence of reliability and validity. The OPHI-II includes information not only on role performance but also on occupational performance tasks, which are the next step of the evaluation process. In conclusion, after patients have identified the roles that they want or need to perform, they more easily can identify the tasks and activities needed to fulfill each role (see Chapter 3).

The second step in the evaluation process is the assessment of occupational performance tasks: activities of daily living (ADL), instrumental ADL (IADL), work, education, and play/leisure (Box 4-2). "Because roles, tasks, activities, and their contexts are unique to each person, a client-centered assessment tool such as the *Canadian Occupational Performance Measure* (COPM)[47] is recommended."[51] The *Canadian Occupational Performance Measure* uses a semistructured interview to measure a patient's self-perception of occupational performance over time. First, patients identify problem areas in self-care, productivity, and leisure. Second, they rate the importance of each problem area, which assists therapists in setting treatment priorities. Third, patients rate their own performance and their satisfaction with their performance on the five most important problem areas. Therapists may use these performance and satisfaction ratings again as outcome measures, measuring change across time. If therapists are concerned that a patient cannot rate performance accurately because of a cognitive impairment or age, therapists may use direct observation of selected activities or a caregiver interview to verify the information. The information elicited by the *Canadian Occupational Performance Measure* is unique to each patient and the individual's environment, which is an essential part of the OT task-oriented approach.

Another recommended measure of occupational performance specific to ADL and IADL is the Assessment of Motor and Process Skills (AMPS). The assessment is patient-centered because the person chooses two or three ADL or IADL tasks to be performed, which ensures that the task or activity is familiar and relevant to the person being evaluated. The purpose of the AMPS is "to determine whether or not a person has the necessary motor and process skills to effortlessly, efficiently, safely and independently perform the ADL tasks needed for community living."[22] The AMPS is appropriate for persons from diverse backgrounds and with diverse needs and interests because it has been standardized internationally and cross-culturally. "A unique feature of the AMPS is that it can adjust, through Rasch analysis, for the difficulty of tasks performed and the severity of the rater who scores the client's performance. In addition, it allows a therapist to compare the performance of clients who performed one set of tasks on initial evaluation with the results of a re-evaluation on a different set of tasks."[51] The primary limitation of the AMPS is that it requires a 5-day training workshop to learn how to administer the assessment in a reliable and valid way. Computer software to score the AMPS is provided as part of the workshop. Finally, the AMPS assists in the next step in the evaluation process, because it requires observation of patients performing occupational performance tasks (see Chapter 20).

While evaluating occupational performance tasks, "therapists need to observe both the outcome and the process (i.e., the preferred movement patterns, their stability or instability, the flexibility to use other patterns, efficiency of the patterns, and ability to learn new strategies) to understand the motor behaviors used to compensate and to achieve functional goals."[51] Determining the stability of the motor behavior is important to determine the feasibility of achieving behavioral change in treatment. "Behaviors that are very stable will require a great amount of time and effort to change. Behaviors that are unstable are in transition, the optimal time for eliciting behavioral change."[51] Thus, when behaviors are more stable, a compensatory approach may be most appropriate; when behaviors are unstable, a remediation

approach may be more successful. Quantitative and qualitative measures are needed to evaluate the process of task performance.

The third step in the evaluation process involves task selection and analysis. The tasks selected for observation should be ones that patients have identified as important but difficult to do. Task analysis requires therapists to observe their patients performing one or more occupational performance tasks. In most cases, observation of performance happens as part of the second step described previously. Therapists use task/activity analysis to evaluate activity demands, context, patient factors, performance skills, and performance patterns to determine whether a match exists that enables persons to perform occupational tasks within a relevant environment. If the person is unable to perform the task, therapists attempt to determine which person or environment subsystems are interfering with occupational performance. "In dynamical systems theory, these are considered the critical control parameters or the variables that have the potential to shift behavior to a new level of task performance."[51] Each person has unique strengths, limitations, and environmental context after a stroke. Therefore the critical control parameters that support or limit occupational performance tasks also are unique. In other words, an intervention strategy that is effective for one person after stroke may not be effective for the next person. Another concept of dynamical systems theory is that critical control parameters also change as persons and their environments change over time. Therefore an intervention that worked well early in a patient's rehabilitation might not work well late in the rehabilitation process or vice versa.

The identification of critical control parameters is the most challenging part of the evaluation process. However, evidence in the research literature indicates that some variables or subsystems of the person and/or environment are potential critical control parameters for persons after stroke. Gresham, Phillips, Wolf, et al[34] reported that psychosocial and environmental factors were significant determinants of functional deficits in persons for the long term after stroke. In a review, Gresham, Duncan, Stason, et al[33] reported that 11% to 68% of persons experience depression after stroke, with 10% to 27% meeting the criteria for major depression. In the cognitive area, Galski, Bruno, Zorowitz, et al[26] reported that for persons after stroke, "deficits in cognition, particularly higher-order cognitive abilities (e.g., abstract thinking, judgment, short-term verbal memory, comprehension, orientation) play an important role in determining length of stay and in predicting functional status at the end of hospital stay." In the sensorimotor area, weakness,[62] fatigue,[41] impaired motor function,[6] and visuospatial deficits[80] are associated with poorer functional outcomes. For example, Bernspang, Asplund,

Eriksson, et al[6] reported that motor function measured with the Fugl-Meyer Assessment[25] was correlated moderately (r = 0.64) with self-care ability.

Practitioners must use the aforementioned literature on potential control parameters with caution. Most of these were correlation studies, which indicate relationships between these variables and functional performance, but they do not prove a causal link. In addition, most correlations were moderate or low, which suggests that any one variable explains a relatively small percentage of the variance associated with functional performance. However, Reding and Potes[66] provided evidence that as the number of performance component impairments increased, functional outcomes decreased. "Thus, multiple variables contribute to functional performance for most persons with central nervous system dysfunction. The challenge is to identify those variables that are most critical to your clients."[51]

Bobath[9] suggested that spasticity is the primary cause of motor deficits in persons after stroke and that weakness and decreased range of motion are due to spastic antagonists. However, evidence is increasing that indicates that spasticity is not a critical control parameter.[10] For example, Sahrmann and Norton[68] reported electromyography findings that indicated movements were not limited by antagonist stretch reflexes (spasticity) but were limited by delayed initiation and cessation of agonist contraction. Similarly, Fellows, Kaus, and Thilmann[21] found no relationship between movement impairments and passive muscle hypertonia in the antagonist muscles. O'Dwyer, Ada, and Neilson[61] found no relationship between spasticity and either weakness or loss of dexterity. "Thus, research evidence challenges the assumption that spasticity causes the weakness and decreased range of motion often seen in persons with central nervous system dysfunction."[51] Recently, the Neuro-Developmental Treatment Association acknowledged this change in thinking: "There is not a direct relationship between spasticity and constraints on motor impairments or functional performance, as the Bobaths first proposed"[39] (see Chapter 10).

After identifying the critical control parameters that support or constrain occupational performance, the therapist must assess the interactions of these systems. Consider two patients who have complete loss of voluntary control of their dominant hand. The role and occupational performance tasks of the patient as a worker may or may not be affected. If the worker were an automobile mechanic, the interaction of this personal limitation with the activity demands of the work environment likely would make the task of repairing a car engine difficult or impossible to perform. However, if the worker were a self-employed writer, the person could learn to use a one-handed keyboard with the nondominant hand. As a result, the person could continue writing because the interaction of performance skills and activity demands would not interfere with role and task performance. This part of the evaluation requires the therapist to use qualitative and quantitative assessments and clinical reasoning to determine how subsystem of the person and the environment might affect occupational performance.

The fourth step in the evaluation process is to perform specific assessments of patient factors, performance skills, and performance patterns, which are thought to be critical control parameters. The critical control variables are the only ones that need to be evaluated. "The evaluation of selected variables according to the OT task-oriented approach contrasts with bottom-up approaches that evaluate all component variables. This selective approach eliminates the need to evaluate variables that have little functional implication and saves therapists' time, which is critical for cost containment."[51]

Occupational therapists use a variety of assessments to evaluate patient factors, performance skills, and performance patterns that support or constrain occupational performance. Some assessments were designed to examine one or more impairments within the context of occupational performance. The Arnadottir OT-ADL Neurobehavioral Evaluation (A-ONE)[3] facilitates evaluation of perceptual and cognitive systems within the context of ADLs (see Chapter 18 for details). From a task-oriented perspective, this is a preferred assessment tool because it links impairments more closely to occupational performance. In contrast, most assessments of impairments are conducted independent of occupational performance.

The fifth step of the evaluation process is evaluation of the environment: context and activity demands. The inclusion of physical, social, and cultural environments in American Occupational Therapy Association[2] uniform terminology acknowledges their important impact on occupational performance. A number of occupational therapy theories[15,19,48,75] emphasize the importance of assessing environmental context as part of the overall evaluation process. See Radomski[64] and Cooper, Letts, Rigby, et al[16] for specific assessments of environmental contexts.

## TREATMENT PRINCIPLES USING THE OCCUPATIONAL THERAPY TASK-ORIENTED APPROACH

### Help Patients Adjust to Role and Task Performance Limitations

Many patients are not able to continue some of the roles and tasks that they performed before their strokes. This is a frustrating and sometimes depressing situation for many persons after stroke. Therapists can help by exploring alternative ways of fulfilling roles and of performing the associated tasks. Therapists also can explore potential new roles and new tasks. For example, in the case study presented at the end of this chapter, an important role for G.W. was continuing to help his son on the farm. The therapist helped the patient identify the tasks with which he had helped in the past and which ones would be impossible or difficult to perform in the future. For G.W., heavy or bilateral tasks (e.g., moving bales of hay and repairing heavy equipment) would fit this category. Brainstorming about alternative tasks that he could do unilaterally or relatively light tasks (e.g., record keeping) that he could still perform would enable him to continue his role as an assistant to his son. Inclusion of the son in this discussion was important, because he had suggestions that G.W. had not considered.

## Create an Environment That Utilizes the Common Challenges of Everyday Life

Therapists need to be creative in creating environments within their clinical settings that provide typical challenges. Some facilities have purchased more real-life environments such as Easy Street, whereas other facilities have remodeled their clinics to simulate environments in which patients typically have to interact. Some have created small apartments to create a more realistic environment, in contrast to a typical hospital room, in which patients can interact before being discharged. Home care settings are ideal situations for following this treatment principle because the patient's own environment and objects can be used for therapy.

A stroke unit provides a more effective environment for improving functional outcomes.[40] The physical environment is set up to enable patients to function more independently. Patients are encouraged to wear their own clothing instead of hospital gowns. Thus, they are confronted with the common clothing of everyday life. In addition, staff members are trained to encourage independent behaviors. In G.W.'s case, nursing staff on the previous unit had assisted him in dressing and bathing. On the rehabilitation unit, nursing staff would encourage him to perform as many self-care tasks as possible. In addition, most rehabilitation units have patients eat together in a dining area instead of in their own rooms. This is a more typical way of eating, plus it facilitates social interaction and support from others struggling with many of the same problems. In addition, dining with others facilitates learning from and problem solving with each other.

## Practice Functional Tasks or Close Simulations to Find Effective and Efficient Strategies for Performance

In all cases the therapist must use the functional tasks and activities that have been identified as important and meaningful to their patients. This demonstrates to patients that the therapist has listened to them and respects their choices and priorities. Patients more easily understand the relevance of therapy to their lives.

Use of functional, natural tasks rather than rote exercise in treatment is important. A number of studies have demonstrated that the kinematics of movement are different when one performs a real task instead of rote exercise.[54,88] A meta-analytic review[49] provided evidence that "engagement in purposeful activity produces better quality of movement than concentration on movement per se." Nelson, Konosky, Fleharty et al[58] demonstrated that after stroke, persons who performed an occupationally embedded exercise had significantly greater supination active range of motion than persons who did a rote exercise. These studies support the idea that the use of functional tasks has beneficial therapeutic effects.

Higgins[37] suggested that persons need to practice functional, everyday activities to find the most effective and efficient way of doing the activity. Because persons are unique, their performance patterns and levels of skill vary. Therefore, therapists should not expect that one way of performing a task would be the most effective and efficient way of performing a task for all patients. Thus, therapists should encourage patients to experiment to find the most effective and efficient way of performing functional tasks.

## Provide Opportunities for Practice Outside of Therapy Time

Therapists need to recognize that the amount of time they have to work with a patient is short relative to the total time in a day. Therefore, enticing patients to continue therapy on their own time is important. Therapists can provide homework assignments for patients to work on their own. If homework is given, follow-up is important, and therapists should ask their patients how their homework went. What worked for the patients, and what did not work for them? Effective communication with other rehabilitation staff and family members is crucial, so that their attempts to be helpful do not reduce the opportunities for patients to practice outside of therapy time. Most important is for therapists to help patients find new ways to use their involved extremity, even if it is only to stabilize objects. A good homework assignment is to challenge the patient to find a new way to use the involved arm each day.[24] Ultimately, the goal is to get the patient to use an involved arm without thinking about it.

## Minimize Ineffective and Inefficient Movement Patterns

As described previously, during observation of a patient performing an occupational performance task, therapists attempt to identify what may be critical personal or environmental factors that are interfering with effective and efficient movement patterns. The following strategies are ways that therapists can intervene to reduce ineffective and inefficient movement.

***Remediate a Person Factor (Impairment) if It Is the Critical Control Parameter.*** When therapists identify person factors in the cognitive, psychosocial, or sensorimotor systems as possible critical control parameters, then they should attempt to remediate those factors, assuming that is possible. For example, Flinn[24] identified decreased strength as one critical control parameter that interfered with occupational performance tasks for a person after stroke. Thus, she attempted to remediate this sensorimotor variable through the use of exercise and increased use of the involved extremity for functional tasks. For this person, the use of exercise was meaningful because she saw a clear connection between her exercise program and her ability to use her involved arm and hand for everyday tasks. The therapist also encouraged her to use her involved extremity whenever possible in therapy and for various homework assignments.

In the case of G.W., decreased strength, impaired sensation, and neglect of the left upper extremity were identified as possible control parameters. Therefore, attempts to remediate these factors was warranted in this case. However, sometimes remediation of a potential control parameter is impossible because of the severity of the disease process or limited time available for therapy. In such cases a more compensatory approach to treatment is indicated.

***Adapt the Environment, Modify the Task, Use Assistive Technology, and/or Reduce the Effects of Gravity.*** For many patients, the quickest and most effective approach to improving occupational performance is to adapt the task and/or the environment. For example, Gillen[29] described a patient with severe limitations in self-care activities following multiple sclerosis and ataxia. Tremor, impaired postural control, paraparesis, and decreased endurance limited his occupational performance. The patient's priority was to gain access to the community and community resources. He did not have adequate motor control to operate a manual chair or to control a standard power chair. Therefore a specialized power chair was prescribed that provided optimal head and trunk stability, allowed independent tilting, included a joystick with tremor-dampening electronics, and a forearm trough to provide maximal stability to the arm controlling the joystick. A volar wrist splint provided additional stability to the wrist. With training in varied environments, the patient improved from total assistance in mobility to minimal supervision. Thus the use of assistive technology, task modification, and training in varied environ-

ments was the most efficient and effective means of improving the mobility independence of this patient.

For G.W., a standard bath chair enabled independent and safe tub transfers. For shoe tying, G.W. preferred the use of Kno-Bows, an adapted device, for fastening his shoes rather than learning one-handed shoe tying. For cutting meat, an enlarged-handled fork was tried to encourage use of the left hand. However, this was not feasible at the time, so a rocker knife was prescribed. Thus a variety of adapted devices increased the ADL independence of G.W.

***Use Contemporary Motor Learning Principles in Training or Retraining Skills.*** Therapists should consider the following three motor learning principles:

- Use random and variable practice within natural contexts in treatment.
- Provide decreasing amounts of physical guidance and verbal feedback.
- Develop task analysis and problem-solving skills of patients so that they can find their own solutions to occupational performance problems in home and community environments.

Although blocked or repetitive practice of the same task normally is not recommended, such practice may be helpful or necessary when a patient is first learning the requirements of a new task.[70] However, therapists should shift to random and variable practice schedules as soon as possible to enhance motor learning. Random practice involves practicing more than one task within a session (i.e., avoiding repetitive practice of the same task). Variable practice involves experimenting with different tools for completing a task, with different location of the tools relative to the person, or with varied environments for performing a task. In addition, patients should practice tasks in their natural context whenever possible. Therefore, ADL tasks normally done in a patient's room should be practiced there rather than in the occupational therapy clinic. Even better would be patients practicing ADL tasks in their own homes.

When therapists are beginning to teach patients new tasks or new ways to perform previously learned tasks, they may need to provide some physical guidance and verbal feedback.[69] However, guidance and feedback should be tapered off quickly so that the person does not become dependent on them. For a therapist not to provide guidance and feedback when a patient is struggling to perform a task is difficult. However, providing physical guidance prevents patients from learning how to use their remaining resources to get the job done, and providing immediate and frequent feedback prevents patients from learning how to use their own feedback mechanisms to monitor and evaluate their own performance. If patients are unaware of a deficit (e.g., neglect to use involved extremity in a task), the use of a videotape of their performance can supplement their usual feedback mechanisms.[65] By the time a patient is approaching discharge, therapists should be providing minimal guidance or feedback. The therapist should remember that the goal of rehabilitation is to train the patient to be independent without the therapist's presence.

In a related issue, patients need to learn how to analyze tasks and to problem solve on their own. If the therapist analyzes tasks for patients and solves all their problems, they will not learn how to do those things themselves. In the limited therapy time available, preparing patients for all possible tasks, activities, and environments that they will confront after they are discharged is impossible. The therapist's role is to train patients how to do task analysis and problem solving during the rehabilitation process, so that by the time they are discharged, they are capable of doing those things on their own. From early in rehabilitation, the therapist should involve patients in task analysis and guide them through the process. As occupational problems are addressed, the therapist should keep patients involved in trying to find solutions to problems. Therapists should encourage experimentation to find the optimal solution for that specific person. The therapist should remember that the same solution does not work for all patients (see Chapter 5).

### For Persons with Poor Control of Movement, Constrain the Degrees of Freedom.

Persons learning a new task initially restrict the degrees of freedom at their joints by self-imposing some form of freezing of body segments.[37] As a result, their performance appears stiff and uncoordinated. With practice the performance becomes smoother and more coordinated as the restrictions on the degrees of freedom decrease. Unfortunately, some persons with central nervous system damage are not able to constrain the degrees of freedom at their joints. For example, Gillen identified poor postural stability and tremor as interfering with the functional performance of a person with multiple sclerosis and ataxia. He speculated "that performance would be improved by increasing postural stability and decreasing the number of joints (decreasing the degrees of freedom) required to participate in chosen tasks."[30] Therefore, he used orthotic devices, assistive technology, and adaptive positioning of the trunk and upper extremity to help his patient constrain the degrees of freedom and to increase stability, which enabled improved ADL performance. Thus the occupational performance of a patient with tremor was enhanced by strategies to decrease the degrees of freedom at those joints.

### For Persons Who Do Not Use Returned Function in Their Involved Extremities, Use Constraint-Induced Therapy.

A growing body of literature supports the beneficial effects of constraint-induced movement therapy (CIMT) for persons after stroke with some active wrist and finger extension.[46,57,76] Constraint-induced movement therapy usually involves intensive therapy (i.e., about 6 hours per day) while the less involved arm is constrained by a sling or glove. As a result, participants are forced to use their involved extremity to complete functional tasks and thus CIMT counteracts the learned nonuse seen in many persons after stroke. Constraint-induced movement therapy is consistent with two assumptions of the OT task-oriented approach: "functional tasks help organize behavior and experimentation with various strategies leads to optimal solutions to motor problems"[51] (see Chapters 6 and 10).

In most clinical settings the CIMT would need to be modified to fit into the current structure of inpatient rehabilitation programs and current reimbursement practices. However, after stroke many persons do not meet the minimal eligibility requirements during their initial rehabilitation. Thus, most CIMT programs are conducted on an outpatient basis for persons who are 6 months or more beyond the stroke and who have sufficient return of function to benefit from CIMT. No evidence indicates that CIMT is effective for persons without some active wrist and finger extension. Thus, in the case of G.W. with neglect of his involved extremity, he would not be a good candidate for CIMT because he does not have sufficient active wrist and finger extension to benefit. At a later time, when that function does return, a trial of CIMT would be indicated. Chapters 6 and 10 contain more detailed discussions of CIMT. For a more detailed discussion of the OT task-oriented approach treatment, see Bass-Haugen, Mathiowetz, and Flinn.[5]

## SUMMARY

This chapter describes an OT task-oriented approach for persons after stroke and describes the theoretical basis for and assumptions of the approach, based on contemporary motor control, motor learning, and motor development literature. The chapter also provides a top-down evaluation framework that emphasizes the importance of evaluating role and occupational performance tasks first and then the selective assessment of personal and environmental factors. In addition, the chapter describes the application of treatment principles to various patient problems and, finally, includes a case study describing the application of the OT task-oriented approach to a specific person after stroke.

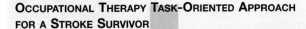

**Case Study**

## OCCUPATIONAL THERAPY TASK-ORIENTED APPROACH FOR A STROKE SURVIVOR

G.W. is a 69-year-old retired farmer who suffered a right cerebral vascular accident with resultant left hemiparesis 5 days ago. He was admitted to the acute care hospital and then was transferred to the rehabilitation unit today.

From the chart, it was learned that he is now medically stable. He is taking angiotensin-converting enzyme inhibitors for high blood pressure and Coumadin for prevention of a second stroke. He has been living in a small town with his wife since moving from their farm 3 years ago. His son, daughter-in-law, and their three children are farming in the local community.

### Initial evaluation

The Role Checklist was administered to evaluate G.W.'s role performance. Although retired, he continued to help out his son part-time as needed on the farm. He did most of the home maintenance, including the yard and a small garden. He attended church regularly, was a member of the men's club, and volunteered for the annual church dinner. In addition to his son who farms, he has another son and a daughter who are married and live within a 2-hour drive. He has eight grandchildren. He and his wife enjoyed traveling with another retired couple from their church.

The *Canadian Occupational Performance Measure* was administered to evaluate occupational performance tasks. The following five tasks were rated as most important to him: dressing, bathing, driving, gardening, and helping his son on the farm. His performance and satisfaction for these tasks were rated low. However, he had not had the opportunity to try the latter three tasks since his stroke, and nursing staff assisted him with dressing and bathing. He reported that he was independent in sink hygiene tasks, feeding (except for cutting meat), and toileting (except for pulling up and fastening trousers). He could ambulate 10 feet with a large, quad-based cane with moderate assistance. His wife did all the grocery shopping and cooking. G.W. had helped his wife with the laundry. He was unsure whether he would be able to play cards in the men's club now.

Dressing and bathing were chosen as tasks to be observed on the following day. G.W. was not able to dress himself independently primarily because of inability to use and/or neglect in using his left upper extremity. When cued to use his left arm, he demonstrated some voluntary control of his left shoulder and elbow and limited movement in the wrist and fingers. He complained of numbness in his left hand. During the bathing assessment, he needed assistance getting into and out of a tub. However, he could transfer in and out of the tub using a standard transfer bench. Once in the tub, he could control the water and bathe himself with one hand. He demonstrated good sitting balance during these activities, and he could stand independently when he could hold onto something with his right arm. He complained about the amount of time and energy it took him to perform self-care tasks. He demonstrated no evidence of cognitive or perceptual deficits except for some neglect of his left arm and left visual space. Based on these observations, it appeared that sensorimotor factors (decreased strength, endurance, range of motion, sensation, and neglect) were potential causes of limitations in occupational performance tasks, so these factors were selected for further evaluation. In contrast, cognitive and psychosocial factors appeared to be potential supports for increased independence. In addition, it appeared that modification of the environment (e.g., use of adaptive equipment such as a bath chair, Kno-Bows for shoe fasteners, and rocker knife) could be used to enable occupational performance tasks. However, more information was needed regarding his home and community environment to prepare for his discharge to home.

Tables 4-1 and 4-2 show the results of manual muscle testing, passive range of motion, and hand strength assessments for the left upper extremity only.

Sensory testing indicated a loss of protective sensation and diminished light touch in the left hand (Semmes-Weinstein monofilaments) and impaired proprioception in the left forearm, wrist, and hand. A line bisection test showed moderate visual neglect of the left side.

### Home environment

G.W. and his wife live in a small two-story home. Their bedroom, bathroom, kitchen, living room, and dining room are on the main floor. The upstairs has two bedrooms, a bathroom, and storage space. The washer and dryer are located in the basement. The front and back of the home have five steps with a handrail on one side only. They have a one-car detached garage that is close to the house. They have a 10-year-old car with a stick shift. They have a 10 × 20 foot vegetable and flower garden in their backyard.

Their home is paid for, and they receive modest checks from Social Security and some farm rental income from their son. If they stay healthy, their income is adequate for what they want to do. However, they are worried that if one or both of them were to become disabled and require nursing home care, then their income would not be sufficient to cover expenses.

## Community environment

Their house is located one block from their church and four blocks from the downtown area, which includes a grocery store, drug store, barber shop, post office, liquor store, and a small café. Their small town has no clothing or hardware store. They must to drive 20 miles to a larger town for these supplies and medical care. Their son's farm is located 5 miles from their house. The church has a split-level entrance with 10 steps to church level and 10 steps to the basement where the men's club meets. Fortunately, the church installed a chair glide to assist persons with mobility problems to get into church. However, no chair glide

is available for the basement level. At this time, he knows that he cannot get up and down 10 steps, and this is a concern.

After a discussion of the evaluation results, the patient and therapist agreed on the following goals.

### Week 1 treatment plan

1. Increase active use of the left upper extremity during activities of daily living (ADL) and leisure tasks (i.e., avoid neglect and learned nonuse of the left arm and hand).
2. Increase independence in ADL and leisure tasks.
3. Begin planning for discharge to home and for possible roles for him on his son's farm.

The patient became aware through the evaluation process that he tended to neglect his left arm and hand and was motivated to improve its function. Thus, he was open to experimenting with using his left upper extremity to assist during functional tasks. He was taught one-handed dressing techniques with reminders to use his left arm and hand as much as possible. For example, G.W. was encouraged to raise his left arm as

## Table 4-1

### Manual Muscle Testing and PROM Assessment

| LEFT UPPER EXTREMITY | MMT | PROM | LEFT UPPER EXTREMITY | MMT | PROM |
|---|---|---|---|---|---|
| Shoulder flexion | 2+ | 0-155 | Pronation | 2− | 0-75 |
| Shoulder abduction | 2+ | 0-155 | Supination | 3− | 0-80 |
| Shoulder external rotation | 2− | 0-45 | Wrist flexion | 2+ | 0-80 |
| Shoulder internal rotation | 2+ | 0-70 | Wrist extension | 1+ | 0-45 |
| Elbow flexion | 3− | 0-150 | Finger and thumb flexion | 3+ | Full |
| Elbow extension | 2− | 0-150 | Finger and thumb extension | 1+ | Full |

*MMT*, Manual muscle test; *PROM*, passive range of motion (units in degrees).

## Table 4-2

### Hand Strength Assessment

| HAND STRENGTH | RIGHT HAND | INTERPRETATION | LEFT HAND | INTERPRETATION |
|---|---|---|---|---|
| Grip | 102# | WNL | 3# | BNL |
| Key pinch | 19# | WNL | 2# | BNL |
| Palmar pinch | 17# | WNL | 1# | BNL |

*WNL*, Within normal limits; *BNL*, below normal limits.

he slid his shirt on and to stabilize his shirt and pants while buttoning. Various options for tying his shoes were explored. He chose to use Kno-Bows because of the ease of using them compared with alternatives. A rocker knife was chosen to enable independent cutting of meat. The therapist communicated with his wife and nursing staff on what he was able to do relative to ADL tasks and what adapted equipment (e.g., bath chair) he needed to be independent. G.W. was independent in bathing himself when the bath chair was available to him. He expressed some concern about slipping and falling when he would get home. Plans were made to order the grab bars, bath chair, and nonskid bath mat.

In addition, various leisure activities including card playing were explored. He was able to pull cards toward himself with his left hand but was unable to pick them up or hold them. A cardholder was prescribed so that he could play cards immediately. Although he only had a mild interest in playing checkers, he found out that he could slide enlarged checkers with his left hand and was willing to work at this activity.

During one session, his son and wife came to discuss his roles at home and on his son's farm. Both of them suggested that they could get help for the things that he could not do. Although G.W. agreed that some tasks he could no longer do or did not care to do, he still wanted to do some gardening and to help with some things on the farm. He did not want just to sit around and watch television. After brainstorming what roles and tasks might still be possible, the discussion shifted to adapted strategies and equipment that might be needed to make these tasks possible.

At the end of the first week, he was able to perform all ADL task with minimal supervision (i.e., reminders to use his left hand and to search his left visual space). He could now walk 30 feet with his cane and was practicing going up and down steps in physical therapy.

**Week 2 treatment plan**

1. Explore the possibility of driving and continued gardening.
2. Finalize plans for discharge to home, including ordering and installing adapted devices.
3. Finalize home program and follow-ups.

The patient was evaluated on some aspects of driving using a modified car. He was able to transfer in and out of the car with moderate supervision. He was discouraged that he was not able to push in the clutch with his left foot. He preferred driving a stick shift but could see that a car with an automatic transmission would be easier for him. He agreed to discuss getting a different car with his wife and son. Other adaptations that might make driving easier and safer were explored. The issue of neglect of his left visual field was discussed and evaluated using a driving simulator. He did have problems (i.e., simulated crashes) because of neglect. It was decided that additional practice with the simulator and other activities to improve his visual scanning were necessary before he could drive again.

G.W. continued to use various leisure and ADL activities to increase active use of his left arm and hand. Setup of the activities was structured to require increased visual scanning as he did these activities.

Although G.W. continued to improve in his walking and stair-climbing ability, it was decided that a second handrail should be installed at both entrances to the home and in the basement and upstairs stairways. His son agreed to arrange for someone to do this. In addition, he agreed to install grab bars in the bathroom and in the hallway between the bathroom and bedroom. Sometimes, G.W. needed to use the bathroom at night. Although he was improving in his performance on the driving simulator, he was told that he was not yet safe to drive. G.W. was referred to a regional driving center, which evaluates and trains persons with disabilities in safe driving. His wife or son would drive him until he could drive again.

A home program was developed with a variety of tasks and activities that required the use of his left arm and hand. He was now approaching the level of function that made him an appropriate candidate for constraint-induced movement therapy. Unfortunately, access to this type of program was not feasible for G.W. because of distance and money. The therapist explained the concept of constraint-induced movement therapy and developed a modified program that G.W. could do on his own. The modified program was adapted from a small study by Page, Sisto, Levine, et al,[63] which provided some evidence that an outpatient program of constraint-induced movement therapy could be beneficial. Five outpatient follow-ups were scheduled to monitor and upgrade his home program.

# REVIEW QUESTIONS

1. What are at least four assumptions of the occupational therapy task-oriented approach?
2. What is the primary focus of an evaluation of persons after stroke using the occupational therapy task-oriented approach?
3. From an occupational therapy task-oriented approach perspective, when is it appropriate to evaluate a performance component?
4. Describe at least four intervention principles of the occupational therapy task-oriented approach and how they could be applied to persons after stroke.
5. Describe at least two ways that contemporary motor learning principles could be applied to persons after stroke.

# REFERENCES

1. American Occupational Therapy Association: Occupational therapy practice framework: domain and process, *Am J Occup Ther* 56(6):609-639, 2002.
2. American Occupational Therapy Association: Uniform terminology for occupational therapy, ed 3, *Am J Occup Ther* 48(11):1047-1054, 1994.
3. Arnadattoir G: *The brain and behavior: assessing cortical dysfunction through activities of daily living*, St Louis, 1990, Mosby.
4. Barris R, Oakley F, Kielhofner G: The role checklist. In Hemphill BJ: *Mental health assessment in occupational therapy*, Thorofare, NJ, 1988, Slack.
5. Bass-Haugen J, Mathiowetz V, Flinn N: Optimizing motor behavior using the occupational therapy task-oriented approach. In Trombly CA, Radomski MV, editors: *Occupational therapy for physical dysfunction*, ed 5, Philadelphia, 2002, Lippincott Williams & Wilkins.
6. Bernspang B, Asplund K, Eriksson S, et al: Motor and perceptual impairments in acute stroke patients: effects on self-care ability, *Stroke* 18(6):1081-1086, 1987.
7. Bernstein N: *The coordination and regulation of movements*, Elmsford, NY, 1967, Pergamon Press.
8. Bobath B: *Adult hemiplegia: evaluation and treatment*, ed 3, Oxford, 1990, Butterworth-Heinemann.
9. Bobath B: *Adult hemiplegia: evaluation and treatment*, ed 2, London, 1978, William Heinemann Medical Books.
10. Bourbonnais D, Vanden Noven S: Weakness in patients with hemiparesis, *Am J Occup Ther* 43(5):313-319, 1989.
11. Brunnstrom S: *Movement therapy in hemiplegia*, New York, 1970, Harper & Row.
12. Burton AW, Davis WE: Optimizing the involvement and performance of children with physical impairments in movement activities, *Pediatr Exerc Sci* 4:236-248, 1992.
13. Carr JH, Shepherd RB: *Neurological rehabilitation: optimizing motor performance*, Oxford, 1998, Butterworth-Heinemann.
14. Carr JH, Shepherd RB: *A motor relearning programme for stroke*, ed 2, Rockville, Md, 1987, Aspen.
15. Christiansen C, Baum C: Person-environment occupational performance: a conceptual model for practice. In Christiansen C, Baum C, editors: *Occupational therapy: enabling function and wellbeing*, Thorofare, NJ, 1997, Slack.
16. Cooper B, Letts L, Rigby P, et al: Measuring environmental factors. In Law M, Baum C, Dunn W, editors: *Measuring occupational performance: supporting best practice in occupational therapy*, Thorofare, NJ, 2001, Slack.
17. Davis WE, Burton AW: Ecological task analysis: translating movement behavior theory into practice, *Adapted Phys Activity Q* 8:1 54-177, 1991.
18. Dean CM, Shepherd RB: Task-related training improves performance of seated reaching tasks after stroke, *Stroke* 28:722-728, 1997.
19. Dunn W: Measurement of function: actions for the future, *Am J Occup Ther* 47:357-359, 1993.
20. Fasoli S, Trombly CA, Tickle-Degnen L, et al: Effect of instructions on functional reach in persons with and without cerebrovascular accident, *Am J Occup Ther* 56:380-390, 2002.
21. Fellows SJ, Kaus C, Thilmann A: Voluntary movement at the elbow in spastic hemiparesis, *Ann Neurol* 36:397-407, 1994.
22. Fisher A: *Assessment of motor and process skills*, ed 3, Fort Collins, Colo, Three Star Press.
23. Fisher AG, Short-DeGraff M: Improving functional assessment in occupational therapy: recommendations and philosophy for change, *Am J Occup Ther* 47(3):199-201, 1993.
24. Flinn N: A task-oriented approach to the treatment of a client with hemiplegia, *Am J Occup Ther* 49(6):560-569, 1995.
25. Fugl-Meyer AR, Jääskö L, Leyman I, et al: The post-stroke hemiplegic patient: a method for evaluation of physical performance, *Scand J Rehabil Med* 7(1):13-31, 1975.
26. Galski T, Bruno RL, Zorowitz R, et al: Predicting length of stay, functional outcome, and aftercare in the rehabilitation of stroke patients: the dominant role of higher-order cognition, *Stroke* 23:1794-1800, 1993.
27. Gibson JJ: *The ecological approach to visual perception*, Boston, 1979, Houghton Mifflin.
28. Gibson JJ: The theory of affordances. In Shaw R, Bransford J: *Perceiving, acting, and knowing*, Hillsdale, NJ, 1977, Erlbaum.
29. Gillen G: Improving mobility and community access in an adult with ataxia, *Am J Occup Ther* 56(4):462-466, 2002.
30. Gillen G: Improving activities of daily living performance in an adult with ataxia, *Am J Occup Ther* 54(1):89-96, 2000.
31. Gleick J: *Chaos: making a new science*, New York, 1987, Penguin Books.
32. Gordon J: Assumptions underlying physical therapy interventions: theoretical and historical perspectives. In Carr JH, Shepherd RB, Gordon J, et al, editors: *Movement science: foundations for physical therapy in rehabilitation*, Rockville, Md, 1987, Aspen.
33. Gresham GE, Duncan PW, Stason WB, et al: *Post-stroke rehabilitation: clinical practice guidelines, No 16*, AHCPR Pub No 95-0662, Rockville, Md, 1995, US Department of Health and Human Services, Public Health Service, Agency for Health Care Policy and Research.
34. Gresham GE, Phillips T, Wolf P, et al: Epidemiologic profile of long-term stroke disability: the Framingham study, *Arch Phys Med Rehabil* 60(11):487-491, 1979.
35. Hanlon RE: Motor learning following unilateral stroke, *Arch Phys Med Rehabil* 77(8):811-815, 1996.
36. Heriza C: Motor development: traditional and contemporary theories. In Lister MJ, editor: *Contemporary management of motor control problems: proceedings of the II STEP conference*, Alexandria, Va, 1991, Foundation for Physical Therapy.
37. Higgins S: Motor skill acquisition, *Phys Ther* 71:123-139, 1991.
38. Horak FB: Assumptions underlying motor control for neurologic rehabilitation. In Lister MJ, editor: *Contemporary management of motor control problems: proceedings of the II STEP conference*, Alexandria, Va, 1991, Foundation for Physical Therapy.
39. Howle JM: *Neuro-developmental treatment approach: theoretical foundations and principles of clinical practice*, Laguna Beach, Calif, 2002, Neuro-Developmental Treatment Association.
40. Indredavik B, Bakke F, Solberg R, et al: Benefit of a stroke unit: a randomized controlled trial, *Stroke* 22(8):1026-1031, 1991.
41. Ingles JL, Eskes GA, Phillips SJ: Fatigue after stroke, *Arch Phys Med Rehabil* 80(2):173-178, 1999.
42. Jongbloed L, Stanton S, Fousek B: Family adaptation to altered roles following stroke, *Can J Occup Ther* 60:70-77, 1993.

43. Kamm K, Thelen E, Jensen JL: A dynamical systems approach to motor development, *Phys Ther* 70:763-775, 1990.

44. Kielhofner G: *User's manual for the OPHI-II*, Chicago, 1988, Model of Occupational Performance Clearinghouse.

45. Knott M, Voss DE: *Proprioceptive neuromuscular facilitation*, ed 2, New York, 1968, Harper & Row.

46. Kunkel A, Kopp B, Muller G, et al: Constraint-induced movement therapy for motor recovery in chronic stroke patients, *Arch Phys Med Rehabil* 80(6):624-628, 1999.

47. Law M, Baptiste S, Carswell A, et al: *Canadian Occupational Performance Measure*, ed 3, Ottawa, 1998, CAOT Publications.

48. Law M, Cooper B, Strong S, et al: Theoretical contexts for the practice of occupational therapy. In Christiansen C, Baum C, editors: *Occupational therapy: enabling function and well-being*, ed 2, Thorofare, NJ, 1997, Slack.

49. Lin K-C, Wu C-Y, Tickle-Degnen L, et al: Enhancing occupational performance through occupationally embedded exercise: a meta-analytic review, *Occup Ther J Res* 17:25-47, 1997.

50. Lister MJ: *Contemporary management of motor control problems: proceedings of the II STEP conference*, Alexandria, Va, 1991, Foundation for Physical Therapy.

51. Mathiowetz V, Bass-Haugen J: Assessing abilities and capacities: motor behavior. In Trombly CA, Radomski MV, editors: *Occupational therapy for physical dysfunction*, ed 5, Philadelphia, 2002, Lippincott Williams & Wilkins.

52. Mathiowetz V, Bass-Haugen J: Evaluation of motor behavior: traditional and contemporary views. In Trombly CA, editor: *Occupational therapy for physical dysfunction*, ed 4, Baltimore, 1995, Williams & Wilkins.

53. Mathiowetz V, Bass-Haugen J: Motor behavior research: implications for therapeutic approaches to CNS dysfunction, *Am J Occup Ther* 48(8):733-745, 1994.

54. Mathiowetz VG, Wade M: Task constraints and functional motor performance of individuals with and without multiple sclerosis, *Ecological Psychology* 7:99-123, 1995.

55. McNevin NH, Wulf G, Carlson C: Effects of attentional focus, self-control, and dyad training on motor learning: implications for physical rehabilitation, *Phys Ther* 80:373-385, 2000.

56. Merians A, Winstein C, Sullivan K, et al: Effects of feedback for motor skill leaning in older healthy subjects and individuals post-stroke, *Neurol Rep* 19:23-5, 1995.

57. Morris DM, Crago JE, Deluca SC, et al: Constraint-induced movement therapy for motor recovery after stroke, *NeuroRehab* 9:29-43, 1997.

58. Nelson DL, Konosky K, Fleharty K, et al: The effects of occupationally embedded exercise on bilaterally assisted supination in persons with hemiplegia, *Am J Occup Ther* 50(8):639-646, 1996.

59. Newell KM: Constraints on the development of coordination. In Wade MG, Whiting HTA, editors: *Motor development in children: aspects of coordination and control*, Dordrecht, Netherlands, 1986, Martinus Nijhoff.

60. Oakley F, Kielhofner G, Barris R, et al: The Role Checklist: development and empirical assessment of reliability, *Occup Ther J Res* 6:157-170, 1986.

61. O'Dwyer NJ, Ada L, Neilson PD: Spasticity and muscle contracture following stroke, *Brain* 119(pt 5):1737-1749, 1996.

62. Olsen TS: Arm and leg paresis as outcome predictors in stroke rehabilitation, *Stroke* 21(2):247-251, 1990.

63. Page SJ, Sisto SA, Levine P, et al: Modified constraint induced therapy: a randomized feasibility and efficacy study, *J Rehabil Res Dev* 38(5):583-590, 2001.

64. Radomski MV: Assessing context: personal, social, and cultural. In Trombly CA, Radomski MV, editors: *Occupational therapy for physical dysfunction*, ed 5, Philadelphia, 2002, Lippincott Williams & Wilkins.

65. Radomski MV, Flinn N: Learning. In Trombly CA, Radomski MV, editors: *Occupational therapy for physical dysfunction*, ed 5, Philadelphia, 2002, Lippincott Williams & Wilkins.

66. Reding MJ, Potes E: Rehabilitation outcomes following initial unilateral hemispheric stroke: life table analysis approach, *Stroke* 19:1354-1358, 1988.

67. Rood MS: Neurophysiological reactions as a basis for physical therapy, *Phys Ther Rev* 34:444-449, 1954.

68. Sahrmann SA, Norton BJ: The relationship of voluntary movement to spasticity in the upper motor neuron syndrome, *Ann Neurol* 2:460-465, 1977.

69. Schmidt RA: *Motor learning and performance: from principles to practice*, Champaign, Ill, 1991, Human Kinetics.

70. Schmidt RA: Motor learning principles for physical therapy. In Lister MJ, editor: *Contemporary management of motor control problems: proceedings of the II STEP conference*, Alexandria, Va, 1991, Foundation for Physical Therapy.

71. Schmidt RA: *Motor control and learning: a behavioral emphasis*, ed 2, Champaign, Ill, 1988, Human Kinetics.

72. Shea JB, Morgan R: Contextual interference effects on the acquisition, retention, and transfer of a motor skill, *J Exp Psychol Hum Learn Mem* 5:179-187, 1979.

73. Shumway-Cook A, Woollacott M: *Motor control: theory and practical applications*, ed 2, Philadelphia, 2001, Lippincott Williams & Wilkins.

74. Shumway-Cook A, Woolacott M: *Motor control: theory & practical application*, Baltimore, 1995, Williams & Wilkins.

75. Spencer J, Krefting L, Mattingly C: Incorporation of ethnographic methods in occupational therapy assessment, *Am J Occup Ther* 47(4):303-309, 1993.

76. Taub E, Miller NE, Novack TA, et al: Technique to improve chronic motor deficit after stroke, *Arch Phys Med Rehabil* 74(4):347-354, 1993.

77. Thelen E: Self-organization in developmental processes: can systems approaches work? In Gunnar MR, Thelen E, editors: *Systems and development*, Hillsdale, NJ, 1989, Erlbaum.

78. Thelen E, Fisher DM: Newborn stepping: an explanation for a "disappearing reflex," *Dev Psychol* 18:760-775, 1982.

79. Thelen E, Ulrich BD: Hidden skills. In *Monograph of the Society for Research in Child Development*, 56 (serial no 223), Chicago, 1991, University of Chicago Press.

80. Titus MN, Gall NG, Yerxa EJ, et al: Correlation of perceptual performance and activities of daily living in stroke patients, *Am J Occup Ther* 45(5):410-418, 1991.

81. Trombly CA: Conceptual foundations for practice. In Trombly CA, Radomski MV, editors: *Occupational therapy for physical dysfunction*, ed 5, Philadelphia, 2002, Lippincott Williams & Wilkins.

82. Turvey MT: Preliminaries to a theory of action with reference to vision. In Shaw R, Bransford J, editor: *Perceiving, acting, and knowing*, Hillsdale, NJ, 1977, Erlbaum.

83. VanSant A: Should the normal motor developmental sequence be used as a theoretical model to progress adult patients? In Lister MJ, editor: *Contemporary management of motor control problems: proceedings of the II STEP conference*, Alexandria, Va, 1991, Foundation for Physical Therapy.

84. VanSant A: Life-span development in functional tasks, *Phys Ther* 70(12):788-798, 1990.

85. Warren WH: Perceiving affordances: visual guidance of stair climbing, *J Exp Psychol Hum Percept Perform* 10:683-703, 1984.

86. Winstein CJ, Schmidt RA: Reduced frequency of knowledge of results enhances motor skill learning, *J Exp Psychol [Learn Mem Cogn]* 16:677-691, 1990.

87. World Health Organization: *International classification of functioning, disability, and health*, Geneva, 2001, World Health Organization.

88. Wu CY, Trombly CA, Lin KC, et al: A kinematic study of contextual effects on reaching performance in persons with and without stroke: influence of object availability, *Arch Phys Med Rehabil* 81(1):95-101, 2000.

joyce shapero sabari

**chapter 5**

# Activity-Based Intervention in Stroke Rehabilitation

## key terms

activity analysis

activity synthesis

blocked practice

brain plasticity

capacity

closed tasks

cognitive strategies

compensatory adaptations

constraint-induced movement therapy

contextual interference

declarative learning

dissociation between body segments

explicit learning

extrinsic feedback

function

generalization of learning

generalized motor programs

implicit learning

intrinsic feedback

kinesiologic linkages

knowledge of performance

knowledge of results

learned nonuse

learning

mechanical constraints to movement

metacognition

open tasks

performance

postural adjustments

postural set

practice

practice challenges

practice conditions

procedural learning

repetitive practice

self-monitoring skills

strategies for community participation

task analysis

training

transfer of learning

variable motionless tasks

## chapter objectives

After completing this chapter, the reader will be able to accomplish the following:

1. Apply principles of the International Classification of Function and the Occupational Therapy Practice Framework to occupational therapy intervention for stroke survivors.
2. Understand implications of neuroscience studies of plasticity and constraint-induced movement therapy to activity-based intervention in stroke rehabilitation.
3. Design effective practice opportunities for stroke survivors to recover motor, cognitive, and participation skills.
4. Understand the basis of interventions designed to enhance stroke survivors' potential to achieve maximal recovery.
5. Apply principles of activity analysis and synthesis when designing occupational therapy intervention for stroke survivors.

With advances in medical intervention and societal attitudes toward persons with disabilities, rehabilitation expectations and outcomes for stroke survivors are improving continuously. This chapter presents concepts from the International Classification of Function,[76] the Occupational Therapy Practice Framework,[2] neuroscience studies of brain plasticity, and theories of motor learning to provide a foundation for the general understanding of activity-based intervention with stroke survivors.

When linear thinking dominated society's views about medicine and rehabilitation, the emphasis of occupational therapy on functional performance in self-selected tasks and roles seemed naive and unfocused. Beyond members of the profession and consumers who benefited from therapy services, few understood that return to a meaningful lifestyle after a stroke was contingent on complex interactions between multiple factors.

## INTERNATIONAL CLASSIFICATION OF FUNCTION

The International Classification of Function (ICF) reflects a current understanding that health status is a measure of far more than the absence of disease (Table 5-1). Function, a dynamic interaction between health conditions and contextual factors, is ICF's yardstick for measuring successful rehabilitation outcomes. According to the classification, function is the integrated totality of one's body function, activity, and participation. The term *disability* is used as the antithesis of function and includes impairment, activity limitation, and activity restriction. In its discussion of activity and participation, the ICF distinguishes between capacity (theoretical potential to perform) and performance (in one's actual, current context). This distinction is crucial in occupational therapy with stroke survivors. Demonstrated improvements within a treatment setting are mere changes in capacity. Clearly, the goal must be to promote generalization of regained skills for actual performance improvements.

The ICF integrates medical and social models of disability (Figure 5-1). Although appreciating the value of the medical model in promoting change within an individual, the ICF also recognizes that social and environmental factors influence performance. Occupational therapists share this dual orientation in the approach to stroke rehabilitation and are uniquely skilled in adapting the environment. Depending on a person's current potential for skill recovery, occupational therapists adapt tasks and environments to promote optimal practice conditions for internal change or to facilitate task performance within constraints of insurmountable physical or cognitive limitations.

**Table 5-1**

**International Classification of Function Key Terminology**

| POSITIVE TERM* | NEGATIVE TERM* |
|---|---|
| **Function** | **Disability** |
| Body functions and structures | Impairment |
| Activity | Activity limitation |
| Participation | Participation restriction |
| **Contextual Factors** | |
| Environmental factors (facilitators) | Environmental factors (barriers/hindrances) |
| Personal factors | No International Classification of Function term |

*The meanings of the terms are as follows:
activity:          execution of a task or action by an individual
body functions: physiologic functions of body systems
body structures: anatomic parts of the body
impairment:     significant deviation or loss in body function or structure
participation:  involvement in a life situation

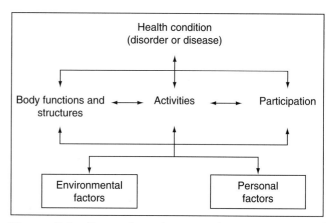

**Figure 5-1** Interactions between the components of International Classification of Function. (From World Health Organization: International classification of functioning, disability, and health (ICF), Geneva, Switzerland, 2001.)

## OCCUPATIONAL THERAPY PRACTICE FRAMEWORK

The occupational therapy profession applauds the vision and semantics of the International Classification of Function. Accordingly, the Occupational Therapy Practice Framework has been structured to synchronize with the ICF and thus highlight that long-standing values within our profession that are consistent with contemporary views about health and quality of life.

The Occupational Therapy Practice Framework provides practitioners with a foundation for designing and implementing multidimensional services that enable patients to participate in self-selected life activities within their homes, families, and communities. The domain of Occupational Therapy requires therapists to include the following components in assessment, planning, treatment, and outcomes:

- Patient factors
- Activity demands
- Context
- Performance patterns
- Performance skills
- Actual performance of tasks and roles in real-life situations

Consistent with the combined medical and social orientation of the International Classification of Function, occupational therapy intervention considers two groups of factors: those within the individual (patient factors, performance patterns, and performance skills) and those within the environment (activity demands and context). Some factors contribute to a particular person's capacity to engage in self-selected occupations; others do not. Some factors are amenable to change, whereas others are not. A patient may wish to change some factors but may have no incentive to change others. For each individual, the skilled occupational therapist determines the unique constellation of effect, potential, and desire. Intervention promotes change in those internal and external factors that the therapist and patient collaboratively have identified as treatment goals (Figure 5-2).

Stroke is a complex condition. Depending on the nature of the cerebrovascular accident and immediate medical care, residual neuropathologic effects varies widely among individuals. Consequently, related impairments and potentials for improvement differ significantly.

Each person has a unique lifetime history of roles, activities, temporal patterns, and culture. Each person and family have unique constraints that govern their willingness to change long-standing routines and environments.

Various chapters in this comprehensive text explore ways occupational therapists intervene to promote change within an individual and to adapt external factors to promote compensation. The ultimate goal of both interventions is participation in valued life activities. A comprehensive occupational therapy program for any stroke survivor artfully targets internal and external factors. The interaction between internal and external factors is complex indeed. Improvements in motor and cognitive skills alone, unaccompanied by adaptations to family structure or physical accessibility, may fail to lead to an outcome of full, meaningful participation. Correspondingly, an overreliance on compensation, without providing stroke survivors with opportunities to improve internal skills, seriously limits patients from reaching their ultimate potentials for engagement in a wide variety of life roles.

## NEUROSCIENCE STUDIES OF BRAIN PLASTICITY

It is common knowledge that necrotic tissue in the mammalian central nervous system does not regenerate.[4] This is the greatest challenge in stroke rehabilitation, compared with rehabilitation of individuals with injuries to the peripheral nervous system or to the musculoskeletal system, for whom ultimate recovery of damaged tissue is expected. Even so, countless stroke survivors experience significant recovery of motor, language, and cognitive function.

Early, spontaneous recovery typically is attributed to resolution of temporary pathophysiologic conditions in regions of the affected hemisphere that have been damaged indirectly by stroke-related sequelae described in Chapter 1. A stroke is a catastrophic physiologic event. In addition to cell death in those neurons that are deprived of oxygen, indirect damage includes changes in cerebral blood flow, cerebral metabolism, edema, and cascading degeneration along neural pathways. The concept of diaschisis, coined by the nineteenth-century Russian neurologist von Monakow, has continued to influence neurologists and neuroscientists.[15,61] Diaschisis, or transient inhibition, spreads to remote sites in the fiber pathways leading from the site of injury. As the diaschisis resolves over time, neural activities return to the temporarily suppressed regions, and the stroke survivor experiences return of function. Diaschisis is a probable explanation for the shift to spontaneous innervation of some flaccid muscles so often seen in the early weeks after a stroke. The phenomenon of learned nonuse, articulated by several authors,[33,35,63,64] represents a person's inability functionally to use this reemerging motor activation. Occupational therapy intervention can prevent or reverse

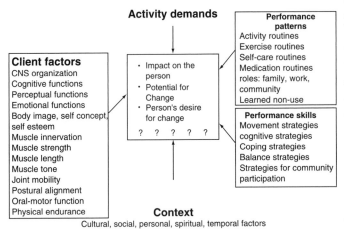

**Figure 5-2** Clinical reasoning process: whether or not to influence domain components during occupational therapy intervention. *CNS*, Central nervous system.

learned nonuse through interventions described later in this chapter.

Neuroscience researchers are actively exploring a variety of potential recovery mechanisms after central nervous system damage. Research at the neuronal level includes studies of dendritic branching, denervation supersensitivity, and axonal sprouting.[41] Although this research holds promise for future pharmacologic management after stroke and spinal cord injury, thus far no evidence indicates that these cellular changes lead to improvements in observable behavior.

The possibility of plasticity, or reorganization of undamaged systems in the brain, has generated a growing body of positive research findings. These studies of human beings and other mammals are providing increasing evidence that recovery of function after brain lesions is associated with recruitment of brain regions not typically activated for a specified function.[41] Studies of human stroke survivors have yielded direct evidence through positron emission tomography, functional magnetic resonance imaging, and transcranial magnetic stimulation that the following regions assume control of generating efferent signals to previously paralyzed muscles after functional recovery: the supplemental motor area, inferior parietal cortex and cerebellum of the hemisphere ipsilateral to the infarct; and the primary sensory-motor cortex of the contralateral hemisphere.[35,41,49] These studies consistently find that the primary influence on central nervous system reorganization is "patterns of use."[12,23] Reorganization of neural mechanisms is a dynamic process that is influenced by the person's active efforts to meet environmental and task demands.[23,24,35] Depending on the extent of neuropathologic damage, all stroke survivors have varying potentials for spontaneous recovery and reorganization of neural mechanisms. Two central questions then must guide the stroke rehabilitation process:

1. How can activity demands be structured and presented to stroke survivors to maximize the inherent potential of their brains to dynamically reorganize?
2. What foundational substrates do stroke survivors need to meet their own internal potential to move, think, and perform desired tasks?

## CONSTRAINT-INDUCED MOVEMENT THERAPY

Constraint-induced movement therapy (CIMT), a promising approach to promoting recovery of functional arm movement after stroke, evolved from the theory of learned nonuse. Studies of laboratory animals[62] and human stroke survivors[38] support the theory that potential motor recovery is limited by a learned overreliance on the unaffected limbs. Immediately after brain injury, contralateral flaccidity limits functional use of the affected

arm and leg. Because motor function remains unaffected on the opposite side, most stroke survivors compensate by relying exclusively on the unaffected limbs to perform tasks. This theory of learned nonuse may explain why upper limb recovery lags behind lower limb recovery. Whereas each attempt to stand or walk requires bilateral activity in the legs, many upper limb activities may be accomplished by using the unaffected side exclusively.

In CIMT, physical constraint to the unaffected upper limb is provided in an effort to reverse the effects of learned nonuse. The typical research protocol has been for subjects who are at least 1 year beyond the stroke to wear a resting hand splint and shoulder sling on the unaffected arm during virtually all waking hours for 12 days. On each of the 8 weekdays, subjects spend 7 hours in a rehabilitation program in which they are challenged with different tasks.[33,64] Functional testing immediately after the 12-day period, and 2 years later, has yielded promising results. Subjects who participated in constraint-induced therapy performed significantly better in the speed and quality of their movement. More importantly, they reported significant differences in the actual amount of use of the affected upper limb compared with control subjects.[38,64] Recent studies have found comparable success using constraint only to the hand, with the shoulder free,[13] with modified constraint schedules,[13,43] and with acute[13,47] and subacute[7] stroke survivors. A note of caution about the use of CIMT in the early stage of stroke recovery emerges from acute animal studies. Studies with lesioned rats[31,44] have found that forced use with these animals during the first 7 days after injury led to degeneration of surrounding, surviving neural tissue.

Proponents of CIMT have never claimed that their approach reverses paralysis. Criteria for participation in constraint programs include the requirement that participants exhibit at least 10 degrees of active extension at the metacarpophalangeal and interphalangeal joints and at least 20 degrees of active extension at the wrist.[33,38] In addition, participants should have intact executive function and problem-solving skills and adequate balance to maintain upright posture without the use of the intact upper limb. Constraint-induced movement therapy is clearly an approach for a select category of stroke patients. In addition the potential exists for combining CIMT with other interventions. Success has been reported in a single case study in which antispasticity medication was paired successfully with constraint. In this case, a 44-year-old male whose recovery in arm movements was limited by residual hypertonicity in finger flexor muscles, had improved hand function after combined treatment with Botox and modified CIMT.[43]

In essence, CIMT "forces" the individual to practice using a paretic limb and thus provides the central nervous system with appropriate challenges for reorganization of motor control. Another aspect of CIMT is never discussed by its proponents and may have significance for occupational therapy intervention with stroke survivors. We can hypothesize a link with Seligman's theory of learned helplessness.[53] First discovered in dogs[54] and later tested in numerous studies of human beings,[42,55] this theory postulates that after repeated exposure to situations in which actions are ineffective, organisms become passive, even when future actions could be effective. After an initial period of flaccidity following a stroke and subsequent relearning of one-handed task performance, many stroke survivors remain essentially unaware of a return of motor potential. Several factors might explain this phenomenon.

- The person has no reason to try to use the arm and thus remains ignorant about emerging motor potential.
- The person notices isolated abilities to perform specific movements but does not know how to use these movements for integrated functional performance.
- The person experiences mechanical constraints that limit the capacity to use the recovering paretic limb in a functional way.

For those stroke survivors who meet the qualifying criteria, CIMT may be an effective way to improve motor performance. For those whose recovery is more limited, the concept of learned nonuse may still be helpful toward structuring effective therapeutic intervention (see Chapter 10).

## PRACTICE AND LEARNING

### Goals of Training and Learning

Learning and training are two distinct phenomena, each with its own required style of practice. The goal of training is to memorize a prescribed solution to a selected task challenge, whereas the goal of learning is to develop one's own solution, which can be applied in a variety of situations. Based on each patient's abilities and role demands, the occupational therapist determines whether the therapeutic goal is to promote training or learning. In thera-

peutic training, practice entails repetitive performance of a designated sequence of behaviors. Task performance must occur in the actual setting in which the individual plans to perform the task because no evidence exists that skills acquired through training can be applied successfully in different environmental contexts.[59,66]

Learning and training are internal phenomena that cannot be observed directly. Therapists assume that training has occurred if performance of a specific task improves and persists over time. Therapists assume learning has occurred when a person demonstrates the two achievements associated with training and also is able to apply a new set of skills within a variety of situations.[50,57] Whenever possible, occupational therapy attempts to promote learning for motor and cognitive skill development that provides the individual with an infinite number of choices for task and role engagement. Practice for learning requires active engagement in tasks that require problem solving and implementation of effective foundational strategies.

### Foundational Strategies for Task Performance

*Appropriate Kinesiologic Linkages for Efficient Control of Balance, Gross Mobility, and Limb Movement.* When the neuromuscular system is functioning optimally, a person can rely on automatic kinematic and kinetic linkages to serve as a foundation for functional movements. Although these linkages are described in a variety of ways,[5,50,57] motor control theorists and kinesiologists agree that they promote optimal mechanical interactions between muscles and body segments. Normal shoulder abduction is an example. Regardless of the task or the environment, kinematic linkages between the scapula and humerus result in the scapulohumeral rhythm that is required to achieve full range of motion and force production (Figure 5-3). In addition, the deltoid and rotator cuff muscles are linked kinetically to

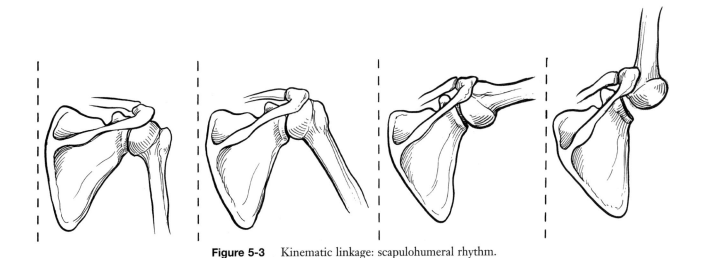

**Figure 5-3** Kinematic linkage: scapulohumeral rhythm.

ensure that the deltoid fibers produce the desired rotary force on the humerus. Without this linkage, an attempt to abduct the shoulder instead results in a nonfunctional upward shrug of the shoulder[40] (Figure 5-4).

Stroke survivors have often lost the automatic kinesiologic linkages associated with efficient movement.[47] Trombly's motion analysis studies of stroke survivors[71,72] reveal these deficits to be disturbances in sensory-motor relationships. Deficits may result from limited mobility of body segments, weakness of specific muscular components, or loss of the motor program that links muscles or joints during a given movement sequence. Several automatic kinematic linkages in addition to the two described previously are commonly observed during normal movement but are often unavailable to stroke survivors. Lumbopelvic rhythm provides for appropriate interactions between movements at the lumbar spine and adjoining pelvis. When rising to stand from a seated position, for example, forward trunk motion is initiated most efficiently at the hips and is accompanied by simultaneous pelvic anterior tilt[40] (see Chapter 14). Glenohumeral external rotation is linked automatically with end-range humeral flexion and abduction. Grasp patterns are automatically linked with wrist extension.

Kinesiologic linkages can be conceptualized as generalized motor programs.[34,50,52] Each of these prestructured sets of central commands governs a particular class of actions. Generalized motor programs are designed to be modified in response to continuous changes in environmental and task parameters. Therefore a unique pattern of activity with core foundational characteristics emerges whenever the generalized motor programs is executed. For illustration purposes, a forehand tennis swing may be conceptualized as a generalized motor program. Foundational kinesiologic relationships comprise the general motor program, but an athlete alters the force characteristics, timing, and spatial details of the forehand swing, depending on the speed, force, and direction of the tennis ball and the player's intentions regarding how to return the ball to an opponent. When designing therapeutic interventions to improve functional motor performance in stroke survivors, therapists determine the generalized motor programs for general categories of movement, such as reach, grasp, balance, standing up, and sitting down. An occupational therapist determines which kinesiologic linkages are impaired and intervenes by assisting with reestablishing these general foundations for normal motor performance. Motion analysis studies of rolling, getting out of bed, standing up from a sitting position, and moving the arms provide useful information that can help an occupational therapist determine which components are essential in a variety of performance contexts.[9,57]

***Cognitive Strategies and Strategies That Compensate for Perceptual Impairments.*** Just as kinematic linkages serve as foundational strategies for efficient movement, cognitive processing strategies provide individuals with a framework for interpreting and acting on complex information in a variety of situations. These strategies are organized approaches that assist a person in selecting relevant cues from the environment and planning the most appropriate response.[66]

Depending on the nature and location of the pathology associated with the cerebrovascular accident, a stroke survivor may demonstrate impairments in selecting and implementing appropriate cognitive strategies for accomplishing complex tasks. If these impairments are severe, they will limit performance of routine self-care tasks. However, the impairments usually become more apparent when the individual attempts to resume more demanding occupations such as home management, work, or school activities. Toglia and Golisz have been particularly influential in designing evaluation and treatment protocols to guide occupational therapists in this aspect of intervention.[19,65-67]

Occupational therapy intervention begins with helping patients develop insight about these deficits through a program that challenges them to estimate task difficulty, predict outcomes, and evaluate personal performance.[68] Then the occupational therapist teaches general processing strategies to be practiced in a variety of contexts.

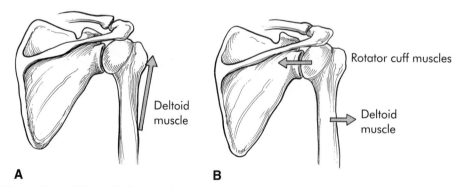

**Figure 5-4** Kinetic linkage: relationship between deltoid and rotator cuff muscles. **A,** Deltoid muscle force acting alone. **B,** Deltoid and rotator cuff muscles working together.

Several examples of cognitive strategies follow. Prioritizing information before beginning a task is a strategy one can apply to activities as varied as grocery shopping (using a list, coupons, and the weekly circular), doing a work-related task, or planning a family outing. Clustering related information together may be a useful strategy for a student who is attempting to master a difficult subject or for a person who is trying to remember what to purchase in the pharmacy. Blocking out irrelevant details is a foundational strategy necessary for reading a map and for managing monthly bills. A person can use a left-to-right scanning strategy to find a certain item in a bathroom cabinet or to check typing for errors. Maintaining a daily notebook of things to do and remember is a strategy with wide applications in a range of situations. Chapters 17, 18, and 19 discuss additional strategies and their applications. Each individual tests the strategies introduced by the therapist to determine whether they are effective and in which situations they can be applied successfully.

***Strategies for Community Participation.*** The social and emotional challenges of coping after a stroke are as demanding as the motor and cognitive challenges (see Chapters 2 and 3). Just as therapeutic interventions can improve strategies essential for moving and for processing information, so too can occupational therapists help stroke survivors develop a core of effective strategies that will help them negotiate their interactions with others and return to full participation within their communities. The therapist should introduce practice of these strategies early in the rehabilitation process, so that stroke survivors clearly understand that it is fully realistic to expect that they will be able to continue engaging in activities and roles that bring quality to their lives, regardless of the amount of motor recovery.

## Types of Learning

***Procedural and Declarative Learning.*** Occupational therapists structure practice opportunities according to the type of learning goal. Declarative learning is needed for tasks in which language skills are used to organize complex sequences of action.[4] Learning a new recipe or a multistep dance routine may require that a person be able consciously to express the processes to be performed. Mental rehearsal is an effective technique for enhancing declarative learning. During mental rehearsal, the individual practices the sequence by reviewing it silently or by verbalizing the steps in the appropriate order. However, most skill development in stroke rehabilitation can be characterized as procedural learning, which is achieved through task practice in a series of varying contexts. For example, a person learns to maneuver a wheelchair through a process of procedural learning. Skill develops through opportunities to experiment with different combinations of arm or arm and leg movements to achieve propulsion in a variety of directions and speeds. Similarly, activities requiring balance or reach and grasp require procedural learning. Chapters 8 and 10 present therapeutic interventions for promoting development of these procedural skills.

***Implicit and Explicit Learning Processes.*** Gentile[16] and colleagues[8,21,74] propose that individuals use two distinct but interdependent processes during the acquisition of functional motor skills. An explicit learning process, which is driven consciously, guides the kinematics of the movement. Gentile hypothesizes that persons use an explicit process to develop a ballpark match between the shape or direction of their movements and the environmental requirements for achieving the goal. External guidance and feedback is likely to have a beneficial effect on the explicit learning process. Schmidt and Lee[50] refer to such intervention as an instructional set, in which the person is given a general idea or image of the task to be learned.

An implicit learning process guides the kinetics of the movement, or the dynamics of force generation. This aspect of movement requires appropriate selection of muscle contraction patterns, determined by accurate predictions of how external forces will affect the movement. Gentile hypothesizes that "the refinement of force dynamics is due to a self-organizing process of implicit learning."[16] This self-organizing process may take longer to develop than explicit learning. Furthermore, implicit learning lies beyond conscious awareness and is unlikely to be augmented by external guidance or feedback.[8,74] Historically, neurorehabilitation interventions that attempted directly to influence implicit aspects of motor performance, such as muscle recruitment or force modulation, have failed to achieve functional outcomes (see Chapter 6). Perhaps attempting to influence only the explicit, or kinematic, features of motor performance through external instructions, guidance, and feedback is wiser. Therapists' contribution to the development of implicit learning may well be achieved best by providing patients with opportunities for effective practice.

## Amount of Practice

Practice is a critical component to learning. Educators, therapists, and neuroscientists universally agree that the amount of practice affects success in skill development.[50,69] "One practice variable dwarfs all the others in terms of importance-practice. Clearly, more learning will occur if there are more practice trials, all other things being equal. Perhaps we do not need to say any more about the amount of practice than this: in structuring the practice session, the number of practice attempts should be maximized."[50] Occupational therapy provides stroke survivors with structured practice opportunities to maximize emerging skills. This is not nearly as simple as it sounds. When persons practice maladaptive strategies, they learn patterns of behavior that may be counterproductive to future improvements in functional performance. To provide appropriate practice opportunities, therapists must be able to envision clearly the intended practice outcomes and to manipulate skillfully a variety of factors within each practice session. These factors include instructions, feedback, activity parameters, salient conditions within the practice environment, and practice schedules. Furthermore, therapists must recognize the importance of practice during daily activities outside of therapy sessions and structure feasible independent practice opportunities for patients. Subsequent chapters emphasize ways occupational therapists structure these factors and their interactions so that stroke survivors can engage in practice that yields desired learning for functional outcomes.

### Promoting Generalization of Learning

Three stages of learning are important in the occupational therapy process:

1. The *acquisition phase* occurs during initial instruction on and practice of a skill (e.g., the initial treatment sessions in which a person learns to use the left arm for functional reach).

2. The *retention phase* occurs after the initial practice period as individuals are asked to demonstrate how well they perform the newly acquired skill; therapists often refer to this as *carryover* (e.g., a patient's ability to perform previously learned reaching activities).

3. In the *transfer phase* the individual must use the skill in a new context (e.g., the patient's ability to perform the reaching strategy when getting dressed or preparing a meal). When a stroke survivor can generalize the strategies learned in the therapy setting and use them in real-life situations, learning has occurred.

Literature about skill acquisition presents several concepts that are helpful in guiding therapeutic intervention that promotes generalization of learning. These concepts can be categorized into three major groups: feedback, strategy development, and practice conditions (Figure 5-5).

*Feedback.* Feedback, or information about a response, can be intrinsic or extrinsic, concurrent or terminal, and can provide knowledge of performance or results. Intrinsic feedback is a result of an individual's own proprioceptive, tactile, vestibular, visual, and auditory sensory systems. After a stroke the somatosensory system often is impaired, which limits the effectiveness of intrinsic feedback about motor performance. Extrinsic feedback from a therapist or feedback technology can provide useful supplementary information to facilitate early awareness and learning. Extrinsic feedback must be decreased gradually for generalization to occur, or the

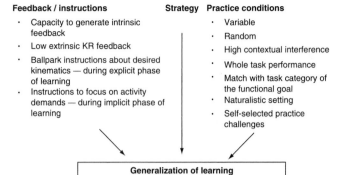

**Figure 5-5** Factors promoting generalization of learning. *KR,* knowledge of results.

person may remain dependent on others for successful task performance.[50]

Concurrent feedback is provided during task performance and includes intrinsic somatosensory feedback and ongoing verbal or manual guidance by a therapist. Terminal, or summary, feedback is given after task completion. No published studies compare the effectiveness of concurrent and terminal feedback, but research has established that excessive external concurrent feedback clearly is distracting to the learner.[51]

*Knowledge of Performance.* Knowledge of performance feedback is information about the processes used during task performance, such as the way a person moves the pelvis or scapula or whether an appropriate cognitive or social strategy has been implemented. Individuals with intact proprioceptive systems receive concurrent, intrinsic knowledge of performance feedback as they move. Stroke survivors, however, often have lost access to this continuous supply of information. Extrinsic knowledge of performance can be provided before a task is initiated. For example, a therapist can guide a person into assuming a postural set that facilitates motor performance or in planning a strategy that enhances performance of a cognitively demanding task. A growing body of research literature examining persons without neurologic impairments[60,81] and stroke survivors indicates that a focus on internal performance factors may be counterproductive to learning. Instructing the learner to focus on relevant information in the environment (such as the distance or shape of a goal object) seems to be more effective than directing the learner's attention internally toward the key elements of a particular movement pattern or sequence.[14] The skillful therapist then must structure selected parameters within the practice tasks to press the individual toward using an intended movement pattern.

*Knowledge of Results.* Knowledge of results is feedback about the outcome of an action in terms of accomplishing a goal. This information can serve as a basis for correcting errors for more effective performance on future trials. Results of laboratory research with normal subjects indicates that frequent, accurate, immediate knowledge of results tends to promote improved performance during the acquisition phase but poorer performance during the retention and transfer stages of learning.[48,75] Similarly, bandwidth knowledge of results, in which feedback is provided only when the performance response is outside a given range of acceptable performance, also leads to better generalization of learning.[75] Schmidt and Lee[50] provide the following theoretical explanation of these findings. Provision of limited knowledge of results during acquisition forces individuals to rely on relevant cues provided by intrinsic mechanisms to improve their performance on future trials. Thus, they tend to develop less dependency on extrinsic feedback. Based on these findings, it is wise for therapists to limit the immediacy and frequency of knowledge of results feedback during stroke rehabilitation. Furthermore, therapists are advised to require that patients determine how effectively they performed therapeutic tasks. To generalize their knowledge for use in situations outside the treatment context, stroke survivors need to learn ways to assess their own performance of functional activities.

***Strategy Development.*** Strategies are organized plans or sets of rules that guide action in a variety of situations. New knowledge is more likely to be generalized for use after the acquisition phase if the individual learns a foundational strategy that can be applied to performance of multiple tasks.[59]

Therapeutic approaches that advocate the importance of strategy formulation during task performance[9,65] seek to develop selected motor or cognitive linkages through engagement in a series of tasks that at a superficial level may seem unrelated. Each task, however, requires use of the selected strategy. To ensure generalization of the strategy, the patient practices the selected underlying skill repeatedly in a variety of contexts during a treatment session. For example, the therapeutic goal may be to develop a selected lumbopelvic linkage as a generalized motor program for forward reach in sitting and standing up from a seated position. The session may begin with the therapist moving the patient's pelvis so that the person understands the kinematic model of action. The therapist then may ask the patient to sit on a therapy ball and rock forward and backward using anterior and posterior pelvic movement. After this, the seemingly unrelated task of reaching for objects from the seated position emphasizes that the patient should tilt the pelvis anteriorly by directing attention to "keeping your back straight" and "bringing your nose over your toes." Finally, the patient practices standing up from and sitting down on a variety of surfaces, with an emphasis on the same lumbopelvic interactions previously practiced in different contexts.

Research findings with normal participants provide support for the use of this approach for learning the invariant structure of a generalized motor program.[18,34] In the terminology of motor learning science, these studies found that a constant or blocked practice schedule of the underlying generalized motor programs, using varied practice parameters, led to enhanced transfer benefits.

Carr and Shepherd's program for optimizing motor function after stroke[9] uses five major techniques to assist patients with developing motor strategies:
1. Verbal instruction
2. Visual demonstration
3. Manual guidance
4. Accurate and timely feedback
5. Consistency of practice

In addition, patients develop skill in providing themselves with intrinsic feedback about the kinematics of their motor performance. Outcome studies[1,10,11] of individuals recovering from stroke provide support for the efficacy of this program.

Toglia[66,67] and Golisz[19,67] developed a systematic approach to promote generalization of cognitive strategies in which the therapist grades treatment by changing certain characteristics of a task but leaving the underlying strategy the same. To illustrate this approach, Chapter 19 discusses the levels of transfer as they relate to treatment designed to facilitate learning and generalization of a strategy for categorizing information.

The initial task is the first activity performed by the patient, such as sorting a deck of playing cards into a red group (hearts and diamonds) and a black group (spades and clubs). Near transfer is an alternate form of the initial task. Using the previous example, the person might be instructed to sort the playing cards into four groups according to their suits or two groups of odd and even numbers.

Intermediate transfer has a moderate number of changes in task parameters but still has some similarities to the initial task. For example, the same person may be asked to create three categories for sorting a stack of photographs for eventual placement in a photo album.

Far transfer introduces an activity that is conceptually the same as but physically different from the initial task. Now the person may be asked to organize a collection of magazines into groups based on general interest areas (e.g., news, sports, and fashion) for display in a clinic waiting room.

Very far transfer requires spontaneous use of the new strategy in daily functional activities. Before traveling to a neighborhood mall, the person may be asked to categorize items on a shopping list based on the type of store in which they most likely can be purchased.

This multicontext approach emphasizes the use of intrinsic knowledge of performance feedback. Before attempting a new task, patients estimate their performance accuracy and efficiency and determine similarities and differences between the current task and previous activities. After completing a task, patients evaluate their performance and identify techniques that may be helpful in the future. The therapist's major roles are to structure the activity progression and guide patients in developing insights and strategies.

**Practice Conditions.** Several aspects of practice conditions have been studied under laboratory and clinical conditions. Occupational therapists can use these findings to structure practice conditions in stroke rehabilitation programs. The key is to structure conditions during the acquisition phase to produce optimal retention and transfer of the learned skills.[32]

*Practice Schedules.* During blocked practice, patients practice one task until they master it. This practice is followed by practice of a second task until it also is mastered. Random practice requires patients to attempt multiple tasks or variations of a task before they have mastered any one of the tasks. In addition, patients perform the various trials in a random order. Subjects who participate in variable practice perform better on transfer tests than subjects who participate in repetitive practice.[22] A study of stroke outpatients found that random practice was more effective than blocked practice for long-term retention of improvements in reach and manipulation skills.[25] These findings typically are explained with the hypothesis that variable practice facilitates generalization by preventing individuals from developing context-dependent inflexibility when using a newly learned skill.

*Contextual Interference.* Contextual interference refers to factors in the learning environment that increase the difficulty of initial learning.[20] One explanation for this finding is that high contextual interference forces a person to "use multiple and variable processes to overcome the difficulty of practice."[32] In addition, persons develop more elaborate memory representations of the underlying strategies that were used for task achievement during the acquisition phase of learning. Limited knowledge of results feedback is one example of contextual interference that has been discussed already. As shown by studies of knowledge of results feedback, these factors tend to promote more effective retention and generalization. Blocked and random practice schedules, described previously, are examples of low and high contextual interference, respectively. Although blocked practice may lead to quicker skill acquisition, random practice results in greater retention and generalization.[22,50]

Motor performance in an open-task context (a setting in which relevant objects in the environment are moving unpredictably) is another example of high contextual interference, which leads to enhanced performance flexi-

bility and skill generalization.[32] Extensive research supports the value of contextual interference during initial learning to future retention and generalization of skills.[20,32,52,56] These findings typically are explained with the hypothesis that initial obstacles to skill acquisition prevent individuals from developing context-dependent inflexibility when using the learned skill in new situations.[6]

*Whole Versus Part Practice.* Therapists may believe intuitively that a patient will find it easier to learn small segments of a task rather than the task in its entirety. However, breaking a task into its component parts for teaching purposes is useful only if the task can be divided naturally into units that reflect the inherent goals of the task.[36,74] One reason for this is that continuous skills (or whole-task performance) are easier to remember than discrete responses. For example, once persons have learned to ride a bicycle or play tennis, they retain these motor skills even without practicing them for many years. However, segmented, laboratory-type motor skills may be acquired easily but are less likely to be retained over time. Therefore, therapists are advised to teach tasks in their entirety rather than in artificial segments. For example, for best retention and generalization the task of putting on a shirt is best taught all at once rather than in different portions during consecutive therapy sessions. If a stroke survivor has difficulty mastering all the steps simultaneously, the therapist can cue the patient or provide manual guidance for selected aspects of the task. The patient will become accustomed to completing the task during each trial. The therapist's assistance can be decreased gradually as practice sessions continue.

*Practice in Natural Settings.* Transferring skills learned during training to real-life situations is influenced significantly by the degree of similarity between the practice environment and the actual environment.[36] Mathiowetz and Wade[37] studied the movement patterns of individuals with and without motor impairments as they performed selected tasks (eating applesauce, drinking from a glass, and turning pages of a book) under three practice conditions. The impoverished condition was the least natural; subjects mimed the tasks with no access to the objects associated with task performance. The partial condition resembled partial simulations that are used often for practice during rehabilitation therapy. Subjects mimed the tasks with a limited array of the objects normally used. In the natural condition, subjects performed the actual tasks. Data collected through the use of a computerized motion analysis system revealed that each of the three practice conditions elicited unique kinematic profiles in individuals with normal motor performance and individuals with movement impairments resulting from multiple sclerosis. This finding indicates that patients may be learning different motor skills when they practice contrived or partially simulated versions of tasks. A motor skill learned during artificial practice sessions is not guaranteed to be generalized by the patient so it can be used for performing the actual task in its natural setting. Wu et al[73,78,79] provided specific support for the value of using real task performance during therapy sessions to improve motor control in stroke survivors. Their motion analysis studies of persons with and without stroke compared the kinematic parameters of reach patterns when participants reached forward to perform a functional task and when they reached forward with no functional goal. Participants in the neurologically intact and poststroke groups performed better when real objects were available to shape the reach performance.

Skills for performing tasks such as dressing or bathing are generalized best when the skills have been acquired in a setting that resembles the environment in which the activity ultimately will be performed. Occupational therapy clinics with simulated home and community environments promote better generalization of performance area skills than clinics in which practice of daily tasks is contrived. However, many stroke survivors can never generalize what they learn in simulated settings; in these cases, home-based occupational therapy is required.

*Different Practice Conditions for Different Task Categories.* Gentile[17] has postulated that motor activities can be classified into four general categories based on environmental pacing conditions and variability between successive trials. Practice conditions for learning vary depending on the task category.

Closed tasks are activities in which the environment is stable and predictable and methods of performance are consistent over time. Brushing teeth or getting into and out of a bathtub are examples of closed tasks that may be goals for stroke survivors. The best strategy for developing skill in a specific closed task is to develop a narrow and consistent method of performance through repetitive practice of the task.

Variable motionless tasks also involve interacting with a stable and predictable environment, but specific features of the environment are likely to vary between performance trials. Drinking is an example of a variable motionless task because the type of mug, glass, or cup used, as well as the amount with which the container is filled, vary in different situations. Dressing is another example because persons' wardrobes consist of clothing of varying fabrics, dimensions, and styles. To achieve independence in a variable motionless task, a patient must learn more than one method of performance. The therapist must provide individuals with opportunities to solve the motor problems of the activity in a wide variety of contexts.

In consistent motion tasks an individual must deal with environmental conditions that are in motion during activity performance; the motion is consistent and predictable between trials. Stepping onto or off of an escalator or moving through a revolving door are examples of consistent motion tasks. Patients need practice that enables them accurately to match the timing of their actions to the predictable changes of the moving objects in the environment.

Open tasks require patients to make adaptive decisions about unpredictable events because objects within the environment are in random motion during task performance. These activities require appropriately timed movements and spatial anticipation of where the relevant objects will be moving. For example, a passenger who is sitting in a moving train must maintain balance when the supporting surface is moving unpredictably. When crossing a street, a person must anticipate the speed and rhythm of pedestrians and oncoming traffic. When playing most ball games, persons must predict the speed and direction of the ball to position themselves in the right place at the right time. Research has shown that the skills required for successful open-task performance cannot be learned through repetitive practice in a stationary environment.[27,28] Natural practice in an unpredictable environment seems to be the best strategy for developing skill in open-task performance.

## OCCUPATIONAL THERAPY AFTER STROKE

An understanding of key concepts from International Classification of Function, the Occupational Therapy Practice Framework, neuroscience studies of brain plasticity, CIMT, and learning principles lead us to ask questions that will guide occupational therapy intervention in stroke rehabilitation.

1. What are the necessary substrates for stroke survivors to meet their maximal potential for recovery? How can therapeutic intervention influence these substrates?
2. How can occupational therapists structure activity demands to provide effective practice opportunities for stroke survivors?

### Necessary Substrates for Meeting Maximal Potential

Depending on the extent of the neuropathologic damage, each stroke survivor has a hypothetical, unknown potential for recovery of function. Although practice is crucial, a variety of factors may impede a person's capacity to benefit from practice opportunities. Fortunately, skilled therapists can identify and influence several necessary substrates for each stroke survivor to meet his or her full recovery potential. These concepts are summarized in Figure 5-6 and introduced later in this chapter. Subsequent chapters discuss specific interventions to influence these substrates for achievement of functional goals.

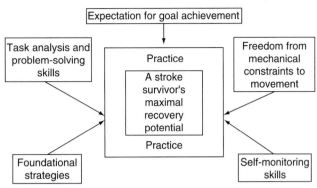

**Figure 5-6** Necessary substrates for meeting maximal recovery potential. NOTE: Each stroke survivor is assumed to have an unknown, hypothetical level of potential for recovery based on the location and extent of neuropathologic damage and potential for cortical reorganization.

## Expectation for Goal Achievement

Stroke is a catastrophic event, often leading to depression and despair. Suddenly, persons find themselves in unfamiliar bodies. Arms and legs no longer respond to willed commands. Small movements pose a threat to balance. Simple tasks are impossible to perform.

Studies of recovery after brain damage consistently show that a drive to perform functional tasks serves as the challenge that may be crucial for cortical remodeling. Most stroke survivors want desperately to move, but in the first few weeks after the cerebrovascular accident, their flaccid muscles prohibit them from acting on this desire. By the time diaschisis begins to subside, many of them have learned not to expect anything of their paretic limbs. They settle for letting others help them perform daily tasks or they settle for accomplishing activities without the contributions of their paretic arm or leg.

Occupational therapists play a critical role in empowering stroke survivors to be active agents in their recovery and return to valued activity engagement. Without making false promises, therapists can challenge patients to be vigilant for incremental returns in function. Without implying that full motor recovery is essential to a meaningful lifestyle, therapists can encourage patients to look for ways to use small improvements in functional ways. Without blaming future limitations in recovery on the stroke survivor, therapists can teach patients ways to prevent secondary impairments and thus to maximize their own potentials for recovery, whatever that potential might be.

A serious error is to present occupational therapy as therapy for the arm. Statistically, far fewer stroke survivors experience significant motor recovery in arm use compared with lower limb function.[26] When the focus of occupational therapy is on the broader goals of returning to independent, safe performance of valued activities, patients can take pride in their reemerging abilities in a variety of physical, cognitive, and social domains. Those who are fortunate enough to detect emerging innervation to muscles of the arm and hand should be challenged to translate this motor recovery into functional performance. Those who do not enjoy such motor return must be presented with other goals toward which they can direct their serious efforts.

## Freedom from Mechanical Constraints to Movement

Stroke survivors encounter several mechanical constraints that limit their ability to move and force them to develop alternative movement strategies. Selected muscle weakness and loss of automatic control over complex postural adjustments are primary impairments directly related to the stroke damage. Other mechanical constraints, such as soft tissue contracture and changes in joint alignment, are secondary changes in posture and loss of mobility associated with stroke.[9,45] As secondary impairments, these losses are preventable and reversible, with timely interventions (see Chapters 10, 12, and 13).

Muscles lose their natural distensibility when they cease to be lengthened passively by antagonist muscles or an external force. This loss of passive muscle length may lead to malalignments in posture that contribute to a continuing spiral of increasing and additional abnormalities in soft tissue flexibility. Without active or passive movement, the person is at risk of developing fixed limitations of joint motion and alignment.[9,45] The problems can be prevented by establishing appropriate postural alignment while lying down, sitting, and standing. In addition, shortly after a stroke, individuals are instructed to follow daily routines to maintain optimal muscle length through the practice of a variety of motor tasks.

Fluid, efficient movement requires a mechanical capacity for dissociation between body segments.[46] In other words, although body segments may be linked kinematically during certain actions, each segment also must be free to move independently of its adjacent structures. Normal scapular-humeral rhythm requires full dissociation between the scapula and thorax. Coordinated shoulder movements require that the humerus be free to move independently of the scapula. A full repertoire of trunk activity requires mobility between the thoracic and lumbar spine and between the pelvis and lumbar spine. Stroke survivors often experience loss of dissociation between adjacent body segments. Dissociation may occur simply because of losses in soft tissue distensibility or may be linked to maladaptive motor strategies persons develop in a subconscious effort to solve other problems. For example, individuals with postural adjustment deficits resulting from stroke often feel insecure about their ability to maintain balance, even in routine sitting or standing positions. The strategy of fixating the pelvis on the lumbar spine or the scapula on the thorax may have the short-term benefit of enhancing a person's sense of postural security. A negative consequence is that these habitual postures lead to difficulty dissociating the pelvis and scapula from adjacent proximal structures. This lack of sufficient limb girdle mobility subsequently limits the normal kinematics of upper and lower extremity movement. Current therapeutic approaches advocate the early introduction of techniques to enhance balance and postural control.[9,45,57] In addition to the inherent advantages of postural security, early recovery of appropriate balance strategies may prevent postural habits that can compromise a stroke survivor's future potential to use reemerging muscle function for functional arm and leg movement.

Other secondary impairments, such as edema and pain, seriously limit a person's potential for movement or functional activity engagement. Therapists are responsible for preventing and minimizing mechanical constraints to movement before introducing practice opportunities for improving motor control.

### Self-Monitoring Skills

Stroke survivors are faced with the challenge of resuming their lives in a body that is different from the one they inhabited before. Sensory information may be difficult to interpret, muscles may no longer work in effortless synchrony, and postural preparation for movement may no longer be automatic.

Before stroke survivors can begin to learn effective strategies for movement and task performance, they need to become acutely aware of the way their bodies work, which movements are possible at different body segments, when their postures are aligned optimally, and when they are efficiently "set" to perform particular activities. These understandings are critical for redeveloping appropriate kinesiologic linkages that serve as motor foundations for task performance.

Metacognition[66,68] is the knowledge and regulation of personal cognitive processes and capacities. Metacognition includes an awareness of personal strengths and limitations and the ability to evaluate task difficulty, plan ahead, choose appropriate strategies, and shift strategies in response to environmental cues. The multicontext approach to cognitive perceptual impairment emphasizes developing insight about personal deficits (and strengths) as a first step toward developing strategies for functional performance after brain injury (see Chapter 19).

Understanding the concept of metacognition is important for understanding movement. Before individuals can generalize the way to use scapulohumeral rhythm in tasks requiring functional reach, they must first understand the amount of mobility their unaffected scapula has. Then they must acknowledge when their affected scapula is not moving freely so that they can develop internal feedback mechanisms that enable them to correct their scapula

movements when they are insufficient for accomplishing a given task. The ultimate goal is to use this personal knowledge of movement to change the foundational strategy used for reaching tasks in a variety of contexts. "The individual's degree of effectiveness in the learning process (and thus in problem solving in general) will be limited by his or her ability for critical self-analysis and environmental analysis in light of the problems encountered and by his or her ability to generate and control the solutions to these problems."[27]

Finally, stroke survivors must know how to monitor their own recovery of motor function. As illustrated in the theory of learned nonuse, many individuals fail to use the hemiparetic arms, even when muscle activity is available. Therapists can teach patients how to check actively for changes in ability to recruit specific muscles. Therapy sessions must be viewed as opportunities for stroke survivors to share their new discoveries with their therapists. In turn, the occupational therapist structures activities for the patient to practice emerging skills, during the therapy session and as "homework" challenges.

### Foundational Strategies

We have previously discussed the value of developing foundational strategies as an intervention approach designed to maximize generalization of learned skills has been discussed previously. Foundational strategies, or generalized motor programs, are critical for a variety of motor actions. In addition, foundational strategies for classes of cognitive and social skills enable stroke survivors to meet current and unanticipated future activity demands. Explicit learning, combined with structured demands to enhance self-monitoring of salient features in a desired strategy, establishes an underlying framework for a foundational strategy. Implicit learning, through participation in selected, graded task challenges, promotes development of higher-order skills associated with the strategy. Practice opportunities for implementing a strategy under varying parameters promotes flexibility in modifying the strategy to accommodate to ever changing environmental demands.

### Task Analysis and Problem-Solving Skills

Occupational therapists have always recognized that the therapist needs to be skillful at analyzing tasks. Task analysis enables an occupational therapist to establish treatment goals, synthesize treatment activities, and develop compensatory strategies.[29] Rehabilitation professionals are increasingly realizing that patients also must learn to analyze activities or be perpetually dependent on their therapists for successful task achievement. A stroke survivor must learn to determine which motor, cognitive-perceptual, and psychological challenges a task presents. Only then can effective strategies be chosen to solve the problems[5] inherent in the infinite variety of tasks encountered while actively engaging in meaningful life roles.

While reading subsequent chapters in this text, one should remember that occupational therapists strive to develop patients' insight and problem-solving skills, regardless of whether the intervention relates to balance, gross motor function, limb movement, visual skills, neurobehavioral performance, or daily living tasks.

## STRUCTURING ACTIVITY DEMANDS TO PROVIDE EFFECTIVE PRACTICE OPPORTUNITIES

Activity-based intervention is a foundation of occupational therapy in stroke rehabilitation. During the evaluation process, an occupational therapist determines which activities are important to the stroke survivor as determined by the individual's roles, interests, and anticipated environment; which activities the stroke survivor can or cannot perform; and which internal and external factors impede the survivor's ability to complete the identified activities.

During treatment, occupational therapists use activities in two major ways. Some activities may be designed to provide structured challenges to improve internal skills. In the occupational therapy literature, this is called purposeful activity[29] or occupation-as-means.[70] For example, an occupational therapist may engage a stroke survivor in a modified card game. Depending on the skill-related goals for this individual, the occupational therapist may structure the activity so that it requires forward reach with a hemiparetic arm. Alternatively, the card game may require the person to place the cards along a wide horizontal surface while standing. This modification in activity parameters provides opportunities for learning balance strategies while shifting the center of gravity in a lateral direction.

Other activities are designed to provide practice of actual task performance in real-life situations. Examples include direct practice in performing a morning self-care routine or getting into and out of an automobile. Practice of individualized roles in real-life situations is critical but typically unfeasible during therapy sessions. Therefore, therapists need to structure homework assignments for stroke survivors to practice at home and discuss at the next therapy session.

### Effectiveness of Activities as Rehabilitation Interventions

A rapidly growing body of research literature by neuroscientists, motor learning theorists, and occupational therapists reinforces the contribution of direct activity engagement to recovery outcomes after brain damage. As discussed in previous sections, activities are powerful modalities for stroke rehabilitation in two major ways: (1) neural reorganization depends on opportunities to confront meaningful environmental challenges, and (2) generalization of learning is facilitated when subjects practice in natural activities that provide opportunities to develop strategies for performance in a variety of contexts.

Nashner's classic studies[39] established that factors in the environmental context of task performance directly influence which motor strategies a person uses. Occupational therapists structure the environment during activity performance to elicit desired motor and cognitive strategies.

Computerized motional analysis studies consistently show that individuals use different movement patterns when actually performing an activity compared with when they pretend to perform.[37,80] More importantly, study results from subjects with and without stroke show that natural activities elicit significantly more efficient organization of movement as evidenced by reach patterns that were faster and straighter, used less force, and showed greater preplanning.[78,79] Additional studies show positive and statistically significant outcomes for improving reach,[58] balance,[30] and symmetrical posture[77] through activity-based treatment after stroke. Evidence-based practice dictates that occupational therapists use the art and science of activity analysis and synthesis in interventions with stroke survivors.

### Activity Analysis

Occupational therapists are experts at analyzing activities and selecting and synthesizing activities that serve as useful rehabilitation modalities. In stroke rehabilitation, occupational therapists use activity analysis as a tool in three major ways:

1. To determine which skills are needed for performance of selected activities (task analysis of selected activities)
2. To assess levels of spared or emerging skills
3. To teach the stroke survivor to develop their own abilities to analyze activities

*Task Analysis of Selected Activities.* An occupational therapist assesses tasks of daily living in the environmental context in which the individual plans to perform each task. The therapist determines which skills are necessary for task performance and compares this analysis to the functional strengths and limitations exhibited by an individual stroke survivor. This task analysis enables the occupational therapist to plan an individualized treatment program that will improve relevant performance skills and enable the person to use compensatory strategies to overcome those limitations that show weak potential for significant improvement. When providing treatment to a stroke survivor, the occupational therapist is most concerned about skills related to balance, motor control, and visuospatial and cognitive skills.

Because the ability to preplan movements often is impaired after stroke, the occupational therapist determines the optimal postural set for performing a selected task. To perform the simple act of standing up, persons must set themselves posturally in several ways. Both feet must be positioned on the floor in an appropriate base of support. Perpendicular angles are established at the ankle and knee and hip joints, and the pelvis is tilted anteriorly to free the lumbar spine for forward movement.[9,57]

When standing, persons automatically change the configuration of their bases of support in anticipation of the direction toward which they expect to shift their body weight. If they plan to shift forward, as is done when reaching ahead, they establish an anterior-posterior base of support. If they plan to shift to the left or right, as is done when stepping laterally to position themselves in front of a bathtub, they establish a medial-lateral base of support. Persons with hemiplegia often assume postural support bases that are inappropriate for the activity in which they are preparing to engage. The occupational therapist facilitates future task performance by determining the appropriate postural sets and then instructing the individual in choosing appropriate postural sets for a performance area activity. For example, assuming the most efficient postural set for standing in front of a toilet can determine whether a man will be able to urinate safely and independently.

Just as appropriate postural sets are important precursors to efficient motor performance, preplanning is also instrumental in determining the success of cognitively or visually challenging tasks. Activity analysis includes a determination of preliminary cognitive strategies that facilitate task performance. For example, a person with right hemisphere dysfunction may experience difficulty in spatially orienting a blouse or slacks for independent dressing. The individual may be unaware that before the stroke a quick and automatic process was used to visualize and orient the garments in relation to the body segments. The occupational therapist's skill in activity analysis enables development of a workable strategy, such as lining up each garment before attempting to complete the additional steps of dressing.

Another aspect of task analysis is when the occupational therapist determines the requirements of each task for shifting body weight in relation to center of gravity. Postural adjustments that normally serve as balance mechanisms during weight shift often are impaired after stroke.[9,45] Understanding the inherent balance challenges of a task is critical for developing treatment goals and compensatory strategies. The therapist can facilitate success in shifting weight during activity performance greatly through the use of appropriate postural sets. The importance of this class of prerequisite skills is important when bathing. If patients are using a tub bench, they need to set themselves posturally for a posterior weight shift from standing next to the bench to sitting on the bench. Once sitting, they need to rotate the pelvis and bring both legs into the tub. The next step is to shift their weight laterally, while sitting, to position themselves on the tub bench.

A forward weight shift often is required to adjust the water, and significant challenges to a lateral weight shift when sitting may occur when patients must wash their genitals. If patients will be stepping into the bathtub and standing under a shower, they must set themselves posturally for a lateral weight shift for entrance and exit to and from the tub or shower. Reaching up and down from the standing position is a critical performance component for safe, independent completion of this activity. Patients may practice these performance component skills in other contexts, such as in activities that require similar balance adjustments while sitting and standing. However, they ultimately must practice them in the context in which the actual bathing activity takes place.

Difficulty with dissociation between body segments is common after stroke.[9,45] The occupational therapist assesses the type and magnitude of such dissociations in each performance area task that is analyzed. For example, to put on shoes and socks, patients must be able to dissociate the pelvis from the lumbar spine to tilt the pelvis anteriorly and posteriorly to cross one leg over the other. They also need to dissociate the lumbar from the thoracic spine to achieve the trunk rotation required to reach the left hand to the right foot. If they are using their paretic arm to assist with the task, disassociation between the scapula and thorax is required, as is disassociation between the humerus and scapula. Determination of these requirements through activity analysis guides treatment and helps the stroke survivor understand the therapist's rationale for choice of treatment methods.

Various tasks require different levels of motor planning and motor sequencing. For patients with impairments in these areas, the therapist determines the nature of each of the challenges within specific performance area activities. Finally, when stroke survivors demonstrate impairments in visuospatial or cognitive skills, the occupational therapist carefully analyzes the unique challenges of each task and assists individuals in developing strategies to meet these specific performance component requirements.

Activity analysis also enables the occupational therapist to determine strategies for task performance that promote efficient movement patterns and are least likely to contribute to the development of secondary impairments. Chapters 10, 12, 13, and 24 describe strategies for relaxing excessive skeletal muscle activity and preventing abnormal postures. The occupational therapist instructs the stroke survivor in the way to incorporate these strategies into the routine performance of daily activities. In addition, activity analysis assists the therapist in determining which compensatory strategies or adaptive equipment are most effective for each individual stroke survivor.

***Assessing Levels of Spared or Emerging Skills.*** Activity analysis enables occupational therapists to evaluate skill levels through observation of patients as they participate in selected tasks. Árnadóttir-Occupational Therapy Neurobehavioral Evaluation (A-ONE)[3] provides a systematic framework for assessing cognitive and perceptual function through structured observations of activities of daily living performance. This tool is discussed further in Chapter 18.

Carr and Shepherd's program for optimizing motor function after stroke[9] describes a therapeutic approach for evaluating motor skills in the context of task performance. The therapist analyzes a patient's performance of a specific task and compares it with the normal kinesiology associated with that task. As in the neurodevelopmental treatment approach,[45] a major focus of this analysis is to identify those factors that serve as obstacles (or blocks) to moving in efficient kinesiologic patterns. For example, when a patient with hemiparesis tries to reach forward to grasp a cup, he or she may tend to use the entire shoulder girdle as one tightly bound unit instead of disassociating the scapula from the thorax or the humerus from the scapula.

Intervention strategies are determined directly from task analysis. In the previous example, the therapist would provide passive mobilization to reduce mechanical constraints and enhance the patient's internal awareness of available scapular motion. The patient then practices reaching forward in a variety of contexts while the therapist provides manual guidance and structures placement of goal objects to maximize appropriate kinematic linkages. Strong backgrounds in kinesiology and movement analysis are helpful to the therapist when implementing a motor relearning approach. In addition, Carr and Shepherd[9] provide descriptions of normal function for selected activities. Occupational therapists may wish to compare their detailed observations of a patient's movement during task performance with these descriptions of normal functions for that activity.

*Skill in Activity Analysis as a Treatment Goal.* As previously mentioned, stroke survivors, as well as occupational therapists, benefit by developing skill in analyzing activities. An ultimate goal in stroke rehabilitation is for individuals to learn the strategy of analyzing activities in reference to their own functional strengths and impairments. During the occupational therapy process, therapists share their strategies for activity analysis and challenge patients to develop their own skills in this area. Midway through the treatment process, therapists present new tasks and require the stroke survivors to analyze the inherent performance requirements of each task. In addition, occupational therapists encourage individuals to develop their own alternative strategies for task performance. The therapist's major role at this stage is to provide feedback about the safety and efficacy of the person's ideas. Before treatment is terminated, stroke survivors

should develop skill in activity analysis so that they have the confidence and capability to attempt an infinite variety of new tasks and roles.

### Activity Selection and Synthesis

Occupational therapists select activities and modify task demands (1) to structure specific practice components within an activity, with the goal of improving internal skills, and (2) to adapt tasks so they are easier or safer to perform, according to each individual's demonstrated internal capacities, limitations, and interests.

The following description of a game of dominoes is an example of modifying activity parameters to elicit specific practice demands. With full knowledge of the patient that the primary purpose of engaging in this game is to practice skills of forward reach and lateral pinch, the therapist modifies the height and distance of the table surface to provide sufficient, but not excessive, challenges to the generalized motor program for forward reach. The therapist purposely places the dominoes on their sides, rather than flat, to encourage external rotation at the glenohumeral joint and supination at the forearm. The therapist also considers the interaction between the person's balance adjustments and ability to control increasing numbers of degrees of freedom in movements of the hemiparetic arm. Based on prior and ongoing assessment, the therapist determines whether the person will perform the task while sitting or standing, and the amount of shift in center of gravity that will be required by positioning of the checkers on the table.

When an occupational therapist modifies an activity to facilitate current performance, the focus is on external adaptations to compensate for unchanging internal limitations. Therapists must understand that both types of activity modification may be appropriate for a single individual. Equally important is that the stroke survivor clearly understands the purpose of each therapeutic activity.

Activity synthesis is unique for each individual. Although the occupational therapist applies carefully considered general foundational concepts when planning treatment for stroke survivors, no textbook can provide specific activity formats that are appropriate for groups of individuals, even if they all have the same diagnosis. Each stroke survivor has an individual constellation of abilities, limitations, interests, roles, and personal goals. Occupational therapists synthesize activities by modifying parameters of specific tasks in specific contexts to provide practice challenges or compensatory adaptations. This requires flexibility, creativity, and sensitivity to individual needs.

## REVIEW QUESTIONS

1. How do the International Classification of Function and the Occupational Therapy Practice Framework

each integrate medical and social models of disability? What interventions do occupational therapists provide to promote internal change within stroke survivors? What interventions do occupational therapists provide to change factors in a stroke survivor's external environment?

2. How do patterns of use influence central nervous system reorganization after injury? What are implications to occupational therapy intervention with stroke survivors?

3. Which stroke survivors are candidates for CIMT? How can the theory of learned nonuse influence occupational therapy intervention for other stroke survivors?

4. From your knowledge of kinesiology, give specific examples of kinematic or kinetic linkages during normal movement.

5. Give two examples of strategies for community participation that are valuable for stroke survivors to develop.

6. What aspects of motor skills are learned through implicit learning processes? What occupational therapy interventions are most effective in facilitating implicit learning?

7. What is contextual interference and how does it affect retention and transfer of learning? Describe three ways an occupational therapist can modify feedback or practice schedules to promote contextual interference.

8. What are the necessary substrates for stroke survivors to meet their maximal potential for recovery? How can therapeutic intervention influence these substrates?

9. Describe the difference between modifying activities to promote practice for skill recovery and modifying activities to help stroke survivors compensate for current limitations.

## REFERENCES

1. Ada L, Westwood P: A kinematic analysis of recovery of the ability to stand up following stroke, *Aust Physiother* 38:135, 1992.
2. American Occupational Therapy Association: The Occupational Therapy Practice Framework: domain and process, *Am J Occup Ther* 56:609-639, 2002.
3. Árnadóttir G: *The brain and behavior: assessing cortical dysfunction through activities of daily living*, St Louis, 1990, Mosby.
4. Bear MF, Connors BW, Paradiso MA: *Neuroscience: exploring the brain*, ed 2, Baltimore, 2001, Lippincott Williams and Wilkins.
5. Bernstein N: *The coordination and regulation of movements*, Elmsford, NY, 1967, Pergamon.
6. Blandin Y, Porteau L, Alain C: On the cognitive processes underlying contextual interference and observational learning, *J Mot Behav* 26:18-26, 1994.
7. Blanton S, Wolf SL: An application of upper-extremity constraint-induced movement therapy in a patient with subacute stroke, *Phys Ther* 79(9):847-853, 1999.
8. Candler C, Meeuwsen H: Implicit learning in children with and without developmental coordination disorder, *Am J Occup Ther* 56(4):429-435, 2002.
9. Carr J, Shepherd R: *Neurological rehabilitation: optimizing motor performance*, Oxford, 1998, Butterworth-Heinemann.
10. Dean CM, Mackey F: Motor assessment scale scores as a measure of rehabilitation outcome following stroke, *Aust Physiother* 38:31, 1992.
11. Dean CM, Shepherd RB: Task-related training improves performance of seated reaching tasks after stroke: a randomized controlled trial, *Stroke* 28(4):722-728, 1997.
12. Donoghue JP: Plasticity of adult sensorimotor representations, *Curr Opin Neurobiol* 5(6):749-754, 1995.
13. Dromerick AW, Edwards DF, Hahn M: Does the application of constraint-induced movement therapy during acute rehabilitation reduce arm impairment after ischemic stroke? *Stroke* 31(12):2984-2988, 2000.
14. Fasoli SE, Trombly CA, Tickle-Degnen LT, et al: Effect of instructions on functional reach in persons with and without cerebrovascular accident, *Am J Occup Ther* 56(4):380-390, 2002.
15. Feeney DM, Baron JC: Diaschisis, *Stroke* 17(5):817-830, 1986.
16. Gentile AM: Implicit and explicit processes during acquisition of functional skill, *Scand J Occup Ther* 5:7-16, 1998.
17. Gentile AM: A working model of skill acquisition with application to teaching, *Quest* 17:3, 1972.
18. Giuffrida CG, Shea JB, Fairbrother JT: Differential transfer benefits of increased practice for constant, blocked, and serial practice schedules, *J Mot Behav* 34:353-365, 2002.
19. Golisz KM: Dynamic assessment and multicontext treatment of unilateral neglect, *Top Stroke Rehabil* 5:11-28, 1998.
20. Goodwin JE, Meeuwsen HJ: Investigation of the contextual interference effect in the manipulation of the motor parameter of overall force, *Percept Mot Skills* 83(3 pt 1):735-743, 1996.
21. Green TD, Flowers JH: Implicit versus explicit learning processes in a probabilistic, continuous fine-motor catching task, *J Mot Behav* 23:293, 1991.
22. Hall KG, Magill RA: Variability of practice and contextual interference in motor skill learning, *J Mot Behav* 27(4):299-309, 1995.
23. Hallett M: Plasticity of the human motor cortex and recovery from stroke, *Brain Res Rev* 36(2-3):169-174, 2001.
24. Hallet M, Wasserman EM, Cohen LG, et al: Cortical mechanisms of recovery of function after stroke, *NeuroRehabil* 10:131, 1998.
25. Hanlon RE: Motor learning following unilateral stroke, *Arch Phys Med Rehabil* 77(8):811-815, 1996.
26. Hendricks HT, van Limbeek J, Geurts AC, et al: Motor recovery after stroke: a systematic review of the literature, *Arch Phys Med Rehabil* 83(11):1629-1637, 2002.
27. Higgins S: Motor skill acquisition, *Phys Ther* 71(2):123-139, 1991.
28. Higgins JR, Spaeth RK: Relationship between consistency of movement and environmental condition, *Quest* 17:61, 1972.
29. Hinojosa J, Sabari J, Pedretti L: Position paper: purposeful activity, *Am J Occup Ther* 47:1081, 1993.
30. Hsieh CL, Nelson DL, Smith DA, et al: A comparison of performance in added-purpose occupations and rote exercise for dynamic standing balance in persons with hemiplegia, *Am J Occup Ther* 50(1):10-16, 1996.
31. Humm, JL, Kozlowski DA, James DC, et al: Use-dependent exacerbation of brain damage occurs during an early post-lesion vulnerable period, *Brain Res* 783(2):286-292, 1998.
32. Jarus T: Motor learning and occupational therapy: the organization of practice, *Am J Occup Ther* 48(9):810-816, 1994.
33. Kunkel A, Kopp B, Muller G, et al: Constraint-induced movement therapy for motor recovery in chronic stroke patients, *Arch Phys Med Rehabil* 80(6):624-628, 1999.
34. Lai Q, Shea CH, Wulf G, et al: Optimizing generalized motor program and parameter learning, *Res Q Exerc Sport* 71(1):10-24, 2000.
35. Liepert J, Bauder H, Wolfgang HR, et al: Treatment-induced cortical reorganization after stroke in humans, *Stroke* 31:1210-1216, 2000.

36. Ma HI, Trombly CA, Robinson-Podolski C: The effect of context on skill acquisition and transfer, *Am J Occup Ther* 53(2):138-144, 1999.

37. Mathiowetz V, Wade MG: Task constraints and functional motor performance of individuals with and without multiple sclerosis, *Ecol Psychol* 7:99, 1995.

38. Miltner W, Bauder H, Sommer M, et al: Effects of constraint-induced movement therapy on patients with chronic motor deficits after stroke: a replication, *Stroke* 30(3):586-592, 1999.

39. Nashner LM: Adaptation of human movement to altered environments, *Trends Neurosci* 5:358, 1982.

40. Neumann DA: *Kinesiology of the musculoskeletal system: foundations for physical rehabilitation*, St Louis, 2002, Mosby.

41. Nudo RJ: Recovery after damage to motor cortical areas, *Curr Opin Neurobiol* 9(6):740-747, 1999.

42. Overmier JB: On learned helplessness, *Interg Physiol Behav Sci* 37(1):4-8, 2002.

43. Page SJ, Elovic E, Levine P, et al: Modified constraint-induced therapy and botulinum toxin A: a promising combination, *Am J Phys Med Rehabil* 82(1):76-80, 2003.

44. Riesdal A, Zeng J, Johansson BB: Early training may exacerbate brain damage after focal brain ischemia in the rat, *J Cereb Blood Flow Metab* 19(9):997-1003, 1999.

45. Ryerson S, Levit K: *Functional movement reeducation: a contemporary model for stroke rehabilitation*, New York, 1997, Churchill Livingstone.

46. Sabari JS: Motor learning concepts applied to activity-based intervention with adults with hemiplegia, *Am J Occup Ther* 45(6):523, 1991.

47. Sabari JS, Kane L, Flanagan S, et al: Constraint induced motor relearning after stroke: a naturalistic case report, *Arch Phys Med Rehabil* 82(4):524-528, 2001.

48. Salmani AW, Schmidt RA, Walter CB: Knowledge of results and motor learning: a review and critical reappraisal, *Psychol Bull* 95(3):355-386, 1984.

49. Schaechter JD, Draft E, Hilliard TS, et al: Motor recovery and cortical reorganization after constraint-induced movement therapy in stroke patients: a preliminary study, *Neurorehabil Neural Repair* 16(4):326-338, 2002

50. Schmidt RA, Lee TD: *Motor control and learning: a behavioral emphasis*, ed 3, Champaign, Ill, 1999, Human Kinetics.

51. Schmidt RA, Wulf G: Continuous concurrent feedback degrades skill learning: implications for training and simulation, *Hum Factors* 39(4):509-525, 1997.

52. Sekiya H, Magill RA, Anderson DI: The contextual interference effect in parameter modifications of the same generalized motor program, *Res Q Exerc Sport* 67(1):59-68, 1996.

53. Seligman ME: Learned helplessness, *Annu Rev Med* 23:407-412, 1972.

54. Seligman ME, Maier SF, Geer JH: Alleviation of learned helplessness in the dog, *J Abnorm Psychol* 73:256-262, 1968.

55. Seligman ME, Weiss J, Weinraub M, et al: Coping behavior: learned helplessness, physiological change and learned inactivity, *Behav Res Ther* 18:459-512, 1980.

56. Shea JB, Morgan RL: Contextual interference effects on the acquisition, retention, and transfer of a motor skill, *J Exp Psychol Hum Learn Mem* 5:179-187, 1979.

57. Shumway-Cook A, Woollacott M: *Motor control: theory and practical applications*, ed 2, Philadelphia, 2001, Lippincott Williams & Wilkins.

58. Sietsema JM, Nelson DL, Mulder RM, et al: The use of a game to promote arm reach in persons with traumatic brain injury, *Am J Occup Ther* 47(1):19-24, 1993.

59. Singer RN, Cauraugh JHL: The generalizability effect of learning strategies for categories of psychomotor skills, *Quest* 37:103, 1985.

60. Singer RN, Lidor R, Cauraugh JH: To be aware or not aware? What to think about while learning and performing a motor skill, *Sport Psychol* 7:19, 1993.

61. Stein DG: Brain injury and theories of recovery. In Goldstein LB: *Restorative neurology: advances in pharmacotherapy for recovery after stroke*, New York, 1998, Futura.

62. Taub E: Movement in nonhuman primates deprived of somatosensory feedback, *Exerc Sport Sci Rev* 4:335-374, 1977.

63. Taub E, Uswatte G, Pidikiti R: Constraint-induced movement therapy: a new family of techniques with broad application to physical rehabilitation—a clinical review, *J Rehabil Res Dev* 36(3):237-251, 1999.

64. Taub E, Wolf SL: Constraint induced movement techniques to facilitate upper extremity use in stroke patients, *Top Stroke Rehab* 3:38-61, 1997.

65. Toglia JP: A dynamic interactional model to cognitive rehabilitation. In Katz N: *Cognition and occupation in rehabilitation: cognitive models for intervention in occupational therapy*, Bethesda, Md, 1998, American Occupational Therapy Association.

66. Toglia JP: Generalization of treatment: a multicontext approach to cognitive perceptual impairment in adults with brain injury, *Am J Occup Ther* 45(6):505-516, 1991.

67. Toglia JP, Golisz K: *Cognitive rehabilitation: group games and activities*, Tucson, 1990, Therapy Skill Builders.

68. Toglia JP, Kirk U: Understanding awareness deficits following brain injury, *NeuroRehabil* 15(1):57-70, 2000.

69. Trombly CA: Foreword. In Smits JG, Smits-Boone EC: *Hand recovery after stroke*, Boston, 2000, Butterworth-Heinemann.

70. Trombly CA: Occupation: purposefulness and meaningfulness as therapeutic mechanisms, *Am J Occup Ther* 49(10):960-972, 1995.

71. Trombly CA: Observations of improvement of reaching in five subjects with left hemiparesis, *J Neurol Neurosurg Psychiatry* 56(1):40-45, 1993.

72. Trombly CA: Deficits of reaching in subjects with left hemiparesis: a pilot study, *Am J Occup Ther* 46(10):887-897, 1992.

73. Trombly CA, Wu CY: Effect of rehabilitation tasks on organization of movement after stroke, *Am J Occup Ther* 53(4):333-344, 1999.

74. Willingham DB: A neuropsychological theory of motor skill learning, *Psychol Rev* 105(3):558-584, 1998

75. Winstein CJ: Knowledge of results and motor learning-implications for physical therapy, *Phys Ther* 71(2):140-149, 1991.

76. World Health Organization: *International classification of functioning, disability, and health (ICF)*, Geneva, Switzerland, 2001.

77. Wu SH, Huang HT, Lin CF, et al: Effects of a program on symmetrical posture in patients with hemiplegia: a single-subject design, *Am J Occup Ther* 50(1):17-23, 1996.

78. Wu CY, Trombly CA, Lin LC, et al: A kinematic study of contextual effects on reaching performance in persons with and without stroke: influences of object availability, *Arch Phys Med Rehabil* 81(1):95-101, 2000.

79. Wu CY, Trombly CA, Lin K, et al: Effects of object affordances on reaching performance in persons with and without cerebrovascular accident, *Am J Occup Ther* 52(6):447-456, 1998.

80. Wu CY, Trombly CA, Lin KC: The relationship between occupational form and occupational performance: a kinematic perspective, *Am J Occup Ther* 48(8):679-687, 1994.

81. Wulf G, Hob M, Prinz W: Instructions for motor learning: differential effects of internal versus external focus of attention, *J Mot Behav* 30:169, 1998.

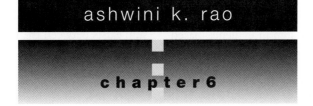

ashwini k. rao

chapter 6

# Approaches to Motor Control Dysfunction: An Evidence-Based Review

### key terms

evidence-based practice          neurotherapeutic approach          task-oriented approach

### chapter objectives

After completing this chapter, the reader will be able to accomplish the following:

1. Understand principles of evidence-based practice and criteria of evaluating research.
2. Understand the rationale behind the various techniques described in this chapter.
3. Evaluate the evidence testing the effectiveness of the approaches in stroke rehabilitation.

The therapeutic professions are in the midst of a paradigm shift in practice for neurologic dysfunction. This chapter examines the evidence, or lack thereof, of some of the historically popular neurotherapeutic approaches. The lack of evidence in their favor has led in part to the articulation of a new clinical paradigm based on a functional task-oriented approach. The evidence for specific therapeutic applications within this task-oriented paradigm are evaluated to determine the best research evidence available for rehabilitation of sensorimotor dysfunction following stroke.

## UNDERSTANDING EVIDENCE-BASED PRACTICE

Evidence-based practice is fast becoming a catchphrase in occupational and physical therapy education and practice.

Its importance stems from the need to use the best (most effective) available techniques, which is a fundamental ethical responsibility of clinical practice. Sackett[45] coined the term *evidence-based medicine* and defined it as "the conscientious, explicit, and judicious use of current best evidence in making decisions about the care of individual patients. The practice of evidence-based medicine means integrating individual clinical expertise with the best available external clinical evidence from systematic research."

Evidence-based practice is the application of the principles of evidence-based medicine to problems in the field of rehabilitation. According to Law,[27] evidence-based practice is based on a self-directed learning model in which practitioners must take responsibility for continuously evaluating their techniques in an effort to improve them.

Mohide[34] identified three basic components of evidence-based practice:

1. Best research evidence: A first step in evidence-based practice is to identify rigorous, clinically relevant research studies that apply to the clinical problem at hand. For this chapter, this would imply an examination of the best available evidence in the rehabilitation of sensorimotor dysfunction following stroke.

2. Clinical expertise: The second step is using one's clinical expertise and experience to identify patients' strengths and weaknesses and the risks and benefits of potential interventions. In other words, once the clinician has identified the best research evidence, the next step is to determine if the techniques described in studies apply to the individual patient, given his or her strengths and weaknesses. A focus on the inclusion and exclusion criteria that the studies used is important to determine if the individual patient in question would benefit from the techniques.

3. Patient values: The final step is to incorporate a patient's values into clinical decision-making.

This chapter examines the best research evidence. To do so requires first defining the criteria by which to evaluate clinical outcome studies.

## CRITERIA FOR EVALUATING RESEARCH ARTICLES

The criteria used for evaluating outcome studies are adapted from the criteria proposed by Sackett.[45] In this framework, research articles are ranked according to the following criteria: I, large randomized controlled trials with low false positives; II, small randomized controlled trials with high false positives; III, nonrandomized concurrent cohort comparisons between subjects that did and did not receive intervention; IV, nonrandomized historical cohort comparisons between current subjects who did receive intervention and former subjects who did not; and V, case series without controls.

Once the studies were classified by the aforementioned criteria, the results of a group of studies on a given treatment technique were summarized. The criteria used in this chapter was that proposed by Sackett[45] in which the evidence is summarized as grade A, B, or C:

Grade A: Recommendations for outcomes are supported by at least one level I study.

Grade B: Recommendations for outcomes are supported by at least one level II study.

Grade C: Recommendations are supported by level III, IV, and V studies.

What follows is a brief description of research designs to help the reader understand the terms used in the evidence tables. For more detailed descriptions of research designs, the reader is referred to Helewa and Walker[18] and Law.[27]

Randomized controlled trials are the most rigorous way of determining whether a cause-and-effect relationship exists between treatment and outcomes. Some of the important features are:

- Subjects are randomly allocated to intervention groups.
- Patients and experimenters should remain unaware of which treatment was given until the study is completed.
- All intervention groups are treated identically except for the experimental treatment.

A cohort study involves studying groups of individuals who share some common characteristics, such as positive history of stroke. In this case, subjects are not allocated to different groups at random, making them less rigorous than randomized controlled trials.

The before-and-after design is a study of one group of patients without a control group. When a control group is included, the design is called *case control design*. Because the control group in this case consists of healthy subjects, the two groups are different at the outset of the study.

Descriptive design is not rigorous but is useful in describing a disorder in detail.

## PARADIGM SHIFTS IN STROKE REHABILITATION

The therapeutic professions of occupational and physical therapy have witnessed two paradigm shifts related to the treatment of neurologic dysfunction. According to Gordon,[16] paradigm shifts within therapeutic practice can occur for two reasons: (1) because the theoretical model underlying a therapeutic approach does not fit with current knowledge and (2) because current approaches do not appear adequate to solve clinical problems. The past 60 years have witnessed two distinct paradigm shifts in the treatment of neurologic disorders, particularly stroke.

The first shift occurred in the years immediately following World War II; at that time the dominant therapeutic paradigm was muscle reeducation, which was used extensively to treat peripheral nerve disorders such as poliomyelitis. Although useful for polio, muscle reeducation was not adequate to treat individuals with disorders of the central nervous system, such as paresis following stroke. As a result, a few therapists began studying how the nervous system controls movements and began to apply these principles into clinical practice. This approach heralded the development of techniques such as proprioceptive neuromuscular facilitation, neurodevelopmental therapy (NDT), Brunnstrom's movement therapy and sensory integration, to name a few of the prominent approaches.

### Neurotherapeutic Approaches: The First Paradigm Shift

*Principles of Neurotherapeutic Approaches.* Although each neurotherapeutic approach is different from each other, all approaches share some common elements.[16,17] This section and the review of the evidence focuses on NDT because this approach historically has been the most widely used in stroke rehabilitation. However, the assumptions also hold true for the other approaches mentioned previously. Some of the common elements of the neurotherapeutic approaches are as follows:

1. The central nervous system is organized hierarchically, with higher centers such as the cerebral cortex controlling the lower centers. When a deficit occurs in the motor system, the more primitive forms of movement, controlled by the lower centers (spinal cord and brainstem), are released from their normal inhibition from the higher centers.[7] Thus, treatment within this framework was aimed at reestablishing control by the higher centers.

2. Normal movement can be facilitated by providing specific patterns of sensory input, particularly through the proprioceptive and tactile sensory systems. Under this assumption, sensory stimulation was proposed to produce long-term effects of reestablishing normal sensorimotor neural connections.

3. Recovery from brain damage follows a predictable sequence that mimics normal development. Treatment used developmental postures in an effort to facilitate recovery.

4. Reflexes were used to facilitate or inhibit motor activity. Experience of normal movement patterns must be provided so that the patient does not learn abnormal patterns of posture and movement after stroke. Reflex inhibitory movement patterns, which were opposite to the pattern of spasticity observed in patients, were used to prevent learning of abnormal movements.

5. Sequelae of stroke can be understood through a neurophysiologic explanation. This assumption means that sensorimotor impairments seen after stroke result primarily from the damaged motor system.

***Outcome Studies on Neurotherapeutic Techniques.*** This section includes an evaluation of the evidence primarily for NDT and limited to an adult population. However, one study was found that examined the effectiveness of proprioceptive neuromuscular facilitation and was included in the review. Table 6-1 shows that 11 studies tested the effect of NDT or compared it with another therapeutic approach, whereas one study examined the effectiveness of proprioceptive neuromuscular facilitation. The studies in the evidence table are rank-ordered based on the rigor of the research design.

*Timing of Therapy.* Of the 11 studies related to NDT, four were conducted on patients in the acute stage and seven in the subacute stage. The only study on the effect of proprioceptive neuromuscular facilitation was conducted in the acute stage.

*Outcomes Measures.* Seven of the 11 studies on NDT measured variables at the impairment and activity limitation levels,* whereas three tested dependent variables only at the impairment level.[20,37,42] One paper measured variables only at the activity limitation level.[30] Dependent variables at the impairment level ranged from range of motion, Arm Research Action Test, Nine or Ten Hole Peg Test, grip strength, gait pattern, weight distribution in sitting and standing, walking velocity, and endurance. The most common outcome measures at the activity limitation level were the Barthel index, Extended ADL Scale, and Rivermead Motor Assessment.

*Study Designs.* The designs included in the review of NDT were eight randomized controlled trials, one retrospective design, and two prospective case series. Of the eight randomized controlled trials, four were classified as level I and four as level II, primarily based on the number of subjects tested. The one study on proprioceptive neuromuscular facilitation was a randomized controlled trial.

*Results of the Review.* Of the eight randomized controlled trials examining the effect of NDT, seven compared NDT with other treatment approaches, such as sham control treatment[13]; task-oriented therapy,[25,36,42] including a behavioral approach[3,51]; and biofeedback training.[37] One study examined the effect of more intensive NDT.[29] Compared with sham treatment, NDT did not show better results; both groups improved at similar rates. In the study comparing biofeedback training with NDT, no stastically significant differences were demonstrated.[37] One of the studies comparing NDT with a behavioral training approach demonstrated a benefit for behavioral training, but this was compromised by the fact that the behavioral training group received more therapy.[51] The other study comparing NDT with a behavioral approach did not demonstrate any differences.[3] Task-oriented treatment demonstrated positive results for functional measures in two studies,[25,36] whereas the third study showed no differences.[42] Increasing the intensity of NDT did not demonstrate positive results either.[29]

The single study testing proprioceptive neuromuscular facilitation compared facilitation with a control treatment of heat and cold therapy.[49] No differences were seen between groups on impairment level or activity limitation level outcome variables.

*Implications for Practice.* The evidence reviewed in this chapter, based on the results of randomized controlled trials, clearly demonstrates (at the grade A level) that neurotherapeutic approaches are at best no more

---

*References 3, 13, 25, 29, 36, 49, 51, 61.

**Table 6-1**

## Evidence for Effectiveness of Neurotherapies

| AUTHORS AND YEAR | AIMS/RATIONALE | DESIGN AND SUBJECTS | INTERVENTION AND OUTCOME MEASURES | RESULTS | COMMENTS | RATING |
|---|---|---|---|---|---|---|
| Stern et al (1970)[49] | Test facilitation exercises based on PNF in acute stroke stage | RCT 62 subjects Daily treatment sessions for duration of hospitalization Subjects with arteriosclerotic or embolic occlusion | Control group: heat/cold therapy, PROM, and ambulation Experimental group: heat/cold therapy, PROM, ambulation, and PNF exercises 1. Motility index 2. Leg strength (cybex) 3. Kenny Institute of Rehabilitation (KIR) scale | No differences found in motility index, leg strength, or functional score on the KIR between groups. | Very good study; duration of training not clear; follow-up testing not specified | I |
| Feys et al (1998)[13] | Test the effect of a neurofacilitation approach in acute stroke stage | Single-blind RCT 100 subjects with ischemic brain damage Training for 5 times a week for 6 weeks Assessment at 1 and 6 weeks, 6 and 12 months | Experimental group: repeated movements, sensory stimulation, and reflex inhibiting postures Control group: sham shock wave therapy 1. Brunnstrom–Fugl-Meyer Test (BFM) 2. Action Research Arm Test 3. Barthel index | Improvement seen in both groups. Experimental group was better on BFM Test at 6 and 12 months. No difference was seen on functional tests. | Well-designed study | I |
| Sunderland et al (1992)[51] | Compare Bobath approach with enhanced behavioral therapy based on motor learning in subacute stroke stage | Single-blind RCT 132 subjects Bobath group: 4 weeks of inpatient and 6 weeks of outpatient therapy; assessments at 1, 3, and 6 months after stroke | Bobath approach: focus on hands-on treatment Behavioral approach: active participation in learning new motor skills with involved arm 1. Extended Motricity Index 2. Subtests of the Motor Club Assessment 3. Passive movement and pain 4. Frenchay Arm Test 5. Nine Hole Peg Test | Behavioral group received more therapy. Behavioral enhanced therapy group showed better strength and range and speed of movement at 6 months for mildly affected patients. No differences were seen in functional skills. | Very good study No control group with enhanced Bobath therapy | I |

| Study | Purpose | Methods | Outcome Measures | Results | Comments | Level |
|---|---|---|---|---|---|---|
| Lincoln, Perry, and Vass (1999)[29] | Compare increased intensity of Bobath therapy with traditional Bobath approach in acute stroke stage | Single-blind RCT 282 subjects independent for feeding Training for 5 weeks Routine PT: 5.75 hours/week Qualified PT: 7.75 hours/week Assistant PT: 5.75 hours/week | All groups received therapy based on Bobath approach by regular therapist, qualified PT, or assistant PT. 1. Rivermead Motor Assessment 2. Action Research Arm test 3. Barthel index 4. Ten Hole Peg Test 5. Grip strength 6. Extended Activities of Daily Living Scale | All groups improved with training; no differences were seen between groups. | Very good study | I |
| Langhammer and Stanghelle (2000)[25] | Compare Bobath approach with motor relearning approach in acute stroke | Double blind RCT 61 subjects with first stroke Groups received training for 40 minutes 5 times a week Assessment at 2 weeks after admission and 3 months after stroke | 1. Motor Assessment Scale 2. Sodring Motor Evaluation Scale 3. Barthel index 4. Nottingham Health Profile | Group trained with motor relearning had shorter stay in hospital and better functional improvement. | Good study Training procedure not described | I |
| Mulder, Hulstijn, and Meer (1986)[37] | Compare electromyographic biofeedback with NDT to improve ankle dorsiflexion | RCT 12 subjects Training 3 times a week for 5 weeks | 1. Range of motion 2. Walking pattern | No differences were seen between groups. | Small sample size | II |

MCA, Middle cerebral artery; NDT, neurodevelopmental therapy; PNF, proprioceptive neuromuscular facilitation; PROM, passive range of motion; PT, physical therapist; RCT, randomized controlled trial.

Continued

**Table 6-1**

## Evidence for Effectiveness of Neurotherapies—cont'd

| AUTHORS AND YEAR | AIMS/RATIONALE | DESIGN AND SUBJECTS | INTERVENTION AND OUTCOME MEASURES | RESULTS | COMMENTS | RATING |
|---|---|---|---|---|---|---|
| Basmajian et al (1987)[3] | Compare two PT approaches: behavioral (including biofeedback) and Bobath in subacute stroke stage | RCT 29 subjects Training 3 times a week for 5 weeks Pretesting and posttesting; 9-month follow-up Subjects with first MCA infarcts | Behavioral group: Electromyographic biofeedback through conceptualization, skill learning, rehearsal, and transfer Bobath group: facilitation with controlled sensory input 1. Upper Extremity Function Test 2. Health Belief Survey 3. Beck's Depression Inventory 4. 16 PF (for mood and affect) | Both groups improved; no differences were seen between groups. Bobath treatment was not superior to behavioral treatment. | Small sample size Good study | II |
| Mudie et al (2002)[36] | Compare task-related, Bobath, and feedback approaches for training weight symmetry in subacute stroke stage | Double-blind RCT 40 subjects Training for 5 times a week for 2 weeks; assessment 1 week before study and 2 and 12 weeks after study | Feedback group: provided visual feedback of symmetry via monitor during reach Task-related group: functional reach in various directions and distances Bobath group: increasing range of motion, normalize tone, improve balance during reach Control group: standard occupational therapy and PT 1. Weight distribution in sitting 2. Weight distribution in standing 3. Barthel index | Bobath group was better at sitting symmetry at 2 weeks; feedback and task-related groups were better at 12 weeks; feedback group was better at standing symmetry at 2 weeks; task-related group was better than Bobath group; and task-related group was better on functional gains. | Good study Small sample size | II |

*MCA,* Middle cerebral artery.

| Study | Purpose | Design | Outcome Measures | Results | Limitations | Level |
|---|---|---|---|---|---|---|
| Pollock et al (2002)[42] | Test effect of independent sitting balance as adjunct to standard therapy based on Bobath approach in subacute stroke stage | RCT with blocked randomization with 2:1 ratio<br>28 subjects<br>Training 5 times a week for 4 weeks; assessment at start and end of training and 2 weeks after training | Experimental group: construction tasks that encouraged balance<br>1. Proportion of patients achieving normal symmetry of weight distribution during standing, sitting, rising to stand, sitting down, and reaching | No differences were seen across groups. | Unequal groups<br>Small sample size<br>One outcome measure | II |
| Lord and Hall (1986)[30] | Compare NDT to traditional therapy | Retrospective study<br>39 subjects | 1. Activities of Daily Living Scale | No differences across groups | Unequal groups | IV |
| Wagenaar et al (1990)[61] | Compare NDT and Brunnstrom approaches in acute stroke stage | Case series<br>Alternating treatment design<br>7 subjects with MCA stroke<br>Training for 5 times a week for 21 weeks; each phase lasted 5 weeks | 1. Action Research Arm Test<br>2. Walking velocity over 8 m<br>3. Barthel index<br>4. VROPSOM List (Dutch version of the Depression Adjective Checklist)<br>5. Neuropsychologic tests | Walking speed was better for only one patient during Brunnstrom treatment; all patients showed some recovery in the first 8 to 10 weeks. | Small sample size<br>No true control group | V |
| Hesse et al (1994)[20] | Test the effect of an NDT-based inpatient program on gait in subacute stroke stage | Case series<br>148 subjects who could walk 20 m independently<br>Training 5 times a week for 4 weeks; assessment at beginning and at 4 weeks | All patients received occupation therapy, speech therapy, and neuropsychologic training as needed.<br>1. Gait measures (peak vertical ground reaction force, loading and deloading rates, time to peak force)<br>2. 10-m walk<br>3. Walking endurance<br>4. Stair climbing | Time for walking and climbing improved, but not endurance; stance duration and symmetry improved. | No control group | V |

effective than traditional therapy and in fact are inferior to training based on a task-oriented approach.

In the past few years, an attempt has been made among proponents of neurofacilitation approaches to integrate established techniques of NDT with the language of newly emerging knowledge in motor control and motor learning. This is readily seen in a recent text describing the theoretic basis of neurodevelopmental treatment (Howle[20a]). Although this is typical during paradigm shifts, the amalgamation of old techniques with new theoretic knowledge is not useful either theoretically (since established NDT techniques are not consistent within the new paradigm of motor control and learning) or for clinical practice (since numerous studies have demonstrated that there is indeed little evidence). The challenge for us as therapists is to move forward and create and subsequently test techniques within the newly emerging paradigm of task-oriented training.

## Functional Task-Oriented Training: The Second Paradigm Shift

The second paradigm shift in the treatment of neurologic disorders began in the 1990s. Therapists have begun to regard neurotherapeutic approaches with less optimism. The dissatisfaction with the neurotherapeutic approaches is due, in part, to the fact that retraining normal movement patterns often did not carry over into the performance of functional daily living skills, which was the ultimate goal of rehabilitation. In addition, demand on therapists has been greater to use interventions that have demonstrated effectiveness. The lack of evidence of the effectiveness of neurotherapeutic approaches, particularly NDT, has led to the development of novel training regimens based on what has been termed the *task-oriented approach*.

### Principles of the Functional Task-Oriented Approach.
The task-oriented approach is based on a systems model of motor control and theories of motor learning. The approach attempts to understand the problems faced by the nervous system to control movements. This field of motor neuroscience represents a multidisciplinary approach to understanding motor control and learning from the perspectives of neurophysiology, biomechanics, and behavioral sciences. Within this framework, motor control is understood as an attempt by the nervous system to adapt movements to the constraints imposed by the mechanics of the motor apparatus (including length, mass of limbs, and intersegmental dynamics) and constraints imposed by the environment (open or closed environment), as well as the behavioral context. Studies on motor control often analyze movements at the biomechanical and behavior levels. See Chapters 4 and 5 for a detailed description.

The previous chapter provides the reader with a more comprehensive description of the task-oriented approach.

What follows is a brief description of some of the incipient principles of treatment, based on suggestions by Carr and Shepherd[8] and Gentile.[15] Within this framework the responsibility of the therapist, as a teacher of motor skills, is to select contextually appropriate functional tasks, vary task parameters to ensure greater transfer of learning, structure practice schedules to encourage active participation of the patients, structure the environment so that all regulatory conditions of a given task are present, and provide feedback. To apply a task-oriented approach to treatment successfully, therapists need to become familiar with analyzing tasks and the processes underlying skill acquisition.

### Outcome Studies Using a Task-Oriented Approach.
For the purpose of this review, the author chose research papers that explicitly tested a task-oriented intervention. The studies included training programs primarily for improving gait, although one study involved sitting balance and reaching tasks.[11] Length of the training programs across the studies was highly variable, ranging from 2 to 20 weeks.

*Timing of Intervention.* Three of the studies tested patients in the acute stage,[24,32,44] one tested patients in the subacute stage,[38] and six tested patients in the chronic stage.*

*Outcome Measures.* Five of the 10 studies only measured outcome variables at the impairment level, whereas the other five measured variables at the impairment and activity limitation levels. Variables at the impairment level commonly tested were gait velocity, endurance, ground reaction forces, kinematic variables in reaching, Action Research Arm Test, and muscle activity. Variables related to activity limitation were measured using the 36-item Short-Form Health Survey, Barthel index, and the Functional Ambulation Classification.

*Study Designs Used.* Of the 10 studies included in the review, six were classified as randomized controlled trials (two of which were level I) and four as case series.

*Results of the Review.* Of the two level I randomized controlled trials, one study demonstrated positive results for the task-oriented approach[24]; these results were not maintained, however, when the groups were tested after 1 year.[23] Of the remaining four level II randomized trials, three demonstrated positive results for task-oriented training.[10,11,44] One study compared brain activation following training and demonstrated greater activation for the task-oriented training group in the contralateral sensorimotor cortex and bilaterally in the parietal cortex.[38] This study provides evidence for a physiologic mechanism for improvement seen following task-oriented training.

*References 5, 10, 11, 23, 35, 47.

All four case series demonstrated improvement following training; however, these results are not conclusive because the task-related training was not compared with a control group (Table 6-2).

*Clinical Implications.* The present review of task-oriented training studies provides some evidence (grade B) of the effectiveness of this approach in comparison with a control group or traditional therapy. Given that this approach is relatively new, more randomized controlled trials with larger number of subjects are needed.

A number of studies were not included under the general category of task-oriented approach but instead were included under specific treatment techniques such as constraint-induced movement therapy (CIMT), treadmill training, and robot-assisted therapy, each of which is reviewed separately next.

### Constraint-Induced Movement Therapy

*Rationale and Principles. Constraint-induced movement therapy.* is a term used for a family of intervention techniques that aim to decrease the effects of learned nonuse of a paretic limb. This family of techniques involves two basic features[55,56]: (1) discouraging the use of the unaffected or less affected limb through verbal prompt but more often by applying some form of restraint to the unaffected limb with a sling, splint, or a mitten, and (2) intensive training of the paretic arm through active participation in functional activities.

Some authors have proposed that the inability to move the paretic limb may arise, at least in part, from a phenomenon termed *learned nonuse.* The proposal is based on experiments in which deafferentation was performed in one limb in primates through dorsal rhizotomy.[52] Following surgery, monkeys did not use their affected limbs because of the lack of sensory feedback, and they preferentially used their unaffected limbs. When the monkeys were forced to use their affected limbs, greater recovery of movement was seen. This indicates that the inability to use the affected limb may be a behavioral learned response to paresis. See Chapters 4 and 10.

*Outcome Studies.* Nine studies were identified in the literature that tested CIMT in patients with hemiparesis following stroke. Of the nine studies, four were randomized controlled trials,[12,40,53,57] and the other five were case series or case reports.[6,22,33,41,63] Training under the CIMT approach typically consists of intensive practice over a period of 2 weeks, including 6 hours of supervised therapy during the week days. During therapy, patients are encouraged to practice functional tasks with the impaired extremity. During the training period, the less impaired extremity is constrained in a sling, mitt, or splint for almost 90% of waking hours.[12,53,57] The exception was the study by Page et al[40] who tested a less intense training program

that more accurately reflects time spent in traditional therapeutic settings.

*Timing of Intervention.* Of the four randomized controlled trials, two were conducted on patients in the chronic stage, whereas one study was conducted in the acute stage and one in the subacute stage. Of the five case studies, three were done at the chronic stage[22,33,63] and two at the subacute stage.[6,41]

*Outcome Measures.* Most of the studies reviewed measured outcome variables at the impairment and activity limitation level. Typical instruments used to measure impairment level measures were the Action Research Arm Test (which measures upper limb dexterity), the Fugl-Meyer Assessment (which measures the ability of the arm to move against the typical synergistic pattern), the Wolf Motor Function Test (which quantifies motor function after stroke), and passive range of motion. Activity limitation was measured by measures such as the Rehabilitation Activities Profile (based on the International Classification of Impairments, Disabilities and Handicaps and which assesses disability and handicap), Motor Activity Log (which measures actual amount of use and quality of movement), Barthel index, and the Functional Independence Measure (which measures activity limitation).

*Results of the Review.* A number of case series provided the initial evidence of a positive effect of CIMT. The limitation of these studies was the lack of a control group. Of the four randomized controlled trials reviewed, only one study was a level I randomized controlled trial.[57] This level I randomized controlled trial demonstrated a modest effect of CIMT compared with the neurodevelopmental therapy. One year after training, only impairment level gains (measured by Action Research Arm Test) were maintained. The results of this study are confounded because the CIMT group performed better at the beginning of training. The two studies testing the typical CIMT training paradigm[12,53] demonstrated a positive benefit for CIMT; the only limitation was the small number of subjects in the study. Constraint-induced movement therapy demonstrated a benefit not only with an intense 2-week training program but also with a modified training program that more accurately reflected current practices[40] (Table 6-3).

*Clinical Implications.* Constraint-induced movement therapy appears to be a beneficial approach, particularly with individuals in the chronic stages. In fact, brain imaging of patients trained with CIMT has shown an increased activation in cortical area of the affected hemisphere.[28] Evidence of its benefit in the early stage after stroke is limited, however.[41] Furthermore, the literature

*Text continued on p.108*

**Table 6-2**

**Evidence for Task-Oriented Approach**

| AUTHORS AND YEAR | RATIONALE | DESIGN AND SUBJECTS | INTERVENTION AND OUTCOME MEASURES | RESULTS | COMMENTS | RATING |
|---|---|---|---|---|---|---|
| Kwakkel et al (1999)[24] | Test effect of different intensity of task-related leg and arm training in acute stroke stage; test whether training produces task-specific improvement | Single-blind RCT 101 subjects randomized in three groups (leg, arm, and control) Training for 5 days/week for 20 weeks Follow-up until 26 weeks | Leg group: sitting, standing, and weight bearing Arm group: leaning, ball pinching, grasping (forced use) Control: leg and arm immobilized 1. Barthel index 2. FAC 3. Action Research Arm Test | Training influenced task-specific improvement. Experimental groups did better than control group on activities of daily living scores, walking ability, and dexterity; leg training generalized better than arm training. | Very good study | I |
| Kwakkel et al (2002)[23] | Test effect of different intensity of task-related leg and arm training 1 year after stroke | RCT Follow-up of 1999 study 86 subjects from original group tested at 6 and 12 months | 1. Barthel index 2. FAC 3. Action Research Arm Test | No differences seen between groups at 6 months and 1 year; improvement was maintained at 1 year. Greater intensity of treatment improved speed of functional recovery in the first 6 months. | Very good study | I |
| Richards et al (1993)[44] | Test effect of early gait-focused therapy | RCT 27 subjects Experimental group: early task-based therapy (1.74 hours/day) Control group 1: early conventional PT (1.79 hours/day) Control group 2: conventional PT (0.73 hours/day) | Experimental group: early standing, weight-shifting, isokinetic exercises, and treadmill training 1. Fugl-Meyer Assessment 2. Barthel index 3. Berg Balance Scale 4. Gait velocity 6-month follow-up | Gait velocity was higher for experimental group. | Benefit in only one variable | II |

| Study | Design | Intervention/Measures | Results | Comments | Level |
|---|---|---|---|---|---|
| Dean and Shepherd (1997)[11] | Test effect of a 2-week program on sitting balance | RCT 20 subjects Experimental group: reaching tasks Control group: sham cognitive tasks 10 sessions over 2 weeks Posttest at 10 weeks | Training sitting balance during reaching tasks. Distance, direction, speed, seat height, and thigh support varied 1. Ground reaction forces 2. Electromyography 3. Reaching distance 4. Movement time | Experimental group performed better on reach distance, reach time, and ground reaction force. | Good treatment and study design Small sample size Few clinical tests given | II |
| Dean, Richards, and Malouin (2000)[10] | Test the effect of task-related circuit training in chronic stroke stage | RCT pilot study 2-month follow-up 9 subjects Exercise for 1 hour, 3 time week for 4 weeks | Experimental group: strengthening and functional activities Control group: functional activities 1. Walking speed and endurance 2. Vertical ground reaction force 3. Step test | Experimental group performed better on walking speed and endurance and on force production. | Small sample size Study only tested added influence of strength training. | II |
| Nelles et al (2001)[38] | Test brain plasticity after task-related training in early stroke stage | RCT 10 subjects after first stroke; early subacute stroke stage Training 4 times a week for 3 weeks | Task-oriented functional reach in different directions and distances Control group: stretching, range of motion 1. Positron emission tomography scan | After training, task-oriented group showed activation of contralateral sensorimotor cortex and bilateral activation of the inferior parietal cortex; control group showed weak activation of only the inferior parietal cortex. | Good study Small sample size | II |
| Malouin et al (1992)[32] | Test application of a task-oriented treatment in improving gait after acute stroke stage | Case series design 10 subjects 2 sessions/day 5 days/week for 8 weeks | Early standing, weight-shifting, isokinetic exercises and treadmill training 1. Treadmill velocity 2. Training duration | Treadmill velocity and training duration increased. | Small sample size No control group Double the typical treatment time in PT | V |

FAC, Functional ambulation category; PT, physical therapy; RCT, randomized controlled trial; SF-36, 36-item Short-Form Health Survey.

Continued

**Table 6-2**

**Evidence for Task-Oriented Approach—cont'd**

| AUTHORS AND YEAR | RATIONALE | DESIGN AND SUBJECTS | INTERVENTION AND OUTCOME MEASURES | RESULTS | COMMENTS | RATING |
|---|---|---|---|---|---|---|
| Smith et al (1999)[48] | Test a task-oriented treadmill exercise program in chronic stroke stage | Case series 14 subjects Training 3 times a week for 3 months | Reflexive and volitional torque generated by dynamometer at different velocities 1. Torque output at different velocities | Torque production for concentric and eccentric contractions increased. | Small sample size No control group | V |
| Monger, Carr, and Fowler (2002)[35] | Test a task-specific home exercise program in chronic stroke stage | Pretest, posttest case series design 6 subjects, 1year after stroke 3-week home exercise program | Intervention was based on motor learning; sit-to-stand and stepping was practiced at different seat heights, speeds, and repetitions. 1. Motor Assessment Scale (MAS) 2. Vertical ground reaction force 3. Walking speed over 10m 4. Grip strength | Scores on the MAS, vertical ground reaction force, and walking speed improved for experimental group; grip force did not improve. | No control group; small sample size Good pilot study | V |
| Bassile et al (2003)[5] | Test effect of a task-related obstacle training program in chronic stroke stage | Case-series Pretraining and posttraining; 1-month follow-up 5 subjects Training 2 times a week for 5 weeks | Subjects walked along a 10-m walkway over obstacles on two thirds of the trials 1. MAS walking section 2. 6-minute walk distance 3. Walking velocity 4. SF-36 | Improvements seen in walking velocity, 6-minute walk distance, MAS, and SF-36. | Good pilot study Small sample size No control group | V |

**Table 6-3**

## Evidence Table for Constraint-Induced Movement Therapy

| AUTHORS AND YEAR | RATIONALE | DESIGN AND SUBJECTS | INTERVENTION AND OUTCOME MEASURES | RESULTS | COMMENTS | RATING |
|---|---|---|---|---|---|---|
| Van der Lee et al (1999)[57] | Evaluate the effectiveness of forced use therapy; compare CIMT with Bobath therapy in chronic stroke stage | RCT 60 subjects Experimental group: immobilization and training Control group: bimanual training based on NDT Training was 6 hours/day 5 days/week for 2 weeks Follow-up for 1 year | Experimental group: splint worn for most of the day; training of functional activities Control group: bimanual activities 1. Rehabilitation Activities Profile 2. Action Research Arm Test (ARAT) 3. Fugl-Meyer Assessment 4. Motor Activity Log (MAL) | CIMT group performed better on ARAT and arm use 1 week after training; gains on ARAT were maintained after 1 year. CIMT group had greater amount of arm use but did not maintain in the long term. | Good study CIMT group performance better at start of training. Modest benefit of CIMT over Bobath approach | I |
| Taub et al (1993)[53] | Test whether forced use of the impaired limb counteracts learned nonuse in chronic stroke stage | RCT 9 subjects in chronic stroke stage Experimental group (4): restraint of the unimpaired limbs for 23 hours; therapy for 6 hours/day 5 days/week for 2 weeks Control group (5): attention control group 2-year follow-up | Limb restrained for 23 hours/day for experimental group. Control group asked to focus on use of impaired limb. 1. Emory Motor Function Test 2. ARAT 3. MAL 4. Passive range of motion | Performance time was quicker for restraint group; quality of movement and functional ability were better for restraint group. | Small sample size Experimental group had much more training. Training massed over 2 weeks No comparison with traditional rehabilitation | II |

*CIMT,* Constraint-induced movement therapy; *RCT,* randomized controlled trial; *NDT,* neurodevelopmental therapy; *PT,* physical therapy.

*Continued*

**Table 6-3**

## Evidence Table for Constraint-Induced Movement Therapy—cont'd

| AUTHORS AND YEAR | RATIONALE | DESIGN AND SUBJECTS | INTERVENTION AND OUTCOME MEASURES | RESULTS | COMMENTS | RATING |
|---|---|---|---|---|---|---|
| Dromerick, Edwards, and Hahn (2000)[12] | Compare CIMT with occupational therapy (OT) in the acute stage | RCT 20 subjects Experimental group (11): mitten worn 6 hours/day, plus OT and CIMT training 2 hours/day for 5 days/week for 2 weeks Control group (9): standard OT and circuit training | Mitten worn 6 hours/day for 14 days 1. ARAT 2. Barthel index 3. Functional Independence Measure (FIM) | CIMT group had better total ARAT scores and upper extremity FIM scores. No other differences were seen. | Little support for benefit of CIMT approach. Small sample size | II |
| Page et al (2002)[40] | Test the efficacy of a modified CIMT protocol in subacute stroke stage | RCT 14 subjects Modified CIMT group: half hour PT and OT 3 times a week for 10 weeks Regular therapy group: half hour PT and OT 3 times a week for 10 weeks Control group: no therapy | Modified CIMT group: restraint for 5 hours/day; training 1 hour/day Traditional group: PNF therapy 1. Fugl-Meyer Assessment 2. ARAT 3. MAL | No change was seen in traditional and control group. Modified CIMT group improved on Fugl-Meyer Assessment, ARAT, and MAL. | Small sample size | II |
| Wolf et al (1989)[63] | First study to test CIMT in chronic stroke stage | Case series Pretreatment and posttreatment 21 subjects Restraint and training 3-month follow-up | 14 days of restraint and 10 days of training 1. Wolf Motor Function Test (WMFT) | Arm function improved following restraint and training. | No control group Small sample size Limited outcome measures | V |

| Study | Purpose | Design | Intervention/Measures | Results | Limitations | Level |
|---|---|---|---|---|---|---|
| Kunkel et al (1999)[22] | Replicate findings of Taub et al[53] | Case series design Pretreatment and posttreatment 5 subjects in chronic stroke stage 3-month follow-up | Limb restrained for 23 hours a day for 14 days 1. MAL 2. WMFT 3. ARAT | Restraint improved MAL, WMFT, and quality of movement. | No control group Small sample size | V |
| Blanton and Wolf (1999)[6] | Test the effectiveness of CIMT in subacute stroke stage | Case report Pretreatment and posttreatment 3-month follow-up 14 days of restraint and 10 days of training | Hand constrained in a mitten for 23 hours a day 1. WMFT 2. MAL | Completion time improved on the WMFT; improvement seen on self report (MAL). | Single patient; limited generalizability | V |
| Miltner et al (1999)[33] | Replicate earlier findings on the benefit of CIMT | Case series 15 subjects in chronic stroke stage Sling on arm for 90% of waking time for 12 days Training for 7 hours/day for 8 days 6-month follow-up | Restraint and shaping with familiar household objects 1. MAL 2. WMFT 3. ARAT | Actual amount of use and quality of movement; functional ability improved and was retained over 6 months. | No control group Small sample size Massed practice | V |
| Page et al (2001)[41] | Test the efficacy of a modified CIMT protocol; compare CIMT embedded in therapy with no therapy in a subacute outpatient setting | Case series 6 subjects 2 subjects: OT/PT 3 times a week for 10 weeks plus sling and mitt for 5 hours/day 5 days/week 2 subjects: OT/PT for 10 weeks 2 subjects: no therapy 10-week follow-up | CIMT and traditional group received 30 minutes of training 3 times week. 1. Fugl-Meyer Assessment 2. ARAT 3. WMFT 4. MAL | CIMT group performed better on Fugl-Meyer Assessment, ARAT, WMFT, and MAL. | Small sample size No statistical analysis of Useful modification CIMT approach to outpatient therapy | V |

needs to address the criticism that the improvements demonstrated may be due to a nonspecific effect of increased intensity of treatment rather than to a specific effect of constrained-induced training.[56] Most of the studies reported in Table 6-3 used a standard CIMT training protocol in which training was massed over a period of 2 weeks and was compared with a control group that received attention training.

According to Taub and Uswatte,[54] the improvements were indeed a result of massing of practice. Given that similar positive results have been obtained by increasing the intensity of traditional physical therapy,[24] van der Lee[56] argues that using traditional therapeutic procedures that often may be less frustrating to patients than CIMT may be just as effective. The one study that compared CIMT with a control group that received a comparable intensity of therapy[57] demonstrated only a modest benefit of the CIMT approach. Thus, in future studies, comparison of CIMT with an equally intense control therapeutic program with a large group of subjects may be useful.

One recent study indicates that the effect of CIMT may not be simply a result of massing practice. Page, Sisto, Johnston, et al[40] tested a less intense CIMT training comparable with traditional intensity of therapy and reported positive results for the CIMT group. This is an encouraging result that needs to be replicated with larger number of subjects. Thus, although CIMT has provided encouraging results, at present the evidence is at best at level B (at least one level II randomized controlled trial).

Finally, the timing of training also may have an influence on outcome; the two randomized controlled trials conducted at the chronic stage[53,57] demonstrated greater benefit at impairment and activity limitation level measures compared with the study that tested CIMT in acute stroke stage.[12] One explanation for this may be that training early after a stroke may be more harmful, as suggested by an animal study that forced rats to use their affected limb early after cortical lesion.[56] However, training in the acute stage thus far has not shown any deleterious effects on patients.[12] Perhaps CIMT is more beneficial once learned nonuse has had time to set in.

### Body Weight Support and Treadmill Training to Improve Gait

*Rationale and Principles.* Approximately half the individuals who suffer a stroke do not recover their ability to walk independently.[4] Given that independent walking is a necessary prerequisite to successful community reintegration, not surprisingly gait training has occupied an important role in physical therapy practice following stroke. Gait training following stroke involves practice of individual segments of walking, practice of walking over ground with assistance of therapists and/or assistive devices, or more recently, practice of walking on a treadmill with partial body weight support.

Experiments on animals have shown that the basic neural circuitry for producing the rhythmic alternating movements of the lower limb is at the spinal cord level. Locomotor training with weight support of the hindlimbs has been shown to improve gait to near normal levels in cats whose spinal cords have been transected at thoracic levels, thereby isolating lower cord segments from the rest of the central nervous system.[2] In fact, patients with spinal cord injury have been shown to improve after treadmill training with body weight support.[62] Apart from the evidence of the benefit of treadmill training in patients with spinal cord injury, the rationale for this approach is that it removes some of the biomechanical and equilibrium constraints of weight bearing and facilitates walking by activation of spinal locomotor circuits.

*Outcome Studies.* A review of studies testing the effectiveness of body weight support training revealed the eight papers listed in Table 6-4. Of the eight studies, five studies were nonrandomized trials[26] or case series,[19,20,48,50] and only three were classified as randomized controlled trials.[9,39,58] Typical training with this approach involves beginning gait training on a treadmill by supporting the body in a harness. The initial support given is generally 40% of the body weight, which is gradually decreased as the patient improves. An exception to this procedure was training on a treadmill with support of the upper extremities.[26] The length of training ranged from 3 to 12 weeks in the studies reviewed.

*Timing of Intervention.* Treadmill training was initiated in the acute stage in one study,[39] in the subacute stage in three studies,[9,26,58] and in the chronic stage in four studies.[19,20,48,50]

*Outcome Measures.* Most of the studies reviewed measured outcome variables at the impairment and activity limitation level. Typical instruments used to assess impairment level measures were the Stroke Rehabilitation Assessment of Movement (which evaluates voluntary movement of the limbs and mobility), Berg Balance Scale (which evaluates balance during sitting and standing activities), walking speed, distance and endurance, the Fugl-Meyer Assessment (which evaluates locomotor function and control, sensory quality, and balance), and kinematic analysis of walking. Instruments used to measure activity limitation were the Functional Independence Measure, Functional Ambulation Classification (which quantifies amount of assistance needed in walking), and the Rivermead Motor Assessment.

*Results of the Review.* As with most intervention approaches, the initial support for treadmill training with weight support came from case series with smaller number of subjects, ranging from 7 to 24 subjects.[19,20,48,50] These

**Table 6-4**

## Evidence Table for Treadmill Training With Body Weight Support

| AUTHORS AND YEAR | RATIONALE | DESIGN AND SUBJECTS | INTERVENTION AND OUTCOME MEASURES | RESULTS | COMMENTS | RATING |
|---|---|---|---|---|---|---|
| Visintin et al (1998)[58] | Test effectiveness of body weight support during treadmill training in subacute stroke stage | RCT<br>100 subjects in subacute stage 6-week training<br>Experimental group: treadmill and body weight support<br>Control group: treadmill only | 1. Berg Balance Scale<br>2. Stroke Rehabilitation Assessment of Movement<br>3. Gait speed<br>4. Gait endurance | Subjects with body weight support had better balance, motor recovery, and walking speed and endurance compared with control group. | Very good study<br>3-month follow-up Large subject pool | I |
| Nilsson et al (2001)[39] | Compare walking training over ground (based on a motor relearning approach) with treadmill training in acute stroke stage | RCT<br>60 subjects<br>Control group: walking training<br>Experimental group: treadmill training with body weight support 30 minutes/day 5 days/week for 2 months | 1. Functional Independence Measure (FIM)<br>2. Fugl-Meyer Assessment<br>3. Functional Ambulation Classification (FAC)<br>4. Walking velocity (10 m)<br>5. Berg Balance Scale | Both groups improved performance on the FIM, walking velocity, FAC, and balance. No differences were seen across groups. | Good study<br>Randomized trial 10-month follow-up | I |
| da Cunha et al (2002)[9] | Compare body weight support treadmill training and typical therapy with only typical therapy | RCT<br>13 patients in subacute stage (<6 weeks)<br>20 minutes/day<br>5 days/week for 3 weeks | 1. FAC<br>2. Gait speed<br>3. Walking distance<br>4. Energy expenditure | Differences were seen in walking energy cost and walking distance. No differences were seen for other outcome measures. | Small sample size<br>No follow-up | II |

*RCT,* Randomized controlled trial; *PT,* physical therapy.

*Continued*

**Table 6-4**

**Evidence Table for Treadmill Training With Body Weight Support—cont'd**

| AUTHORS AND YEAR | RATIONALE | DESIGN AND SUBJECTS | INTERVENTION AND OUTCOME MEASURES | RESULTS | COMMENTS | RATING |
|---|---|---|---|---|---|---|
| Laufer et al (2001)[26] | Compare walking training over ground with treadmill training | Nonrandomized trial 25 subjects in subacute stage Training for 3 weeks Control group: over ground ambulation and PT Experimental group: treadmill ambulation with railing support and PT | 1. Functional walking ability (FAC) 2. Walking speed (10-m walk) 3. Stride length (foot switch) 4. Temporal gait features 5. Electromyographic activation | Treadmill training improved functional ambulation, stride length and paretic single stance. | Small sample size No randomization | III |
| Hesse et al (1994)[20] | Test partial body weight support for trunk stabilization, eliminate the need for equilibrium reflexes, and focus training on stepping patterns | Single group pretreatment and posttreatment design (case series design) 9 subjects Mean of 129 days after stroke 3 weeks of PT before training; multiple test sessions | 1. FAC gait ability 2. Standing balance test (posture) 3. Rivermead Motor Assessment score (motor functions) 4. Motricity Index | Gait, standing balance, and overall motor performance improved in all patients. Muscle tone and strength remained stable. | Small sample size No control group | V |

| Study | Purpose | Design/Subjects | Measures | Results | Limitations | Level |
|---|---|---|---|---|---|---|
| Hesse et al (1995)[19] | Test effectiveness of body weight support training to conventional PT (Bobath approach) in chronic stroke stage | Case series design 7 subjects A-B-A design (A, treadmill; B, Bobath approach) | 1. FAC 2. Rivermead Motor Assessment 3. Motricity Index 4. Modified Ashworth Spasticity Scale 5. Walking velocity | Treadmill training was better for functional ambulation, walking velocity, cadence, and stride length compared to Bobath treatment. | Small sample size | V |
| Smith et al (1999)[48] | Test whether treadmill training increases muscle strength and decreases reflexes in chronic stroke stage | Case series design 14 subjects Low-intensity treadmill walking 3 times a week for 3 months | 1. Reflexive and volitional torque (dynamometer) | Volitional torque production improved after training for after training for concentric and eccentric contractions. | Small sample size No control group No follow-up No correlation with functional tests | V |
| Sullivan, Knowlton, and Dobkin (2002)[50] | Effect of treadmill speed during body weight support training | Case series design; repeated measures 24 chronic stroke subjects 12 training sessions (20 minutes each) over 4-5 weeks | 1. Fugl-Meyer Assessment 2. Self-selected walking speed over ground (10-m walk) | Training at speeds comparable to normal walking velocity were more effective in improving self-selected walking velocity. Gains were maintained over 3 months. | Small sample size No control group | V |

studies demonstrated improvements in walking velocity[19,50] and cadence,[19] balance,[20] and functional ambulation.[19] However, the strength of the results was limited by the small number of subjects and the lack of a control group. The results of the randomized controlled trials provide clearer support for treadmill training. Walking on a treadmill with the body weight supported by a harness[58] produced positive results compared with training that emphasized walking over ground for patients in subacute stroke. When treadmill training was compared with ambulation over ground in the acute stage, no differences were seen; both groups improved a similar amount.[39] When treadmill training was provided in addition to typical rehabilitation, positive results were reported.[9] Supporting the weight of the body seems to be critical in improving functional ambulation; this was confirmed in a randomized controlled trial in which one group was given body weight support while walking on a treadmill, whereas the control group simply trained at walking on the treadmill.[58]

*Clinical Implications.* The evidence for treadmill training with body weight support, although positive, is not conclusive. Two of the four randomized controlled trials used a small number of subjects, limiting the generalizability of the studies.[9,26] Of the two larger randomized trials, one demonstrated support for body weight support training,[58] whereas the other did not show a benefit larger than gait training over ground based on principles of motor learning.[39] Thus the evidence is at the grade B level and requires additional randomized controlled trials with large numbers of subjects.

### Robot-Aided Motor Training

*Rationale and Principles.* A recent addition to the arsenal of techniques for stroke rehabilitation is the use of robotic manipulators for providing training of arm movements. Robot manipulators have been used successfully in experimental paradigms that attempted to elucidate the mechanisms underlying normal motor control and learning[14,46] and also to elucidate mechanisms underlying disorders of upper limb movements in patients with movement disorders.[47]

The rationale for using a robotic device in rehabilitation is to decrease the labor-intensive nature of therapy and to provide a device that could be used for quantitative evaluation and treatment.[59] These authors contend that current therapeutic evaluations are usually subjective and that therapists spend much time on one-on-one interaction with patients. The idea is to have devices available at rehabilitation centers for use when the patient is not in therapy sessions. Given that patients spend a large percentage of time outside therapist interaction, an attempt at facilitating practice during this time should be beneficial. Robot-assisted training attempts to provide intensive practice of repetitive and stereotyped movements.

*Outcome Studies.* A review of studies testing the effectiveness of robot assisted training revealed six papers, as listed in Table 6-5. Of the six studies, one was a case series,[43] two were nonrandomized case control experiments,[1,60] and three were classified as level II randomized controlled trials.[21,31,59] Typical training with this approach involves the patient making horizontal plane movements while grasping the handle of the robot manipulator. Target locations and patient movement are displayed on a computer screen in front of the patient. Typically, patients are trained to produce movements of the shoulder and elbow joints while the wrist and hand joints and the trunk are immobilized with restraints. The robot is typically programmed to produce an assistive force or resistive force during movements.

*Timing of Intervention.* Three studies tested the effectiveness of robot training in the subacute stroke stage,[1,21,59] and three tested its effectiveness in the chronic stroke stage.[31,43,60]

*Outcome Measures.* Most of the studies reviewed measured outcome variables at the impairment and activity limitation levels. A typical instrument used to measure impairment level measures was the Fugl-Meyer Assessment (which evaluates locomotor function and control, motor power, and motor status score and provides kinematic analysis of pointing movements). Instruments used to measure activity limitation were the Functional Independence Measure and the Barthel index.

*Results of the Review.* Subjects who were trained with active, active-assistive, passive, and resistive movements improved on impairment level measures such as movement speed and distance. However, the study was confounded by the lack of a control group.[43] All the randomized controlled trials demonstrated an improvement that was specific to shoulder and elbow movements, which is not surprising because training involved extensive practice of elbow and shoulder movements. Only one study demonstrated beneficial transfer of training to functional skills.[59] This study was confounded by the fact that the control group had much less training with the robot than the experimental group. Long-term follow-up (at 3 years) indicated that only impairment level measures maintained improvements; no benefit was seen for activity limitation level measures.[60]

*Clinical Implications.* The results of robot-assisted training are inconclusive at present. Before larger randomized controlled trials are implemented, however, the rationale and experimental procedures need to be clarified. For instance, at present, robot training provides practice of pointing movements (movements of the shoulder and elbow) on the horizontal plane. In an effort

**Table 6-5**

## Evidence Table for Robot-Assisted Therapy

| AUTHORS AND YEAR | THEORETICAL RATIONALE | DESIGN AND SUBJECTS | TREATMENT AND OUTCOME MEASURES | RESULTS | COMMENTS | RATING |
|---|---|---|---|---|---|---|
| Krebs et al (1998)[21] | Test the use of a robot manipulator in stroke rehabilitation Test whether neurore-habilitation can be less labor intensive on therapists | RCT 20 subjects in subacute stroke stage Control group: regular rehabilitation and sham robot training (1 hour/week) Experimental group: regular rehabilitation and robot training (4-5 hours/week) Training for 7 weeks | Patients moved the robot actively or with assistance; the training was to make movements that required motion at shoulder, elbow, or both joints. 1. Functional Independence Measure (FIM) 2. Fugl-Meyer Assessment 3. Motor Status Score 4. Motor Power Scale (to assess strength) 5. Kinematic variables | The experimental group showed improvement in shoulder and elbow movements only. No differences were seen in the other measures. | Small sample size Experimental group had more training. | II |
| Volpe et al (2000)[59] | Test whether additional sensorimotor training of the paretic limb enhances motor outcome in subacute stroke stage | RCT 56 patients in subacute stage 1 hour/day 5 days/week for a total of 25 sessions Experimental group: 5 hours/week on robot Control group: 1 hour/week on robot | Subjects pointed to a series of targets that required motion at shoulder, elbow, or both joints. 1. Fugl-Meyer Assessment 2. Motor Status Score 3. Motor Power Score 4. FIM | Experimental group had better motor outcome related to shoulder and elbow movements and better FIM scores than control group. | Control group had much less robot training. Limited functional transfer | II |

*RCT,* Randomized controlled trial; *PT,* physical therapy; *NDT,* neurodevelopmental therapy.

*Continued*

**Table 6-5**

## Evidence Table for Robot-Assisted Therapy—cont'd

| AUTHORS AND YEAR | THEORETICAL RATIONALE | DESIGN AND SUBJECTS | TREATMENT AND OUTCOME MEASURES | RESULTS | COMMENTS | RATING |
|---|---|---|---|---|---|---|
| Lum et al (2002)[31] | Compare robotic manipulation of an impaired limb with conventional PT (NDT) in chronic stroke stage | RCT 6-month follow-up 27 subjects, chronic hemiparesis Experimental group: robot-assisted training of shoulder and elbow movements Control group: NDT and robot exposure at each session 24 1-hour sessions | Experimental group: standard rehabilitation and robot-aided therapy Control group: standard rehabilitation and sham robot therapy 1. Fugl-Meyer Assessment 2. Barthel index 3. FIM (self-care and transfer sections) 4. Strength measured through force transducer 5. Reaching kinematics | Robot-assisted group performed better on the proximal Fugl-Meyer Assessment and on the 6-month follow-up on the FIM and had greater reach extent. | Small sample size for RCT | II |
| Aisen et al (1997)[1] | Test whether robotic manipulation of an impaired limb influences motor recovery in early stroke stage | Nonrandomized control group 20 subjects in subacute stage Experimental group: 4 to 5 hours/week of robot training in addition to standard rehabilitation. Control group: Weekly to biweekly session with robot | 1. Upper extremity subsection of Fugl-Meyer Scale 2. Functional Independence Measure 3. Motor power 4. Motor status score | Experimental group improved more than the control group. | Small sample size No randomization | III |

| Study | Purpose | Design | Outcome Measures | Results | Level | Comments |
|---|---|---|---|---|---|---|
| Volpe et al (1999)[60] | Long-term follow-up to test whether robotic manipu-lation of an impaired limb influences motor recovery in chronic stroke stage | Nonrandomized control group trial 12 subjects 3-year follow-up | 1. FIM 2. Fugl-Meyer Assessment 3. Motor Status Score 4. Motor Power Scale | Experimental group retained advantage on Motor Status Score for the shoulder and elbow movements. No differences were seen in the Fugl-Meyer Assessment scores. | III | Patients in the robot treatment group were younger. Small sample size Training benefit was specific to elbow and shoulder muscles. |
| Reinkensmeyer et al (2000)[43] | Explore the effect of active-assistive therapy using robot in chronic stroke stage | Case series 3 subjects (chronic stroke patients) 3 sessions per week for at least 1 month | Subjects pointed to a series of targets as fast as possible 1. Reaching distance 2. Velocity 3. Muscle tone | All subjects improved movement velocity and reaching distance and decreased tone. | V | Small sample size No statistical analysis No control group Robot therapy is similar to passive movement, guiding the limb through simple spatial paths. |

to isolate movements to these two joints, the trunk and distal extremities often are stabilized by constraints producing rather unnatural conditions for practice of arm movements. Functional reaching movements involve coordinated movement of the trunk-arm complex and of the wrist-hand complex. Whether practice of isolated components of the shoulder-elbow complex would transfer to real-world situations is unclear, given the task-specific nature of transfer of training. The responsibility of therapists is to select appropriate, challenging functional tasks, vary task parameters, progress to more difficult tasks, and test for transfer. Given the complexity of therapeutic training, robot manipulators can perhaps serve best by providing quantitative evaluation of impairments rather than as a therapeutic tool.

## SUMMARY

A challenging yet exciting period for stroke rehabilitation is occurring as occupational and physical therapists are being asked to provide training based on sound scientific principles and with demonstrated effectiveness. The lack of support for traditional neurotherapeutic approaches such as NDT, recent advances in understanding of motor control and dyscontrol, and emerging technologies have facilitated a second paradigm shift toward a functional task-oriented approach. The challenge for the next decade is to develop more creative, functional, task-oriented intervention techniques that will maximize best the independent functioning of patients within their natural contextual settings[8] and to test these techniques in a systematic manner at different stages of the recovery process, in different practice settings, and at different intensities. Most likely, no one technique will offer a panacea for stroke rehabilitation given the varied nature of impairments and activity limitations.

## ACKNOWLEDGMENTS

The author acknowledges Glen Gillen and Clare Bassile for helpful discussions. This work was supported in part by a VIDDA Foundation grant to the Department of Rehabilitation Medicine.

## REVIEW QUESTIONS

1. What is evidence-based practice?
2. What are the principles of evidence-based practice?
3. What are the criteria for reviewing articles on treatment outcomes?
4. Describe the most common research designs used in outcome studies.
5. What are some of the basic principles of neurotherapeutic approaches?
6. Is there evidence to support the application of neurotherapeutic approaches?
7. What are some of the basic principles of the functional task-oriented approach?
8. Describe the evidence to support the task-oriented approach, CIMT, treadmill training and body weight support, and robot-assisted training.

## REFERENCES

1. Aisen ML, Krebs HI, Hogan N, et al: The effect of robot-assisted therapy and rehabilitative training on motor recovery following stroke, *Arch Neurol* 54(4):443-446, 1997.
2. Barbeau H, Rossignol S: Recovery of locomotion after chronic spinalization in the adult cat, *Brain Res* 412(1):84-95, 1987.
3. Basmajian JV, Gowland CA, Finlayson JA, et al: Stroke treatment: comparison of integrated behavioral-physical therapy vs traditional physical therapy programs, *Arch Phys Med Rehabil* 68(5 pt 1):267-272, 1987.
4. Bassile CC, Bock C: Gait training. In Craik RL, Oatis CA, editors: *Gait analysis: theory and practice*, St Louis, 1995, Mosby.
5. Bassile CC, Dean C, Boden-Albala B, et al: Obstacle training programme for individuals post stroke: feasibility study, *Clin Rehabil* 17(2):130-136, 2003.
6. Blanton S, Wolf SL: An application of upper-extremity constraint-induced movement therapy in a patient with subacute stroke, *Phys Ther* 79(9):847-853, 1999.
7. Bobath B: *Adult hemiplegia: evaluation and treatment*, ed 3, Oxford, 1990, Butterworth-Heinemann.
8. Carr JH, Shepherd RB: *Stroke rehabilitation: guidelines for exercise and training to optimize motor skill*, Oxford, 2003, Butterworth-Heinemann.
9. da Cunha IT Jr, Lim PA, Qureshy H, et al: Gait outcomes after acute stroke rehabilitation with supported treadmill ambulation training: a randomized controlled pilot study, *Arch Phys Med Rehabil* 83(9):1258-1265, 2002.
10. Dean CM, Richards CL, Malouin F: Task-related circuit training improves performance of locomotor tasks in chronic stroke: a randomized, controlled pilot trial, *Arch Phys Med Rehabil* 81(4):409-417, 2000.
11. Dean CM, Shepherd RB: Task-related training improves performance of seated reaching tasks after stroke: a randomized controlled trial, *Stroke* 28(4):722-728, 1997.
12. Dromerick AW, Edwards DF, Hahn M: Does the application of constraint-induced movement therapy during acute rehabilitation reduce arm impairment after ischemic stroke? *Stroke* 31(12):2984-2988, 2000.
13. Feys HM, De Weerdt WJ, Selz BE, et al: Effect of a therapeutic intervention for the hemiplegic upper limb in the acute phase after stroke, *Stroke* 29(4):785-792, 1998.
14. Flash T, Hogan N: The coordination of arm movements: an experimentally confirmed mathematical model, *J Neurosci* 5(7):1688-1703, 1985.
15. Gentile AM: Skill acquisition: action, movement and neuromotor processes. In Carr J, Shepherd RB, editor: *Movement science: foundations for physical therapy in rehabilitation*, Gaithersburg, Md, 2000, Aspen.
16. Gordon J: Assumptions underlying physical therapy intervention: theoretical and historical perspectives. In Carr J, Shepherd RB, editor: *Movement science: foundations for physical therapy in rehabilitation*, Gaithersburg, Md, 2000, Aspen.
17. Hafsteinsdottir TB: Neurodevelopmental treatment: application to nursing and its effects on the hemiplegic stroke patient, *J Neurosci Nurs* 28(1):36-47, 1996.
18. Helewa A, Walker JM: *Critical evaluation of research in physical rehabilitation*, Philadelphia, 2000, Saunders.
19. Hesse SA, Bertelt C, Jahnke MT, et al: Treadmill training with partial body weight support compared with physiotherapy in nonambulatory hemiparetic patients, *Stroke* 26(6):976-981, 1995.

20. Hesse SA, Bertelt C, Schaffrin A, et al: Restoration of gait in non-ambulatory hemiparetic patients by treadmill training with partial body-weight support, *Arch Phys Med Rehabil* 75(10):1087-1093, 1994.

20a. Howle JM: Neuro-developmental treatment approach: theoretical foundations and principles of clinical practice. Laguna Beach, Calif, 2002, Neuro-Developmental Treatment Association.

21. Krebs HI, Hogan N, Aisen ML, et al: Robot-aided neurorehabilitation, *IEEE Trans Rehabil Eng* 6(1):75-87, 1998.

22. Kunkel A, Kopp B, Muller G, et al: Constraint-induced movement therapy for motor recovery in chronic stroke patients, *Arch Phys Med Rehabil* 80(6):624-628, 1999.

23. Kwakkel G, Kollen BJ, Wagenaar RC: Long term effects of intensity of upper and lower limb training after stroke: a randomised trial, *J Neurol Neurosurg Psychiatry* 72(4):473-479, 2002.

24. Kwakkel G, Wagenaar RC, Twisk JW, et al: Intensity of leg and arm training after primary middle-cerebral-artery stroke: a randomised trial, *Lancet* 354(9174):191-196, 1999.

25. Langhammer B, Stanghelle JK: Bobath or motor relearning programme? A comparison of two different approaches of physiotherapy in stroke rehabilitation: a randomized controlled study, *Clin Rehabil* 14(4):361-369, 2000.

26. Laufer Y, Dickstein R, Chefez Y, et al: The effect of treadmill training on the ambulation of stroke survivors in the early stages of rehabilitation: a randomized study, *J Rehabil Res Dev* 38(1):69-78, 2001.

27. Law M: *Evidence-based rehabilitation: a guide to practice*, Thorofare, NJ, 2002, Slack.

28. Liepert J, Bauder H, Wolfgang HR, et al: Treatment-induced cortical reorganization after stroke in humans, *Stroke* 31(6):1210-1216, 2000.

29. Lincoln NB, Parry RH, Vass CD: Randomized, controlled trial to evaluate increased intensity of physiotherapy treatment of arm function after stroke, *Stroke* 30(3):573-579, 1999.

30. Lord JP, Hall K: Neuromuscular reeducation versus traditional programs for stroke rehabilitation, *Arch Phys Med Rehabil* 67(2):88-91, 1986.

31. Lum PS, Burgar CG, Shor PC, et al: Robot-assisted movement training compared with conventional therapy techniques for the rehabilitation of upper-limb motor function after stroke, *Arch Phys Med Rehabil* 83(7):952-959, 2002.

32. Malouin F, Potvin M, Prevost J, et al: Use of an intensive task-oriented gait training program in a series of patients with acute cerebrovascular accidents, *Phys Ther* 72(11):781-793, 1992.

33. Miltner WH, Bauder H, Sommer M, et al: Effects of constraint-induced movement therapy on patients with chronic motor deficits after stroke: a replication, *Stroke* 30(3):586-592, 1999.

34. Mohide EA: What is EBP: how do we facilitate its use? In Wong R, editor: *Evidence-based healthcare practice: general principles and focused applications to geriatric physical therapy*, Arlington, Va, 2002, Marymount University.

35. Monger C, Carr JH, Fowler V: Evaluation of a home-based exercise and training programme to improve sit-to-stand in patients with chronic stroke, *Clin Rehabil* 16(4):361-367, 2002.

36. Mudie MH, Winzeler-Mercay U, Radwan S, et al: Training symmetry of weight distribution after stroke: a randomized controlled pilot study comparing task-related reach, Bobath and feedback training approaches, *Clin Rehabil* 16(6):582-592, 2002.

37. Mulder T, Hulstijn W, Meer J: EMG feedback and the restoration of motor control: a controlled group study of 12 hemiparetic patients, *Am J Phys Med Rehabil* 65(4):173-178, 1986.

38. Nelles G, Jentzen W, Jueptner M, et al: Arm training induced brain plasticity in stroke studied with serial positron emission tomography, *Neuroimage* 13(6 pt 1):1146-1154, 2001.

39. Nilsson L, Carlsson J, Danielsson A, et al: Walking training of patients with hemiparesis at an early stage after stroke: a comparison of walking training on a treadmill with body weight support and walking training on the ground, *Clin Rehabil* 15(5):515-527, 2001.

40. Page SJ, Sisto SA, Johnston MV, et al: Modified constraint-induced therapy after subacute stroke: a preliminary study, *Neurorehabil Neural Repair* 16(3):290-295, 2002.

41. Page SJ, Sisto SA, Levine P, et al: Modified constraint induced therapy: a randomized feasibility and efficacy study, *J Rehabil Res Dev* 38(5):583-590, 2001.

42. Pollock AS, Durward BR, Rowe PJ, et al: The effect of independent practice of motor tasks by stroke patients: a pilot randomized controlled trial, *Clin Rehabil* 16(5):473-480, 2002.

43. Reinkensmeyer DJ, Kahn LE, Averbuch M, et al: Understanding and treating arm movement impairment after chronic brain injury: progress with the ARM guide, *J Rehabil Res Dev* 37(6):653-662, 2000.

44. Richards CL, Malouin F, Wood-Dauphinee S, et al: Task-specific physical therapy for optimization of gait recovery in acute stroke patients, *Arch Phys Med Rehabil* 74(6):612-620, 1993.

45. Sackett DL: *Clinical epidemiology: a basic science for clinical medicine*, ed 2, Boston, 1991, Little, Brown.

46. Shadmehr R, Donchin O, Hwang E-J, et al: Learning to compensate for dynamics of reaching movements. In Vaadia E, editor: *Motor cortex and voluntary movements*, Boca Raton, Fla, 2003, CRC Press.

47. Smith MA, Brandt J, Shadmehr R: Motor disorder in Huntington's disease begins as a dysfunction in error feedback control, *Nature* 403:544-549, 2000.

48. Smith GV, Silver KHC, Goldberg AP, et al: "Task-oriented" exercise improves hamstring strength and spastic reflexes in chronic stroke patients, *Stroke* 30(10):2112-2118, 1999.

49. Stern PH, McDowell F, Miller JM, et al: Effects of facilitation exercise techniques in stroke rehabilitation, *Arch Phys Med Rehabil* 51(9):526-531, 1970.

50. Sullivan KJ, Knowlton BJ, Dobkin BH: Step training with body weight support: effect of treadmill speed and practice paradigms on poststroke locomotor recovery, *Arch Phys Med Rehabil* 83(5):683-691, 2002.

51. Sunderland A, Tinson DJ, Bradley EL, et al: Enhanced physical therapy improves recovery of arm function after stroke: a randomised controlled trial, *J Neurol Neurosurg Psychiatry* 55(7):530-535, 1992.

52. Taub E: Movement in non-human primates deprived of somatosensory feedback, *Exerc Sport Sci Rev* 4:335-374, 1977.

53. Taub E, Miller NE, Novack TA, et al: Technique to improve chronic motor deficit after stroke, *Arch Phys Med Rehabil* 74(4):347-354, 1993.

54. Taub E, Uswatte G: Constraint-induced movement therapy and massed practice, *Stroke* 31(4):983-986, 2000.

55. Taub E, Wolf SL: Constraint induced movement techniques to facilitate upper extremity use in stroke patients, *Top Stroke Rehabil* 3(4):38-61, 1997.

56. van der Lee JH: Constraint-induced therapy for stroke: more of the same or something completely different? *Curr Opin Neurol* 14(6):741-744, 2001.

57. van der Lee JH, Wagenaar RC, Lankhorst GJ, et al: Forced use of the upper extremity in chronic stroke patients: results from a single-blind randomized clinical trial, *Stroke* 30(11):2369-2375, 1999.

58. Visintin M, Barbeau H, Korner-Bitensky N, et al: A new approach to retrain gait in stroke patients through body weight support and treadmill stimulation, *Stroke* 29(6):1122-1128, 1998.

59. Volpe BT, Krebs HI, Hogan N, et al: A novel approach to stroke rehabilitation: robot-aided sensorimotor stimulation, *Neurology* 54(10):1938-1944, 2000.

60. Volpe BT, Krebs HI, Hogan N, et al: Robot training enhanced motor outcome in patients with stroke maintained over 3 years, *Neurology* 53(8):1874-1876, 1999.

61. Wagenaar RC, Meijer OG, van Wieringen PC, et al: The functional recovery of stroke: a comparison between neuro-developmental treatment and the Brunnstrom method, *Scand J Rehabil Med* 22(1):1-8, 1990.

62. Wernig A, Muller S: Improvement of walking in spinal cord injured persons after treadmill training. In Wernig A, editor: *Plasticity of motoneuronal connections*, Berlin, 1991, Elsevier.

63. Wolf SL, Lecraw DE, Barton LA, et al: Forced use of hemiplegic upper extremities to reverse the effect of learned nonuse among chronic stroke and head-injured patients, *Exp Neurol* 104(2):125-132, 1989.

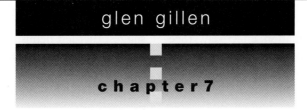

glen gillen

chapter 7

# Trunk Control: A Prerequisite for Functional Independence

**key terms**

activities of daily living          postural control          trunk
hemiplegia

**chapter objectives**

After completing this chapter, the reader will be able to accomplish the following:

1. Understand the functional anatomy of the trunk.
2. Understand the control requirements for various movement patterns and activities.
3. By activity analysis, understand key components of trunk control required for independence in various activities of daily living.
4. Understand treatment activities to improve and compensate for loss of trunk control.

Loss of trunk control commonly occurs in patients who have had a stroke. Impairment in trunk control may lead to the following:

- Dysfunction in upper and lower limb control
- Increased risk of falls
- Potential for spinal deformity and contracture
- Impaired ability to interact with the environment
- Visual dysfunction resulting from head/neck malalignment
- Symptoms of dysphagia because of proximal malalignment
- Decreased independence in activities of daily living (ADL) and other meaningful tasks
- Decreased sitting and standing tolerance, balance, and function

For a comprehensive review of this topic, see Chapters 4 and 5 for incorporating task-oriented, learning and environmental strategies into treatment plans focused on improving trunk control, Chapter 8 for a complete overview of the multiple variables that affect balance skills, Chapter 10 for a review on the interdependence of trunk control and upper extremity function, and Chapter 14 for an overview of mobility impairments.

Regaining trunk control has been a major focus of stroke rehabilitation for many years. The majority of the literature that focuses on trunk control/postural control is based on expert clinicians' observations of and treatment philosophies about trunk dysfunction after stroke. The traditional approaches to treatment[6,7,14,18,29] have emphasized improved trunk control as a key element of focus in the stroke population, and this focus continues as therapists integrate current models of motor control and learning (see Chapters 4 and 6).

Well-controlled studies that specifically examine the effect of decreased trunk control on independence in ADL are lacking in the rehabilitation literature. Thus, another goal of this chapter is to serve as an impetus for more studies that ultimately will enhance therapists' ability to treat the stroke population effectively. (See Chapter 10 for the available research related to trunk control during upper extremity tasks and Chapter 8 for research concerning trunk control and posture in relation to balance dysfunction.)

Bohannon, Cassidy, and Walsh[10] have studied trunk muscle strength impairments after stroke (specifically forward and lateral trunk flexion strength). Their study included 20 patients with stroke and resultant hemiparesis and 20 control subjects. Trunk strength was measured with a handheld dynamometer; subjects were seated upright during the study. Results indicated that trunk strength, whether lateral or forward, was significantly decreased in the patients relative to controls. The greatest difference in strength was in forward flexion strength. The patients demonstrated trunk weakness on the paretic side relative to the nonparetic side. The conclusion was that trunk muscle strength was impaired multidirectionally in the stroke population.

Bohannon[9] studied 11 stroke patients and evaluated lateral trunk flexion strength and the effect of trunk muscle strength on sitting balance and ambulation. His results indicated that the mean lateral flexion force on the paretic side was 32.1%, which was significantly less than the mean lateral flexion force on the nonparetic side. His study further demonstrated a statistically significant correlation between sitting balance and strength of the lateral trunk flexors.

Bohannon[8] also studied the recovery of trunk muscle strength after stroke in 28 subjects. Subjects' strength was tested in a variety of directions, including forward flexion, movement toward the paretic side, and movement toward the nonparetic side. Statistical analysis demonstrated that trunk muscle strength increased significantly over time. The greatest recovery was in the direction of forward flexion. This study again verified a strong correlation between trunk muscle strength and sitting balance at the initial and final assessments.

In addition to the mentioned studies, several studies have focused on documenting electromyographic activity in normal subjects during a variety of tasks including trunk displacements.* See Basmajian's and DeLuca's[4] text for a comprehensive review of electromyographic studies performed during functional tasks.

Esparza et al[19] examined hemispheric specialization and the coordination of arm and trunk movements during pointing in subjects with strokes. They concluded that arm and trunk timing was disrupted compared with healthy controls, temporal coordination of trunk and arm recruitment is mediated bilaterally by each hemisphere,

and that the differences they found in the range of trunk displacement between subjects with right and left lesions suggest that left hemisphere plays a greater role than the right in controlling complex arm-trunk movements.

## FUNCTIONAL TRUNK ANATOMY

### Skeletal System

This section reviews the bony components of trunk anatomy, including articulations and range of motion.

*Vertebral Column.* The vertebral column is made up of 26 vertebrae, which are classified as follows:

Cervical: 7
Thoracic: 12
Lumbar: 5
Sacral: 5 (fused into one bone, the sacrum)
Coccygeal: 4 (fused into one or two bones, the coccyx)

As a whole the vertebral column from sacrum to skull is equivalent to a joint with three degrees of freedom[26] in the directions of flexion and extension, right and left lateral flexion, and axial rotation. Kapandji[26] has documented the range of motion (ROM) throughout the vertebral column (Box 7-1).

An understanding of spinal alignment is necessary for effective evaluation and treatment planning. Normal alignment of the vertebral column implies that the appropriate spinal curvatures are present. In the sagittal plane the vertebral column shows four curvatures[26] (Box 7-2 and Figure 7-1).

---

**Box 7-1**

**Range of Motion of the Vertebral Column**

**FLEXION**

Cervical: 40 degrees
Thoracolumbar: 105 degrees
Total: 145 degrees

**EXTENSION**

Cervical: 75 degrees
Thoracolumbar: 60 degrees
Total: 135 degrees

**LATERAL FLEXION**

Cervical: 35 to 45 degrees
Thoracic: 20 degrees
Lumbar: 20 degrees
Total: 75 to 85 degrees

**ROTATION**

Cervical: 45 to 50 degrees
Thoracic: 35 degrees
Lumbar: 5 degrees
Total: 85 to 90 degrees

---

*References 1, 4, 16, 21, 38, 40.

### Box 7-2

### Spinal Curvatures

Sacral curvature (fixed curvature): convex posteriorly
Lumbar curvature: concave posteriorly
Thoracic curvature: convex posteriorly
Cervical curvature: concave posteriorly

***Pelvis.*** According to Kapandji,[26] "The bony pelvis constitutes the base of the trunk. It supports the abdomen and links the vertebral column to the lower limbs. It is a closed osteo-articular ring made up of three bony parts and three joints." The three bony parts include the two iliac bones and the sacrum. The three joints of the pelvis include two sacroiliac joints and the symphysis pubis.

To remember that because of the firmness of the sacroiliac and lumbosacral junctions, every pelvic movement is accompanied by a realignment of the spine predominantly in the lumbar region is critical.[35]

Pelvic tilt can occur anteriorly or posteriorly. In an anterior tilt the anterior superior iliac spines of the ilia migrate anteriorly to the foremost part of the symphysis pubis. This pelvic motion accentuates the lumbar curve and results in increased hip flexion. In contrast, posterior pelvic tilt results in a "flattening" of the lumbar curve and an increase in hip extension.

Lateral pelvis tilting results in a height discrepancy of the iliac crests and is accompanied by lateral spine flexion and a lateral rib cage displacement.

***Rib Cage.*** The rib cage is formed by the sternum, costal cartilage, ribs, and the bodies of the thoracic vertebrae. The rib cage protects the organs in the thoracic cavity, assists in respiration, and provides support for the upper extremities. During inspiration the ribs are elevated, and during expiration the ribs are depressed.

Although each rib has its own ROM (occurring primarily at the costovertebral joint), rib cage shifts occur with movement of the vertebral column. During column extension, the rib cage migrates anteriorly and the ribs are elevated. During spinal flexion, the rib cage moves posteriorly and the ribs are depressed. Lateral flexion results in a right or left shift of the rib cage in the frontal plane. Finally, rotation of the vertebral column results in one side of the rib cage moving posteriorly and movement of the opposite side anteriorly in the transverse plane.

### Muscular System

#### Muscles of the Abdominal Wall

The general functions of the abdominal muscles are as follows:

■ Abdominal viscera support
■ Respiration assistance
■ Trunk control in the directions of flexion, lateral flexion, and rotation

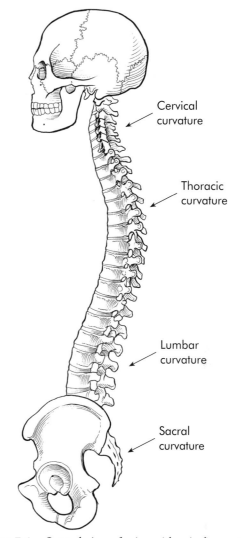

**Figure 7-1**    Lateral view of spine with spinal curvatures.

Although these muscles are situated primarily on the anterior aspect of the trunk, they also are situated laterally and slightly posteriorly, forming a girdle around the abdomen. The abdominal muscles consist of three groups: the rectus abdominis, the obliques (internal and external), and the transversus abdominis (Figure 7-2).

***Rectus Abdominis.*** The rectus abdominis consists of right and left sides that are separated by a fibrous band called the *linea alba*, which runs from the xiphoid process to the pubis.

The proximal attachment is the xiphoid process of the sternum and adjacent costal cartilage, whereas the distal attachments are the pubic bones near the pubic symphysis.[35]

The muscle is palpated easily in the following two cases:

1. When the subject is supine and is asked to lift the head and shoulders off the support surface in a straight plane (sit-up)

2. During backward sway in sitting or standing position

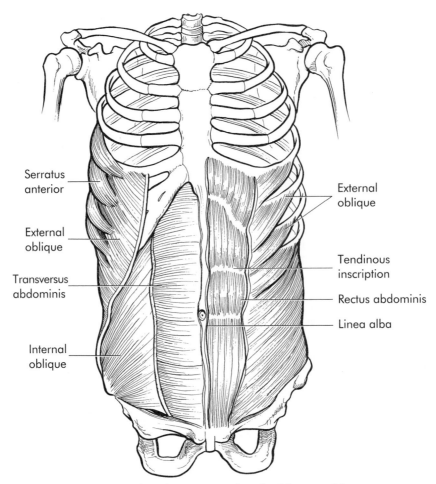

**Figure 7-2**    Anterior anatomy of trunk with resected layers.

When this muscle is activated and not opposed by the extensors, the pelvis and sternum are approximated, the pelvis is pulled into a posterior tilt, and the lumbar curves flatten. Because of its multisegmental arrangement, the rectus abdominis can contract in part or as a whole, making a variety of postures possible. De Troyer's work[16] demonstrated that "abdominal muscle recruitment which naturally occurs in response to posture in most individuals does not uniformly involve the whole of the muscles."

The rectus abdominis (and the other muscles of the trunk) require a stable origin to function efficiently.[14] This stable origin can be the pelvis or thorax, depending on the posture and which part of the trunk is moving. Davies[14] further explains, "The pelvis is stabilized in lying, sitting, and standing by the activity of the muscles around the hips, and in sitting and lying the stabilization is helped by the weight of the legs themselves. Stabilization of the thoracic origin for activities in which the abdominals contract to move or prevent movements of the pelvis requires selective extension of the thoracic spine." Davies further points out that the abdominal muscles cannot function effectively when their origin and

insertion are approximated (e.g., in patients with an exaggerated thoracic kyphosis). Winzeler-Mercay and Mudie[39] noted weakness based on electromyographic recordings in the rectus abdominis after stroke during dynamic trunk movements such as donning shoes. The weakness was noted particularly on the involved side. Similarly, Tanaka, Hachisuka, and Ogata[37] found that peak torque of the flexors was significantly less than in healthy controls.

The rectus abdominis can be self-palpated by assuming a recumbent posture in a chair (slumping in the chair) and then pulling up and forward to an aligned position. One should notice that the burst of activity diminishes when leaning forward (shoulders move in front of hips).

*Obliques.* The obliques consist of three interwoven muscles: internal obliques, external obliques, and transversus abdominis.

The external oblique forms the superficial layer of the abdominal wall. Its fibers run an oblique course superoinferiorly and lateromedially.[26] The muscle is lateral to the rectus abdominis and covers the anterior and lateral regions of the abdomen. The attachments are as follows[35]:

*Proximal attachment:* Anterolateral portions of ribs where the muscle interdigitates with serratus anterior and slips from latissimus dorsi

*Distal attachment:* Upper fibers run down and forward and attach to an aponeurosis that connects them to the linea alba; lower fibers attach to the crest of the ilium

If the external oblique contracts unilaterally, the trunk rotates to the opposite side. Therefore, if one rotates to the left, the right external oblique is active and vice versa. Bilateral contraction assists in trunk flexion and a resultant posterior pelvic tilt. This muscle is also active during straining and coughing.[35] The muscle is palpated easily while rotating the trunk to the opposite side.

The internal obliques also are located laterally and are covered by the external obliques. In essence, the internal obliques constitute the second layer of muscles on the abdominal wall. This muscle basically covers the same area as the external oblique, but its fibers cross those of the external oblique. Attachments are as follows[35]:

*Proximal attachment:* Inguinal ligament, crest of ilium, and thoracolumbar fascia

*Distal attachments:* Pubic bone, an aponeurosis connecting to linea alba, and last three or four ribs

This muscle groups is activated during trunk rotation, but contraction occurs toward the same side (i.e., rotation to the left occurs following contraction of the left internal oblique). Clearly the external and internal obliques are synergists in the action of trunk rotation. The right external and left internal oblique work together to rotate the trunk to the left and vice versa. "The efficient action of the muscles of one side of the abdominal wall is therefore very much dependent upon the fixation or anchorage provided by the activity of the muscles on the other side, particularly for activities involving rotation of the trunk."[13]

Tanaka, Hachisuka, and Ogata[37] examined trunk rotation performance in poststroke hemiplegic subjects and found significantly lower muscle performance in the subjects compared with the health controls. No differences were found when comparing right and left rotation in terms of angular velocities, the side of hemiplegia, or gender, but muscle performance in both directions was decreased compared with controls.

The internal obliques are difficult to palpate. However, the therapist may feel tension under the fingertips when palpating the lateral abdominal wall on the side toward which the trunk is rotating. This tension is due in part to activation of the internal obliques.

*Transversus Abdominis.* The transversus abdominis is the deepest layer of the abdominal wall. Its fibers run transversely, and the muscle has been called the *corset muscle* because it encloses the abdominal cavity like a corset. Attachments are as follows[35]:

*Proximal attachments:* Lower ribs, thoracolumbar fascia, crest of the ilium, and inguinal ligament

*Distal attachments:* Via an aponeurosis fuses with other abdominal muscles into linea alba

The main action of the transversus abdominis is forced compression; the muscle acts like a girdle to flatten the abdominal wall and compress the abdominal viscera. Weakness of this muscle permits bulging of the anterior abdominal wall, thereby indirectly leading to an increase in lordosis.[27] The therapist may palpate this muscle between the lower ribs and the crest of the ilium during forced expiration.

***Posterior Trunk Muscles.*** The posterior trunk muscles include the quadratus lumborum, the erector spinae group, and latissimus dorsi (Figure 7-3). The actions of this group of muscles include trunk extension, lateral flexion, rotation of the trunk, and assistance with balancing the vertebral column.

*Quadratus Lumborum.* The quadratus lumborum is lateral and posterior (i.e., on the posterior abdominal wall); it lies between the psoas major and the erector spinae group. The attachments are as follows[35]:

*Proximal attachment:* Crest of ilium

*Distal attachments:* Twelfth rib and transverse processes of first to third lumbar vertebrae

The main action of this muscle is to assist in "hip hiking." Therefore the muscle is active during lateral trunk flexion. The easiest way to palpate the quadratus lumborum is to have the subject prone, to palpate superior and lateral to the iliac crest, and to ask the subject to hike the hip.

*Erector Spinae Group.* The erector spinae group of muscles is a large mass that fills the spaces between the transverse and spinous processes of the vertebrae and extends laterally covering a large portion of the posterior thorax. Multiple muscles make up this group, and they are named according to attachments, shape, and action. Muscles such as the transversospinales, the interspinales, the longissimus, and the iliocostalis are included in this group.

Collectively, these muscles connect the back of the skull to the posterior iliac crest and sacrum. Unopposed contraction of the back extensors approximates the head and the sacrum. The pelvis is pulled into an anterior tilt (accentuating the lumbar curve), and the ribs are forced to flare. These muscles also contract during lateral flexion (to balance the abdominals), and they may assist in trunk rotation during unilateral contraction (e.g., assist the trunk with rotating to the ipsilateral side). The therapist easily can palpate this muscle group with patients in

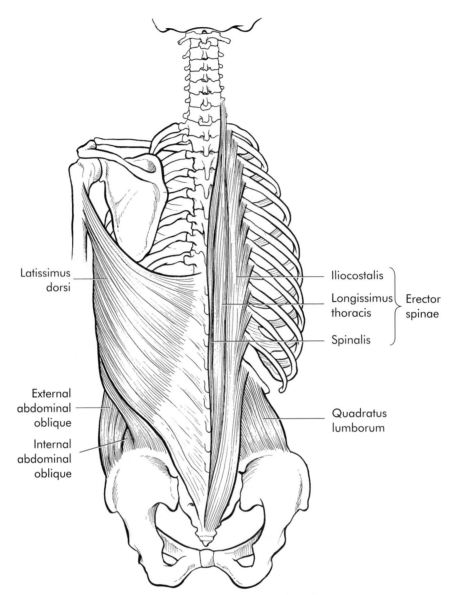

Latissimus
dorsi

Iliocostalis

Longissimus
thoracis

Erector
spinae

Spinalis

External
abdominal
oblique

Quadratus
lumborum

Internal
abdominal
oblique

**Figure 7-3**    Posterior anatomy of trunk.

the prone position if the head and shoulders are lifted from the support surface[35]; palpation also is possible during forward sway in sitting or standing. The therapist easily can palpate the lower back extensors during low back extension (accentuating the lumbar curve) while the patient is sitting.

Winzeler-Mercay and Mudie[39] found increased activity in the erector spinae on both sides during work activities (such as reaching and donning shoes) and at rest. This increased activity was particularly evident on the involved side. They hypothesized that this abnormal response might reflect a disruption of cortical influences on motor unit activity. Similarly, Tanaka, Hachisuka, and Ogata[36] found that peak torque of the extensors was significantly less than in healthy controls.

*Latissimus Dorsi.* The latissimus dorsi is superficial and covers the posterior/lateral trunk. Its attachments include the following[35]:

*Proximal attachments:* Spinous processes of T6 down, dorsolumbar fascia, posterior crest of ilium, lower ribs, interdigitations with external oblique; fibers converge toward axilla, passing over the inferior angle of the scapula.

*Distal attachments:* Tendon attaches to crest of lesser tubercle of humerus, proximal to the teres major.

Acting unilaterally, the latissimus dorsi adducts, extends, and internally rotates the humerus and laterally flexes the trunk (approximates the shoulder and the pelvis). Bilateral contraction helps hyperextend the spine and anteriorly tilt the pelvis.

## MOTOR CONTROL CONSIDERATIONS

### Trunk Muscle Contractions

To achieve full trunk control and use this control during functional tasks, patients must regain the ability to contract their trunk muscles under three different circumstances outlined by Davies.[14] The task of lower extremity bathing from a seated position illustrates these points:

1. Contracting to move opposite the pull of gravity: When the trunk is moving in a direction that is opposite to gravitational pull, the muscles on the uppermost side of the trunk are contracting concentrically. For example, after washing feet, the trunk is straightened from a bent-over position by concentric contraction of the back extensors (the uppermost muscles). Therefore the muscles are shortening actively. The one exception to the rule that the uppermost muscles are active during this type of contraction is bridging. In this case, movement does occur in a direction opposite the pull of gravity (back and buttocks moving away from the support surface), but the underside muscles (the extensors) are contracting concentrically and are responsible for the success of this task. Concentric contractions are used functionally to reposition the trunk during or after task completion.

2. Preventing movement that would occur because of gravitational pull: This type of muscle contraction (usually isometric) prevents falling toward the pull of gravity, stabilizes the trunk for successful completion of tasks, and forms the basis of many balance reactions. During lower extremity washing, the back extensors contract to stabilize (isometrically hold) the trunk as one washes the lower leg, allowing proximal stabilization for distal function. As a note, when one leans all of the way forward (extreme flexion), the back extensors become inactive, and the vertebral ligaments become responsible for holding the trunk in this posture.[4]

3. Controlling the speed of trunk movements in the direction of gravitational pull: In this type of contraction the muscles are contracting eccentrically (in controlled and active elongation). The muscles responsible for this contraction are on the side of the trunk that is opposite the pull of gravity. When one leans forward to wash the feet during lower body washing, the back extensors contract eccentrically to control the speed and range of the forward trunk movement. This muscle contraction has a braking effect as the large mass of the trunk moves into the pull of gravity.

The previous examples show that functional independence requires control of all three trunk muscle contractions and combinations. Successful treatment plans must include activities that elicit a variety of trunk muscle contractions. Self-care training inherently challenges a variety of trunk postures and muscle contractions.

### Musculoskeletal Components

Control of the trunk depends on several musculoskeletal variables including ROM, biomechanical alignment, strength, and muscle length. These variables are interdependent and can create a vicious circle in stroke patients.

### Postural Malalignment

Stroke patients commonly assume postural malalignments that include the following:

- Posterior pelvic tilt
- Pelvic obliquity characterized by unequal weight bearing through the ischial tuberosities
- Lumbar spine flexion (loss of the lumbar curve)
- Increased kyphosis
- Lateral spine flexion
- Rib cage rotation (following loss of abdominal control)
- Head/neck malalignment (rotation away from and lateral flexion toward the involved side)

Prolonged postural malalignment results in muscle shortening on one side of the trunk and muscle overstretching on the opposite side. For example, a posterior pelvic tilt with lumbar flexion results in shortening of the anterior musculature and elongation (overstretching) of the posterior muscles. Lateral flexion on the right side results in muscle shortening on the right side and muscle elongation on the left side of the trunk.

Postural malalignment may occur because of unilateral weakness (specifically around the pelvis), unbalanced skeletal muscle activity, perceptual dysfunction and an inability to perceive midline, and soft tissue shortening.

Prolonged postural malalignment can result in soft tissue shortening, loss of ROM, and an inability to generate enough force to contract the muscle group in question. The total force of muscle (active tension) is high at the rest length of the muscle (i.e., when the trunk is aligned properly) and less when the muscle is tested at shorter lengths. Therefore the force-generating mechanism within the muscle works optimally at the rest length of the msucle[27] (i.e., a symmetrical and aligned trunk).

### Dissociation

Mohr[29] states, "Normal control in any body part demands the ability to dissociate (separate) different parts of the body." She gives the examples of dissociating the head from the body, one side of the body from the other, and the upper trunk from the lower trunk.

Examples of dissociation during functional tasks include upper trunk rotation with lower trunk stability while reaching for toilet paper, counterrotation of the trunk during ambulatory activities, and upper trunk rotation with concurrent lower trunk lateral flexion to increase the range of reach beyond the arm span when reaching for a phone positioned on the left side of a desk with the right hand.

Difficulty with dissociation may result from soft tissue tightness, bony contracture, or efforts by the patient to decrease the degrees of freedom in the trunk[33] during functional activities.

## Motor Adaptation

Concerning motor adaptation, Smith, Weiss, and Lehmkuhl[35] state, "Normal postural control requires the ability to adapt responses to changing tasks and environmental demands. This flexibility requires the availability of multiple movement strategies and the ability to select the appropriate strategy for the task and environment. The inability to adapt movements to changing task demands is a characteristic of many patients with neurological disorders. Patients become fixed in stereotypical patterns of movement, showing a loss of movement flexibility and adaptability."

Motor adaptation can occur in response to an external perturbation or in anticipation of potentially destabilizing forces. Unexpected external perturbations include bumping into someone in a crowded lobby, being in a vehicle that unexpectedly turns or decelerates, and being on a moving platform, such as an escalator, that stops unexpectedly.

Activities that lead to trunk movements in anticipation of destabilizing forces include reaching for a heavy book off of a shelf, reaching beyond the arm span, and preparing to push or pull a chair into place. Shumway-Cook and Woollacott[34] point out that anticipatory postural control depends heavily on previous experience and learning. Research focusing on anticipatory postural responses during reach activities is presented in Chapter 10.

## GENERAL CONSIDERATIONS FOR EVALUATION AND TREATMENT OF THE TRUNK

Therapists should consider the following points during evaluation of the trunk and treatment planning:

1. Proper evaluation and treatment of the trunk result from use of keen observational skills. Patients should be undressed (shirtless or in sports bra or bathing suit top) so that movements are more easily observed during functional tasks. Clothing folds, wrinkles, and crooked seams can lead to incorrect observations.
2. The therapist must realize that the slightest change in posture can change trunk muscle activity and alignment completely.[13] For example, a subtle anterior shift of the shoulders results in extensor activation, whereas a subtle posterior shift of the shoulders results in trunk flexor activation.
3. The therapist should evaluate the trunk in a variety of postures that coincide with ADL. Trunk adjustments are task specific; therefore a trunk evaluation of a patient who is supine should include activities such as

rolling and bridging. Evaluations of seated patients should include activities such as upper and lower extremity dressing, scooting, and bathing; evaluations of standing patients should include reaching for items in medicine cabinets, on bookshelves, and in kitchen cabinets.

## EVALUATION PROCESS

### Subjective Interview

Therapists should question patients about their perceived stability limits. *Stability limits* have been defined as the "boundaries of an area of space in which the body can maintain its position without changing the base of support."[35] Patients' perceived stability limits may or may not be consistent with their actual limits. If patients' perceived limits of stability are greater than their actual limits, they are at risk for falls. If their perceived limits of stability are less than their actual limits, they may be reluctant to attempt tasks with progressively greater demands on their postural system (e.g., lower extremity dressing without assistive devices and picking up objects from the floor without a reacher).

Perceived stability limits may have a direct correlation with observed neurobehavioral deficits. Body scheme disorders commonly occur in the stroke population. These deficits include body neglect, somatoagnosia, and impaired right/left discrimination.[2] Ayres[3] has defined body scheme as a postural model on which movements are based. Knowledge of body parts and their relationships are necessary for deciding what and where to move and in what way to perform.[2] Spatial relation deficits including spatial neglect, depth perception, and spatial relation disorders also may have an effect on patients' perceived stability limits (gaining and regaining midline orientation and position in space) (see Chapter 18).

Other components of the subjective interview include determining patients' insights into their trunk malalignments and their ability to perceive and assume midline positions. The therapist's goal in this interview is to gain insight into the patients' ability to make accurate observations about their postural dysfunction. This is difficult for many patients because trunk control does not occur at a conscious level in the majority of daily tasks.

### Standardized Assessments

The use of valid and reliable tools is always recommended. The following section reviews available measurement instruments related to trunk control.

*Trunk Control Test.* The Trunk Control Test[12] examines four movements: roll from supine to the weak side, roll from supine to the strong side, sitting up from supine, and sitting on the edge of the bed for 30 seconds (feet off the ground). Each of the four tasks are scored as follows:

0, unable to perform with assistance, 12, able to perform but in an abnormal manner, and 25, able to complete movement normally. The range of scores is 0 to 100.[22]

The Trunk Control Test has been shown to be sensitive to change in assessing recovery of stroke patients, to correlate with the Functional Independence Measure, predict motor Functional Independence Measure items at discharge better than motor Functional Independence Measure scores at admission alone,[22] and predict walking ability by 18 weeks.[12] In addition, Duarte et al[17] found that the Trunk Control Test significantly correlated with length of stay, discharge motor Functional Independence Measure scores, gait velocity, walking distance, and the Berg Balance Scale. They also found that the Trunk Control Test predicted 52% of the variance in length of stay and 54% of the discharge Functional Independence Measure.

*Postural Assessment Scale for Stroke Patients.* The Postural Assessment Scale for Stroke Patients includes items related to trunk control. Overall, the scale contains 12 four-point items graded from 0 to 3. Items include sitting without support, standing with and without support, standing on the nonparetic leg, standing on the paretic leg, supine to affected side, supine to nonaffected side, supine to sit, sit to supine, sit to stand, stand to sit, and standing and picking up a pencil from the floor. The Postural Assessment Scale for Stroke Patients has been found to be highly valid and reliable during the first 3 months after stroke.[5]

Five items have been suggested[24] to measure trunk control: sitting without support, supine to affected side, supine to nonaffected side, supine to sitting on the edge of the bed, and sitting to supine.

*Motor Assessment Scale.* The Motor Assessment Scale[11] is a comprehensive assessment of motor behavior and includes items related to trunk control. Overall the scale consists of eight items: supine to side-lying (onto intact side), supine to sit, balanced sitting, sit to stand, walking, upper arm function, hand movements, and advanced hand activities. Each item is scored on seven-point scale from 0 to 6.

*Fugl-Meyer Assessment.* The Fugl-Meyer Assessment[23] evaluates five areas: joint motion and pain, balance, sensation, upper extremity motor function, and lower extremity motor function. The balance subscale includes seven functions related to postural control: sit without support, protective reactions on affected and nonaffected sides, stand with support, stand without support, stand on nonaffected leg, and stand on affected leg.

Mao et al[28] compared the psychometric properties of the balance subscale of the Fugl-Meyer Assessment, the Berg Balance Scale (see Chapter 8), and the Postural Assessment Scale for Stroke Patients. They concluded that all three tests showed acceptable levels of reliability, validity, and responsiveness with the Postural Assessment Scale for Stroke Patients showing slightly better psychometric characteristics. The reader is referred to Chapter 8 for a review of other standardized assessments of postural control. In addition the reader should review Chapter 20 concerning use of the Assessment of Motor and Process Skills. The assessment includes motor skill items such as stabilizes, aligns, and positions. The Assessment of Motor and Process Skills is unique and highly recommended, for the therapist can gather information related to motor skills during ADL performance.

## Observations of Trunk Alignment/Malalignment

For the purposes of this chapter, observations concern the seated posture.

The patient's trunk should be exposed as much as possible, and the patient should be asked to "Sit up nice and straight and gently rest your hands in your lap." (Table 7-1 outlines the ideal alignment of the trunk and extremities and common asymmetries observed after stroke during static sitting.)

**Table 7-1**

### Normal Alignment and Common Malalignments after Stroke

| NORMAL ALIGNMENT | COMMON MALALIGNMENT |
| --- | --- |
| **Pelvis** | |
| Equal weight bearing through both ischial tuberosities | Asymmetrical weight bearing |
| Neutral to slight anterior tilt | Posterior pelvic tilt |
| Neutral rotation | Unilateral retraction |
| **Vertebral Column** | |
| Straight from posterior view | Scoliosis |
| Appropriate curves from lateral view | Loss of lumbar curve; increased thoracic kyphosis |
| | Shortening on one side; elongation on opposite side |

*Continued*

**Table 7-1**

## Normal Alignment and Common Malalignments after Stroke—cont'd

| NORMAL ALIGNMENT | COMMON MALALIGNMENT |
|---|---|
| **Rib Cage** | |
| Neutral in terms of lateral tilt | Lateral tilt |
| Neutral rotation | Flaring on one side |
| Alignment over pelvis and under shoulders | Unilateral retraction |
| **Shoulders** | |
| Symmetrical height | Asymmetrical height |
| Alignment over pelvis | Unilateral retraction |
| **Head/Neck** | |
| Neutral | Protraction |
| | Flexion to weak side |
| | Rotation away from weak side |
| **Upper Extremities** | |
| Resting in lap; if weight bearing, effortless and symmetrical | Use of stronger extremity as postural support to maintain alignment |
| | Too little or too much activity in more involved extremity |
| **Lower Extremities** | |
| Hips at 90 degrees | Hips toward extension because of posterior pelvic tilt |
| Knee aligned with hips | Hip adduction resulting in knee contact |
| Feet in full contact with floor, accepting weight; feet under knees | "Windswept" hips |
| | Feet not equally bearing weight, or "pushing"; foot placed in front of knee |

Following the evaluation of postural malalignments during static sitting, the therapist should begin to hypothesize the cause of these malalignments. Causes may include increased skeletal muscle activity on one side of the trunk, inability to recruit muscle activity or weakness, soft tissue shortening, fixed deformity, body scheme disorder, and inability to perceive midline.

The therapist must remember that observed postures may be caused by more than one impairment. For example, stroke patients tend to sit in a posterior pelvic tilt position with resultant hip extension and thoracic spine flexion. This posture may result from one of or a combination of the following:

1. Weakness or lack of activity in the trunk extensors, especially in the lower back
2. Fixed contracture of the hamstrings and/or thoracic spine
3. Abdominal weakness: The mentioned posture changes the center of gravity and decreases the potential to fall backward. The abdominal muscles are primarily responsible for preventing backward sway, therefore assuming a flexed posture reduces the chance of having to activate the abdominals to prevent falls.

Another example of a commonly observed malalignment is trunk shortening on the side affected by the stroke. The patient may assume this posture for several reasons:

1. Inactive shoulder elevators on the side affected by the stroke that let the shoulder depress[13]
2. Increased muscle activity of the scapula depressors that pull the shoulder down on the affected side
3. Perceptual dysfunction resulting in an inability to find midline, bearing the most weight on the stronger side and resulting in a shortening of the affected side
4. Increased muscle activity or shortening of the affected lateral flexors resulting in a shortening response
5. Fear of shifting weight to the affected side, with the majority of weight on stronger side, resulting in shortening of the affected side

Following the observation of the patient in a static posture, the occupational therapist must observe trunk responses during functional activities. The two most effective methods of making these observations are observing patients during self-care and mobility in a variety of positions (Table 7-2) and controlled reach pattern activities.

During functional reach patterns, trunk responses are required to provide proximal stability for distal function, enhance the ability to interact with the environment by increasing reaching distance (i.e., extend the arm span with an appropriate trunk response), and prevent falls.

**Table 7-2**

## Effects of Object Positioning on Trunk Movements and Weight Shifts During Reaching Activities*

| POSITION OF OBJECT | TRUNK RESPONSE/WEIGHT SHIFT |
|---|---|
| Straight ahead at forehead level, past arm's length | Trunk extension, anterior pelvic tilt<br>Anterior weight shift |

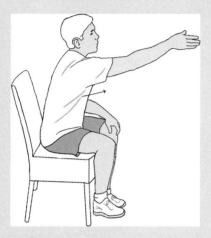

| On floor, between feet | Trunk flexion<br>Anterior weight shift |
|---|---|

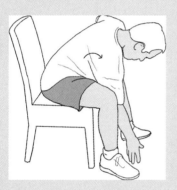

| To side at shoulder level, past arm's length | Left trunk shortening, right trunk elongation, left hip hiking<br>Weight shift to right |
|---|---|

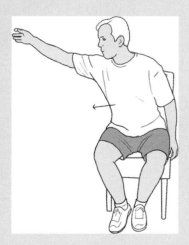

*These examples are for a patient with left hemiplegia. The left-hand column indicates where to position objects during a reaching task (using the right upper extremity). The right-hand column indicates the resultant trunk position and weight shift.

**Table 7-2**

**Effects of Object Positioning on Trunk Movements and Weight Shifts During Reaching Activities—cont'd**

| POSITION OF OBJECT | TRUNK RESPONSE/WEIGHT SHIFT |
|---|---|
| On floor, below right hip | Right trunk shortening, left trunk elongation<br>Weight shift to right |

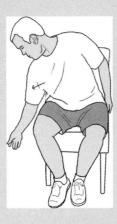

| | |
|---|---|
| Behind right shoulder, at arm's length | Trunk extension and rotation (right side posteriorly)<br>Weight shift to right |

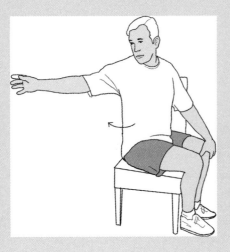

**Table 7-2**

**Effects of Object Positioning on Trunk Movements and Weight Shifts During Reaching Activities—cont'd**

| POSITION OF OBJECT | TRUNK RESPONSE/WEIGHT SHIFT |
| --- | --- |
| At shoulder level, to left of left shoulder | Trunk extension and rotation (left side posteriorly)<br>Weight shift to left |

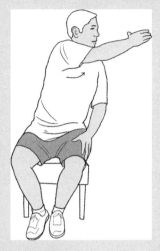

| POSITION OF OBJECT | TRUNK RESPONSE/WEIGHT SHIFT |
| --- | --- |
| On floor, to left of left foot | Trunk flexion and rotation (left side posteriorly)<br>Weight shift to left |

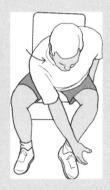

| POSITION OF OBJECT | TRUNK RESPONSE/WEIGHT SHIFT |
| --- | --- |
| Above head, directly behind | Trunk extension, shoulders move behind hips<br>Posterior weight shift |

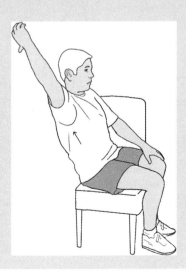

An individual's reaching ability is limited by static trunk postures. As soon as an object is placed beyond arm's length (e.g., on a floor, across a dining table, or under a sink), a trunk response is required to pick up the object successfully.

In general, picking up an object from the floor or from in front of an individual requires an anterior trunk shift. Picking up objects placed beyond the arm span to the right or left of the individual requires a lateral weight shift from the trunk primarily onto one of the ischial tuberosities. Retrieving objects placed behind the trunk requires a posterior weight shift. Rotational trunk responses result from reaching across the midline or for objects posterior to the shoulders or hips.

The therapist's goals while observing the patient perform functional reach patterns are the following:

1. Ensure that trunk and upper extremity patterns are coordinated to result in successful task completion.
2. Note any fall potential.
3. Note asymmetries during reaching.
4. Objectively evaluate the perceived and actual stability limits of the patient.
5. Note in which directions the patient is or is not able to reach beyond the arm span.
6. Note factors such as trunk stiffness and decreased ROM.

### Evaluation of Specific Trunk Movement Patterns

In addition to performing each movement pattern, the reader should refer to the appropriate figures while reading this section. The following evaluation procedures are based on the work of Mohr,[29] Boehme,[7] Davies,[13] and Basmajian and DeLuca.[4]

*Trunk Flexor Control.* The trunk flexors are evaluated by the five different methods that follow:

1. Patients assume a seated, upright position. The therapist asks them to move their shoulders behind their hips slowly and with control (Figure 7-4, *A*); this movement pattern occurs in the sagittal plane, is initiated from the upper trunk,[29] and elicits an eccentric contraction of the trunk flexors.[21,38] Holding the end range of this posture results in an isometric contraction of the trunk flexors. Observations should include resistance to movement, fall potential, and symmetry of the posterior weight shift. Unilateral weakness causes the weak side to become posterior to the stronger side (i.e., it results in rotation of the trunk).
2. From the end position of the first movement pattern, the therapists asks patients to move their shoulders forward so that they are sitting in proper alignment within the sagittal plane (Figure 7-4, *B*); this movement pattern is achieved by a concentric contraction of the trunk flexors.[21] The therapist should note symmetry during the movement pattern. Unilateral weakness causes the stronger side to lead the pattern.

3. In an aligned, seated position, patients assume a controlled lumbar flexion posture (posterior tilt with flattening of the lumbar curve and spinal flexion) (Figure 7-4, *C*). Mohr[29] states that this movement pattern is initiated by the lower trunk and pelvis. If this pattern is performed actively, the final posture is assumed by concentric flexor contraction. Patients also may achieve this posture by a relaxation response of the low back extensors, so the therapist should palpate the flexors to ensure the pattern is a result of active movement. At the end range of this pattern—posterior tilt and spinal flexion (a recumbent posture)—little to no muscle activity exists, and patients maintain this posture by support of their vertebral ligaments.[4]
4. The therapist also should evaluate control of the trunk flexors when the patient is supine (during rolling and bed mobility activities). While the patient is in a supine position, the therapist asks the patient to sit up in a straight plane. This movement pattern, which is

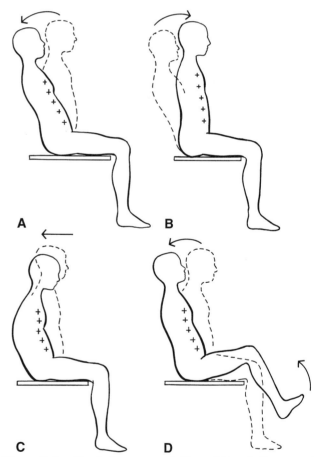

**Figure 7-4**    Trunk flexor control. Dotted lines indicate trunk starting position, solid lines indicate trunk final position, arrows indicate movement direction, and plus signs indicate muscle groups primarily responsible for control of pattern. (Skeletal muscle activity occurs on both sides of the trunk; that is, reciprocal innervation.)

controlled primarily by the rectus abdominis, allows the therapist to evaluate antigravity control of the trunk flexors. The therapist also can ask the patient to roll by lifting one shoulder up and across the trunk in a position of trunk flexion and rotation. This movement pattern also gives the therapist insight into the antigravity control of the flexors (primarily the obliques).[27]

5. Although the first four movement patterns to test flexor control were initiated by the patient, testing the response of the flexors to being moved by the therapist also is useful. The therapist lifts the lower legs of the patient into a position of increased hip flexion. For the patient to refrain from falling backward, the trunk flexors must be activated isometrically (Figure 7-4, D).

As a rule of thumb the trunk flexors are activated in the seated position when the shoulders move posterior to the hips (backward sway), when the trunk is moving away from the support surface (supine starting point), and during rotational activities.

***Trunk Extensor Control.*** The following four movement patterns are used to evaluate trunk extensor control during seated activities and bridging.

1. To start this movement pattern, the patient assumes a flexed spine posture with a posterior pelvis tilt (the resting posture for many stroke patients). The patient initiates the movement with the lower trunk and pelvis[29] and assumes an extended spine posture with a neutral to slight anterior tilt, which accentuates the lumbar curve (Figure 7-5, A). The patient completes the movement pattern by a concentric contraction of the trunk extensors, which is the trunk pattern required for forward reach.

2. Patients assume an aligned, seated starting position and are asked to keep their spine straight as they lean forward, keeping the shoulders in front of the hips in the sagittal plane (Figure 7-5, B). They assume this posture by an eccentric contraction of the trunk extensors,[4,21,38] and if they hold the posture between the middle to end range, the back extensors isometrically contract. The patient has unilateral weakness if the trunk moves forward asymmetrically. Unilateral weakness causes the weaker side to lead the movement pattern (e.g., to fall into gravity). If the movement continues in a forward direction (e.g., patient reaches down to the floor), the back extensors become inactive at the end range, and the tension of the vertebral ligaments maintains the position.[4]

3. While patients are in the end posture of the second movement pattern, the therapists asks them to move their shoulders back to assume a seated, aligned position (Figure 7-5, C). To assume this posture, the trunk extensors contract concentrically, although the hip extensors initiate the movement[4,38]; this movement occurs in the sagittal plane.

4. The therapist also should test the back extensors by observing the patient in a bridge posture. While the patient is in a supine position with the hips and knees flexed, the therapist asks the patient to assume a bridge position, which is accomplished by a concentric contraction of the back and hip extensors[13] and is maintained by an isometric contraction of the same muscles. The release of the posture is controlled by eccentric contraction of the back and hip extensors.

As a rule of thumb, in the seated posture the back extensors are active during anterior weight shifts (in which the shoulders move in front of the hips), during

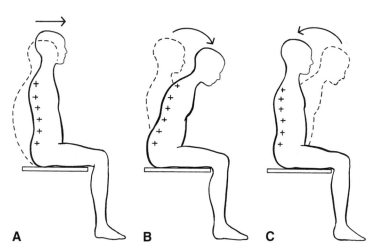

**Figure 7-5** Trunk extensor control. Dotted lines indicate trunk starting position, solid lines indicate trunk final position, arrows indicate movement direction, and plus signs indicate muscle groups primarily responsible for control of pattern. (Skeletal muscle activity occurs on both sides of the trunk; that is, reciprocal innervation.)

correction of posture to a position of alignment from an anterior weight shift, and during bridging activities.

***Control of the Lateral Flexors.*** Lateral flexion occurs in the coronal plane; therefore a balance of control between the flexors and extensors is required to maintain movement. Electromyographic studies have demonstrated that dorsal and ventral muscles coactivate during lateral flexion.[38] Electromyographic activity of the right and left erector spinae has been documented during lateral trunk flexion.[4,21]

Mohr[29] states, "Two different movement strategies occur when you reach down to the side: (1) the initiation may occur in the upper trunk and the ipsilateral spine shortens, or (2) the movement can be initiated with your lower trunk and pelvis, resulting in ipsilateral elongation." Three movement patterns are used to evaluate control of lateral trunk flexion:

1. The first movement pattern is initiated from an aligned, seated position. The pelvis remains stable, and the upper trunk initiates lateral flexion toward the floor with the shoulder approximating the hip (Figure 7-6, *A*). The end posture (one of ipsilateral trunk shortening) occurs by an eccentric contraction of the side of the trunk that is elongating.[29,38] In Figure 7-6, *A*, the right side of the trunk is shortening, but the predominant control is on the left side, which is elongating eccentrically. Holding this posture between the middle and end ranges allows evaluation of isometric lateral flexion control. Therapists should evaluate both sides of the trunk using this movement pattern.

2. While patients are in the end position of the first movement pattern, the therapist asks them to realign themselves by sitting up straight (Figure 7-6, *B*). The trunk is realigned by a concentric contraction

of the lateral flexors[38] (the left lateral flexors in Figure 7-6, *B*).

3. The last movement pattern evaluates lateral flexion, which initiates the movement from the lower trunk and pelvis.[29] This movement pattern allows reach beyond the arm span in the frontal plane. During this movement the majority of weight is shifted to one ischial tuberosity; the shoulder and hip approximate in this pattern. In the resulting posture the trunk is elongated on the weight-bearing side, and trunk shortening occurs on the non–weight-bearing side (Figure 7-6, *C*). The predominant control comes from concentric contraction of the lateral flexors on the shortening side. Figure 7-6, *C*, illustrates the contraction on the right side of the trunk. The therapist must evaluate both sides of the trunk.

***Rotation Control.*** Concerning rotation control, Kapandji[26] states, "Rotation of the vertebral column is achieved by the paravertebral muscles and the lateral muscles of the abdomen. Unilateral contraction of the paravertebral muscles causes only weak rotation. . . . During rotation of the trunk, the main muscles involved are the oblique muscles. Their mechanical efficiency is enhanced by their spiral course around the waist and by their attachments to the thoracic cage away from the vertebral column, so that both the lumbar and lower thoracic vertebral columns are mobilised." During rotation of the trunk to the left, the right external and left internal obliques are activated (Figure 7-7). The fibers of both of these muscles run in the same direction and are synergistic. Basmajian's[4] review of the literature on electromyography demonstrates that bilateral activity in the extensors at the thoracic level is evident during rotation.

Mohr[29] states, "Stroke patients will very rarely rotate because normal rotation requires extensors and flexors to be active simultaneously on opposite sides of the trunk." Rotational trunk control depends on muscle fixation on one side of the trunk, resulting in efficient muscle action on the opposite side.

Trunk rotation can occur in two positions: flexion with rotation and extension with rotation.[6] Mohr[29] points out that rotation can be initiated by the upper trunk or the lower trunk/pelvis. Rotation control is evaluated by five movement patterns[7,29]:

1. In the first movement pattern the patient sits upright, and the pelvis remains stable on the support surface. The patient reaches across midline so that the shoulder moves toward the opposite hip (e.g., reaching with the right arm across the body toward the floor). The result is a position of flexion and rotation. The primary control is by concentric contraction of the obliques and contraction of the back extensors (especially at the thoracic level). The therapist must evaluate both sides of the trunk.

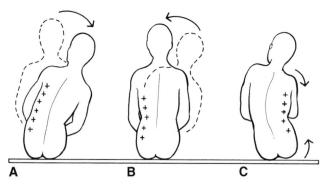

**Figure 7-6**    Lateral flexor control. Dotted lines indicate trunk starting position, solid lines indicate trunk final position, arrows indicate movement direction, and plus symbols indicate muscle groups primarily responsible for control of pattern. (Skeletal muscle activity occurs on both sides of the trunk; that is, reciprocal innervation.)

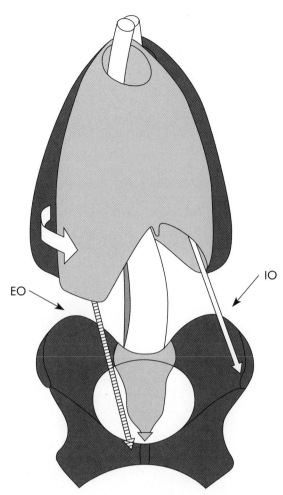

**Figure 7-7**    Rotation control. *IO,* Internal oblique; *EO,* external oblique. (From Kapandji IA: *The physiology of the joints,* vol 3, *The trunk and vertebral column,* New York, 1974, Churchill Livingstone.)

2. In the second movement pattern the upper trunk remains stable, and the lower trunk and pelvis initiate a forward movement on one side (e.g., scooting forward). The result is a position of extension with rotation.

3. In the third movement pattern the patient reaches behind at the shoulder level (upper trunk initiation), and the resulting posture is rotation and extension.

4. The fourth movement pattern involves initiating a backward shift with the lower trunk and pelvis (scooting backward) while shifting to one side and rotating the opposite side posteriorly; this posture is flexion with rotation.

5. The final movement pattern is similar to a pattern reviewed in the section on trunk flexion control. The patient is supine and initiates a segmental roll by lifting the shoulders up from the support surface and toward the opposite side of the body. This pattern is controlled by a concentric contraction of the abdominal muscles (the obliques).

## Trunk Control During Activities of Daily Living

Franchignoni, Tesio, and Ricupero[22] state that trunk control appears to be obvious prerequisite for the control of more complex limb activities that in turn constitute a prerequisite for complex behavioral skills.

Hsieh et al[24] concluded that strong evidence exists for the predictive value of trunk control on comprehensive ADL, and they recommended early assessment and management of trunk control after stroke.

The previous section focused on select movement patterns of the trunk. Evaluating the trunk in this manner is useful for identifying specific problem areas and focusing treatment plans. However, the impact that impaired trunk control has on functional tasks is more relevant to all rehabilitation professionals. Most, if not all, of the reviewed movement patterns (and combinations of them) are used during ADL performance. Therefore the evaluation of trunk control can take place during skilled observations of ADL.

For clarification, an infinite number of variations are observed in movement patterns during task performance. Therefore the focus of evaluation and treatment should be on observing, evaluating, and treating the patient in a variety of different environments and with tasks that include multiple variables. The situational context and task demands determine which components of trunk control are necessary for successful task performance. Box 7-3 has an example of task variables that affect trunk control patterns.

The list of trunk control variations during ADL performance in the following section are not considered exhaustive but are guidelines for observing trunk patterns and inherent variations during various tasks. The reader should mimic performing each task to ensure understanding of the posture descriptions.

### Upper Extremity Dressing

*Pullover Shirt.* Putting on a pullover shirt requires the following movements:

---

**Box 7-3**

**Variables of Eating That Affect Required Trunk Control Patterns**

- Size of table
- Type of seating surface (e.g., presence of armrests or backrest, cushions, chair height, distance person is from table)
- Placement of items such as condiments, utensils, and serving bowls (e.g., near or far, right or left)
- Type of food (e.g., hot soup, cold fruit)
- Solitary or group dining (e.g., may get assistance with passing needed items)
- Errors (e.g., dropping fork, spilling beverage)

- *Trunk flexion:* Required for the patient to manipulate the shirt in the lap and reach down toward the lap to insert an arm into the sleeve.
- *Trunk extension:* Observed as the patient realigns the trunk, continues to pull up the sleeve, and inserts the head into the shirt.
- *Trunk rotation with extension:* May be necessary for reaching posteriorly and adjusting the orientation of the shirt and/or tucking the shirt into the pants.

*Button-Down Shirt.* Putting on a button-down shirt requires the following movements:
- *Trunk flexion:* Used to orient the shirt correctly on the lap for preparation of donning and to guide the arm into the sleeve when the trunk is inclined forward.
- *Trunk extension:* Required to realign the trunk from the previous position.
- *Trunk rotation with extension:* Used to reach with the more functional arm behind the head and to the opposite shoulder to grasp the collar of the shirt and pull it to the opposite side (Figure 7-8); also used to move the second arm through the sleeve and tuck the shirt into the pants.
- *Trunk flexion:* Used as the patient attempts to button the shirt; more often used as relaxation position (a slumped posture) rather than an active flexion pattern.

***Lower Extremity Dressing (Seated).*** Putting on pants, underwear, shoes, and socks requires the following movements:
- *Trunk flexion:* Required to reach down toward the feet (Figure 7-9).
- *Trunk rotation with flexion:* Required to reach the more functional arm toward the opposite foot.
- *Trunk extension:* Required to realign the trunk from the previous positions.

- *Lateral flexion:* Required when using a crossed-leg method to don/doff pants, underwear, or footwear (the crossed-leg position shifts the patients' center of gravity posteriorly, placing increased demand on the abdominal muscles [i.e., controlling the trunk in flexion while preventing a posterior fall]) (Figure 7-10); also required to pull pants and underwear up or down over the buttocks and hips successfully.

### Grooming
*Oral Care.* Hygiene of the mouth requires the following movements:
- *Trunk flexion:* Isometric control commonly used to position the head over the sink to preventing spillage of toothpaste and saliva onto clothing; increased trunk

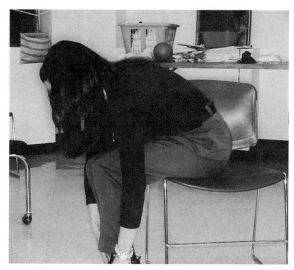

**Figure 7-9**   Trunk control during lower extremity dressing.

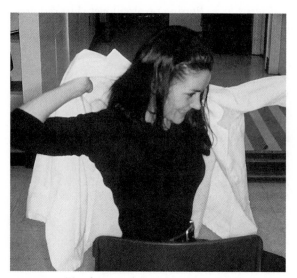

**Figure 7-8**   Trunk control during upper extremity dressing.

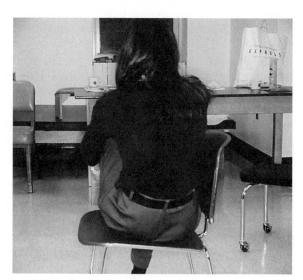

**Figure 7-10**   Trunk adjustments during lower extremity dressing.

flexion for expectorating (toothpaste and mouthwash) after completion of tooth brushing.

■ *Trunk extension:* Used to realign body from previous position; also used to reach for supplies in a medicine cabinet over a sink and during gargling.

■ *Trunk rotation with flexion:* May be used to reach toward and adjust the faucet opposite the arm being used.

*Hair Care.* Hair care requires the following movements:

■ *Trunk flexion or extension:* May be used isometrically during hair washing; trunk flexion is used if patients prefer to lean forward and allow the lather to be rinsed off in front of them; trunk extension (and head/neck extension) is used if patients prefer to lean back and allow the lather to be rinsed off behind them; both may be used during hair combing to accentuate the position of the head and optimally position the brush or comb to make contact with the scalp.

■ *Lateral flexion:* May be used during hair washing or combing (initiated by upper trunk) as the head is tilted to the right or left side; also may be used for optimal head placement.

*Eating.* Eating requires the following movements:

■ *Trunk flexion and extension:* Used in varying degrees with a hand-to-mouth pattern in which an anterior weight shift of the trunk toward the table occurs (Figure 7-11) to position the mouth over the plate as food enters. (The degree to which this weight shift occurs depends on the type of food being eaten. Food that is hot or liquid requires increased flexion toward the plate or bowl. The increased flexion reduces the distance the food must be transported, thereby reducing spillage opportunities.)

■ *Trunk rotation:* May be used in flexion and extension to reach for condiments that are across the midline of the trunk.

■ *Lateral flexion:* Lower trunk initiation may be used in reaching for condiments that are positioned to the side of the place setting and beyond arm's length and also may be used with trunk rotation postures (Figure 7-12); upper trunk initiation may be used when reaching for an object that drops on the floor to the side of the patient.

***Bathing (Seated on a Tub Seat or Bench).*** Bathing requires the following movements:

■ *Trunk flexion and extension:* Required to reach toward the lower extremities and then realign.

■ *Trunk rotation:* Trunk rotation with flexion is used to reach down toward the opposite lower extremity for lower leg and foot washing; trunk rotation with extension may be used when reaching posteriorly to wash back and neck. (In general, trunk rotation is used when reaching across the midline of the trunk. The amount of flexion and extension depends on the area of the body being washed [e.g., flexion for lower body washing; extension for upper body washing].)

■ *Lateral flexion:* Lower trunk initiation is required to wash the perineum and rectal areas; upper trunk initiation may be used to wash the sides of the lower legs or to pick up a bar of soap from the bottom of the tub. (Bathing activities place extra demands on trunk control because of the slippery nature of the support surface.)

***Toileting.*** Using the toilet requires the following movements:

■ *Lateral flexion:* Lower trunk initiation may be used depending on the sequence of clothing management

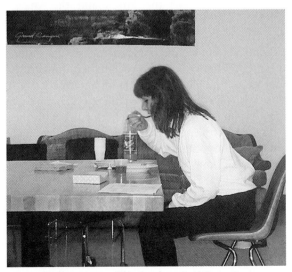

**Figure 7-11**   Trunk control while eating.

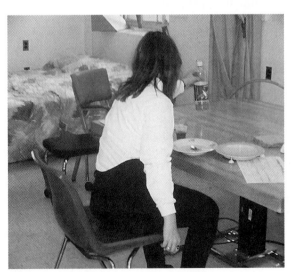

**Figure 7-12**   Trunk adjustments while reaching for utensils or condiments.

for toileting and the type of transfer being used (For example, if patients are performing a sit-pivot transfer, clothing usually is managed from the seated position. Therefore, lateral flexion is necessary so that pants and underwear can clear the hips/buttocks.); may also be used for wiping after toileting.

- *Trunk rotation with extension:* Used to reach across the body for toilet paper.
- *Trunk flexion:* May be used for self-catheterization, application of a condom-style catheter, management of feminine hygiene products, and wiping after toileting.

*Bridging.* Bridging requires trunk extension, which is necessary at the trunk and hips to assume a functional bridge position. (The height of the bridge depends on the task. For example, bridging to use a bedpan requires more extension than bridging to don/doff pants.) See Chapter 14.

*Scooting.* Scooting requires the following movement:

- *Trunk flexion and extension:* Must be balanced for successful scooting. (The efficiency of the scooting pattern is compromised if the patient maintains a flexed trunk with a posterior pelvic tilt or a hyperextended trunk.)
- *Lateral flexion:* Lower trunk initiation is used to clear the buttocks from the support surface, which is required to advance the hip forward.
- *Trunk rotation with extension:* Lower trunk initiation allows the patient to achieve the goal of scooting forward.

## TREATMENT TECHNIQUES TO ENHANCE TRUNK CONTROL DURING TASK PERFORMANCE

### Assuming an Appropriate Starting Posture

Before initiation of tasks and retraining of trunk control the trunk must be in a proper biomechanical alignment. Therapists should observe patients anteriorly, posteriorly, and laterally to detect deviations from normal alignment (see Table 7-1).

Physically or verbally cueing patients to assume an appropriate starting posture should place them in a position of readiness for function-optimal symmetry in the trunk that is usually in midline, depending on the task (Box 7-4).

This starting posture is similar to the position the trunk and lower extremities assume when a person begins a typing task.

An aligned and upright trunk posture has been shown to recruit muscle activity in the trunk. Floyd and Silver's electromyographic studies[21] demonstrated that a "slumped" position while sitting (simultaneous trunk flexion and extension of the hip joint) resulted in trunk extensor relax-

---

**Box 7-4**

**Seated Position of Readiness for Function**

Pelvis is in neutral to anterior tilt
Equal weight bearing on both ischial tuberosities
Trunk erect and midline with appropriate spinal curves
Shoulders symmetrical and over the hips
Head/neck neutral
Hips slightly above the level of the knees
Knees in line with the hips
Feet equally weight bearing and underneath the knees

---

ation. In contrast, sitting upright in a chair without a backrest resulted in increased activity of the erector spinae muscle group. This muscle activity persisted as long as the trunk remained in extension despite adjustments of the head and shoulders. A "slumped" posture, which consists of trunk flexion, posterior pelvic tilt, and resulting hip extension, is observed commonly during evaluation of posture in the stroke population; the position requires minimal skeletal muscle activity.

Andersson and Ortengren's review of the literature[1] demonstrated that the position of the feet had an effect on the myoelectric activity of the trunk extensors. Knee flexion (causing the feet to come toward the chair) increased muscle activity in the trunk, whereas knee extension resulted in a decrease in muscle activity. Stroke patients commonly assume a seated posture in which their feet (especially the more affected lower extremity) are positioned on the floor in front of their knees (e.g., in knee extension). The position of the feet tends to have an effect on pelvic tilt and resultant trunk postures. When the feet are positioned under the knees and toward the chair, an anterior pelvic tilt and trunk extension are enhanced. The opposite is also true: when the feet are positioned in front of the knees and the knees are extended, a posterior pelvic tilt and resulting trunk flexion are enhanced.

Patients should be encouraged to feel the difference between an aligned and a malaligned posture. The patient should be able to assume an appropriate posture automatically. Demonstration of the effect that a slumped posture has on reaching activities performed with the side less affected by the stroke may be helpful. Patients may realize that the distance and quality of their reach is enhanced when they are sitting in a proper alignment.

Although the use of mirrors for visual feedback may be appropriate for some patients, mirrors should be used with caution for patients with neurobehavioral deficits. Another technique for assisting patients with gaining symmetry is to have the therapist positioned in front of the patient and to assume the patient's postures to provide feedback for the patient. Therapists should slowly correct their posture, instructing the patient to mimic the movement. The therapist may state, "Keep your shoulders in line with mine" or "Keep your forehead at the same level as mine."

Mohr[29] emphasizes use of activities that encourage rotation and lateral flexion to gain midline control: "the active movements of the trunk into rotation and lateral flexion are caused by the same muscles that flex and extend the trunk. The different movements occur as a result of different interactions of these muscles with each other...In order for patients to achieve midline postural control, the therapist must work with the patient in the higher levels of lateral and rotational planes of movement."

## Maintaining or Increasing Trunk Range of Motion Through Mobilization and Movement

Concerning range of motion in the trunk, Mohr[29] states, "If there is not full range in all trunk movements (flexion extension, lateral flexion, and rotation), it will be more difficult to gain full control of the trunk. Any lack of range of motion in the trunk will lead to decreased function."

Although limited ROM in the extremities commonly is evaluated and treated, the ROM in the spine often is overlooked. After acute strokes, patients lose the ability to shift their weight and make postural adjustments. Evaluating patients who have trunks that are influenced completely by gravity and who demonstrate only static trunk postures is common. In these cases, prolonged immobilization of the trunk because of loss of control can result in loss of soft tissue elasticity, joint play, and ultimately function. These problems, compounded by inappropriate trunk positioning and support in upright postures, lead to a cycle of immobility, soft tissue changes, loss of range, and impaired functional abilities.

Specific trunk mobilization techniques are beyond the scope of this chapter but are discussed in the literature.[7,13,18,29] Just as therapists train patients to perform self-ROM activities for their extremities, therapists must promote patient awareness of trunk mobility and educate them about specific movement patterns that maintain and/or increase their trunk ROM. Following are examples of movement patterns that patients can perform to meet this goal:

1. While supine, patients flex their hips and knees as if preparing to bridge. Patients are instructed to keep their shoulders flat on the bed and simultaneously allow their knees to fall slowly from one side and then the other. This movement pattern encourages dissociation from the upper and lower trunk (*rotation*).
2. While supine, patients keep their hips and knees straight while cradling their more affected upper extremity. The goal is to lift and rotate the upper trunk as if initiating a roll with the upper trunk (*rotation*).
3. While sitting, patients cradle their more affected upper extremity against their chest. The therapist encourages

patients to move the upper trunk in a twisting motion without letting the pelvis move (*rotation*).
4. While sitting, patients practice moving from an upright posture to a posture of lateral flexion on one side so that they are bearing weight on their forearm to the side of their trunk. The pelvis should remain stable on the support surface for optimal stretch (*lateral flexion*).
5. While sitting, patients hold their more affected wrist and reach to the floor between their feet. The therapist also encourages them to allow their head to drop and dangle (*flexion*).
6. While supine, patients assume a bridge posture and hold the position as able (*extension*).
7. While sitting, patients practice lifting their hip from the support surface. This movement can be enhanced by having the patient reach up and to the side with the opposite upper extremity. Reaching beyond the arm span in this posture requires lateral flexion for the reach pattern to be successful (*lateral flexion*).

## Using Various Postures

Therapists may use various postures as an adjunct treatment during patients' performance of functional tasks. Therapists should select postures based on specific patient needs. The chosen posture should accentuate and challenge the movement and control patterns that are interfering with independent performance of life activities. As a note, if the patient is not engaging in a specific activity (self-care tasks, games, and adapted sports), the use of these postures in isolation is not encouraged. Examples of varying postures include the following:

1. Seated with legs crossed: Use of this posture is appropriate for patients whose inability to control lateral flexion and flexion patterns and to shift their weight is preventing functional independence. Working with patients in this posture encourages weight transference to one ischial tuberosity and has the added effect of challenging abdominal control. This occurs because the crossed leg is in a position of hip flexion. When the hips are flexed, the traction on the hamstrings tends to tilt the pelvis posteriorly,[26] resulting in a posterior shift in the center of gravity. Abdominal control therefore is required to prevent a posterior loss of balance. Participation in tasks such as lower extremity dressing, lower body washing, and activities such as modified volleyball place extra demands on patients who are in this position.
2. Sitting in front of a table while bearing weight on both forearms: Ryerson and Levit[32] recommend this posture during the acute stage of hemiplegia when little postural control is evident. In this posture, patients use their upper extremities as a point of proximal stability. The therapist should stress that the arm should

be active and the trunk should not be allowed to "hang" on an inactive arm.

Patients are encouraged to practice anterior, posterior, and lateral shifting in this posture to reestablish postural control; coordinate trunk, scapula, and humerus patterns; and establish weight bearing of the upper extremities. Because both arms are engaged in a weight-bearing activity, patient participation in functional tasks is difficult. Immediately following use of this posture, the therapist must engage the patient in a follow-up activity such as reaching to ensure the postures can be incorporated into daily living activities.

3. Prone on elbows: Although effective for gaining trunk extension, this position should be used with caution. The position may compromise respiratory status, cause shoulder pain if upper extremity alignment is not considered, and be generally uncomfortable for older stroke patients. The position may be effective for some patients and may be a required posture for some transitional movements such as floor-to-chair transfers.

4. Kneeling: This posture is appropriate for patients who are experiencing difficulty in gaining trunk/hip extension. Patients also may find this posture uncomfortable, but it may be necessary for transitional patterns.

5. Variations on the degree of hip flexion while seated: Changing the position of the lower extremities can challenge the performance of specific trunk patterns. Being in a position with the knees below the hips, such as sitting on a high stool, decreases the amount of hip flexion and has a tendency to place the trunk in increased extension.

Conversely, positioning the patient with the knees above the hips (increasing the amount of hip flexion) results in a position of trunk flexion and a posterior weight shift, which places greater demands on the trunk flexors.

## Treating the "Pusher Syndrome"

The "pusher syndrome" is a phrase coined by Davies,[14] who derived the name from what she felt was the most striking aspect of this syndrome: the patient pushes heavily toward the hemiplegic side in all positions and resists any attempt at passive correction (i.e., a correction that would bring the weight toward or over the midline of the body to the unaffected side).

Perennou et al[31] investigated whether the pusher syndrome affects only the trunk for which gravitational feedback is given by somesthetic information, or the head as well (gravitational information given by the vestibular system). The results of their pilot study indicated that that the pusher syndrome does not result from disrupted processing of vestibular information but from a higher-order disruption in the processing of somesthetic information originating in the left hemibody, which could be

an extinction phenomenon. The authors felt that this disruption leads pushers actively to adjust their body posture to a subjective vertical bias to the side opposite the lesion.

Currently only one study[30] has focused on the rehabilitation of patients with the pusher syndrome. The study examined the incidence of the syndrome, the relation of this syndrome to neurobehavioral deficits, and the effect of the syndrome on the rehabilitation process in 327 patients. The study revealed a 10% incidence and also found no significant differences in hemineglect or anosognosia in patients with and without ipsilateral pushing. The study also found that patients who demonstrated ipsilateral pushing required 3.6 weeks longer to reach the same final outcome as patients who did not demonstrate ipsilateral pushing. Of note in this study are the Barthel index scores at admission and discharge. On admission, patients who demonstrated ipsilateral pushing scored an average of 13.7 on the Barthel index compared with 46.8 for patients without evidence of pushing. On discharge the average score for pushers was 43.9 compared with 66.8 for patients without pushing. In other words the discharge scores (in terms of ADL function) of the patients who were pushers were still below the admission scores for patients who did not push.

Davies[14] summarizes the typical signs of the pusher syndrome as the following:

- Head turned away from affected side and laterally flexed toward stronger side
- Decreased ability to perceive stimuli from affected side
- Lack of facial expression
- Poor breath control with monotone, hypophonic voice
- An elongated affected side
- Evidence of pushing with stronger leg while supine
- Holding onto side of bed or mat as if falling
- Shortening of stronger side of trunk with elongation of hemiplegic side while sitting
- Marked resistance to attempts to transfer weight to stronger side
- Pushing with stronger arm and leg to more affected side
- Difficulty transferring, especially to stronger side
- All weight shifted to affected side while standing; leaning against therapist's supporting arm or flexing forward at hips
- Hemiplegic leg adduction (scissors) when walking; difficulty taking a step with affected leg because of an inability to shift weight to stronger side

Davies[14] recommends the following specific treatments for the pusher syndrome:

- Restore head movements: maintain full passive range of motion, stretch, and encourage active range of motion by scanning activities.
- Activate the side flexors (see activities described in previous sections).
- Use functional activities to regain midline while standing.

A hands-on approach does not seem to be effective with patients who have the pusher syndrome; therapists' attempts to assist patients with gaining midline by handling is met by further patient resistance. Manipulating the environment and providing external cues (verbal) seem to be more effective. Examples include the following:

- Have patients reach with their stronger upper extremity for objects beyond their arm span to encourage a weight shift to the stronger side.
- Provide verbal cues to realign the trunk, such as, "Bring your head toward mine" and "Bring your left shoulder toward the wall."
- Provide a target toward which patients can move their trunk and maintain the position as long as possible. For example, place a bolster on patients' stronger side, and cue them to lean against the bolster and hold the position.

### Engaging in Reaching Tasks

Therapists can use placement of objects in reaching activities as a way to place a variety of demands on the trunk. The key to eliciting a trunk response is to place the object slightly beyond the arm's reach. Fisher[20] observes that when subjects without brain injuries reach, they anteriorly tilt the pelvis, slightly extend the upper back, and move the trunk in the direction of the arm. Patients with brain injuries do not incorporate trunk movements into arm movements and reach only to arm's length as they maintain a slumped posture.

Therapists have the ability to control the desired response by the way they set up the activity. Setting up the activity includes placing items required during ADL in specific places, choosing the appropriate environment (e.g., kitchen with upper and lower shelves, bookcase, desk space, meal table), deciding how far beyond the arm span the activity should be placed, and deciding on the characteristics of the objects the patient is reaching for (number of objects, weight of the objects, and whether objects require one or two hands). Table 7-2 includes examples of activity placement and resulting trunk response.

Dean and Shepard[15] investigated, via a randomized placebo-controlled trial of task-related training after stroke, the effect of a training program designed to improve the ability to balance in sitting after stroke. The training program was designed to improve sitting balance and involved emphasis on appropriate loading of the affected leg while at the same time practicing reaching tasks using the unaffected hand to grasp objects located beyond arm's length. The reaching tasks were performed under varied conditions. Changing the location of the object that the subject was reaching for varied the distance and direction of reach. Seat height, movement speed, object weight, and extent of thigh support also were varied. Increasing the number of repetitions and complexity of the tasks advanced the training. The authors found that after training, subjects were able to reach faster and farther, increase load through the affected foot, and increase activation of affected leg muscles compared with the control group (highlighting the critical contribution of the lower extremities in promoting sitting balance). The experimental group also improved in sit to stand. The control group did not improve in reaching or sit to stand, and finally, neither group improved in walking. See Table 7-3 for suggestions to grade reaching tasks.

### Using Movable Surfaces

Several authors have advocated the use of movable surfaces to challenge trunk control.[7,13,25] Movable surfaces used in treatment include items such as therapy balls, bolsters, and rocker boards. Movable surfaces can be used in treatment in a variety of ways, including the following:

- To grade the difficulty of the task
- To challenge the patient to maintain control of the surface without outside assistance (challenge isometric patterns)
- To allow the patient to respond to the therapist's perturbation of the movable surface
- To allow the patient to initiate moving the surface
- To enhance stretching and mobilization of the trunk by using a particular surface such as a large ball

**Table 7-3**

### Examples of Grading Activities during Reaching Tasks

|  | EASIER | MORE DIFFICULT |
|---|---|---|
| Sitting surface: | Firm surface | Cushioned or unstable surface |
|  | Full thigh support | Partial thigh support |
| Object: | Within arm's reach | Beyond arm's reach |
|  | Light (e.g., a pencil) | Heavy (e.g., bag of flour) |
| Use of arms: | Reach with one arm | Reach with both arms |
| External support: | Maximum via therapist, bolsters, and so on | None |
| Prediction: | Predictable (e.g., lift stationary object) | Unpredictable (e.g., catch a ball) |

- To add variety to treatment sessions
- To focus on isolated trunk control

Although movable surfaces are used commonly in the clinic, research concerning the effectiveness of this type of treatment compared with other types is lacking. One may argue that when patients master trunk control on a movable surface (a difficult situation), their control will improve on less demanding surfaces (surfaces that do not move). Unfortunately, this argument is not supported by current research that advocates task-specific training.

Use of movable surfaces may be appropriate for patients who are experiencing difficulty controlling their trunk in environments with external perturbations (e.g., trains, automobiles, and buses).

## Adapting the Environment

Some patients may have little improvement in trunk control. Environmental adaptations are necessary for these patients to enhance independent performance. Examples include the following:

- Use of outside supports can help maintain trunk stability while the extremities are engaged in functional tasks. Supports such as lateral supports, anterior chest straps, arm chairs, pillows and cushions for propping, and lap trays are examples of equipment used to compensate for compromised trunk control (see Chapter 24).
- Rearrangement of the environment can decrease demands on the trunk. Placing required equipment within the patient's reach (arm reach) not only increases independence but also may prevent falls. Storing dishes on the counter instead of in a cabinet, placing utensils in front of the patient, and keeping grooming items on top of the sink instead of in a medicine cabinet are examples of this strategy.
- Provision of adaptive equipment is a common strategy to increase independent performance and minimize safety risks. Activities of daily living equipment issued to compensate for poor trunk control may include the following: long-handled shoe horns, elastic laces, adapted bath brushes, soap on a rope, reachers, tub seats, and commodes. See Chapter 27 for more information on adaptive devices.
- Home modifications such as grab bars and bed rails also may be indicated. See Chapter 25 for a full review of home adaptations and equipment recommendations.

## Handling

Handling is a common technique used in the clinic. This intervention commonly is associated with neurodevelopmental therapy.[6] Handling may allow the patient to feel the desired movement pattern, gain range, assist weak movement patterns, and provide external support to prevent falls. To be effective, the patient must be aware of the goal associated with handling, and the therapist should use handling within the context of a functional task. In addition, the handling from the therapist should be graded to allow the patient to perform as much of the movement pattern as possible. A variety of texts* are available that review specific techniques of handling. Although commonly used, research does not support use of this technique (see Chapter 6).

## Using Activities of Daily Living and Mobility Tasks

Clearly the most effective tools that occupational therapists can use to help patients regain trunk control are self-care, instrumental ADL, and mobility tasks.

The therapist first must perform a thorough evaluation as described in previous sections. Following the evaluation, therapists and patients should identify the most problematic movement patterns that occur during the patients' daily activities. At this point, therapists use their activity analysis skills to choose appropriate tasks that incorporate the desired patterns and postures. For example, if the identified problematic patterns are lateral flexion and lateral weight shifts, therapists may choose the following activities for the patient to practice:

- Lower extremity dressing
- Weight shifting for pressure relief
- Scooting
- Assuming a sitting position from side-lying position
- Reaching for objects that are positioned above and to the side of the patient opposite the side where lateral flexion is desired
- Reaching for objects on the floor that are on the side of the patient

The majority of ADL and mobility tasks encompass a variety of postures and movements. For the mentioned strategies to be effective, therapists initially should focus patients' attention on the desired components of trunk movements. As the patient progresses, the obvious goal is for the trunk responses to be relearned and become automatic.

---

*References 6, 7, 13, 14, 18, 25.

---

## Case Study

### REGAINING TRUNK CONTROL AFTER A STROKE

S.G. is a 64-year-old female who came to the rehabilitation unit after a right middle cerebral artery cerebrovascular accident. The following data were collected from the initial evaluation (specific to the trunk):

- Sensation was intact.
- Static postural malalignments included posterior pelvic tilt, retracted left rib cage, and increased weight bearing on left ischial tuberosity.
- Dynamic posture was difficult to assess because the patient was afraid to move. The patient could not

reach beyond her arm span when reaching with her right arm. She had a tendency to fall backward and to the left during lower extremity dressing and when reaching for objects behind her.

■ S.G.'s personal occupational therapy goals were to be able independently to don her shoes, be able to reach for objects she had dropped without falling, and decrease the amount of spillage that occurred during meals.

The initial treatment plan included adapting her wheelchair with lateral supports (which were removed when she was supervised by friends, family, and staff) and a lumbar roll to maintain optimal alignment while functioning in the wheelchair, trunk mobilizations (specifically in the directions of extension and lateral flexion to both sides), activities to recruit abdominal activity (rolling, games that encouraged trunk rotation, reaching for objects positioned overhead and behind her), and activities that presented unexpected challenges to her trunk control (e.g., balloon volleyball and catch). During the initial stages of treatment, the therapist sat behind S.G. in a straddle position, which increased feelings of security and allowed the therapist to provide outside assistance with difficult patterns and to prevent falls. S.G. was observed while eating, and the therapist noted that she did not shift her weight anteriorly when bringing food to her mouth. Instead she kept her trunk supported against the back of the chair. Because of the increased distance the food had to travel to reach her mouth, spillage was considerable, especially of liquids on a spoon (e.g., soup and cereal milk). S.G. was trained to shift her weight forward as she brought food to her mouth. Although spillage still occurred, it happened less frequently, with the food falling to the plate or table and not in her lap.

As S.G. progressed, the therapist was able to sit next to or in front of her during activities. She engaged in graded reaching activities in which the distance S.G. was required to reach was increased progressively. Activities included reaching to lower shelves in the refrigerator and reaching for objects positioned at specific levels (e.g., knee level, midshin level, and floor level).

On discharge from inpatient rehabilitation, S.G. was able to perform all basic activities of daily living with distant supervision and without assistive devices, reach to the floor when she propped her upper trunk with her more affected forearm against her knees, and eat independently by using a rocker knife to cut her food, with spillage occurring only 10% of the time.

## REVIEW QUESTIONS

1. What is considered an aligned posture in preparation for engagement in functional tasks? What are the common deviations from this posture after stroke?
2. Name three activities of daily living tasks that require control in the rotation plane.
3. What are advantages and disadvantages of using movable surfaces in trunk control treatment?
4. What are appropriate treatment activities for patients who lack trunk extensor control?
5. Explain the reason an appropriate starting alignment is considered a prerequisite for initiating functional activities.
6. Which trunk patterns are required for donning a button-down shirt?

## REFERENCES

1. Andersson BJ, Ortengren R: Myoelectric back activity during sitting, *Scand J Rehabil Med Suppl* 3:73-90, 1974.
2. Árnadóttir G: *The brain and behavior: assessing cortical dysfunction through activities of daily living*, St Louis, 1990, Mosby.
3. Ayres AJ: *Developmental dyspraxia and adult onset apraxia*, Torrance, Calif, 1985, Sensory Integration International.
4. Basmajian JV, DeLuca CJ: *Muscles alive: their functions revealed by electromyography*, ed 5, Baltimore, 1985, Williams & Wilkins.
5. Benaim C, Perennou DA, Villy J, et al: Validation of a standardized assessment of postural control in stroke patients, *Stroke* 30(9):1862-1868, 1999.
6. Bobath B: *Adult hemiplegia: evaluation and treatment*, ed 3, London, 1990, Butterworth-Heinemann.
7. Boehme R: *Improving upper body control: an approach to the treatment of tonal dysfunction*, Tucson, 1988, Therapy Skill Builders.
8. Bohannon RW: Recovery and correlates of trunk muscle strength after stroke, *Int J Rehabil Res* 18(2):162-167, 1995.
9. Bohannon RW: Lateral trunk flexion strength: impairment, measurement reliability and implications following unilateral brain lesion, *Int J Rehabil Res* 15(3):249-251, 1992.
10. Bohannon RW, Cassidy D, Walsh S: Trunk muscle strength is impaired multidirectionally after stroke, *Clin Rehabil* 9:47, 1995.
11. Carr JH, Shepherd RB, Nordholm L, et al: Investigation of a new motor assessment scale for stroke patients, *Phys Ther* 65(2):175-180, 1985.
12. Collin C, Wade D: Assessing motor impairment after stroke: a pilot reliability study, *J Neurol Neurosurg Psychiatry* 53(7):576-579, 1990.
13. Davies PM: *Right in the middle: selective trunk activity in the treatment of adult hemiplegia*, New York, 1990, Springer-Verlag.
14. Davies PM: *Steps to follow: a guide to the treatment of adult hemiplegia*, New York, 1985, Springer-Verlag.
15. Dean CW, Shepard RB: Task-related training improves performance of seated reaching tasks after stroke: a randomized controlled trial, *Stroke* 28(4):722-728, 1997.
16. De Troyer A: Mechanical role of the abdominal muscles in relation to posture, *Respir Physiol* 53(3):341-353, 1983.
17. Duarte E, Marco E, Muniesa JM, et al: Trunk control test as a functional predictor in stroke patients, *J Rehabil Med* 34(6):267-272, 2002.
18. Eggers O: *Occupational therapy in the treatment of adult hemiplegia*, New York, 1983, Springer-Verlag.
19. Esparza DY, Archambault PS, Winstein CJ, et al: Hemispheric specialization in the co-ordination of arm and trunk movements during pointing in patients with unilateral brain damage, *Exp Brain Res* 148(4):488-497, 2003.

20. Fisher B: Effect of trunk control and alignment on limb function, *J Head Trauma Rehabil* 2:72, 1987.

21. Floyd WF, Silver PHS: The function of the erector spinae muscles in certain movements and postures in man, *J Physiol* 129:184, 1955.

22. Franchignoni FP, Tesio L, Ricupero C, et al: Trunk control as an early predictor of stroke rehabilitation outcome, *Stroke* 28(7):1382-1385, 1997.

23. Fugl-Meyer AR: Post-stroke hemiplegia: assessment of physical properties, *Scand J Rehabil Med* 7(suppl):85-93, 1980.

24. Hsieh CL, Sheu CF, Hsueh IP, et al: Trunk control as an early predictor of comprehensive activities of daily living function in stroke patients, *Stroke* 33(11):2626-2630, 2002.

25. Hypes B: *Facilitating development and sensorimotor function: treatment with the ball*, Hugo, Minn, 1991, PDP Press.

26. Kapandji IA: *The physiology of the joints*, vol 3, *The trunk and vertebral column*, New York, 1974, Churchill Livingstone.

27. Kendall FP, McCreary EK, Provance P: *Muscles testing and function*, ed 4, Baltimore, 1993, Lippincott William & Wilkins.

28. Mao HF, Hsueh IP, Tang PF, et al: Analysis and comparison of the psychometric properties of three balance measures for stroke patients, *Stroke* 33(4):1022-1027, 2002.

29. Mohr JD: Management of the trunk in adult hemiplegia: the Bobath concept, *Top Neurol* 1:1-12, 1990.

30. Pedersen PM, Wandel A, Jorgensen HS, et al: Ipsilateral pushing in stroke: incidence, relation to neuropsychological symptoms, and impact on rehabilitation: the Copenhagen stroke study, *Arch Phys Med Rehabil* 77(1):25-28, 1996.

31. Perennou DA, Amblard B, Laassel el M, et al: Understanding the pusher behavior of some stroke patients with spatial deficits: a pilot study, *Arch Phys Med Rehabil* 83(4):570-575, 2002.

32. Ryerson S, Levit K: The shoulder in hemiplegia. In Donatelli RA, editor: *Physical therapy of the shoulder*, ed 2, New York, 1991, Churchill Livingstone.

33. Sabari JS: Motor learning concepts applied to activity-based intervention with adults with hemiplegia, *Am J Occup Ther* 45(6):523-530, 1991.

34. Shumway-Cook A, Woollacott M: *Motor control: theory and practical applications*, Baltimore, 1995, Williams & Wilkins.

35. Smith LK, Weiss EL, Lehmkuhl, LD: *Brunnstrom's clinical kinesiology*, ed 5, Philadelphia, 1996, FA Davis.

36. Tanaka S, Hachisuka K, Ogata H: Muscle strength of trunk flexion-extension in post-stroke hemiplegic patients, *Am J Phys Med Rehabil* 77(4):288-290, 1998.

37. Tanaka S, Hachisuka K, Ogata H: Trunk rotary muscle performance in post-stroke hemiplegic patients, *Am J Phys Med Rehabil* 76(5):366-369, 1997.

38. Thorstensson A, Oddsson L, Carlson H: Motor control of voluntary trunk movements in standing, *Acta Physiol Scand* 125:309, 1985.

39. Winzeler-Mercay U, Mudie H: The nature of the effects of stroke on trunk flexor and extensor muscles during work and rest, *Disabil Rehabil* 24(17):875-886, 2002.

40. Woodhull-McNeal AP: Activity in torso muscles during relaxed standing, *Eur J Appl Physiol* 55(4):418-424, 1986.

susan m. donato
karen halliday pulaski

**c h a p t e r 8**

# Overview of Balance Impairments: Functional Implications

## key terms

| | | |
|---|---|---|
| balance | center of mass | limits of stability |
| base of support | gaze stabilization | posture |

## chapter objectives

After completing this chapter, the reader will be able to accomplish the following:

1. Identify the systems involved in balance, and review the assessment and evaluation of component balance skills and balance during functional activity.
2. Provide examples of treatment plans and ideas based on specific balance dysfunctions to allow the therapist to implement focused intervention.
3. Participate in the development of goals and documentation systems with emphasis on the setting for service delivery and the effect of the current health care environment.

## THEORY

Balance is the ability to control the center of mass over the base of support within the limits of stability; balance results in the maintenance of stability and equilibrium. A person's ability to maintain balance in any position depends on a complex integration of multiple systems. Many theories have been proposed to explain the ability to maintain balance. In the reflex or hierarchical model, balance is considered the interaction of reflexes and reactions, which are organized hierarchically, that result in the support of the body against gravity.[17,24] In this model, balance deficits result from eliminating higher central

nervous system control, resulting in the release of spinal and supraspinal reflexes. This model has declined in popularity in recent years because common opinion embraces the idea that the nervous system more likely is comprised of complex interactions of multiple systems rather than organized as a distinct hierarchy.

The systems or distributed control model introduced by Bernstein describes balance as a complex interaction of musculoskeletal and neural systems.[35] The ability to maintain balance is specific to and modified around the constraints of the environment and task. Within this system a disruption of balance (or instability) results from a malfunction in or disruption of any one or more of the elements of the postural control system. Likewise, balance is maintained through the interaction of sensory organization and postural control systems. The information is combined and integrated in the central nervous system.

## SENSORY ORGANIZATION

According to the systems model, information from three sensory systems is used for maintaining balance. Information from the visual, vestibular, and somatosensory systems is critically important.

The visual system (see Chapter 16) provides information regarding vertical orientation and visual flow. Visual or optical flow information, which describes movement of an image on the retina, is important input that aids detection of personal and environmental movement. Information provided by the visual system can be ambiguous and must be compared with other sensory information to determine accuracy. For example, a person sitting in a stationary car next to another stationary car at a red light then may receive optical flow information that indicates the other car is moving backward. This information alone is not adequate for determining which vehicle is moving; it only reveals relative movement. The information must be compared with the other sensory information to determine which car has moved.

Somatosensory information is comprised of cutaneous and pressure receptors on the soles of the feet and of muscle and joint receptors. This information helps determine characteristics of and the relationship of the individual to the support surface. During most tasks, somatosensory information may be the most heavily relied on input in the adult population. Like visual input, somatosensory input can be ambiguous. For example, dorsiflexion at the ankle indicates that the body is displaced anteriorly over the base of support. However, when standing on an incline, this ankle position may coincide with midline posture. The individual must take other senses into consideration to determine which position is accurate.

Information from the vestibular system helps determine head position and head motion in space relative to gravity. This information generally plays a minor role in balance control, unless somatosensory and visual input are inaccurate or unavailable. The vestibular system is the only sensory reference that is not ambiguous because it depends on gravity, which is consistent in the environment.

The vestibular system (see Chapter 9) is composed of the otolith and semicircular canals. The semicircular canals sense angular acceleration, which is a change in velocity along a curved path (e.g., shaking or nodding the head). The canals are capable of detecting movement in all planes because all three are oriented in different planes (Figure 8-1). Input from the semicircular canals influences postural responses and drives compensatory eye movements.

The otolith is composed of the utricle and saccule. Together they are responsible for determining changes in head position in the linear plane or translational movement of the head. Specifically the utricle responds to head tilt and translations along the horizontal plane. In addition, the utricle appears to play an important role in producing small, torsional eye movements, which keep the eyes level when the head is tilted laterally. This helps with maintaining postural control and vertical orientation in space. The saccule appears to be instrumental in detecting vertical translations of the head.

In addition to these three systems, individuals' internal representations or perceptions influence the interactions of information. Each individual possesses an internal

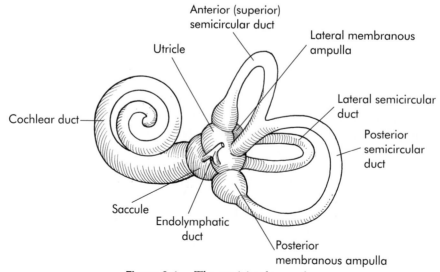

**Figure 8-1**    The semicircular canals.

perception related to the task, themselves, and the environment, which in turn influences sensory interactions and responses.

To use sensory information appropriately, each individual develops what is referred to as a *sensory strategy*. A sensory strategy is formulated when the central nervous system integrates, evaluates, and selects information received from the visual, somatosensory, and vestibular systems. The information is evaluated according to internal and external constraints, including availability of sensory information and the accuracy of environmental information. Information evaluation also may depend on the movement strategy that is occurring. The development of a sensory strategy results in a sensory-motor interaction. The central nervous system determines the most efficient use of sensory input, which then allows for generation of appropriate motor output to complete the necessary task or reach a desired goal. This is a rapid process that is not detectable when no deficits exist.

## POSTURAL CONTROL

An individual's ability to maintain equilibrium depends not only on accurate evaluation and use of sensory information but also on the implementation of effective movement strategies. Movement strategies are stereotyped or synergistic patterns used to maintain the center of mass over the base of support; they are characterized as automatic, not reflexive or voluntary. Movement strategies occur too quickly to be under voluntary control but are too slow to be considered reflexive. Synergistic movement patterns are useful in that they reduce the degrees of freedom, thus decreasing the response time. Postural actions are reduced or absent when an individual uses an external support such as a cane or countertop to help maintain postural control. Automatic postural responses include ankle, hip, and stepping strategies.[33]

An ankle strategy is used to maintain the center of mass over the base of support when movement is centered around the ankles. Knee, hip, and trunk stability is necessary for this strategy to be effective. Ankle strategies are used to control small, slow swaying motions. They are effective when the surface area is firm and long in relation to foot length. Muscular activation while using the ankle strategy occurs in a distal to proximal sequence. Timing of muscular contractions is important to generate sufficient torque about the ankles and maintain adequate stability at the hips, knees, and trunk. Ankle strategies frequently are used during "quiet" standing. For example, this strategy is effective in controlling the small, slow swaying motions that occur when a person stands in line (e.g., at a bank or grocery store).

Hip movement that maintains or restores equilibrium is a hip strategy. This strategy is most effective in maintaining stability when the support surface is short in relation to foot length or is compliant. Hip movement is used to control large or rapid swaying motions or when an ankle strategy is ineffective (i.e., unable to occur rapidly enough or generate adequate torque). Muscle activation while using hip strategies occurs in a proximal to distal sequence. This strategy is used more frequently than ankle strategies when the center of mass approaches the outer limits of the base of support and is more effective because of the ability to generate greater speed and range. An example of a situation in which persons would use a hip strategy would be a circumstance that requires them to stand on a narrow beam.

When ankle and hip strategies are or are perceived to be ineffective, the base of support is expanded in the direction of center of mass movement, resulting in the use of what is referred to as a *stepping strategy*. In this case the person takes a step to widen the base of support. This is the strategy that is used effectively when taking each step while walking. The person shifts weight outside the existing base of support and takes a step to bring the base of support back under the center of mass.

Each of the preceding movement strategies is a reactive response to center of mass movement. Anticipatory control is postural muscular activity that precedes and decreases center of mass movement. Previous experience weighs heavily in the determination of the appropriate sequence and degree of muscle activity required to maintain stability when anticipating a perturbation. Because anticipatory activities precede destablization, misperceiving the needed amount of muscle activity may result in too much or too little correction. For example, when persons pull a door open, they initiate a posterior weight shift to counteract the weight of the door. If the weight of the door is lighter than anticipated, too much correction might occur and may result in a posterior perturbation of balance.

## CENTRAL NERVOUS SYSTEM STRUCTURES

Maintaining equilibrium involves the precise integration of sensory information and the generation of appropriate and effective motor responses. Specific central nervous system structures are responsible for performing these complex tasks.

The cerebellum is the primary integrating and modulating force in balance control. The cerebellum receives information from structures such as the cortex, basal ganglia, spinocerebellar tract, vestibular nuclei, and vestibular pathways. Input is modulated, interpreted, and sent out to the cortex; basal ganglia; thalamus; fourth, fifth, and sixth cranial nerves; vestibular nuclei and pathways; and indirectly to the spinal cord, providing the regulatory input needed to control movement. Damage to any one of these structures can result in difficulties with balance and postural control. Through this complex network of central nervous system interactions the cerebellum facilitates smooth coordination of movement. The cerebellum influences the timing and synergy of muscle groups during synergistic movements as well as muscle tone or stiffness. Symmetrical, appropriate, balanced skeletal muscle activity is necessary for maintaining postural alignment and is required for smooth, coordinated movements and stability. An example of a disorder involving the cerebellum is ataxia (poor coordination of agonist and antagonist muscles that results in jerky, poorly controlled movements). An individual with cerebellar dysfunction might have an unsteady gait or visual disturbances.

The basal ganglia also are involved in integrating information used for postural control. They are involved in a series of complex pathways, much of the exact nature of which is uncertain. The basal ganglia receive information from the cortex and cerebellum and then output information to the motor cortex via the thalamus. The basal ganglia work closely with the cerebellum and are believed to influence the sequencing of automatic postural reactions including the ankle, hip, and stepping strategies previously discussed. The continuous postural adjustments that play a role in smooth, coordinated movement also are controlled by the basal ganglia. Examples of disorders involving the basal ganglia include but are not limited to rigidity, bradykinesia (slowness of movement), akinesia, resting or intention tremors, chorea, and athetosis.

The brainstem also is involved in balance control because it houses the vestibular nuclei, which receive input from the cerebellum and the vestibular system. Information is output to the vestibulospinal tract, oculomotor complex, cerebellum, and parietal lobe. The brainstem is instrumental in the integration of the vestibular input and influences compensatory eye movements (Table 8-1).

## COMPREHENSIVE EVALUATION

A comprehensive evaluation is crucial in helping the therapist understand specific balance problems patients may be experiencing. A comprehensive evaluation always should include a subjective client interview, an assessment of balance component skills, and an assessment of balance skills within the context of meaningful functional tasks. Evaluations may vary depending on the acuteness of the neurologic insult, severity of the cerebrovascular accident (CVA), and setting in which care is provided (e.g., inpatient rehabilitation, outpatient rehabilitation, or home health care).

### Subjective Interview

Patients who have had an acute CVA may not be able to provide accurate information during the interview process. They may be able to provide more information later in treatment when they are outpatients or are functioning in the home and community.

Subjective patient interviews allow patients to describe in their own words the way the CVA has affected their

**Table 8-1**

### Central Nervous System Structures Involved in Balance Control

| STRUCTURE | INPUT | OUTPUT | FUNCTION | INDICATION OF DYSFUNCTION |
|---|---|---|---|---|
| Cerebellum | Cortex<br>Basal ganglia<br>Spinocerebellar tract<br>Vestibular nuclei<br>Vestibular pathways | Cortex<br>Basal ganglia<br>Thalamus<br>Cranial nerves: IV, V, VI<br>Vestibular nuclei<br>Vestibular pathways | Integrates and modulates information.<br>Regulates input to control movement.<br>Influences muscle tone/stiffness.<br>Inputs timing and synergy of muscle groups during synergistic movements. | Ataxia<br>Unsteady gait<br>Visual disturbance |
| Basal ganglia | Cortex<br>Cerebellum | Motor cortex<br>Thalamus | Sequences automatic postural reactions. | Rigidity<br>Bradykinesia<br>Akinesia<br>Tremors (resting/intention)<br>Chorea<br>Athetosis |
| Brainstem | Cerebellum<br>Vestibular system | Vestibulospinal tract<br>Oculomotor complex<br>Cerebellum<br>Parietal lobe | Integrates vestibular input.<br>Initiates compensatory eye movements. | Dysfunctional compensatory eye movements<br>Vestibular dysfunction |

level of functioning. The interview should allow the therapist to obtain the following information about the patient:

1. Premorbid health history

   The patient's premorbid health history can have a significant impact on prognosis and thus appropriate goals. Having a thorough understanding of any premorbid conditions that could affect a patient's balance functioning is important for the therapist. Examples include diabetic neuropathies, vision disturbances, vertigo, prior CVA or head injuries, prior lower extremity range of motion or strength problems, or other orthopedic issues.

2. Prior lifestyle

   As more details are added to this portion of the interview, the therapist will be better equipped to create an individualized treatment plan to meet the individual patient needs. The interview should include information such as the following:

   - Waking time each morning
   - Schedule of tasks used to prepare for the day
   - Whether a bath, shower, or sponge bath is taken
   - Bathing time
   - Other household chores for which the patient is responsible

   Outlining a schedule of a typical day at home may be helpful (if the patient is able). The therapist's attendance to the specifics of performing tasks and to the order in which tasks occur is important.

3. *Prior functional status*

   The therapist needs to have a thorough understanding of the patient's functional level before the CVA. This portion of the interview should include information such as the following:

   - Whether the patient ambulated independently and what device if any was necessary for ambulation
   - Whether the patient required any assistance with performing daily tasks
   - Whether the patient was able to function independently in the community (including specifics about activities) and whether any change in activity was experienced in the past 6 months

4. Patient's perspective of current functioning

   This area may be difficult for patients who have just had a CVA, but understanding what patients consider as problems resulting from balance deficits is important for the therapist. Early in the rehabilitation process, patients may cite self-care and mobility as problem areas. Later, when patients are receiving home health or outpatient services, they may no longer experience difficulty in these basic areas but may cite problems with household or community activities. This portion of the interview is important for determining patients' awareness level about the way their balance deficit limits their participation in normal activities and for determining appropriate and meaningful goals.

## Component Assessment

When the subjective interview has been completed, the therapist should collect objective data. Evaluation of the component parts of balance control is important before introduction of more complex tasks. Thorough range of motion testing of active and passive range of motion, particularly of the trunk and lower extremities, must be completed and helps determine whether a patient has any biomechanical constraints that might have an effect on postural control. The therapists must evaluate the patient's strength and appropriate patterns of skeletal muscle activity, particularly of the lower extremities and trunk, to determine neuromotor influences on postural control. The therapist also must examine the sensory systems that play a role in maintaining equilibrium. One such system is the visual system (see Chapter 16) and includes visual acuity and oculomotor function assessments. Oculomotor function is eye movements such as voluntary movements and gaze stabilization. Assessment of sensation is also critical and should include light touch, deep pressure, proprioception, and kinesthesia assessments. Sensation in the lower extremities is clearly one of the most critical factors affecting balance control. Vestibular system function is difficult to evaluate in isolation but is discussed further in the context of sensory organization (see Chapter 9).

After evaluating balance components, the therapist must examine more complex tasks that integrate the components. The therapist should evaluate patients' postural alignment while they are seated and standing. Observation skills are critical in performing these and subsequent assessments. Symmetrical alignment and appropriate positioning of body parts over the base of support are the goals. The therapist should note any asymmetry in alignment or bias over the base of support. In general, the posture should be symmetrical; the head should be in midline, centered over the shoulders; the shoulders should be centered and aligned over the pelvis; under "normal" conditions the feet should be approximately hip distance apart; and the pelvis should be centered over the base of support created by the feet (Figures 8-2 and 8-3).

Each individual possesses an area about which the center of mass may be moved over any given base of support without disrupting equilibrium. This is referred to as the *limits of stability*. Assessment of patients' ability to move within their limits of stability and noting the symmetry and extent of those limits is important. Because of the biomechanical constraints of the foot and ankle, the limits are greatest in the anterior/posterior direction and smaller in the lateral direction. The greatest degree of movement can occur anteriorly. The area created by the limits of stability is in the form of an ellipse (Figure 8-4). The limits of stability may be measured in a number of ways. An experienced evaluator with a strong understanding of typical limits of stability might ask patients to shift

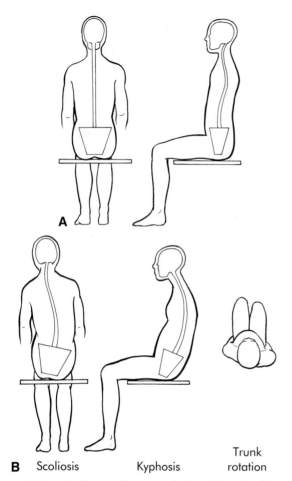

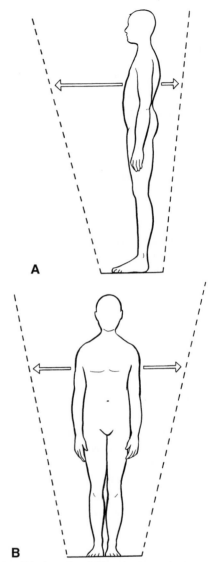

**Figure 8-2**   **A,** Correct alignment during sitting. **B,** Common asymmetries assumed after stroke.

**Figure 8-4**   Limits of stability. **A,** Lateral view. **B,** Anterior view.

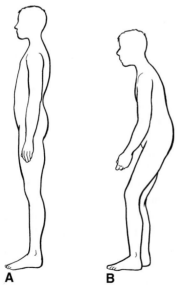

**Figure 8-3**   **A,** Correct alignment during standing. **B,** Flexed posture. (Note hip/knee flexion, kyphosis, forward head posture, and change in center of gravity.)

their weight as far as they can in all directions and then observe and note the patients' ability to move over their base of support. The therapist also may ask patients to perform a task that requires the center of mass to move over the base of support while observing their performance. Several computerized pressure plate systems on the market are able to compute an individual's "normal" limits of stability based on height by force plate analysis. The therapist then can compare normal and actual figures. These pieces of equipment are costly and are not available in all clinics.

***Postural Control System.***   Information regarding biomechanical and neuromuscular parameters available to the patient has been established through the comprehensive component evaluation. Integration and the effectiveness of these capabilities in the central nervous system are

therapists in determining whether their hypotheses are substantiated. For example, patients may lose their balance when attempting to put on their pants while standing. Therapists may hypothesize that the loss of balance results from a poor ability to shift weight accurately, poor postural alignment when attempting to shift weight, and a lack of lateral hip strategy use when standing on one leg. These hypotheses can be supported by testing patients' limits of stability, evaluation of their postural alignment, and assessment of whether they are using an available hip strategy. These steps allow therapists to develop individualized treatment plans and set realistic short- and long-term goals for each patient.

To remember that therapists do not treat balance deficits separately from other deficits a stroke survivor may have is important. The treatment of balance dysfunction obviously is affected by any existing cognitive or visual perceptual deficits such as memory deficits or left neglect. For example, patients with cognitive deficits undoubtedly benefit more from a treatment program that incorporates familiar, repetitive functional tasks than an exercise program with activities that are meaningless to them. Therapists should incorporate multiple goals into each treatment session.

Because of current, ongoing changes in health care reimbursement, therapists' collaboration with patients to focus treatment around goals for the home or at work is crucial. This approach allows patients to transition as quickly as possible to less restrictive environments. Failure to focus on goals may result in patients being discharged to more restrictive environments that allow less independent lifestyles (e.g., to a nursing home instead of home). Therapists should also focus on treating specific balance deficits to develop an individualized treatment plan that will assist patients with becoming independent as soon as possible.

## ESTABLISHING GOALS AND TREATMENT PLANS

Setting goals for patients with balance disorders can be difficult. Therapists must have a thorough understanding of patients' specific CVA neuropathologic condition. Although complete neuroanatomy review is beyond the scope of this chapter, appropriate resources are listed in the references. Several factors contribute to whether patients receive a positive or poor prognosis and may include size and location of the lesion and any secondary factors that have developed, such as extensions of the original CVA, brain edema, and anoxia. The previous medical history also is important for determining eventual functional outcomes. Factors to consider include any prior CVAs, a history of alcohol use, any head trauma, diabetic neuropathies, age-related changes (such as the loss of inner ear hairs), and balance problems (such as

vertigo). Prior problems may interfere with a patient's ability to compensate for the new neurologic insult.

Ideally, a treatment team consists of an otolaryngologist or neurologist, a physical therapist, an occupational therapist, the patient, and the patient's family (if applicable). The occupational therapist is not responsible for prognosticating, but to set realistic goals and design an appropriate treatment plan, the therapist must have input from the otolaryngologist or neurologist concerning prognosis. If therapists are not fortunate enough to work directly with an otolaryngologist, they should contact the neurologist treating the patient for the CVA. Occupational therapists also must work closely with physical therapists to ensure that the treatment plans of both disciplines support and reinforce each other rather than work against each other.

After receiving the prognosis, the therapist must decide whether to design a treatment plan that focuses on remediation, compensation, or both. The plan may be affected greatly by the setting in which the therapist provides treatment. If the prognosis indicates considerable improvement within 3 to 4 weeks, a therapist providing inpatient services may decide to emphasize remediation for the first few weeks and then compensation just before discharge to ensure that the patient is functional in basic tasks. A therapist providing outpatient treatment for the same patient may focus solely on remediation because the patient already has established a safe way to function in the environment and is now focusing on improving balance deficits. If a patient has a poor prognosis for recovery of balance function, the therapist may emphasize compensation early in treatment to ensure success. A patient's cognitive status also significantly affects when compensatory devices are introduced into treatment. A patient with memory loss requires more repetition and time to learn to use a walker while performing kitchen tasks than a patient with no memory loss. Introducing devices and training the patient in their use early in treatment is more likely to facilitate learning specific techniques.

Therapists need to understand the implications of prescribing use of compensatory devices for patients with balance deficits. When a walker or cane is introduced into treatment before a patient is even given a chance to function without it, the therapist cannot assess accurately the patient's ability to remediate the balance deficits. A walker or cane instantly increases the base of support and thus decreases the demand on the patient's balance system to improve. A walker or cane also greatly changes the way in which a patient moves during functional activities and alters normal movement. The patient no longer has to shift weight in a normal way. Instead, weight is shifted through the upper extremities during ambulation. Postural muscle activity has been shown to be altered even with light upper extremity support.

Therapists must make informed decisions about using equipment during treatment. They must take into consideration all of the factors discussed previously when choosing a treatment plan. Tub seats and reachers may be appropriate for patients with orthopedic limitations or who have a poor prognosis for recovery of balance function; however, introducing too many devices too early in treatment in fact may hinder recovery of balance function. For example, if patients are given tub benches or shower seats before being given the opportunity to attempt to stand in the shower, they may not be able to reach their full level of independence. This is not to suggest that devices should not be considered or recommended—numerous patients are able to function only because of their adaptive equipment and devices—it is only to suggest that when planning treatment, therapists should be aware of the implications of using each device. Therapists may consider allowing patients to use devices outside of therapy that provide greater independence but limit their use during actual therapy sessions. Patients then can maintain their independence while still working toward improving their balance. Therapists may be able to help patients function more safely and become more active, even if they are using a device.

Using functional activities and emphasizing functional outcomes always have been basic principles of occupational therapy, and they are now beginning to be embraced by many other disciplines. Hsieh et al[20] stated that using added-purpose occupation is motivating during performance. They add that numerous studies suggest that using meaningful tasks in treatment improves movement and performance.* Traditional treatment of balance disorders has been focused on exercise with the hope and assumption that patients would carry over what they learned in exercise into daily function. Although occupational therapists always have centered treatment around functional activities, during the past few decades therapists may have treated daily activities as secondary in their attempt to integrate older neurophysiologic treatment approaches. Currently available information supports the use of functional tasks as primary intervention tools (Boxes 8-1 and 8-2). The tasks specifically should address the balance component disturbances that have been identified during evaluation so that occupational therapists can provide treatment that is individualized and functional.

## TREATING ASYMMETRICAL WEIGHT DISTRIBUTION

Patients who have had a CVA often have an impaired ability to control their center of mass over their base of

---

*References 4, 19, 21-23, 27-29, 31, 36, 37, 42, 43.

**Box 8-1**

### Sample Treatment Activities and Goals While in Standing Postures

- Static standing (no engagement in activity) graded by timed tolerance for the posture
- Static standing while holding a glass of water
- Standing while fastening shirt closures
- Retrieving an object (graded by size and weight of object) from a shelf at chest level
- Retrieving an object from a shelf at knee level (graded by weight and size of object)
- Pulling up pants from ankles while standing
- Setting table, including covering table with table cloth
- Opening refrigerator and retrieving object from top shelf
- Opening refrigerator and retrieving object from bottom shelf
- Removing shoes while standing
- Donning pajama pants while standing
- Picking up phone book from floor
- Placing full pet food bowl on floor
- Retrieving pot or pan from lower cabinet

These treatment activities do not necessarily represent a progression of difficulty.

**Box 8-2**

### Sample Treatment Activities and Goals for Ambulatory Patients

- Carrying empty shopping bag 30 feet (graded by distance and surface)
- Carrying bag of groceries 30 feet (graded by weight, distance, and surface)
- Carrying a half-full glass of water 30 feet
- Carrying a full glass of water 30 feet
- Carrying a full cup on a saucer 30 feet
- Walking upstairs without upper extremity support
- Walking upstairs carrying laundry basket

These treatment activities do not necessarily represent a progression of difficulty.

support. These patients often assume an asymmetrical posture during activities that require static and dynamic balance skills. Asymmetrical posture and poor upright stability have been correlated with an increased risk for falls.[41] In addition, an unstable upright posture also has been correlated with functional assessment on the Barthel index.[25] Wu et al[41] state the "one functional goal in rehabilitating persons with hemiplegia should be . . . to improve symmetrical characteristics of postural control." The most common form of treatment for asymmetrical weight bearing and poor postural control is using passive and active weight shifting. This treatment traditionally has been provided in the form of exercise or introduction of outside perturbations to encourage postural reactions. The underlying assumption is that practicing the repetition of postural adjustments will result in long-term improvements in balance during ambulation and functional activities.[12] Numerous authors have advocated the use of passive and active weight shifting as a viable treatment approach.[5-7,39] If patients are not able actively to shift their weight, they initially may need guidance from the therapist and assistance with moving in effective patterns. Patients also must be able actively to shift their weight. Active weight shifting requires postural adjustments that are intrinsic to the activity being performed.[12] Patients must be able to initiate and execute a skilled weight shift that is an appropriate response to the perturbation actually experienced to maintain balance. Patients who experience difficulty with perceiving weight shifts and limits of stability may overestimate or underestimate the amount of weight shift required to adjust to the perturbation. Other patients may know the needed weight shift but may not be able to execute the coordinated motor movements and timing to make it effective.

Treatment for patients should focus on value-added occupations specific to individual patients. The therapist can use information gained during the patient interview to determine in which performance areas a patient is experiencing balance deficits (e.g., donning pants while standing or reaching into a lower cabinet during meal preparation) and which activities the patient values. Occupational therapists must perform task analyses to determine which weight shifts are required to complete the tasks patients want to perform. The therapist also should consider information from the component evaluation (e.g., poor ability to shift center of mass laterally and anteriorly when reaching up to a high cabinet in the kitchen) when making the treatment plan.

Incorporating active weight shifting into a specific activity allows patients to learn more normal postural responses to particular activities; therapists do not have to assume training has transferred from an exercise to an activity. Therapists also can be sure that the type of weight shifting they are asking patients to do is appropriate for particular tasks. Patients then are able to incorporate an anticipatory set based on the specific task, an important component of motor learning. Activities can be graded by the amount of weight shifting required, size of the base of support, and complexity of the task. Weight shifting can occur as a result of present anticipatory controls (e.g., shifting the center of gravity laterally to prepare to don pants while standing) or outside perturbations (e.g., getting on or off an escalator). Weight shifts also can occur in response to movement that is initiated by the upper extremities (e.g., putting a table cloth on a table). The therapist can make these activities more difficult by gradually increasing the force required by the upper extremities to perform the task (e.g., picking up an empty suitcase and then a full suitcase). The therapist can break down activities into a hierarchy of tasks ranging from simple to more complex and should select tasks based on patients' abilities and their typical daily activities. For example, the task of making a bed requires numerous weight shifts but would not be an appropriate activity for a patient who did not make beds before the CVA.

Patients may be able to use a variety of feedback mechanisms to improve symmetrical postural alignment. Therapists can instruct them to use somatosensory information about pressure they receive through their feet while weight shifting (if sensation is intact). If patients have a lateral bias, the therapist needs to cue them. For example, a therapist can cue a patient with an anterior or posterior bias to locate foot pressure in relation to the balls of the feet.

The therapist also may instruct patients to use visual information. Therapists may need to use a mirror for patients with a posterior bias so that the patients can see they are drifting away from the mirror. This method may be most appropriate when performing self-care tasks that normally involve the use of a mirror.

## TREATMENT PLANNING

As stated previously, the central nervous system uses information from the visual, vestibular, and somatosensory systems to maintain balance. Shumway-Cook and Horak[34] state that the central nervous system uses this feedback to monitor the relationship between the position of the body in space and the forces acting on it. The therapist must incorporate information obtained from the component balance assessment (specifically, from the test of sensory organization) into the treatment planning process. The therapist usually will be able to establish a correlation between functional observations and assessments from the test for sensory organization. Therapists should be able to identify functional tasks that place patients at risk for loss of balance; these activities can become part of the treatment plan (Table 8-3). Patients who lose their balance while transitioning from linoleum to carpet in their house usually perform poorly under testing conditions forcing them to maintain balance on uneven surfaces. Likewise, patients who lose their balance while walking in a mall or busy area with a great deal of peripheral movement usually perform poorly under the testing conditions forcing them to maintain their balance while receiving conflicting visual input. Therapists need to observe patients' performances during component testing and functional tasks. Therapists also must determine possible compensations or strategies patients may use when one or more systems are impaired. Patients with somatosensory dysfunctions usually become visually dependent, whereas patients with visual disturbances

**Table 8-3**

**Correlation of Component Testing and Functional Activities**

| SENSORY INFORMATION* | STRATEGIES | TASK |
|---|---|---|
| 1. Difficulty with 4, 5, and 6 (sway reference support) | Absent hip strategy | Standing on carpet while opening a lower drawer with flexed hips and knees; walking outside on grass or beach and picking up object off ground; getting on or off escalator or moving sidewalk |
| 2. Difficulty with 2, 3, 5, and 6 (visual conflict) | Excessive ankle/step strategies | Walking in mall; scanning items in kitchen cabinets; scanning items in grocery store; hanging clothes on line out of basket; rinsing shampoo out of hair while in shower with eyes closed and head tipped backward |
| 3. Difficulty with 5 and 6 (must rely on vestibular input) | Delayed strategies | Getting up at night to go to bathroom (e.g., walking in low light down carpeted hallway and transitioning to linoleum in bathroom); walking in dark movie theater down incline while searching for seat |
| 4. Difficulty with 4, 5, and 6 | None or delayed lateral hip strategies | Standing on one foot to don pants; standing in near tandem to reach up or down into cabinet; walking from one point to another; standing in near tandem to pick something up off of floor (e.g., cat's dish) |

*Numbers refer to test conditions (see Table 8-2).

usually become dependent on surfaces. Patients with vestibular dysfunctions may become visually or surface dependent. These compensatory strategies can work for patients in isolated environments but prevent true independence and result in a higher risk for falls for patients who are active in the home and/or community. Patients often limit their participation in home activities or simply stop going out into the community as a way to compensate for balance deficits, resulting in social isolation or depression. The therapist can obtain this information from the initial patient interview.

After determining which systems are impaired, therapists should identify activities that are important to the patient and involve those systems. Those impaired systems can be challenged gradually to relearn adaptation by controlling the conditions in which the activities are performed. Surface-dependent patients may be more likely to lose their balance when transitioning from one surface to another in the home (e.g., from the kitchen linoleum to the living room carpet). Carrying an object from the kitchen into the living room may be a functional task that places patients at risk for loss of balance. Therapists can develop a treatment plan that initially requires patients to practice holding an item while standing on an uneven surface. The next step would be to have patients reach for an item while standing on an uneven surface. Patients would then carry an item as they transitioned from an uneven surface to an even surface and vice versa. These particular patients also would be at risk for loss of balance during other functional tasks that required community (beyond the household) ambulation. Curbs,

sidewalks, gravel, grass, and sand are all uneven surfaces. The somatosensory information received from the feet of surface-dependent patients tells the central nervous system that the patients are falling. A balance reaction that is inappropriate to the task (e.g., walking on an uneven surface) but appropriate to the information the central nervous system receiving and processing may result. Therapists first should have patients practice simple functional tasks on uneven surfaces and then increase the challenge by asking them to engage in more complex tasks while transitioning to and from uneven and even surfaces. The tasks should be meaningful to patients and related to their lifestyles.

Visually dependent patients often are at risk for loss of balance when their vision is obscured for any reason (e.g., when they are in the dark or poorly lit areas) or the central nervous system receives "false" visual information (e.g., peripheral images of persons walking past patients telling the central nervous system they are falling forward when they are not).

Patients may be at risk for losing their balance when getting up in the middle of the night to get a drink or go to the bathroom, walking in a movie theater, or taking a nighttime stroll outside if they are too reliant on their vision. Treatment plans can be developed that require patients to perform various activities in low lighting or with obscured vision. Common examples of this include closing the eyes in the shower while rinsing out shampoo, stepping from a brightly lit environment into a darker environment, and carrying a glass of liquid while walking (patients must keep their eyes on the glass rather than on the floor and the environment to make sure they do not spill the contents). Even walking while engaged in conversation can be difficult for visually dependent patients because persons normally look at one another rather than the environment while talking.

Patients also may lose their balance during functional activities if they have difficulty with head-eye coordination and gaze stabilization. Activities such as walking in a busy mall, scanning the grocery store shelves for items, and placing groceries on various shelves can cause loss of balance. The central nervous system is unable to override the false visual information that results from these tasks, and thus the patients feel like they are losing their balance. Patients then institute postural reactions that are incongruent with the actual events that are occurring. Therapists can develop treatment plans that challenge patients' ability to maintain gaze stability during functional activities requiring coordinated head-eye movements.

Patients with impaired vestibular function are generally visually and surface dependent, although they usually rely more heavily on one system. Patients with premorbid health issues may be more reliant on one system for a predetermined reason. For example, patients with diabetic neuropathies may be more visually dependent because they do not have access to somatosensory information through their lower extremities. Most traditional treatment approaches have relied on graded, repetitive head movements in the form of exercise to improve vestibular functions.[8,11] Cohen et al[10] outline a treatment approach that incorporates this basic premise into functional activity. They stress that treatment activities must include head movements and positions that elicit the vestibular dysfunction during assessment. They also stress that activities must be interesting to patients; their use may assist patients with relating to real-life experiences. Suggested activities include retrieving towels in a basket on the floor and hanging them on an overhead clothesline, ambulating in the hallways while scanning and describing objects placed at various heights, playing badminton, and dribbling a basketball back and forth across the room. A thorough and accurate assessment of the specific impaired balance deficit is necessary to design the most efficacious treatment plan.

## RETRAINING BALANCE STRATEGIES

As discussed previously, part of the balance assessment is assessing what patients do to regain their balance. Three strategies were outlined as normal balance strategies: ankle, hip, and step strategies. A component assessment allows therapists to determine whether a strategy is being used, the amount of delay in strategy use (and therefore its effectiveness), and whether the appropriate strategy is being used. Therapists must be able to complete skilled, accurate task analyses to determine which strategy should be used in particular activities. Therapists should see a cor-

relation between functional activity observations and the results of component testing. This information can be used to determine which functional activities may place patients at risk for loss of balance. The identified activities then may become part of the treatment plan (see Table 8-3).

Therapists also can design treatment plans to elicit the use of appropriate balance strategies. Therapists can elicit ankle strategies by asking patients to engage in tasks requiring small weight shifts on solid support surfaces that are larger than their feet. For example, patients could reach up into a cabinet to put away groceries or put away laundry on a shelf in a closet. They can elicit hip strategies by asking patients to engage in tasks requiring larger weight shifts on narrow bases of support. These tasks could include playing toss and catch on a balance beam. Therapists also can elicit hip strategies by asking patients to reach into drawers or cabinets without locking their knees in extension; hip flexion is necessary to counteract the resulting anterior weight shift (Figure 8-5). Therapists

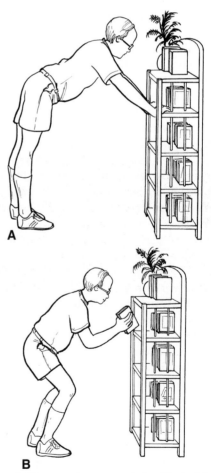

**Figure 8-5** **A,** Knees are hyperextended and locked during functional activity, with weight shifted forward onto the upper extremities. Upper extremities are used as a base of support rather than for function. **B,** Hips and knees are flexed (as during hip strategy use) to allow center of mass to remain over lower extremity base of support. Upper extremities are free to be used for function.

can elicit step strategies by engaging patients in activities that require them to make weight shifts outside of their base of support, such as hitting a tennis ball against a wall or reaching out of their base of support to pick up work boots off the floor.

## OTHER FACTORS AFFECTING TREATMENT PLANNING

Therapists must consider other factors that may impair patients' balance while functioning. A common factor that often is overlooked, especially in inpatient rehabilitation, is endurance. When patients are treated in an inpatient setting, they often are not asked to complete tasks entirely. For example, when bathing or dressing, the therapist unintentionally may "help" patients who are bathing or dressing by gathering their clothes or getting towels. Inpatients also often have large periods of time between therapy sessions when they are not engaged in activity. Therefore a rehabilitation day may have a great deal of therapy hours, but it does not accurately reflect patients' daily home life.

In the hospital, patients usually have breakfast brought to them and often eat it in bed. They then may have a break before occupational therapists arrive to address self-care tasks. Patients then may have another break before physical therapists arrive to address mobility activities. This type of schedule can result in an inaccurate picture of patients' independence and clearly does consider whether patients' endurance levels will affect their balance at home. Therapists need to devise a treatment plan that resembles the patients' typical day at home as closely as possible.

Other factors that can influence a patient's balance during functional activities are cognitive and visual perception impairments. Familiar, functionally based activities can help to reduce the effects of these impairments, but clearly occupational therapists must address these issues during treatment as well.

Medical factors such as infections, metabolic disturbances, and medications also can affect a patient's balance skills. Any significant changes that therapists observe should be reported immediately to the physician.

## DOCUMENTATION

Accurate documentation should include a full evaluation, description of the treatment plan, short- and long-term goals, and patient outcomes, which must be functional and measurable. Because of the current climate of managed health care, documentation should be as streamlined as possible and easily understood by any person who accesses the information, including other team members, case managers, third-party payers, patients, and family members. The documentation format should span the continuum of care and should be adjusted easily to meet the patient's needs and for the setting in which intervention is being provided (e.g., inpatient rehabilitation or outpatient clinic).

Documentation can help structure thought processes and reinforce clinical reasoning skills in the areas of assessment, treatment planning, and establishment of goals. Documentation tools should be reliable, valid, sensitive, and specific and should reflect real-life situations. If possible, the therapist should use one multipurpose form.

Specific balance component assessments can be accomplished by using any of the assessments discussed previously, including sensory organization, balance strategy, and actual and perceived limits of stability testing. Documentation also should include an evaluation of physical status (e.g., range of motion and strength).

One documentation tool is the functional independence day (FID) form.[14] Figure 8-6 is an example of a FID form that was used in an inpatient rehabilitation program. The FID form is used to generate a list of activities that can be adapted and individualized for patients based on one of their typical days. The example given in Figure 8-6 involves getting up in the morning, bathing, dressing, and carrying out simple homemaking tasks. The activity can be rated simply as pass or fail; that is, patients either are able to accomplish a task without losing their balance or are not. In this manner, the FID form could serve as the initial evaluation for function.

Therapists could complete assessments of function weekly, biweekly, or monthly, depending on the setting in which services are being provided. Four weeks of progress are included in Figure 8-6, so the FID information also could be the functional status portion of a weekly or monthly progress note. Therapists could document progress further by distinguishing whether an activity was completed in a wheelchair or while ambulating level. A space for comments could be provided for observations, such as the number of times patients lose their balance, any devices used (such as a walker or tub bench), and cues provided during the task.

A FID form should be structured to measure the effect fatigue may have on patients' balance over a period of time. Therapists can adapt the FID form to reflect a typical day for an individual patient (this information should have been gained during the patient interview). The order in which activities occur should reflect the order in which they normally occur for patients. Activities can be added and deleted based on patients'

Functional Independence Day

Patient name: _____

Diagnosis: _____

General comments (including general observations of balance, consistent direction of bias, reactions or loss of balance, cognitive/perceptual status, interfering factors): _____

_____

_____

_____

_____

| Activity    Evaluation date: Level: wheelchair (WC) or ambulatory (amb) | | | | Comments (Note cues, assistive device, assistance, or # of loss of balance/posture) |
|---|---|---|---|---|
| Rolling | | | | |
| Moving from supine to sitting | | | | |
| Transferring out of bed | | | | |
| Gathering necessary items for dressing | | | | |
| Going to shower | | | | |
| Undressing | | | | |
| Transferring into shower | | | | |
| Showering | | | | |
| Transferring out of shower | | | | |
| Drying off | | | | |
| Dressing | | | | |
| Going to room | | | | |
| Putting away items | | | | |
| Stripping bed | | | | |
| Going to laundry | | | | |
| Returning to room | | | | |
| Making bed | | | | |
| Gathering breakfast items | | | | |
| Preparing meal | | | | |
| Placing tablecloth | | | | |
| Setting table | | | | |
| Cleaning up (loading dishwasher) | | | | |
| Vacuuming rug | | | | |
| Going back to room | | | | |

**Figure 8-6**  Functional independence day form. (Courtesy Susan Donato, Karen Pulaski, Diane MacKenzie, Karen McManus, and Eileen Wusteny.)

daily activities. The FID format could be appropriate for inpatient, outpatient, home health, and even extended care settings.

A FID form also allows therapists to see quickly which activities are difficult for the patient. Combined with the diagnosis, prognosis, and data from the evaluation, this information could assist the therapist in determining appropriate short- and long-term goals. The environment for therapy services also has an influence on the choice of goals. Because of shorter lengths of stay, patients leaving inpatient settings may not even have independent goals for basic activities such as bathing and dressing if a family member is available to assist. Outpatient and home health therapists and clinicians providing treatment in subacute or extended care settings may be assisting the patient with basic activities and household management and community tasks. A FID form could readily assist the therapist with identifying specific problematic activities and allow the therapist to address these activities directly without spending extensive time and effort to reassess the patient.

A FID form also could be used for patient and family education. The form is easy for patients and families to understand and clearly identifies activities the patient can complete independently or those in which the patient requires assistance. The therapist could use the form during a hands-on demonstration of these tasks and show the family the way to assist the patient.

Families and patients could be given a copy of this form so that they can see the progress that has been made and the type of assistance required. A FID form also could be used for the discharge evaluation. The form clearly tracks a patient's progress toward goals and status on discharge. The form then could be forwarded to the next care setting in the continuum and used as a source of information not only about initial evaluation and discharge status but also weekly or monthly progress. Specific skill component assessment information also should be forwarded.

One potential problem with using a FID format is the amount of time necessary to complete the assessment, especially if tasks are performed in the time frame described by the patient. One way to address the issue of time and ensure that all team members are working toward consistent, patient-centered goals is to share the responsibility of the evaluation among team members. They can accomplish this task by arranging back-to-back therapy sessions (i.e., blocking off a large amount of time to assess one patient). Because task performance is rated on a pass/fail basis (and therefore the subjectivity involved when grading a test is not an issue), the assessment can be carried out by many team members. Once the assessment is complete, team members can collabo-

rate to determine the treatment focus for the next week, set short- and long-term goals, and arrange discharge plans.

Another potential problem is that in some settings, such as subacute or extended care, performance of specific relevant tasks may be limited by space and/or equipment. Occupational therapists must improvise as much as possible to simulate a patient's typical day and work within the confines of the treatment setting.

The FID form is just one example of a documentation system that meets previously discussed criteria for documentation tools. Every setting is unique, so therapists should develop documentation formats that meet the needs of the patients served in each particular setting and must ensure that documentation is focused on functional outcomes.

## BALANCE ASSESSMENTS

In addition to those mentioned, numerous other functional balance assessments have been developed.[16,18,26,32] A brief overview of several of these assessments follows.

- The "get up and go" test requires the patient to stand up from a chair with armrests, walk a short distance, turn around, return to the chair, and sit again.[26] Performance is rated on a somewhat nonspecific 5-point scale. This test is used with the older adult population and because of its vague rating criteria, the criteria should be established in a facility if used as an assessment tool.[30]

- The clinical test of sensory organization and balance,[34] which was described previously, uses six test conditions to assess an individual's ability to access, use, and organize sensory information. Within this formalized procedure, the therapist times the tests, measures the amount of sway, and records complete loss of balance falls. This test is also appropriate for use in children, patients with hemiplegia,[13] and patients with vestibular disorders.[9]

- The functional reach test[16] requires the patient to stand next to a wall with a yardstick placed parallel to the floor. The patient is asked to reach as far forward as possible, and the reach length is measured. This test is quick and easy to perform and does not require expensive equipment. Test/retest and interrator reliability are high.[16,40] The test has been used with a variety of populations spanning children through the elderly.[15,16,40] The disadvantage of this examination is that it only measures one functional task and only assesses skills in the anterior direction.[30]

- The Tinetti test[38] assesses balance and gait. A specific scoring method is used, and some education about the test is needed to administer it. For example, gait rating involves observation of several aspects of gait, including step symmetry and step length. This test is also fairly quick and is easy to administer. The test has been developed for and is used primarily with older adults.

- The Berg Balance Scale[2] is more time consuming. The test examines a number of factors, such as unsupported sitting and standing, transfers, reaching forward, picking objects up from the floor, turning 360 degrees, and standing on one foot, and each is graded on a 5-point scale. The assessment outlines the specific scoring criteria. This test examines many aspects of balance and has been shown to have high interrelator reliability and validity in older adults.[1-3,30] This test has been developed primarily for and used with the older population and stroke patients.[2,3]

The assessment and treatment of balance disorders for recovering stroke patients are complex. Therapists need to understand the balance system and have a comprehensive way to assess balance function and dysfunction. They then determine realistic short- and long-term goals that are appropriate for each patient based on diagnostic and evaluation information. The therapist should devise a comprehensive treatment plan to improve specific balance deficits and ultimately assist the patient with transitioning to a more independent lifestyle.

## Case Study

### IMPROVING FUNCTION THROUGH BALANCE RETRAINING

M.J. is 58-year-old female who was diagnosed with a right middle cerebral artery cerebrovascular accident. She was assessed first by an inpatient rehabilitation occupational therapist who determined that the patient had difficulty controlling her balance during bathing, grooming, and dressing. The patient stated that she wanted to perform all of these activities independently. The therapist noted that M.J. had a postural bias to the right with static and dynamic balance, used a wide base of support during functional tasks, and was unable to control her center of gravity when shifting her leg to the left to complete a task. Component testing revealed left hemiplegia, but M.J. was able to support weight on her left lower extremity. Sensation was impaired but not absent in her left lower extremity. M.J.'s perceived limits of stability

were not congruent with her actual limits of stability. She underestimated her ability to shift weight to the left and thus could not complete tasks that required her to shift weight to the left. When assisted with a left weight shift, M.J. was not able to control the shift because of poor coordination and timing of muscle activation. Because she lost control whenever she shifted weight to the left, M.J. compensated by maintaining an asymmetrical postural alignment. When asked to shift her weight actively to the left, M.J. altered her postural alignment by attempting to shift her shoulders rather than her center of mass.

Treatment initially centered on assisting M.J. passively and then actively to achieve and maintain a symmetrical postural alignment during static standing tasks. The therapist selected parts of self-care tasks that did not require large weight shifts (e.g., combing her hair, washing her face, and selecting clothing from her closet) and focused on maintaining midline. The therapist helped M.J. learn to use visual and somatosensory information when possible to provide information about her position in space.

As M.J. improved her ability to achieve and maintain midline during additional static standing tasks, the therapist began to introduce tasks requiring a more significant weight shift from right to left (e.g., putting on her shirt while standing, reaching for objects on the sink, and getting objects out of the closet that were placed to elicit a left weight shift). Emphasis was placed on assisting M.J. with developing an awareness of her actual limits of stability. As M.J.'s control improved, the therapist also focused on narrowing her base of support to the more normal site dictated by particular activities. M.J. improved to the point that she could maintain midline and actively shift weight laterally during self-care activities without assistance from the therapist.

## REVIEW QUESTIONS

1. Name the three sensory systems involved in balance control and describe their roles.
2. What purpose do automatic postural responses serve in balance control?

3. What is the role of the cerebellum in balance control?
4. What composes a component assessment of balance skills?
5. Describe three balance assessments.
6. Why should a therapist observe a patient during functional activity? What information should be gathered?
7. In what way does a therapist determine the focus of treatment (e.g., remediation or compensation)?
8. In what way does the treatment of balance deficits by occupational therapy differ from traditional physical therapy treatment?
9. Describe the concept and benefits of using a functional independence day flow sheet.

## REFERENCES

1. Berg KO: Balance and its measure in the elderly: a review, *Physiother Can* 41:240, 1989.
2. Berg KO, Maki BE, Williams JI, et al: Clinical and laboratory measures of postural balance in the elderly population, *Arch Phys Med Rehabil* 73(11):1073-1080, 1992.
3. Berg KO, Wood-Dauphinee S, Williams J: The balance scale: reliability assessment with elderly residents and patients with an acute stroke, *Scand J Rehabil Med* 27(1):27-36, 1995.
4. Block MW, Smith DA, Nelson DL: Heart rate, activity, duration and affect in added-purpose versus single-purpose jumping activities, *Am J Occup Ther* 43(1):25-30, 1989.
5. Bobath B: *Adult hemiplegia: evaluation and treatment*, ed 2, London, 1978, William Heinemann.
6. Brunnstrom S: *Movement therapy in hemiplegia*, New York, 1970, Harper & Row.
7. Carr J, Shepherd R: *Physiotherapy in disorders of the brain*, Rockville, Md, 1980, Aspen.
8. Cawthorne T: The physiological basis for head exercises, *Charter Soc Physiother* 29:106, 1994.
9. Cohen H, Blatchly CA, Gombash LL: A study of the clinical test of sensory interaction and balance, *Phys Ther* 73(6):346-351, 1993.
10. Cohen H, Miller LV, Kane-Wineland M, et al: Vestibular rehabilitation with graded occupations, *Am J Occup Ther* 49(4):362-367, 1995.
11. Cooksey F: Physical medicine, *Practitioner* 155:300, 1945.
12. Daleiden S: Weight shifting as a treatment for balance deficits: a literature review, *Physiother Can* 42:81, 1990.
13. DiFabio RP, Badke MB: Extraneous eye movement associated with hemiplegic posture sway during dynamic goal-directed weight distribution, *Arch Phys Med Rehabil* 11:365, 1990.
14. Donato S, Pulaski K, MacKenzie D, et al: Functional independence day. Paper presented at the CanAm Occupational Therapy Association Annual Conference, Boston, 1994.
15. Duncan PW, Studenski S, Chandler J, et al: Functional reach: predictive validity in a sample of elderly male veterans, *J Gerontol* 47(3):93-98, 1992.
16. Duncan PW, Weiner DK, Chandler J, et al: Functional reach: a new clinical measure of balance, *J Gerontol* 45(6):192-197, 1990.
17. Easton T: On the normal use of reflexes, *Am Sci* 60(5):591-599, 1972.
18. Fregly A, Graybiel A: An ataxia battery not requiring rails, *Aerosp Med* 39(3):277-282, 1968.
19. Heck S: The effect of purposeful activity on pain tolerance, *Am J Occup Ther* 42(9):577-581, 1988.
20. Hsieh C, Nelson DL, Smith DA, et al: A comparison of performance in added-purpose occupations and rote exercise for dynamic standing balance in persons with hemiplegia, *Am J Occup Ther* 50(1):10-16, 1996.
21. Kircher M: Motivation as a factor of perceived exertion in purposeful versus nonpurposeful activity, *Am J Occup Ther* 38:165, 1984.
22. Lang E, Nelson D, Bush M: Comparison of performance in materials-based occupation, imagery-based occupation, and rote exercise in nursing home residents, *Am J Occup Ther* 46:607, 1992.
23. Licht B, Nelson D: Adding meaning to a design copy task through representational stimuli, *Am J Occup Ther* 44:408, 1990.
24. Magnus R: Some results of studies in the psychology of posture, *Lancet* 2:531, 1926.
25. Mahoney FI, Barthel DW: Functional evaluation: the Barthel index, *Md State Med J* 14:61, 1965.
26. Mathias S, Nayak USL, Isaacs B: Balance in the elderly patient: the "get up and go test," *Arch Phys Med Rehabil* 67:387, 1986.
27. Miller L, Nelson D: Dual-purpose activity vs. single-purpose activity in terms of duration on task, exertion level, and effect, *Occup Ther Ment Health* 7:55, 1987.
28. Morton GG, Barnett DW, Hale LS: A comparison of performance measures of an added-purpose task versus a single-purpose task for upper extremities, *Am J Occup Ther* 46(2):128-133, 1992.
29. Mullins C, Nelson D, Smith D: Exercise through dual-purpose activity in the institutionalized elderly, *Phys Occup Ther Geriatr* 5:29, 1987.
30. Poole JL, Whitney SL: Can balance assessments predict falls in the elderly? Presentation at the American Occupational Therapy Association Annual Meeting and Conference, Denver, April 9, 1995.
31. Riccia C, Nelson D, Bush M: Adding purpose to the repetitive exercise of elderly women through imagery, *Am J Occup Ther* 44:714, 1990.
32. Shumway-Cook A, Horak FB: Balance disorders assessment, *NERA* 1992.
33. Shumway-Cook A, Horak FB: Balance rehabilitation in the neurological patient, *NERA* 1992.
34. Shumway-Cook A, Horak FB: Assessing the influence of sensory interaction on balance, *Phys Ther* 66(10):1548-1550, 1986.
35. Shumway-Cook A, Olmscheld R: A systems analysis of postural dyscontrol in traumatically brain-injured patients, *J Head Trauma Rehabil* 5:51, 1990.
36. Steinbeck TM: Purposeful activity and performance, *Am J Occup Ther* 40(8):529-534, 1986.
37. Thibodeaux CS, Ludwig FM: Intrinsic motivation in product-oriented and non-product-oriented activities, *Am J Occup Ther* 42(3):169-175, 1988.
38. Tinetti ME: Performance-oriented assessment of mobility problems in elderly patients, *J Am Geriatr Soc* 34(2):119-126, 1986.
39. Voss D: Proprioceptive neuromuscular facilitation, *Am J Phys Med* 46:838, 1985.
40. Weiner DK, Duncan PW, Chandler J, et al: Functional reach: a marker of physical frailty, *J Am Geriatr Soc* 40(3):203-207, 1992.
41. Wu S, Huang HT, Lin CF, et al: Effects of a program on symmetrical posture in patients with hemiplegia: a single-subject design, *Am J Occup Ther* 50(1):17-23, 1996.

42. Yoder RM, Nelson DL, Smith DA: Added-purpose versus rote exercise in female nursing home residents, *Am J Occup Ther* 43(9):581-586, 1989.

43. Yuen H: *The purposeful use of an object in the development of skill with a prosthesis*, master's thesis, Kalamazoo, Mich, 1988, Western Michigan University.

helen s. cohen

**chapter 9**

# Vestibular Rehabilitation and Stroke

## key terms

endolymph

otoliths

semicircular canals

vestibular labyrinth

vestibular rehabilitation

vestibuloocular reflex

Wallenberg's syndrome

## chapter objectives

After completing this chapter, the reader will be able to accomplish the following:

1. Understand key components of the anatomy and physiology of the vestibular system.
2. Understand stroke syndromes that are associated with vestibular signs and symptoms.
3. Understand general concepts of vestibular rehabilitation.

The vestibular system is one of the special senses; that is, it has receptors on the head and signals the brain via a cranial nerve. The end organs for the vestibular system, the vestibular labyrinths, detect head acceleration, or a change in the rate at which the head is moving. This information is converted to a velocity signal (velocity is speed plus direction), so the signal received by the brain really represents the speed and direction at which the head moves. The labyrinths are located within cavities inside the temporal bones of the skull, on either side of the head, so the end organs are inaccessible from the outside world. One cannot see the end organ or otherwise examine it without drilling into the temporal bone to expose it. Because the end organ is not obvious and because the roles of the vestibular system—contributions to postural control (see Chapter 8), oculomotor control, spatial orientation, and modulation of some autonomic function—the vestibular system was the last of the special

senses to be discovered, and many persons still do not understand it.

## OVERVIEW OF THE VESTIBULAR SYSTEM

### Peripheral Vestibular Labyrinth

A discussion of the anatomy and physiology of the vestibular system is beyond the scope of this chapter but has been reviewed in many journal articles and textbooks. For excellent reviews, readers are encouraged to review other texts.[2,10,17,26] To put the topic of this chapter in context requires a brief review of some main points about the vestibular system.

The vestibular labyrinth has two sets of detectors, three semicircular canals (lateral, posterior, and superior) that act as rotary accelerometers to detect rotary motions of the head and two saclike otoliths (utricle and saccule) that act as linear accelerometers to detect linear acceleration of the head (Figure 9-1). Because gravity is a fixed linear acceleration, the otoliths also detect static tilt with reference to gravity. This gravitational signal is important for spatial orientation because it acts as an earth-fixed reference.

So, why is all of this information and the complex anatomic structures associated with it needed? It is needed to keep the head erect and see where one is going while moving through space, to plot a course for movement, and to generate appropriate autonomic responses when encountering a perturbation; that is, when one is thrown off balance inadvertently. These motor skills help some lower animals capture and eat their prey and help other animals avoid becoming prey. The vestibular system serves similar purposes in human beings as they move through space while avoiding or encountering obstacles and performing purposeful activities that involve manipulating objects while they move their heads through all planes in space. Persons with impaired vestibular systems complain of vertigo and poor spatial navigation skills, impaired postural control, nausea, and other signs of autonomic involvement

***Inertial Mechanism.*** The mechanism of the vestibular labyrinth is based on the principle of inertia, that is, that an object remains at rest until an asymmetrical force acts on it and then it continues to move until another asymmetrical force acts on it to stop it. The semicircular canals are narrow (imagine a curved tube approximately the width of a hair on your head), so they provide a lot of resistance to the fluid, known as *endolymph*, that fills them. Endolymph has a high specific gravity, so it has high inertia. The combined inertial properties of endolymph and the high resistance of the canals mean that the vestibular system is not sensitive to extremely slow head movements. The system is somewhat responsive to slow head movements but responds most accurately to moderate to rapid head movements, in the range of 0.1 to 7.0 Hz. Not surprisingly, this frequency bandwidth is the range of most normal head movements. When a person rotates his or her head, for example, while shaking the head "no," tiny cilia attached to specialized hair cells located on a miniscule hillock that blocks one end of the canal bend backward in response to movement of the endolymph over the gelatinous cup or cupula into which they protrude. This motion of the cilia starts a chain of events within the hair cells in which ions are exchanged, the cell membrane polarization changes, neurotransmitter may be released, and if so, the adjoining vestibular nerve fires, signaling to the related neurons in the vestibular nuclei, located in the medulla, that the person turned the head.

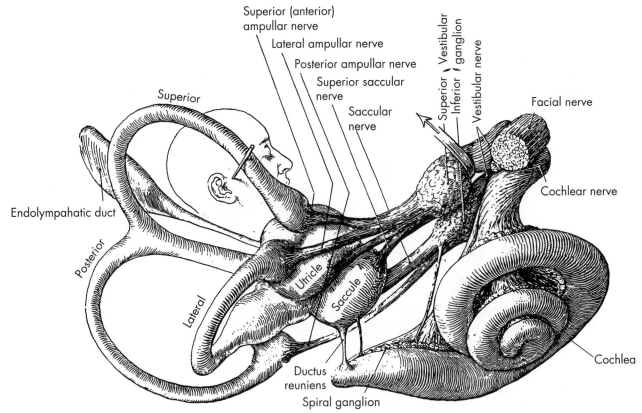

**Figure 9-1**  Gross anatomy of the vestibular labyrinth. (From Brödel M: *Three unpublished drawings of the anatomy of the human ear,* Philadelphia, 1946, WB Saunders.)

In the otoliths the hair cells are located in patches in the base of the utricle or on the side of the saccule. The otolithic cilia protrude into the otoconial membrane, which is a protein matrix containing many microscopic crystals of calcium carbonate known as otoconia. The otoconia act as an inertial mass. In other words, the otoconial membrane slides back and forth over the cilia in response to linear acceleration; for example, when a person accelerates a car going forward, the otoconial membrane slides backward over the underlying cilia, bending them backward and commencing the transduction process described in the preceding paragraph.

***Innervation and Blood Supply.*** All of this hardware in the temporal bone is supplied by nerves and arteries. The vestibular labyrinth is innervated by the vestibular nerve, which is half of cranial nerve VIII. The vestibular nerve has two branches. The superior branch innervates the superior and horizontal semicircular canals and the utricle. The inferior branch innervates the posterior canal and the saccule.

The arterial supply to the vestibular labyrinth is similar to the innervation. The entire labyrinth receives its blood supply from one artery, the anterior inferior cerebellar artery, which is a branch off the basilar artery. A major branch from the anterior inferior cerebellar artery, the labyrinthine artery supplies the entire inner ear. Inside the inner ear, this artery bifurcates to form the common cochlear artery and anterior vestibular artery. The anterior vestibular artery supplies the area primarily innervated by the superior vestibular nerve, that is, the superior and horizontal semicircular canals and the utricle. These areas drain into the anterior vestibular vein. The common cochlear artery bifurcates and forms the cochlear artery and the posterior vestibular artery. The posterior vestibular artery innervates the posterior semicircular canal and the saccule. These areas drain into the posterior vestibular vein. Both veins join with the vein from the round window, elsewhere in the inner ear, and form the vestibulocochlear vein, eventually draining into the cochlear aqueduct and then the inferior petrosal sinus. Other small veins from the semicircular canals join to form the vein of the vestibular aqueduct, eventually draining into the lateral venous sinus (Figure 9-2).

Interruption of the blood supply to the vestibular labyrinth can cause the usual manifestations of vestibular weakness, including vertigo, disequilibrium, blurred vision, and nausea. Ischemia or infarction can interrupt the blood supply. When the anterior vestibular artery is involved, the patient does not have hearing loss because the loss of blood supply is distal to the bifurcation of the labyrinthine artery. When the labyrinthine artery is involved, hearing loss is more likely. During the acute phase of sudden, dramatic, and incapacitating symptoms, which may last hours to days, patients are treated medically with palliative care. After the acute phase is over,

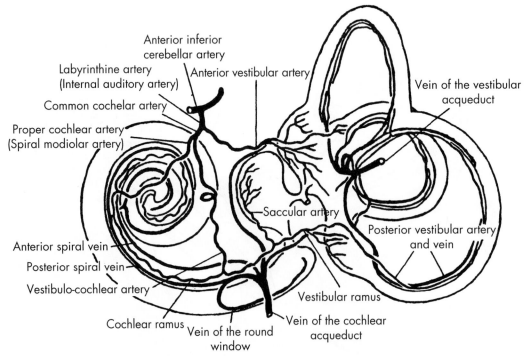

**Figure 9-2** Arterial supply to the vestibular labyrinth. (Modified from Nabeya D: Study in comparative anatomy of blood-vascular system of internal ear in mammalia and in homo, *Acta Schol Med Imp Kioto* 6:1, 1923.)

patients who have not compensated spontaneously may be referred for vestibular rehabilitation. These patients often are rehabilitated successfully.

## Central Projections

The vestibular nerve projects to the vestibular nuclei in the rostral medulla (Figure 9-3). The projection has some spatial specificity in that different nerves project to different areas of the vestibular nuclei. From there, projections go to the dentate and fastigial nuclei of the cerebellum. Eventually those signals make their way to the flocculus, nodulus, and ventral uvula in the cerebellar vermis, that is, the so-called vestibulocerebellum. Projections out of the cerebellum return to the vestibular nuclei. From there, some signals descend the vestibulospinal tracts to cervical and lumbosacral levels of the spinal cord. Those pathways are involved in postural control and are especially important in the absence of vision. Patients with vestibular weakness caused by peripheral or central lesions often have impaired balance.

Other tracts, after receiving input from oculomotor-related neurons in other nuclei, ascend the medial longitudinal fasciculus in a complex set of crossed and uncrossed pathways to synapse on the nuclei from cranial nerves III, IV, and IV. Those cranial nerves control the extraocular muscles of the eyes, so those vestibuloocular pathways control the vestibuloocular reflex. The vestibuloocular reflex is an eye movement made in response to head movement to stabilize the position of the eye in space. The head is relatively large and sits atop a flexible neck, so as a person moves his or her body through space, the head moves. To see clearly while moving the head, a person generates the vestibuloocular reflex in the direction opposite the head movement. Patients with unilateral vestibular weakness caused by peripheral or central lesions often complain of blurred vision during head movement because of decreased amplitude of the vestibuloocular reflex. Some patients with central vestibular lesions also have other unusual or abnormal eye movement patterns. Neurologists sometimes use these patterns of eye movements to help localize cerebellar and brainstem lesions.

A few pathways, which still are mapped poorly, ascend via the thalamus to some poorly defined areas in the cerebral cortex, mostly around some auditory projection areas in the temporal lobe near the junction of the temporal

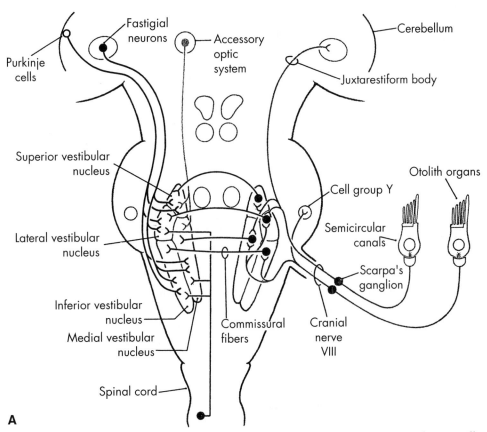

**Figure 9-3**   Central vestibular projections. Closed cell bodies are excitatory and open cell bodies are inhibitory. **A,** Afferent projections of the vestibular nerve. Projections mediating the horizontal vestibuloocular reflex

*Continued*

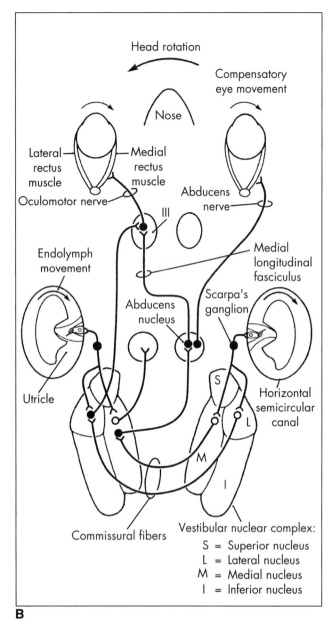

**B**

**Figure 9-3 cont'd** (B), vestibulocortical projections

and parietal lobes and into the insula (see Figure 9-3).[5,15] The functions of these projections are not clear, but they may mediate the conscious perception of motion or the vestibular contributions to spatial orientation. For example, one report in human beings has shown that stimulation to those brain regions in patients undergoing neurosurgery elicits a sense of motion.[25] Lesions to the posterolateral thalamus impair upright body orientation.[20] Lesions to the putative vestibular cortex impair spatial perception by affecting perception of the subjective visual vertical.[28]

A fourth set of projections, also poorly understood, are involved in mediating some aspects of autonomic function.[27] Therefore, some patients with vestibular weakness complain of autonomic signs such as nausea, sweating, or increased heart rate.

## Central Arterial Supply

The vestibular nuclei receive their blood supply from the anterior and posterior cerebellar arteries (anterior inferior cerebellar artery and posterior inferior cerebellar artery, respectively). The anterior inferior cerebellar artery arises from the basilar artery and supplies the cerebellopontine angle, part of the anterior cerebellum, part of the vermis and the vestibulocerebellum, part of the rostral pons, the middle cerebellar peduncle, cranial nerve VII (facial nerve), and cranial nerve VIII. The posterior inferior cerebellar artery is a branch off the rostral section of the vertebral artery and supplies the lateral medulla and part of the cerebellum, including part of the vermis, where the nodulus and ventral uvula are located (Figure 9-4). The vestibular cortical projection is probably supplied by the middle cerebral artery off the branches that supply the temporal lobe. Because the vestibular cortex still is being investigated, the exact blood supply may be a matter for some debate.

## STROKE SYNDROMES

In approximately 20% of patients who complain of vertigo, in general the cause is vascular (stroke, vertebrobasilar migraine headache, or transient ischemic attack).[24] However, vestibular lesions in stroke patients, as indicated by complaints of vertigo, are rare. In one study of 474 confirmed strokes in which patients were hospitalized, only 2% of patients complained of vertigo.[22] More than half of all brainstem strokes are in the pons,[16] and strokes in that area can cause lesions of the vestibular nuclei.

### Wallenberg's Syndrome

The most common stroke of the vestibular system, first reported in the late nineteenth century,[21] is Wallenberg's syndrome, also known as lateral medullary syndrome.[1,4] This stroke is a cerebrovascular accident of the posterior inferior cerebellar artery or anterior inferior cerebellar artery. In other words, this is a lateral brainstem stroke. Because both arteries that supply the vestibular nuclei also supply other areas, lateral medullary syndrome is manifested by mixed sensory and motor loss, including vertigo, lateropulsion, disequilibrium, ataxia, contralateral loss of pain and temperature sensation in the trunk and limbs, and the following ipsilateral signs: facial numbness, Horner's syndrome (drooping of the upper eyelid, constriction of the pupil, and decreased sweating), and dysphagia. Involvement of the posterior inferior cerebellar artery also includes hoarseness and skew deviation of the eyes. Involvement of the anterior inferior cerebellar artery also includes ipsilateral tinnitus, hearing

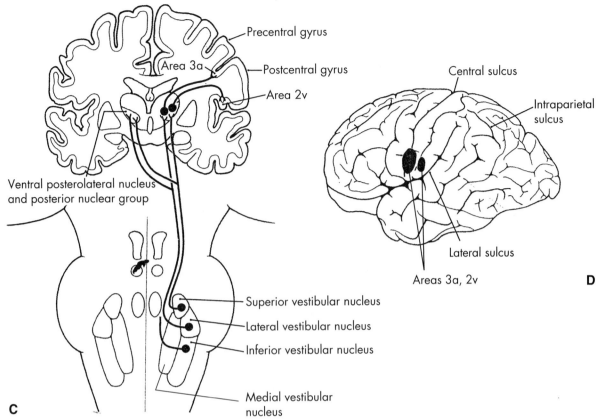

**Figure 9-3 cont'd**    (**C**), and likely vestibular projection areas (**D**) in the cerebral cortex. (From Dickman JD: The vestibular system. In Haines DE, editor: *Fundamental neuroscience*, New York, 1997, Churchill Livingstone.)

loss, facial weakness, and reduced peripheral vestibular responses on objective diagnostic tests. In other words, these patients have vertigo, difficulty standing and walking, sensory loss on the ipsilateral side of the face and on the contralateral side of the body, difficulty speaking and swallowing, abnormal eye movements, and hearing impairments. In addition to thrombosis and ischemia, dissection of the vertebral artery caused by sports injuries or by chiropractic manipulation of the neck can cause this syndrome.[23]

Wallenberg's syndrome is common. Patients with this syndrome may be referred for rehabilitation, although many of them recover spontaneously. No studies have evaluated the effectiveness of rehabilitation in this population, but Furman and Whitney[18] have commented that these patients usually respond well to therapy. Therapy should involve functional skills, balance therapy, and habituation exercises to reduce vertigo, that is, the kinds of exercises used to reduce vertigo in patients with peripheral vestibular disorders.[13]

## Cerebellar Infarcts

Cerebellar lesions without involvement in the brainstem can be caused by occlusion of the posterior inferior cere-bellar artery, anterior inferior cerebellar artery, or vertebral artery. Patients with these lesions rarely are seen for vestibular rehabilitation. According to noted authorities Baloh and Harker,[3] the acute episodes of vertigo, disequilibrium, and nausea accompanied by typical cerebellar signs of ataxia, disdiadochokinesia, and gaze nystagmus often are followed by edema of the cerebellum. Cerebellar edema can be fatal because, when the cerebellum becomes compressed, the nearby brainstem structures can be damaged unless the area is surgically decompressed.

## Lesions of Vestibular Areas in Cerebral Cortex

Strokes affecting just the insular cortex are rare. One paper reported that of 4800 new strokes in a database, 4 (<0.001%) were restricted to the insula. The three patients with anterior insula lesions had transiently poor balance, and some had transient aphasia and dizziness.[7] These persons recovered spontaneously. More frequently, vertigo and balance problems can be part of the syndrome seen in large middle cerebral artery cerebrovascular accidents. In that case, therapists should incorporate general principles of vestibular rehabilitation in the rehabilitation treatment plan as needed.

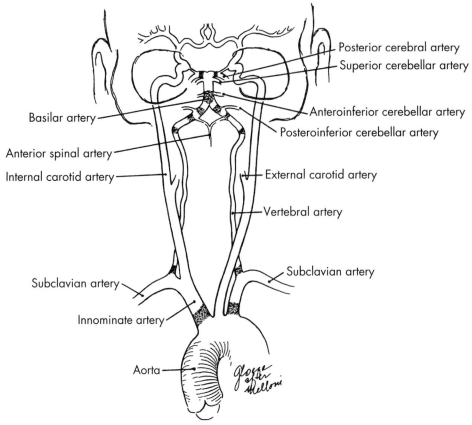

**Figure 9-4**    Arterial supply to the subcortical central vestibular areas. (From Baloh RW: *Dizziness, hearing loss, and tinnitus: the essentials of neurotology*, Philadelphia, 1983, FA Davis.)

## VESTIBULAR REHABILITATION

Although isolated central vestibular impairments are unusual, patients with strokes sometimes have symptoms of vestibular disorder along with their other symptoms. Any patient who complains of vertigo should be evaluated to determine whether the problem is central or peripheral. A detailed discussion of vestibular rehabilitation is beyond the scope of this chapter, but many reviews of this topic have been published.

The American Occupational Therapy Association has defined the necessary entry-level skills for this subspecialty.[8] An overview of this topic follows.

Interventions such as habituation exercises and activities for vertigo,[12-14] balance therapy, repositioning maneuvers for benign paroxysmal positional vertigo,[6,11,19] functional skills training, adaptive safety equipment, and home modifications can be incorporated into the treatment plan for stroke rehabilitation as needed.[9] The goals of vestibular rehabilitation are usually to reduce or eliminate vertigo when it is present, to reduce oscillopsia (illusory movement of the visual world) when it is present, to improve safety and decrease falls, and as in all rehabilitation, to increase independence. Habituation exercises and activities involve repetitive rotations of the head to elicit vertigo in an attempt to desensitize the system to the sensation. Current practice incorporates a visual target; that is, the patient should be looking at something while moving the head. Therefore, tasks involving repetitive head movements, for example, sorting tasks in which the containers are on different sides, are therapeutic.

Graduated balance training exercises and activities are used when patients complain of disequilibrium. These programs usually increase in difficulty from standing still to standing on an unstable surface, to moving through space while moving the head about and manipulating objects. Therapy should incorporate movement in anteroposterior, mediolateral, and off-axis planes.

Patients with vertigo and balance problems are at risk for falling, so therapy should involve some discussion of home modifications such as bathtub seats, bathroom grab bars, night-lights, and the tacking down of throw rugs. Therapists can incorporate these issues into discharge planning for most stroke patients seen as inpatients or during routine discussions during outpatient care.

# REVIEW QUESTIONS

1. What is the most common stroke to disrupt the function of the vestibular system? List the symptoms associated with this stroke.
2. What are the signs and symptoms of a cerebellar stroke?
3. What are the two major goals of a vestibular rehabilitation program after a stroke?
4. What are the specific interventions used to improve function during a vestibular rehabilitation program?

# REFERENCES

1. Baloh RW: Vertebrobasilar insufficiency and stroke, *Otolaryngol Head Neck Surg* 112(1):114-117, 1995.
2. Baloh RW, Halmagyi GM: *Disorders of the vestibular system*, New York, 1996, Oxford University Press.
3. Baloh RW, Harker LA: Central vestibular disorders. In Cummings CW, Fredrickson JM, Krause CJ, et al, editors: *Otolaryngology: head and neck surgery*, ed 3, St Louis, 1998, Mosby.
4. Baloh RW, Harker LA: Central vestibular system disorders. In Harker LA, editor: *Ear and cranial base*, ed 2, St Louis, 1993, Mosby.
5. Brandt T, Dieterich M, Danek A: Vestibular cortex lesions affect the perception of verticality, *Ann Neurol* 35(4):403-412, 1994.
6. Brandt T, Steddin S, Daroff RB: Therapy for benign paroxysmal positioning vertigo, revisited, *Neurology* 44(5):796-800, 1994.
7. Cereda C, Ghika J, Maeder P, et al: Strokes restricted to the insular cortex, *Neurology* 59(12):1950-1955, 1996.
8. Cohen HS: Specialized knowledge and skills in adult vestibular rehabilitation for occupational therapy practice, *Am J Occup Ther* 55:661-665, 2001.
9. Cohen HS: Vestibular and balance disorders: vestibular rehabilitation, *Occup Ther Pract* 5:14-18, 2000.
10. Cohen H: *Neuroscience for rehabilitation*, ed 2, Philadelphia, 1998, Lippincott Williams & Wilkins.
11. Cohen HS, Jerabek J: Efficacy of treatments for posterior canal benign paroxysmal positional vertigo, *Laryngoscope* 109(4):584-590, 1999.
12. Cohen H, Kane-Wineland M, Miller LV, et al: Occupation and visual/vestibular interaction in vestibular rehabilitation, *Otolaryngol Head Neck Surg* 112(4):526-532, 1995.
13. Cohen HS, Kimball KT: Increased independence and decreased vertigo after vestibular rehabilitation, *Otolaryngol Head Neck Surg* 128(1):60-70, 2003.
14. Cohen H, Miller LV, Kane-Wineland M, et al: Case reports of vestibular rehabilitation with graded occupations, *Am J Occup Ther* 49:362-367, 1995.
15. Fasold O, von Brevern M, Kuhberg M, et al: Human vestibular cortex as identified with caloric stimulation in functional magnetic resonance imaging, *Neuroimage* 17(3):1384-1393, 2002.
16. Fritschi JA, Reulen HJ, Spetzler RF, et al: Cavernous malformations of the brain stem: a review of 139 cases, *Acta Neurochir* 130(1-4):35-46, 1994.
17. Furman JM, Cass SP: *Balance disorders: a case study approach*, Philadelphia, 1996, FA Davis.
18. Furman JM, Whitney SL: Central causes of dizziness, *Phys Ther* 80(2):179-187, 2000.
19. Herdman SJ, Tusa RJ, Zee DS, et al: Single treatment approaches to benign paroxysmal positional vertigo, *Arch Otolaryngol Head Neck Surg* 119:450-454, 1993.
20. Karnath HO, Ferber S, Dichgans J: The neural representation of postural control in humans, *Proc Natl Acad Sci USA* 97(25):13931-13936, 2000.
21. Lanska DJ: Classic articles of 19th-century American neurologists: a critical review, *J Hist Neurosci* 11(2):156-173, 2002.
22. Rathore SS, Hinn AR, Cooper LS, et al: Characterization of incident stroke signs and symptoms: findings from the atherosclerosis risk in communities study, *Stroke* 33(11):2718-2721, 2002.
23. Saeed AB, Shuaib A, Al-Sulaiti G, et al: Vertebral dissection: warning symptoms, clinical features and prognosis in 26 patients, *Can J Neurol Sci* 27(4):292-296, 2000.
24. Solomon D: Distinguishing and treating causes of central vertigo, *Otolaryngol Clin North Am* 33(3):579-601, 2000.
25. Tasker RR, Organ LW: Stimulation mapping of the upper human auditory pathway, *J Neurosurg* 38(3):320-325, 1973.
26. Wilson VJ, Melvill Jones G: *Mammalian vestibular physiology*, New York, 1979, Plenum Press.
27. Yates BJ, Miller AD: *Vestibular autonomic regulation*, Boca Raton, Fla, 1996, CRC Press.
28. Yelnik AP, Lebreton FO, Bonan IV, et al: Perception of verticality after recent cerebral hemispheric stroke, *Stroke* 33(9):2247-2253, 2002.

glen gillen

**chapter 10**

# Upper Extremity Function and Management

### key terms

| | | |
|---|---|---|
| biomechanical alignment | impingement | postural control |
| complex regional pain syndrome | learned nonuse | reaching |
| constraint-induced movement therapy | manipulation | shoulder supports |
| contracture | motor control | spasticity |
| deformity | orthopedic injuries | subluxation |
| function | pain | weakness |
| | positioning | weight bearing |

### chapter objectives

After completing this chapter, the reader will be able to accomplish the following:

1. Develop treatment plans to regain upper extremity function through the use of functional tasks.
2. Understand the application of adjunct treatments for the upper extremity after stroke, including treatments such as positioning, shoulder supports, biofeedback, and stretching programs.
3. Choose functional treatment activities appropriate to the level of available motor control.
4. Understand evaluation and treatment procedures for patients with symptoms of pain syndromes and implement pain prevention protocols into current treatment plans.
5. Identify the common biomechanical malalignments of the upper extremity and trunk after stroke and recognize their effect on function.

Impaired upper extremity function is one of the most common and challenging sequelae of a cerebrovascular accident (CVA). The Copenhagen stroke study included 515 stroke patients, 71% of whom received occupational and physical therapy and 69% of whom had mild to severe upper extremity dysfunction on admission; all treatment plans included a focus on upper extremity function.[95] Obviously, numerous hours of therapy are spent on this area, as are numerous dollars. This chapter highlights problems associated with upper extremity function after a CVA, research that has been published on upper extremity function/dysfunction after stroke, and suggested evaluation and treatment techniques that focus on acquiring functional use of the extremity and preventing pain syndromes and deformities. Readers should review the concepts in Chapters 4 to 9 for a complete overview of topics related to motor control.

## OVERVIEW OF OCCUPATIONAL THERAPY PERSPECTIVE

"I want to use my arm again" is a goal that occupational therapists hear from stroke survivors during almost every evaluation. For therapists to assist patients with meeting this goal, a thorough understanding of the various problems associated with upper extremity dysfunction after stroke is required. The therapist has the responsibility to stay informed of (and contribute to) the new developments in and information about upper extremity function.

Current models of motor control encompass a variety of neuromotor, biomechanical, behavioral, cognitive, environmental, and learning processes. Mathiowetz and Bass-Haugen[87] have compared and contrasted the various models of motor control therapy in the past and present. Research comparing the effectiveness of various approaches is lacking. However, clearly the current motor behavior research supports a treatment technique well known to occupational therapists: the use of function-based tasks (see Chapter 6).

The use of functional activities has formed the basis of occupational therapy since its inception.[90] However, the complex problems that interfere with upper extremity function may require an integrated treatment approach that uses functional tasks as the intervention foundation and hands-on approaches/modalities (e.g. mobilization, soft-tissue elongation, and biofeedback) as adjuncts to intervention.

As the body of knowledge concerning motor behavior continues to grow, therapists must analyze research findings critically as well as their own clinical practices. Burgess[25] reminds us that "A danger in times of transition and rapid change is a distraction from basic principles. When faced with a choice between conventional and new approaches, the occupational therapist should consider the following questions: Is this treatment really effective? How does it work and on what principles is it based? Is it accomplishing what is needed for this patient? Are some of the older treatment methods more solidly based, more effective, or cheaper? Are there other better ways to meet this patient's needs?"

## DEFINITIONS AND CLASSIFICATIONS

A review of the literature on upper extremity function reveals a consistent problem: the lack of a definition for the word *function*. This may be attributed to the fact that a variety of disciplines are contributing information. From an occupational therapy perspective, *function* refers to using the upper extremity to support engagement in meaningful occupations. The International Classification of Function of the World Health Organization is a helpful classification system that includes the following categories:

- Impairment of body systems and body structure: examples include paresis, sensory loss, and decreased postural control
- Activity limitations: dysfunction in task performance such as activities of daily living and leisure tasks
- Participation restrictions: factor that limits or prevents fulfillment of a role (e.g., parent or worker)[136]

Hughlings Jackson's classification of observed symptoms after a central nervous system lesion is another system that is helpful for evaluating and treating the upper extremity after stroke. Jackson, a nineteenth-century neurologist, classified symptoms as positive or negative.

Positive symptoms are spontaneous, exaggerated disturbances of normal function and react to specific external stimuli. Positive symptoms include spasticity, increased deep tendon reflexes, and hyperactive flexion reflexes.

In contrast, the negative symptoms are deficits of normal behavior or performance. Negative symptoms include loss of dexterity, loss of strength, and restricted ability to move.[78,79]

In the past the major focus of therapeutic interventions was to decrease the positive symptoms associated with brain lesions. Therapists worked under the assumption that a cause-and-effect relationship existed between the two groups of symptoms. More recently, researchers have demonstrated that the alleviation of positive symptoms (e.g., spasticity) does not automatically result in an increased ability to move. Therapists therefore must take a broader view when identifying and treating upper extremity problems. A focus on only the positive symptoms (e.g., normalizing tone) does not result directly in increased function (see Chapter 6).

## ACTIVITY ANALYSIS OF SELECT UPPER EXTREMITY TASKS

The following examples illustrate the complexity of upper extremity function and should assist in the evaluation process.

### Reaching Task

The reaching task described requires the patient to reach for a book on a shelf that is at forehead level. First and foremost, initiation of any movement pattern requires a motivational drive to perform; therefore the activity must have an inherent purpose. The motivation behind and purpose of this activity may be to further knowledge, enhance leisure time, or pass a midterm examination. To complete this activity successfully, the patient must process appropriately the visual/perceptual information collected during the scanning process before initiating the reach pattern. Because the item is above eye level, neck extension with concurrent right and left lateral head and neck rotation and sufficient ocular range of motion (ROM) are required. A person collects a variety of visual information during visual scanning that helps identify particular characteristics of the book (e.g., call number, title, color, and size). This information is interpreted by several visual/perceptual processes (e.g., figure ground, color discrimination, and depth perception) (see Chapters 16 and 18).

Before initiation of the reach pattern the lower extremities and trunk undergo several postural adjustments to provide stabilization. The antigravity shoulder muscles prepare to bring the arm to shelf level, and the hand is prepositioned and oriented to prepare for grasping. While the reach pattern is being performed, the scapula protracts and rotates upward by the combination actions of the serratus anterior and upper and lower trapezius muscles. The rotator cuff keeps the humerus in a position biased toward external rotation and seats the head of the humerus in the glenoid fossa. The lower extremities and trunk stay active and stable during the performance of the pattern and may assist with a weight shift toward the shelves depending on the body position.

When the hand makes contact with the book, it is molded to the spine of the book, and the pattern of function is reversed (eccentrically) to return the book to the side of the body. After the person removes the book from the shelf, the grasp and pattern of skeletal muscle recruitment may be adjusted depending on the weight of the book. Although this activity pattern is preplanned based on prior experience, the book may be lighter or heavier than anticipated, so adjustments must be made in response to the feedback. (For example, attempting to pick up a supposedly full suitcase that is actually empty results in an exaggerated lifting motion that may cause a loss of balance.) While the book is being returned to the side, a variety of adjustments may have to be made to allow visualization of the cover of the book or call number (Figure 10-1).

### Weight-Bearing Task

The weight-bearing task described requires the patient to use one arm as a postural support (i.e., extended-arm weight bearing) on a kitchen table while the other arm and hand wipe the table. As mentioned previously, motivation and purpose are required. The motivation may be hunger (so the table must be cleaned in preparation for a meal), extrinsic (e.g., visitors), or work-related (e.g., table space needed to balance the checkbook or prepare a lecture). Because the weight-bearing arm is being used as a postural support, a variety of postural adjustments occur in the arm. The weight-bearing arm is active during the task; the active skeletal muscles include (but are not lim-

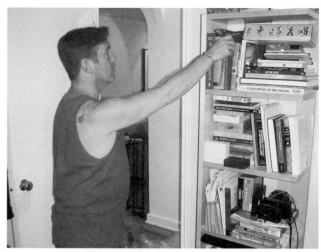

**Figure 10-1**    Reaching task.

ited to) the scapula muscles biased toward protraction, the elbow extensors, the lower extremities, and the trunk muscles. The amount of skeletal muscle activity in the arm may decrease because of fatigue, resulting in a "locked" elbow, an inactive scapula biased toward an elevated position and retraction, and the trunk inactive and "hanging" on the arm.

The arm that is wiping the table must stay active and endure the entire activity if the task is going to be successful. The shoulder complex of this arm glides the hand and sponge along the table surface, so the upper extremity is supported by the environment and is moving simultaneously. The amount of force and pressure exerted on the hand depends on the demands of the task (e.g., wiping crumbs or cleaning off dried syrup).

A variety of weight shifts occur during this activity, and they are affected by the size of the table and amount of pressure needed by the wiping hand to accomplish the task. The degree and variety of motor output is specific to the demands of the task.

As with all upper extremity tasks, multiple visual/perceptual processes are required for successful completion of this task. These processes are used to locate the crumbs on the table, clean both sides of the table, and determine when the task is complete (i.e., when the table is clean) (Figure 10-2).

## SELECTED EVALUATION TOOLS

Evaluation tools that are standardized, reliable, and valid can be overlooked no longer. Many therapists continue to use piecemeal evaluations that do not incorporate the use of functional tasks and rely too heavily on evaluation of impairments.

Beyond validity and reliability, when choosing assessments, clinicians must consider time factors, level of motor function, the purpose of the evaluation (clinical,

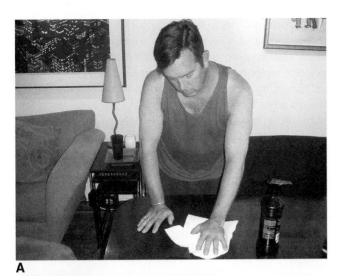

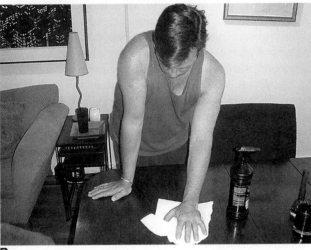

**Figure 10-2**   **A,** Using the right upper extremity as a postural support while the left upper extremity is supported by the table but moving. Intervention for the involved upper extremities should include engaging the patient in activities that use the upper extremities to support task performance. **B,** An alignment that fosters minimal upper extremity activity. Compare with *A.*

research, or both), and the environment in which the assessment will take place. Many available assessments such as the Fugl-Meyer Assessment only evaluate the impairment level and do not include information regarding how the upper extremity is used during daily occupations. Some assessments are exceptions to this statement, such as the Assessment of Motor and Process Skills.

### Assessment of Motor and Process Skills

The therapists evaluates motor and process skills[46,47] within the context of basic activities of daily living and instrumental activities of daily living (IADL). This evaluation allows the occupational therapist to assess a variety of motor (and process) skills within the context of occu-

pational performance, specifically during observation of basic activities of daily living and IADL. Examples of evaluated motor skills include posture, mobility, coordination, strength, reach, manipulation, grip, lifting, effort, and energy expenditure. This is a model occupational therapy evaluation (see Chapter 20).

### Arm Motor Ability Test

The Arm Motor Ability Test has been used to determine the effectiveness of constraint-induced movement therapy and includes 13 unilateral and bilateral tasks. Sample items include tying a shoe, opening a jar, wiping up spilled water, using a light switch, using utensils, and drinking. The therapist times task performance and rates movement quality on a six-point scale.[75]

### Wolf Motor Function Test

The Wolf Motor Function Test has been used to document the outcomes related to constraint-induced movement therapy and includes a variety of tasks such as reaching and manipulative tasks. The therapist times task performance and qualitatively grades movement.[133]

### Jebsen Test of Hand Function

The Jebsen Test of Hand Function[70] includes the performance of seven test activities: writing a short sentence, turning over index cards, picking up small objects and placing them in a container, stacking checkers, simulating eating, moving empty large cans, and moving weighted large cans during timed trials. The original paper is based on data collected from 360 normal subjects and patients, including patients with hemiparesis resulting from a CVA. The mean times and standard deviations for normal subjects (with their dominant and nondominant hand) are published in the paper. The test is standardized and reliable and does not have a practice effect. Therapists must be aware that some of the tasks are simulated activities and some tasks cannot be considered ADL tasks.

### Motor Activity Log

The Motor Activity Log is a self-report questionnaire (report by patient or family) related to actual use of the involved upper extremity outside of structured therapy time. Quality and amount of use are graded on a six-point scale.[124]

### Fugl-Meyer Assessment (Upper Extremity Motor Function)

Familiarity with this impairment-based test is helpful because the test is used in many research papers to document improvement in function. The assessment is based on the motor recovery model developed by Twitchell and on Brunnstrom's idea that motor recovery occurs in a specific sequence of steps. Improved motor function is considered a deviation from stereotypical synergies defined by Brunnstrom in this test. The test does not involve the use of functional tasks. Sections include range of motion, sensation, balance, upper extremity, and lower extremity. Items are graded on a three-point scale.[49]

### Action Research Arm Test

The Action Research Arm Test consists of 19 items in four categories: pinch, grasp, grip, and gross movement. The test is short (approximately 10 minutes). Items are graded on a four-point scale. The tasks included are contrived.[84]

### Motor Assessment Scale

Developed by Carr and Shepherd, the Motor Assessment Scale[30] has been found to be highly reliable, with an average interrater correlation of 0.95 and a 0.98 average test/retest correlation. This evaluation includes sections on upper arm function, hand movements, and advanced hand activities. The upper arm function section includes movement patterns without tasks; the hand sections incorporate the use of objects.

### Functional Test for the Hemiplegic/Paretic Upper Extremity

Although this evaluation[131] is based on Brunnstrom's view that motor recovery takes place in a specific sequence, it does involve functional tasks associated with daily living. This test has been found to be highly correlated with scores on the Fugl-Meyer Assessment. The test requires approximately 30 minutes to administer. Examples of tasks evaluated include folding a sheet, stabilizing a jar, hooking and zipping a zipper, screwing in a light bulb, and placing a box on a shelf.

### Frenchay Arm Test

This test includes five items, such as hair combing with the weak arm and drinking water. Items are graded as successful or unsuccessful.[62]

## USE OF THE INVOLVED UPPER EXTREMITY TO SUPPORT TASK PERFORMANCE: SUGGESTIONS FOR INTERVENTION

The foundation of occupational therapy is built on patients taking an active role in their own recovery by participating in functional activities. In the recent past, many therapists, while attempting to apply neurophysiologic principles to treatment, have limited their use of this modality in favor of more passive techniques that are applied to the patient (e.g., brushing, icing, and neurodevelopmental treatment-based handling techniques performed separately from functional tasks). Occupational therapy now has come full circle, with the most current research on motor control supporting the use of tasks performed in context-specific situations. (See Chapters 4 through 6.) Functional tasks in therapy include occupations that require upper extremity weight bearing for postural support, reaching, carrying, lifting, grasping, and manipulating of common objects. These types of activities clearly carry over into daily life tasks and are comprehensive enough to treat a variety of problem areas. The importance of using occupation-embedded interventions as opposed to rote exercise has been established.[82,138]

### Reaching and Manipulation

The events leading up to a simple voluntary movement such as reaching for a glass of water involve multiple complex processes. Ghez[51] classifies these processes as follows.

First, the person needs to identify the glass and its position in space. This first step encompasses a variety of visual and perceptual processes. Second, the person needs to select a plan of action to bring the glass to the mouth. Ghez points out that this step involves specifying which body parts are needed and in which direction they should move. To do this, the person must evaluate the location of the glass in relation to the position of the hand and body. The information collected allows the motor system to determine the appropriate trajectory of the hand. The last step is the execution of the response. Multiple commands are sent to the motor neurons specifying the temporal sequence of muscle activation, the forces to be developed, the changes in joint angles, the orientation of the hand to fit the glass, and the coordination of the shoulder with the distal arm to ensure that the glass will be grasped on contact and without delay. Multiple problems can interfere with these three steps, including the issues discussed in the previous section, visual dysfunction, and praxis deficits.

Two components of upper extremity function have been described by Jeannerod[68,69]: the transportation component, which includes the trajectory of the arm between the starting position and the object, and the manipulation component, which is the formation of grip by combined movements of the thumb and the index finger during arm movement.

In her study of reaching deficits in subjects with left hemiparesis, Trombly[123] used kinematic analysis and electromyography to document impairments in voluntary arm movements. Her analysis demonstrated that the ability to reach smoothly and with coordination was significantly less in the impaired arms than in the unimpaired arms. The continuous movement strategy used during reaching activities was lost, movement time was longer, peak velocity occurred earlier, and indications of weakness were present.

In a follow-up study, Trombly[122] documented the observed improvements in her subjects' reaching abilities.

Her findings indicated that the amplitude of peak velocity improved over time. The level of muscular activity did not improve, but the discontinuity of movements decreased. From her findings, Trombly hypothesized that therapy that allows relearning of sensorimotor relationships is warranted for some patients. She stated that the "level and pattern of muscle activity of these subjects depended on the biomechanical demands of the task rather than any stereotypical neurological linkages between muscles."

Van Vliet et al[127] studied subjects in the early months after a stroke. The subjects were able to improve their reaching kinematics during a 3- to 4-week period; they progressed toward normal performance. Providing the subjects with a meaningful task (e.g., drinking from a cup) helped them perform the reach-to-grasp movement.

Jeannerod[69] states that "Formation of the finger grip during the action of grasping a visual object involves two main functional requirements, the fulfillment of which will determine the quality of the grasp. First, the grip must be adapted to the size, shape, and use of the object to be grasped. Second, the relative timing of the finger movements must be coordinated with that of the other component of prehension by which the hand is transported to the spatial location of the object." Jeannerod observes that finger posturing anticipates the real grasp and occurs during transportation of the hand. This shaping of the hand is a mechanism that is independent of the manipulation itself. If treatment programs focused on improved function of the upper extremity are to be designed, then they must include a variety of common objects with different shapes, sizes, and textures to affect this reaching component.

Exner,[44] who defines *in-hand manipulation* as the process of adjusting objects being grasped in the hand, has developed a classification system that can assist the therapist in activity choice despite its not being standardized on stroke survivors. (Box 10-1 outlines Exner's classification system.)

Wu, Trombly, and Lin[137] demonstrated that using material-based occupation (e.g., picking up a pen and preparing to write one's name) enhanced quality of movement performance more than imagery-based occupation (e.g., pretending to pick up a pen and preparing to sign one's name) and exercise (e.g., moving the arm forward). Their data suggest that material-based occupation resulted in decreased reaction time, movement time, and movement units. Although this study was performed on normal subjects, they inferred that material-based occupation may be used to elicit efficient and economical pre-programmed movement for performing tasks.

In a study of fine motor coordination training, Neistadt[96] examined the effects of constructing puzzles and performing kitchen activities on fine motor coordination in a group of brain-injured men. Her results demonstrated that the subjects in the functional meal

## Box 10-1

### Exner's Classification of Manipulation Tasks

**TRANSLATION**

The object in the hand moves from the finger surface to the palm or vice versa.

**SHIFT**

Movement occurs at the finger and thumb pads by alternating thumb and radial finger movements (e.g., moving a coin near the distal interphalangeal joints farther out to the pads of the fingers).

**SIMPLE ROTATION**

The object is turned or rolled between the finger pads and thumb pad by alternating thumb and finger movements (e.g., unscrewing a jar lid).

**COMPLEX ROTATION**

The object is rotated, which requires isolated, independent movements of the finger or thumb. The object is turned between 180 degrees and 360 degrees (e.g., turning a paper clip so that correct end can be placed on a piece of paper).

preparation group showed significantly greater improvements in dominant hand dexterity, which is used for picking up small objects, than the subjects in the tabletop puzzle activity group. Her findings suggest that functional activities are more effective (not to mention more meaningful) than tabletop activities for fine motor coordination training in the brain-injured population.

Sietsema et al[116] studied brain-injured patients engaged in rote exercise tasks and occupationally embedded tasks (e.g., reaching out to control a computer game). Their subjects had "mild to moderate spasticity" on evaluation. Their results indicated that the game elicited significantly more ROM during the reach pattern performance than the rote exercise. Their study supports the hypothesis that occupationally embedded interventions promote increased performance. The authors hypothesized that the game provided motivating feedback that enhanced performance.

At this point, research has confirmed that the demands and goals of the task influence motor output. For example, the characteristics of an item being carried across a kitchen influence factors such as how fast a person moves, whether one or two hands are used to grip the object, how close to the body the item is carried, and how stable the arms are held. In daily life there are many examples of the ways in which movement in daily activities is influenced by the environment (e.g., carrying empty ice trays or full trays, a half-glass of wine or a full cup of coffee, one paper plate or a stack of china plate).

Rosenbaum and Jorgensen[107] have demonstrated that the goal of the task influences motor output. Their subjects were asked to reach for a cylinder and stand it on one end or the other. Depending on the goal of the task (i.e., which side they were to stand the cylinder on), subjects reached with a pronated or supinated grasp pattern. Box 10-2 provides sample activities used to retrain reach patterns. (See Chapters 4 and 5.)

### Weight Bearing

The use of weight-bearing tasks has long been advocated in patients after stroke. Upper extremity weight bearing has been suggested anecdotally for achieving a variety of therapeutic goals, including inhibiting hypertonus by moving the body proximally against the distal upper extremity[36] and stimulating upper extremity extension during protective responses.[9] Brouwer and Ambury[24] concluded that upper extremity weight bearing normal-

---

### Box 10-2

### Activities to Retrain Reach Patterns

- With the patient positioned in a supine posture, the therapist supports the weight of the distal extremity with a handhold position. The patient attempts to hold various positions and/or to follow the movements of the therapist's hand. This activity is appropriate for the early motor recovery stage. The degrees of freedom are minimized (with trunk and scapula being supported by the supine posture), and the therapist eliminates the weight of the patient's extremity, maximizing the potential for skeletal muscle recruitment. This activity is easily taught to family members.
- The patient stands or sits in front of a table with a hand resting on a dust cloth that is on top of the table. The patient focuses on gliding the hand across the table. The critical pattern consists of humeral flexion, scapula protraction, and elbow extension. The cloth reduces friction, and the weight of the arm is supported on the table (e.g., reach with support).
- The patient is seated, and objects are positioned on the floor in front of patient. The patient reaches for objects on the floor. This downward reach pattern enhances scapula protraction, humeral flexion, and elbow extension by nature of the position of the objects. As the patient gains more control, the objects are raised up to the midshank level, then the knee level, and then the waist level, systematically increasing the motor demands of the task.
- The patient is engaged in the foregoing reach patterns while therapist provides resistance to the functional pattern by tying an elastic band around the palm. The therapist is behind the patient holding the opposite end of the band and is able to grade the level of resistance.
- During the reach activities the demands of the distal components of movement are systematically increased (e.g., increasing manipulation requirements). Examples include pouring water and opening jars.

---

izes corticospinal facilitation of motor units in stroke patients. They hypothesized that the mechanism responsible for their results was a sustained increase in motor cortical excitability through augmented afferent input.

McIllroy and Maki[88] and Marsden, Merton, and Morton[85] documented that if the upper extremity is used as a postural support (e.g., during weight bearing), postural responses to the movements of the opposite arm occur throughout the weight-bearing upper extremity and to other perturbations of posture. Their paper also demonstrated that postural responses from the triceps only occurred when the hand was in contact with a firm object.

Although from a neurophysiologic perspective the effect of weight bearing on upper extremity control (i.e., the "normalization of tone" and "inhibition of spasticity") remains controversial and unproven, the use of weight-bearing patterns is still necessary for treating the upper extremity after a stroke if the goal of treatment is to improve functional performance. Examples include using the more affected upper extremity in a weight-bearing pattern and as a postural support while manipulating clothing during toileting activities or to enhance participation in IADL (e.g., using the more affected extremity as a postural support during activities requiring standing such as doing the laundry or preparing a meal).

Therapists also can use weight-bearing activities to address impairments that interfere with function. The problem of soft tissue shortening in the long flexors can be prevented or reversed by bearing weight on extended wrists with extended digits to maintain or increase tissue length. If evaluation reveals that weakness in the extremity is having a limiting effect on function, the therapist can use extended-arm weight-bearing activities to strengthen the triceps and scapula musculature (i.e., the protractors) if the weight-bearing activities are performed in appropriate alignment and the weight-bearing pattern remains active during the activity.

To ensure appropriate alignment, the therapists should avoid severe internal rotation, forced elbow extension, and an inactive trunk in patients.[111] During weight-bearing activities, maintenance of palmar hand arches is important for maintaining biomechanical alignment and enhancing active patterns. The points of contact between the weight-bearing surface and the hand include the thenar eminence, hypothenar eminence, metacarpal heads, and palmar surfaces of the phalanges.[73] The arch should be maintained so that therapists can insert a finger between the web space and the first metacarpal head and slide it under the hand until they make contact with the hypothenar eminence.

Although the more affected arm is in a weight-bearing position, the less involved extremity should be engaged in activities that promote weight shifting in all directions (Figure 10-3). Weight-bearing activities can be per-

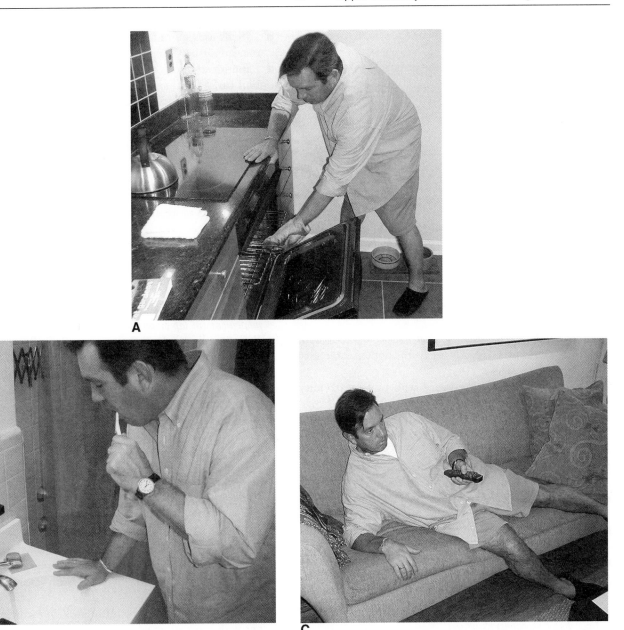

**Figure 10-3**    **A** to **C**, Weight-bearing during daily occupations.

formed by the forearm or an extended arm, depending on the demands of the task and the level of available motor control.

## SAMPLE GOALS AND ACTIVITY CHOICES

The following goals are examples of treatment activities for different levels and combinations of functional recovery. Using goals and treatments interchangeably ensures a task-specific approach to intervention. These examples should not be interpreted as progression in recovery. Although previous assumptions were that proximal recovery of abilities precedes distal recovery of abilities, this is not always the case. The following activities are graded by increasing the degrees of freedom (e.g., increasing the number of planes of movement that are controlled and integrating hand use), the level of anti-gravity control, and the objects used in the task. An important note is that the cognitive demands of the task have a substantial effect on the level of upper extremity function. Readers should not consider this list to be hierarchical. For example, weight-bearing is not a prerequisite to reaching, because the neurologic and biomechanical demands are different. Patients need to be engaged in a variety of tasks that require the use of the upper extremity in a variety ways and engaged in task-specific training.

*Focused attention on the more affected upper extremity (no active movement)*

■ Patient washes upper extremity during upper body bathing activities.

■ Patient attends to upper extremity while rolling by passively guiding upper extremity across trunk when preparing to roll.

■ Patient prevents arm from dangling while seated in chair.

■ Patient positions upper extremity on table during mealtime.

*Prevention goals*

■ Patient stretches arm correctly by reaching to floor and maintaining this position after difficult tasks result in arm posturing.

■ Patient's family demonstrates proper guarding techniques for a mobile patient.

■ Patient's caretaker demonstrates proper positioning of patient in bed.

*Forearm weight bearing as a stabilizer*

■ Patient stabilizes checkbook with upper extremity while writing checks.

■ Patient stabilizes cutting board with upper extremity during meal preparation.

■ Patient holds magazine open with upper extremity while doing crossword puzzle.

*Using upper extremity for assistance during transitions*

■ Patient uses upper extremity for assistance with assuming sitting position from side-lying position.

■ Patient uses upper extremity to push up into standing position.

■ Patient uses upper extremity to reach back before sitting.

■ Patient uses upper extremity to lower trunk to mat when assuming supine posture from sitting posture.

*Incorporating upper extremity as a postural support when sitting and standing (extended arm weight bearing with stabilized hand on support surface)*

■ Patient uses upper extremity to assist with lateral shifting while relieving pressure.

■ Patient stabilizes upper body with affected upper extremity while wiping and dusting table or ironing with less affected upper extremity.

■ Patient uses more affected upper extremity as a stabilizer on a grab bar while manipulating clothing with less affected upper extremity during toileting.

■ Patient stabilizes upper body with upper extremity while grooming at sink.

*Weight bearing with superimposed motion (i.e., hand does not leave support surface but slides and pulls objects)*

■ Patient irons and dusts with more affected upper extremity while stabilizing upper body with less affected upper extremity.

■ Patient uses affected upper extremity to lock wheelchair brakes with brake extensions.

■ Patient uses more affected upper extremity to smooth out laundry.

■ Patient uses more affected upper extremity to wax and buff car.

■ Patient uses more affected upper extremity to push shopping cart or rolling walker.

*Antigravity shoulder movements without hand function*

■ Patient initiates roll with more affected upper extremity.

■ Patient lifts more affected upper extremity into shirt sleeve.

■ Patient lifts more affected upper extremity to countertop.

■ Patient pushes drawer closed with back of more affected hand.

■ Patient turns off light switch with side of more affected hand.

*Initial hand movement (static grasp) with limited shoulder movement (in lap or on work-surface activities)*

■ Patient adjusts shirt cuff with more affected upper extremity.

■ Patient holds book in lap with both hands while reading.

■ Patient stabilizes fruits or vegetables with affected hand while cutting with less affected hand.

■ Patient holds shopping bag with more affected upper extremity during ambulation.

■ Patient holds washcloth with more affected upper extremity and washes mid to lower body.

*Reach patterns with hand activity*

■ Patient picks up sock from floor with more affected upper extremity.

■ Patient retrieves item from under sink cabinet with more affected upper extremity.

■ Patient opens medicine cabinet with more affected upper extremity.

■ Patient retrieves item from top shelf of medicine cabinet with more affected upper extremity.

■ Patient drinks out of a cup with more affected upper extremity.

*Advanced hand activities*

■ Patient holds coins in affected palm and slides them to finger tips.

■ Patient types 15 words per minute with both upper extremities.

■ Patient signs check with more affected upper extremity.

■ Patient picks up and reorients paperclip with affected upper extremity.

Wilson[130] suggested the use of functional descriptors related to level of usage. This classification system may be of use to clinicians to choose activities and develop goals (Box 10-3). Table 10-1 provides further suggestions for choosing tasks for a variety of levels of function.

**Box 10-3**

## Levels of Usage

### NONASSISTIVE

Patient is unable to use the limb in any functional activities because of pain, range of motion limitations, apraxia, and neglect. Compensatory techniques and assistive devices are necessary to improve function. See Chapter 27.

### MINIMAL STABILIZING ASSIST

Patient uses limb passively to hold objects, such as stabilizing paper while writing.

### MINIMAL ACTIVE ASSIST

Patient uses the shoulder and elbow actively to place the limb on the lap or through the sleeve of the shirt or to stabilize the trunk when upright. No active hand use occurs.

### MAXIMAL ACTIVE ASSIST

Patient uses the arm actively with the shoulder, elbow, and gross grasp and release. Fine motor function is not present.

### INCORPORATION INTO BILATERAL ACTIVITIES

Patient uses the impaired hand and arm in all bilateral activities associated with activities of daily living and mobility.

From Wilson DJ: Stroke rehabilitation: setting realistic occupational therapy goals, *Physical Disabilities Special Interest Section Quarterly* 1980.

## Constraint-Induced Movement Therapy

The term *learned nonuse* was coined by Taub.[118] The learned nonuse phenomenon originally was identified in primate studies and later was applied to chronic stroke patients. With deafferentation of a single forelimb of a monkey, the animal would not use that limb in an unrestricted (free) environment. The monkey's initial attempts to use the limb resulted in failures (e.g., dropping food, losing balance, and falling). The monkeys in this study soon found that they could function in their environment with three limbs instead of four. Continued attempts to use the affected limb led to repeated failures at attempted tasks; the effect was suppression of any desire to use that limb. The monkeys *learned* not to use the limb to avoid failure, which masked any future recovery of limb function. Taub et al[118] pointed out that in a free situation, the monkeys did not learn that they could regain use of the forelimb as they recovered function. When the intact forelimb was restrained, the monkeys were forced to use the affected side. This technique converted a useless limb into one capable of extensive movement.

Taub[118] hypothesized that the nonuse or limited use of an affected upper extremity in human beings after stroke could in some cases result from a similar phenomenon of learned suppression.

To test this hypothesis, Taub[118] studied nine patients with chronic (i.e., greater than 1 year after stroke) hemiplegia. To be included in this study, patients had to demonstrate the ability to extend the metacarpalphalangeal and

**Table 10-1**

## Suggestions for Categorizing Upper Extremity Tasks

| CATEGORY | TASKS |
| --- | --- |
| No functional use | Teach shoulder protection |
| | Self range of motion |
| | Positioning |
| Postural support/weight bearing (forearm or extended arm) | Bed mobility assist |
| | Support upright function (work, leisure, activities of daily living) |
| | Support during reach with opposite hand |
| | Stabilize objects |
| Supported reach (hand on work surface) | Wiping a table |
| | Ironing |
| | Polishing |
| | Sanding |
| | Smoothing out laundry |
| | Applying body lotion |
| | Washing body parts |
| | Vacuuming |
| | Locking wheelchair brakes |
| Reach | Multiple possibilities to engage upper extremity into activities of daily living, leisure, and mobility; grade tasks by height/distance reached, weight of object, speed, and accuracy |

interphalangeal joints at least 10 degrees, extend the wrist 20 degrees, and walk without an assistive device. They had to have grossly intact cognitive function, no excess spasticity, be right-arm dominant, and be less than 75 years old.

Patients were assigned to a control or an experimental group. The experimental group underwent forced-use/constraint-induced movement therapy (CIMT) in which the intact limb was placed in a sling and resting-hand splint. The restraint was worn at all times during waking hours except when toileting, when napping, and at times when balance might be compromised. The restraint was worn for 14 days. Each weekday, patients received therapy and were given a variety of tasks—such as eating with utensils, playing ball, playing Chinese checkers and dominoes, writing, and sweeping—to perform with the paretic limb for 6 hours throughout the day.

The treatment of the control group focused on increasing attention to the paretic limb. This group was told that they had more potential in their extremities than they were using. Therapists performed passive ROM activities, and patients performed ROM activities daily for 15 minutes. The affected limb was not given any training for active movement.

Each group was evaluated before and after intervention with a variety of arm function evaluations and a self-reported Motor Activity Log. The restraint group had significantly faster mean performance speeds from the evaluations, increased quality of movement, and an increased ability to use the extremity in ADL. These improvements were reevaluated 2 years later; they were at least maintained if not increased. Although the comparison group made subtle gains after intervention, the gains were not retained for the follow-up evaluation. Taub et al[118] concluded that the motor ability of stroke patients who met their inclusion criteria could be increased significantly by the interventions effective for overcoming learned nonuse.

Wolf et al[134] researched forced-use treatment in 25 chronic hemiplegic and stroke patients with minimal to moderate extensor muscle function. The CIMT program lasted for 2 weeks, with the intact limb being restrained during waking hours. The authors noted significant changes in performance of 19 of the 21 tasks that were evaluated, with most changes persisting for 1 year after the study. The authors concluded that learned nonuse does occur in select patients with neurologic deficits and that this behavior can be reversed through application of a CIMT paradigm.

Van der Lee et al[125] completed an observer-blinded randomized clinical trial with 66 chronic stroke patients who were randomized to 2 weeks of CIMT or a comparison of equally intensive bimanual training based on 2 weeks of neurodevelopmental therapy. One week after the last treatment session, the authors found a significant difference in effectiveness in favor of CIMT group compared with the neurodevelopmental therapy group, after correction for baseline differences, on the Action Research Arm Test and the Motor Activity Log amount of use score. One-year follow-up effects were observed only for the Action Research Arm Test. The authors also found that the differences in treatment effect for the Action Research Arm Test and the Motor Activity Log amount of use scores were clinically relevant for patients with sensory disorders and hemineglect, respectively.

Page et al[99] examined the feasibility and efficacy of a modified CIMT protocol administered on an outpatient basis. Their protocol was developed to be more consistent with therapy scheduling and reimbursement patterns, in other words, more user friendly and feasible from the therapist's perspective. They examined six patients who were in a subacute stage of stroke recovery and who exhibited learned nonuse. The patients were assigned to one of three groups: two patients received half-hour physical and occupational therapy sessions 3 times/week for 10 weeks while they simultaneously had their unaffected arms and hands restrained 5 days per week during 5 hours identified as times of frequent use, two patients received regular therapy, and two control patients received no therapy. Outcomes were measured by the Fugl-Meyer Assessment of motor recovery, the Action Research Arm Test, the Wolf Motor Function Test, and the Motor Activity Log. Patients receiving modified CIMT exhibited substantial improvements on the Fugl-Meyer Assessment, Action Research Arm Test, the Wolf Motor Function Test and reported increases in amount and quality of use of the limb based on the Motor Activity Log. Patients receiving traditional or no therapy exhibited no improvements. The author concluded that modified CIMT may be an efficacious method of improving function and use of the affected arms of patients exhibiting learned nonuse.

Dromerick, Edwards, and Hahn[42] questioned whether a CIMT program could be implemented in the acute stroke population (2 weeks after stroke) and whether this intervention was more effective than traditional upper extremity interventions (control group) during the acute period. The research team enrolled 23 subjects a pilot randomized, controlled trial that compared CIMT with traditional therapies. Treatment plans were designed to make sure that patients in both groups received equivalent time and intensity of treatment directly, and an occupational therapist supervised the program. The subjects received routine interdisciplinary stroke rehabilitation, except for the CIMT that occurred during the regularly scheduled occupational therapy sessions. Individualized and circuit-training techniques were used in both groups. All subjects received study treatment for 2 hours per day, 5 days per week, for 2 consecutive weeks. Twenty subjects completed the trial. The CIMT group had significantly higher scores on the Action Research Arm Test and pinch subscale scores. Differences in the mean grip, grasp, and gross movement subscale scores of the Action Research Arm Test did not reach statistical significance. Activities of daily living performance was not significantly different between groups. No subject withdrew because of pain or frustration. The authors concluded that CIMT during acute rehabilitation is feasible. Furthermore, CIMT was associated with less arm impairment at the end of the trial. The authors warned that long-term studies are needed to determine whether CIMT in the acute stage of stroke is superior to traditional therapies.

In addition to the apparent functional improvements in the select group of patients who are appropriate for a trial of CIMT, researchers have demonstrated that CIMT produces long-term alteration in brain function. This is the first documented cortical-level change associated with a therapy-induced improvement in the rehabilitation of movement after neurologic injury. Liepert et al[81] investigated whether CIMT could produce treatment-induced plastic changes/reorganization of the motor cortex in the human brain. Using focal transcranial magnetic stimulation, the authors mapped cortical motor output area of a hand muscle on both sides in 13 stroke patients in the chronic stage of their illness before and after a 12-day-period of CIMT. The authors found the following:

- Before treatment, the cortical representation area of the affected hand muscle was significantly smaller than the contralateral side.
- After treatment, the muscle output area in the affected hemisphere was significantly enlarged, corresponding to a greatly improved motor performance of the paretic limb.
- Shifts of the center of the output map in the affected hemisphere suggested the recruitment of adjacent brain areas.
- In follow-up examinations up to 6 months after treatment, motor performance remained at a high level.
- At follow up, the cortical area sizes in the two hemispheres became almost identical, representing a return of the balance of excitability between the two hemispheres toward a normal condition.

Taub et al[118] summarized by stating that if the "neural substrate for a movement is destroyed by CNS injury, no amount of intervention designed to overcome learned nonuse can be successful in helping recover lost function. However, many stroke patients...have considerably more motor ability available than they utilize. The suppression of this additional motor capacity is set up by unsuccessful attempts at movement in the acute post-stroke phase...increased motor activity should then become increasingly possible, but the suppression of movement remains unabated and inhibits use of the limb. However, if individuals are correctly motivated to use this unexpressed ability, they will be able to do so."

In his review of the CIMT research, Dromerick[41] suggests that multicenter trials that randomize subjects to CIMT or another active motor treatment of equal time and intensity are needed to determine effectiveness. In addition, studies should include subjects with chronic and acute hemiparesis (Box 10-4). (See Chapter 6.)

## Managing Inefficient and Ineffective Movement Patterns

Being unable to move effectively and therefore unable to interact with the environment is one of the most devastating sequelae of stroke. The loss of the ability to move effectively is a negative stroke symptom.

### Box 10-4

### Summary of Constraint-Induced Movement Therapy

- **Use to counteract learned nonuse.** Hypothesized causes of learned nonuse include therapeutic interventions implemented during the acute period of neurologic suppression after stroke, an early focus on adaptations to meet functional goals, negative reinforcement experienced by the patients as they unsuccessfully attempt to use the affected limb, and positive reinforcement experienced by using the less involved hand and/or use of successful adaptations.
- **Motor inclusion criteria.** Control of the wrist and digits is necessary to engage in this type of intervention. Current and past protocols have used the following inclusion criteria: 20 degrees of extension of the wrist and 10 degrees of extension of each finger; or 10 degrees extension of the wrist, 10 degrees abduction of the thumb, and 10 degrees extension of any two other digits; or able to lift a wash rag off a table using any type of prehension and then release it.
- **Main therapeutic factor.** Massed practice and shaping of the affected limb during repetitive functional activities appears to be the therapeutic change agent. "There is thus nothing talismanic about use of a sling or other constraining device on the less-affected limb."[119]
- **Activity choices and therapist's interventions.** Select tasks that address the motor deficits of the individual patient, assist the patient to carry out parts of a movement sequence if they are incapable of completing the movement on their own at first, providing explicit verbal feedback and verbal reward for small improvements in task performance, use modeling and prompting of task performance, use tasks that are of interest and motivating to the patient, ignore regression of function, and use tasks that can be quantified related to improvements.
- **Outcome measures.** The Motor Activity Log (actual use outside of structured therapy or "real-world use"), Arm Motor Ability Test, Wolf Motor Function Test, and the Action Research Arm Test have been used to document outcomes.

*Continued*

**Box 10-4**

**Summary of Constraint-Induced Movement Therapy—cont'd**

- Cortical reorganization. Constraint-induced movement therapy is the first rehabilitation intervention that has been demonstrated to induce changes in the cortical representation of the affected upper limb.
- The continued rigorous research that has been and continues to be carried out to demonstrate the effectiveness/efficacy of constraint-induced movement therapy should be used as a gold standard for other rehabilitation interventions that are used traditionally (e.g., neurodevelopmental therapy) but have little or no research support.
- Based on available evidence, constraint-induced movement therapy appears to be an effective intervention for stroke survivors who have learned nonuse and who fit the motor inclusion criteria.

The movement patterns of CVA patients have long been discussed in the literature. Controversy continues over the nature of these patterns. These movement patterns have been described as reflex based, a release of abnormal synergies, the result of reversed inhibition or the release of lower patterns of activity from higher inhibitory control, and as learned patterns of movement. Mathiowetz and Bass-Haugen[87] point out that more contemporary models of motor control describe patterns developing after central nervous system damage as results of attempts to use remaining resources to achieve occupational performance. They give the example of a typical flexor pattern (scapula retraction, internal rotation, elbow/wrist/digit flexion) in the upper extremity; the pattern can stem from factors other than spasticity, such as the inability to recruit appropriate muscles, weakness, soft tissue tightness, and perceptual deficits.

Carr and Shepherd[28] state that "muscles that are held persistently in a shortened position not only develop contracture but also appear 'easier' for the patients to activate.... In the stroke patient such activity appears to become habitual, certain muscle groups, apparently those whose mechanical advantages are greatest (because of their shortened length), contracting persistently to the disadvantage of others." The therapist can observe this phenomenon if a patient is reaching out to a target. Many patients have difficulty with the protraction, elbow extension, and wrist and digit extension patterns of this task. If the therapist observes the patients who have been in a resting posture (e.g., seated in a wheelchair) for a prolonged time period, the shortened muscles include the retractors, elbow flexors, and wrist and digit flexors.

Ada et al[1] hypothesize that muscle weakness or paralysis effectively immobilize the upper limb, which results in soft tissue contracture. The immobility causes length-associated changes in muscles, and persistent positioning results in contracture. These changes in the upper limb result in compensatory movements that generate strong neural connections after frequent repetition, ensuring that the compensatory or adaptive movement patterns become learned rather than more effective and efficient.

A Russian neurologist, Nicoli Bernstein, emphasized a early task-oriented view of motor performance and introduced the concept that purposeful movement is organized to solve motor problems.[112] Bernstein introduced the concept of degrees of freedom. He hypothesized that the principal problem faced by the central nervous system was the large number of joints and muscles in the human body and the infinite combinations of muscle action. For example, the upper extremity has multiple degrees of freedom if the number of planes through which each joint moves are combined. When contemplating the combinations of degrees of freedom in the trunk, scapula, and shoulder to the hand, it becomes evident that task of controlling them is phenomenal. Bernstein states that "The coordination of a movement is the process of mastering redundant degrees of freedom of the moving organ, that is, its conversion to a controllable system."[112] Bernstein views motor control as a person's ability to coordinate kinematic linkages that limit degrees of freedom (see Chapter 5).

Flinn[48] uses the example of gymnasts learning a new maneuver to apply the concept of degrees of freedom to a task. Gymnasts limit the degrees of freedom in the task by holding some joints rigid while focusing on one specific body part (e.g., foot placement). Although the gymnasts initially may appear stiff, as they become able to control more degrees of freedom, the stiffness disappears and movement relaxes. This example can be applied to learning how to roller-blade, ice-skate, or perform a new swimming stroke. Sabari[112] discusses a patient with hemiplegia who does not dissociate the pelvis from the lumbar spine or scapula from the thorax, which may be an effort to decrease the degrees of freedom.

With this concept in mind, many of the ineffective movement patterns observed in patients can be attributed to attempts to control the degrees of freedom. Therapists need to consider this during treatment planning when choosing activities. The degrees of freedom must be controlled carefully by stabilizing or eliminating use of some of the joints and therefore decreasing the number of joints involved (e.g., supporting the distal extremity on a table or substituting flat-hand stabilization for a hand grasp).[48] Gillen[53,54] has demonstrated a variety of methods to improve task performance in clients with central nervous system dysfunction by manipulating the degrees of freedom via positioning, splinting, movement retraining, and equipment. Further research is required with the stroke population (see Table 10-1).

Many of the inefficient movement patterns in CVA patients may result from attempting tasks beyond their level of motor control (Figure 10-4). Many therapists have watched patients with newly developed motor control proudly show how they can "lift their arm." Of course, the resulting movement is a stereotypical pattern used by CVA patients. Mathiowetz and Bass-Haugen[87] suggest that the use of these movement patterns is evidence of attempts to use remaining systems to complete tasks. They give the example of a patient with weak shoulder flexors trying to lift an arm. The patient flexes the elbow when trying to raise the arm because this movement strategy shortens the lever arm and makes shoulder flexion easier.

Based on these concepts, the roles of the occupational therapist in treating inefficient and ineffective upper extremity patterns are the following:

- To use skills of activity analysis to guide patients' participation in functional upper extremity tasks that correspond to their level of motor control
- Through this process, to enable patients to interact with the environment using their more affected upper extremity

- To use evaluation skills to determine which impairments (e.g., loss of postural control, weakness, pain, or a combination of components) related to upper extremity function are blocking improvements in occupational performance (e.g., ADL, IADL, work, and leisure)
- To provide function-based activities that focus on improving the identified problem area in an effort to improve task performance
- To provide opportunities to use available motor control throughout the day (Figure 10-5)

In terms of treatment, Mathiowetz and Bass-Haugen[87] suggest that therapists help the patients "find the optimal strategy for achieving functional goals." Goals can be achieved by altering the task requirements, altering the environmental context, and by guiding remediation of the component deficits that interfere with functional performance. The most powerful tools occupational therapists have for intervention are functional activities. Although functional activities have formed the basis of treatment since the profession was developed, only recently has the true impact of functional tasks been evaluated in this area of intervention (Figure 10-6). (See Chapter 4.)

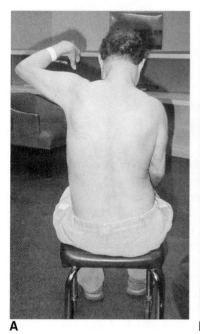 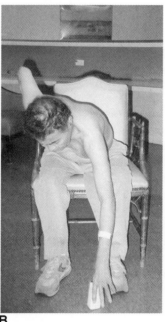 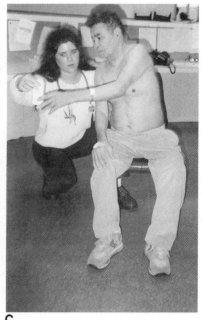

**A**                    **B**                    **C**

**Figure 10-4**    **A,** When asked to reach, this patient uses a stereotypical flexor pattern. Note trunk lateral flexion, scapula adduction, humeral abduction, and distal flexion. **B,** When the position of the activity is changed to correspond with the available motor control and the patient is given a goal (e.g., "Pick up the bottle"), movement pattern is more effective and efficient. **C,** Another position change of same activity results in forward reach with less impact of compensations seen in **A.** The patient reaches with wrist extension, and his hand is prepositioned for successful task completion. The purpose of the activity drives motor output.

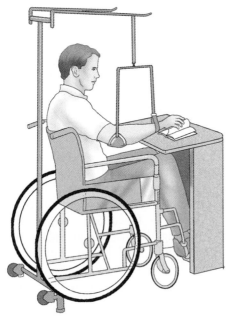

**Figure 10-5** Suspension arm sling. Unweighting the upper extremity may promote increased use during the day. The therapist must consider ways in which the patient can move and use the upper extremity outside of therapy. Caution: When evaluating patients using this device, the therapist must make sure that the movement is being generated by the upper extremity as opposed to swinging the arm by moving the trunk.

## SELECTED ADJUNCT INTERVENTIONS USED WITH A TASK-ORIENTED APPROACH

### Mental Practice/Imagery

The use of imagery in treatment has received an increasing amount of support in the literature. Using imagery and mental practice has been shown to do the following:

- Activate the cortical representation and musculature the correlates with the imagined movements
- Improve learning and performance
- Reorganize the motor cortex

Yue and Cole[139] proposed a method for increasing skeletal muscle strength. Healthy subjects were separated into three groups: those receiving imagining training (i.e., training in which the person imagines a muscle is contracting but is not activating the muscle), those receiving contraction training, and a control group. Training resulted in a maximum voluntary contraction force increase of 22% in the imagining group, 30% in the contraction group, and 3.7% in the control group. This study demonstrated that strength increases can be achieved without muscle activation. Early strength increases appear to result from practice efforts on central motor programming. This study adds to the increasing evidence that the neural origin of strength increases before muscle hypertrophy.

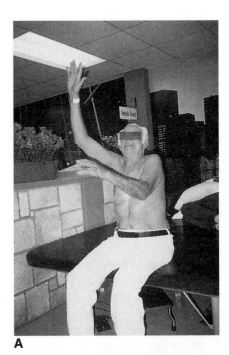

**A**

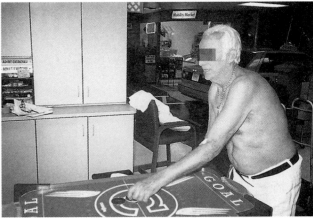

**B**

**Figure 10-6** Reaching activities used to challenge available motor control appropriately. **A,** When attempting to lift both arms, this gentleman uses an ineffective and inefficient movement pattern. He is recruiting his available scapula elevators, elbow flexors, trunk extensors, and head/neck extensors. Although it may appear that he lacks elbow extension or that his elbow flexors are "spastic" or "overactive," muscle testing in supine yields a grade of 4 out of 5 for all elbow musculature. His lack of ability to use elbow extension in this movement may indicate an attempt to shorten the lever arm and control the degrees of freedom. **B** and **C,** Using leisure and work tasks that are more appropriate to this gentleman's level of motor control. Both activities are considered supported reach because the hand is in contact with the work surface. Note that the upper extremity patterns are more effective and efficient.

*Continued*

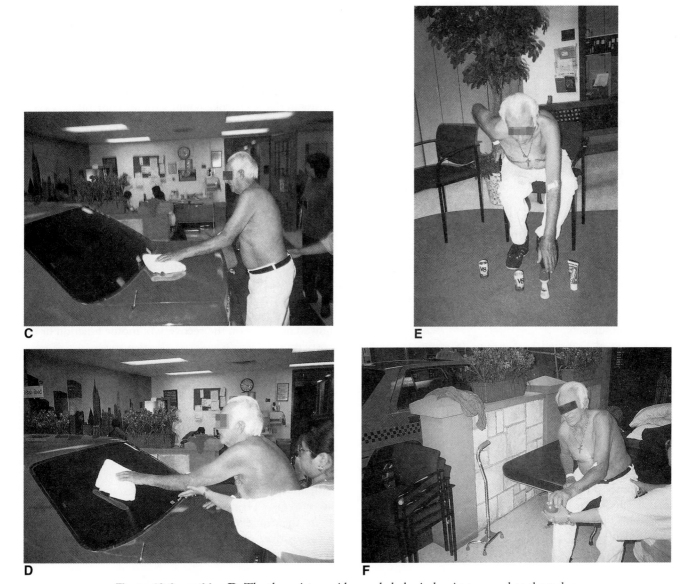

**Figure 10-6 cont'd    D,** The therapist provides graded physical assist to complete the task as increased biomechanical demands are made using the incline of the car. **E** and **F,** Grading the reaching in space activity using gravity to make the task progressively more difficult.

Page[98] hypothesized that imagery use combined with traditional occupational therapy could enhance motor recovery in patients with upper extremity hemiparesis. He provided eight chronic stroke patients with a 4-week course of occupational therapy and imagery (a 20-minute audio tape that consisted of relaxation followed by cognitive visual images related to the upper extremity being used in weight-bearing tasks and functional tasks that were practiced in occupational therapy). This group was compared with eight controls that received only occupational therapy. He concluded that the patients who received occupational therapy and imagery had significantly more improved function as measured by the upper extremity section of the Fugl-Meyer Assessment.

## Biofeedback

Electromyographic biofeedback shows promise and should be studied further for its potential use in treating upper extremity dysfunction after stroke. Biofeedback is provided by electronic instruments that measure and give information about neuromuscular or autonomic activity in the form of auditory or visual feedback signals.

Tries' review[121] of the literature includes a variety of rationales for integrating this noninvasive modality, including training voluntary inhibition of spastic muscles and restoring muscle balance, into an upper extremity program. Tries[121] outlines specific techniques for scapula mobility and stability, humeral rotation, integrating scapular and humeral rotation with a forward reach pattern, and reinforcement of functional patterns in the elbow, forearm, and hand.

Tries[121] presents a case study outlining the applications of biofeedback for a left-sided hemiplegic patient. Her case study illustrated that despite sensory, cognitive, and perceptual impairments, this patient had significant clinical upper limb functional improvements when combining electromyographic biofeedback and traditional occupational therapy.

Greenberg and Fowler[57] compared kinesthetic biofeedback (feedback information pertaining to actual movement of a body part rather than the activity of muscle fibers) to conventional occupational therapy. Their results indicated that kinesthetic biofeedback was equally as therapeutic as but no more effective than conventional occupational therapy for increasing elbow extension in hemiplegic subjects.

Crow et al[34] studied two groups (a group receiving biofeedback and a control group) of 20 patients. The patients were studied before and after 6 weeks of treatment and during a follow-up visit 6 weeks later. Although the groups did not differ significantly before treatment, the biofeedback group improved significantly on arm-function evaluations. At the 6-week follow-up, the beneficial effects were discovered not to have persisted in the experimental group.

Schleenbaker and Mainous[115] concluded from their meta-analysis that biofeedback is an effective tool in neuromuscular reeducation for executing ADL. The use of electromyographic biofeedback warrants further investi-gation into its use as an adjunct tool to enhance upper extremity function in select patients with hemiparesis.

### Electrical Stimulation

The use of functional electrical stimulation and transcutaneous electrical nerve stimulation has been advocated for use in the poststroke population for controlling a variety of symptoms including subluxation, pain, and delayed motor responses. In Price and Pandyan's evidenced-based review[105] of electrical stimulation for the hemiplegic shoulder, they concluded that the evidence from randomized controlled trials does not confirm or refute that electrical stimulation around the shoulder after stroke influences pain but that benefits appear to be related to increasing passive humeral external rotation, possibly from the reduction of glenohumeral subluxation. Specifically, they concluded that no significant change in pain incidence or pain intensity occurred, a significant increase in pain-free external rotation was found, the severity of subluxation was reduced, and treatment showed no effect on the recovery of motor function or on spasticity.

The authors pointed out that further trials are needed before a prudent clinical decision can be made regarding the effectiveness of this modality.

## IMPAIRMENTS TO CONSIDER DURING EVALUATION AND INTERVENTION

Evaluation and intervention of the upper extremity are complex tasks that require an understanding of multiple systems. Therapists need to remain open-minded about their interventions and consider the complexity of causes that interfere with upper extremity use (Figure

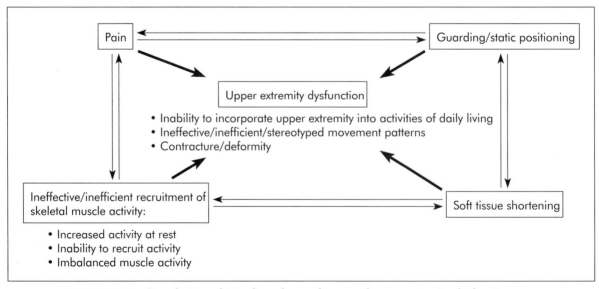

**Figure 10-7** Complexity and interdependence of causes of upper extremity dysfunction.

10-7). Many of the various problems associated with upper extremity function overlap and build on each other. The following paragraphs review common impairments in stroke survivors that may or may not interfere with integrating the upper extremity into daily occupations.

## Impaired Postural Control

Improving proximal stability to enhance distal mobility has long been a tenet of occupational therapy interventions. Postural adjustments stabilize supporting body parts while other parts (i.e., the upper extremities) are being moved.[50] The following studies describe the effect of postural adjustments on arm function.

In the classic study by Belenkii, Gurfinkle, and Paltsev,[7] unimpaired subjects who were evaluated while standing were asked to raise their arm to a horizontal position after they heard an external signal. Various electromyographic studies were performed to trace the pattern of muscle activation. The results demonstrated that the postural muscle synergies of the trunk and lower extremities were activated *before* (by 90 ms) the anterior deltoid, the primary muscle used to perform this motion. The subjects then were evaluated in the supine position while performing the same task. No lower extremity activation was detected in this position (i.e., a different pattern of postural adjustments). The following conclusions can be inferred from this study:

1. Postural adjustments are task specific.
2. Training of the upper extremity in the supine position does not automatically carry over to activities performed while sitting or standing (if postural control is a limiting factor).
3. Having different disciplines treat one particular half of the body is detrimental to patients' progress because upper extremity function depends on postural support from the lower extremities and trunk.

Bouisset and Zattara[17] replicated the previous study and demonstrated that an upward and forward trunk movement resulting from spine and/or lower limb extension precedes upper limb movement. This movement pattern is familiar to therapists who cue their patients to focus on spinal extension and the associated anterior pelvic tilt while treating arm function.

Horak et al[63] compared postural adjustments of subjects with and without hemiplegia during a variety of tasks with different parameters. The hemiplegic subjects demonstrated the same sequence of muscle activation as the subjects without hemiplegia, although activity on the hemiparetic side was delayed. In addition, the hemiparetic individuals were not capable of making rapid movements with the unimpaired arm. This was hypothesized to result from a delay in the anticipatory activity of the contralateral hemiplegic muscles. This study dispels the myth of "good" and "bad" sides after a stroke, especially when postural control is compromised.

In their study of postural adjustments during arm movements, Cordo and Nashner[33] were able to demonstrate that when subjects' postural stability was increased (e.g., by outside shoulder support or placing a finger lightly on a support rail), postural activity was reduced, and voluntary movement enhanced. This concept is crucial to understand when treating upper extremity dysfunction. As support is increased, the postural demands of the task are decreased and vice versa. The therapist can control the patient's level of postural stability by manipulating the following treatment environment factors: positioning—supine to sitting to standing; type of support surface—stationary or unstable surfaces; positioning of objects used in activities—near or far, base of support, and amount of external stability.

Cordo and Nashner[33] also make a critical distinction between associated postural adjustments that *precede* voluntary movements (e.g., reaching) and automatic postural adjustments that *follow* external perturbations (e.g., standing on a bus that stops at a light or being moved by the therapist). Training in one type of adjustment cannot be assumed to carry over into other types of adjustments.

Woollacott, Bonnet, and Yabe[135] demonstrated that their subjects' postural activity varied depending on the task being performed (pushing, pulling) and whether they received information in advance regarding the goal of the task.

Massion[86] points out that voluntary movements are "accompanied by postural adjustments which show three main characteristics: (1) they are 'anticipatory' with respect to movement and minimize the perturbations of posture and equilibrium due to the movement, (2) they are adaptable to the conditions in which the movement is executed, and (3) they are influenced by the instructions given to the subject concerning the task to be performed."

Postural control disorders in stroke patients have been well documented. Lee[80] emphasized the detrimental impact that postural dysfunction has on free arm movements and therefore ADL. Although a variety of muscles can serve as postural stabilizers, postural control of the trunk is critical for upper extremity function[9] (see Chapter 7).

Occupational therapists must use their activity analysis skills to help patients develop the missing trunk control components. (See Table 7-2 for examples of the effects of object positioning on trunk control and weight shifting during reaching activities.) Functional mobility patterns requiring increased trunk control (e.g., scooting) should be incorporated into treatment plans for upper extremity function (see Chapter 14).

Postural control evaluations should be performed within the context of upper extremity tasks such as reaching or performing ADL and IADL. Evaluating postural control separately does not provide the therapist with

## Spasticity

Spasticity, which is a positive symptom according to Jackson's classification system, has been a subject of debate by various authors. Although an abundance of research has been done on spasticity, disagreements still exist about its definition, physiologic basis, treatment, and evaluation. Glenn and Whyte[52] define spasticity as "a motor disorder with persistent increase in the involuntary reflex activity of a muscle in response to stretch. Four specific phenomena may be variably observed in the constellation of spasticity: hypertonia (frequently velocity dependent and demonstrating the clasp-knife phenomenon), hyperactive (phasic) deep tendon reflexes, clonus, and spread of reflex responses beyond the muscle stimulated." In addition, Babinski's sign is characteristic, and hyperactive tonic neck or vestibular reflexes may be present.[83]

Several different phenomena commonly observed in stroke rehabilitation including hyperactive stretch reflexes, increased resistance to passive movement, posturing of the extremities, excessive cocontraction, and stereotypical movement synergies are clumped together in the category of spasticity. Spasticity has become a catchall term for a variety of problems. Rather than being a specific symptom, spasticity is related to a variety of neural and nonneural factors. Therefore, spasticity cannot be treated uniformly by surgical, physical, or pharmacologic procedures. *Spastic paresis* is a commonly used term that implies a cause-and-effect relationship (i.e., a cause-and-effect relationship between positive and negative symptoms). This belief has been challenged recently.

Preston and Hecht[102] provide further information regarding the clinical presentation of spasticity to include the following:

■ Patients having difficulty initiating rapid alternating movements
■ Abnormally timed electromyographic activation of the agonist and antagonist
■ Fluctuation of spasticity as a result of a change in position
■ Usual patterns include upper extremity flexion and lower extremity extension

Bobath[8] stated that there is "An intimate relationship between spasticity and movement . . . spasticity must be held responsible for much of the patient's motor deficit." Treatment techniques were based on "helping the patient gain control over the released patterns of spasticity by their inhibition." Patients were treated under the assumption that "Weakness of muscles may not be real, but relative to the opposition by spastic antagonists." A variety of studies have been published that refute these assumptions (see Chapter 6).

Sahrmann and Norton[113] studied normal subjects and subjects with upper motor neuron symptoms. The movement pattern studied was alternating flexion and extension of the elbow. The analysis of their electromyographic findings showed that the primary cause of impaired movement was not antagonist stretch reflexes but limited and prolonged agonist contraction recruitment and delayed cessation of agonist contractions after movement had stopped. Rather than focusing treatment on inhibiting spasticity, therapists should train patients to perform alternating movement patterns (e.g., hand-to-mouth patterns) efficiently.

Fellows, Kaus, and Thilmann[45] studied the importance of hyperreflexia and paresis on voluntary arm movements in normal subjects and subjects with spasticity resulting from a unilateral ischemic cerebral lesion. The subjects with spasticity showed a lower maximum movement velocity; the more marked the paresis, the greater the reduction in maximum velocity. No relationship was found between the degree of voluntary movement impairment and level of passive muscle hypertonia in the antagonist. The conclusion was that agonist muscle paresis, rather than antagonist muscle hypertonia, had the most significant effect on impaired voluntary movement.

In their study on overcoming limited elbow movement in the presence of antagonist hyperactivity, Wolf et al[132] concluded that functional elbow improvements could be made without first training the patient specifically to inhibit hyperactivity.

Landau[79] performed pharmacologic interventions that effectively abolished the hyperactive stretch reflexes in his patients. This intervention did not result in a corresponding improvement in motor behavior.

In the traditional evaluation of spasticity, the therapist moves the patient's limb. The therapist moves the limb quickly in a direction opposite to the pull of the muscle group being tested, and the examiner feels for a resistance to the movement. The gold standard for rating resistance is the Ashworth Scale[3] or the Modified Ashworth Scale[14] (Box 10-5).

The response of a spastic muscle to stretch has been argued not to be the same during passive and active movement. In addition, spasticity is a multidimensional problem that incorporates neural and nonneural components (e.g., altered soft tissue compliance). Therefore, some authors have questioned the usefulness of test measures such as the Ashworth Scale and are investigating a more comprehensive evaluation of spasticity.

Although the research on spasticity does not support focusing treatment on suppressing stretch reflexes, it does support treatment focusing on preventing secondary structural muscle changes in patients with spasticity.

Hufschmidt and Mauritz's study[64] suggests that spastic contracture is the result of degenerative changes (e.g., atrophy and fibrosis) and changes of the passive and contractile muscle properties.

In their study on spastic and rigid muscles, Dietz, Quintern, and Berger[40] concluded that the actual muscle fibers undergo changes, which explains the increased muscle tone in spastic patients.

For treating patients with spasticity, Perry[100] emphasizes early mobilization and assistance with developing evolving motor control into effective function. These two interventions result in minimal contractures and prevent improper use of patients' available control mechanisms. Hummelsheim et al[65] studied the results of sustained stretch in spastic patients. They found that sustained muscle stretch of approximately 10 minutes led to significant reduction in the spastic hypertonus in the elbow, hand, and finger flexors. They hypothesized that this benefit is a result of stretch receptor fatigue or adaptation to the new extended position.

Little and Massagli[83] also emphasize using a stretching program incorporating nociception prevention and patient education focusing on the adverse effects of spasticity (contracture), use of slow movements, and importance of daily stretching.

In addition to the mentioned techniques, specific modalities and their physiologic bases have been described anecdotally in the literature and include local cooling, vibration therapy, and electrical stimulation.

Perry[100] summarizes the effective rehabilitation of a patient with spasticity by using five categories: contracture minimization, realistic planning, muscle strength preservation and restoration, enhancement of returning control, and substitution for permanent functional loss.

Carr, Shepherd, and Ada[29] summarized their treatment approach based on the assumption that clinical spasticity is a manifestation of length-associated muscle changes and disordered motor control: "The development of spasticity will be less severe if soft tissue length can be maintained and if motor training emphasizes elimination of unnecessary muscle force and training muscle synergies as part of specific actions."

Again, the point must be emphasized that many of the observed phenomena that occur during treatment should not be attributed automatically to spasticity and require more in-depth evaluations and treatment plans (Box 10-6; Table 10-2).

Preston and Hecht[102] have comprehensively reviewed the literature related to spasticity management, including topics such as oral and intrathecal medications, nerve blocks, orthopedic surgery, and neurosurgical interventions.

Nerve blocks are being used increasingly as an adjunct therapy in the rehabilitation process. Preston and Hecht[102] differentiate between short-term blocks such as procaine, lidocaine, and bupivacaine used to diagnose and assist in the evaluation process and long-term blocks such as phenol and botulinum toxin type A (Botox).

## Box 10-5

### The Ashworth Scales

**ASHWORTH SCALE***

1 Normal tone
2 Slight hypertonus; noticeable catch when limb is moved
3 More significant hypertonus, but affected limb still moves easily
4 Moderate hypertonus; difficulty with passive movement
5 Severe hypertonus; rigid limb

**MODIFIED ASHWORTH SCALE†**

0 No increase in muscle tone
1 Slight increase in muscle tone, manifested by a catch and release or by minimal resistance at the end of the range of motion when the affected part is moved in flexion or extension
1+ Slight increase in muscle tone, manifested by a catch, followed by minimal resistance throughout the remainder (less than half) of range of motion
2 More significant increase in muscle tone throughout most of the range of motion but affected part is moved easily.
3 Considerable increase in muscle tone; difficult passive movement
4 Affected part in rigid flexion or extension

---

*From Ashworth B: Carisoprodol in multiple sclerosis, *Practitioner* 192:540, 1964.
†From Bohannon RW, Smith MB: Interrater reliability of a modified Ashworth scale of muscle spasticity, *Phys Ther* 67(2):206-207, 1987.

## Box 10-6

### Treatment of Spasticity

■ Prevent pain syndromes.
■ Guide *appropriate* use of available motor control.
■ Maintain soft-tissue length.
■ Avoid using excessive effort during movement.
■ Encourage slow and controlled movements.
■ Teach specific functional synergies during tasks.
■ Avoid use of repetitive compensatory movement patterns.
■ Keep spastic muscles on stretch via positioning or orthotics to prevent contracture.
■ Teach the patient or caretaker specific stretching techniques targeted at the spastic muscles.
■ Use activities to enhance the agonist/antagonist relationship.
■ Refer when appropriate for pharmacologic or surgical interventions.[102]

**Table 10-2**

## Suggested Interventions for Problems Commonly Thought to Be Caused by Spasticity*

| OBSERVATIONS DURING TREATMENT | SUGGESTED INTERVENTIONS |
| --- | --- |
| Posturing of upper extremity—usually consisting of retraction, posterior trunk rotation, internal rotation, elbow flexion, and wrist and digit flexion—during difficult tasks (e.g., gait, transfers, and dressing) | Upper extremity posturing indicates that the task is difficult for the patient. Treatment should include increasing the efficiency of task performance by building in trunk and lower extremity control, incorporating the upper extremity into the task (e.g., by bilateral ironing or using arm as postural support), and teaching the patient to relax the upper extremity after difficult tasks. |
| Stereotypical flexor patterns when attempting to move arm against gravity | Evaluate components of movement pattern and identify factors that limit efficient movement (e.g., weakness, postural dysfunction, malalignment, and inappropriate task choice). Provide activities that elicit the missing components of movement pattern. |
| Flexion posture when resting | Implement a contracture prevention program. Provide adequate positioning and teach safe, self range-of-motion exercises. |
| "Catch" felt during quick-stretch evaluation of upper extremity | Do not assume that this phenomenon is resulting in observed movement dysfunction. Instead, interpret it as a red flag warning that soft tissue shortening may be present or developing. |

*This table represents a variety of functional limitations and problems traditionally considered to be the direct result of spasticity. Although sometimes interconnected, these problems stem from different sources and must be treated accordingly.

Rousseaux, Kozlowski, and Froger[108] assessed the efficacy of Botox treatment on disability, especially in manual activities, and attempted to identify predictive factors of improvement in 20 patients with stroke. They concluded that botulinum toxin A is efficient in improving hand use in patients with relatively preserved distal motricity and in increasing comfort in patients with severe global disorders. Similarly, Bakheit et al[4] completed a randomized controlled trial to assess the efficacy of Botox in decreasing spasticity in stroke survivors. They concluded that treatment with Botox reduced muscle tone in patients with poststroke upper limb spasticity.

As spasticity increases, the risk for soft tissue shortening is heightened, which in fact may lead to a vicious circle of problems such as spasticity, soft tissue shortening, overrecruitment of shortened muscles, and increased stretch reflexes. Secondary problems that may occur if the spasticity is not managed in a therapy program include the following:

- Deformity of the limbs, specifically the distal upper limb (elbow to digits)
- Impaired upright function caused by soft tissue contracture (e.g., plantar flexion contractures resulting in a loss of the ankle strategies required to maintain upright stance)
- Tissue maceration of the palm
- Pain syndromes resulting from loss of normal joint kinematics. These syndromes are usually related to soft tissue contracture blocking full joint excursion. A typical example of this issue is the loss of full passive external rotation of the glenohumeral joint. Attempts at forced abduction in these cases results in a painful impingement syndrome of the tissues in the subacromial space.
- Impaired ability to manage basic activities of daily living tasks, specifically upper extremity dressing and bathing of the affected hand and axilla when flexor posturing is present
- Loss of reciprocal arm swing during gait activities
- Risk for falls because of postural malalignment[55]

In summary, although reducing spasticity does not appear to result in automatic improvements related to function, therapists must manage spasticity to prevent soft tissue contracture, prevent deformity, and maintain a flexible and mobile arm.

### Loss of Soft Tissue Elasticity (Contractures and Deformities)

Contracture in stroke patients results from immobilization and may be attributed to spasticity, flaccidity, improper positioning, postural malalignment, a lack of variation in limb postures (e.g., prolonged sling use), or a combination of various factors. The formation of contractures indicates a poor prognosis for limb function.

Perry[100] discusses the vicious circle of contracture and spasticity: "contractures stiffen tissues, immobility creates contractures. Spasticity preserves the contracture by excluding the intramuscular fibrous tissues from the stretching force."

Botte, Nickel, and Akeson[16] have reviewed the literature correlating spasticity and contracture. As the stroke patient progresses to a state of spasticity, the increased activity of the spastic muscles may result in characteristic posturing of the limb, resulting in increased stiffness of the soft tissue surrounding the joint and the eventual formation of fixed contracture. The authors further point out that contracture is associated with loss of elasticity and fixed shortening of involved tissues. Contracture may occur in a variety of soft tissues including the following: skin, subcutaneous tissue, muscle, tendon, ligament, joint capsule, vessels, and nerves.

Halar and Bell[59] categorize contracture as arthrogenic (resulting from cartilage damage, joint incongruency, or capsular fibrosis), soft tissue related (skin, tendons, ligaments, subcutaneous tissue), and myogenic (shortening of the muscle by intrinsic or extrinsic factors). The therapist must consider the difference between myogenic and joint contracture, especially if the muscle spans two or more joints (e.g., the wrist and hand). The therapist can differentiate contractures by flexing the proximal joint and noting the resulting position of the distal joints. Joint contracture is not affected by changes in proximal joint position (see Chapter 12).

Booth[15] has reviewed the physiologic and biochemical effects of immobilization on muscle. His findings indicate that muscle strength rapidly declines during limb immobilization because of a decrease in muscle size; muscle fatigability increases rapidly after immobilization. His observations also indicate that muscle atrophy in immobilized limbs begins rapidly, and a decrease in muscle size is greatest in the early phases of immobilization.

***Passive Range of Motion.*** Soft tissue and joint mobilization are the treatments of choice for preventing contracture. The benefits of mobilization include maintenance of joint lubrication,[16] prevention of secondary orthopedic problems (impingements), maintenance of soft tissue length, and possible reduction of spasticity by acting on the nonneural components of spasticity.

Contracture is prevented by deliberate and frequent limb movement, with active movement being preferred over passive when possible. Perry[100] points out that it is essential to move the patient through complete ranges of motion and not just the middle ranges. Therapists must determine what is a full ROM for each patient and so must consider age-related factors. Determining the full ROM on the less affected side may be helpful. A joint that moves or is moved through its full ROM once daily develops almost no deformities. Although the therapist should maintain the patient's ability to participate in all ranges of trunk and upper extremity activities, the therapist should pay particular attention to the following ranges:

- The mobility of the scapula on the thoracic wall with emphasis on protraction and upward rotation should be maintained because this range is critical in the prevention of soft tissue impingement in the subacromial space during overhead movements of the arm and in preparation for forward reach patterns. Overhead ranges should not be attempted unless the scapula is freely gliding in upward rotation.

- Maintaining external (lateral) rotation of the glenohumeral joint allows abduction of the arm as the humerus rotates laterally to permit the greater tuberosity of the humerus to clear the acromial process. Bohannon et al,[12] Ikai et al,[67] and Zorowitz et al[140] concluded that loss of external rotation range of motion was the factor most significantly correlated to shoulder pain.

- Elbow extension is important because the majority of stroke patients favor elbow flexion as a rest posture.

- The therapists also should maintain wrist extension with concurrent radial deviation. During wrist ROM exercises, therapists must realize that the range of wrist deviation is at a maximum when the wrist is slightly flexed and a minimum when the wrist is fully flexed. Wrist extension is at a maximum during neutral deviation and a minimum during ulnar deviation.[73]

- Composite flexion of the digits leads to collateral ligament elongation. Therapists must maintain this length to prevent deformity and prepare the hand for return of motor function.

- Composite extension of the wrist and digits results in long flexor elongation.

- Digits ranged in intrinsic plus (metacarpophalangeal flexion and interphalangeal extension) and intrinsic minus (metacarpophalangeal extension and interphalangeal flexion).

Halar and Bell[59] recommend active ROM and passive ROM combined with a terminal stretch at least twice per day if contracture is beginning to develop. Therapists must use low-load prolonged stretch if a contracture has developed (see Chapters 12 and 13). During the terminal stretch, the therapist should stabilize the proximal body part well. The therapist may distract slightly the joint during the stretch to prevent soft tissue impingement. The therapist must monitor scapula position during passive ROM activities. If necessary the therapist should support the scapula in a position of protraction and upward rotation. In addition, the therapist must support the humerus in an external rotation position. The elbow crease should be facing up (not medially toward the trunk) to ensure proper alignment (Figure 10-8).

***Positioning.*** Positioning is another effective means of maintaining soft tissue length and can be used to promote low-load, prolonged stretch. Therapists must address positioning needs of patients while they are in bed or wheelchairs/armchairs (see Chapter 24) and anytime they are in a recumbent position. Effective positioning encourages proper joint alignment, variations in joint position, comfort, and the maintenance of stretch in areas at risk for contracture. Common areas of concern

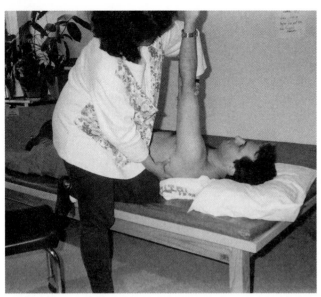

**Figure 10-8** Passive range of motion activities with strict attention to the biomechanical alignment of the scapulothoracic and glenohumeral joints. Therapist's right hand assists with mobilization (upward rotation) of the scapula, while left arm keeps humerus externally rotated.

during patient positioning include head and neck alignment, trunk alignment, glenohumeral joint alignment, scapula alignment, maintenance of abduction, external rotation, elbow extension, and maintenance of long flexor length.

A thorough literature review comparing authors' strategies on bed positioning has been published.[27] This review found no consensus on some issues and multiple discrepancies on strategies. Many of the positioning protocols are based on the principle of inhibiting primitive reflexes, a topic of considerable debate.

Patients are engaged in therapy only a portion of the day. Studies have shown that patients in rehabilitation units spend almost half of their days engaged in passive pursuits including sitting unoccupied and lying in bed.[6] Therefore, patients at risk for developing contracture because of limb immobilization are good candidates for participation in a positioning program in addition to therapy.

The positioning suggestions in Box 10-7 are based on Carr and Kenney's review[27] of the positioning literature and highlights the consensus of reviewed authors.

Although the positioning suggestions in Box 10-7 represent the consensus of many authors, major areas of intervention are missing, which result in the controversies surrounding this area of intervention. For example, glenohumeral joint support remains controversial. Although most authors agree that the scapula should be protracted with a pillow, no consensus exists about support of the humerus. If only the scapula is protracted with a pillow, the humerus takes on a position of relative

**Box 10-7**

**Suggested Bed Positioning**

**POSITIONING OF PATIENT ON UNAFFECTED SIDE**

Head/neck: neutral and symmetrical
Affected upper limb: protracted and forward on pillow-wrist neutral, fingers extended, and thumb abducted
Trunk: aligned
Affected lower limb: hip forward, flexed, and supported; knee forward, flexed, and supported

**POSITIONING OF PATIENT ON AFFECTED SIDE**

Head/neck: neutral and symmetrical
Affected upper limb: protracted forward with elbow extended, hand supinated, wrist neutral, fingers extended, and thumb abducted
Trunk: straight and aligned
Affected lower limb: knee flexed
Unaffected lower limb: knee flexed and supported by pillows

**POSITIONING PATIENT IN SUPINE**

Head/neck: slight flexion
Affected upper limb: protracted and slightly abducted with external rotation with wrist neutral and fingers extended
Trunk: straight and aligned
Affected lower limb: hip forward on pillow; nothing against soles of the feet

extension. Therefore, only support of both the scapula and humerus achieves the original goal of proper joint alignment (Figure 10-9).

At this point, no definitive studies support one type of positioning more than another. Occupational therapists must decide what their intervention goals are and critically analyze their effectiveness. Therapists should not use general, generic strategies for bed positioning; instead, they should evaluate each patient's positioning needs individually.

*Patient Management of the Extremity.* Strategies to teach patients safe ROM activities they can perform themselves need to be initiated as soon as patients are medically stable. Although the clasped-hand position followed by overhead movements of both extremities has been advocated by some authors, this position may not be the most effective, especially for trauma prevention. This movement pattern does not account for factors such as scapula-humeral rhythm (especially if weakness, malalignment, or tightness around the scapula exists), overzealous patients who do not or cannot respect their pain, or critical shoulder biomechanics. Many patients observed performing this type of ROM activity have their trunk hyperextended, scapula retracted, and humerus internally

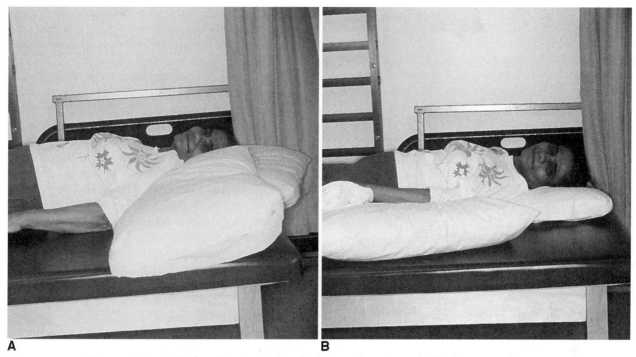

**A**                                    **B**

**Figure 10-9**    **A,** Bed positioning with only the scapula supported. The humerus takes on a position of relative extension, with the head of the humerus migrating anteriorly. **B,** Proper support of scapula and humerus ensures proper biomechanical alignment of shoulder joint.

rotated. This type of alignment does not correspond with an ROM pattern that emphasizes forward flexion of the humerus; it promotes proximal patterns (e.g., retraction) that should be discouraged (Figure 10-10). Recommended techniques for patients performing ROM activities by themselves safely include the following:

1. "Towel on table": The patient is seated at a table with both arms on top of a towel. The less affected arm guides the towel around the table, with the majority of movement occurring in the trunk and from hip flexion. The patient's goal is to "polish the table" while holding positions at the end of desired ROM. The farther the patient's chair is positioned from the table, the greater the ROM. This technique not only enhances the range of the glenohumeral and elbow joint but also encourages scapula protraction and weight shifting. Excessive effort is minimized because the towel assists the movement (Figure 10-11).

2. "Rock the baby": The patient's less affected arm cradles the more affected arm, lifts it to 90 degrees, and places it into positions of horizontal abduction and adduction. Increased horizontal adduction on the more affected side encourages scapula protraction. This technique also encourages trunk rotation (Figure 10-12).

3. While seated or standing, the patient reaches down to the floor and allows both arms to dangle. This position encourages extension of the elbow, wrist, and digits and forward flexion of the humerus with scapula protraction. The activity is an especially useful

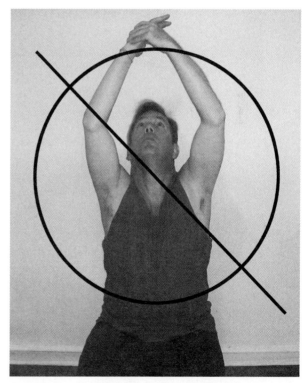

**Figure 10-10**    Because of multiple biomechanical concerns (e.g., impingement), self-overhead range of motion is discouraged.

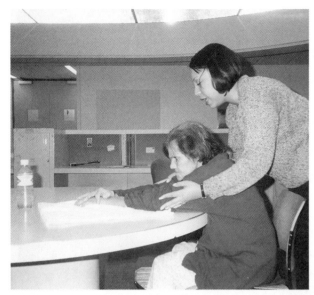

**Figure 10-11**    "Towel on table." Therapist is training patient to perform safe self range of motion activity. As the patient pushes the towel toward bottle, range of motion is gained in humeral flexion, scapular protraction, and elbow extension (which are ranges required for functional reach). Much of the range is gained by hip and trunk flexion.

technique for patients after they have performed an excessively difficult activity (e.g., gait, transfer, or dressing) that results in stereotypical arm posturing (Figure 10-13).

4. While seated or standing, the patient places the more affected extremity onto a table or counter so that the forearm is bearing the weight. With the extremity in this position, the patient turns the trunk away from the supported extremity. As the trunk turns farther away and is enhanced by the posterior reach of the less affected arm, the external rotation of the more affected shoulder increases (Figure 10-14).

5. Davis[38] has advocated rolling over the protracted scapula (from supine to side lying) several times to mobilize the scapula.

6. If the scapula of a patient is mobile and stays mobile, the range of abduction and external rotation may be increased by having the patient lie supine, placing the hands behind the head, and allowing the elbows to fall toward the bed (Figure 10-15). This is a common resting position for an individual who has unimpaired upper extremity function. This technique should be used judiciously and only for patients who move slowly, respect pain, and have a mobile scapula. Therapists may use the five techniques outlined previously for almost all patients because they inherently follow biomechanical principles.

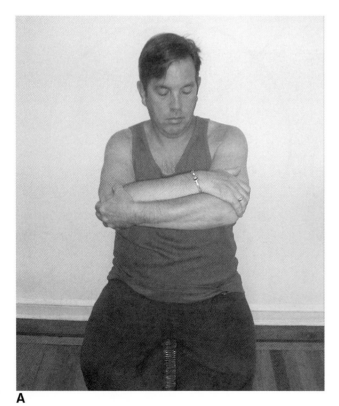

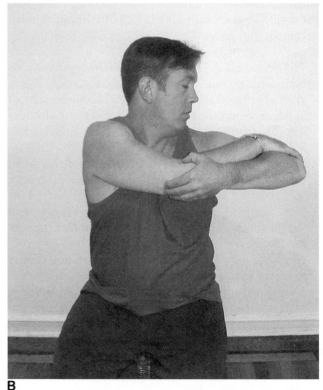

**A**                                                                                          **B**

**Figure 10-12**    "Rock the baby." The patient lifts upper extremity to chest level **(A)** and abducts **(B)** and adducts

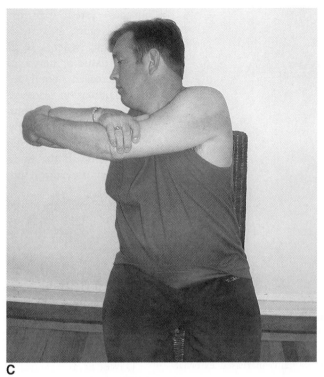

**C**

**Figure 10-12, cont'd**    (**C**) horizontally, allowing trunk rotation.

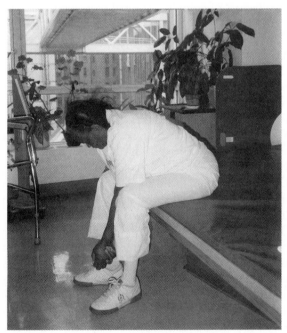

**Figure 10-13**    Patient performs self range of motion activity by reaching to floor. This pattern is especially effective after a difficult task that results in stereotypical posturing.

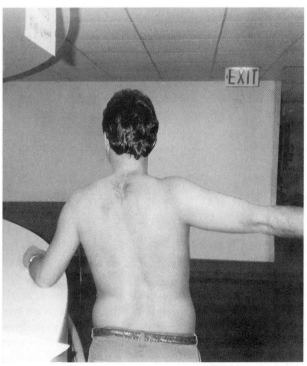

**Figure 10-14**    External rotation of the left glenohumeral joint is achieved by reaching to side and behind with opposite arm.

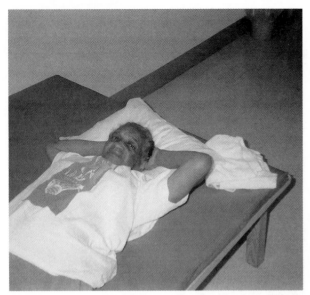

**Figure 10-15** External rotators stretch to be used judiciously for patients who respect their own pain. This rest posture is effective at maintaining external rotation and abduction of the glenohumeral joint. If range is lacking, the humerus can be supported with a towel until patient gains increased external rotation and horizontal abduction.

The ultimate strategy used to decrease contracture and maintain ROM is encouraging functional use of the trunk and upper extremity. A person who has never had a stroke maintains ROM of an extremity by incorporating it into ADL. Activities that eliminate maladaptive positions during activities, improve balanced muscle activity on both sides of the joints, and focus on activities that encourage ROMs that are commonly decreased in stroke patients (e.g., external rotation, forward flexion, abduction, and protraction) should be incorporated into a comprehensive upper extremity program. (See Chapters 12 and 13 for other adjunct treatments to prevent or correct short tissue shortening.)

## SHOULDER-HAND SYNDROME/COMPLEX REGIONAL PAIN SYNDROME TYPE I

Shoulder-hand syndrome (SHS) is classified as a reflex sympathetic dystrophy disorder or complex regional pain syndrome type I. The painful lesion that precipitates SHS is a proximal trauma such as a shoulder, neck, or rib cage injury or a visceral source such as stroke. The syndrome begins with severe pain and progresses to stiffness in the shoulder and pain throughout the extremity. Other symptoms include moderate to considerable swelling of the wrist and hand, vasomotor changes, and atrophy.[77] If untreated, SHS may result in a frozen shoulder and permanent hand deformity.[21]

Although the cause of SHS remains obscure, most authors associate it with a change in the autonomic nervous system (primarily sympathetic).[32] A study by Braus, Krauss, and Strobel[21] suggests that the SHS in hemiplegic patients is initiated by a peripheral lesion (e.g., a tissue or nerve injury). The authors hypothesize that increased neural activity after a peripheral injury or inflammation leads to a central sensitization that is responsible for the severe pain associated with SHS. Autopsy data collected by the authors confirmed microbleeding in the area of the suprahumeral joint of the affected side. If the underlying cause is in fact peripheral, then prevention programs theoretically would be effective.

The reported incidence of SHS varies from 27%[21] to 25%[120] to 12.5%[39] to 1.56%.[101] Males seem to be slightly more affected than females.[39,120] The majority of patients with SHS symptoms have partial motor loss, moderate or severe sensory loss, and varying degrees of spasticity.[39] Associated risk factors include subluxation, considerable weakness, moderate spasticity, deficits in confrontational field testing (following hemianopia or neglect), and altered shoulder biomechanics that may compromise the suprahumeral joint structures.[21]

Daviet et al[37] examined 71 patients with hemiplegia; 34.8% had a complex regional pain syndrome type I. They identified four main clinical factors in the prognosis of complex regional pain syndrome type I as motor deficit, spasticity, sensory deficits, and initial coma. They also concluded that shoulder subluxation, unilateral neglect, and depression did not seem to be determinant predictive factors of complex regional pain syndrome type I severity.

Three stages of SHS have been described (Box 10-8). Davis et al[39] outlined the major diagnostic criteria for SHS based on the following clinical symptoms:

- Shoulder: loss of ROM and pain during abduction, flexion, and external rotation movements
- Elbow: no signs or symptoms
- Wrist: intense pain during extension movements, dorsal edema, and tenderness during deep palpation
- Hand: edema over metacarpals and no tenderness
- Digits: moderate fusiform edema, intense pain during flexion of the metacarpophalangeal and proximal interphalangeal joints, and loss of skin lines

The Tepperman et al[120] study concluded that metacarpophalangeal tenderness during compression was the most valuable clinical sign of reflex sympathetic dystrophy, with a predictive value of 100%. Vasomotor changes and interphalangeal tenderness had the next highest predictive value at 72.7%. Therapists must remember that many of the mentioned signs and symptoms can be found in stroke patients without SHS. If a patient has several characteristic signs and symptoms, one safely can make a diagnosis on clinical grounds alone.[32] Although the diagnosis for SHS is primarily clinical, the most effective way to confirm its presence is to use a differential neural

**Box 10-8**

**Stages of Shoulder-Hand Syndrome/Complex Regional Pain Syndrome Type I**

**STAGE 1**

The patient complains of shoulder and hand pain, tenderness, and vasomotor changes (with symptoms of discoloration and temperature changes). Chances of reversal are high at this stage.

**STAGE 2**

The patient has early dystrophic limb changes, muscle and skin atrophy, vasospasm, hyperhidrosis (increased sweating), and radiographic signs of osteoporosis. At this stage, should-hand syndrome becomes increasingly difficult to treat.

**STAGE 3**

Patients rarely have pain and vasomotor changes, but they do have soft tissue dystrophy, contracture (including a frozen shoulder and clawed hand), and severe osteoporosis. At this stage, shoulder-hand syndrome is irreversible.

---

blockade. The therapist may use a stellate ganglion block to alleviate the symptoms. The block interrupts the abnormal sympathetic reflex; the diagnosis of SHS is confirmed if the block alleviates symptoms.

Therapists should prevent SHS so that it will not have to be treated. Davis[38] has developed a prevention protocol that focuses on the following:

- Therapists gaining full understanding of the anatomy and physiology of normal and hemiplegic shoulders
- Proper handling of the upper extremity, including avoiding arm traction during mobility, ADL, and gait activities; supporting the arm as necessary, preventing prolonged arm dangling, and using the trunk and scapula rather than the arm as support during transitional movements
- Staff education focusing on the mentioned handling techniques
- Mobilizing the scapula to ensure gliding when raising or performing ROM activities with the arm
- Family education focusing on proper extremity handling and transfer techniques; training families not to guard at the affected upper extremity during ambulation (because a balance loss would result in an automatic reflex—grabbing the patient's arm)
- Edema control that begins as soon as signs of it are observed (see Chapter 11)
- Training patients to take responsibility for protecting their affected arm

Davis et al[39] hypothesize that therapists can control certain factors contributing to SHS. One factor is the extravasation of intravenous fluids. Therapists should infuse intravenous fluids into the less affected arm if possible; if not, therapist should infuse fluids proximal to the wrist on the affected side. This strategy prevents infiltration around the needle and a possible edema syndrome. Another contributing factor is poor positioning. Therapists should position patients so that they cannot roll over onto the affected arm, pin it down, and compromise circulation. The other factor is immobilization of a painful shoulder by the patient. Davis[38] writes, "In this sense, a painful shoulder (but not necessarily SHS) can evolve into SHS through immobility and consequent circulatory problems. Therefore, proper management of the hemiplegic patient in order to prevent trauma to the shoulder is critical."

In a recent prospective, two-part study performed by Braus, Krauss, and Strobel,[21] a prevention protocol was implemented that focused on protecting the affected upper extremity from trauma. All patients, relatives, and members of the therapy and medical teams received detailed instructions when patients initially were hospitalized to avoid peripheral injuries to the affected limb. Wheelchair and bed positioning were modified to ensure no pain resulted from improper positioning. Passive movements of the upper extremity were not made unless the scapula was fully mobilized. Any activity or position that caused pain was changed immediately, and no infusions into the veins of the hemiplegic hands were performed. These strategies alone decreased the incidence of SHS from 27% to 8%.

If symptoms of SHS begin to develop, therapists should make an early diagnosis and begin aggressive treatment. In the study by Braus, Krauss, and Strobel,[21] patients who already had definite SHS symptoms were placed in an experimental group (that received a 14-day treatment with low doses of orally administered corticosteroids and daily therapy) or a placebo group (that received placebo medication and daily therapy). Of the 36 patients in the experimental group, 31 were free of symptoms after 10 days of treatment. Chu, Petrillo, and Davis[32] and Davis[38] also have advocated use of orally administered corticosteroids with therapy.

Therapy intervention should be symptom specific. Therapists must alleviate edema immediately and maintain joint mobility while preventing pain.[77,129] Davies[36] advocates using activities that result in increased upper extremity ROM but actually result from trunk and hip flexion (e.g., towel exercises, pushing away a therapy ball while seated, and reaching to the floor). Mobilizing the scapula, which can be accomplished by the therapist or having the patient roll onto the protracted scapula from the supine to the side-lying position, also has been described.

Research is beginning to show that peripheral lesions are the cause of SHS in stroke patients, so interventions should incorporate this knowledge. Inappropriate ROM exercises (e.g., overhead ROM activities in patients without scapula mobility or overzealous exercise) and mishandling during ADL (e.g., pulling on the affected arm during transfers, bathing, dressing, and bedtime activities) are factors to consider. In addition to evaluating and treating SHS, occupational therapists play a major role in staff education. All staff and family members who physically move patients need to be aware of appropriate techniques so as to prevent injuries.

## Weakness

The impact of weakness (a negative symptom) on stroke patients' functional status has long been ignored. The motor control deficits in patients previously were attributed exclusively to spasticity, which resulted in treatment focused on inhibiting the spasticity. Many therapists considered upper extremity muscle tests for strength difficult to interpret because of common "synergy patterns." Bourbonnais et al[19] demonstrated that the patterns of activity in the elbow flexor muscles were not consistent with established synergistic patterns. Weakness of the upper extremity musculature plays a major role in upper extremity dysfunction, probably more than the positive symptoms after stroke. Muscle weakness is reflected by the inability of patients to generate normal levels of muscle force.[18] Stroke survivors who have written about their experiences focus on the difficulty in force production. Brodal[22] reflected on his own stroke: "It was a striking and repeatedly made observation that the force needed to make a severely paretic muscle contract is considerable.... Subjectively this is experienced as a kind of mental force, a power of will. In the case of a muscle just capable of being actively moved the mental effort needed was very great."

Bourbonnais and Vanden Noven[18] reviewed the physiologic changes in the nervous system that contribute to muscle weakness in patients with hemiparesis. They summarized specific changes at the motor neuron and muscle levels that decrease a patient's ability to produce force. Box 10-9 summarizes these changes.

### Box 10-9

### Physiologic Changes Contributing to Weakness

- Motor neuron changes: loss of agonist motor units, changes in recruitment order of motor units, and changes in the firing rates of motor units
- Nerve changes: changes in peripheral nerve conduction
- Muscle changes: changes in the morphologic and contractile properties of motor units and in the mechanical properties of muscles

Bohannon et al[11] found that static strength deficits of the shoulder medial rotator and elbow flexor muscles did not correlate with antagonist muscle spasticity. They concluded that therapists might determine the capacity for force production for an agonist muscle based on its own tone rather than that of its antagonist.

Gowland et al[56] studied agonist and antagonist activity during upper limb movements in stroke patients and concluded that treatment should be aimed at improving motor neuron recruitment rather than reducing antagonist activity. In their study, patients who could not perform select upper extremity tasks had electromyographic values that were significantly and consistently lower than those of patients who were successful at the task.

Bohannon and Smith[13] analyzed strength deficits in stroke patients and verified that muscle strength improves in stroke patients with hemiplegia who are undergoing rehabilitation. The most effective means of increasing muscle strength needs to be researched.

Flinn[48] presented a case study of a young female with left-sided hemiplegia. Her treatment program focused on participating in graded functional tasks that systematically increased the motor demands on the more affected upper extremity. Her task-oriented treatment program was augmented by resistive exercises using elastic tubing. Substantial results after 6 months of therapy included improved level of occupational performance in ADL and IADL, improved manual muscle test scores (which increased from 2/5 to the 4/5 and 5/5 ranges), improved hand function, and improved grip strength scores. Identifying the underlying problems (in this case, weakness and an inability to control excess degrees of freedom) is of utmost importance when planning treatment strategies.

The debate about which type of muscle contraction (eccentric, concentric, or isometric) is the most effective in strengthening patients has been long-standing. Muscle groups need to contract in a variety of ways to complete functional tasks successfully. For example, when a person reaches for a can of soup on a high shelf, the shoulder musculature must contract (concentrically) to bring the hand to the level of the shelf, maintain the contraction (isometrically) to locate the correct item, and control the weight of the arm and item in gravity (eccentrically) as the can is placed with control on the countertop.

In a study of dynamic muscle strength training in stroke patients, Engardt et al[43] found that eccentric contractions were more effective than concentric contractions. Twenty patients with hemiparesis resulting from strokes participated in activities that elicited concentric or eccentric contractions. After the treatment, significant improvements resulted in the relative strength of paretic muscles during eccentric and concentric actions in the group that was trained solely with eccentric contractions (i.e., eccentric training increased the strength of both types of contractions); this was not true for the group that only received concentric contraction training. Therefore the authors determined eccentric contraction training to be more advantageous and efficient (Box 10-10).

### Superimposed Orthopedic Injuries

Orthopedic problems associated with stroke have been well documented. These complications have a negative impact on functional outcomes, prolong rehabilitation, and are one of the main causes of upper extremity pain syndromes after stroke.

*Rotator Cuff and Biceps Tendon Lesions.* The rotator cuff guides and leads the movements of the shoulder joint. The cuff supplies the strength needed to complete the ROM in the shoulder joint and seats the head of the humerus into the glenoid fossa.

Najenson, Yacubovic, and Pikielni[94] studied 32 hemiplegic patients with severe upper limb paralysis; 18 patients served as controls by having their less affected side evaluated. Forty percent of the patients had a rotator cuff tear on the affected side. None of the patients had complaints about the affected shoulder before the stroke. Only 16% of the patients in the control group had ruptured rotator cuffs on the less involved side; all three seemed to be long-standing tears.

Najenson, Yacubovic, and Pikielni[94] also discussed the pathophysiology of a rotator cuff tear in hemiplegic patients. Many older patients are predisposed to rotator cuff ruptures because of degenerative changes associated with aging. Cuff tears commonly result from impingement of the cuff between the greater tuberosity and acromial arch (Figure 10-16), which occurs when the humerus is forced into abduction without external rotation (e.g., during inappropriate passive ROM activities or activities that are not sensitive to shoulder biomechanics [e.g., reciprocal pulleys]). Therapists who have a thorough understanding of joint alignment can prevent impingement during treatment.

Nepomuceno and Miller[97] found seven rotator cuff tears and one a transverse bicipital tendon tear in 24 subjects with painful hemiplegic shoulders. None of the patients had premorbid pathologic conditions of the shoulder. With

one exception, all patients with soft tissue lesions had left-sided hemiplegia. (This study did not evaluate the presence of visual field loss or neglect.)

Therapists should note that a relationship between rotator cuff age and wear has been documented. After age 50, the percentage of lesions significantly increases, reaching 60% after 60 years of age.[102]

*Adhesive Changes.* Adhesive changes in the hemiplegic shoulder are considered to result from immobilization, synovitis, or metabolic changes in joint tissue. Hakuno et al[58] studied adhesive changes in hemiplegic shoulders and found that hemiplegia had a significant influence on the prevalence of adhesive changes in the shoulder. Adhesive changes were found in 30% of patients' affected glenohumeral joints as opposed to 2.7% on the less involved side.

Rizk et al[106] examined 30 hemiplegic patients by arthrography of the shoulder and found that 23 patients had capsular constriction typical of frozen shoulder (adhesive capsulitis). Therefore the authors advocated early passive ROM for the shoulder.

Roy, Sands, and Hill[109] use the following clinical criteria for adhesive capsulitis: shoulder pain, external rotation of less than 20 degrees, and abduction of less than 60 degrees. Ikai et al[67] concluded that adhesive capsulitis is a main cause of shoulder pain.

*Brachial Plexus Injury.* Kaplan et al[74] identified brachial plexus injury in 5 of 12 patients in their study. All five had electromyographic evidence indicating neuropathy of the upper trunk of the brachial plexus on the side affected by the stroke. The deltoid, biceps, and infraspinatus muscles were involved. Moskowitz and Porter[93] also summarized the findings in five CVA patients with

### Box 10-10

**Task Parameters That Can Be Manipulated to Increase Strength**

- Gravity: eliminated, assisted, against
- Weight of objects used during tasks
- Amount of external support (e.g., slide hand across table versus reach into space)
- External resistance (e.g., weights, elastic bands, resistance from therapist's hands)

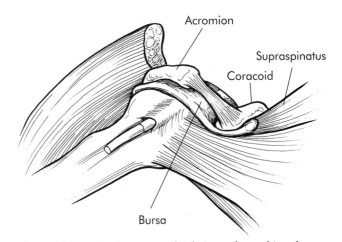

**Figure 10-16** Impingement of soft tissues located in subacromial space. Impingement occurs between the head of humerus and acromion/coracoid. Impingement occurs during forced humeral flexion/abduction without concurrent upward rotation of scapula and/or external rotation of humerus.

"traction neuropathies" of the upper trunk of the brachial plexus.

Merideth, Taft, and Kaplan[89] reviewed the diagnostic and treatment procedures for CVA patients with brachial plexus injuries. Physical examination findings included flaccidity and atrophy of the supraspinatus, infraspinatus, deltoid, and biceps muscles in the affected upper extremity with increased muscle tone or distal movement (an atypical pattern of recovery). Electromyographic criteria for diagnosing brachial plexus injuries include the finding of fibrillation potentials in the muscles innervated by the upper trunk of the brachial plexus.

Treatment of these patients included positioning and passive and active ROM activities. During active ROM activities, effects of gravity were monitored to prevent further traction. Using a positioning pillow, the affected upper extremity was positioned as follows: externally rotated 45 degrees, 90 degrees of elbow flexion, and forearm neutral. Patients used slings while ambulating and were educated not to sleep on their affected side, which could result in compression and traction injuries to the upper trunk. (Many authors encourage sleeping on the affected side if this pathologic condition is not present.) A major component of the treatment program was the education of the patient, staff, and families regarding proper care and positioning of the upper extremity.

## Pain Syndromes

Although pain syndromes have been discussed previously in the context of orthopedic injuries and SHS, their impact on functional recovery is significant, so this section specifically reviews the literature on hemiplegic shoulder pain.

The incidence of shoulder pain in hemiplegic patients has been reported to be as high as 72%.[12,109,126] Roy, Sands, and Hill[109] identified strong associations between hemiplegic shoulder pain and prolonged hospital stays, arm weakness, poor recovery of arm function, ADL, and lower rates of discharge to the home. Those responsible for stroke patients have the onus to be aware of hemiplegic shoulder pain and to diagnose, relieve, and prevent this syndrome. Although shoulder pain is obviously not the only variable leading to prolonged hospital stays, it is a potentially preventable variable over which occupational therapists have some control.

Pain can limit patient's activities, such as rolling in bed, transferring, putting on a shirt or blouse, and bending to reach the feet to put on shoes and socks. The occurrence of shoulder pain also has been linked to depression.[114]

The literature concerning hemiplegic shoulder pain is confusing at times and often contradictory. The following review was obtained from a selection of articles from a variety of disciplines. The focus of the review is clinical correlations associated with hemiplegic shoulder pain.

In their study of 55 patients, Roy, Sands, and Hill[109] found positive correlations between hemiplegic shoulder pain and "glenohumeral malalignment without descent of the humeral head" and between hemiplegic shoulder pain and reflex sympathetic dystrophy (SHS). The study did not confirm a strong association between spasticity (measured by the Ashworth Scale) and hemiplegic shoulder pain.

Joynt[72] found significant correlations between loss of motion and shoulder pain and questioned the relationship between neglect/perceptual dysfunction and pain. His left-sided hemiplegic subjects had a higher incidence of shoulder pain, which led him to question whether the incidence of trauma was increased. He found no correlation between shoulder pain and subluxation, spasticity, strength, or sensation.

Joynt[72] identified the subacromial area as a pain-producing location in a significant number of cases. Of 28 patients who received a subacromial injection of 1% lidocaine, more than half obtained moderate or significant pain relief and improved ROM. The author suggested that physical agent modalities, steroid injections, and careful ROM activities focusing on impingement prevention were significant in reducing pain.

The subacromial area is prone to trauma during therapy and patient handling. The subacromial space includes the supraspinatus tendon, long head of the biceps, and subacromial bursa[26] (Figure 10-17). All of these structures are prone to impingement and inflammation. Structure impingement can develop easily in hemiplegic patients during ROM activities because the normal scapulohumeral rhythm becomes impaired. If the scapula is not rotated upward (by therapist's manipulation or active control), the humerus becomes blocked by the acromion and causes impingement, inflammation, and pain (see Figure 10-16). Combined motions of scapula retraction with forward flexion should be avoided to prevent impingement. Instead, the scapula should glide freely and be protracted and upwardly rotated during upper extremity activities. Objects for reaching activities should be placed in front or below waist level of the patient to encourage humeral forward flexion with scapular protraction.

Some patients may develop inflammation around the biceps tendon and supraspinatus insertion because of impingements. Palpation skills are important for determining which structures are involved (Figure 10-18). To palpate the biceps tendon, the therapist palpates the acromion and drops one finger to the anterior shoulder; the biceps tendon lies in the groove between the greater and lesser tuberosities of the humerus. If the patient feels pain on application of pressure, the biceps tendon probably has been affected. (Passively rotating the humerus while palpating assists the therapist with locating the tuberosities.)

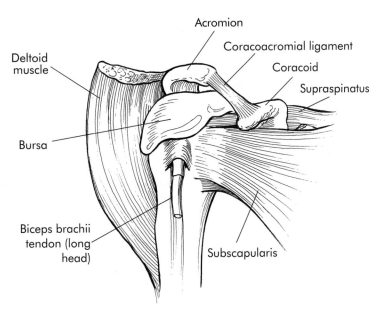

**Figure 10-17**  Subacromial space.

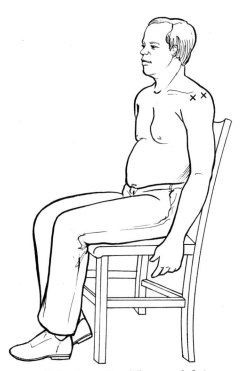

**Figure 10-18**  Palpation point. The *x* on left (more anterior) is palpation point for long head of biceps. The *x* on right (more lateral) is palpation point for supraspinatus tendon.

To palpate the supraspinatus tendon, the therapist palpates the acromion, but this time drops one finger to the lateral shoulder right below the center of the acromion. If pressure or slight friction elicits pain, the supraspinatus most likely has been affected.

Bohannon et al[12] studied the relationship of five variables (age, time since onset of hemiplegia, range of external rotation of the hemiplegic shoulder, spasticity, and weakness) to shoulder pain. In their study of 50 patients, 36 had shoulder pain. Range of shoulder external rotation was considered the factor related most significantly to shoulder pain. They hypothesized that hemiplegic shoulder pain was in part a manifestation of adhesive capsulitis. In this study only patients with full external rotation were free of pain. The suggested treatment was elimination of inflammation and maintenance of ROM.

Hecht[61] treated 13 patients with limited ROM and shoulder pain with percutaneous phenol blocks to the nerves of the subscapularis (a major shoulder internal rotator). Immediate and significant improvements were observed in the flexion, abduction, and external rotation ROMs; pain relief also was noted. This study indicates that the subscapularis is a key muscle and should be addressed during treatment focusing on maintaining soft tissue length. The subscapularis muscle may tighten in patients with the previously mentioned pain syndrome. If the humerus resists external rotation with the arm at the side during evaluation, the therapist can presume the subscapularis to be a factor contributing to the deformity. This study adds more support to the concept of focusing on maintaining the range of humeral external rotation to prevent resulting complications.

Bohannon and Andrews[10] studied 24 patients in an effort to establish a relationship between subluxation and pain. Despite the emphasis placed on reduction of subluxation, the relationship between shoulder pain and subluxation has not been established. Their study did not find an association between shoulder pain and subluxation (which was defined in this study as the separation between the acromion and the humeral head). A study by Arsenault et al[2] also found no significant relationship between subluxation and shoulder pain.

A more recent study by Zorowitz et al[140] also focused on the correlation between subluxation and pain. Results showed that shoulder pain did not correlate with age, vertical or horizontal subluxation, shoulder flexion, abduction, or Fugl-Meyer Assessment scores, but it did correlate with the degree of shoulder external rotation. Wanklyn, Forster, and Young[128] also found an association between reduced external rotation and hemiplegic shoulder pain, with an incidence as high as 66%. This association was believed to be due to abnormal muscle tone or structural changes, namely adhesions. Similarly, Ikai and othes[67] evaluated 75 subjects and found no correlation between subluxation and pain.

Kumar et al[76] demonstrated a positive correlation between shoulder pain and therapy programs that did not consider biomechanical shoulder alignment during treatment. Patients were assigned to one of three exercise groups: ROM initiated by the therapist, skateboard treatment, and overhead pulley treatment. Of the patients who developed pain during the treatment programs, 8% were in the ROM group, 12% in the skateboard group, and 62% in the overhead pulley group. The probable cause of this discrepancy was soft tissue damage resulting from forced abduction without external rotation. This study showed that poorly prescribed activities by the therapist could be the cause of pain syndromes. This study found no significant relationship between subluxation and pain.

In a 3-year study of 219 hemiplegic patients, Van Ouwenaller, Laplace, and Chantraine[126] found that 85% of the patients who developed pain had spasticity (an increased myotatic reflex) compared with 18% of flaccid patients. They also found that 50% of the patients who developed pain had anteroinferior subluxations (which were not defined). The authors advocated use of muscle relaxation techniques for the shoulder girdle.

Jensen[71] attributes shoulder pain to traumatic tendonitis resulting from unskilled and strenuous joint treatment during ADL (e.g., bathing, dressing, and bed mobility) and bilateral ROM activities of more than 90 degrees resulting in "jamming [of] soft tissue against the acromion resulting in lesions" (see Figure 10-10). Jensen suggests the following precautions: educating all staff members, placing signs over patients' beds to warn staff of the shoulder instability, supporting the arm during the acute stage, avoiding treatment that may cause soft tissue impingement, having a thorough understanding of shoulder anatomy, and dissuading use of pulley exercises and self-ROM activities.

Lastly, Wanklyn, Forster, and Young[128] found a 27% increased incidence of shoulder pain in dependent patients after discharge, which may reflect improper handling at home by caregivers. They suggested a greater emphasis on patient and caregiver education regarding proper transfer techniques and correct handling of the hemiplegic arm (Box 10-11).

## Box 10-11

### Hemiplegic Shoulder Pain Prevention

- Maintain and/or increase passive glenohumeral joint external rotation.
- Maintain scapula mobility on the thorax.
- Avoid passive or active shoulder movements beyond 90 degrees (flexion and abduction) unless the scapula is gliding toward upward rotation and sufficient external rotation is available. These two movements are necessary to prevent shoulder impingement.
- Educate the patient, family, and staff about potential complications related to an unstable shoulder.
- Teach patients and caregivers proper management during activities of daily living to avoid shoulder traction and forced overhead movements. Specific activities that should be addressed include applying deodorant, transfers, guarding during ambulation, bathing the axilla, and upper body dressing.
- Educate patients regarding different types (e.g., stretch versus sharp) of pain. Avoid sharp pain during any shoulder movements or activities.
- Provide positioning to prevent a dangling upper extremity. Assess shoulder positions in bed, in wheelchair, and during upright function.
- Avoid activities that may cause impingements such as use of overhead pulleys, forced overhead self range of motion, or overaggressive passive range of motion by the therapist.

## Loss of Biomechanical Alignment

Immediately after a stroke, patients lose their ability to maintain upright control and become malaligned because of the effects of gravity, weakness, and muscle imbalance.

Occupational therapists must be able to identify malalignments to treat upper extremity dysfunction effectively. The following section discusses common trunk and upper extremity alignment problems and reviews activities to counteract the adverse effects of malalignment.

***Loss of Pelvic/Trunk Alignment.*** After a stroke, patients commonly lose their ability to perform postural adjustments and maintain postural alignment because of weakness, a loss of equilibrium, and righting reactions; the trunk assumes an asymmetrical posture.[8,9,36]

The first area to observe is the patient's pelvis and its effect on spinal alignment. Patients typically bear weight asymmetrically through their pelvis (by one ischial tuberosity accepting more weight than the other), which results in lateral spine flexion. This lateral flexion causes the trunk musculature to become shortened on the non–weight-bearing side and lengthened on the weight-bearing side[36] (Figure 10-19). At the same time, patients tend to assume a posterior pelvic tilt, which results in spinal flexion. Again the result is a muscle imbalance, with the anterior musculature (abdominals) becoming

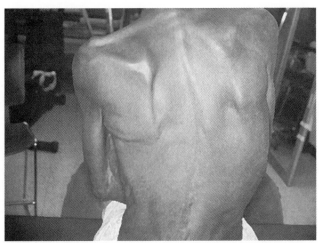

**Figure 10-19** Asymmetrical trunk posture in patient with left hemiplegia. Note the left trunk shortening, right trunk elongation/overstretching, rib cage shift, loss of scapula stability on rib cage, relative downward rotation of scapula, increased weight bearing on right ischial tuberosity, and shoulder asymmetry (left hemiplegia).

shortened and the posterior muscles (extensors) becoming elongated. Davies[36] hypothesizes that patients sit with posterior pelvic tilt to compensate for weak abdominals. Patients assume this "safe" posture to prevent themselves from falling backward. The spinal flexion that results from the posterior tilt leads to loss of natural lumbar spine lordosis and accentuated thoracic spine kyphosis.

Abdominal weakness (especially the obliques) results in a destabilization of the rib cage. A lack of balance between the obliques results in trunk and rib cage rotation[73] (see Chapter 7).

***Loss of Scapula Alignment.*** Upper extremity malalignment commonly results from pelvic and trunk malalignments. When in a resting position, the scapula is flush on the rib cage (the scapulothoracic joint) and upwardly rotated. When one palpates the scapula, the distance between the inferior angle and the vertebral column should be greater than the distance between the medial border of the scapular spine and the vertebral column[73] (Figure 10-20). In the resting position the glenoid fossa of the scapula faces upward, forward, and outward. Therefore the trunk and rib cage must be stable to support the scapula properly. In hemiplegic patients the scapula loses its orientation on the thoracic wall and assumes a position of relative downward rotation.[26]

Cailliet[26] describes several events that result in a downwardly rotated scapula (Figure 10-21), such as lateral flexion toward the hemiparetic side. The lateral flexion may be a result of trunk weakness, perceptual dysfunction that results in an inability to perceive midline, or excess activity in unilateral trunk flexors (i.e.,

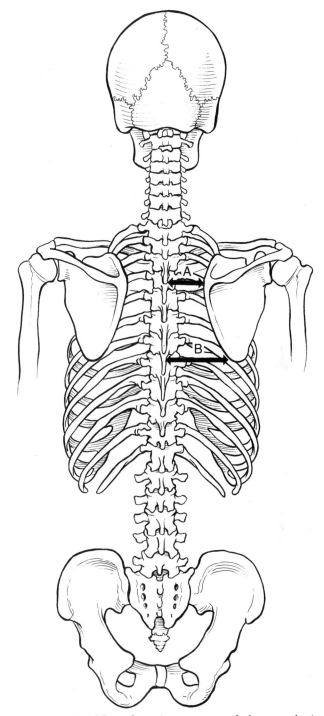

**Figure 10-20** Normal resting posture of the scapula in upward rotation. *A* is the distance (in finger breadths or centimeters) from the medial border of the spine of the scapula to the vertebral column. *B* is the distance from the inferior angle of the scapula to the vertebral column. Distance *B* should be greater than distance *A* if the scapula is aligned appropriately. If *A* equals *B* or *A* is greater than *B*, then the scapula has assumed a position of relative downward rotation.

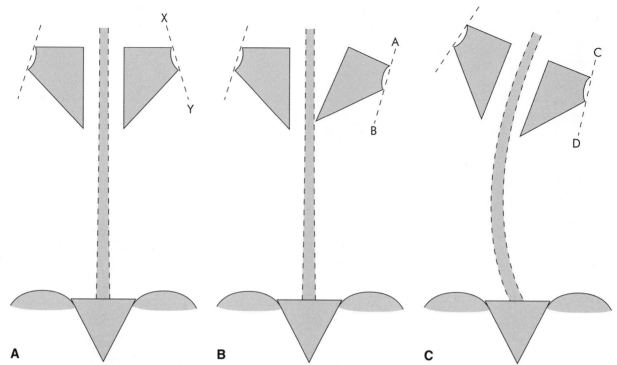

**Figure 10-21**    **A,** Scapular alignment with a straight spine (*xy* glenoid angle). **B,** Paresis with downward rotation of scapula (*AB* glenoid angle). **C,** Relative downward rotation of scapula with functional scoliosis (*CD* glenoid angle). (From Cailliet R: *The shoulder in hemiplegia,* Philadelphia, 1980, FA Davis.)

latissimus dorsi). Downward rotation also can be caused by unopposed muscle activity that depresses and downwardly rotates the scapula (i.e., rhomboids, levator scapulae, and latissimus dorsi) or by generalized weakness in the muscles that orient the scapula in a position of upward rotation (i.e., serratus anterior, upper and lower trapezius).

***Loss of Glenohumeral Joint Alignment.*** Thus far the loss of pelvic/trunk, rib cage, and scapula control have been reviewed. All of the aforementioned alignment changes have an effect on the stability and alignment of the glenohumeral joint. The mechanisms of glenohumeral joint subluxation remains controversial. As reviewed by Cailliet[26] and Basmajian,[5] the following factors assist in maintaining glenohumeral joint stability: the angle of the glenoid fossa when facing forward, upward, and outward; the support of the scapula on the rib cage; the seating of the humeral head in the fossa by the supraspinatus; possible support from the superior capsule; and contraction of the deltoid and cuff muscles when passive support is eliminated by slight abduction of the humerus.[26] Cailliet states that any change in these factors may play a role in causing subluxation (Figure 10-22). Basmajian's electromyographic studies[5] confirm that the supraspinatus prevents downward migration of the humeral head when a downward load is applied to the

upper extremity (e.g., when a person holds a briefcase). Authors previously believed that the deltoid performed this function, but the deltoid actually shows no activity during this function. The author points out that the supraspinatus is a horizontally positioned muscle that runs through the supraspinous fossa and can be effective only if the scapula is oriented correctly on the thorax.

The upward orientation of the glenoid fossa creates a "cradle" for the humeral head. As the humerus is pulled downward, it is forced to move laterally by the slope of the fossa.[5] The supraspinatus (and superior portion of the capsule) prevents this lateral movement and therefore downward migration. Basmajian[5] also points out that this mechanism is not effective if the humerus is abducted. This position predisposes patients to subluxation by eliminating the described mechanism. Many patients are positioned so that their humerus is abducted slightly because of the lateral trunk flexion toward the more affected side or as a result of passive positioning.

The relationship between scapula rotation and inferior subluxation has been challenged. Prevost et al[103] evaluated both shoulders of 50 stroke survivors with inferior subluxations using tridimensional x-ray. Results included the following:

- The affected and nonaffected shoulders were different in terms of the vertical position of the humerus vis-a-vis the scapula.

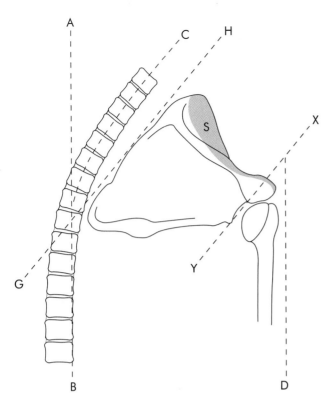

**Figure 10-22** Possible biomechanics of subluxation from malalignment. Line *AB* indicates an aligned spine (the goal of treatment). Instead the spine assumes a position of lateral flexion (curve *CB*). The scapula downwardly rotates (*GH*), resulting in a downward angulation of the glenoid fossa (*XY*). Because of the scapula position, the supraspinatus (*S*) loses its mechanical line of pull, making it ineffective and prone to overstretching. The final result is a subluxation of the glenohumeral joint. (Modified from Cailliet R: *Shoulder pain*, Philadelphia, 1990, FA Davis.)

- The orientation of the glenoid cavities was also different; the subluxed one faced less downward.
- The angle of abduction of the arm of the affected side was significantly greater than on the nonaffected side, but the relative abduction of the arm was on the same order of magnitude for both sides.
- No significant relationship existed between the orientation of the scapula and the severity of the subluxation.
- The abduction of the humerus was weakly ($r = 0.24$) related to the subluxation, which partly explained the weak association found between the relative abduction of the arm and the subluxation.

Overall, the authors concluded that the position of the scapula and the relative abduction of the arm cannot be considered important factors in the occurrence of inferior subluxation in hemiplegia.

Similarly, Culham, Noce, and Bagg[35] examined 17 subjects with high tone and 17 subjects with low tone based on the Ashworth Scale. Linear and angular measures of scapular and humeral orientation were calculated from tridimensional coordinates of bony landmarks collected using an electromagnetic device with subjects in a seated position with arms relaxed by their sides. Glenohumeral subluxation was measured from radiographs. They found the following:

- The scapula was farther from the midline and lower on the thorax on the affected side in the low-tone group.
- Glenohumeral subluxation was greater in the low-tone group.
- The scapular abduction angle was significantly greater on the nonaffected side in the low-tone group compared with the affected side in this group and with the nonaffected side in the high-tone group.
- In the high-tone group, no differences were found between the affected and nonaffected sides in the angular or linear measures.
- No significant correlation was found between scapular or humeral orientation and glenohumeral subluxation in either group.

Chaco and Wolf[31] confirmed that the supraspinatus did not respond to loading in the hemiplegic patients they studied. Although not immediate, subluxation did develop later in the study in the patients who remained flaccid. They inferred that the joint capsule holds the head of the humerus in relation to the glenoid foss, but unless the supraspinatus starts responding, it cannot prevent subluxation indefinitely. Therefore, subluxation appears to be caused by the weight of the arm and mechanical stretch to the joint capsule and traction to unresponsive shoulder musculature.

Ryerson and Levit[110,111] have described three patterns of subluxation in the glenohumeral joint. They emphasize that the therapist must assess trunk posture, determine the position of the scapula on the trunk, evaluate scapular mobility and rhythm, and examine the alignment and mobility of the glenohumeral joint before setting treatment goals for the shoulder. Table 10-3 reviews Ryerson and Levit's subluxation classifications, including inferior, anterior, and superior subluxations.

Hall, Dudgeon, and Guthrie[60] assessed the validity of three clinical measures (palpation, arm length discrepancy, and thermoplastic jig measurement) for evaluating shoulder subluxation in adults with hemiplegia resulting from a stroke. These measures were combined with anterior/posterior radiographic examinations of the hemiplegic shoulder; results indicated that palpation had the highest correlation with successful subluxation evaluation. In their technique for palpating subluxation, the patient is seated with the upper extremity unsupported at the side in neutral rotation; trunk stability was maintained during the evaluation. During palpation, the therapist measured subluxation by palpating the subacromial space (the distance between the acromion and the superior aspect of

**Table 10-3**

## Subluxation/Malalignment Patterns in the Upper Extremity After Stroke

| | TRUNK ALIGNMENT | SCAPULA ALIGNMENT | HUMERAL ALIGNMENT | DISTAL EXTREMITY ALIGNMENT | MOVEMENT AVAILABLE |
|---|---|---|---|---|---|
| Inferior subluxation | Lateral flexion to weak side | Downwardly rotated | Relative abduction and internal rotation; humeral head below inferior lip of fossa | Elbow extension and pronation | Scapula elevation and internal rotation |
| Anterior subluxation | Increased extension, lateral flaring, or rotation of rib cage | Downwardly rotated and elevated, winging | Hyperextension and internal rotation; humeral head inferior and forward relative to fossa | Elbow flexion and pronation or supination | Shoulder elevation, humeral internal rotation and hyperextension, and elbow flexion |
| Superior subluxation | Elements of flexion and extension; rib cage flaring | Elevated and abducted | Internal rotation and abduction; humeral head lodged under coracoid | Supination and wrist flexion | Shoulder elevation, abduction, and internal rotation; elbow/wrist flexion |

Data from Ryerson S, Levit K: Glenohumeral joint subluxations in CNS dysfunction, *NDTA Newsletter* Nov 1988; and Ryerson S, Levit K: The shoulder in hemiplegia. In Donatelli RA, editor: *Physical therapy of the shoulder*, ed 2, New York, 1991, Churchill Livingstone.

the humeral head) with the index and middle fingers. The authors concluded that their findings provided cautious optimism in terms of measuring and identifying subluxation. Prevost et al[104] also validated that palpation is a reliable measurement tool in the evaluation of subluxation. One should note that the evaluator should palpate both shoulders for comparison.

Hall, Dudgeon, and Guthrie[60] used a 0 (no subluxation) to 5 (2½ finger widths of subluxation) scale during their study. Bohannon and Andrews[10] used a three-point scale to demonstrate interrater reliability for measuring subluxation: none, 0; minimal, 1; and substantial, 2.

***Loss of Distal Alignment.*** Shoulder alignment problems directly effect the alignment and control of the distal extremity. Boehme[9] states that rotational movements of the forearm "occur at the proximal end with the radius rotating on a vertical axis . . . the ulnar head is displaced, . . . the mechanics are made possible by concurrent external rotation of the humerus." The typical alignment of the humerus after stroke is one of internal rotation, which blocks forearm rotation.

Kapandji[73] states that when the elbow is flexed (a typical posture), pronation is reduced to 45 degrees. Boehme[9] points out that when the wrist is bound by flexion and ulnar deviation (the typical posture of the CVA patient), control of forearm rotation also is blocked.

Wrist motion can become limited by virtue of its own alignment. The range of deviation is at its minimum when the wrist is in flexion and at its maximum when the wrist is in a neutral position or slight flexion. Flexion and extension ranges of the wrist are at a minimum when the hand has an ulnar deviation and at a maximum when the hand has a neutral deviation.[73]

A loss of palmar arches in the hand results in an inferior movement of the metacarpals followed by a distal hyperextension of the metacarpophalangeals and flexion of the proximal interphalangeal joints and distal interphalangeal joints, the typical claw-hand posture (see Chapter 12).

***Interdependence of Trunk and Limb Alignment.*** Anatomically, therapists must remember that only one bony attachment connects the entire limb to the axial skeleton, the sternoclavicular joint. (The scapulothoracic joint is not a true joint; the scapula rides on the thoracic cage and is maintained by muscular attachments only.) Therefore the clavicle serves as an anatomic link between the shoulder complex and trunk. This point should solidify the interdependence between the trunk and upper extremity. Any malalignments in the proximal segments have deleterious effects on the upper extremity (Figure 10-23).

The musculature acting on the shoulder has proximal points of attachment. A group of upper extremity muscles (the trapezius, rhomboids, serratus anterior, and levator scapulae) runs between the trunk and scapula, and another (the pectoralis and latissimus dorsi) runs between the trunk and humerus. Another group of muscles (the deltoid, rotator cuff, and coracobrachialis) attaches from

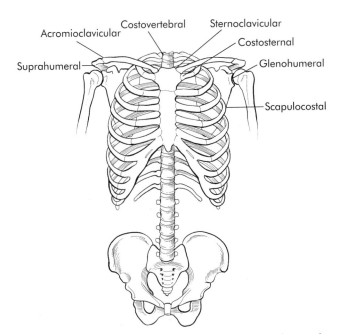

**Figure 10-23** Shoulder anatomy. Seven joints make up the shoulder complex. The sternoclavicular joint is the only bony attachment of the shoulder to the trunk, with the clavicle serving as a bridge between the trunk and shoulder. Skeletal alignment of the shoulder joint depends on trunk alignment and stability. For example, if the pelvis becomes malaligned (pelvic obliquity), the vertebral column, the rib cage, and other components lose their alignment (see Figure 10-19).

the humerus to the scapula. These attachments emphasize the interdependence of trunk alignment and extremity control.

Mohr[91] points out that biomechanical malalignment produces a pattern of movement that looks like stereotypical patterns used by patients with spasticity. For example, patients who gain early control of scapula elevation and humeral abduction continue to use this pattern and also flex the trunk, resulting in more elevation and abduction. As the scapula tips forward, it predisposes the humerus to internal rotation and extension because of its position in the fossa. The distal arm follows into elbow flexion, pronation, and wrist and digit flexion. The author points out that if a normal individual only activates the scapula elevators with humeral abductors, the resulting pattern looks similar to the patterns used by CVA patients.

These alignment problems need to be addressed before and throughout the treatment session. Therapists should correct them by mobilization techniques, positioning, and appropriate activity choices. The therapist needs to ensure alignment during ROM activities and maintain appropriate alignment during functional activities. For example, the alignment of the trunk and pelvis of patients who are

trying to feed themselves has a direct effect on the quality of the extremity movement pattern. Even in persons without a known neuropathologic condition, the quality of the eating activity clearly is compromised if they assume a forward flexed and laterally flexed static posture rather than an aligned and active trunk posture.

Ryerson and Levit[110] suggest patients perform activities that maintain enhanced trunk alignment and simultaneously coordinate movements of the scapula, trunk, and humerus.

## Shoulder Supports

Shoulder supports include any devices used to align, protect, or support an affected proximal limb. Shoulder supports include bed-positioning devices, adaptations to seating systems, and slings. The use of shoulder supports, especially slings, has been debated in the literature for at least 30 years.

Much of the debate is fueled by the variety of available slings, the controversy regarding their effectiveness, when and how they should be used, and whether they add to the already numerous complications resulting from an extremity affected by stroke.

Boyd and Gaylard[20] published the results of their survey of Canadian occupational therapists who prescribe slings. The respondents most frequently indicated that the goals of using a sling were to decrease and prevent subluxation and pain. The respondents frequently measured the effectiveness of their interventions by the level of resulting pain relief, subluxation assessments, and the amount of hand swelling. Less frequent measures of effectiveness included ROM, spasticity, and body awareness.

In light of the previously proposed cause of subluxation (see Loss of Biomechanical Alignment), Cailliet[26] suggests that if the goal of treatment is to provide glenohumeral joint stability, then the device must support the scapula on the rib cage with the glenoid fossa facing upward, forward, and outward and must compensate for a lack of support by the rotator cuff and possibly the superior capsule. At this point, no slings are available on the market that assist in realigning the scapula on the rib cage. Therefore, slings cannot be prescribed to "reduce a subluxation." They may lift the head of the humerus to the level of the glenoid fossa, but the scapular and trunk alignments (the key to correcting shoulder malalignment) remain impaired. This reduction may be seen as treating a symptom of a larger problem. The therapist must realize that they may find cases in which treating this symptom is appropriate. Analysis is critical for determining which goals certain interventions are achieving. Palpating the subluxation before and after the sling is donned is not sufficient. The therapist must evaluate the effect (if any) of the sling on the more proximal segments.

In their review of the literature, Smith and Okamoto[117] identified desirable and undesirable features of slings. Proper positioning of the humeral head in addition to humeral abduction, external rotation, and elbow extension are cited as desirable positions as opposed to humeral adduction, internal rotation, and elbow flexion. The latter positions typically cause problems in the maintenance of tissue length in the stroke population. The sling also should permit the impaired extremity to provide postural support when the patient is seated and should allow self-ROM. In terms of positioning, the sling should provide neutral wrist support, unobstructed hand function, finger abduction, and scapula protraction and elevation.

Smith and Okamoto[117] emphasize that if a therapist expects compliance with sling use, comfort, cosmetic appeal, and easy donning and doffing are crucial. The authors published a checklist to assist therapists in analyzing the slings they provide.

The percentage of therapists using slings has been reported to be as high as 94%,[20] despite the fact no definitive studies support or reject the use of slings.

Several studies have compared and contrasted the effectiveness of various supports. Zorowitz et al[141] compared the following four supports:

1. The single-strap hemisling: The strap has two cuffs that support the elbow and wrist. The arm is held in a position of adduction, internal rotation, and elbow flexion.
2. The Bobath roll: This strap includes a foam roll that is placed in the affected axilla beneath the proximal humerus. The shoulder is maintained in a position of abduction and external rotation with elbow extension.
3. The Rolyan humeral cuff sling: This figure-eight strap system has an arm cuff that is sized to fit distally on the humerus of the affected arm. The shoulder is positioned in slight external rotation.
4. The Cavalier shoulder support: This type of support provides bilateral axillary support and consists of bilateral straps that are positioned along the humeral head and integrated posteriorly into a brace that rests between the scapula.

In this study, 20 patients were evaluated in the listed supports with anteroposterior shoulder radiography. The authors evaluated the vertical, horizontal, and total asymmetries of glenohumeral joint subluxation compared with the opposite shoulder. In terms of vertical asymmetry, the single-strap hemisling corrected the vertical displacement, the Cavalier support did not alter vertical displacement, and the remaining supports significantly reduced but did not correct vertical displacement.

Although as a group, the subjects had no significant horizontal asymmetry when no supports were used, the Bobath roll and the Cavalier support produced a signifi-

cant lateral displacement of the humeral head of the more affected shoulder. This fact is of interest because one proposed goal of a sling is to decrease or prevent subluxation; this study demonstrated that equipment that is not well researched actually may cause shoulder asymmetry in patients who previously had none.

In terms of total asymmetry, the Rolyan humeral cuff sling was the only support that significantly decreased (although it did not eliminate) total subluxation asymmetry.

Moodie, Brisbin, and Grace Morgan[92] evaluated the effectiveness of five shoulder supports: the Bobath roll, an acrylic plastic lap tray on a wheelchair, a wheelchair-mounted arm trough, a conventional triangular sling (which is much like an arm cast support), and the Hook Hemi Harness (which has two adjustable shoulder cuffs with a suspension strap that are tightened while the affected arm is lifted, resulting in shoulders of equal height). Anteroposterior radiographs of 10 subjects demonstrated that the conventional sling, lap tray, and arm trough were effective in decreasing the width of the glenohumeral space to normal. The Bobath roll and the Hook Hemi Harness were not effective in reducing the subluxation. The authors pointed out that although the conventional sling decreased the subluxation, it reinforced the flexor pattern found in the upper extremity.

Brook et al[23] compared the effects of three supports: the Bobath sling, an arm trough/lap board, and the Harris hemisling (which has two straps and cuffs that cradle the elbow and wrist, holding the arm in a position of adduction, internal rotation, and elbow flexion). The Harris hemisling resulted in good vertical correction; in comparison the Bobath sling did not correct the subluxation as well, the arm trough/lap board was less effective and tended to overcorrect, and the Bobath sling tended to distract the joint horizontally.

An important note is that none of the mentioned studies discussed scapular or trunk alignment; they only addressed the glenohumeral joint.

Hurd, Farrell, and Waylonis[66] alternately placed 14 patients into a control group (which used no sling) or treatment group (which used a sling). These patients were treated identically in all other respects. The patients were evaluated initially and again 2 to 3 weeks later and 3 to 7 months later. No appreciable difference in shoulder ROM, shoulder pain, or subluxation was found between the treated or control groups. No evidence of increased incidence of peripheral nerve or plexus injury was noted in the control group. The authors concluded that the hemisling does not need to be used uniformly by all patients with a flaccid limb after a CVA. They suggested that a sling might be useful when used with discrimination but did not elaborate on this point.

Some authors have suggested that slings be prescribed to prevent overstretching of soft tissue. Chaco and Wolf[31] suggested that permanent subluxation of the gleno-humeral joint could be prevented by avoiding loading on the joint when the limb is flaccid. They concluded that the joint capsule holds the head of the humerus in relation to the fossa when the supraspinatus is not responding but cannot prevent subluxation for an unlimited time unless the cuff responds.

If the joint capsule is prevented from stretching during the stage in which the limb is flaccid, patients may have a better opportunity to develop adequate muscle function to maintain joint alignment. Kaplan et al[74] suggest using a sling during the flaccid stage to prevent distraction of the joint resulting in a possible brachial plexus injury.

Some therapists have suggested that sling use may increase body neglect and interfere with body image, although this hypothesis has not been researched. Although they have not been specifically related to sling use, the learned nonuse studies of Taub, Uswatte, and Pidikiti[119] may influence therapists' decisions about whether to prescribe a sling, especially for a patient in the acute phase.

Zorowitz[141] states that "although supports are commonly used during the rehabilitation of stroke survivors, there is no absolute evidence that supports prevent or reduce long-term shoulder subluxation when spontaneous recovery of motor function occurs, or that a support will prevent supposed complications of shoulder subluxation. Without proper training in the use of a support, stroke survivors may face potential complications such as pain and contracture." Although the literature does not give definitive answers about when or whether to use slings, one can infer the following guidelines:

- Therapists should minimize sling use during the rehabilitation process.
- Slings may be useful for supporting the more affected extremity during initial transfer and gait training.
- Slings that position the extremity in a flexor pattern should never be worn unless the patient is in an upright posture; in these cases, they should be worn only for select activities (initial mobility training) and short time frames. This type of sling should never be worn by patients in recumbent postures.
- Therapists must evaluate each patient's clinical picture. Therapists need to weigh the pros and cons of slings and clarify the goal of sling use (Box 10-12). Following prescription of the sling, the therapist must reevaluate the effectiveness of the sling (i.e., determine whether the sling truly is meeting the predetermined goal).
- Therapists must become familiar with a variety of slings. One particular sling will not meet the needs of every patient (Figure 10-24).
- Therapists should continue to investigate the use of alternative means to support the more affected extremity during activities performed in the upright position, such as putting the hand in a pocket, receiving support from an over-the-shoulder bag, adding scapular taping

## Box 10-12

### Considerations When Prescribing a Sling

**PROS**

- Protects patient from injury during transfers.
- Allows therapist freedom to control trunk and lower extremities during initial gait, transfer, and upright function training.
- May prevent soft tissue stretching (e.g., supraspinatus and capsular stretching).
- Prevents prolonged dangling of extremity.
- May relieve pressure on neurovascular bundle (brachial plexus/brachial artery).
- Supports weight of arm.

**CONS**

- May contribute to neglect of body scheme disorders.
- May contribute to learned nonuse.
- May hold upper extremity in a shortened position (e.g., internal rotators, adductors, and elbow flexors).
- Fosters dependence on passive positioning.
- May initiate shoulder-hand syndrome development (i.e., immobility leading to swelling, shortening, and pain)
- May predispose patient to shoulder pain from shortened internal rotators.
- Does not reduce the amount of subluxation because the alignment of the scapula and trunk are not affected.
- Approximates head of humerus to malaligned scapula.
- Prevents reciprocal arm swing while walking.
- Prevents arm function (e.g., postural support and carrying) in upright postures.
- Blocks sensory input.
- Prevents balance reactions of the upper extremity.
- May block spontaneous use of the upper extremity.
- Places no motor demands on the upper extremity.

protocols to present treatment plans, or using functional electrical stimulation (Figure 10-25).

One may infer from the literature that the most effective way to reduce the level of subluxation is to provide the patient with activities that enhance trunk and scapula alignment, activate the rotator cuff, and enhance functional use of the extremity during weight-bearing and reach patterns.

## GENERAL TREATMENT PRINCIPLES

Therapists should consider the following treatment principles:

- Maintain a client-centered approach to the treatment of upper extremity dysfunction.
- Evaluate and plan treatments that focus on improving occupational performance.
- Focus treatment on task-specific training.

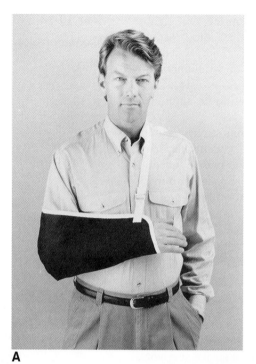

**A**

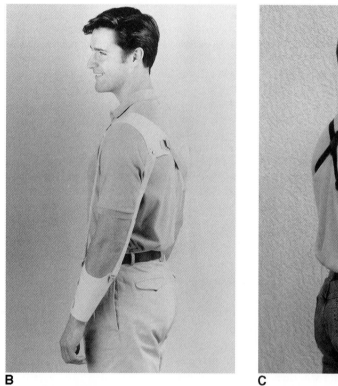

**B**

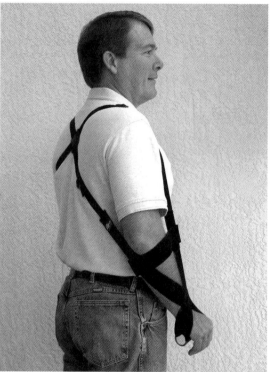

**C**

**Figure 10-24**    **A,** Pouch sling. Sling is only to be used for short periods with patients in upright postures and frees therapist's hands to control trunk and lower extremities. This sling may be appropriate for initial phases of walking, transfer, and upright function training. **B,** Shoulder saddle sling. Sling supports distal weight of extremity and can be worn under clothing. This style of sling can be worn all day because it does not block distal function or hold extremity in a flexor pattern. **C,** The GivMohr Sling (www.givmohrsling.com, 505-292-1144). (**A** and **B** courtesy of Sammons Preston Rolyan, Inc, Bolingbrook, Ill.)

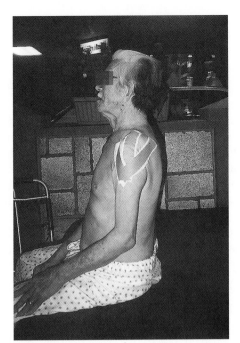

**Figure 10-25** Taping is being used more commonly to treat shoulder instability. Further research is required to determine its effectiveness.

■ Maintain mobility (upward rotation and protraction) of the scapula and humeral external rotation to prevent pain syndromes and prepare for return of function.

■ Maintain soft tissue length and joint mobility in the trunk, head and neck, and more affected upper extremity.

■ Provide appropriate positioning strategies for times when patients are not involved in activities and are in recumbent postures.

■ Provide opportunities for patients to use the upper extremity outside of structured therapy time.

■ Train all caregivers (staff and family) in the appropriate handling of the more affected upper extremity during ADL and mobility.

■ Evaluate and treat any pain syndrome immediately and consistently until symptoms are alleviated.

■ Guide appropriate usage of available motor control by providing functional activities that correspond to the patient's level of recovery. Discourage participation in activities that require extra effort.

■ Grade activities systematically and with control to increase level of control and functional use.

■ Prevent learned nonuse by incorporating the upper extremity into daily life immediately after the stroke.

■ Encourage patients to take responsibility for the protection, maintenance, and improvement of their more affected upper extremity.

## Case Study

### UPPER EXTREMITY FUNCTION AFTER STROKE

J.C. is a 60-year-old male who suffered a right middle cerebral artery cerebrovascular accident 1 week before referral. J.C. was in his usual state of good health until he experienced a sudden onset of left-sided weakness. Before this incident, J.C. had just sold his antique store to enjoy retirement. J.C. lives alone, and his interests include reading, gardening, watching movies, wine tasting, and restoring furniture. J.C.'s evaluation and occupational therapy treatment plan (focusing on improved upper extremity function for this study) were as follows.

### INITIAL EVALUATION

J.C. was alert and oriented, followed complex commands, had no evidence of cognitive-perceptual deficits with the exception of questionable difficulty with activities incorporating spatial relations components, and had intact sensation. His resting sitting posture consisted of a posteriorly tilted pelvis with minimal functional kyphosis, increased weight bearing on the left ischial tuberosity, right trunk shortening, and a posteriorly rotated left rib cage. J.C. required minimal assistance with postural adjustments while performing reaching tasks with the right upper extremity. At rest, his left scapula was rotated downward and had minimal winging. The left glenohumeral joint had an anterior-inferior subluxation.

When asked to demonstrate any arm function, J.C. attempted to lift his arm against gravity with a resulting pattern of active lateral trunk flexion to the right, active scapula retraction and elevation, and active humeral abduction; during this attempted movement, the distal extremity fell passively into gravity with a resulting pattern of humeral internal rotation, pronation, and wrist flexion.

Passive range of motion was within normal limits after the scapula was mobilized and gliding with the exception of lacking 20 degrees of external rotation. No evidence of spasticity was found on quick stretch. J.C.'s muscle grades were grossly 2 out of 5; scapula and humerus (except external rotation), 0 out of 5; elbow, 3 out of 5; forearm, 2 out of 5; wrist, 1 out of 5; finger flexion, 3+ of 5; finger extension, 2 out of 5; and finger abduction/adduction, 1 out of 5. J.C. did not have selective control of his extremity; instead he moved in gross patterns. He was not able to incorporate his left upper extremity into his activities of daily living on initial evaluation. Limitations to J.C.'s ability to use his upper extremity were identified as inefficient

**UPPER EXTREMITY FUNCTION AFTER STROKE—cont'd**

movement patterns ("stereotypical") as a result of loss of postural control, weakness, and trunk and upper extremity malalignments.

## WEEK 1 GOALS AND TREATMENTS

Treatment goals for the first week were as follows:
1. Roll independently while protecting the left upper extremity.
2. Stretch independently (using the towel-on-table program).
3. Independently position the left upper extremity on a table while eating and performing leisure activities.
4. Independently relieve pressure by lateral weight shifting in the wheelchair. (J.C. was instructed to perform this in front of the dining table with both forearms supported on the table.)

At this stage, J.C. also was provided with a half swing-away lap tray and bed positioning items, including a pillow for under his left scapula and left elbow.

Treatment focused on left upper extremity protection during transitional movements and reaching activities using the right upper extremity in all directions, with a focus on trunk responses and inclusion of rotational activities to recruit abdominal muscle activity. Activities such as repotting plants were used because they required a variety of reach patterns and were previously enjoyed by J.C. At this point the left upper extremity was used to stabilize objects (e.g., the bag of soil).

J.C. was given a polystyrene plastic cup and asked to support his forearm on his lap tray, place the cup upside down into his left hand, and practice releasing it. As the task became easier, he turned the cup right side up to increase the difficulty level. During therapy, treatment focused on controlling the distal arm from the mouth to the table (eccentrically) with his elbow supported on the table and the therapist supporting the humerus with J.C.'s hand empty.

## WEEKS 2 AND 3 GOALS AND TREATMENTS

Treatment goals for the second and third weeks were as follows:
1. Independently hold a toothpaste tube in the left hand while unscrewing the cap with the right hand.
2. Lift the arm from the lap to the lap tray without the right upper extremity assisting.

3. Independently stretch the left wrist and digits into extension.

At this stage, J.C. progressed to assuming standing postures in front of a work surface. Activities included buffing tables and sliding papers across the table past arm's length with the left upper extremity to encourage scapula protraction. Wiping the table (hand-over-hand) and focusing on patterns to the far left were used to maintain soft tissue length and encourage external rotation. As the task became easier, J.C. held the towel in his left hand and wiped the table using only his left upper extremity.

## WEEKS 3 AND 4 GOALS AND TREATMENTS

Treatment goals for the third, fourth, and fifth weeks were as follows:
1. Locking wheelchair brakes independently with the left upper extremity.
2. Use both upper extremities to pull pants up from midthigh to waist while standing with close supervision.
3. Independently support the left upper extremity in the pants pocket while walking.

Week 4 (the final week of inpatient treatment) goals and treatment activities included the following:
1. Independently opening a kitchen drawer with the left upper extremity while standing.
2. Holding an over-the-shoulder bag with the left upper extremity while walking.
3. Using both hands to don a sock.
4. Turning sink faucets on and off with the left upper extremity while standing.

The goals and treatment activities were not considered different entities. Treatment was task and goal specific.

When discharged from inpatient rehabilitation, J.C. was able to use his left upper extremity as a postural support during forearm and extended arm weight-bearing activities, integrate use of his left upper extremity during self-care activities (but limited to movement patterns below chest level [e.g., in lap activities and reaching below the hips]), integrate use of his left hand into fine motor activities, and carry items in his left hand while walking. Movement patterns that required further antigravity shoulder patterns, increased hand control, and strengthening with resistance were the focus of outpatient occupational therapy.

# REVIEW QUESTIONS

1. Which factors contribute to glenohumeral joint subluxation?
2. Which factors contribute to a painful shoulder condition after a stroke?
3. In what way does biomechanical malalignment of the trunk and upper extremity contribute to ineffective and inefficient movement patterns?
4. Describe the learned nonuse phenomenon and treatments aimed at its prevention or reversal.
5. Which factors contribute to a malaligned scapula?
6. Describe a treatment progression aimed at increasing manipulation patterns.

## REFERENCES

1. Ada L, Canning CG, Call JH, et al: Task-specific training of reaching and manipulation. In Bennett KMB, Castiello U, editors: *Insights into the reach to grasp movements*, Amsterdam, 1994, Elsevier Science.
2. Arsenault AB, Bilodeau M, Dutil E, et al: Clinical significance of the V-shaped space in the subluxed shoulder of hemiplegics, *Stroke* 22(7):867-871, 1991.
3. Ashworth B: Carisoprodol in multiple sclerosis, *Practitioner* 192:540, 1964.
4. Bakheit AM, Thilman AF, Ward AB, et al: A randomized, double blind, placebo-controlled study of the efficacy and safety of botulinum toxin type A in upper limb spasticity in patients with stroke, *Eur J Neurol* 8:559, 2001.
5. Basmajian JV: The surgical anatomy and function of the arm-trunk mechanism, *Surg Clin North Am* 43:1471, 1963.
6. Bear-Lehman J, Bassile CC, Gillen G: A comparison of time-use on an acute rehabilitation unit: subjects with and without stroke, *Phys Occup Ther Geriatr* 20:17, 2001.
7. Belenkii VY, Gurfinkle VS, Paltsev YI: Elements of control of voluntary movements, *Biophysics* 12:135, 1967.
8. Bobath B: *Adult hemiplegia: evaluation and treatment*, ed 3, Oxford, 1990, Butterworth-Heinemann.
9. Boehme R: *Improving upper body control: an approach to assessment and treatment of tonal dysfunction*, Tucson, 1988, Therapy Skill Builders.
10. Bohannon RW, Andrews AW: Shoulder subluxation and pain in stroke patients, *Am J Occup Ther* 44(6):507-509, 1990.
11. Bohannon RW, Larkin PA, Smith MB, et al: Relationship between static muscle strength deficits and spasticity in stroke patients with hemiparesis, *Phys Ther* 67(7):1068-1071, 1987.
12. Bohannon RW, Larkin PA, Smith MB, et al: Shoulder pain in hemiplegia: a statistical relationship with five variables, *Arch Phys Med Rehabil* 67(8):514-516, 1986.
13. Bohannon RW, Smith MB: Assessment of strength deficits in eight paretic upper extremity muscle groups of stroke patients with hemiplegia, *Phys Ther* 67(4):552-555, 1987.
14. Bohannon RW, Smith MB: Interrater reliability of a modified Ashworth scale of muscle spasticity, *Phys Ther* 67(2):206-207, 1987.
15. Booth FW: Physiologic and biochemical effects of immobilization on muscle, *Clin Orthop* 219:15-20, 1987.
16. Botte MJ, Nickel VL, Akeson WH: Spasticity and contracture: physiologic aspects of formation, *Clin Orthop* 233:7-18, 1988.
17. Bouisset S, Zattara M: A sequence of postural movements precedes voluntary movement, *Neurosci Lett* 22:263, 1981.
18. Bourbonnais D, Vanden Noven S: Weakness in patients with hemiparesis, *Am J Occup Ther* 43(5):313-319, 1989.
19. Bourbonnais D, Vanden Noven S, Carey KM, et al: Abnormal spatial patterns of elbow muscle activation in hemiparetic human subjects, *Brain* 112(pt 1):85-102, 1989.
20. Boyd E, Gaylard A: Shoulder supports with stroke patients: a Canadian survey, *Can J Occup Ther* 53:61, 1986.
21. Braus DF, Krauss JK, Strobel JS: The shoulder-hand syndrome after stroke: a prospective clinical trial, *Ann Neurol* 36(5):728-733, 1994.
22. Brodal A: Self-observations and neuro-anatomical considerations after a stroke, *Brain* 96(4):675-694, 1973.
23. Brooke MM, de Lateur BJ, Diana-Rigby GC, et al: Shoulder subluxation in hemiplegia: effects of three different supports, *Arch Phys Med Rehabil* 72(8):582-586, 1991.
24. Brouwer BJ, Ambury P: Upper extremity weightbearing effect on corticospinal excitability following stroke, *Arch Phys Med Rehabil* 75(8):861-866, 1994.
25. Burgess MK: Motor control and the role of occupational therapy: past, present, and the future, *Am J Occup Ther* 43:345, 1989.
26. Cailliet R: *The shoulder in hemiplegia*, Philadelphia, 1980, FA Davis.
27. Carr EK, Kenney FD: Positioning of the stroke patients: a review of the literature, *Int J Nurs Stud* 29(4):355-369, 1992.
28. Carr JH, Shepherd RB: *A motor relearning programme for stroke*, ed 2, Rockville, Md, 1982, Aspen.
29. Carr JH, Shepherd RB, Ada L: Spasticity: research findings and implications for intervention, *Physiotherapy* 81:421, 1995.
30. Carr JH, Shepherd RB, Nordholm L, et al: Investigation of a new motor assessment scale for stroke patients, *Phys Ther* 65(2): 175-180, 1985.
31. Chaco J, Wolf E: Subluxation of the glenohumeral joint in hemiplegia, *Am J Phys Med* 50(3):139-143, 1971.
32. Chu DS, Petrillo C, Davis SW, et al: Shoulder-hand syndrome: importance of early diagnosis and treatment, *J Am Geriatr Soc* 29(2):58-60, 1981.
33. Cordo PJ, Nashner LM: Properties of postural adjustments associated with rapid arm movements, *J Neurophysiol* 47(2):287-302, 1982.
34. Crow L, Lincoln NB, Nouri FM, et al: The effectiveness of EMG biofeedback in the treatment of arm function after stroke, *Int Disabil Stud* 11(4):155-160, 1989.
35. Culham EG, Noce RR, Bagg SD: Shoulder complex position and glenohumeral subluxation in hemiplegia, *Arch Phys Med Rehabil* 76(9):857-864, 1995.
36. Davies PM: *Steps to follow: the comprehensive treatment of patients with hemiplegia*, New York, 2000, Springer-Verlag.
37. Daviet JC, Preux PM, Salle JY, et al: Clinical factors in the prognosis of complex regional pain syndrome type I after stroke, *Am J Phys Med Rehabil* 81(1):34-39, 2002.
38. Davis J: The role of the occupational therapist in the treatment of shoulder-hand syndrome, *Occup Ther Pract* 1:30, 1990.
39. Davis SW, Petrillo CR, Eichberg RD, et al: Shoulder-hand syndrome in a hemiplegic population: a five year retrospective study, *Arch Phys Med Rehabil* 58(8):353-356, 1977.
40. Dietz V, Quintern J, Berger W: Electrophysiological studies of gait in spasticity and rigidity: evidence that altered mechanical properties of muscle contribute to hypertonia, *Brain* 104(3): 431-449, 1981.
41. Dromerick A: Evidence-based rehabilitation: the case for and against constraint-induced movement therapy, *J Rehabil Res Dev* 40(1):vii-ix, 2003.
42. Dromerick A, Edwards DF, Hahn M: Does the application of constraint-induced movement therapy during acute rehabilitation reduce arm impairment after ischemic stroke? *Stroke* 31(12):2984-2988, 2000.
43. Engardt M, Knutsson E, Jonsson M, et al: Dynamic muscle strength training in stroke patients: effects on knee extension

torque, electromyographic activity, and motor function, *Arch Phys Med Rehabil* 76(5):419-425, 1995.

44. Exner CE: In-hand manipulation skills. In Case-Smith J, Pehoski C, editors: *Development of hand skills in the child*, Rockville, Md, 1992, American Occupational Therapy Association.

45. Fellows SJ, Kaus C, Thilmann AF: Voluntary movement at the elbow in spastic hemiparesis, *Ann Neurol* 36(3):397-407, 1994.

46. Fisher AG: *Assessment of motor and process skills*, ed 4, Fort Collins, Colo, 2001, Three Star Press.

47. Fisher AG: The assessment of IADL motor skills: an application of many-faceted Rasch analysis, *Am J Occup Ther* 47(4):319-329, 1993.

48. Flinn N: A task-oriented approach to the treatment of a client with hemiplegia, *Am J Occup Ther* 49(6):560-569, 1995.

49. Fugl-Meyer AR, Jaasko L, Leyman I, et al: The post stroke hemiplegic patient: a method for evaluation of physical performance, *Scand J Rehabil Med* 7(1):13-31, 1975.

50. Ghez C: Posture. In Kandel ER, Schwartz JH, Jessell TM, editors: *Principles of neural science*, ed 3, New York, 1991, Elsevier.

51. Ghez C: Voluntary movements. In Kandel ER, Schwartz JH, Jessell TM, editors: *Principles of neural science*, ed 3, New York, 1991, Elsevier.

52. Glenn MB, Whyte J: *The practical management of spasticity in children and adults*, Philadelphia, 1990, Lea & Febiger.

53. Gillen G: Improving mobility and community access in an adult with ataxia: a case study, *Am J Occup Ther* 56(4):462-466, 2002.

54. Gillen G: Improving activities of daily living performance in an adult with ataxia, *Am J Occup Ther* 54(1):89-96, 2000.

55. Gillen G: Managing abnormal tone after brain injury, *Occup Ther Pract* Sept 1998, pp 18-24.

56. Gowland C, deBruin H, Basmajian JV, et al: Agonist and antagonist activity during voluntary upper-limb movement in patients with stroke, *Phys Ther* 72(9):624-633, 1992.

57. Greenberg S, Fowler RS: Kinesthetic biofeedback: a treatment modality for elbow range of motion in hemiplegia, *Am J Occup Ther* 34(11):738-743, 1980.

58. Hakuno A, Sashika H, Ohkawa T, et al: Arthrographic findings in hemiplegic shoulders, *Arch Phys Med Rehabil* 65(11):706-711, 1984.

59. Halar EM, Bell KR: Contracture and other deleterious effects of immobility. In DeLisa JB, editor: *Rehabilitation medicine: principles and practice*, Philadelphia, 1993, JB Lippincott.

60. Hall J, Dudgeon B, Guthrie M: Validity of clinical measures of shoulder subluxation in adults with poststroke hemiplegia, *Am J Occup Ther* 49(6):526-533, 1995.

61. Hecht JS: Subscapular nerve block in the painful hemiplegic shoulder, *Arch Phys Med Rehabil* 73(11):1036-1039, 1992.

62. Heller A, Wade D, Wood V, et al: Arm functions after stroke: measurement and recovery over the first three months, *J Neurol Neurosurg Psychiatry* 50(6):714-719, 1987.

63. Horak FB, Esselman P, Anderson ME, et al: The effects of movement velocity, mass displaced, and task certainty on associated postural adjustments made by normal and hemiplegic individuals, *J Neurol Neurosurg Psychiatry* 47(9):1020-1028, 1984.

64. Hufschmidt A, Mauritz KH: Chronic transformation of muscle in spasticity: a peripheral contribution to increased tone, *J Neurol Neurosurg Psychiatry* 48(7):676-685, 1985.

65. Hummelsheim H, Munch B, Butefisch C, et al: Influence of sustained stretch on late muscular responses to magnetic brain stimulation in patients with upper motor neuron lesions, *Scand J Rehabil Med* 26(1):3-9, 1994.

66. Hurd MM, Farrell KH, Waylonis GW: Shoulder sling for hemiplegia: friend or foe? *Arch Phys Med Rehabil* 55(11):519-522, 1974.

67. Ikai T, Tei K, Yoshida K, et al: Evaluation and treatment of shoulder subluxation in hemiplegia: relationship between subluxation and pain, *Am J Phys Med Rehabil* 77(5):421-426, 1998.

68. Jeannerod M: The formation of finger grip during prehension: a cortically mediated visuomotor pattern, *Behav Brain Res* 19(2):99-116, 1986.

69. Jeannerod M: The timing of natural prehension movements, *J Motor Behav* 16:235, 1984.

70. Jebsen RH, Taylor N, Trieschmann RB, et al: An objective and standardized test of hand function, *Arch Phys Med Rehabil* 50(6):311-319, 1969.

71. Jensen EM: The hemiplegic shoulder, *Scand J Rehabil Med* 7(suppl):113-119, 1980.

72. Joynt RL: The source of shoulder pain in hemiplegia, *Arch Phys Med Rehabil* 73(5):409-413, 1992.

73. Kapandji IA: *The physiology of the joints*, vol 1, *The upper limb*, New York, 1982, Churchill Livingstone.

74. Kaplan PE, Meridith J, Taft G, et al: Stroke and brachial plexus injury: a difficult problem, *Arch Phys Med Rehabil* 58(9):415-418, 1977.

75. Kopp B, Kunkel A, Flor H, et al: The arm motor ability test: reliability, validity, and sensitivity to change of an instrument for assessing disabilities in activities of daily living, *Arch Phys Med Rehabil* 78(6):615-620, 1997.

76. Kumar R, Metter EJ, Mehta AJ, et al: Shoulder pain in hemiplegia: the role of exercise, *Am J Phys Med Rehabil* 69(4):205-208, 1990.

77. Lankford LL: Reflex sympathetic dystrophy. In Hunter JM, Schneider L, Mackin E, et al, editors: *Rehabilitation of the hand: surgery and therapy*, ed 3, St Louis, 1990, Mosby.

78. Landau WM: Spasticity: what is it? what is it not? In Feldman RG, Young RR, Koella WP, editors: *Spasticity: disordered motor control*, Chicago, 1980, Year Book.

79. Landau WM: Spasticity: the fable of a neurological demon and the emperor's new therapy, *Arch Neurol* 31:217, 1974.

80. Lee WA: A control systems framework for understanding normal and abnormal posture, *Am J Occup Ther* 43(5):291-301, 1989.

81. Liepert J, Bauder H, Wolfgang HR, et al: Treatment-induced cortical reorganization after stroke in humans, *Stroke* 31(6):1210-1216, 2000.

82. Lin K: Enhancing occupational performance through occupationally embedded exercise: a meta-analysis, *Occup Ther J Res* 17:25, 1997.

83. Little JW, Massagli TL: Spasticity and associated abnormalities of muscle tone. In DeLisa JA, editor: *Rehabilitation medicine: principles and practice*, ed 2, Philadelphia, 1993, JB Lippincott.

84. Lyle R: A performance test for assessment of upper limb function in physical rehabilitation treatment and research, *Int J Rehabil Res* 4(4):483-492, 1981.

85. Marsden CD, Merton PA, Morton HB: Human postural responses, *Brain* 104(3):513-534, 1981.

86. Massion J: Postural changes accompanying voluntary movements: normal and pathological aspects, *Hum Neurobiol* 2(4):261-267, 1984.

87. Mathiowetz V, Bass-Haugen J: Motor behavior research: implications for therapeutic approaches to central nervous system dysfunction, *Am J Occup Ther* 48(8):733-745, 1994.

88. McIllroy WE, Maki BE: Early activation of arm muscles follows external perturbation of upright stance, *Neurosci Lett* 148(3):177-180, 1995.

89. Merideth J, Taft G, Kaplan P: Diagnosis and treatment of the hemiplegic patient with brachial plexus injury, *Am J Occup Ther* 35(10):656-660, 1981.

90. Meyer AZ: The philosophy of occupational therapy, *Am J Occup Ther* 31(10):639-642, 1977.

91. Mohr JD: Management of the trunk in adult hemiplegia: the Bobath concept, *Top Neurol* 1990, pp 1-12.

92. Moodie NB, Brisbin J, Grace Morgan AM: Subluxation of the glenohumeral joint in hemiplegia: evaluation of supportive devices, *Physiother Can* 38:151, 1986.

93. Moskowitz E, Porter JI: Peripheral nerve lesions in the upper extremity in the hemiplegic patient, *New Engl J Med* 269:776, 1963.

94. Najenson T, Yacubovic E, Pikielni SS: Rotator cuff injury in shoulder joints of hemiplegic patients, *Scand J Rehabil Med* 3(3):131-137, 1971.

95. Nakayama H, Jorgensen HS, Raaschou HO, et al: Recovery of upper extremity function in stroke patients: the Copenhagen stroke study, *Arch Phys Med Rehabil* 75(4):394-398, 1994.

96. Neistadt ME: The effect of different treatment activities on functional fine motor coordination in adults with brain injury, *Am J Occup Ther* 48:877, 1994.

97. Nepomuceno CS, Miller JM: Shoulder arthrography in hemiplegic patients, *Arch Phys Med Rehabil* 55(2):49-51, 1974.

98. Page SJ: Imagery improves upper extremity motor function in chronic stroke patients: a pilot study, *Occup Ther J Res* 20:201, 2000.

99. Page SJ, Sisto SA, Levine P, et al: Modified constraint induced therapy: a randomized feasibility and efficacy study, *J Rehabil Res Dev* 38(5):583-590, 2001.

100. Perry J: Rehabilitation of spasticity. In Feldman RG, Young RR, Koella WP, editors: *Spasticity: disordered motor control*, Chicago, 1980, Year Book.

101. Petchkrua W, Weiss DJ, Patel RR: Reassessment of the incidence of complex regional pain syndrome type 1 following stroke, *Neurorehabil Neural Repair* 14(1):59-63, 2000.

102. Preston LA, Hecht JS: *Spasticity management: rehabilitation strategies*, Bethesda, Md, 1999, American Occupational Therapy Association.

103. Prevost R, Arsenault AB, Drouin G, et al: Rotation of the scapula and shoulder subluxation in hemiplegia, *Arch Phys Med Rehabil* 68(11):786-790, 1987.

104. Prevost R, Arsenault AB, Drouin G, et al: Shoulder subluxation in hemiplegia: a radiologic correlational study, *Arch Phys Med Rehabil* 68(11):782-785, 1987.

105. Price CIM, Pandyan AD: Electrical stimulation for preventing and treating post-stroke shoulder pain (Cochrane review). In *The Cochrane Library Issue 3*, Oxford, 2002, Update Software.

106. Rizk TE, Christopher RP, Pinals RS, et al: Arthrographic studies in painful hemiplegic shoulders, *Arch Phys Med Rehabil* 65(5):254-256, 1984.

107. Rosenbaum DR, Jorgensen MJ: Planning macroscopic aspects of manual control, *Hum Mov Sci* 11:61, 1992.

108. Rousseaux M, Kozlowski O, Froger J: Efficacy of botulinum toxin A in upper limb function of hemiplegic patients, *J Neurol* 249(1):76-84, 2002.

109. Roy CW, Sands MR, Hill LD: Shoulder pain in acutely admitted hemiplegics, *Clin Rehabil* 8:334, 1994.

110. Ryerson S, Levit K: The shoulder in hemiplegia. In Donatelli RA, editor: *Physical therapy of the shoulder*, ed 2, New York, 1991, Churchill Livingstone.

111. Ryerson S, Levit K: Glenohumeral joint subluxations in CNS dysfunction, *NDTA Newsletter* Nov 1988.

112. Sabari JS: Motor learning concepts applied to activity-based intervention with adults with hemiplegia, *Am J Occup Ther* 45(6): 523-530, 1991.

113. Sahrmann SA, Norton BJ: The relationship of voluntary movement to spasticity in the upper motor neuron syndrome, *Ann Neurol* 2(6):460-465, 1977.

114. Savage R, Robertson L: Shoulder pain in hemiplegia: a literature review, *Clin Rehabil* 2:35, 1988.

115. Schleenbaker RE, Mainous AG: Electromyographic biofeedback for neuromuscular reeducation in the hemiplegic stroke patient: a meta-analysis, *Arch Phys Med Rehabil* 74(12):1301-1304, 1993.

116. Sietsema JM, Nelson DL, Mulder RM, et al: The use of a game to promote arm reach in persons with traumatic brain injury, *Am J Occup Ther* 47(1):19-24, 1993.

117. Smith RO, Okamoto G: Checklist for the prescription of slings for the hemiplegic patient, *Am J Occup Ther* 35(2):91-95, 1981.

118. Taub E, Miller NE, Novack TA, et al: Technique to improve chronic motor deficit after stroke, *Arch Phys Med Rehabil* 74(4):347-354, 1993.

119. Taub E, Uswatte G, Pidikiti R: Constraint-induced movement therapy: a new family of techniques with broad application to physical rehabilitation, *J Rehabil Res Dev* 6(3):237-251, 1999.

120. Tepperman PS, Greyson ND, Hilbert L, et al: Reflex sympathetic dystrophy in hemiplegia, *Arch Phys Med Rehabil* 65(8):442-447, 1984.

121. Tries J: EMG feedback for the treatment of upper extremity dysfunction: can it be effective? *Biofeedback Self Regul* 14(1):21-53, 1989.

122. Trombly CA: Observations of improvements of reaching in five subjects with left hemiparesis, *J Neurol Neurosurg Psychiatry* 56:40, 1993.

123. Trombly CA: Deficits of reaching in subjects with left hemiparesis: a pilot study, *Am J Occup Ther* 46(10):887-897, 1992.

124. Uswatte G, Taub E: Constraint-induced movement therapy: new approaches to outcome measurement in rehabilitation. In Stuss DT, Winocur G, Robertson IH, editors: *Cognitive neurorehabilitation: a comprehensive approach*, Cambridge, 1999, Cambridge University Press.

125. van der Lee JH, Wagenaar RC, Lankhorst GJ, et al: Forced use of the upper extremity in chronic stroke patients: results from a single-blind randomized clinical trial, *Stroke* 30(11):2369-2375, 1999.

126. Van Ouwenaller C, Laplace PM, Chantraine A: Painful shoulder in hemiplegia, *Arch Phys Med Rehabil* 67(1):23-26, 1986.

127. Van Vliet P, Sheridan MR, Fentem P, et al: The influence of functional goals on the kinematics of reaching following stroke, *Neurol Rep* 19:11, 1995.

128. Wanklyn P, Forster A, Young J: Hemiplegic shoulder pain (HSP): natural history and investigation of associated features, *Disabil Rehabil* 18(10):497-501, 1996.

129. Waylett-Rendall J: Therapist's management of reflex sympathetic dystrophy. In Hunter JM, Schneider L, Mackin E, et al, editors: *Rehabilitation of the hand: surgery and therapy*, ed 3, St Louis, 1990, Mosby.

130. Wilson DJ: Stroke rehabilitation: setting realistic occupational therapy goals, *Physical Disabilities Special Interest Section Quarterly* 1980.

131. Wilson DJ, Baker LL, Craddock JA: Functional test for the hemiparetic upper extremity, *Am J Occup Ther* 38(3):159-164, 1984.

132. Wolf SL, Catlin PA, Blanton S, et al: Overcoming limitations in elbow movement in the presence of antagonist hyperactivity, *Phys Ther* 74(9):826-835, 1994.

133. Wolf SL, Catlin PA, Ellis M, et al: Assessing Wolf motor function test as outcome measure for research in patients after stroke, *Stroke* 32(7):1635-1639, 2001.

134. Wolf SL, Lecraw DE, Barton LA, et al: Forced use of hemiplegic upper extremities to reverse the effect of learned nonuse among chronic stroke and head-injured patients, *Exp Neurol* 104(2): 125-132, 1989.

135. Woollacott MH, Bonnet M, Yabe K: Preparatory process for anticipatory postural adjustments: modulation of leg muscles reflex pathways during preparation for arm movements in standing man, *Exp Brain Res* 55(2):263-271, 1984.

136. World Health Organization: *International classification of function*, Geneva, 2002, The Organization.

137. Wu CY, Trombly CA, Lin KC: The relationship between occupational form and occupational performance: a kinematic perspective, *Am J Occup Ther* 48(8):679-687, 1994.

138. Wu S, Trombly CA, Lin K, et al: Effects of object affordances on movement performance: a meta-analysis, *Scand J Occup Ther* 5:83, 1998.

139. Yue G, Cole KJ: Strength increases from the motor program: comparison of training with maximal voluntary and imagined muscle contractions, *J Neurophysiol* 67(5):1114-1123, 1992.

140. Zorowitz RD, Hughes MB, Idank D, et al: Shoulder pain and subluxation after stroke: correlation or coincidence? *Am J Occup Ther* 50(3):194-201, 1996.

141. Zorowitz RD, Idank D, Ikai T, et al: Shoulder subluxation after stroke: a comparison of four supports, *Arch Phys Med Rehabil* 76(8):763-771, 1995.

ann burkhardt

## chapter 11

# Edema Control

## key terms

| | | |
|---|---|---|
| congestive heart failure | entrapment | pain syndromes |
| deep venous thrombosis | lymphatic | renal failure |
| edema | massage | vascular |

## chapter objectives

After completing this chapter, the reader will be able to accomplish the following:

1. Describe causes and underlying medical conditions that result in clinical symptoms of edema.
2. Provide clinical reasoning for edema treatment.
3. Describe types of evaluations used to detect edema and the success of edema treatment.
4. Describe types of treatments for edema and provide specific information concerning possible indications and contraindications for the use of specific treatments.

Edema is a condition that results in an enlargement of a body part such as a limb or one of the various compartments of the body. Edema that develops after a stroke may be related to sequelae of the stroke underlying organ dysfunction. Therefore, for therapists to use their clinical reasoning skills to determine the following is important: (1) which factors may be causing the edema, (2) whether the underlying cause of the edema is related to failure or decreased functioning of an organ or system of the body (such as the heart, lungs, circulatory system, or kidneys), (3) whether contributing factors are present (such as a blood clot) that could worsen the patient's condition if treated in certain ways, and (4) whether the edema treatment will increase the patient's function and quality of life.

## PATHOPHYSIOLOGY AND MEDICAL MANAGEMENT

Upper extremity edema first seen unilaterally in a limb may result from (1) an entrapment from a postural change that causes impingement; (2) decreased activity of the vascular muscle pump, which is normally active during movement and functional use; (3) development of an abnormal sympathetic nerve response (e.g., reflex sympathetic dystrophy); or (4) a blood clot in the involved limb. Although rare, if the patient has another malignant condition such as cancer that obstructs the lymphatic vessels, the unilateral upper extremity condition may result from tumor involvement.

A meta-analysis of the rehabilitation literature conducted in 2000 examined research studies regarding the cause and treatment of poststroke hand edema and shoulder-hand syndrome that were published between January 1973 and August 1998. Based on systematic analysis of the literature, the authors concluded the following: the shoulder is involved in only half of the cases with painful swelling of wrist and hand, suggesting a "wrist-hand syndrome" between simple hand edema and shoulder-hand syndrome; hand edema following stroke and lymphedema are not the same; shoulder-hand syndrome generally occurs in patients who have increased arterial blood flow in the affected limb; idiopathic trauma causes aseptic joint inflammations in the limbs of persons who have stroke-related shoulder-hand syndrome; no specific treatment has yet proved advantageous over other physical methods for reducing hand edema; and orally administered corticosteroids are the most effective treatment for shoulder-hand syndrome when poststroke edema in a limb is caused by shoulder-hand syndrome.[6]

Another study suggests that peripheral microcirculation tends to be more pronounced in the edematous than in the nonedematous extremities.[12] Fifty-three hemiplegic patients (28 men, 25 women; mean age 58.2 ± 3.8 years) were studied. Subjects were divided into edema and nonedema groups. The edema group included 29 hemiplegic patients with edematous paretic upper extremities. Twenty-four hemiplegic patients in the nonedema group did not suffer from limb edema in the paretic upper extremity. Cutaneous microvascular perfusion responses to three grade levels of iontophoretically applied 1% acetylcholine, 1% acetylcholine plus 1% N(G)-monomethyl-L-arginine, and 1% sodium nitroprusside in the skin of subjects' forearms were determined by laser Doppler perfusion measurements. Hemodynamic characteristics in the arterial and venous vessels were measured by impedance plethysmography. Cutaneous microcirculatory function in the paretic upper extremity after stroke may be impaired. The impairment may occur because of decreased endothelium-dependent dilation in skin vasculature.

Several entrapment syndromes can result in upper extremity edema, including scalenus anticus syndrome, first rib syndrome (costoclavicular syndrome), thoracic outlet syndrome, and reflex sympathetic dystrophy (RSD). These syndromes may develop with postural changes after stroke. The alleviation of some of these disorders through treatment may focus on changing seating behaviors through positioning, exercise, and modifications of activity performance.

Scalenus anticus syndrome[12] is characterized by neck and shoulder discomfort and a tingling sensation in the hand and fingers. The pain is vague and achy, and although the person occasionally may complain of shooting pain, such pain is not the prominent complaint associated with this condition. The scalenus anticus muscle is a strap muscle of the neck that originates on the cervical vertebrae (3 through 6) and inserts on the scalenus tubercle of the first rib. The subclavian artery and brachial plexus are normally behind the muscle. The scalenus anticus often is used for minor postural adjustments of the head such as nodding during a conversation. The muscle assists with suspending the head over the trunk and is also an accessory muscle used during breathing, but its dysfunction is never life threatening from a respiratory perspective. The most significant clinical test for scalenus anticus syndrome is one that tests the patient's response to manual pressure on the muscle while the patient's head is rotated, laterally flexed, and posteriorly tilted to the opposite side. The area is tender to palpation.[8] The person may feel warmth or an exacerbation of the tingling as the muscle is stretched (during palpation). These symptoms are vascular in origin and are related to neurovascular bundle impingement. The scalenus anticus syndrome evolves because the person assumes a position in which the shoulders are rotated internally (commonly referred to as *round shouldered*), the head is flexed forward, and the cervical spine is hyperextended. Although the scalenus anticus muscle attaches to the first rib, this condition is different than first rib syndrome because it does not result in rotation of the first rib.

The first rib syndrome is characterized by shoulder pain radiating proximally to distally. The first rib may impinge the neurovascular bundle as well, but impingement is less likely to occur than with scalenus anticus syndrome. The first rib normally is tilted down and forward. If the person develops an abnormal posture of the cervical spine, the soft tissues accommodate over time, causing the anterior end of the rib to migrate into a position of upward rotation,[11] which impinges on the thoracic inlet of the neurovascular bundle. The symptoms usually arise later in the course of the disease because the body tends to adapt initially when the soft tissues are pliable and may be stretched. Over time, as contracture of the soft tissues occurs, the condition worsens.

Thoracic outlet syndrome after a stroke may result from a narrowing of the space through which the neurovascular structures leave the chest cavity (the thorax) and descend to the peripheral structures in the arms. Thoracic outlet syndrome may be associated with trauma or repeated trauma of the thoracic outlet at the shoulder. After repeated transient compressions, the brachial plexus may become scarred (i.e., develop neurofibrosis). Thoracic outlet syndrome is a compression syndrome and may result when a person with a hemiparetic upper extremity and decreased proprioceptive and kinesthetic sensation bears weight on the extended limb while the shoulder girdle is unsupported. The syndrome also could be exacerbated by bilateral overhead lifting, which often occurs when a person with hemiparesis is advised passively to assist the arm affected by the stroke with the other arm, especially when the affected arm has no protective position sense; that is, a lack of normal arm suspension occurs as the head of the humerus glides down into overhead flexion and abduction with external rotation. The humeral head slides down so far that the normal counterbalance provided by the shoulder depressors is disturbed, resulting in impingement on the thoracic outlet. Repeated banging of the humeral head against the clavicle could narrow the thoracic outlet and irritate and inflame the brachial plexus.[1] Over time and with repeated trauma the acute inflammatory response, the cytokine reaction (which at the cellular level results in abnormal collagen formation and a loss of elastin in soft tissue), evolves into a chronic condition with permanent hypertrophic scarring of the nerves and permanent narrowing of the thoracic outlet.[1,10] The usual clinical complaints associated with thoracic outlet syndrome are pain, paresthesia, and arm weakness that worsens with activities requiring overhead reaching (overhead activities). This complaint also usually is associated with persons who had a history of being sedentary and then suddenly or abruptly increased their overhead activities. The usual pain distribution is tingling and numbness in the ulnarly innervated hand digits (the ulnar border of the middle, ring, and little fingers). The underlying cause for this clinical symptom is the direct trauma to the medial cord of the inferior trunk of the brachial plexus.

Reflex sympathetic dystrophy is a pain disorder that results from an injury but clinically appears to be out of proportion to the extent of the injury. The dystrophy usually results from trauma, fractures, crush injuries, and sprains but also has been known to develop after a myocardial infarction; after a stroke; in patients with cervical disk disease, phlebitis, tuberculosis infection, or cancer; and after animal bites or frostbite. The dystrophy also has been observed in a patient who received an intramuscular influenza vaccine in a hemiparetic extremity and in another patient who had a repetitive strain injury after overusing an upper extremity bilateral exerciser. Typically, the patient first is seen with recalcitrant pain that worsens when the limb is touched or moved. Although a number of studies have attempted to link laboratory findings with the presence of RSD, the only laboratory anomaly that appears to be consistent is an elevated erythrocyte sedimentation rate in 70% of patients in one group. The results of one animal study suggested that this anomaly may be linked to an increased number of Langerhans' cells in the skin, resulting in altered capillary innervation and eventual degeneration of motor end plates.[11] This anomaly has not yet been demonstrated in human beings. Reflex sympathetic dystrophy is a complex disorder and probably is formed by intricate neurophysiologic pathways that form an organic basis for the disorder. A preexisting psychologic condition once was thought to cause or predispose a person to RSD. Current thought is that chronic pain and debilitating body changes probably cause psychologic responses.

Reflex sympathetic dystrophy is a systemic disease that usually begins in an affected extremity (e.g., an extremity affected by a stroke). Reflex sympathetic dystrophy has three stages. Stage I is characterized by burning pain that worsens in severity and paresthesia resulting from light touch. Pitting edema of the dorsum of the hand is also common.[5] Digital and wrist motions progressively decrease, in part as a result of the edema, which acts as an internal splint and prevents full active motion, possibly resulting in overstretching of the extensor muscles of the hand and a loss of extrinsic muscle-generated power (tenodesis). Motion also is diminished when the patient avoids using the limb because of anticipated pain exacerbation. The hand color is initially pale to bluish (cyanotic), but erythema of the metacarpal phalange joints eventually develops at the conclusion of stage I. The typical trophic changes of the skin are increased sweating and coolness. Vasospasm and peripheral vasoconstriction are common in this stage. Osteoporotic changes may be detectable after 3 weeks and are characterized by the moth-eaten appearance of the bones on x-ray films. This stage usually lasts approximately 3 months[5] (Figure 11-1).

Stage II may last for 9 months and is characterized by worsening pain, decreases in the sweating response, shiny skin, erythema, and increased localized heat in the portion of the limb where the pain is most intense. Progressively worsening stiffness is a prominent feature. Osteoporotic changes may affect the long bones of the arm. Edema persists, but rather than being fluid and causing pitting, it changes and causes the limb to become firm and brawny.[5]

Stage III, sometimes referred to as the *atrophic stage*, may last more than 2 years. The edema progresses from brawniness to periarticular thickening of the joint lining. For example, the digital ligaments and joint capsules may become thick and scarred as the soft tissues lose elastin after a cytokine response to a chronic inflammation. The

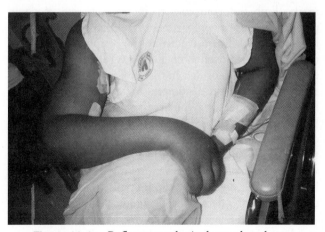

**Figure 11-1**    Reflex sympathetic dystrophy edema.

fingertips take on a typical pencil-point appearance as the subcutaneous tissue and muscles atrophy. Osteoporosis is profound at this stage[5] (see Chapter 10).

In contrast to the entrapment syndromes, a stroke survivor also may develop peripheral edema associated with deep venous thrombosis (DVT) or phlebitis.[6] These conditions usually develop in individuals who have clots or vascular disorders and often have embolic stroke syndromes. Blood clots form when the number of platelets (blood cells that assist with blood clotting) is increased. A thrombus often forms in a blood vessel region that has had vessel wall trauma. Areas with more plaque are prone to developing clots (e.g., carotid arteries). However, limbs are also prone to clot formation when trauma to their vascular structures is related to prolonged vessel compression (e.g., resulting from bed rest, being unconscious, or being immobile during surgery. The intraoperative use of pneumatic pumps is a method used to prevent the development of DVT during or after surgery. Thromboembolic disease stockings also help prevent clots from developing in sedentary persons. Persons with hemiparesis of an upper extremity also may develop DVT in the arm.

Deep venous thrombosis in any limb may result in edema. The most common clinical sign of DVT in the lower extremity is calf tenderness and in any extremity is tenderness when a muscle compartment is squeezed lightly.[6] Initially the edema accompanying DVT is compartmentalized. If undetected for a day or two, the edema progresses distally to the clot. The person may experience distal vasomotor changes because the vascular flow is diminished mechanically by the loss of intravessel space caused by obstruction by the clot. The goal in the overall management of a blood clot is to dissolve and not cause movement of the clot because the clot may travel to life-sustaining body organs and result in a secondary complication. For example, if a clot migrates to the heart, it may result in a heart attack. If the clot migrates to the lungs, it may result in a pulmonary embolus and perhaps respiratory distress. If the clot migrates to the brain, it may result in repeated cerebrovascular accidents. If the clot remains in the limb but continues to increase in size, it could potentially cause a compartment syndrome (i.e., the circulation may be fully obstructed to the peripheral portion of the limb). The distal limb loses oxygen, and the tissue begins to necrose, or die. In this situation, surgical extraction of the clot and decompression of the intramuscular limb compartment may be necessary, or the patient could lose the limb or die. The most frequent clinical sign of a compartment syndrome is acute loss of motor function followed by vascular signs such as cyanosis. Additional weakness in a person with preexisting hemiparesis could be difficult to detect, yet the therapist is often the first team member to detect the change in functional status.

Generalized edema that involves the trunk of the body or edema that involves bilateral limbs of the body may be a result of major organ dysfunction rather than the aforementioned impingement syndromes. Most commonly, patients with generalized edema are seen first with bilateral pedal edema involving both feet. In a patient with no history of stroke, pedal edema may develop for a number of reasons that are completely unrelated to stroke risk. For the purposes of this chapter, the edema discussion is limited to edema in stroke survivors.

Bilateral pedal edema (Figure 11-2)—swelling of the feet and ankles—may be a sign of preexisting peripheral vascular disease, congestive heart failure, chronic renal failure, diabetic-related small vessel disease, inactivity resulting in understimulation of the internal large muscle pumps, or lymphedema tarda (an edema to which the person is predisposed genetically and that develops in adulthood). Peripheral vascular disease may involve the venous or arterial systems of the limbs, or both.[6] When a person is sitting with the legs in a dependent position, such as when the person is sitting on a bed with the feet resting on the floor, gravity encourages interstitial fluid to circulate toward the feet. If vascular disease is present, the vessels are narrowed by plaque (e.g., from hypercholesterolemia), damaged by tar and nicotine (e.g., from cigarette smoking), or atrophied because of hyperglycemic circulation (e.g., from diabetes). Whether the dysfunction results from vascular valve dysfunction, atrophy of vessel musculature atrophy, or internal vessel flow resistance (from a number of factors that result in vessel constriction), the edema results from impaired hemodynamics. One concern is the lack of assisting muscle pumping. A simple increase in active muscle contraction of the legs is sometimes sufficient to decrease pedal edema. Regardless of whether activity level has increased, if edema persists, further evaluation and treatment may be indicated. When patients have heart and lung or kidney dysfunction, medications may allow them to be able to use activity to resolve the edema. For example,

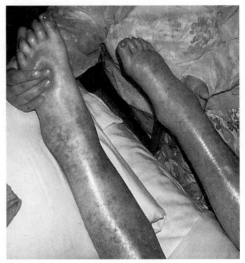

**Figure 11-2**   Bilateral pedal edema.

diuretic medications may improve kidney function and mobilize the fluids abnormally retained by the body.[2]

If major organ system dysfunction persists or septicemia develops (a widespread infection in the bloodstream), the edema may develop in the trunk (*ascites*) or throughout the entire body (*anasarca*). Treatment for ascites usually includes medications to enhance organ function and mobilize the fluids.[2] A patient with ascites or anasarca may have to stay in bed because the body may need all its energy for central hemodynamic and homeostatic processes rather than for the peripheral mechanical hemodynamic function potential that may be gained through gross mobilization and stimulation of cardiopulmonary function. When septicemia is the main cause of anasarca or ascites,[2,6] an antibiotic may be the most important treatment of the underlying cause of the edema. In this situation the edema is caused by a lymphatic response to the potentially unbeatable antigen (bacteria, fungus, or virus) resulting in a white blood cell, protein-rich edema, rather than a fluidlike blood plasma. In today's hospital environment, decades of fighting infections with broad-spectrum antibiotic agents has resulted in increasing numbers of resistant infections that are tougher to control until more effective drugs or methods are devised.

In addition to diuretics, other drugs that enhance function of specific organs may be used to mobilize fluid as well. For example, patients with congestive heart failure may be receiving a diuretic (e.g., furosemide) while they also are receiving a drug to stabilize blood pressure (e.g., a β-blocker) and possibly even a drug to stabilize their arrhythmia (e.g., digoxin). Therefore, internal medicine physicians often attempt to achieve homeostasis in an individual who has major organ failure by many methods. Rehabilitation may be only a small part of the initial treatment picture for these individuals.

## EVALUATION METHODS

The most commonly used method to measure edema is taking circumferential measurements. The method for taking circumferential measurements often is not standardized from clinic to clinic, possibly resulting in haphazard approaches to measuring edema and its response to treatment. Therapists who work in settings in which edema is measured or treated consistently usually choose one of two methods of measurement: (1) measuring the limb consistently a certain distance (in centimeters) above and below an anatomic landmark (e.g., an upper extremity such as the elbow) and (2) measuring the limb at certain anatomic landmarks (e.g., the insertion of the triceps or the midbelly of the biceps), the distance of which varies according to the anatomic distribution in the individual. As with goniometry and manual muscle testing the outcomes of these measurements probably are most consistent when the same therapist measures and remeasures the person each time (i.e., relies on intrarater versus interrater reliability). A specific type of tape measure also may be appropriate to control the degree of pull against the tape (e.g., a measurement made with a weighted pull).

Another method used to measure the girth of a limb is volumetrically displacing water by submersing the limb in water that is contained in an enclosed space. The container has a spill-off valve from which the displaced water is collected and measured. Commercial volumeters may be purchased for the clinical setting. If volumetric measurements are used, consistent positioning must be used each time, and the limb always must be submerged to the same point; otherwise the measurement is skewed.

Computer-generated measurements also have been developed but are currently too expensive for most clinics to own. These are probably the most reliable forms of volumetric measurement, but they presently are not consistently applicable.

Tonometry is another method used to detect or measure edema in a limb. The difficulty with using tonometry is that it does not accommodate for quality differences in edema. For example, a brawny limb may have measurements that are similar to a normal limb because the tone of the soft tissue is firmer, like toned muscle. In contrast, fluid and pitting edemas would result in greater girth.

Clinical observations also are useful for evaluation of edema. Examples of observations include the following:

- Skin temperature
- Skin moisture: moist or dry
- Skin color: red (erythema), pale, or cyanotic (bluish tint)
- Firmness on palpation (soft, fluidlike, pitting, brawny, firm, and woody)
- Presence, quality, and distribution of pain (tingling, numbness, coolness, heaviness, cramping, electrical, or shocking)
- Weeping of the edema through the skin
- Loss of mobility or motion by increased girth versus motor weakness
- Blood pressure (although the therapist should take care to avoid inflating a blood pressure cuff on a limb suspected of having DVT or phlebitis or that has had a lymphatic impairment)

Monitoring blood tests also may be helpful in the overall management of the edema. Erythrocyte sedimentation rate,[11] platelet level, white blood cell count, prothrombin time,[6] blood glucose levels, and creatinine and bilirubin counts may be helpful to follow, depending on the underlying medical conditions. Platelet levels and prothrombin time indicate the possible presence of or response to treatment of clotting disorders. White blood cell counts indicate the possible presence of an infection by stimulation of an immune response. Blood glucose levels in a diabetic patient are elevated greatly if the white blood cell count is elevated. Creatinine and bilirubin counts are indicators of renal function.

One study[9] suggests that many clinical symptoms and the main features of sympathetic dysfunction in complex regional pain syndrome could be explained by central nervous system pathophysiology. In their article the authors observed the pattern of autonomic symptoms in patients with complex regional pain syndrome I compared with patients a few days after stroke. Autonomic failure in the latter group is assumed to represent definite central nervous system origin. Seventeen stroke patients, 21 patients in the acute and late stages of complex regional pain syndrome I, and a control group of 23 healthy subjects were investigated. The authors performed detailed neurologic examinations, induced sweating centrally (thermoregulatory sweating [TST]) and peripherally by carbachol iontophoresis (QSART), and quantified sweating by evaporation hygrometry. They assessed skin temperature by infrared thermography. The incidence of motor-sensory dysfunction (without pain) and the incidence of edema was strikingly similar in patients with stroke and complex regional pain syndrome. Furthermore, stroke patients had increased TST but not QSART responses on the contralesional limb ($p < 0.05$), and skin temperature was decreased ($p < 0.001$). The same pattern of autonomic failure was found in late complex regional pain syndrome (TST, $p < 0.02$; skin temperature, $p < 0.01$), whereas in acute complex regional pain syndrome additional, presumably peripheral mechanisms, contribute to sympathetic symptoms.

Sensory assessment is a key component in the determination of the level of the entrapment[8] (i.e., the nerve root, following the distribution of the dermatome, the plexus, following the sensory loss of the pattern of the plexus trunk; or the peripheral nerve). In addition, diabetic patients may have entrapment neuropathies of rapidly adapting nerve fibers (A fibers: moving two point and vibratory sense) superimposed on a limb that has a diabetic large fiber (C fiber: pain and temperature sense) neuropathy. If patients have a lesion affecting the cerebellum, their position sense also may be impaired. If sensation is impaired, patients may tend to avoid or underuse the involved limb. The inactivity can generate edema through understimulation of the internal muscle pumps in the limb.[2] In addition, trauma caused by imperception of pain in the involved limb could result in posttraumatic edema. Documentation of type, distribution, and quality of pain perceived in the limb may provide clues to potential pain syndrome evolution (e.g., RSD). Cramping muscle pain is common at the proximal attachment of the extremity of the limb and is common intracompartmentally in the extremity, especially in the forearm and lower leg when edema is present.

Active range of motion assessment is also important because distention of a limb area may decrease the available range of motion through overstretching one group of muscles (e.g., the extensors of the hand and wrist in a person with an edematous hand). Increased girth of a limb also limits full active movement of the limb into flexion (e.g., the elbow in an arm or the knee in a leg). Passive range of motion activities should not be aimed at forcing an edematous compartment through full range of motion because it could result in additional chronic deformity. For example, overstretching the extensor digiti minimi can result in ulnar slippage and displacement of the tendon over time.

## TREATMENT METHODS

Therapists may relieve edema associated with entrapment syndromes—scalenus anticus syndrome, first rib syndrome, and thoracic outlet syndrome—by treating the posture, positioning, and habits that have contributed to the development of these conditions. Strengthening of weak muscles also may assist in correcting imbalances, which result in assuming positions of comfort that may contribute to decreased function by limiting ability to participate in activities. For example, a person with hemiparesis who sits in a posterior tilt may have flattening of their lumbar and thoracic curves and abducted scapulae, internally rotated and adducted humeri, and a hyperextended cervical spine. As a result of this posture the soft tissues (e.g., muscles, tendons, nerves, ligaments, blood and lymphatic vessels, fascia, and skin) have assumed a shortened position. Prolonging this position results in reflex muscle spasms to accommodate overstretching or shortening. As the muscles contract, the fascia tightens and the skin shortens, all entrapping the nerves and vascular structures and causing sensory changes and edema.

If the person shifts weight into a neutral pelvic tilt, the spinal curves often are restored, the head is suspended up over the spine, the scapulae adduct, and the humeri abduct and externally rotate.[3] Once repositioned, the individual can inhale more deeply, possibly enough to rotate the rib into a normal position. Teaching the person to self-cue and adjust the posture using techniques such as the Alexander technique also may improve postural habits.

With release of the soft tissues, hemodynamic flow improves because other structures such as overstretched, reflex-spasming, posturally compromised muscles were impinging the vessel flow. Impingement on vascular structures results in restriction of hemodynamic flow. Impaired vascular return results in local backflow, venous and lymphatic stasis, and edema. Myofascial release is a manual technique that is often helpful for stretching out and elongating (restoring normal length to) the soft tissue structures.

Positional elevation, compression and gentle massage techniques, pneumatic compression, and compression bandaging and gradient compression garments may be indicated for edemas resulting from impingement syndromes and major organ dysfunction. Indications for and contraindications to the use of some of these techniques exist that should influence clinical reasoning and treatment modality choice. Awareness of the way the treatment causes change may provide the necessary underpinnings of the clinical reasoning process.

Positional elevation uses gravity to assist the hemodynamic flow in the limb backward and down toward the heart. The right side of the heart propels deoxygenated blood from the peripheral vascular system into the left side of the heart, where it becomes reoxygenated. Therefore, if the stroke survivor has any right-sided heart failure, this technique would not be advisable. Encouraging backflow may overstress the heart and contribute to a life-threatening event. A person who has DVT also would not be encouraged to elevate the limb. Elevation could transport the clot toward the central organs: the heart, lungs, and brain in particular. A person with arterial dysfunction cannot tolerate positional elevation because it produces Raynaud's phenomenon and can decrease viability of the distal ends of the limb (the fingers or toes); the person develops dysesthesia within a short time.

When used, elevation only needs to suspend the distal portion of an extended limb 9 cm above the right side of the heart.[2] The person's extremity needs to remain elevated for 45 minutes to an hour at a time. Active movement is encouraged to prevent limb stiffness and stimulate the muscle pump to return the excess fluid to central circulation. Elevating the limb too much can contribute to traction or compression of the brachial plexus if the limb is positioned improperly, which could result in a change in the sensory and motor status of the limb and prolong the rehabilitative period. Elevation can help to mobilize fluid, but the edema returns when the limb returns to a dependent position.

Compression garments or wraps must be used to prevent backflow and limb refilling. Temporary compression garments, such as tubular support bandages, Isotoner gloves, self-adherent (e.g., Coban) wraps, and compression wrapping bandages (e.g., Ace bandage and Comprilan) are useful. Stroke survivors are more prone to cyanotic changes when using compression wrapping. Changes in capillary refill and subtle somatic complaints of tingling and numbness may necessitate removal of the support. When patients tolerate compression wraps, the wraps assist in stimulating the internal muscle pump while the person is using the limb actively. The wraps also provide neutral warmth, which can help relax the skeletal muscle response. Gracies et al[7] did a crossover study of outpatients and inpatients who had spasticity and edema of their arms and hands. They used Lycra garments designed as dynamic splints to exert directional pull on certain limb segments, which were worn for 3 hours by hemiplegic patients. Assessments were performed at the start and end of a 3-hour period during a standard rehabilitation day when the patients were and were not wearing the garment ($n = 16$ patients). The authors found a decrease in edema with the use of the Lycra garments: digit circumference decreased by 4% ($p < 0.01$). They concluded that Lycra garments have rapid splinting and antispastic effects on wrist and fingers in patients with hemiplegia and that these garments may help severely affected patients with major spasticity or painful swollen limbs.

Although not yet supported by research evidence, a new method of treatment is growing in popularity: kinesiotaping. Kinesiotape is a hypoallergenic skin tape that has a circular, elasticized weft. The tape was invented by a doctor from Japan and is manufactured in Japan. The tape has a dynamic component to its composition and lifts skin and soft tissue in a line of pull. Kinesiotape is believed to promote retrograde flow in a limb and thus reduce edema. From the author's own anecdotal clinical use of kinesiotape, some dramatic results have occurred in edema reduction in clients who have poststroke edema in a flaccid, dependent limb.

Therapists also can use external supports such as air splints (which are static) and pneumatic massage pumps (which are dynamic-sequential or gradient sequential) to create a pressure gradient in the limb. These devices use air-filled sleeves to provide the pressure gradient. Inflation of the splint is by mouth or pump while the limb is in the sleeve; a valve retains the pressure in the device. Pneumatic pumps rely on a continuous airflow system generated by a motor (an air compressor), which inflates the pneumatic sleeve. Some pumps have one chamber or cell that inflates and then deflates around the limb; other pumps have multiple cells per sleeve. The distal cell fills first, and the remaining cells continue to fill distally to proximally, creating a "milking" motion that dynamically decongests the edematous limb. Pneumatic massage and air splints should not be used by stroke survivors who have DVT or active phlebitis; are receiving anticoagulant medications that drop their platelet levels below 120,000 $mm^3$; have active, untreated, moderate to severe congestive heart failure; or chronic renal failure.

Manual massage also may help decrease limb edema. The most popular massage technique in current use is manual lymphatic massage. The superficial lymphatics in the trunk and uninvolved extremity are stimulated first. The involved extremity then is massaged lightly using a combination of scooping, vibratory, and wedging strokes. The proximal extremity is massaged first, the middle portion second, and the distal portion last. Other popular techniques that also may be helpful are retrograde massage and accupressure massage (Figure 11-3).

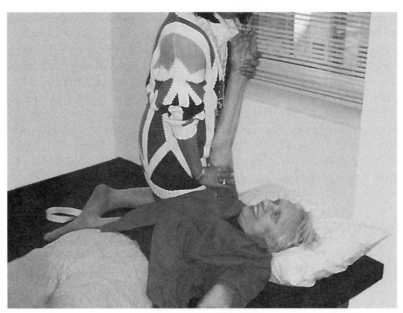

**Figure 11-3**    Manual massage techniques may assist with decreasing edema in a limb.

The treatment of RSD is more complex because edema stemming from RSD may stimulate the pain response and increase the intensity of, while decreasing the tolerance for, the recalcitrant pain. Techniques that may be useful in treating RSD include stress-loading an activity, combining rehabilitative treatment with nerve blocks (saline, Baer, lidocaine and/or bupivacaine ganglion blocks), and pharmacologic treatment (e.g., amitriptyline, nortriptyline, carbamazepine, phenytoin). Electrical ganglion blocks, such as high-voltage galvanic stimulation or transcutaneous nerve stimulation, also may be helpful as long as the affected limb is not ipsilateral to the region of a pacemaker or the individual does not have active, suboptimally controlled arrhythmia. Acupuncture also may be helpful in treating RSD pain. In stage II or stage III RSD, heavy sedation may be indicated to begin treatment depending on the patient's pain and psychologic response.[4]

Reflex sympathetic dystrophy also may be treated with ice baths and contrast baths. One technique is to plunge the limb with RSD into an ice-slush bath for 3 to 5 seconds and repeat 2 to 3 times (Figure 11-4), causing quick vasomotor restriction. The ice bath should be followed by active or active assistive overhead motion (with respect for the patient's pain). The activities should be graded over time and progressed to include stress-loading activities within the context of activities of daily living. No single technique works for every person with RSD. Knowledge of and training in the aforementioned techniques may provide more options for the therapist and the patient with edema and pain to try until they determine the correct combination of techniques or modality. Creativity, ingenuity, and compassion are important for effectively treating persons with pain syndromes.

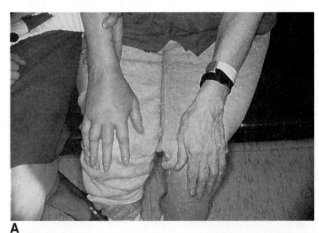

A

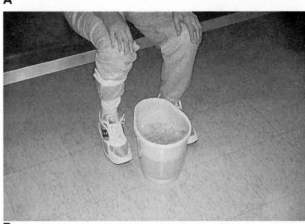

B

**Figure 11-4**    Limbs affected by reflex sympathetic dystrophy (**A**) may be treated with ice baths (**B, C,** and **D**) for a noticeable decrease in edema (**E**).

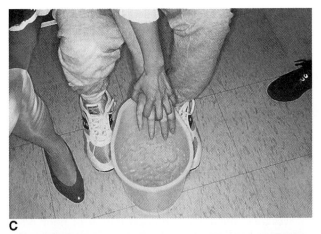

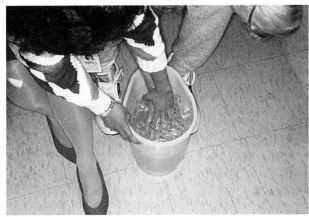

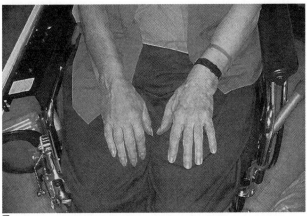

C

D

E

**Figure 11-4 cont'd**

## Case Study

### TOO MUCH TOO FAST

V.L. is a 52-year-old woman who developed edema and worsening pain during a rehabilitation unit stay after a stroke that caused residual right hemiparesis. A "go-getter," V.L. performed 5 times the number of repetitions of all exercises and activities prescribed by her therapist. She says she assumed that "doing more and more would make her better sooner."

V.L. (who was right-hand dominant) complained of pain in her right shoulder that increased in intensity whenever she used the upper extremity bilateral exercise machine. She was instructed to use the machine 3 times per day. In hopes of speeding up her recovery, she had been doing her repetitions 6 times per day.

V.L. is married and has a young child. Before her stroke, she worked full time as a manager. Her avocational activities included skiing, ice skating, and walking. She enjoyed going to the theater, visiting museums, and trying new restaurants.

On evaluation, V.L. complained of middeltoid and clavicular pain. After obtaining a brief history, it was revealed that she had neck and shoulder discomfort for more than a decade before to her stroke. Her arm was moderately edematous, dusky in color, and cool in the distal portion. During active, overhead range of motion activities, she experienced a stabbing feeling that progressed to burning pain in the middeltoid. She also complained of reflex muscle spasm in her neck and shoulder girdle. Her active range of motion of her elbow was within functional limits, but she had an incomplete grasp/release and nonfunctional fine motor skills; for example, she could not hold money, a pen, or a piece of paper. If she tried to continue to move, she felt a cramping sensation. She was unable to use her arm for any self-care activities, such as washing or brushing her hair, toileting, fastening her brassiere, writing, holding utensils and cups, and handling her child.

*Continued*

## Case Study

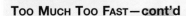

### TOO MUCH TOO FAST—cont'd

Her evaluation included measurement of her active range of motion, documentation of the circumferential measurements of both upper extremities, observations of the trophic changes in her skin and her right arm circulatory status, and documentation of functional strength and skill level.

Treatment included active assistive range of motion activities for the neck and entire right arm; lymphatic massage; compression bandaging; elevation and distal muscle pumping; stress-loading activities (e.g., using her arm as a support and cleaning the table with her affected arm); massage of and myofascial release techniques for the neck, trunk, and right upper extremity; guided imagery to decrease her anxiety about treatment possibly exacerbating her pain, and activities of daily living (basic and instrumental).

Within a month, V.L. could use both arms to embrace her child when she sat on V.L.'s lap. V.L. also could prepare a cup of tea and carry a plate from the kitchen to the dining room table and could brush the right side of her hair with her arm supported on a table. Her edema decreased significantly with a combination of elevation, massage, and improved vascular return resulting from functional use of the arm. The relaxation response evoked by the guided imagery helped to decrease her concern about potential pain. Her therapy, combined with acupuncture treatment and high-voltage galvanic stimulation on acupuncture meridians on days when she did not receive acupuncture treatment, contributed to a positive outcome for this patient with RSD.

## SUMMARY

Edema after a stroke may be caused by a number of underlying pathologic conditions, poor posture or positioning, or trauma to a limb that is weak or has diminished sensation or may accompany major organ failure. Knowledge of the underlying conditions and the side effects of their treatment helps the therapist make an informed recommendation for and implement a treatment plan.

Edema treatment is tied closely to the medical model. Rehabilitative strategies contribute to the resolution of the condition but not without the medical and other complementary techniques that may assist recovery. Patience, creative problem solving, and perseverance are characteristics that commonly contribute to successful treatment of persons with edema. More qualitative and quantitative research is needed to document successful functional outcomes in the management of edema and pain in the stroke population. Reflex sympathetic dystrophy is an expensive and disabling condition when not treated early and when treatment choices are not grounded in procedural clinical reasoning.

## REVIEW QUESTIONS

1. Explain the differences between scalenus anticus syndrome, first rib syndrome, and thoracic outlet syndrome. Discuss sensory findings and patterns of weakness including the contribution of poor posture to the development of these syndromes and the edema that results.
2. If a stroke survivor has symptoms of bilateral pedal edema, how would you choose the rehabilitation treatment?
3. Which drugs are used to treat neuropathic pain?
4. Describe the stages of reflex sympathetic dystrophy.
5. How would you treat hand edema in a person who has deep venous thrombosis in the hemiparetic upper extremity? Which precautions would you take?

## REFERENCES

1. Barbis J: Therapist's management of thoracic outlet syndrome. In Mackin EF, Callahan AO, Osterman L, et al, editors: *Rehabilitation of the hand: surgery and therapy*, ed 3, St Louis, 1990, Mosby.
2. Brunwald E: Edema. In Wilson JD, et al, editors: *Harrison's principles of internal medicine*, ed 12, New York, 1991, McGraw-Hill.
3. Davis PM: *Steps to follow: a guide to the treatment of hemiplegia*, Heidelberg, Germany, 1985, Springer-Verlag.
4. Davis J: The role of the occupational therapist in the treatment of shoulder hand syndrome, *Occup Ther Pract* 1:30, 1990.
5. Lankford LL: Reflex sympathetic dystrophy. In Mackin EF, Callahan AO, Osterman L, et al, editors: *Rehabilitation of the hand: surgery and therapy*, ed 3, St Louis, 1990, Mosby.
6. Geurts AC, Visschers BA, van Limbeek J, et al: Systematic review of aetiology and treatment of post-stroke hand oedema and shoulder-hand syndrome, *Scand J Rehabil Med* 32(1):4-10, 2000.
7. Gracies JM, Marosszeky JE, Renton R, et al: Short-term effects of dynamic Lycra splints on upper limb in hemiplegic patients, *Arch Phys Med Rehabil* 81(12):1547-1555, 2000.
8. Post M: *The shoulder: surgical and non-surgical management*, Philadelphia, 1988, Lea & Febiger.
9. Riedl B, Beckmann T, Neundörfer B, et al: Autonomic failure after stroke—is it indicative for pathophysiology of complex regional pain syndrome? *Acta Neurol Scand* 103(1):27-34, 2001.
10. Rote NS: Inflammation. In McCance KL, Heuther SE, editors: *Pathophysiology: the biological basis for disease in adults and children*, ed 2, St Louis, 1994, Mosby.
11. Shelton RM, Lewis CW: Reflex sympathetic dystrophy: a review, *J Am Acad Dermatol* 22(3):513-520, 1990.
12. Wang JS, Yang CF, Liaw MY, et al: Suppressed cutaneous endothelial vascular control and hemodynamic changes in paretic extremities with edema in the extremities of patients with hemiplegia, *Arch Phys Med Rehabil* 83(7):1017-1023, 2002.

stephanie milazzo
and glen gillen

chapter 12

# Splinting Applications

**key terms**

| | | |
|---|---|---|
| alignment | function | prevention |
| biomechanics | low-load prolonged stress | splinting |
| clinical reasoning | neurophysiologic approach | thermoplastics |
| contracture | orthotics | |

**chapter objectives**

After completing this chapter, the reader will be able to accomplish the following:

1. Identify a variety of splinting options.
2. Review positive and negative aspects of commonly used splints.
3. Summarize the research that has been published regarding splinting and persons who have had strokes.
4. Present rationales for splinting that consider current concepts of motor control, including biomechanical principles.
5. Critically analyze and reconsider the present approach to splinting, evaluating, and developing interventions for each extremity based on individual findings.

Any discussion of splinting of the upper extremity after stroke produces debate among occupational therapists. The use of splints after stroke can be traced as far back as 1911.[32] Since then the debate about whether to splint and about the rationales for splinting has continued.

The following principles guide splinting decisions for patients after stroke:

- Splints are used to maintain or increase the length of soft tissues (e.g., muscles, tendons, and ligaments) by preventing or lengthening shortened tissues and preventing overstretching of antagonist soft tissue.
- Splints are used to correct biomechanical malalignment, restoring muscles to normal resting length and protect-

ing joint integrity. This biomechanical correction may result in a decrease in excessive skeletal muscle activity.
- Splints are used to position the hand to assist in functional activities.
- Splints may be used to promote independence in specific areas of occupation.
- Splints compensate for weakness by providing external support, blocking the pull of muscle groups that have lost a balanced agonist-antagonist relationship, and altering the resting alignment of the joints to enhance functional postures.

The use of one rationale (i.e., never splinting, always splinting, or only using resting splints) for splinting patients after stroke cannot be effective because of the variety of problems that occur after stroke. The sequelae of stroke are multilayered, encompassing a variety of symptoms and problem areas. The complexity of these problems has served as fuel for the splinting debate and the controversies surrounding splinting.

## HISTORICAL PERSPECTIVE

Neuhaus et al[32] have published a review of the splinting literature covering a 100-year period. Their review has documented two different approaches to splinting: the biomechanical approach and the neurophysiologic approach.

The biomechanical perspective considers issues such as soft tissue lengthening, prevention of contracture and deformity, maintenance of biomechanical alignment, and effects on the nonneural components of spasticity. In contrast, the neurophysiologic perspective considers reflex inhibition, effects on the neural basis of spasticity, facilitation through sensory input, and inhibition through positioning and sensory input.

Earlier publications (from the early 1900s to the 1950s) emphasized a biomechanical approach, whereas literature after World War II emphasized a shift toward the neurophysiologic frame of reference. During this time, therapists (Rood, Bobath, Knott, Voss) developed theories based on neurophysiologic principles. Many of the neurophysiologic theorists clearly were opposed to splinting; others did not mention splinting at all as part of their treatment regimens. Rood (as cited by Stockmeyer[40]) stated that spasticity may be increased "by activating sensory stimuli of touch, pressure, and stretch, which result in undesirable contraction of muscle."

The neurophysiologic perspective currently is being seriously questioned because of a lack of research support, and a shift is occurring toward a more comprehensive and current understanding of motor behavior. Nevertheless, many styles of splints and rationales are still based on neurophysiologic principles.

To date, research does not support one style of splint as superior to another. Many of the statements and principles documented by the originators of the neurophysiologic theories have been accepted as fact. In light of current understanding of motor control, these statements need to be analyzed and researched critically before further splinting interventions are based on these concepts. See Chapter 6 for a comprehensive review of these issues.

## DORSAL VERSUS VOLAR SPLINTING

Splint fabrication and points of contact are areas of continuing debate. The following studies have investigated this controversy.

Zislis[46] compared the effects of two different wrist-hand splints on a patient with spastic hemiplegia. The author used simultaneous electromyographic recordings of the flexors and extensors in the forearm to provide an objective measure of muscle activity. Electromyographic readings were taken with no splint, with a dorsal-based splint (which kept the wrist neutral, fingers adducted and extended, and thumb free) used in hopes of facilitating the extensors, and with a volar-based splint (which kept the wrist neutral, fingers extended and abducted, and thumb free).

Zislis' results[46] indicated that extensor muscle activity was not altered in any of the three situations, although flexor activity was varied. With no splint, flexor activity was exaggerated compared with extensor activity. The dorsal splint greatly increased the flexor activity, even more so than when no splint was worn. Finally, the volar-based splint diminished flexor activity and achieved a state of "balanced physiologic activity between flexor and extensor muscle groups."

Zislis[46] drew the following conclusions from the patient he studied:

- Dorsal facilitation of the extensor was not evident, although dorsal facilitation of the flexors did occur.
- Flexor inhibition from volar cutaneous receptors may occur.
- Abduction and extension of the fingers may produce flexor inhibition.

Therefore, Zislis[46] recommended the use of volar-based splints with extension and abduction of the fingers.

Charait[7] observed 20 patients in her study of dorsal versus volar "functional position splints." In the splinted position the wrist varied from less than neutral to 30 degrees, the thumb was abducted and opposed, and the fingers were positioned at 45 degrees of finger flexion at the metacarpophalangeal (MP) and proximal interphalangeal (PIP) joints.

Charait[7] observed the amount of spasticity and voluntary movement in both groups. In the group wearing volar splints, four patients showed no change in spasticity or voluntary motion and six experienced increased spasticity. In the group wearing dorsal splints, one patient showed no change, one experienced a considerable increase in spasticity, and eight had decreased spasticity (four of these also exhibited increased active finger and wrist extension). The author drew the following conclusions from her observations:

- Volar pressure facilitates flexor muscles.
- Dorsal pressure with decreased volar contact facilitates the extensors.
- Prolonged stretch enhances inhibition.

Charait[7] recommended splinting using dorsal-based appliances.

McPherson et al[27] compared dorsal and volar resting splints for the reduction of hypertonus. They assigned

10 subjects with hypertonic wrist flexors to the dorsal or volar group. For the purposes of the study, the authors defined *hypertonus* as "the plastic, viscous, and elastic properties of the muscle resistant to stretch and with a tendency to return a limb to a particular abnormal resting posture." They used a spring-weighted scale to take measurements to assess the effectiveness of the splints in reducing hypertonicity. The results indicated no significant difference between the volar and dorsal splints in the reduction of hypertonus. As an aside, the authors found a correlation between age and reduction in hypertonus. The older subjects in the study demonstrated gradual but not statistically significant decline in hypertonus, whereas the younger adults demonstrated significant decline in hypertonus over 6 weeks.

Other studies have not compared dorsal and volar splinting specifically but instead have evaluated the effects of one or the other. Kaplan[20] evaluated 10 patients who wore dorsal wrist splints. His study set out to "determine whether prolonged therapy with a dorsal splint will inhibit or diminish hyperreflexia or stretch reflex and at the same time increase muscular power by sensorimotor stimulation." The splint used in this study positioned the wrist and fingers in extension and supported the thumb in abduction. Most of the subjects wore the splints at least 8 hours per day, and Kaplan noted that many patients required several serial splints to increase the stretch on the flexors gradually. Patients were evaluated with electromyographic, strength testing, and hand function evaluation before and after splint application. The subjects in this study demonstrated "improvement in strength and function of muscle, with a decrease in the stretch reflex and spasticity . . . when a dorsal splint was properly applied in treatment of hemiplegia involving an upper extremity."

Brennan[5] studied the effects of volar-based splints on his subjects. At the end of his study the patients who wore the volar-based wrist and hand splints demonstrated increased range of passive movement in which no resistance to stretch could be felt.

In their study of positioning devices on normal and spastic hands, Mathiowetz, Bolding, and Trombly[25] demonstrated that a volar-based resting splint increased electromyographic activity as the subjects performed a grasping activity on the contralateral side. They noted that the volar splint "is the least desirable positioning device while the hemiplegic subject is doing any activity that requires a comparable effort to squeezing 50% maximal voluntary contraction of grip."

The variability in the aforementioned studies makes decisions regarding dorsal- versus volar-based treatment difficult to reach based on available research. Therapists must still evaluate each patient individually to determine the effect of variables on splinting outcomes. Moreover, the studies discussed in this chapter used a variety of outcome measures, varied in their methodologies, and implemented variable definitions and styles of splints.

## REVIEW OF SPLINTS COMMONLY USED FOR PATIENTS AFTER STROKE

This section reviews positive and negative aspects of splints frequently used by occupational therapists; available research is discussed. Several of the following splints were developed based on a now outdated understanding of motor function. Some of the splints still may be useful and effective, although the rationale for their use may no longer be based on the original purpose of the splint.

### Finger Spreader (Finger Abduction Splint)

The finger spreader (finger abduction splint) is fabricated of foam rubber and positions the fingers and thumb in abduction. According to Bobath[3] the purpose of the splint is to "obtain extension of wrist and fingers. . . . Abduction not only facilitates extension of the fingers, but also reduces flexor spasticity throughout the whole arm. . . . It has a better and more dynamic effect than the use of a (standard) splint and reduces the possibility of edema." One should note that Bobath's rationale is not consistent with the current understanding of motor control and related neurologic principles.

A sturdier version of this splint (fabricated of low-temperature plastic) was proposed by Doubilet and Polkow.[9] They recommended wearing the splint only during the day. Their paper includes anecdotal evidence of the effectiveness of the splint:

> The finger abduction splint is presently being worn by fifteen patients who are two to six months post CVA, these patients exhibited moderate to severe spasticity of the fingers and wrist, decreased range of motion, and edema in the wrist and hand. After one week of using the splint plus standard treatment in the therapy sessions a moderate reduction of spasticity was seen in these patients.

Doubilet and Polkow[9] concluded that the splint results are promising and warrant continued trial and experimentation.

Mathiowetz, Bolding, and Trombly[25] objectively evaluated the finger abduction splint in a study investigating the effects of a variety of splints on the distal muscle activity of normal and hemiplegic subjects. Subjects wore the splints while performing resistive activities with the opposite hand. The results indicated "significantly *greater* EMG activity for the finger spreader compared to no device in the flexor carpi radialis of normal subjects during grasping" with the contralateral hand. In hemiplegic subjects the finger spreader did not evoke less electromyographic activity than no device. According to the authors, the belief that this splint decreases spasticity shortly after application needs to be questioned seriously.

The finger spreader may be useful in maintaining the length of the flexors; however, wrist position is not considered with this splint, and the therapist must be aware of the wrist position. To control for this problem, the therapist may combine the finger spreader with a standard wrist extension splint. Because the splint is subtle in terms of corrective forces, it may be indicated for patients with low tolerance for other, more cumbersome devices and for patients with low pain thresholds. Donning and doffing procedures are straightforward for the confused patient (Figure 12-1).

### Firm Cone

The firm cone can be fabricated of low-temperature plastic or purchased commercially; it is based on the traditional theories of Rood. Rood's theory (as interpreted by Stockmeyer[40]) states that firm and prolonged pressure over the flexor surface of the palm and fingers results in an inhibition of the long flexors. A more current understanding of the mechanism of this splint from a biomechanical and functional perspective is that the cone is positioned to place stretch on the shortened long flexors and is graded progressively to increase stress to the soft tissues to promote a more normal resting length. The cone initially is positioned with the narrow end of the cone toward the radial side of the hand in the web space if the hand is excessively tight. As the hand begins to relax from the directed stress, the ideal *biomechanical* position is for the cone to be positioned opposite to the initial position; that is, the wide end of the cone is placed in the radial side of the hand in the web space and the narrow end is placed in the ulnar side of the hand (Figure 12-2). The therapist can use strapping material to hold the cone in place. This device was included in the study by Mathiowetz, Bolding, and Trombly[25]; the researchers found that the cone did not evoke significantly less electromyographic activity during contralateral resisted function.

Neurophysiologic principles aside, the cone may be an effective positioning device for patients who have developed contracture in the long flexors. Combined applications of the cone with a standard wrist-extension splint, controlling the stretch on the wrist and digit flexors separately, are feasible. The size of the cone and the angle of wrist extension can be graded as the patient's status improves.

Another practical use of the cone is in the prevention of maceration of tissue in patients with moderate to severe flexion of the digits. The maintenance of flexor length is required for hygiene and cosmesis. Similar to the use of the finger abduction splint, the use of the cone in isolation does not provide wrist support, thus predisposing the wrist to a flexed posture. Donning and doffing procedures are straightforward.

### Orthokinetic Orthotics

According to Neeman and Neeman,[29] the term *orthokinetic orthosis* "describes a cuff-shaped dynamic orthopaedic appliance which does not include rigid polymer or metal components. It does not apply any extraneous modulating force or constraint, in contrast to the typical splint." The orthokinetic cuffs designed by Blashy and Fuchs-Neeman[1] have been used for almost 40 years for patients with muscle weakness, muscle paresis, and resulting agonist-antagonist imbalance. The action of these orthoses is "exerted through internal restoration of neuromuscular balance between agonist and antagonist musculatures, by input of mild neural stimuli to mechanoreceptors in specifically targeted skin areas."[1] The designers state that the neurophysiologic mechanism involves activation of

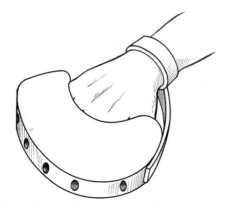

**Figure 12-1**    Bobath finger spreader (finger abduction splint).

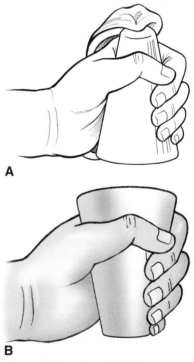

**A**

**B**

**Figure 12-2**    **A** and **B**, Firm cone.

paretic agonist muscles and reciprocal inhibition of antagonist musculature.

The orthokinetic cuffs are fabricated of ribbed elastic bandage material applied circumferentially around various aspects of the patient's upper extremity. The cuffs are held on the arm by fasteners. Half of the cuff is designed to be elastic (the active field), and the other half of the cuff is sewn to reduce the stretch (the inactive field). The active field is worn over the muscle belly to be activated, and the inactive field is placed over the antagonist.

Neeman and Neeman have published several studies[28-31] on the effectiveness of these cuffs in the rehabilitation of the upper extremity after stroke. They concluded that use of the cuffs results in pronounced restoration of agonist-antagonist muscle balance, increased active range of motion throughout the extremity, and increased ability to participate in functional tasks.

The orthokinetic cuffs have been subjected to the greatest number of efficacy studies, all showing positive results. Fabrication guidelines are stated clearly in the cited studies, and the cuffs are applied easily and are comfortable.

The neurophysiologic rationale for the orthokinetic cuff has not been established fully. The active field may produce cutaneous stimulation and activate the exteroceptors of the skin and Ia afferent neurons of the muscle spindle. The inactive field seems to provide sustained deep pressure, which may produce an inhibitory response (Figure 12-3).

### Orthokinetic Wrist Splint

The dynamic design of the orthokinetic wrist splint is based on the concepts of Rood (as cited in Stockmeyer[40]). Components of the splint include a firm cone in the palm of the hand, a volar-based forearm support, elastic straps to secure the forearm support by acting as orthokinetic cuffs, and a wrist hinge.[21] This splint has been recommended for patients with flexor hypertonicity who have at least minimal voluntary extensor activity. However, no data support the effectiveness of this splint (Figure 12-4).

### Spasticity Reduction Splint

The spasticity reduction splint was developed by Snook[38] and is based on the Bobath[3] principle of reflex-inhibiting

patterns that has not been supported by current research. The splint is fabricated of low-temperature plastic. The forearm support is dorsal based and continues into a volar-based finger support. The wrist is positioned in 30 degrees of wrist extension; the metacarpophalangeal joints are at 45 degrees of flexion. The interphalangeal joints are extended fully, the fingers are abducted with separators, and the thumb is positioned in abduction and extension. Snook[38] notes that if a flexion contracture is present, the wrist may be positioned at neutral or slightly less than neutral without producing a significant effect on the effectiveness of the splint.

Snook[38] recommends an intermittent wearing schedule, observing that "a decrease in tone is usually seen almost immediately upon splint application; however, after an extended period of wearing time, tone tends to gradually increase."

Snook's original article describes fabrication and provides clinical observations and case studies. Research was not included in this article. Snook[38] concluded that based on preliminary findings, the spasticity reduction splint has an effect "on the reduction and normalization of tone" and should be considered as a therapeutic tool when the therapist is dealing with a spastic hand.

McPherson[26] evaluated the effect of this splint on five severely and profoundly handicapped subjects (no patients who had strokes were included in this study). His results demonstrated a significant reduction in hypertonicity after 4 weeks of splint use. He further stated that the effects of the splint were not permanent; after the splints were removed, hypertonicity increased. The author measured "the force of spastic wrist flexors in pounds of pull on a spring weighted scale."

The fabrication guidelines for this splint are outlined in Snook's article.[38] Compliance in wearing schedules may be problematic because the splint is bulky and the wrist and hand are held in an extreme range. Many patients require assistance donning the splint, depending on the level of flexion posturing in their hands.

Although the principles that this splint was based on originally are out of date, this splint maintains a stretch to the musculature that traditionally becomes shortened in patients after stroke. It may be useful as an adjunct to treatment focusing on the maintenance of soft tissue length. Further research is required on patients after cerebrovascular accident to document this splint's effectiveness (Figure 12-5).

### Inflatable Pressure Splints (Air Splints)

The use of inflatable pressure splints as adjuncts to therapy was first advocated by Johnstone.[18] These splints are commercially available and exert continuous or intermittent pressure to the area to which they are applied. The

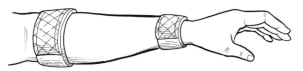

**Figure 12-3**    Orthokinetic orthotics.

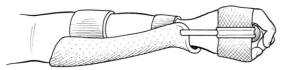

**Figure 12-4**    Orthokinetic wrist splint.

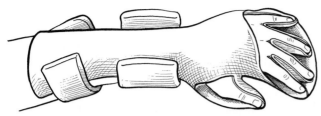

**Figure 12-5** Spasticity reduction splint.

pressure of the splints should not exceed 40 mm Hg.[37] According to Poole et al,[37] "inflatable splints have been used with patients who have had a stroke to reduce tone, facilitate muscle activity around a joint, facilitate sensory input, control edema, and reduce pain." Their article includes a review of the neurophysiologic rationales for the use of inflatable splints.

Three studies have been published of investigations of the effectiveness of inflatable splints on patients who have had strokes. The earliest was a case study by Bloch and Evans[2]; its results indicated a reduction in spasticity and an increase in hand range of motion.

Nicholson[33] (as cited by Poole and Whitney[36]) treated patients for 1 week with inflatable splints along with weight-bearing patterns. At the end of the treatment protocol, no improvements had occurred in sensation, strength, and range of motion.

Likewise, Poole et al[37] treated 18 persons and assigned them to splint or no-splint treatment protocols. The splinted group wore the splint for 30 minutes 5 days a week for 3 weeks. The splinted patients did not perform activities with the splinted extremity. The authors' results indicated no statistically significant differences in mean change in upper extremity sensation, pain, and motor function between the splinted and nonsplinted groups.

Although inflatable pressure splints do not seem to elicit the effects originally proposed, some therapists may consider using this style of splint to enhance functional performance during weight-bearing activities (Figure 12-6). In essence, this splint can be used to control the degrees of freedom in the upper extremity, thereby promoting functional use during daily activities.

## Resting Splints

The resting splint can be dorsal or volar based. The suggested position is 20 to 30 degrees of wrist extension, metacarpophalangeal joints at 40 to 45 degrees of flexion, interphalangeal joints in 10 to 20 degrees of flexion, and thumb in opposition to the index finger.[24]

One of the most important aspects of clinical reasoning is that each patient must be evaluated and treated individually, and these goniometrics should be used as a guideline only. The goal is to adjust the splint to promote a low-load prolonged stress to achieve a more advantageous biomechanical position as necessary.

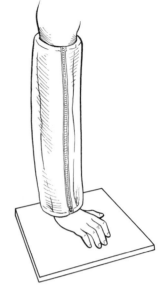

**Figure 12-6** Inflatable pressure splint.

The resting splint is used commonly in clinics. Although the splint may be effective in the long term for patients after stroke, therapists must analyze critically the effects of this splint on the patient with acute and subacute impairments. This splint blocks any automatic and voluntary attempts at movement, thereby promoting learned nonuse, because it completely covers the surface of the hand (thus preventing sensory input) and gives full passive support to the wrist and digits, which may be contrary to treatment programs attempting to train patients to be responsible for the positioning and ranging of their hands. Therapists need to consider alternatives to this splint.

Mathiowetz, Bolding, and Trombly[25] demonstrated that the use of a volar-based resting splint increased electromyographic activity in hemiplegic subjects who were performing grasping tasks with the opposite extremity. They concluded that this type of volar splint "is the least desirable positioning device while the hemiplegic subject is doing any activity that requires a comparable effort to squeezing fifty percent maximal voluntary contraction of grip."

Resting splints can be custom fabricated; they also are available commercially. The therapist may consider nighttime use of the resting splint for prevention of soft tissue contracture, but this style of splint should not be worn during daytime because it completely blocks spontaneous function, sensory input, and self-management of the hand and may promote learned nonuse (Figure 12-7).

## Tone and Positioning Splint

The tone and positioning splint is semidynamic and is commercially available from Smith & Nephew Rolyan. The splint supports the thumb in abduction and exten-

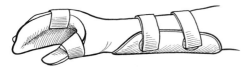

**Figure 12-7**    Resting pan splint and submaximal range splint.

sion with a neoprene glove. The tone and positioning splint includes an elastic strap that is wrapped spirally up the forearm, providing a dynamic assist into pronation and supination. Data supporting the effectiveness of this splint are not available.

Casey and Kratz[6] have published a paper on the thumb abduction supinator splint. This splint is similar in design to the commercially available tone and positioning splint. Their paper includes fabrication guidelines and recommends a wearing schedule of 3 to 4 hours on then 30 minutes to 1 hour off to allow the skin to be exposed to the air. They recommend using the splints on patients with mild to moderate spasticity without severe contractures: those who posture in a pattern of forearm pronation, with a fisted hand, and with the thumb in the palm.

The tone and positioning splint and thumb abduction supinator splint may present difficulties to patients learning to don and doff splints independently. These splints are designed to be used to enhance positioning and to be worn during functional activities. They may be particularly effective if worn during activities that result in stereotypical posturing of the limb (e.g., gait and transfers). They also may be effective during upper extremity activities because the digits are free to move (Figure 12-8).

### Thumb Loop and Thumb Abduction Splint

Variations of the thumb abduction splint have been proposed by several authors.[8,15,39] The papers cited in the references include fabrication guidelines; the splint is commercially available.

The thumb abduction splint is considered a semidynamic splint, and the focus of positioning is on thumb and wrist alignment. The strapping material used in the fabrication of this splint positions the thumb in abduction and aligns the wrist in a position of slight radial wrist extension. The hand is placed in a position that enhances prehension, manipulation, and release of objects and provides the freedom of movement needed for bilateral coordination.[15]

Stern[39] states that another indication for use is during any activity involving effort, particularly when performing fine activities with the unaffected limb results in increased thumb adduction on the affected side. Therefore, this splint has been suggested for positioning and enhancement of functional performance.

Stern[39] cautions that "For this splint to be of any value, the patients must be able to use the affected hand for grasp and release, their main problem being adduction of the thumb, which prevents sufficient opening of the hand to allow for palmar grasp." Patients with fixed adductor contracture are less likely to benefit.

Research evaluating the effectiveness of this splint in the adult population is lacking. Currie and Mendiola[8] evaluated the effectiveness of a variation of this type of splint on five children with "mild to moderate spastic hemiplegic cerebral palsy." These children exhibited a cortical thumb (adducted thumb) at rest, and their hand function was limited to a "raking" ulnar type of prehension pattern.

With the use of this splint, all five children's resting thumb patterns were enhanced, and their prehension patterns improved to a radial grasp, usually in a three jaw chuck or large cylindrical prehension pattern, depending on the size of the object being manipulated (Figure 12-9).

### Hand-Based Thumb Abduction Splint

If the patient has controlled wrist movement in flexion and extension (not necessarily full wrist range of motion,

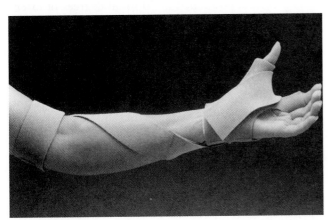

**Figure 12-8**    Tone and positioning splint. (Courtesy Smith & Nephew Rolyan, Germantown, Wis.)

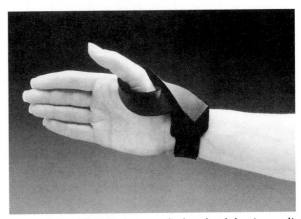

**Figure 12-9**    Thumb loop and thumb abduction splint. (Courtesy of Smith & Nephew Rolyan, Germantown, Wis.)

but some isolated control) but continues to have flexor activity influencing the digits, a hand-based thumb abduction C-spacer splint may be useful during functional activities. The splint is custom fabricated from thermoplastic material. The thumb abduction splint positions the thumb in an enhanced prehension pattern for manipulation of objects during grasp and release activities (Figure 12-10).

### MacKinnon Splint

Although the MacKinnon splint was developed for the pediatric population, it may be indicated at times for the adult population. The splint includes a dorsal-based forearm support that wraps three fourths of the distal half of the forearm, a dowel placed in the palm of the hand to provide pressure on the metacarpophalangeal heads, and rubber tubing attaching the dowel to the dorsal forearm support; the fingers are left free to assume functional patterns.

The goal of this splint is to release the overactive finger flexors and adductor pollicis to gain balanced muscle action of the wrist. The paper by MacKinnon, Sanderson, and Buchanan[23] includes fabrication guidelines and observations of approximately 30 children who used the splint and gained improved hand awareness, increased use, and decreased spasticity when the splint was removed. Research regarding the effectiveness of this splint is not available, and it has not been documented for use with the adult patient recovering from cerebrovascular accident (Figure 12-11).

### Submaximal Range Splint

The submaximal range splint was described by Peterson[35]; its design is based on the clinical observation

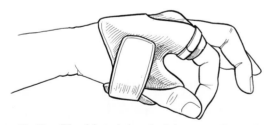

**Figure 12-10**    Hand-based thumb abduction splint to be used when wrist control returns; thumb requires abduction assistance for functional opposition activities.

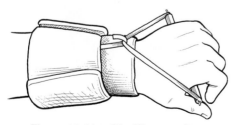

**Figure 12-11**    MacKinnon splint.

that muscles splinted on full stretch or maximal range of motion increased in tightness.

The splint is fabricated in the fashion of a resting hand splint. The splint should position the distal extremity with the thumb in partial opposition to the index finger, the metacarpophalangeal and PIP joints in 45 degrees of flexion, with distal interphalangeal (DIP) joint extension, and the wrist in 10 to 20 degrees of extension; the splint should provide pressure to the palmar arch. If the patient cannot achieve this ideal range, each joint should be positioned in 5 to 10 degrees less than the available range.[10] Fabrication guidelines are the same as those for a resting hand splint.

No research is available that evaluates the effectiveness of this splint, but the precautionary statements about the resting hand splint are similar to those for this splint design (see Figure 12-7).

### Serpentine Splint

The serpentine splint must be custom fabricated from thermoplastic materials. The splint originally was designed for use with pediatric patients with cerebral palsy who had difficulty grasping objects. The splint is adapted easily to the adult with neurologic impairments. The serpentine splint provides sufficient thumb abduction support, positions the hand and wrist in a more optimal position for function, and allows "active wrist function in the child with moderately increased tone."[41] The designers of the splint feel that the serpentine splint inhibits the thumb-in-palm reflex by using the thumb abduction position.

The authors have used an adaptation of the serpentine splint with several patients after cerebrovascular accident, with positive outcomes. The serpentine splint can be used for patients with mild to moderate increased skeletal muscle activity (it is not recommended for the flaccid hand). This splint is never recommended for hands that exhibit severe increases in skeletal muscle activity for the reasons outlined previously in this chapter.

The wrist is positioned in 20 to 30 degrees of extension, the thumb is positioned in 30 to 40 degrees of abduction, and the material continues two thirds of the length proximally up the forearm. The splint positions the hand in a more functional position for grasping exercises and activities.[41] The splint is worn during the day for activities and wrist support and is removed at night. The serpentine splint requires maximal assistance for application and moderate assistance for removal and is a practical alternative to more conventional static splints. Because the splint is an open splint, it is less confining; it also is lightweight and allows for air circulation, which results in decreased perspiration, decreased skin maceration, and reduced potential for skin breakdown. When fabricating this splint, the therapist places the roll in the palm, then wraps it around the ulnar aspect of the hand, forms it over the dorsum of the hand through the web space, brings the roll over the thenar eminence and under the base of the thumb, and continues wrapping the material two thirds of the way up the forearm. The seam made by rolling the splint material should face away from the skin to prevent skin irritation and breakdown (Figure 12-12).

### Drop-Out Splint

The drop-out splint is a custom-fabricated splint designed to decrease elbow contractures that may be common in the patient after stroke. The splint is designed from thermoplastic material positioned volarly on the humerus, distal to the axilla; it extends into the palm of the hand proximal to the distal palmar crease. The splint is fabricated with the shoulder and humerus externally rotated and the forearm in as much supination as possible. The splint is customized with a gentle stretch to the contracted elbow joint (not to the point of discomfort) using the low-load prolonged stress principles in the section Treatment of Joint Contractures with Low-Load Prolonged Stress. The splint is used during rest periods to maximize the low-load prolonged stretch to the elbow. The elbow contracture is measured with a goniometer before application of the splint and checked weekly to allow appropriate adjustments of the splint for increased extension as needed. As with all splints used in the patient who has had a stroke, but especially for splints using the low-load prolonged stretching principles, the therapist must monitor the upper extremity frequently for skin maceration and breakdown (Figure 12-13) (see Chapter 13).

### Belly Gutter Splint for Proximal Interphalangeal Joint Flexion Contractures

The belly gutter splint is a static PIP extension splint custom fabricated from thermoplastic material. Many PIP extension splints are commercially available: Joint Jack, LMB Wire-foam, and safety-pin splints, which apply two points of volar pressure to make a perpendicular pull on the involved segments, are a few. If the flexion contracture is greater than 35 degrees, these splints are not effective. Dynamic extension splints and the belly gutter splint provide traction tension at a 90-degree angle to the phalanx. The belly gutter splint provides the 90-degree angle pull by incorporating a convex belly in the middle of the gutter.[45] When fabricating and applying this splint, the therapist must place the Velcro strap directly under the PIP joint; the belly of the splint must be directly under the PIP joint axis for the splint to be effective. The authors have found this splint to be effective for flexion contractures of the PIP joint from approximately 15 degrees of contracture to 35 degrees of contracture. A PIP joint contracture of more than 35 degrees requires dynamic splinting.[11] The belly gutter splint is used at the beginning of treatment for 1 hour on and 1 hour off. Gradually, as the contracture decreases, the time may be extended to as much as 4 hours, but as always, close monitoring of the splint is mandatory (Figure 12-14).

### Inflatable Hand Splint

The inflatable hand splint, which is commercially available, is marketed for contracture management of the population in the chronic stages of stroke rehabilitation. The splint consists of an adjustable volar-based wrist support that is adjusted easily to achieve the desired range of

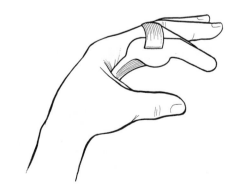

**Figure 12-13** Drop-out splint.

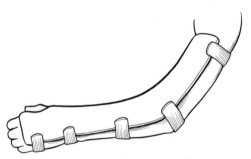

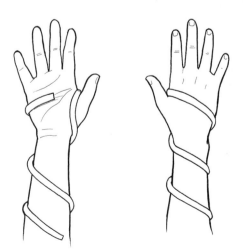

**Figure 12-12** Serpentine splint.

**Figure 12-14** Belly gutter splint for proximal interphalangeal joint flexion contractures.

extension. The palmar aspect of the splint is an air bladder that can be inflated or deflated easily, depending on the desired stretch and level of contracture. The splint is donned easily and is comfortable (Figure 12-15).

The therapist must consider many issues when prescribing or designing a splint for use on persons after stroke. The following section exposes therapists to the complexity of issues to be considered during the splinting evaluation.

## CONSIDERATIONS IN PRESCRIBING AND DESIGNING A SPLINT FOR THE DISTAL EXTREMITY AFTER STROKE

### Spasticity

Many commonly used splints are applied in the hope that they will inhibit spasticity with an end result of improved function. As outlined in Chapter 10, the cause-and-effect relationship between spasticity and function has not been supported in available research.

The link between spasticity and contracture has been well documented; see Chapter 10. Therefore, splinting of patients who are experiencing distal spasticity may be indicated to prevent painful contractures and loss of tissue length. This differentiation is important if therapists are to analyze objectively the effectiveness of the splints provided.

Hummelsheim et al[16] have demonstrated that prolonged stress resulted in "a significant reduction in the spastic hypertonus in elbow, hand and finger flexors" of the 15 patients they studied. Spasticity was measured by the Ashworth Scale. The electromyographic recordings included in their study objectively demonstrated that late electromyographic potentials are reduced or disappear after sustained muscle stretch. The authors hypothesized that "the beneficial effect resulting from sustained muscle stretch is due to stretch receptor fatigue or adaptation to the new extended position."

Although this study was based on manual stretching techniques, the same principles may be applied to splinting. Therefore, splinting may be used as an adjunct to interventions aimed at relaxing the distal extremity.

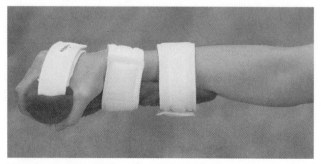

**Figure 12-15** DeRoyal's Pucci Air-T Inflatable Hand Orthosis. (Manufactured and distributed by DeRoyal.)

Feldman[10] recommends early splinting interventions for patients with spasticity; treatment should begin before the spasticity becomes severe. She states that "the longer tonal influences are left to bear on the joints, the greater the risk for contractures and other complications." Feldman also warns that patients with severe spasticity should not be considered for splinting programs. These patients are at risk for skin breakdown, edema, and circulatory impairment. Instead, Feldman recommends interventions with spasticity medication and nerve blocks for these patients (see Chapter 10).

### Soft Tissue Shortening

Many of the wrists and hands that therapists evaluate are immobilized. This immobilization may be because of weakness, static splinting for prolonged periods, excessive skeletal muscle activity, or contracture. The deleterious effects of immobilization begin to occur soon after immobilization is initiated.

Consequences of prolonged positioning following immobilization include anatomic, biochemical, and physiologic changes. Specific changes include changes in the number of sarcomeres, changes in protein content, loss of muscle weight, changes in the amount of passive and active soft tissue tension, decreased aerobic function and type I and II fiber atrophy.[13]

From their review of the literature, Gossman, Sahrman, and Rose[13] concluded that "evidence from experimental studies and clinical observations clearly indicates that muscle is an extremely mutable (prone to change) tissue. Change is more pronounced when a muscle is shortened than when it is lengthened. The changes can be deleterious, but they are reversible, a condition that can be used in correcting movement dysfunction."

Halar and Bell[14] state that if mild contractures have formed, prolonged stretches for 30 minutes are effective. More severe contractures may require longer sustained stretch through splinting. They recommend application of heat before splinting to decrease the viscous properties of connective tissue and maximize the effects of stretching.

During the splinting evaluation, the therapist must assess the differences between extrinsic and intrinsic tightness and joint contractures. Therapists must understand the biomechanical mechanism of the extrinsic flexors and extensors. To review, when the wrist and digits are in composite flexion (i.e., all joints are flexed), the extensors are stretched fully and the flexors are slack. In contrast, when the wrist and digits are in composite extension (i.e., all joints are extended), the flexors are stretched fully and the extensors are slack (Figure 12-16).

Fess and Philips[11] suggest altering wrist posture to detect extrinsic soft tissue involvement. If extrinsic tightness is evident, changing the wrist posture from slight extension to flexion results in an increase in the range of

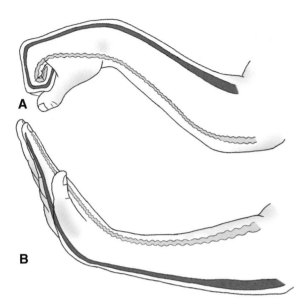

**Figure 12-16** Normal excursion of the flexor and extensor muscles acting on the wrist and hand. **A,** Wrist and digits flexed: extensors are fully stretched (elongated) and the flexors are slack (shortened). **B,** Wrist and digits extended: flexors are fully stretched (elongated) and extensors are slack (shortened).

motion of the digits (the tenodesis effect). In contrast, if range of motion limitations are caused by a pathologic condition of the joint, an altered wrist position does not affect the range of motion. Evaluation procedures for assessing extrinsic tightness are as follows: (1) extend the wrist with the digits flexed, and (2) maintain the wrist in extension and attempt to extend the digits. If composite extension can be achieved, then the extrinsic flexors have full excursion. If the digits cannot be extended while the wrist is in extension, the evaluation must continue to determine whether the limitation is related to a pathologic joint condition or extrinsic flexor tightness. The evaluation continues as follows: (3) flex the wrist and determine if the excursion of the digits toward extension (tenodesis) is increased. If so, the limitation is due to extrinsic flexor tightness. If no change in available digit extension occurs, the pathologic condition of the joint is the limiting factor[42] (Figure 12-17).

In terms of the biomechanics of the intrinsic mechanism, when the metacarpophalangeal joints are flexed and the interphalangeal joints are extended (intrinsic plus), the intrinsic muscles are shortened. In contrast, when the metacarpophalangeal joints are extended and interphalangeal joints are flexed, the intrinsic muscles are fully stretched (Figure 12-18).

Fess and Philips[11] suggest evaluating intrinsic tightness by holding the metacarpophalangeal joint in extension and attempting to flex the PIP joint; full passive flexion of the PIP joint is absent if the intrinsic muscles

have become tight. With intrinsic tightness, however, one may possibly attain full passive PIP joint flexion with the metacarpophalangeal joint in flexion (Figure 12-19).

Many patients also develop contracture of the extensor tendons. Therapists must determine whether the alteration of the position of the metacarpophalangeal joint affects the amount of flexion obtained at the PIP joint. If shortening or adhesion of the extensor has occurred, the therapist is able to flex the PIP joint further with the metacarpophalangeal joint extended than with it flexed.[42] This phenomenon occurs because extension relaxes the extensor system, whereas flexion builds up the passive tension.

Collateral ligament tightness of the PIP joint limits PIP joint motion regardless of the position of the metacarpophalangeal joint.[17] The testing is performed by flexing the PIP joint with the metacarpophalangeal joint extended and again with it flexed; if PIP joint motion is limited in both testing positions, the collateral ligaments of the PIP joint have shortened (Figure 12-20) and splinting of the PIP joint is indicated. A dynamic PIP extension splint is used if the contracture is greater than 35 degrees; a static PIP extension splint is used if the contracture is less than 35 degrees.[11] A combination of both splints sometimes is used; the dynamic splint is applied for the more severe contracture, and a static extension splint is worn after the contracture is reduced to less than 35 degrees.

Loss of active flexion of the DIP joint may be caused by joint contracture or contracture of the oblique retinacular ligament. The therapist performs the oblique retinacular ligament tightness test by passively flexing the DIP joint with the PIP joint in extension and then repeating the test with the PIP joint in flexion. If more motion occurs when the PIP joint is flexed than when it is extended, a shortening or contracture of this ligament has occurred (Figure 12-21). If equal loss of flexion occurs with the PIP joint flexed or extended, a joint contracture is evident.[17] Contracture of the DIP joint with decreased DIP flexion can be treated with the use of a flexion strap with the metacarpophalangeal, PIP, and DIP joints in as much flexion as possible. This strap can be fabricated from Velcro strapping and is commercially available (Figure 12-22). The patient can use the strap intermittently during the day for 1 hour on and 1 hour off.

### Treatment of Joint Contractures with Low-Load Prolonged Stress

Neuromuscular dysfunction is a common cause of physiologic joint restriction and contractures.[22] Splints are used to maintain or lengthen soft tissues and maintain joint integrity. If a joint has become contracted, the joint capsule becomes stiff, the synovial fluid becomes thickened from nonmovement, and the ligaments around one side of the joint become shortened, whereas the ligaments on the other side become lax. Soft tissue involvement in contractures includes shortened tendons and skeletal muscle. High-load brief stretch manual therapy alone does not achieve plastic elongation of tissues over time.[12] Low-load prolonged stress (LLPS) involves holding the tissues in a low-lengthened position for a total end range time. A low-lengthened position is a passive position with a low-load stress (in which the patient feels a slight stress but one that he or she can tolerate for a significant amount of time—for example, 3 to 4 hours total end range time). The total end range time increases over time to an ideal of 6 to 8 hours. The soft tissue grows, not stretches, to the new lengthened position.[22]

Current literature supports LLPS as the preferred method of lengthening shortened tissues. The common clinical practice of stretching contractures manually with high brief-load periods for 1 to 2 minutes is contraindicated in the literature.[22] The elongation accomplished by manual stretch alone shortens when the force is relaxed.

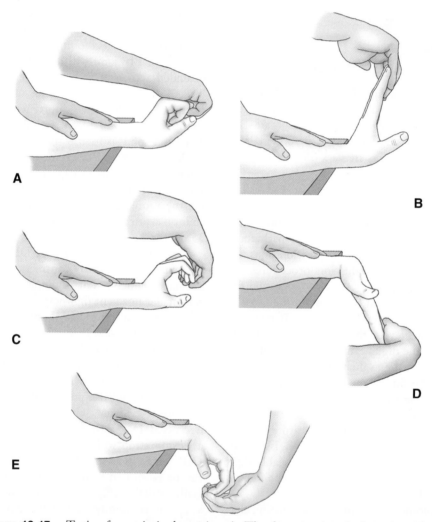

**Figure 12-17** Testing for extrinsic shortening. **A,** The therapist extends the wrist with the digits flexed. This position partially elongates the long flexors. **B,** The therapist maintains the wrist in extension and extends the digits. If composite extension can be achieved, the extrinsic flexors have full excursion and the evaluation is complete. **C,** If the therapist cannot extend the wrist and digits fully simultaneously, the evaluation must continue to determine whether the limitation is related to a pathologic joint condition or extrinsic flexor tightness. **D,** The therapist flexes the wrist to determine if excursion of the digits toward extension (tenodesis) is increased. If so, the limitation is due to extrinsic flexor tightness. **E,** If no change in available digit extension occurs while the wrist is flexed, the pathologic joint condition (i.e., bony contracture) is the limiting factor.

Manual therapy prepares tissues but must be followed with splinting and activities to effect permanent changes.[12]

A study by Light et al[22] tested knee contractures using high-load brief stretch or LLPS on 11 geriatric patients. All subjects had bilateral knee contractures; high-load brief stretch was the treatment for one knee, and LLPS was the treatment for the other. The LLPS in this study was accomplished by traction. Low-load prolonged stress produced a greater overall increase in passive range of motion than did the high-load brief stretch.

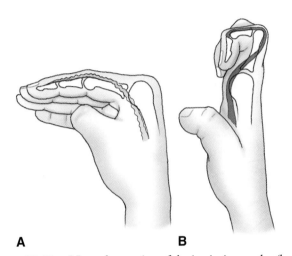

**Figure 12-18**  Normal excursion of the intrinsic muscles (lumbricales). **A,** When the metacarpophalangeal joints are flexed and the interphalangeal joints are extended ("intrinsic plus"), the intrinsic muscles are in a shortened position. **B,** When the metacarpophalangeal joints are extended and the interphalangeal joints are flexed ("intrinsic minus"), the intrinsic muscles are elongated.

Splinting to provide an LLPS is a noninvasive, nonstressful, and ideally painless treatment.[22] The treatment for joint stiffness and contracture is stress, which involves intensity (amount of effort), duration (amount of time), and frequency (amount of repetition).[12] Although all these stress factors are important, duration is the most important for LLPS, the optimal time being 6 to 8 hours. This optimal duration usually must be built up slowly, beginning with 1 to 2 hours. As the joint contracture decreases, the splint must be readjusted regularly (usually weekly) to increase prolonged stress. Low-load prolonged stress is the principle used in some of the splints mentioned previously in this chapter, including the elbow drop-out splint, the belly gutter splint, and any dynamic splinting. As with all splinting, but especially in using LLPS splinting for patients with sensory impairments, therapists must monitor patients using these splints for skin breakdown.

### Injury to the Extremity

Because of decreased motor control and perceptual dysfunction (e.g., body neglect and somatoagnosia), many patients are at risk for injuries to the already compromised extremity. Many times these patients assume malaligned upper extremity patterns for prolonged periods. A common example may be observed during bed mobility training. Patients assume sitting postures from side lying and end up bearing their weight through the dorsum of their hands with the wrist flexed. This posture puts patients at risk of developing traumatic synovitis, increased edema, and pain. The patient, depending on the level of awareness, may maintain this maladaptive posture during the next task (e.g., dressing) before noticing the problem, resulting in the potential for tissue damage.

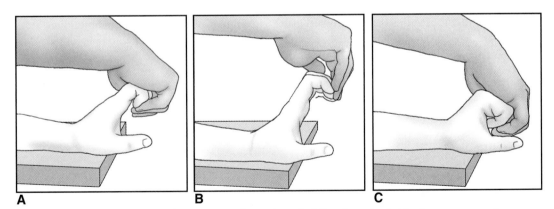

**Figure 12-19**  Testing for intrinsic shortening. **A,** The therapist holds the metacarpophalangeal joints in extension and attempts to flex the proximal interphalangeal joints. If the therapist can achieve this position, then full excursion of the intrinsic muscles is present. The evaluation is complete. **B,** If therapist cannot achieve full passive flexion of the proximal interphalangeal joint while the metacarpophalangeal joints are extended, the intrinsic muscles have become tight. **C,** With intrinsic tightness, however, the therapist possibly may attain full passive proximal interphalangeal flexion with the metacarpophalangeal joint in flexion.

Another common alignment problem that puts patients at risk for injury occurs if upper extremity positioning devices are ineffective. Many patients are prescribed half or full lap trays to provide upper extremity support while they are seated in their wheelchairs. In many cases the supported extremity slides between the lapboard and the patient's trunk, pinning the wrist in extreme flexion. Depending on patient and staff awareness, this position unfortunately may be maintained for prolonged periods. Injury also can lead to pain and swelling, which in turn may trigger the initial symptoms of shoulder-hand syndrome.

### Biomechanical Alignment

The position a hand assumes at rest (the resting posture) has been documented by several authors. A summary of this posture is as follows:

- Forearm midway between pronation and supination[24]
- Wrist at 10 to 15 degrees of extension[11]
- Thumb in slight extension and abduction with the metacarpophalangeal and interphalangeal joints flexed approximately 15 to 20 degrees
- Digits posture toward flexion, exhibiting greater composite flexion toward the ulnar side of the hand
- Second metacarpal aligned with the radius
- Palmar arches maintained (see the following section)
- Hand exhibiting "dual obliquity"

The therapist must consider the concept of dual obliquity when evaluating the alignment of the hand. Because of a successive decrease in the length of the metacarpals from the radial to the ulnar side, objects held in the hand assume two oblique angles.[34] For example, if a pencil is held in the palm across the metacarpal heads (eraser toward the ulnar side) and the forearm is held in pronation resting on the table, the examiner can identify two

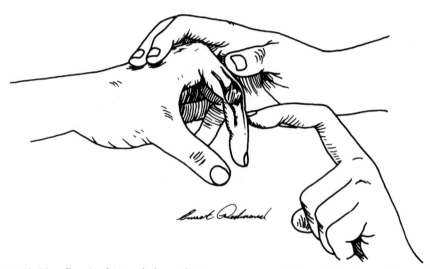

**Figure 12-20**    Proximal interphalangeal joint contracture. Collateral ligament tightness limits proximal phalangeal joint motion, regardless of the position of the metacarpophalangeal joint. (From Hunter JM, Mackin E, Callahan A: *Rehabilitation of the hand: surgery and therapy,* ed 4, St Louis, 1995, Mosby.)

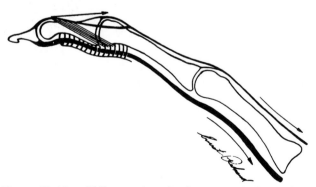

**Figure 12-21**    Oblique retinacular ligament. (Redrawn from Tubiana R: *The hand,* Philadelphia, 1981, Saunders.)

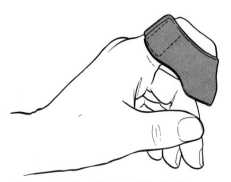

**Figure 12-22**    Flexion ("Buddy") strap.

oblique angles. The first angle is observed with the pencil point angled upward in relation to the wrist joint axis. The second oblique angle is observed on examination of height of each end of the pencil. The radial side is held higher than the ulnar side, that is, the pencil is not parallel to the table (Figure 12-23).

The obliquity of the palmar transverse arch follows a line from "the second to the fifth metacarpal head and forms an angle of seventy-five degrees with the axis of the third ray."[42] Therefore, from a biomechanical perspective, the firm cone splint discussed earlier for a moderately relaxed hand should be placed with the narrow end in the ulnar side and the wide end on the radial side, following the normal obliquity.

The therapist must note deviations from the resting posture; they assist in the design of the splint. Therapists must consider that patients may differ slightly from the normal resting posture because of heredity, habits, and job descriptions; examining the opposite hand is helpful in determining the "normal" resting posture for each patient.[21]

The distal extremity assumes several typical alignment deviations after stroke. These deviations and their consequences include the following:

1. Wrist flexion following decreased skeletal muscle activity. This common posture (most often observed in the flaccid stage) produces a variety of pathologic processes. A hand positioned in wrist flexion results in the following: flattening of the palmar arches, passive extension of the fingers as a result of tenodesis action, shortened collateral ligaments because of the extended digits, narrowing of the web space,[11] inability to perform the grasping function (flexor action of the thumb and digits reinforced by extension of the wrist),[42] blockage of ulnar and radial deviation of the wrist when it is in flexion,[19] overstretching of the

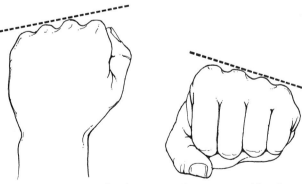

**Figure 12-23**    Dorsally, the consecutive metacarpal heads create an oblique angle to the longitudinal axis of the forearm. Distally, the fisted hand exhibits an ulnar metacarpal descent that creates an oblique angle in the transverse plane of the forearm. (From Fess EE, Philips CA: *Hand splinting: principles and methods*, ed 2, St Louis, 1987, Mosby.)

wrist extensors and dorsal ligaments,[42] shortening of the long flexors, and a tendency to develop an edema syndrome.

2. Extreme ulnar deviation. The posture of ulnar deviation results in a variety of compounded problems. A wrist positioned in extreme ulnar deviation produces the following: effective blockage of wrist extension,[19] shortening of the ulnar deviators and overstretching of the radial deviators, and shifting of the proximal and distal rows of carpal bones.[42]

3. Wrist and digit flexion. This posture may occur following excessive skeletal muscle activity and soft tissue shortening. This posture results in the following: loss of normal tenodesis function (wrist extension with digit flexion and adduction, wrist flexion with digit extension and abduction), shortening of the extrinsic flexors with resultant overstretching of the extensors, potential for skin maceration, and painful contracture and deformity.

### Loss of Palmar Arches

A familiar alignment problem in patients after stroke is the loss of palmar arches, or the development of a "flattened hand." The maintenance of the palmar arches is crucial for hand function.[4] Kapandji[19] outlines the arches of the hand as follows (Figure 12-24):

■ Transverse arch: This structure consists of two arches and includes the carpal arch, which corresponds to the concavity of the wrist and is continuous with the distal metacarpal arch formed by the metacarpal heads. The carpal arch is rigid, whereas the metacarpal arch is mobile and adaptable. The long axis of the transverse arch crosses the lunate, capitate (the "keystone" of the carpal arch[11]), and the third metacarpal bones. Boehme[4] states that the functional significance of this arch stems from its forming the hand into a gutter, bringing together the radial and ulnar borders of the hand. This arch can widen or narrow the surface area of the hand.

■ Longitudinal arch: This arch includes the carpometacarpophalangeal arches. These arches are formed for each finger by the corresponding metacarpal bones and phalanges. Kapandji[19] notes that the arches are concave on the palmar surface; the "keystone" of each arch lies at the level of the metacarpophalangeal joint. According to Boehme,[4] in its simplest form this arch supports a basic cylindrical grasp. If the arches are expanded, the hand is longer. This arch allows the palm to flatten and cup itself around objects.[11]

■ Oblique arches: These arches are formed by the thumb during opposition with the other fingers. Kapandji[19] states that the most important of these arches is the one linking the thumb and index finger; the most extreme is the one linking the thumb and the little finger. These arches are obviously crucial in the opposition of the digits.

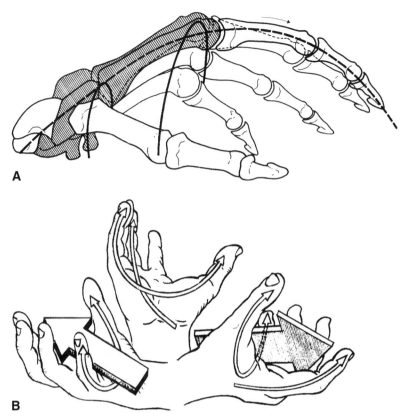

**Figure 12-24**    **A,** Side view of the longitudinal and transverse arches of the hand. The shaded areas show the fixed part of the skeleton. **B,** The thumb forms, along with the other digits, four oblique arches of opposition. The most useful and functionally important arch is between the thumb and index finger, used for precision grip. The farthest arch, between the thumb and little finger, ensures a locking mechanism on the ulnar side of the hand in power grips. (From Tubiana R, Thomine JM, Mackin E: *Examination of the hand and wrist,* St Louis, 1996, Mosby.)

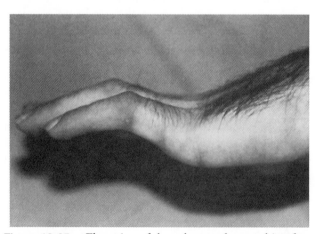

**Figure 12-25**    Flattening of the palmar arches resulting from hand paralysis. Hyperextension of the metacarpophalangeal joints and flexion of the proximal and distal interphalangeal joints occur because of an imbalance of the extrinsic flexor and extensor systems. (From Hunter JM, Mackin E, Callahan A: *Rehabilitation of the hand: surgery and therapy,* ed 4, St Louis, 1995, Mosby.)

Patients lose their arches after stroke for a variety of reasons, including edema in the dorsum of the hand that biomechanically forces the metacarpals inferiorly, inactivity of the wrist and hand, prolonged and extreme wrist flexion (resulting in a flattening of the arches), and inappropriate support of the hand during weight-bearing activities.[4]

During evaluation of splinting, therapists should examine the arches of the hand and compare them with those of the unaffected hand. In the dorsal surface of a normal hand at rest, the metacarpophalangeal joints form an arch with the apex at the third metacarpal (i.e., the third metacarpal head is higher than the others) (see Figure 12-24). Many patients have a flattened arch (i.e., the metacarpophalangeal joints lose their arches), and in response the proximal phalanges hyperextend. This posture puts the patient at risk for developing a permanent claw-hand deformity and effectively blocks opposition of the thumb (Figure 12-25).

In these cases, splinting may be indicated to give outside support to the arches through upward pressure on the palmar surface of the hand. To be effective and give full support to the metacarpals, the splint must conform to the arches and be contoured to the individual's hand. Commercially available splints are not effective for this type of intervention because they do not take into account the variability of arches.

For patients with hyperextended metacarpophalangeals and flexed PIP joints (i.e. claw-hand deformity), a dorsal metacarpophalangeal extension restriction splint can be fabricated in thermoplastic material to eliminate deformity and increase function (Figure 12-26).

### Learned Nonuse

Current research (see Chapter 10) has demonstrated the existence of a component of upper extremity dysfunction resulting from a learned phenomenon of nonintegration of the hand into functional tasks. This process likely begins in the early stages after stroke, before any functional recovery has commenced. Patients learn to compensate with their unaffected sides, thereby repressing any return of function on the hemiplegic side.

Many cerebrovascular accident protocols call for splinting immediately after stroke. Some facilities have standing orders for splinting in their acute services. Current research indicates that early splinting in the early poststroke phase may be detrimental. The splint gives a message that an outside device is responsible for the maintenance and improvement of the affected hand. Because the hand is supported and aligned through outside means, the patient does not attend to the hand, stretch the wrist and hand, or attempt to integrate it into functional tasks. In other words, early splinting may predispose patients to a learned nonuse phenomenon. A sign that a patient is predisposed to learned nonuse is the observation that a patient, after cueing, can integrate functional return during a therapy session but does not integrate this new function outside the sessions. The therapist must balance interventions for contracture prevention with activities that encourage functional use of the hand, thereby negating the effects of learned nonuse. Splinting for contractures can be used at night instead of during the day to prevent learned nonuse behavior patterns.

## DECISION-MAKING PROCESS

The therapist must evaluate all of the following areas when deciding whether to splint and choosing the type of splint to fabricate. This section is designed to help guide the therapist's clinical reasoning in making splinting decisions.

1. Evaluate cognitive and perceptual status: Does the patient attend to the extremity during the day (attending includes self-ranging, rubbing, positioning, and protecting)? Is the patient alert for the greater portion of the day?

   If the answer is yes, the patient may be able to maintain range of motion and alignment in the extremity without the use of splints; the therapist should consider not splinting.

   If the answer is no, neglect, decreased attention, somatoagnosia, and decreased alertness and arousal may place the patient at risk for contracture and malalignment; splinting therefore may be indicated.

2. Evaluate soft tissue tightness: Does the patient have full composite flexion and extension? Can the patient be ranged into a full intrinsic minus/intrinsic plus position? Does the patient have full and pain-free range of wrist motion, especially extension and radial deviation?

   If the answer is yes, the therapist should consider not splinting. Treatment should focus on teaching the patient and family techniques to maintain this range and prevent pain and contracture.

   If the answer is no, splinting may be indicated to improve or at least maintain soft tissue length. The splint should be designed to place the shortened soft tissues on prolonged stress.

3. Evaluate joint contracture: Splinting is necessary to ameliorate joint contracture and prevent further deformity.

4. Evaluate learned nonuse: Does the patient integrate the extremity into functional tasks in the clinic without carryover into nontherapy hours?

   If the answer is yes, the therapist should consider not splinting. In this situation the patient does have distal function; this function should not be impeded by splinting. The splint may in fact feed into the learned nonuse cycle.

5. Evaluate function: Does the patient exhibit distal motor control (including gross patterns) that can be integrated into activities of daily living and instrumental activities of daily living?

   If the answer is yes, the therapist should consider not splinting or should choose a splint that enhances the functional return (e.g., a basic wrist extension splint to provide a stable proximal segment for the digits to work from or a simple opponens splint to improve fine motor control).

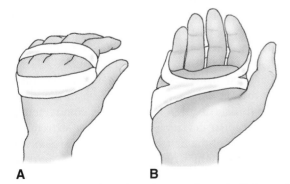

**A**        **B**

**Figure 12-26**   Anticlaw splint. **A,** Dorsal view. **B,** Palmar view.

If the answer is no, splinting may be indicated, although the therapist must consider that splinting a hand without functional recovery may block the initial motor return (sometimes automatic reactions and protective responses) or the patient's initial attempts at function.

6. Evaluate potential for soft tissue injury: Is evidence of skin maceration and laceration in the palm of the hand and lateral aspect of the thumb from extreme flexion apparent?

   If the answer is yes, the therapist seriously must consider splinting to prevent further damage and enhance the healing process; wrist extension splints with distal cones or palm guards are recommended.

   If the answer is no, the therapist should consider not splinting.

7. Evaluate biomechanical alignment: Are deviations from the standard resting position of the hand evident? Does realigning the hand result in increased relaxation?

   If the answer is yes, the therapist should consider splinting to improve resting alignment of the extremity to prevent shortening and overstretching of soft tissue.

   If the answer is no, the therapist should consider not splinting.

8. Evaluate sensation: Does the patient have sensory impairments?

   If the answer is yes, the therapist should consider the amount of cutaneous surface area that is covered by splinting. The splint may end up blocking the little sensory input the hand is receiving. A general goal for the involved extremity is to maximize sensory input. If sensation is impaired, extra precautions are necessary for careful, custom splint fabrication and diligent, ongoing monitoring of the skin condition by the therapist, patient, and family for any breakdown or maceration, which the patient may not detect. This is especially important if cognitive deficits are present.

9. Evaluate edema: Does the patient have distal edema? If the answer is yes, the therapist should consider whether a splint will support a flexed wrist with the goal of counteracting the dependent positioning of the hand, thereby decreasing or preventing further edema. Will the immobilization of the splint increase the edema by blocking the "pumping action" of muscles generated by active range of motion? Patients with edema tend to lose digit flexion, thereby keeping the collateral ligaments in a shortened position. Will the splint block digit flexion, thereby exacerbating this problem? Will the splint impinge on neuromuscular structures and further limit hemodynamic function?

10. Evaluate posturing: Does the patient posture in persistent flexion?

- If the answer is yes, the therapist should consider splinting to maintain stress on soft tissues. Rechecking of biomechanical alignment is essential; proximal realignment may relax the hand.
- If the answer is no, the therapist should consider not splinting.

## GENERAL SPLINTING GUIDELINES

Therapists should consider the following guidelines regarding splinting:

1. Check for abnormal pressure points, especially over bony prominences (e.g., ulnar head).
2. Decide during which activities and periods the patient will wear the splint. The splint must be evaluated or fabricated while the patient is in the most difficult posture and performing the most stressful activities if the effectiveness of the splint is to be evaluated. For example, fabricating a splint while the patient is seated and relaxed may result in a good fit with a relaxed hand. However, if the patient then leaves therapy to prepare a meal at home, the therapist may find the patient's hand "clawing" and flexing out of the splint. If the splint was fabricated with the patient standing and with the appropriate level of stretch, this phenomenon may not be a problem.
3. Splint for comfort. Pain and pressure responses may increase the patient's bias toward stereotypical posturing.
4. Patients need to experience full range of motion. Use positioning splints only as adjuncts to a comprehensive upper extremity program.
5. Monitor full range of motion. Many patients have been provided with resting hand splints to prevent flexion contractures only to end up with extension contractures, or "intrinsic lock."
6. Make wearing schedules practical to ensure patient compliance.
7. Therapists must have reasonable expectations for splints. An extremely tight hand may require several serial splints to achieve a desired position. Splints designed to provide correction at more than one joint can lead to added deformity if excessive skeletal muscle activity is present. For example, attempting to position the wrist and digits into extension may create a clawing effect in the digits as a result of the amount of stretch at the wrist and digits.[43] A severely malaligned hand may respond best if the therapist only focuses on one particular aspect of the malalignment (proximal first). For example, counteracting the extreme ulnar deviation in this type of extremity may be the goal of the first splint, followed by neutral deviation with slight wrist extension for the next splint. The therapist must remember that with an extremely tight or contracted hand, all deformities cannot be

addressed simultaneously; if simultaneous correction is attempted, compliance with splinting may be jeopardized because of the discomfort level and skin breakdown.

8. Educate patients about the realistic goals and expectations of the use of a splint. Many patients wear their splints for prolonged periods with the hope that the splint will "make their hand better." Most patients interpret "better" as a return in function. However, this may not be the case for all patients; therefore the patient should be aware of the reasons that the splint was prescribed. No splint should be worn continuously.

## GENERAL FABRICATION GUIDELINES

Many splinting materials are commercially available today. They are basically thermoplastic materials; some have more rubber content base than others. The rubber content base materials tend to have increased conformability and drape compared with pure thermoplastic materials, but they may be more difficult to handle because of their draping quality.

Thermoplastic materials generally have a greater memory capacity than do the rubber-based thermoplastics. Memory indicates the capability of the material to return to its original shape after the reheating that occurs during fabrication of the splint. Some therapists prefer the thermoplastics because of the memory capacity. The thermoplastics are available in perforated and solid forms. Perforated materials are recommended to allow for breathability and decrease the possibility of skin maceration (especially with patients with sympathetic nerve changes and sensory impairments). The therapist must take care when using maxiperforated thermoplastics to eliminate sharp edges after cutting the material. The edges must be heated with a heat gun and turned down to smooth the edging; the edges also may be covered with $1/16$-inch solid material cut into 1-inch wide but long pieces, heated in water, and then applied to the edging. The therapist also may use a thin layer of moleskin to smooth the edges of perforated material.

The thermoplastic materials and rubber-based thermoplastics are available in various thicknesses ranging from $1/8$ inch, $3/32$ inch, $1/12$ inch, and $1/16$ inch; the most common width is $1/8$ inch. Some of the splinting materials are available in a wide range of colors; these may help draw attention to the involved limb and prevent the splint from being lost in hospital bedding. Color also may enhance compliance. Several vendors offer precut splint blanks and kits. These products can be cut to size for customization and to decrease the amount of splinting time required for fabrication. Prefabricated splints also are available for many splinting needs, but some may be difficult to customize. The authors do not recommend some of the commercially available spring wire splints for patients with sensory impairments because these splints may apply too much pressure that the patient will not be able to detect. Custom-fabricated splints are the splints of choice for patients with sensory impairments.

Velcro strapping materials are now available in multiple colors. Velfoam, a padded strapping material, is highly recommended for the patient with sensory impairments because it is a softer strapping material.

Splint padding does not compensate for a poorly fitted splint and increases the pressure within the splint. Splint padding is recommended to cushion fingers at the point of contact of the thermoplastic material in dynamic splints only. Splint padding is available under different trade names. Splint padding materials only increase the pressure of an ill-fitting splint. Splint padding materials used in this way also may be hot and uncomfortable for the patient and may increase the possibility of skin maceration because of the increased perspiration that the padding may cause in a patient.

Splinting the extremity of a patient with neurologic involvement is sometimes difficult if severely increased skeletal muscle activity is evident in the upper extremity. Maintaining the desired alignment and molding the splinting material may be almost impossible. The assistance of another person for positioning usually is indicated for a proper fit. Pattern-making also may be difficult with this type of patient. The fabrication of a gross pattern on the unaffected hand and reversal of the pattern for transfer to the splinting material are helpful at times.

The therapist must make allowances for bony prominences by cutting around or flaring the splinting material over the prominence. A helpful hint for flaring out the material is to place a spot of dark lipstick over the bony prominence (on the patient's skin); place the cooled, already formed splint on the patient; and remove the splint. The lipstick now will be on the splint in the exact spot at which the splint requires flaring.

During the use of thermoplastic materials in splinting, the placement of curve in the material increases the tensile strength of the material to approximately 20 times that of straight material. This is helpful to remember in the fabrication of dynamic outriggers from thermoplastic material or the creation of an additional roll in the material as a spine or support.

## SPECIFIC FABRICATION GUIDELINES

### Forearm Support

If the splint prescribed for a patient includes a forearm trough, basic splinting principles call for the trough to cover two thirds of the forearm. To compensate for the weight of the hand and the excess force created by increased distal flexor activity, the forearm trough should be two thirds of the length of the forearm to provide a sufficient lever.

## Palmar Support

Many patients with neurologic involvement have flattened arches at the metacarpophalangeal joints, with resultant clawing of the digits. This malalignment usually occurs in patients with little or no skeletal muscle activity in the affected hand. In molding the splint into the palmar arch in these cases, the therapist can use the thumb to mold a letter T pattern over the palmar surface of the splint. The base of the T runs longitudinally through the center of the palm, whereas the top of the T runs across the metacarpal heads. The base of the T should connect to the top of the T at the third metacarpophalangeal head. The T shape is molded into the palm to enhance the arch. To ensure sturdy arch support, the splint must progress distal to the distal palmar crease and does not need to clear the thenar eminence in a hand without movement. The therapist should reevaluate the patient frequently for returning motor control and should adjust the splint as needed. If the patient exhibits controlled digit flexion, the distal end of the splint needs to be rolled back proximal to the distal palmar crease so that returning function is not blocked. If the patient begins to exhibit thumb function, the palmar support surface of the splint must again be rolled back to clear the thenar eminence and therefore not block active movement.

After splint fabrication, the therapist evaluates the palmar support section of the splint by checking that the dual obliquity of the hand is maintained, the third metacarpal head is the apex of the arch formed by the metacarpal heads, and the hand is not "flattened" in the splint (Figures 12-27 and 12-28).

## Wrist Support

When molding and evaluating the wrist component of a splint for the patient after stroke, the therapist must consider alignment:

- The third metacarpal should lie midway between the radius and ulna in a neutral deviated hand. Many hands with neurologic involvement have a tendency to assume a position of ulnar deviation. Splint modifications to the wrist component include raising the border of the splint that lies lateral to the fifth metacarpal. This modification effectively blocks the ulnar deviation (Figure 12-29).
- The wrist should be supported between 0 and 20 degrees of extension. The final decision depends on which angle allows the maximal amount of function or (if the hand is not functional) which angle in this range decreases the usual abnormal flexor activity in the digits. (Many patients' digits relax if they are realigned proximally.) In some cases the splint may be fabricated in some degree of flexion. This may be required if contracture

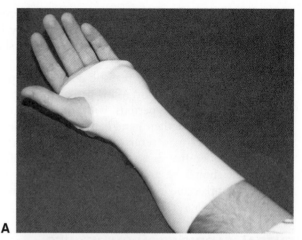

**A**

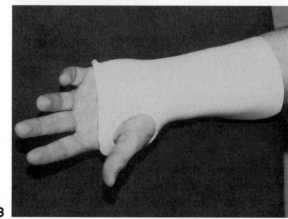

**B**

**Figure 12-27**    Variations on palmar support fabrication. **A,** Full palmar support (material progresses past the distal palmar crease and gives the thumb support over the first metacarpal). **B,** As function returns, the distal and thenar aspects of the splint are rolled back to allow for joint excursion during functional tasks. The T shape is molded into the palmar aspect of the splint.

of the extrinsic flexors is evident and the goal is systematically to lengthen the flexors with serial splinting. In these cases each subsequent splint should be molded with an increased stretch on the flexors. For example, the first splint may be molded in 20 degrees of wrist flexion; the next in 10 degrees of flexion, neutral wrist; and finally in some degree of extension. Therapists must remember that if the goal is to lengthen the extrinsic flexors, wrist and digit support is required.

- After molding the splint, the therapist should check that the hand is not in a position of medial or lateral rotation (neutral) compared with the forearm. Many patients who exhibit excessive skeletal muscle activity develop a tendency for the hand to rotate medially or laterally in relation to the forearm. The hand should be positioned in the splint so that the fifth metacarpal is aligned with the ulna instead of lying inferior to the ulna (the hand is laterally rotated in relation to the

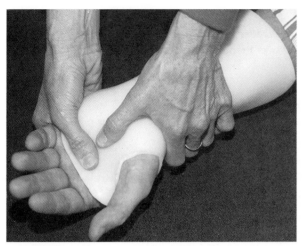

**Figure 12-28**   Molding the T support into the splint. The base of the T runs longitudinally through the palm, whereas the top of the T supports the metacarpal arch. The base of the T intersects the top of the T at the third metacarpal head. Palmar support is accurate if the arches of the hand are maintained and the third metacarpal head is superior to the metacarpal heads of digits two and four.

forearm) or lying superior to the ulna (the hand is medially rotated in relation to the forearm).

### Digit Support

The therapist should use a digit support platform only as a last resort. The therapist must include a digit support platform in the splint if the patient exhibits excessive flexor activity in the digits that cannot be otherwise controlled and if the patient is being splinted for contracture management. If the splint includes a digit platform, daytime use of the splint is discouraged.

If a patient exhibits excessive flexor activity, the therapist first should try a forearm and wrist splint that enhances

alignment. In many patients a proximal realignment of the joints and a prolonged state of accommodation of muscles to their resting length relaxes the hand. Therapists can evaluate this phenomenon by manually realigning the joints with their hands and evaluating whether a relaxation response occurs.

If a digit support platform is necessary, the digits should not be overstretched to the point that a "clawing" of the hand or a "bottoming out" of the metacarpals occurs. The therapist must ensure that the palmar arch remains intact when the digits are stretched onto the platform (Figure 12-30).

### Thumb Support

In the nonfunctional hand the thumb should be supported in a position midway between palmar and radial abduction. This position can be maintained by the previously described palmar support, which also supports the first metacarpal; if the splint is rolled back to clear the thenar eminence, the thumb cannot be supported in this position (see Figure 12-27).

If the thumb is functional, the splinted position is dictated by evaluation of the position of thumb that is the most effective at enhancing function with the thumb in opposition. Figure 12-31 describes the clinical reasoning process followed for deciding on the type and style of splint to fabricate.

### Prefabricated Splints

In cases in which prefabricated splints are indicated, therapists must take great care to assure proper fitting. Patients should not be encouraged to purchase splints "off the shelf" without a therapist's input because of the potential complications. Examples of commonly used and useful prefabricated splints include air-assist splints for LLPS (see Figure 12-15), a multipodus ankle/foot orthosis (Figure 12-32), and elbow splints to provide stretch (Figure 12-33).

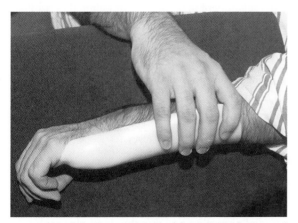

**Figure 12-29**   The lateral aspect of the splint is built up along the fifth metacarpal effectively to block ulnar deviation.

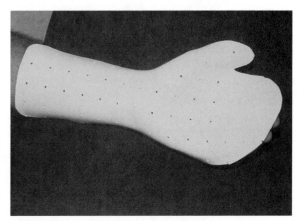

**Figure 12-30**   Full support provided to the distal extremity. This style of splint is recommended only if alternative attempts of proximal realignment do not relax the hand. This splint is recommended for night use only.

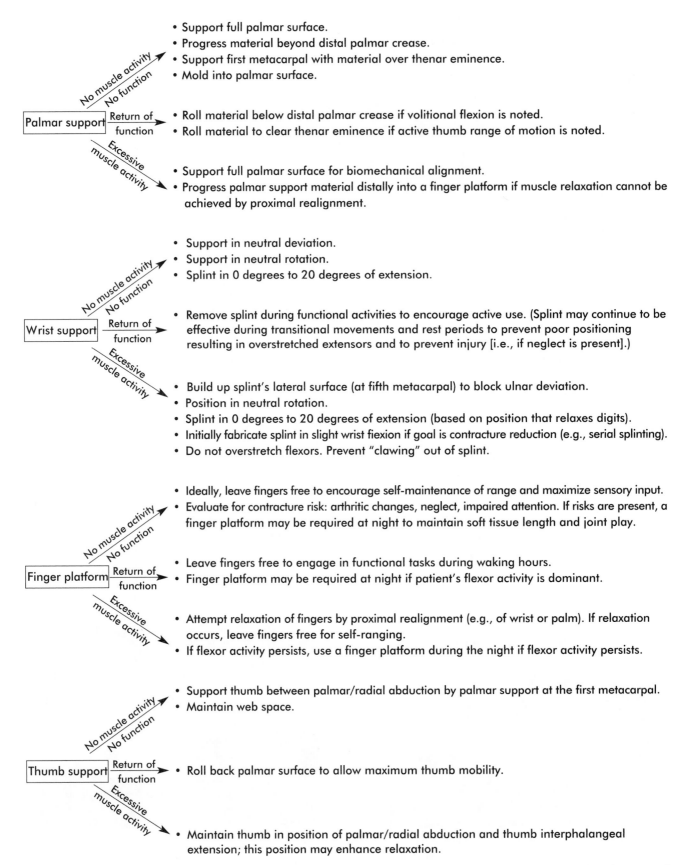

**Palmar support**

*No muscle activity / No function*
- Support full palmar surface.
- Progress material beyond distal palmar crease.
- Support first metacarpal with material over thenar eminence.
- Mold into palmar surface.

*Return of function*
- Roll material below distal palmar crease if volitional flexion is noted.
- Roll material to clear thenar eminence if active thumb range of motion is noted.

*Excessive muscle activity*
- Support full palmar surface for biomechanical alignment.
- Progress palmar support material distally into a finger platform if muscle relaxation cannot be achieved by proximal realignment.

**Wrist support**

*No muscle activity / No function*
- Support in neutral deviation.
- Support in neutral rotation.
- Splint in 0 degrees to 20 degrees of extension.

*Return of function*
- Remove splint during functional activities to encourage active use. (Splint may continue to be effective during transitional movements and rest periods to prevent poor positioning resulting in overstretched extensors and to prevent injury [i.e., if neglect is present].)

*Excessive muscle activity*
- Build up splint's lateral surface (at fifth metacarpal) to block ulnar deviation.
- Position in neutral rotation.
- Splint in 0 degrees to 20 degrees of extension (based on position that relaxes digits).
- Initially fabricate splint in slight wrist flexion if goal is contracture reduction (e.g., serial splinting).
- Do not overstretch flexors. Prevent "clawing" out of splint.

**Finger platform**

*No muscle activity / No function*
- Ideally, leave fingers free to encourage self-maintenance of range and maximize sensory input.
- Evaluate for contracture risk: arthritic changes, neglect, impaired attention. If risks are present, a finger platform may be required at night to maintain soft tissue length and joint play.

*Return of function*
- Leave fingers free to engage in functional tasks during waking hours.
- Finger platform may be required at night if patient's flexor activity is dominant.

*Excessive muscle activity*
- Attempt relaxation of fingers by proximal realignment (e.g., of wrist or palm). If relaxation occurs, leave fingers free for self-ranging.
- If flexor activity persists, use a finger platform during the night if flexor activity persists.

**Thumb support**

*No muscle activity / No function*
- Support thumb between palmar/radial abduction by palmar support at the first metacarpal.
- Maintain web space.

*Return of function*
- Roll back palmar surface to allow maximum thumb mobility.

*Excessive muscle activity*
- Maintain thumb in position of palmar/radial abduction and thumb interphalangeal extension; this position may enhance relaxation.

**Figure 12-31**    Fabrication decisions: clinical reasoning. A volar-based forearm trough that supports two thirds of the forearm with sides parallel to the radius and ulna serves as the base splint in this decision-making process.

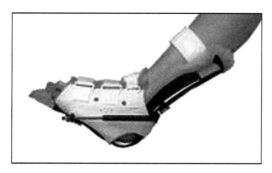

**Figure 12-32** Multi Podus Phase II System (Restorative Care of America Inc.). This orthosis allows the ankle to be positioned incrementally towards neutral. The total range is from 40 degrees of plantar flexion to 10 degrees of dorsiflexion.

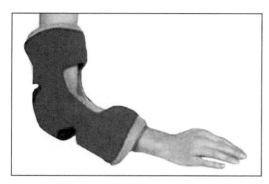

**Figure 12-33** Arm-Respond Range of Motion Elbow Orthosis (Restorative Care of America Inc.). This orthosis allows the elbow to be positioned in 10-degree increments of flexion or extension.

## SUMMARY

When designing or fabricating a splint for a patient after stroke, the therapist must consider each patient individually; no set of rules applies to all patients with neurologic impairments. No definitive answers or protocols are available. The reader is encouraged to consider the questions in the decision-making section of this chapter to guide clinical reasoning, because the therapist must consider so many factors in treatment.

Any hand with a malalignment or deformity results in an overstretching of the soft tissues (muscles, ligaments) on one side of the joint and shortening of the soft tissues on the opposite side. All treatment, including splinting, should be instituted after consideration of this phenomenon and should aim to preserve the length and balance of soft tissue on either side of the joint. This treatment prepares the hand for possible future integration into functional activities and prevents permanent deformity.

All splints applied to patients after stroke, especially patients with increased skeletal muscle activity and decreased sensation who are being treated with the principles of LLPS, must be monitored continually by therapists, nursing staff, and family members to assess for skin integrity. This concept is particularly crucial for patients with cognitive and perceptual deficits. Factors in the monitoring of skin integrity include signs of skin discoloration, maceration, edema, and breakdown.

Splinting for patients after stroke that combines the principles of biomechanical positioning and the neurophysiologic concepts of facilitation and inhibition may lead to the most favorable components of function.[44]

Realistic outcomes must be the guiding forces in the decision-making process in the fabrication of splints for patients after stroke. Clinicians working with this population who use splinting as an adjunct treatment should strive to gain a solid understanding of anatomy, biomechanics, and motor control theories.

Finally, therapists have a responsibility not only to stay current on research regarding this area of intervention but also to add to the literature through research, from single-subject case studies to qualitative trend analyses to large subject-sample qualitative studies. Until more definitive and well-designed research studies are available concerning this treatment, the splinting controversy for patients after stroke will continue, and therapists may be providing patients with less than optimal care.

## REVIEW QUESTIONS

1. What is the normal resting posture of the hand? What are the common malalignments observed after a stroke?
2. What precautions should be followed when splinting a patient after stroke?
3. What is the recommended rationale for splinting the patient after stroke?
4. How does the therapist differentiate among intrinsic tightness, extrinsic tightness, and joint contracture when evaluating for a splint?
5. What are the advantages of low-load prolonged stress versus high-load brief stretch?

## REFERENCES

1. Blashy MRM, Fuchs-Neeman RL: Orthokinetics: a new receptor facilitation method, *Am J Occup Ther* 13:226-234, 1959.
2. Bloch R, Evans MG: An inflatable splint for the spastic hand, *Arch Phys Med Rehabil* 58(4):179-180, 1977.
3. Bobath B: *Adult hemiplegia: evaluation and treatment*, ed 3, Oxford, 1990, Butterworth-Heineman.
4. Boehme R: *Improving upper body control: an approach to assessment and treatment of tonal dysfunction*, Tucson, 1988, Therapy Skill Builders.
5. Brennan J: Response to stretch of hypertonic muscle groups in hemiplegia, *Br Med J* 1:1504-1507, 1959.
6. Casey CA, Kratz EJ: Soft splinting with neoprene: the thumb abduction supinator splint, *Am J Occup Ther* 42(6):395-398, 1988.
7. Charait SE: A comparison of volar and dorsal splinting of the hemiplegic hand, *Am J Occup Ther* 22(4):319-321, 1968.
8. Currie DM, Mendiola A: Cortical thumb orthosis for children with spastic hemiplegic cerebral palsy, *Arch Phys Med Rehabil* 68(4):214-217, 1987.
9. Doubilet L, Polkow LS: Theory and design of a finger abduction splint for the spastic hand, *Am J Occup Ther* 21(5):320-322, 1977.

10. Feldman PA: Upper extremity casting and splinting. In Glenn MB, Whyte J, editor: *The practical management of spasticity in children and adults*, Philadelphia, 1990, Lea & Febiger.

11. Fess EE, Philips CA: *Hand splinting: principles and methods*, ed 2, St Louis, 1987, Mosby.

12. Flowers K: Orthopaedic assessment and mobilization of the upper extremity, *Scar Wars I & II*. Seminar conducted in New York City, 1992.

13. Gossman MR, Sahrman SA, Rose SJ: Review of length associated changes in muscles: experimental evidence and clinical implications, *Phys Ther* 62(12):1799-1808, 1982.

14. Halar EM, Bell KR: Contracture and other deleterious effects on immobility. In Delisa JA, editor: *Rehabilitation medicine: principles and practice*, ed 2, Philadelphia, 1993, JB Lippincott.

15. Hill SG: Current trends in upper extremity splinting. In Boehme R, editor: *Improving upper body control: an approach to assessment and treatment of tonal dysfunction*, Tucson, 1988, Therapy Skill Builders.

16. Hummelsheim H, Munch B, Butefisch C, et al: Influence of sustained stretch on late muscular responses to magnetic brain stimulation in patients with upper motor neuron lesions, *Scand J Rehabil Med* 26(1):3-9, 1994.

17. Hunter JM, Mackin E, Callahan A: *Rehabilitation of the hand: surgery and therapy*, ed 4, St Louis, 1995, Mosby.

18. Johnstone M: *Restoration of motor function in the stroke patient: a physiotherapist's approach*, New York, 1983, Churchill Livingstone.

19. Kapandji IA: *The physiology of the joints*, vol 1, *Upper limb*, ed 5, New York, 1982, Churchill Livingstone.

20. Kaplan N: Effect of splinting on reflex inhibition and sensorimotor stimulation in treatment of spasticity, *Arch Phys Med Rehabil* 43:565-569, 1962.

21. Kiel JH: *Basic hand splinting: a pattern-designing approach*, Boston, 1983, Little, Brown.

22. Light KE, Nuzik S, Personius W, et al: Low-load prolonged stretch vs high-load brief stretching in treating knee contractures, *Phys Ther* 64(3):330-333, 1984.

23. MacKinnon J, Sanderson E, Buchanan J: The MacKinnon splint: a functional hand splint, *Can J Occup Ther* 42(4):157-158, 1975.

24. Malick MH: *Manual on static hand splinting*, ed 5, Pittsburgh, 1985, Harmarvile Rehabilitation Center.

25. Mathiowetz V, Bolding DJ, Trombly CA: Immediate effects of positioning devices on the normal and spastic hand measured by electromyography, *Am J Occup Ther* 37(4):247-254, 1983.

26. McPherson JJ: Objective evaluation of a splint designed to reduce hypertonicity, *Am J Occup Ther* 35(3):189-194, 1981.

27. McPherson JJ, Kreimeyer D, Aalderks M, et al: A comparison of dorsal and volar resting hand splints in the reduction of hypertonus, *Am J Occup Ther* 36(10):664-670, 1982.

28. Neeman RL, Liederhouse JJ, Neeman M: A multidisciplinary efficacy study on orthokinetics treatment of a patient with post-CVA hemiparesis and pain, *Can J Rehabil* 2:41-52, 1988.

29. Neeman RL, Neeman M: Efficacy of orthokinetic orthotics for post-stroke upper extremity hemiparetic motor dysfunction, *Int J Rehabil Res* 16(4):302-307, 1993.

30. Neeman RL, Neeman M: Orthokinetic orthoses: clinical efficacy study of orthokinetics treatment for a patient with upper extremity movement dysfunction in late post-acute CVA, *J Rehabil Res Dev* 29(ann suppl):41-53, 1992.

31. Neeman RL, Neeman M: Rehabilitation of a post stroke patient with upper extremity hemiparetic movement dysfunction by orthokinetic orthoses, *J Hand Ther* 5:147-155, 1992.

32. Neuhaus BE, Ascher ER, Coullon BA, et al: A survey of rationales for and against hand splinting in hemiplegia, *Am J Occup Ther* 35(2):83-90, 1981.

33. Nicholson DE: The effects of pressure splint treatment on the motor function of the involved limb in patients with hemiplegia, master's thesis, University of North Carolina, 1984, Chapel Hill.

34. Pedretti LW: Hand splinting. In Pedretti LW, Zoltan B, editors: *Occupational therapy: practice skills for physical dysfunction*, ed 3, St Louis, 1990, Mosby.

35. Peterson LT: Neurological consideration in splinting spastic extremities, unpublished paper, 1980.

36. Poole JL, Whitney SL: Inflatable pressure splints (airsplints) as adjunct treatment for individual with strokes, *Phys Occup Ther Geriatr* 11(1):17-27, 1992.

37. Poole JL, Whitney SL, Hangeland N, et al: The effectiveness of inflatable pressure splints on motor function in stroke patients, *Occup Ther J Res* 10(6):360-366, 1990.

38. Snook JH: Spasticity reduction splint, *Am J Occup Ther* 33(10):648-651, 1979.

39. Stern GR: Thumb abduction splint, *Physiotherapy* 66(10):352, 1980.

40. Stockmeyer S: An interpretation of the approach of Rood to the treatment of neuromuscular dysfunction, *Am J Phys Med* 46(1):900-961, 1967.

41. Thompson-Rangel T: The mystery of the serpentine splints, *Occup Ther Forum* pp 4-6, Sept 20, 1991.

42. Tubiana R, Thomine JM, Mackin E: *Examination of the hand and wrist*, St Louis, 1996, Mosby.

43. Wilson D, Caldwell C: Central control insufficiency. III. Disturbed motor control and sensation: a treatment approach emphasizing upper extremity orthoses, *Phys Ther* 58(3):313-320, 1978.

44. Woodson AM: Proposal for splinting the adult hemiplegic hand to promote function. In Cromwell FS, editor: *Hand rehabilitation in occupational therapy*, Redding, Calif, 1988, Hawthorne Press.

45. Wu SH: A belly gutter splint for proximal interphalangeal joint flexion contracture, *Am J Occup Ther* 45(9):839-843, 1991.

46. Zislis JM: Splinting of hand in a spastic hemiplegic patient, *Arch Phys Med Rehabil* 45:41-43, 1962.

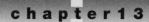

# lauren joachim

## chapter 13

# Casting Applications

## key terms

| | | |
|---|---|---|
| anteroposterior splint | drop-out cast | plaster |
| bivalve cast | fiberglass | reflexes |
| casting | heterotopic ossification | resting cast |
| cerebrovascular accident | holding cast | serial casting |
| contracture | inhibitory casting | spasticity |

## chapter objectives

After completing this chapter, the reader will be able to accomplish the following:

1. List objectives of casting a patient who has survived a stroke.
2. List indications for casting a patient who has survived a stroke.
3. List precautions when casting.
4. List contraindications to casting.
5. Describe what to consider clinically when evaluating a patient for casting.
6. Compare and contrast plaster and fiberglass.
7. Compare and contrast various types of casts, their associated indications, and their pros and cons.
8. Develop an understanding of casting progression guidelines.
9. Describe cast application and removal procedures.
10. Describe fabrication of various casts including drop-out and bivalve casts.
11. Describe clinical issues relating to casting a patient who has survived a stroke.

Little documentation exists in the literature regarding the use of serial and inhibitory casting for patients who have had a stroke. Most of the literature published is developed for use with patients diagnosed with traumatic head injury, cerebral palsy, and quadriplegia.* Patients who have survived a stroke may be at risk for developing soft tissue contracture or severe spasticity. Casting may be

necessary when traditional methods of treatment have failed and the patient is at risk for contracture because of severe spasticity. If not treated, a variety of dysfunctions and problems may develop, such as functional limitations in self-care and instrumental activities of daily living; inability for caregivers to assist patients with bathing, hygiene, and dressing; and an unpleasant appearance, skin breakdown, or a negative perception of body image. Traditional therapeutic interventions include using passive

---

*References 1, 4, 7, 9, 10, 16, 17, 19, 21, 23, 25, 29, 31, 32, 34, 36, 37.

range of motion (PROM) activities, generalized and localized inhibitory handling techniques, splinting, positional devices, myofascial release, acupressure, physical agent modalities, a tilt table, positioning, nerve blocks, and pharmacologic intervention.* Serial casting has been demonstrated to be effective in reducing spasticity and contractures.†

Anesthetic and phenol nerve blocks, drugs, and topical anesthesia have been used for treating and diagnosing spasticity. Procaine or lidocaine hydrochloride anesthetic nerve blocks may be used before cast application to relax spastic muscles. Repeated use of nerve blocks may reduce spasticity enough to improve function. For example, an obturator nerve block may aid a patient who has a scissoring gait. Anesthetic nerve blocks can be used to differentiate spasticity from fixed contracture. In addition, nerve blocks provide a preview of more permanent phenol nerve blocks and tendon-lengthening procedures.

Phenol nerve or phenol motor point injections enable further rehabilitation during recovery. Peripheral phenol nerve blocks may be used for severe spasticity because complete cessation of muscle activity occurs. A therapist performing an open peripheral nerve injection of nerves containing motor and sensory branches should inject only the motor branches to prevent dysesthesia and loss of sensation after the nerve block. Therapists may perform phenol motor point injections at the bedside for patients with minimal spasticity that is interfering with function. The block lasts 1 to 2 months; repeat blocks may be performed. Spastic muscles are not relaxed as completely as they are with peripheral nerve blocks.[12]

Drugs may benefit patients with spasticity resulting from a stroke. Medications more commonly used to treat spinal cord–injured patients with spasticity may be used in the stroke population. However, presently no uniform treatment is known for this population. Therapists use drugs on each patient individually until achieving a satisfactory effect. Therapists must consider side effects. Drugs most effective in reducing spasticity include baclofen, diazepam, dantrolene, chlorpromazine, clonidine, and progabide.[5,12] Baclofen (Lioresal) may be used orally or intrathecally. Baclofen is less sedating than diazepam and equally effective. The effects of baclofen on cerebral forms of spasticity are presently not clear. In the brain-injured population, baclofen may interfere with attention and memory. Baclofen has been demonstrated to be safe for long-term use and has a low incidence of side effects. Orally administered diazepam (Valium) is generally not appropriate for patients with brain injuries because of its negative effects on attention and memory. Intellectual impairment and reduction in motor coordination are possible side effects, and physiologic addiction is possible.

Withdrawal symptoms may appear if diazepam is tapered too quickly. Orally administered dantrolene (Dantrium) is the preferred drug for cerebral forms of spasticity such as spastic hemiplegia. Dantrolene is less likely to cause lethargy or cognitive dysfunction than baclofen or diazepam. Dantrolene is likely to decrease clonus and muscle spasms from innocuous stimuli. Dantrolene has been suggested to "weaken" muscles; however, its effect on spasticity does not affect motoric function. Hepatotoxicity (liver toxicity) may occur in approximately 1% of the population. The therapist also may try orally administered chlorpromazine, orally and transdermally administered clonidine, and orally administered progabide in an effort to decrease spasticity in cerebral forms of edema.[5] No spasticity-reducing drugs are given intravenously.

Topical anesthesia (20% benzocaine sprayed for 15 seconds) applied to the patient's skin is an additional treatment that has been used successfully to decrease hypertonicity resulting in increased active range of motion, PROM, and improved gait pattern.[28] An example of the use of this form of topical anesthesia is the "spray and stretch technique."

Casting can be done on upper and lower extremities. Tissues shorten in time if not lengthened regularly. These tissues can lengthen if undergoing constant, prolonged stretching.[23] Through animal studies, Tabary et al[31] have demonstrated that changes in muscle fiber and sarcomere length and number occur with prolonged stretch. Although the same process is suggested to occur in human beings, it has not been proved.

Serial casting is based on the biomechanics of muscle length. Casts are used with contracted muscles to provide prolonged stretch in a lengthened position to allow for changes in sarcomere distribution, increased muscle or tendon length, or both. Multiple casts are applied gradually to increase range of motion (ROM) until full ROM is restored or maximum attainable range occurs. Inhibitory casting uses positioning to relax muscles and pressure to decrease excessive skeletal muscle activity.[17] This mechanism remains unclear. Some rationales include neutral warmth and constant pressure, an increase in muscle or tendon length, and inhibition of Golgi tendon organs and muscle spindles.[1,3,23,30] Neutral warmth is a local inhibitory technique that may cause a decrease in γ–motor neuron activity.[8] Continuous, slow stretching places the contracted muscle of the casted limb in a prolonged position at maximal tolerable length. Maintaining this position causes cutaneous stretch receptors to adapt rapidly, thus causing inhibition by preventing additional stimuli from entering the system.[8,33] Continuous pressure is inhibitory; it activates the pacinian corpuscles, which are rapidly adapting receptors. Pressure on a tendon insertion activates deep receptors by applying pressure across the longitudinal axis of a tendon.[33] Sometimes casting combines serial casts and positioning.

---

*References 1, 8, 12, 17, 19, 23, 27.
†References 1, 4, 16, 17, 19, 21, 23, 25, 31, 34, 36, 37.

When performing serial or inhibitory casting, the therapist must consider the effects of long-term immobilization. In 1982, Booth[3] documented that when a muscle was immobilized in a shortened position, the muscle atrophied. However, when the muscle was in a lengthened position, the muscle enlarged. After weeks of immobilization, muscles composed of predominately slow-twitch fibers took on characteristics of fast-twitch muscles. Electromyographic activity of immobilized limbs was reduced 5% to 15% compared with controls. In addition, the resting membrane potential of immobilized limbs did not change or decrease.

The effectiveness of prolonged stretch has been documented since as early as 1959 in a study of 14 hemiplegic patients with spasticity for an average duration of 18 months from onset.[6] The author studied the responses to stretch of 19 flexor muscle groups, 18 upper extremities, and 1 lower extremity for 3 years. Each flexed limb was stretched constantly in extension with a polythene-polyurethane splint for an average of 3 months. When increased active extension was demonstrated and the flexor spasm terminated for at least 1 month, the splint was worn for shorter daily periods of time. The splint was removed twice daily for bathing. At that time, the patient was encouraged to move the limb actively. Most of the patients demonstrated decreased spasticity and increased active range of motion. A follow-up visit revealed that the gains were maintained with an increase in function. However, the length of the period before the follow-up and the amount of increase in function were not specified. Those patients who did not improve in their functional abilities did at least demonstrate improved body appearance resulting from improved limb posture. The author of this study suggests the following time guideline for prolonged stretching that will abolish different degrees of spasticity with lasting effects: 12 weeks of constant stretching followed by 8 weeks of intermittent stretching for moderate spasm. This time should be adjusted for lesser and greater amounts of spasm.

In 1989, MacKay-Lyons[24] reported that low-load prolonged stretching with the Dynasplint successfully reduced elbow flexion contracture following head trauma. A Dynasplint is a dynamic elbow splint that consists of two adjustable cuffs with medial and lateral struts hinged at the joint axis. By varying the tension of the springs housed in each of the distal struts, one can alter the amount of force applied across the joint. After a trial of the splint, the contracture decreased from −67 degrees of elbow extension to −15 degrees of elbow extension, a gain of 52 degrees. Range of motion gains were still present at follow-up evaluations conducted 2 and 6 months after treatment. Average splint wear was 8 to 12 hours per day at a tension setting of 10. Positive outcomes included decreased flexion contracture, an increase in bilateral upper extremity use for activities of daily living, and the ability to ambulate short distances with a walker.

The use of serial and inhibitory casting for patients who have had a stroke has been documented in the literature.[1] The literature is inconsistent regarding which factors are necessary if casting is used to decrease excessive muscle activity. A point that has been suggested but not demonstrated is that the cast maintains the limb with excessive muscle activity in a reflex-inhibiting position. Reflex-inhibiting postures are defined by Bentzel as positions that inhibit spasticity by passively elongating spastic muscles.[2] The effectiveness of reflex-inhibiting postures has not been demonstrated in the research literature. In addition, the roles of total even pressure and neutral warmth in reducing spasticity have been claimed and reported. The combination of the static position of the joint and muscle and neutral warmth and constant pressure has been postulated to cause thermal and rapidly adapting tactile receptors to turn off, thus reducing the influence on the excitability of interneurons, motor neurons, or both.[1] Barnard et al[1] reported the use of early cylindrical, short leg plaster casts on an 11-year-old who sustained a closed-head injury and could not be treated with traditional therapies. Positive results were achieved: the patient's overall increased muscle activity decreased, and spontaneous movement of the left extremities and ankle ROM increased.

A 1994 study by Hill[16] compared casting to traditional treatment techniques, which included PROM activities, stretching, and splinting for severe brain-injury patients whose upper extremities had increased muscle activity. Fifteen subjects with brain injury were assigned randomly to receive one of two treatments: (1) 1 month of casting followed by 1 month of traditional therapy, or (2) 1 month of traditional therapy followed by 1 month of casting. The subjects were evaluated before intervention, after the first month of intervention, and after the second month of intervention for ROM, clinical indications of spasticity, and functional use. All but one patient's ROM improved with casting rather than with traditional therapy. Decreased spasticity with casting occurred in 11 of the 15 subjects; however, the decrease did not translate into improved function with either group.

In 1990, Yasukawa[34] casted a 15-month-old patient who was first seen with spastic hemiparesis. Initially, four short arm serial casts were each used for 1 week. In the second phase, the unaffected extremity was casted to encourage active use of the involved extremity. In the third phase a bivalve, long arm splint was used at night on the affected arm. Increased scapular stability and humeral flexion, use of the affected limb during transitions, and spontaneous use of the involved limb during bilateral tasks were reported after 1 ½ years.

Law et al[21] examined the use of a short arm cast on 73 children with cerebral palsy. The children were divided into four treatment groups: (1) regular neurodevelopmental treatment, (2) regular neurodevelopmental treatment and a cast, (3) intensive neurodevelopmental treatment, and (4) intensive neurodevelopmental treatment and a cast. Quantitative differences were not found between the groups. However, quality of movement and wrist extension were found to be improved in casted groups.

King[19] discussed treatment of a 46-year-old patient who had suffered a subarachnoid hemorrhage and intraventricular bleeding following aneurysm clipping. Traditional inhibitory techniques along with purposeful activity had been unsuccessful in reducing spasticity. A series of plaster drop-out casts were fabricated. A full circumferential portion enclosed the upper arm from axilla to the olecranon process; a volar forearm portion was added to prevent elbow flexion. The elbow was placed in maximum achievable extension. Ranging and bilateral upper extremity activities were implemented. Later a bivalve cast was worn for 12 hours at night for 2 weeks until the patient could actively and passively maintain range. Passive ROM increased from −90 degrees of elbow extension to −20 degrees of elbow extension, a 70-degree gain. Once discharged from the inpatient rehabilitation unit, the patient was followed up biweekly for 4 months. The patient was monitored for an increase in independence with activities of daily living and maintenance of active use of the impaired extremity with no return of spasticity. Specific gains regarding functional use were not reported. Gains were maintained and attributed to a reduction in elbow spasticity.

Smith and Harris[29] used casting to prevent an increase in elbow flexion contracture of a 5 ½-year-old girl with spastic quadriplegia. They initially observed a sharp decrease in elbow flexion contracture and then a slight increase.

Tona and Schneck[32] compared short-term upper extremity inhibitive casting with encased thermoplastic splinting on an 8 ½-year-old girl with upper extremity spasticity. Increased quality of movement, increased awareness and use of the casted extremity, and decreased spasticity and resistance to passive movement were noted but only lasted for 3 days.

Kaplan[18] examined the use of dorsal splinting on the surface opposite the spastic muscles to provide prolonged stretching for hemiplegic upper limbs. A light splint consisting of three to four layers of plaster and one external layer of fiberglass impregnated with resin on the outside were used. Velcro straps held the splint in place. Patients wore the splint as long as it was tolerable. Range of motion and gross motor activity improved. The study did not report whether the patients were followed up.

Zachazewski, Eberle, and Jefferies[37] described the use of short leg inhibitory casts on a 25-year-old man who sustained a head injury in a motor vehicle accident. The patient had a positive support reaction in bilateral lower extremities, which was elicited during weight-bearing activities, transfers, and standing. Medications were not successful because of resulting drowsiness. Ice placed on the gastrocnemius and soleus muscles was also not effective. Bilateral lower extremity inhibitory casts were fabricated and left in place for 4 weeks. When the casts were removed, the patient's gait had improved. The positive support reaction was decreased in the right lower extremity and absent in the left. Several days after cast removal the positive support reaction reappeared in the right lower extremity during ambulation. The casts were made bivalve and used at night but were ineffective. A molded polypropylene "tone-inhibiting ankle foot orthosis" then was fabricated for the right lower extremity. The patient's gait improved, and the positive scissoring was reduced enough to allow the patient to use a rolling walker to ambulate with supervision or minimal assistance. The authors of the study suggest that an inhibitory cast should be used to assess the patient for gains before fabricating a tone-inhibiting ankle-foot orthosis because it is quicker, cheaper, and less complex to fabricate. In addition, casting may be needed to increase the patient's ROM and static stretching before fabrication of the tone-inhibiting ankle-foot orthosis.

In summary, the serial casting has been demonstrated to be successful in increasing active and passive ROM, decreasing increased muscle activity, decreasing pressure, and less so at improving function in some cases. If the therapist chooses this technique as an intervention, the goals must be clear (i.e., increasing function, improving cosmesis, and improving hygiene) and the benefits must outweigh the risks.

## CAUSES OF SOFT TISSUE CONTRACTURES

A patient who has had a stroke with resultant spasticity, cognitive and perceptual deficits (e.g., body neglect), hemiparesis, or hemiplegia is at risk for developing soft tissue contracture.[15] Tissues may shorten if not stretched over a period of time.[8] Traditional treatments to prevent soft tissue shortening include use of PROM activities, splinting, and other techniques.[1,23] A patient with a decreased level of alertness and poor attention, concentration, initiation, memory, or cooperation may not be able volitionally to perform the ROM activities necessary to maintain full joint range. This potentially could result in soft tissue contracture(s).[27] In addition, a patient with unilateral body neglect may not acknowledge the affected side; therefore the patient usually cannot perform self-ROM activities. A patient with hemiparesis may not have the motor control to move the joint actively through full ROM, thus contributing to soft-tissue contracture. A patient with hemiplegia also may not be able to take the joint through full ROM as a result of pain or inability to perform self-ROM effectively. Patients who have had a stroke may develop spasticity to varying degrees.

Patients with severe spasticity may develop reduced joint mobility as a result of ineffective treatment modalities to maintain joint ROM or reduce spasticity.

## CASTING OBJECTIVES

The therapist should consider the following objectives when planning for casting therapy:
1. Improve ROM.
2. Decrease influence of excessive skeletal muscle activity.
3. Lengthen or maintain soft tissue contracture.
4. Obtain or maintain proper joint alignment.
5. Increase efficiency of available movement.
6. Increase functional use of an extremity.
7. Enable fit of a more definitive orthosis by improving ROM and positioning and decreasing spasticity.
8. Evaluate for "hidden" potential for motion.
9. Decrease joint posturing.

## CASTING INDICATIONS

The therapist should consider the following indications for casting therapy:
1. Spasticity[3,4,10,14,36]
2. Soft-tissue contracture[3,14]
3. Active and passive ROM limitations*
4. Pathologic reflexes
5. At least a 10-degree limitation of ROM at a joint
6. Severe spasticity resulting in potential joint contracture or deformity that is not responding well to traditional medical or physical treatment
7. Demonstrated neurologic recovery when loss of ROM is a result of spasticity and not other factors, such as heterotopic ossification, healing fracture, or ligamentous injury[25]
8. A need for fit of a more definitive orthosis
9. A need to evaluate for "hidden" potential for motion

## CASTING PRECAUTIONS

When casting a patient, observation of safety precautions is imperative. The therapist must consider the following:
1. Avoid poor casting technique, insufficient padding, or poor patient positioning, all of which may result in imperfect casting.[23]
2. Agitated patients are at risk for skin breakdown from cast abuse.[23] Fiberglass generally is not recommended because it splinters, leaving sharp edges.[4]
3. Use flat rather than flexed fingers and precise hand placement. Minimize indentations within the cast while the patient is being positioned during cast formation. Abnormal pressure points may cause skin breakdown.

4. Bony prominences such as the olecranon process, malleoli, and calcanei are common sites of skin breakdown. Bony prominences should be well padded.[4,23]
5. Cast cutters can abrade or cut the skin during cast removal. Have the safety of the unit checked periodically.
6. Improper casting procedures can cause late-onset peripheral neuropathy resulting from nerve compression from the cast. Ulnar and peroneal nerves are most at risk for compressive neuropathy.[23]
7. Wrapping a limb too tightly in a cast can obstruct venous return and result in edema. Remove a cast that results in discoloration of toes or fingers of a casted limb for more than 20 to 30 minutes or when capillary refill is not observed from the outset. However, temporary skin discoloration during casting is not uncommon[3,4,23,25] and may be associated with peripheral circulatory changes or in response to heat generated as the cast sets.
8. Do not initiate weight-bearing activities for 24 hours after cast application to promote hardening of casting material, prevent skin breakdown, prevent deformities of the interior plaster, and prevent indentations.[4,10,23,25]
9. Patients may not tolerate multiple casts well.[3] They can be heavy and limit function. In addition, they may interfere with homeostasis by elevating body temperature, and they limit limb access for monitoring vital signs or intravenous use.
10. Discomfort is expected within the first 24 hours after cast application. Analgesic medications usually alleviate this discomfort. Discomfort should not be severe.[3,9]
11. Casting can cause edema, which can result in decreased circulation because of cast compression of the vascular and lymphatic structures of the limb. Elevating the casted extremity can decrease the amount of occurrence of edema.[3,10]
12. Impaired sensation may place the patient at risk for skin breakdown.[10]
13. The therapist must consider dermatologic conditions such as cellulitis, fungus growth, open wounds, and those caused by drug reactions when deciding whether to cast the patient. Skin maceration may occur if moisture builds up in the cast.
14. Patients with impaired communication abilities may not be able to express that they are experiencing pain and discomfort.
15. Patients who have difficulty tolerating stress on related musculoskeletal areas may be prone to development of tendonitis or trigger points.
16. Perform a plaster sensitivity test before cast application if the patient has sensitive skin.
17. After cast application, check for red areas, pulse at points distal to cast, pain, temperature comparison of

---

*References 3, 4, 10, 14, 17, 22, 36.

both extremities, swelling, discoloration of hand or foot and nail beds, and dusky veins.

18. Check the patient's position before cast application.

19. Check whether the patient has a known allergy to a casting material.

20. Check whether the patient has adherent scar tissue.

21. The cause of heterotopic ossification is not known. Heterotopic ossification is the formation of bone in abnormal sites. The literature reports that heterotopic ossification can develop in patients who have had a STROKE. Heterotopic ossification most commonly develops in limbs with spasticity or those that have experienced trauma.[11] Clinical signs of heterotopic ossification include pain, decreasing ROM, and mildly swollen joints. Joints may be warm. The patient's alkaline phosphatase blood level will be elevated. Diagnosis is by radiographs and bone scans. The role of PROM with heterotopic ossification remains controversial. Some authors report maintenance or increases in PROM with joint manipulation or judicious ROM. Other authors report PROM or manipulation enhances the heterotopic ossification process.[12] Literature does not document specifically the role of PROM or joint manipulation for the patient who has survived a stroke. Generally, the therapist may use active and active assistive ROM. When heterotopic ossification is present, controversy surrounds whether aggressive joint ROM or manipulation should be performed or whether it worsens the situation.[13] Management of major heterotopic ossification may include aggressive joint manipulation while under general anesthesia. When the patient is under anesthesia, spasticity can be differentiated from bony ankylosis. Surgical excision has not always been successful.[12] Documentation regarding whether serial casting is contraindicated is inconsistent throughout the literature.[3,13] In cases of heterotopic ossification, the therapist should stretch gently, change casts more frequently, range joints between cast changes to prevent solidification or fusion, and alternate bivalve casts between flexion and extension to prevent loss of ROM in either direction.

22. Plaster of Paris casts can burn a patient's skin. Lavalette, Pope, and Dickstein[20] found that skin could be burned under certain circumstances: (1) the water in which to dip the casting material is greater than 24° C, (2) the cast is greater than eight ply, (3) a pillow is used over the cast while setting and prevents dissipation of heat from the cast, and (4) the casting material is not dipped in water for an adequate amount of time. Rapid, intense, localized heat may penetrate deep into the cast, which prevents dissipation of heat and places the patient at risk for being burned.

## CASTING CONTRAINDICATIONS

The literature regarding contraindications to casting is inconsistent. Following is a list of contraindications that are found most consistently in the literature.*

1. Severe heterotopic ossification of the joint(s) may be enhanced[13] by casting.[23,25]

2. Fluctuating muscle activity may not be responsive to serial casting.

3. Skeletal muscle rigidity is not responsive to serial casting.[22,35] These limbs already resist passive stretch in both directions. Static positioning of a limb with a cast for 5 to 7 days may exacerbate the stiffness. An alternative may be to alternate bivalve casts in submaximal flexion and extension to reduce skeletal muscle rigidity and gradually increase joint ROM in both directions.[35]

4. Skin conditions (open wounds, abrasions, blisters, lacerations, skin graft) are contraindications.[4,17,23,25,26] Using bivalves and windows may be options to open access to compromised skin in some circumstances.

5. Edema in the extremity may impair distal circulation, place the patient at risk for a compartmental syndrome, or have a tourniquet effect. A compartmental syndrome is a condition in which circulation to a structure such as a nerve or tendon is being constricted in an enclosed space. The structure may no longer be able to move freely in the compartment. The intracompartment pressure rises, and circulation ceases. The tissues eventually necrose in the enclosed space.

6. Occurence of subluxation of the carpal bones or other orthopedic deformities that may require specialized interventions such as surgery.

7. Impaired circulation indicated by pale skin color, low skin temperature, trophic changes, significant edema, and low distal pulse of the extremity to be casted may cause the casted limb to become cyanotic.[26] The patient may develop a compartmental syndrome.

8. Severe spasticity may cause microtears in the soft tissues resulting from improper fit, overstretching, and poor positioning.[7] Bleeding may result and cause a compartmental syndrome.

9. Extreme wrist extension can cause carpal tunnel syndrome because pressure is placed on the tunnel and magnifies the symptoms. Circulatory problems also may cause cyanosis of the limb.

10. Uncontrolled hypertension may result because the cast causes an isometric contraction and may increase blood pressure.[26]

11. Patient, physician, or family does not provide consent.[26]

---

*References 4, 7, 17, 22, 25, 26, 34, 35.

12. Sensory or motor changes of the extremity to be casted may indicate circulatory problems, compartmental syndromes, or nerve impingement.[10,26]
13. Unstable fractures that exist in the extremity to be casted.[4,26] Do not serial cast until fractures are healed and stable, because the patient may resist the cast and displace the fracture. Dislocation of the fragments or fixation is possible.
14. Presence of pathologic inflammatory conditions, including arthritis of the joints proximal and distal to the casted joints, and gout.[26]
15. Limb access is required for an intravenous line or to monitor vital signs.[4,23,25]
16. Patients are in danger of abusing themselves or getting injured.[26]
17. Intracranial pressure is unstable[4,14,23] because the cast is an isometric contraction and may increase intracranial pressure.
18. Diaphoresis, as well as the isometric effects of the cast, produce the potential for the skin to macerate under the cast.[23]
19. Contracture existing longer than 6 to 12 months.[3,4,23]
20. Poor compliance and/or attendance as an outpatient.
21. Internal fixation devices that limit ROM.
22. Metastatic disease with a risk of fracturing.

## PRECASTING ASSESSMENT

When traditional methods for maintaining and improving range of motion or managing spasticity have failed and casting is being considered, a precasting assessment is advisable. Initially, the therapist reviews the patient's hospital course and present medical status for potential contraindications to casting and notes baseline skin integrity, mental status, circulation, orthopedic conditions, course of rehabilitation therapy, and potential length of stay. The therapist may evaluate circulation by checking capillary refill; the therapist applies pressure and withdraws pressure from the fingertip or toe. The area touched initially should blanch (turn white) on application of pressure and immediately return to its usual color on removal of pressure. If the patient is an outpatient, the therapist should review compliance, the attendance record, and the support from caregivers. The therapist must weight the risks and benefits of casting and must consider the cost, time, disposition, and goal of casting.

The patient must be medically stable and without medical contraindications to casting (see Casting Contraindications) if a casting program is to be initiated. Additionally, the patient and/or caregiver, as well as the physician, must consent to the casting program. Following is a list of initial evaluation considerations:

1. Skin integrity: Observe skin for open wounds; irritation; skin breakdown; edema; and excessively dry, moist, or sweaty skin. Is skin fragile or thin? If casting will be used despite skin irritation or breakdown, photograph skin before and after casting to compare skin integrity.[22] Consider using extra padding, T-foam, and drop-out casts. If skin is macerated, identify and manage the source of maceration before casting. Sources of maceration may include incontinence, vascular insufficiency, or sweating. Do not cast over an infection or wound. The wound would be enclosed and not have proper aeration and could not be accessed for wound care.
2. Sensation: Does the patient have absent or impaired proprioception; graphesthesia; two-point discrimination; or perception of sharp and dull, light touch, and pressure?[22] If a patient's sensation perception is absent, function may be compromised severely; therefore casting may not be appropriate unless the goal is to increase ROM.[3]
3. Circulation: Is blanching occurring? What are the color and temperature of nailbeds and extremities? Are pulses distal to the cast strong (e.g., radial for elbow and pedal for knee)? Is capillary refill good? Are trophic changes present?
4. Continence: Hygiene and cleanliness within the cast are affected in an incontinent patient who requires lower extremity casting.
5. Joints: Assess active and passive ROM,[3] temperature, soft tissue restrictions, and end feel. End feel is the feeling at the completion of range of motion of a joint.[22] End feel may be empty, gradual, abrupt, nonyielding bony, or painful. When end feel is empty, nothing indicates an ending has been reached, but the therapist realizes that further pushing may cause damage. When end feel is gradual, it allows the therapist to feel a gradual tightening of soft tissues as end range is approached. When end feel is abrupt, end range is reached without any tapering. A bony end feels as if the therapist has hit one bone against another. A patient may complain of pain as the end of range is approached (a painful end feel). The therapist may use a local anesthetic nerve block when necessary to differentiate spasticity from fixed contracture. Nerve blocks eliminate spasticity but do not affect muscle-tendon length. The therapist can use an anesthetic nerve block to allow normal joint position if the only cause of the deformity is spasticity.[3] The therapist must differentiate soft tissue contracture from joint contracture if the muscle crosses two joints. To evaluate for the type of contracture, flex the proximal joint and note the resultant position of the distal joints. Joint contracture is not affected by change in position of the proximal joint. If the deformity is soft tissue contracture, a procaine nerve block will not correct the joint deformity. A hard end feel often indicates a bony block, which is usually not responsive to serial casting.[22] Do joints or soft tissues

require mobilization before casting? What is the patient's active control, selective, or patterned movement?[3] What is patient's hand function?

6. Contracture: What is the duration of the contracture? Contractures of shorter duration tend to be more responsive to serial casting.[3,4,22]

7. Glenohumeral joint subluxation: If such subluxation is present, will the weight of the cast affect the proximal glenohumeral joint and pull the humerus into subluxation?

8. Position of scapula: What is the position of the scapula on the thorax (e.g., is subluxation evident)? Will the added weight of the cast adversely affect the position of the scapula on the thorax?

9. Effects on joints: In what way will the additional stress from the cast affect other joints proximal and distal to the cast?[22]

10. Joint stretching: Can one joint be stretched in isolation without other joints being stretched?[22]

11. Cast requirements: Will the cast require a plantigrade surface or wedge for ambulation or weight-bearing activities?

12. Muscle activity responsiveness: Does the patient respond to relaxation and handling techniques that optimize position for casting? Patients with muscle activity that is responsive to handling should benefit from casting. Rigid, unchanging skeletal muscle activity probably will not be responsive. Are abnormal reflexes present that will affect casting?[22] For example, if an asymmetrical tonic neck reflex is present, will this affect application of the cast?

13. Mental status: Is the patient self-abusive or abusive to others? Is the patient combative? What is the patient's level of alertness? Can the patient communicate with others? Can the patient follow directions?[3] Are caregivers able to manage the patient with a cast?

14. Orthopedic considerations: Are fracture(s) present? Heterotopic ossification may preclude casting.[3,22] Consider the option of using drop-out casts.

15. Sedatives: Will the patient require sedation and/or muscle relaxants before casting?

16. Goals: Will casting meet the patient's goals and result in gains in function? Will expected gains outweigh the cost and time required to cast the patient?[3]

17. Cast selection: Determine type of cast and type of material (plaster or fiberglass) required (Box 13-1).

## CASTING MATERIALS

The following materials are needed for fabrication of casts. Materials should be gathered before initiating the casting process.

1. Plaster or fiberglass casting material: 2-, 3-, 4-and/or 6-inch, depending on the cast to be fabricated[4,9]

2. Cast padding in the size corresponding to the casting material[3,4]

3. Stockinette: 3-inch for upper extremity casts, 4-inch for lower extremity casts[4]; on occasion, 2-inch for a small adult or adolescent

4. Bucket for water[3,4]

5. Water: warm if using plaster and cool if using fiberglass[4]

6. Cast spreader[3,4]

7. Cast-cutter scissors[3]

8. Cast saw[3,4]

9. Trimming knife[4]

10. Sticky-back foam padding

11. Plastic or rubber gloves

12. Sheets, newspaper, or plaster drapes to protect the patient, floor, and equipment

13. Petroleum jelly, liquid soap, or lotion if working with fiberglass

**Box 13-1**

### Comparison of Plaster and Fiberglass Casting Materials

**PLASTER**

- Longer drying time[3] (approximately 24 hours)[9]
- Longer period before patient can bear weight (24 hours)
- More prone to indentations that may lead to areas of high compression and cause skin breakdown[3,14]
- Stronger[3]
- Heavier[3,17]
- Reinforceable[3]
- Easier to adjust[3]
- More difficult to clean up after casting patient[3]
- More difficult to keep clean[3]
- More absorbent[3]
- Less expensive[10]
- Better when frequent cast changes are indicated
- More variability in setting time; setting can be varied according to the needs of the situation

**FIBERGLASS**

- Shorter drying time[3,14] (approximately 30 minutes)[14]
- Shorter period before patient can bear weight (20 to 30 minutes)[10]
- Higher risk of splintering[3,14]
- Harder[3]
- Lighter[3,10,17]
- More resilient[3]
- More soil resistant[10]
- Better when no further gains in range of motion are achieved[10] because final cast is usually a bivalve cast, which is usually made of fiberglass
- More adherence to skin or nonlubricated gloves[10]
- Less variability in setting time: must prevent a layer from hardening because subsequent layers will not bond well[10]
- More expensive[10]
- More durable[10]
- May be better for patients with neglect because bright-colored casts may assist with cueing strategies

## TYPES OF CASTS

Several types of serial casts are available. Each has its own implications for outcome (Table 13-1).

1. Resting cast: This cast is cylindrical and is left on for 7 to 10 days. The cast is the initial one in a casting program and is applied with the limb positioned at the end of easily attainable ROM.4
2. Drop-out cast: This cast consists of a series of cylindrical casts that have a portion of the cast cut out to allow for further range and stretching in the intended direction of stretch while preventing movement in the contracted direction. Casts are changed weekly and reapplied, with the cast accommodating the limb in an improved position. An average of three to four drop-out casts are used to achieve maximally attainable ROM.
3. Holding cast: This cylindrical cast holds the limb in place for 7 to 10 days to maintain the newly acquired ROM; it is also known as a *final cast.*4
4. Bivalve cast: This type of cast is a holding cast that is cut lengthwise into two pieces (anterior and posterior), with the top portion comprising one third of the cast and the bottom portion comprising two thirds of

the cast. The edges of the cast may be finished with padding or tape. The two pieces of the cast are held together around the extremity with straps. Patients are gradually weaned from wearing this cast as they become more active. If patients continue to have increased muscle activity, they continue to wear the bivalve cast at night.

The following are specific examples of casts:

- *Rigid circular elbow cast* (Figure 13-1): This rigid circular cast encloses the forearm and humerus and can be used to increase elbow ROM gradually in an elbow with contracture or increased muscle activity. In addition, the cast may be used for an elbow with fluctuating muscle activity because the cast can provide equalized pressure throughout the arm. A gradual increase in elbow ROM is a result of the stabilizing effect of the cast, which neutralizes abnormal muscle activity.[17,35]
- *Drop-out cast with humeral portion enclosed* (Figure 13-2): This type of cast is effective for treating severe elbow flexion contracture.[35]
- *Drop-out cast with forearm portion enclosed* (Figure 13-3): Enclosing the forearm increases elbow ROM while incorporating the wrist and forearm.

**Table 13-1**

### Comparison of Cast Types

| CAST | PROS | CONS |
|---|---|---|
| Serial | Provides a constant prolonged stretch. Provides an intimate fit. Can help to maintain biomechanical alignment. | May interfere with ADL and mobility. Does not allow access to a joint or extremity to monitor skin and provide other therapy (e.g., ROM, modalities, joint mobilization, weight bearing). |
| Bivalve | Ensures compliance. Allows access to joint and extremity to monitor skin. Allows access to joint and extremity for other interventions. Allows removal of cast for ADL and mobility. May be used as a night or resting splint. Allows quick removal of cast in emergencies. | Impossible for cast to fit exactly together again once it is cut. Can be difficult to maintain a wearing schedule. Provides an intermittent stretch. Has potential to pinch or cause soft tissue trauma. |
| Drop-out | Gravity aids in stretching. Allows enhanced active or passive movement in the desired direction while preventing further contracture. Allows access to joint for mobilization, stretching, and soft tissue mobilization. Allows active ROM in desired range that may strengthen weak muscles opposing contracture. Allows active movement that may increase patient's perception of movement via kinesthetic responses/stimulation if neglect is present. | If cast is not precisely made and cut, has potential for movement within cast and subsequent skin breakdown and/or patient removal. |

*ADL,* Activities of daily living; *ROM,* range of motion.

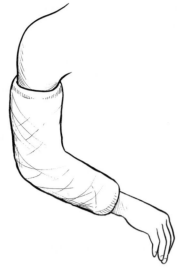

**Figure 13-1**    Rigid circular elbow cast.

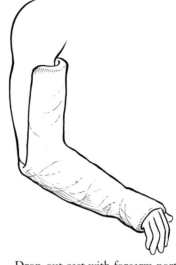

**Figure 13-3**    Drop-out cast with forearm portion enclosed.

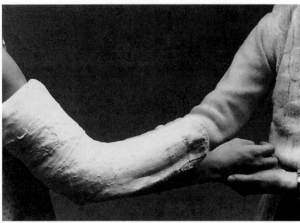

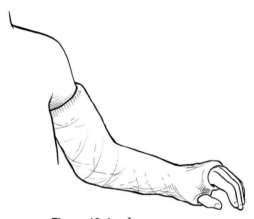

**Figure 13-4**    Long arm cast.

This cast can be applied on a patient with skin breakdown in the humeral region.[35]

■ *Long arm cast* (Figure 13-4): The long arm cast manages problems of the elbow, wrist, and forearm simultaneously. The cast effectively can control increased muscle activity in the forearm muscles.[17,35]

■ *Reverse drop-out cast* (Figure 13-5): A reverse drop-out cast is used when increased muscle activity causes an elbow extension contracture that results in decreased elbow flexion ROM. The cast also puts weak biceps in a mechanically advantageous shortened position. The humerus is enclosed during fabrication. Casting application is most effective when the patient is in a supine or side-lying position, which allows gravity to assist the forearm into a position of elbow flexion.[17,35]

■ *Elbow drop-out cast with wrist included* (Figure 13-6; see also Figure 13-5): This type of cast permits passive and active elbow extension while maintaining

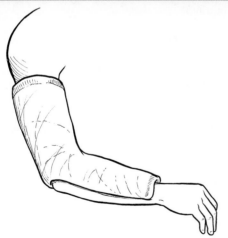

**Figure 13-2**    Drop-out cast with humeral portion enclosed. (From Hill J: Management of abnormal tone through casting and orthotics. In Kovich KM, Bermann DE, editors: *Head injury: a guide to functional outcomes in occupational therapy*, Gaithersburg, Md, 1988, Aspen.)

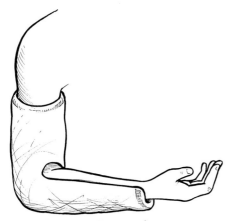

**Figure 13-5** Reverse drop-out cast.

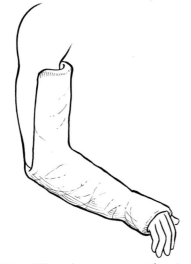

**Figure 13-6** Elbow drop-out cast with wrist included.

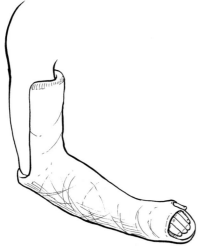

**Figure 13-7** Elbow drop-out cast with hand included.

already attained elbow extension ROM. The weight of the cast acts with gravity to provide a passive stretch when the patient is seated or in an upright

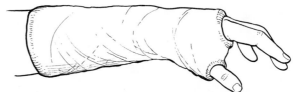

**Figure 13-8** Wrist cast.

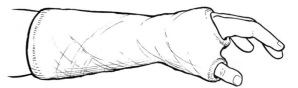

**Figure 13-9** Short arm cast with thumb post.

position. The wrist can be included. The forearm is casted in neutral.[4]

- *Elbow drop-out cast with hand included* (Figure 13-7): This drop-out cast is similar to the previously mentioned elbow drop-out cast with wrist included, except that it can include the hand. Its functions are the same.
- *Wrist cast* (Figure 13-8): A wrist cast is indicated when the wrist exhibits increased muscle activity, contractures, and general weakness. The problems may originate in the wrist only or in a combination of other joints. This cast facilitates functional movement by increasing wrist ROM, decreasing abnormal muscle activity, and isolating wrist movement from hand movement. The cast controls the wrist movements but leaves the digits free. This cast effectively influences distal hand function when the patient has active digit motion.[17,35]
- *Short arm cast with thumb post* (Figure 13-9): A wrist cast with the thumb enclosed manages the thumb-in-palm deformity caused by increased muscle activity of the thumb flexor and adductor. This deformity can decrease the effectiveness of hand functions such as grasp, pinch, and release. Thumb contracture or increased muscle activity may result in web-space shortening, joint subluxation, an unstable metacarpophalangeal joint, or an overstretched extensor pollicis. A wrist cast with the thumb enclosed can enhance grasp or improve overall range and normalize muscle activity in the hand.[17,35]
- *Platform cast* (Figure 13-10): The platform cast is used when the patient has isolated muscle control but still is limited by increased flexor muscle activity that interferes with efficient and precise small muscle blend patterns. A platform cast can improve function with or without the thumb enclosed.[17,35]
- *Finger shell* (Figure 13-11): Severe wrist and digit contractures greatly impair function. Muscle activity

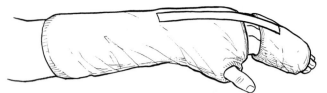

**Figure 13-11**    Finger shell.

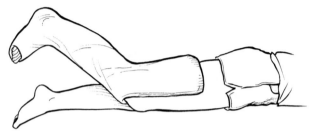

**Figure 13-12**    Knee drop-out cast with anterior portion removed above the knee.

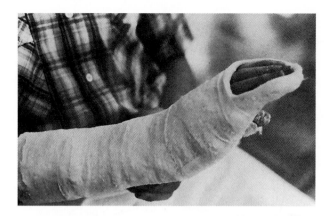

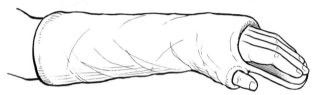

**Figure 13-10**    Platform cast. (From Hill J: Management of abnormal tone through casting and orthotics. In Kovich KM, Bermann DE, editors: *Head injury: a guide to functional outcomes in occupational therapy*, Gaithersburg, Md, 1988, Aspen.)

is increased in the wrist and digit flexors and the intrinsic muscles. A finger shell is attached to a wrist cast to stretch the fingers into extension slowly and gradually.[17,35]

- *Knee drop-out cast with anterior portion removed above the knee* (Figure 13-12): This type of cast is indicated for a knee flexion contracture. The anterior portion is removed to act as a knee flexion stop. Gravity can provide a prolonged stretch to tight flexors.[25]
- *Knee drop-out cast with anterior portion removed below the knee* (Figure 13-13): This knee drop-out cast has the same functions as the previously mentioned knee drop-out cast, except that the anterior portion removed is below instead of above the knee.[25]

## CASTING PROGRESSION

Initially, a resting cast is applied with the limb in submaximal range for 7 to 10 days.[3,4] Then a series of dropout or positional casts are applied weekly in the improved position to increase ROM and decrease spasticity. The therapist performs PROM activities between casts to stretch tissues and avoid reverse contractures.[3,4,17] The therapist should evaluate ROM, sensation, and motor control between cast changes to monitor improvements[3,10,17] also should check skin integrity.[3,17] This process is repeated until no further gains are obtained or full ROM is achieved.[3,10,22,26] Montgomery states that three to four cast changes typically are required to achieve a casting goal.[4]

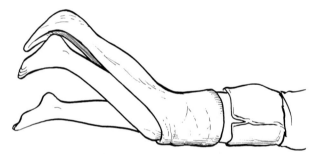

**Figure 13-13**    Knee drop-out cast with the anterior portion of cast removed below the knee.

A final/holding cast then is applied for 1 to 2 weeks to maintain the maximum range that has been achieved.[10] The holding cast then is made bivalve and converted to an anteroposterior splint.[3] The bivalve cast is used to maintain ROM and decrease spasticity. Initially the cast is worn at all times except during therapy sessions. The patient gradually is weaned from this splint until activity is increased.[4] Some patients cannot be weaned fully; for example, if a patient continues to have increased spasticity or weakness, the patient will wear the splint at night[3,4] (Table 13-2).

## GUIDELINES FOR CAST APPLICATION

The following are guidelines for cast application:
1. Obtain physician's orders.[17]
2. Perform the initial evaluation.
3. Pretreat the patient with sedatives, if needed.[10,17,25]
4. Explain the procedure to the patient and what is expected of the patient.
5. Protect the floor with newspaper or plastic. Cover the mat, plinth, chair, and other things with plastic or

**Table 13-2**

## Purpose of and Wearing Times for Different Cast Types

| TYPE OF CAST | GOAL | WEARING TIME |
| --- | --- | --- |
| Resting cast positioned at end of easily obtainable range | To hold the extremity in a painless maximum range and decrease the influence of spasticity | 7-10 days |
| Repeated series (often three to four) of serial or drop-out casts | To increase the ROM gradually of the joint and decrease the influence of spasticity | Weekly intervals with full passive ROM to immobilize joints between cast changes |
| Holding cast | To maintain the gained ROM and decrease the influence of spasticity | 7-10 days |
| Anteroposterior splint (a holding cast made bivalve and converted into a splint) | To maintain the gained ROM | Gradually decreased to night wear and discontinued when no longer needed |

From Garland D, Doyle MM, Booth BJ: *Early management of spastic deformities*, Downey, Calif, 1979, Ranchos Los Amigos Medical Center, Adult Brain Injury Service.
*ROM*, Range of motion.

sheets. Protect the patient's skin, face, and clothing with towels and sheets.[10]

6. Evaluate and document the patient's skin integrity, noting scars, open wounds, and discoloration.

7. If applicable, cut foam padding to size if the patient is at risk for skin breakdown over bony prominences. If fabricating a drop-out cast, cut straps.

8. Precut stockinette 4 to 6 inches longer than the length of the cast on each end so it can be rolled back over the ends of the cast.[10] This pads the ends of the cast and improves the final appearance.

9. Measure and record joint ROM.[10]

10. Mobilize the joint and soft tissue as needed.[26]

11. Fill the bucket with water.

12. Clean and dry the skin thoroughly.[10]

13. Apply the stockinette to the limb to be casted. Smooth out wrinkles to avoid skin breakdown.[3,4,10,17,25] Cut a slit for the thumb if necessary. A stockinette is not always required; however, a stockinette is needed for bivalve or anteroposterior casts to protect the cotton padding from fraying during frequent cast removal. The stockinette is easily replaceable if it becomes stained.[4]

14. Determine the cast length.

    *a. Elbow or elbow and wrist cast*

    The upper arm length should be 1 to 2 inches below the axilla and allow a sufficient lever arm. The distal end of an elbow cast should terminate just proximal to the ulnar styloid.

    A wrist cast should reach 1 to 1 ½ inches from the elbow joint and allow a sufficient lever arm. The distal end should terminate just proximal to the metacarpal phalangeal joints.

    *b. Knee or knee and ankle cast*

    A thigh-length cast should allow 3 to 4 inches from the groin and allow sufficient lever arm.

    The distal end of a knee cast should be 3 inches above the malleoli or 1 to 2 inches below the fibular head.

    The distal end of a cast incorporating the ankle should support the metatarsal heads fully.

    If the patient is ambulatory or weight bearing, the plantar surface of the cast should include a wedge.

15. Open the casting materials: cotton padding, fiberglass or plaster rolls, and foam or felt padding. Fiberglass should be opened one package at a time and applied within 1 minute. Fiberglass will harden and not bond when left exposed to the air.[10]

16. The patient's extremity is casted in submaximal range (5 to 10 degrees less than easily achievable range) initially and at end range with minimal stretching for subsequent casts.[10,17,23] Instruct helper in how and where to position the extremity to be casted.[10]

17. Apply one layer of cotton padding in a spiral fashion with ½ inch overlapping layers in a figure eight around the elbow or knee. Avoid wrinkles to prevent pressure sores. The top and bottom ends should be cylindrical.[3,4,10,17,25]

18. Apply felt or foam padding to bony prominences.[3,4,10,17,25]

19. Add another two or three layers of cotton padding, and hold the felt or foam padding in place.[3,4,17,25] Apply padding 1 to 2 inches above and below the desired cast length to ensure a soft edge.

20. Don plastic gloves. Petroleum jelly, lotion, or liquid soap should be applied to gloves initially and

throughout the procedure. Without lubrication, the gloves will be difficult to remove, and fiberglass may adhere to the patient's skin.[10] Gloves protect the therapist's nailbeds during use of plaster.

21. Apply plaster or fiberglass proximally to distally in a spiral fashion with the extremity positioned so that it has the correct amount of stretch.[3] Fiberglass should overlap itself by half a tape width.[10] Leave 1 inch of padding exposed (and do not cover it with plaster) to create soft cast edge. Keep the roll of material close to the limb to avoid pulling and decrease tension. If applying plaster, dip plaster roll in water while holding the end of the roll; dip it 5 or 6 times until it bubbles.[10] Crimp the end of the rolls to avoid wringing when removing excess water.[4] Removing too much water can cause the plaster to dry too rapidly before it bonds with the gauze. Additional water can be applied but only before the plaster dries. Avoid denting plaster to avoid pressure points. Fiberglass is submerged in cool water and gently squeezed 5 or 6 times, removed from the water, and applied immediately. The assistant should stretch the joint without holding the cast by placing the hands proximal and distal to the cast.[10] After applying each roll (if using plaster), smooth the plaster material into the gauze. As layers are applied, rub the cast in circular motions to smooth the material.[3,10] If using fiberglass, applying petroleum jelly, liquid soap, or lotion to the top of the finished cast helps the material adhere to itself instead of the therapist.[10] Wrapping a wet Ace bandage around the cast also can shorten drying time and ensure a smooth cast.[3] The limb is held in position until the material is set or begins to harden.[3,4] Four to five layers of plaster or three to four layers of fiberglass casting material should be applied.[10]

22. While the cast is setting, insert one or two fingers between the stockinette and padding, and pull them out around the full circumference of cast at proximal and distal ends without applying a counterpressure with the thumbs. This ensures that the ends are not too tight, which may decrease the patient's circulation.[10]

23. Before applying the last layer of casting material, turn the ends of the stockinette back onto the cast to give a smooth, finished edge to the cast. Apply the last layer of casting material just below this edge.[10,17]

24. Allow the cast to set.

25. Write the patient's name, therapist's name, date of cast application, and anticipated date of cast removal on the cast with a permanent marker when it has dried.[17]

26. Draw lines on the cast in case emergency bivalving or removal is necessary.

27. Remove any plaster that may have dripped onto the patient's skin.[10]

28. Elevate the patient's casted extremity 10 to 20 cm above the patient's heart to prevent edema or decrease developing edema.

29. Check patient's circulation.

30. Communicate with medical staff, and post instructions above patient's bed and in nurses' cardex regarding wearing schedule, precautions, positioning, therapist's name and extension, and location of cast cutter for emergency cast removal in an "off hour."

## FABRICATING A DROP-OUT CAST

Following is the procedure for converting a resting or holding cast into a drop-out cast:

1. If removing the posterior aspect of an upper arm cast, draw a line on the medial and lateral aspects of the cast. Connect the two lines with a horizontal line just distal to the olecranon process.

2. If removing the posterior aspect of a forearm cast, draw a line on the medial and lateral aspects of the cast. Connect the two lines with a horizontal line just proximal to the olecranon process.

3. If removing the anterior aspect of a lower leg cast to increase knee extension, draw lines on the medial and lateral aspects of the cast. Connect the two lines with a horizontal line just proximal to the patella.

4. If removing the posterior aspect of a lower leg cast to increase knee flexion, draw lines on the medial and lateral aspects of the cast. Connect the two lines with a horizontal line 2 to 3 inches proximal to the popliteal fossa.

## GUIDELINES FOR CAST REMOVAL

The following are guidelines for removing casts:

1. Explain to the patient the way the cast cutter operates. Tell the patient that the cast cutter does not cut the skin. The blade oscillates back and forth. The blade can be touched to the skin lightly while in motion without cutting the skin.

2. Determine the line the cut will follow (which depends on the plan to bivalve the cast) according to the mechanical force of pull and ability to clear bony prominences.

3. Drape the patient and surrounding area with sheets and newspaper.

4. Put goggles on the patient; the therapist and the holder also should wear goggles.

5. If a patient has pulmonary problems or a tracheostomy, consider using masks or careful draping to protect the patient from breathing in the dust from the cast as it is being cut.

6. Cut through the casting material. Cut with direct inward pressure in one place at a time. Do not lift the cast cutter until you feel the blade drop into the

space that it has created. Do not move the cast saw proximally to distally along the length of the cast; searing can occur. Casts with severe angles require two cuts.

7. Spread cast apart with the cast spreader.
8. Use bandage shears to cut through the padding and stockinette.
9. Completely separate and remove the cast.
10. Check the patient's skin for red areas, edema, or breakdown.
11. Record measurements and clinical observations.
12. Clean and dry the extremity. Moisturize the skin.[10]

## FABRICATING A BIVALVE CAST

When the maximum gain in ROM has been achieved, the therapist may create a bivalve cast and use it to maintain gains.

1. The cast usually is fabricated from fiberglass but can be fabricated from plaster.[10]
2. Drape the patient and surrounding area with sheets and newspaper.
3. Cut the cast into anterior and posterior portions using the cast saw. (See number 6 in the previous section for the correct technique.)
4. Create a bivalve portion in the cast at the medial and lateral aspects of the forearm so that one third of cast is on top and two thirds is on the bottom. For a lower extremity splint, create a bivalve portion in the cast at the medial and lateral aspects, slightly anterior to the medial and lateral malleolus so that one third of the cast is on top and two thirds is on the bottom. The blade cutter will not easily cut through the stockinette and padding, which should be taken into consideration. For example, do not double back the stockinette when cutting a bivalve.
5. Use the cast spreader to spread the cast apart. Use cast scissors to cut the padding and stockinette; discard the padding and stockinette.
6. Realign the cast halves with cotton padding using same amount required for the original cast fabrication. Extend the padding over the edges and sides of the shells. Do not cause ripples; the interior must be smooth. If necessary, rip the padding edges off to create a smooth surface. Replace the stockinette if it does not fit the splint.
7. Use adhesive tape or moleskin to secure the padding edges, which should be folded over the shells.
8. Cut the stockinette 4 to 6 inches longer than the length of each shell. Line each shell with a stockinette, and use adhesive tape to secure. NOTE: If too much underpadding is added, the cast angle will be reduced or shifted.
9. Secure bivalves on patient with Ace bandages or straps. Straps can be fabricated using 1- to 3-inch

wide webbing and buckles that can be riveted, taped, glued, or sewn onto the stockinette. Webbing also can be attached using casting material (i.e., plaster or fiberglass).

## CAST MONITORING

The patient, caregivers, and staff should monitor the cast every 2 hours[17,25,35] for the first 24 hours for the following:

1. Pain, discomfort
2. Edema
3. Sensory changes such as numbness, tingling, and "pins and needles"
4. Circulatory changes such as coldness and changes in nailbed color
5. Increased or decreased movement inside the cast
6. Skin integrity including reddened or broken skin
7. Severe itching
8. Dents or cracks in or softening of the cast

## CAST CARE

The patient can bathe in a tub or shower while wearing a cast but should avoid wetting the cast. The cast can be covered with a plastic bag or a commercially available cast cover. Tape the edges down to prevent the cast from getting wet. However, sponge bathing is preferred. Cover the cast when it is near water (e.g., when washing dishes).

## CLINICAL ISSUES

Patients with diminished cognitive status may be casted if a caregiver assumes responsibility for safety. However, if the patient is acutely ill, medical needs and contraindications may preclude casting. For example, a patient may require the insertion of an intravenous line in the limb that needs to be casted. A cast can have a window around a line, which may be left open for Doppler ultrasound to check distal circulation. However, this is not optimal. In addition, poor skin integrity or fractures may preclude casting. Casting a cognitively impaired patient may allow the therapist to concentrate on improving the patient's positioning and motor function, so when the patient's cognitive status improves the patient can focus on performing functional tasks using maximum joint ROM and more normal movement patterns. In addition, casting can be used as an early intervention to work on a patient's cognitive status. For example, standing a patient with a lower extremity cast in a tilt table may improve the patient's level of alertness because of the maintenance of the upright position. The therapist also can focus on motor control of the pelvis, trunk, and shoulder girdle, which may result in improved abilities to move from sitting to standing, transfer, and position the wheelchair.

Attempting to decrease excessive extension or flexion and enhance dissociated movements results in better positioning.

A patient may require multiple casts, which may affect the patient's nursing care and rehabilitation by other therapists. The therapist may need to consider alternate methods of positioning and nonverbal communication. The benefits of multiple-extremity casting for improved ROM or motor control must outweigh the risks, potential complications, and potential for improvement. The patient may not tolerate multiple casts well. Combining bivalve splints and casts may improve the patient's tolerance. Casts should be applied to the extremity in a way that severely limits ROM and spasticity. Bivalve splints can be applied to an extremity with minimal spasticity or ROM deficits and allow for increased function by easy removal.[36]

Casts should be changed as functional gains are achieved. For example, a long leg cast may interfere with sitting activities that are being used to encourage trunk control and trunk alignment. A long leg cast encourages a posterior pelvic tilt, kyphotic posture, and neck flexion positions that do not lend themselves to developing effective postural control. A short leg cast with a removable splint for knee extension or a long leg cast with a hinged locking joint to permit knee flexion while sitting or extension to increase ROM may better suit the patient's functional status.[36]

Booth, Doyle, and Montgomery[4] suggest that agitated patients' treatment often is directed at encouraging rather than restricting limb movement. Although serial casting inhibits movement, it is recommended because agitated patients' movements are random, and contractures can form easily. A cast also protects the limb from injury if the patient should become agitated. When choosing the casting material, the therapist should consider several factors. Fiberglass dries quickly, which may be beneficial for patients who are agitated. The cast is less likely to be dented,[4] and it is harder, lighter, and more resilient than plaster.[36] However, fiberglass can splinter if patients strike a hard object. Edges may be rough, and patients may be in danger of hurting themselves. Plaster, however, may be better for the agitated or combative patient because additional layers may be added to increase the durability of the cast. However, increasing layers of plaster increases the overall weight of the cast. Regardless of the material selected, additional padding should be added to bony prominences to protect the patient from skin breakdown.

As motor control improves, the therapist must decide if the focus of treatment should be to continue to improve ROM or motor control. The goal is to have ROM and motor control but not one at the expense of the other. If motor control is gained without sufficient range, the limb will not be functional. If ROM is gained at the expense of

motor control, functional mobility will be difficult to maintain. The residual contracture, mental status, skin integrity, and severity of spasticity can aid in determining treatment priorities. If the patient cannot follow directions and carry out an exercise program or incorporate gains into functional activities, casting should be discontinued. Casting may be discontinued on patients who can follow directions and actively use their contracted limb for functional tasks so that they actively can maintain the function of their contracted limb. A bivalve splint is recommended for easy access to the limb for therapy and to maintain ROM. A patient whose cognition is good but who has remaining severe contracture or spasticity, may need to stay in a cast for a longer period of time until a bivalve splint is indicated. However, if a drop-out cast is indicated, electrical stimulation can be used on the antagonist of the contracted muscle. Electrical stimulation of the antagonist of the contracted muscle combined with a drop-out cast can also be used if the joint is amenable to contracture management. Active participation of the patient is not required. Electrical stimulation also may facilitate motor control of the stimulated muscle.[36]

## SUMMARY

Casting can be used effectively for patients who have suffered a stroke when traditional methods have failed to improve ROM and decrease spasticity. The therapist carefully must consider the goals of casting, type of casts, material to be used, time and cost of therapists, precautions, and contraindications before initiating a casting program.

**Case Study 1**

### SERIAL CASTING AFTER STROKE

L.P. is a 72-year-old man who suffered a stroke that resulted in severe bilateral upper extremity spasticity in the elbow flexors. He was independent in activities of daily living before admission. L.P. lived with his wife and daughter. Traditional methods of therapy had been unsuccessful during his brief time in the acute care service. L.P. had become dependent in all aspects of self-care. He was cognitively intact. There were no contraindications to a casting program. While in the rehabilitation unit, L.P. consented to being casted. He was casted with bilateral long arm casts that were left in place for 8 days. The spasticity reduced enough to allow the patient to perform hand activities, including self-feeding, shaving, and brushing his teeth. In addition, the spasticity decreased enough to allow traditional methods of therapy to be used. L.P. eventually was discharged back to his previous living arrangement, where he was again independent in all aspects of self-care.

## Case Study 2

### SERIAL CASTING AFTER STROKE II

S.D. is an 80-year-old female who suffered a stroke that resulted in soft tissue contracture of the elbow flexors to 90 degrees of elbow flexion, severely increased skeletal muscle activity in the wrist and finger flexors, resulted in difficulty maintaining the web space following the thumb posturing in flexion and adduction, and resulted in spasticity in the intrinsic muscles of the hand. S.D. did not have functional use of the extremity. She was globally aphasic and demonstrated ideational and motor apraxia. Sensation and skin integrity were intact. There were no contraindications to casting. S.D. was unable to consent to casting; however, her son consented. Initially, S.D. was fitted with a long arm resting cast with full hand and thumb portions. The cast was left in place for 10 days. The spasticity in her wrist and hand reduced. She then was fit with a cylindrical elbow extension holding cast for 10 days to maintain maximum elbow extension. The cast then was made into a bivalved anteroposterior cylinder splint and was worn at night. The extremity did remain nonfunctional; however, S.D. then was able to be maintained with traditional therapies.

## REVIEW QUESTIONS

1. List five indications for serial casting.
2. List 10 precautions for serial casting.
3. List 10 contraindications to serial casting.
4. Describe the initial evaluation process for serial casting.
5. Describe the purpose of the following casts: resting, holding, anteroposterior/bivalved.
6. Compare and contrast plaster and fiberglass casting materials.
7. Describe the cast application procedure.
8. Describe the cast removal process.

## REFERENCES

1. Barnard P, Dill H, Eldredge P, et al: Reduction of hypertonicity by early casting in a comatose head-injured individual: a case report, *Phys Ther* 64(10):1540-1542, 1984.
2. Bentzel K: Remediating sensory impairment. In Trombly CA, editor: *Occupational therapy for physical dysfunction*, ed 4, Baltimore, 1995, Williams & Wilkins.
3. Booth FW: Effect of limb immobilization on skeletal muscle, *J Appl Physiol* 52(5):1113-1118, 1982.
4. Booth BJ, Doyle M, Montgomery J: Serial casting for the management of spasticity in the head-injured adult, *Phys Ther* 63(12):1960-1966, 1983.
5. Katz RT: Management of spasticity. In Braddom RL, editor: *Physical medicine & rehabilitation*, Philadelphia, 1996, WB Saunders.
6. Brennan JB: Response to stretch of hypertonic muscle groups in hemiplegia, *Br Med J* pp 1504-1507, 1959.
7. Bronski B: Serial casting for the neurological patient, *Physical Disabilities Special Interest Section Newsletter* 18:4, 1995.
8. Cherry DB: Review of physical therapy alternatives for reducing muscle contracture, *Phys Ther* 60(7):877-881, 1980.
9. Davies PM: Overcoming limitation of movement, contracture and deformity. In *Starting again: early rehabilitation after traumatic brain injury or other severe brain lesion*, New York, 1994, Springer-Verlag.
10. Feldman PA: Upper extremity casting and splinting. In Glenn MB, Whyte J, editors: *The practical management of spasticity in children and adults*, Philadelphia, 1990, Lea & Febiger.
11. Garland DE, Blum CE, Waters RL: Periarticular heterotopic ossification in head-injured adults, *J Bone Joint Surg Am* 62(7):1143-1146, 1980.
12. Garland DE, Keenan MAE: Orthopedic strategies in the management of the adult head-injured patient, *Phys Ther* 63(12):2004-2009, 1983.
13. Garland DE, Razza BE, Waters RL: Forceful joint manipulation in head-injured adults with heterotopic ossification, *Clin Orthop* 169:133-138, 1982.
14. Giorgetti MM: Serial and inhibitory casting: implications for acute care physical therapy management, *Neurol Rep* 17:18, 1993.
15. Grossman MR, Sahrmann SA, Rose SJ: Review of length-associated changes in muscle, *Phys Ther* 62(12):1799-1808, 1982.
16. Hill J: The effects of casting on upper extremity motor disorders after brain injury, *Am J Occup Ther* 48(3):219-224, 1994.
17. Hill J: Management of abnormal tone through casting and orthotics. In *Head injury: a guide to functional outcomes in occupational therapy*, Rockville, Md, 1988, Aspen.
18. Kaplan N: Effect of splinting on reflex inhibition and sensorimotor stimulation in treatment of spasticity, *Arch Phys Med Rehabil* 43:565-569, 1962.
19. King TI II: Plaster splinting as a means of reducing elbow flexor spasticity: a case study, *Am J Occup Ther* 36:671, 1982.
20. Lavalette R, Pope MH, Dickstein H: Setting temperatures of plaster casts, *J Bone Joint Surg Am* 64(6):907-911, 1982.
21. Law M, Cadman D, Rosenbaum P, et al: Neurodevelopmental therapy and upper extremity inhibitive casting for children with cerebral palsy, *Dev Med Child Neurol* 33(5):379-387, 1991.
22. Leahy P: Precasting work sheet: an assessment tool—a clinical report, *Phys Ther* 68(1):72-74, 1988.
23. Lehmkuhl LD, Thoi LL, Baize C, et al: Multimodality treatment of joint contractures in patients with severe brain injury: cost, effectiveness, and integration of therapies in the application of serial/inhibitive casts, *J Head Trauma Rehabil* 5:23, 1990.
24. MacKay-Lyons M: Low-load, prolonged stretch in treatment of elbow flexion contractures secondary to head trauma: a case report, *Phys Ther* 69(4):50-56, 1989.
25. Nash DL: Serial casting. In Lennard TA, editor: *Physiatric procedures in clinical practice*, Philadelphia, 1995, Hanley & Belfus.
26. Orest MR: Casting protocol for patients with neurological dysfunction, *PT Magazine*, pp 51-55, 1993.
27. Ough JL, Garland DE, Jordan C, et al: Treatment of spastic joint contractures in mentally disabled adults, *Orthop Clin North Am* 12(1):143-151, 1981.
28. Sabbahi MA, De Luca CJ, Powers WR: Topical anesthesia: a possible treatment method for spasticity, *Arch Phys Med Rehabil* 62(7):310-314, 1981.
29. Smith LH, Harris SR: Upper extremity inhibitive casting for a child with cerebral palsy, *Phys Occup Ther Pediatr* 5:71, 1985.
30. Stockmeyer S: An interpretation of the approach of Rood to the treatment of neuromuscular dysfunction, *Phys Med* 26(1):900-961, 1967.
31. Tabary JC, Tabary C, Tardiev C, et al: Physiological and structural changes in the cat's soleus muscle due to immobilization at different lengths by plaster casts, *J Physiol* 224:231, 1972.

32. Tona JL, Schneck CM: The efficacy of upper extremity inhibitive casting: a single-subject pilot study, *Am J Occup Ther* 47(10):901-910, 1993.

33. Umphred DA: Classification of treatment techniques based on primary input systems. In Umphred DA, editor: *Neurological rehabilitation*, ed 3, St Louis, 1995, Mosby.

34. Yasukawa A: Upper-extremity casting: adjunct treatment for the child with cerebral palsy. In Case-Smith J, Pehoski C, editors: *Development of hand skills in the child*, Rockville, Md, 1992, American Occupational Therapy Association.

35. Yasukawa A, Hill J: Casting to improve upper extremity function. In Boehme R, editor: *Improving upper body control: an approach to assessment and treatment of tonal dysfunction*, Tucson, 1988, Therapy Skill Builders.

36. Zablotny C, Forte Andric M, Gowland C: Serial casting: clinical applications for the adult head-injured patient, *J Head Trauma Rehabil* 2:46, 1987.

37. Zachazewski JE, Eberle ED, Jefferies M: Effect of tone-inhibiting casts and orthoses on gait, *Phys Ther* 62(4):453-455, 1982.

## SUGGESTED READING

Preston LA, Hecht JS: *Spasticity management: rehabilitation strategies*, Bethesda, Md, 1999, American Occupational Therapy Association.

leslie a. kane
and karen a. buckley

**chapter 14**

# Functional Mobility

**key terms**

bed mobility
environmental conditions
mobility

scooting
task-specific training
transfers

transitional movements
trunk control
upright function

**chapter objectives**

After completing this chapter, the reader will be able to accomplish the following:

1. Recognize the impact of impairment on mobility tasks.
2. Analyze specific movement patterns observed during mobility tasks and common compensatory strategies.
3. Use a function-based approach to retraining mobility patterns.
4. Understand the impact of environmental changes on mobility tasks.

## TERMINOLOGY

Many terms have been used in occupational therapy practice to describe an individual's ability to change the position of the body in space and move within the environment. *Mobility* broadly refers to movements that result in a change of body position or location. The term *bed mobility* has been used interchangeably with *gross mobility* within the rehabilitation setting and traditionally has included tasks such as rolling to both sides, rolling to side lying, moving from a sitting to a supine position and vice versa, and moving from sitting to standing. *Transfer* refers to movement from one surface to another such as from a bed to a wheelchair, from a wheelchair to a toilet, or from a wheelchair to a car, and involves varied methods of achievement.

## OVERVIEW OF THE LITERATURE

Within the literature, numerous studies carefully have examined mobility functions of the adult in relation to gait and locomotion. Unfortunately, few studies have examined functional mobility tasks. The analysis of the normal sit-to-stand sequence of movement has received attention and is reviewed later in this chapter.[17,18,28,76,77] Rising from bed has been examined in relation to age differences and the most common movement strategies selected.[30] This research demonstrates that age-related trends occur across the life span, but great variety remains evident in the selection of specific movement strategies. A limitation of this study is that the oldest age group examined was the 50- to 59-year-old group; thus, information concerning older adults most at risk for cerebrovascular accident (CVA) was not included. A study of normal adult rolling patterns also has shown that adults exhibit great variability in the selection of movement patterns. In addition, the authors of this study have noted indications that a developmental sequence of movement patterns exists but is not inclusive of all individuals. Clearly many aspects of functional mobility still warrant further investigation.[82]

## FUNCTIONAL MOBILITY: RELATIONSHIP TO ACTIVITIES AND PARTICIPATION

Occupational therapists have always approached functional mobility from the perspective that individual elements involved in changing the position of the body were necessary to achieve competency in broad areas of occupation. Improvement in activities of daily living, instrumental activities of daily living, education, work, play, leisure, and social participation always has been the ultimate goal of occupational therapy. The American Occupational Therapy Association, in "Practice Framework: Domain and Process," describes functional mobility as "moving from one position or place to another (during performance of everyday activities), such as in-bed mobility, wheelchair mobility, transfers (wheelchair, bed, car, tub, toilet, tub/shower, chair, floor). Performing functional ambulation and transporting objects."[4]

Within the Practice Framework, functional mobility is presented as a separate activity category of basic activities of daily living, in which mobility functions occur relative to taking care of one's own body.

Alternatively, in the *International Classification of Functioning, Disability and Health*, the World Health Organization presents mobility as a separate domain under the broader category of Activities and Participation. Mobility "is about moving by changing body position or location or by transferring from one place to another, by occupying, moving or manipulating objects, by walking, running or climbing, and by using various forms of transportation."[88]

In this more global perspective, mobility is presented as much more than a function of personal self-care. Mobility is viewed as essential to enabling an individual to engage in a full range of life areas and is central to enabling the individual to participate in life situations.

In planning comprehensive treatment programs, the occupational therapist should be mindful that functional mobility is not just relevant to performing self-care tasks but is necessary to permit engagement in education, work opportunities, community life, recreation, leisure, religious pursuits, and domestic life. In practice the extent to which these areas are addressed may be limited by time constraints imposed by the venue of treatment. Clinicians working within an acute care setting often emphasize basic bed mobility tasks to prepare the patient for inde-

pendence in grooming, bathing, and dressing activities. Within a rehabilitation setting, occupational therapists may have the opportunity to approach functional mobility more comprehensively in relation to more advanced tasks such as community mobility and tasks related to specific work and home-management requirements. The occupational therapist determines goals of treatment with the patient, contingent on imminent and future plans to resume responsibility for activities demanding advanced mobility.

The task-related approach of occupational therapy to intervention to improve functional mobility is consistent with present motor learning research emphasizing the important role environment plays in the organization of movement to solve motor problems (see Chapters 4 to 6).[8,33]

Impairments of body functions and structures and performance skills have been used as the basis for assessing abilities in the patient with hemiplegia. Each patient has different strengths, abilities, and impairments that affect the performance of functional mobility. A patient may have strong neuromusculoskeletal and movement-related functions but demonstrate significant impairment in mental functions of sequencing complex movements (e.g., apraxia). Alternately, a patient may have several problems affecting the neuromusculoskeletal system, including decreased alignment and postural stability that interfere with the ability to roll efficiently toward the nonaffected side. Nevertheless, such a patient may demonstrate the ability to learn new strategies to sequence movement to accomplish the task.

## INFLUENCE OF CONTEXTUAL FACTORS ON FUNCTIONAL MOBILITY

Contextual factors represent a variety of interrelated conditions and situations, which may influence an individual's ability to become proficient in performing mobility tasks. Personal and environmental factors affect the patient with hemiplegia and may support or impede performance.

Personal factors are unique to the individual's life and living situation and influence the selection of mobility interventions. The occupational therapist considers factors such as age, gender, race, and social background.

When considering the age of an individual who has sustained a CVA and assessing expectations of the potential for functional mobility, the therapist must use caution. Many factors besides age contribute to the differences in the abilities older adults exhibit in functional mobility. The reader is encouraged to explore the literature examining the effect of aging on postural control and life span mobility.

Certainly the patient's stage in the life cycle more clearly guides assessment and interventions in the consideration of overall mobility needs. The young patient with hemiplegia who attends college has specific mobility needs. Sit-to-stand movements must be accomplished in changing environments and under varying conditions. For example, using public transportation, which may be moving or stationary; rising from a low seat at a football stadium; sitting down in a crowded and darkened movie theater; and getting into a truck present different challenges. These mobility tasks are not unique to young persons, however. The retired person who enjoys traveling frequently and visiting family members also has special mobility needs.

Social and cultural variations also have an effect on the success of functional mobility interventions. The therapist must consider culturally derived boundaries of interaction,[51] because the therapist frequently must work within an intimate distance during mobility retraining.[36] The physical environment in which interventions occur also affects the patient's willingness to participate actively. Some patients prefer treatment to occur in the privacy of their hospital rooms, whereas others are more comfortable with these "close encounters" occurring in the open space of a therapeutic gymnasium. The patient, family, significant individuals, and therapist have perceptions and beliefs founded on their cultural conditionings. Similarities and differences of belief may occur in three areas influencing the success of functional mobility retraining: the perceived state of health and illness; the perceived relevance of therapeutic interventions; and the belief that functional mobility is relevant to resuming previous occupations.[53]

The therapist's ability to listen to personal needs and appreciate individual values helps ensure success.[53] The degree of independence a patient finds acceptable must be self-determined. The therapist must remember that cultural variations influence compliance with home programs.[4,53,58]

Environmental factors are external to the individual and are considered at two levels, individual and societal. Individual environmental factors include the immediate environment of the individual, which can be viewed as the hospital or clinical venue, and the expected environments. Environment determines a patient's function. The patient with hemiplegia may be able to roll to either side and come to a seated position on a mat or plinth within the clinical setting and engage in donning and doffing of upper extremity clothing. However, in bed within a home setting the patient may not be able to roll as efficiently or come to a seated position without some assistance. Grooming and dressing tasks may not be practical because of changes in the height and firmness of the supporting surface. These occurrences and the reasons underlying the performance deficits are well represented in the current motor learning literature. The postural adjustments necessary to roll and come to a seated position to engage in self-care tasks can be learned only in the context of task performance[1,19] and in the expected environment.[33,34]

The treatment of a patient with hemiplegia often occurs on a continuum that directly influences the physical treatment environment. Many treatment environments impose constraints that limit the therapist's interventions. Ideally the relearning of motor skills and tasks should occur in the actual environment in which the task will be performed.[20,63]

Societal environmental factors directly influence the patients' ability to resume participation in instrumental activities of daily living and include systems within the community or society that can assist the individual to resume an active lifestyle outside of one's immediate living situation (see Chapter 3).

## FUNCTIONAL MOBILITY: THE OUTCOME OF MULTIPLE PROCESSES

Functional mobility requires the successful interaction of a number of systems. Carrying out skilled rolling, sitting, and standing does not depend solely on the integrity of the neuromusculoskeletal system. Occupational therapists must be mindful of the interdependence of various sensory, perceptual, and cognitive functions in the execution of these tasks and create evaluation tools that respect this relationship such as the Árnadóttir Occupational Therapy Neurobehavioral Evaluation (see Chapter 18). This awareness ensures more appropriate treatment planning for the "total person" than do evaluations that look at motor behaviors in isolation. Occupational therapists' knowledge and expertise in task analysis render them uniquely qualified to evaluate and plan treatment to improve functional mobility skills while keeping all the patient's needs in mind.

Individual differences and variations in movement strategies may be related to factors such as the patient's build (short, tall, obese, thin) and history of activity before the CVA (i.e., the patient was a trained athlete, dancer, physically inactive, occasional exerciser, or physical laborer). Additionally, each patient comes to a therapist with a history of customs and habits that influence movement.[27] A patient's psychological state may indeed be reflected in movement (e.g., inhibitions or lack of them and reactive depression about the current situation). Pain before or after the stroke may affect movement patterns. These individual differences and their effects on functional mobility have been explored in the literature.[82] The occupational therapist must be cognizant of these factors and others in assessment and treatment planning.

## IMPAIRMENT OF BODY FUNCTIONS AND STRUCTURES AND SKILLS

Many sequelae associated with a CVA may produce difficulties in the carrying out functional mobility tasks. The occupational therapist uses basic knowledge of body functions and structures, performance skills, and impairments as a means to organize assessment of an individual's capacity for functional mobility. The following sections review impairments resulting from CVA and their effects on performance of functional mobility skills.

## Sensory Processing

*Vision.* Warren[84] presented a hierarchical model for understanding visual perceptual dysfunction in adults with brain injury. This model asserts that visual perceptual skill is comprised of lower- and higher-level skills interacting and subserving with each other. Lower-level skills such as visual fields, visual acuity, and oculomotor control form the foundation on which visual attention, scanning, pattern recognition, memory, and visual cognition can be developed and integrated.

Visual field deficits are common after CVA and traumatic brain injuries. The most common visual field defect is a homonymous hemianopsia caused by involvement of the striate cortex or geniculocalcarine tract and usually is congruent (the same for both eyes). With or sometimes without cueing, patients can shift their eyes to compensate for such a defect. Hemianopsia often can coexist with visual inattention, but these are two distinct phenomena. According to Warren,[84] functional visual attention requires an efficient intrahemispheric and interhemispheric network for visual information processing to take place. An individual with visual inattention ignores objects in one visual field while attending to objects in the other field. Inattention usually occurs in patients with large right cerebral lesions involving the parietal and temporal lobes, which are supplied by posterior cerebral arteries, or the parietal and frontal lobes, which are supplied by the middle cerebral arteries.

Many patients with homonymous hemianopsia learn to compensate using gaze by turning the head a sufficient amount to bring the affected visual field into the unaffected one. With visual inattention, heightening the patient's awareness to the problem is instrumental to success in using compensatory strategies. Visual inattention can affect functional mobility skills significantly because the ability to scan the environment while moving is inconsistent at best. Decreased visual attention to one side may render transfers from bed to wheelchair difficult or even dangerous in cases in which awareness of the problem is poor (see Chapter 16).

*Somesthetic Sensation.* Disturbances of sensation are frequent in patients who have had acute strokes and are observed in 46% of 1000 consecutive patients, usually in association with other neurologic deficits; in only 2% of those cases did the disturbances occur in isolation. The sensory involvement most commonly shows a face-arm-leg distribution (55.5% of cases) and less commonly a face-arm (29%) or arm-leg (7%) distribution. Rarely only one of these three areas is affected in isolation (arm, 6%; face, 2%; leg, 0.5%).[12]

Diminished or absent somesthetic sensation resulting in hemisensory loss can account for difficulties with functional mobility tasks. Proprioceptive loss particularly can contribute to difficulties with purposeful movement, even if motor strength is intact. Sensory loss in the affected extremities necessitates cognitive vigilance to that side during bed mobility and transfers of any kind. Additionally, decreased pain sensation is a risk factor for injuries to the patient.

The use of peripheral feedback in the control of movement has long been debated. The research suggests that many gross motor activities involving the limbs may be achieved in the absence of somatosensory feedback. Researchers theorize that in the adult, many stored motor programs have been learned through a variety of experiences, giving the individual an extensive repertoire of movement possibilities.[54]

Pain can limit severely the extent to which a patient can work on functional mobility skill training. For example, many techniques in bed mobility and transfers require a pain-free arc of motion at the hemiplegic shoulder to be carried out easily. Addressing pain in this case may be the key to promoting function (see Chapter 10).

*Perceptual Processing.* Right-left disorientation (e.g., the patient gives the incorrect response to the command "show me your right hand") usually is associated with left hemisphere damage. In general these individuals have difficulty differentiating between the right and left halves of their bodies or the bodies of others.[46]

Disturbances of body image may cause an individual to fail to perceive stimuli on the left side, confuse body positional and spatial relationships, misperceive left-sided stimulation as occurring on the right, and fail to realize that the extremities or other body organs are in some way compromised.[47]

Damage to the right hemisphere alters many aspects of visual-spatial and perceptual functioning. Disturbances can vary individually; however, typically these patients display difficulty with the analysis of geometric space, depth perception, distance, shape, orientation, position, perspective, and figure-ground recognition. The patient may misplace things, have difficulty with balance, stumble and bump into the walls and furniture, and become easily lost, confused, and disoriented while walking or driving. Attempting functional mobility skills training with these patients requires the therapist to be mindful that with each change of position patients undergo, the perception of position in relation to supporting surfaces and surfaces to which they are to move may be disrupted. These patients often misperceive the distance between themselves and the furniture toward which they are moving. Additionally, these patients may experience fear when attempting to move; this may result in a "poverty of movement" because staying in one spot is less threatening (see Chapters 17 to 19).

## Neuromusculoskeletal and Movement-Related Functions

Motor weakness is found in 80% to 90% of all patients after stroke.[12] Hemiparesis with uniform weakness of the hand, foot, shoulder, and hip is the most frequent motor deficit profile, constituting at least two thirds of all cases.[57] Flaccidity may be evident early on; however, spasticity may develop in the acute phase as well. Limb flaccidity may be associated with retained reflexes; not infrequently reflexes remain normal or even increase. Although many authors have tried to find differences in frequency, severity, and profile of the hemiparesis in right- and left-sided lesions, the majority of such studies showed no significant differences.[57]

Patients after stroke typically experience changes in muscle tone, contralateral weakness (although ipsilateral weakness also is sometimes evident), and poor endurance. Left unattended over time, muscle stiffness and learned nonuse[80] are likely to occur. An extensive review of the causes of weakness in hemiplegia appears in the occupational therapy literature. Although further study clearly is needed in this area, this review substantiates the notion that far too much emphasis has been placed on the role of spasticity in producing the inability to activate affected muscles. An increasing body of knowledge points to alterations in the physiology of motor units, particularly regarding changes in firing rates and muscle fiber atrophy, and the contribution of other factors results in mechanical restraint of agonist muscles by their antagonists.[14] Early intervention aimed at avoiding contractures and facilitating activation of the more involved side is crucial even if consensus is lacking on the most effective means of management.

Many motor assessments used in the past emphasized the patient's limitations rather than the patient's abilities and created an emphasis on the quality of movement rather than on the actual movement accomplished by the patient. The inability to perform movements correctly can result from other neurobehavioral sequelae related to the stroke, not only from hemiparesis. Patients with motor neglect show a lack of initiation moving their limbs even in the presence of preserved strength, and patients with motor impersistence are unable to maintain voluntary action. Apraxia has been a challenging sequela to treat and is defined as a disorder of skilled, purposeful movement in the absence of impaired motor functioning and comprehension (see Chapter 19).[5]

Apraxic abnormalities usually are associated with left hemisphere damage, in particular injuries involving the left frontal and inferior parietal lobes.[46] Currently the shift in emphasis to appropriate task analysis is influencing occupational therapists in their assessments and is broadening these assessments to include perceptual, cognitive, and behavioral features of the task.

Difficulties with postural control become evident for a variety of reasons after stroke. Shumway-Cook and Woollacott[78] view "postural control as the ability to control the body's position in space for the dual purposes of stability and orientation." They define postural stability as "the ability to maintain the position of the body (specifically the center of mass) within the specific boundaries of space, referred to as stability limits." They further explain postural orientation: "Stability limits are boundaries of an area of space in which the body can maintain its position without changing the base of support. Postural orientation is defined as the ability to maintain an appropriate relationship between the body segments and between the body and the environment for a task."

Multiple sensory systems, including the vestibular, somatosensory, and visual systems, allow the individual to receive reference cues about gravity, the supporting surface, and the relationship of the body to objects in the environment, respectively. Disruption to any of these systems can occur after a stroke and must be accounted for in the evaluation process (see Chapters 8 and 9).[78]

## Cognitive Integration

### Arousal and Attention.
Disorders of arousal and confusional states, not infrequently in combination, are the most common disorders of consciousness in patients who have suffered acute strokes. Arousal refers to the general state of readiness of an individual to process sensory information and organize a response.[83] This often is referred to as the orienting reaction and as the arousal reaction. The orienting response should be understood as divided into two phenomena: a general arousal effect and a selective orienting of attention to the source of the information.[65] Of note is that selective orienting is important to vision and has a distinct subcortical circuit mediating this function.[83] Arousal undergoes slow fluctuations throughout the day (tonic arousal) and is influenced by factors such as sleep, food intake, and endogenous neural and endocrine circadian rhythms. Rapid fluctuations in arousal (phasic arousal) occur in response to the presentation of challenging cognitive and physical tasks and signals indicating that an event requiring a response is about to occur (warning signals).[85]

The patient's level of arousal has an effect on readiness to participate in treatment and must be factored into the evaluation of performance of mobility skills. This necessity requires treatment planning in and of itself. The occupational therapist in the acute care or rehabilitation setting may have ample skills to monitor the patient's arousal through 24-hour nursing reports. In the home care setting, family members and other caretakers need to be educated about arousal and its fluctuation.

The neural structures mediating arousal are the reticular activating system, which has fibers of noradrenergic, dopaminergic, cholinergic, and serotonergic types; hypothalamus; limbic system; and cerebral cortex. The neurotransmitter fibers of the reticular activating system have a broad distribution to the cortex, and the reticular activating system receives direct and indirect feedback from the cortical regions to which it projects. Large areas of the cortex are alerted during arousal; however, other parts of the cortex must be inhibited to allow for selective orientation and attention to specific stimuli. The reticular activating system is able to alert the cortex, but cortical processing also is able to increase activity in the reticular activating system.[66]

The right hemisphere appears to be dominant for tonic arousal and has greater noradrenergic and serotonergic content than does the left.[64] Right hemisphere lesions produce significant slowing of reaction time, particularly in unwarned tasks. Phasic arousal appears to be less significantly impaired by brain damage, including right hemisphere injury.

Selective attention can be thought of as the way and the direction in which the energy supplied by arousal is channeled. Selective attention refers to the ability to select and focus on one type of information to the exclusion of others. From a survival perspective the role of location in selective attention is formidable in accurately detecting food and predators. Posner, Inhoff, and Friedrich[64] suggest that spatial selective attention can be divided into three sets of operations: disengagement of attention from its current location, movement of attention to a new location, and engagement of attention onto a new stimulus.

Many forms of neuropathology can impair spatial selective attention. Lesions in the cerebral hemispheres (particularly the right) can produce transient or long-lasting unilateral inattention. *Unilateral neglect* or *inattention* has been defined as a failure to orient to, respond to, or report stimuli presented on the side contralateral to the cerebral lesion in patients who do not have primary sensory or motor deficits; this neglect may become manifest in a variety of ways with varying degrees of specific sensory, motor, and visual components.[48]

The effect of attention on evaluation and treatment is profound. Attention affects the ability to learn and remember. Disorders of attention manifest in a variety of ways and may include distractibility, impulsivity, hypersensitivity to stimuli, and decreased attention span. A distractible patient, for example, may cue into external stimuli (i.e., anything in the environment) or internal stimuli (i.e., the patient's own thoughts, hunger, or pain) and consequently "tune out" the interventions the therapist is attempting with them. Therapists initially may have to work with such patients in a distraction-free environment, if possible. In the patient's hospital room, bed mobility training can be begun with the curtain pulled around the bed to screen out potential distractions.

Most if not all assessments of functional mobility fail to take this most important cognitive ability into account in assessing the ability to perform functional mobility skills. If the patient's attention to task is poor, learning cannot take place. In fact, attention can be thought of as the prerequisite on which learning occurs.

***Awareness.*** Awareness of disability is crucial in treatment planning and outcome. Awareness is a distinct phenomenon from denial (which is characterized by overrationalization), although each may be present to varying degrees. A significant proportion of brain-injured adults have demonstrated a lack of awareness of their deficits. Hartman-Maeir et al[37] have examined the frequency of awareness of disabilities after stroke rehabilitation. In addition, they explored the relationship of unawareness with neuroanatomic lesion sites and the impact on functional outcomes. Their findings indicate that unawareness of disabilities that persists to discharge from rehabilitation appears to correlate with neuroanatomic findings, specifically lesion sites in the right frontal and temporal lobes and size of lesion (the larger the lesion, the more likely one is to be unaware). In addition, their research indicated that unawareness was a negative predictor of outcome.

A model of awareness has been developed to aid the therapist's evaluation of the patient. This model is hierarchical and describes different levels of awareness in the following order[22]:
1. Intellectual awareness
2. Emergent awareness
3. Anticipatory awareness

Patients tend to fall into one of these three categories, and one goal in therapy becomes helping the patient progress through these levels. The rehabilitation process only proves useful if the patient understands that a problem exists.

Although a greater tendency exists for patients to acknowledge deficits in motor areas, facilitating recognition of deficits in the cognitive and behavioral realms is far more difficult. Impulsivity (action not conditioned by reasoning), for example, which is exemplary of attention disorder, typically is not acknowledged as a problem by patients in the safe performance of functional mobility tasks. The ramifications of this in planning for a safe environment on discharge after hospitalization are obvious.

***Memory and Learning.*** *Learning* can be defined as the acquisition of information and skills, and *memory* is the retention and storage of that knowledge. Learning can occur in the absence of overt behavior, but its occurrence can be inferred only from changes in behavior. Short-term memory (also referred to as *working memory*) describes the conscious retention and manipulation of information for recent, brief periods. *Declarative memory* refers to long-term memory amenable to conscious retrieval. Declarative memory includes the learning of facts and experiences that can be reported verbally. Procedural, or nondeclarative, memory comprises a number of functions expressed in motor, perceptual, and cognitive skills and habits.[89] These skills and habits cannot be expressed verbally and are connected with pavlovian conditioning. A special form of nondeclarative memory is priming, the preparation of a cognitive process by a previous task. Nondeclarative memory typically is spared in patients with amnesia because the memory individuals have of motor tasks is separate from the memories they have of other events in life.

Disruption of the underlying mechanisms subserving memory function occurs frequently after CVAs. Declarative memory skill relies on the hippocampi, whereas the basal ganglia play a major role in procedural memory skills. The cerebellum probably plays a role in pavlovian conditioning. To evaluate memory function, the therapist must assess whether the individual is taking in information efficiently by noting attention, association, organization, and other cognitive skills.

How much is understood about the way learning takes place? Studies on the neurobiology of learning after brain injury suggest that functional reorganization and plasticity possibly play roles in the recovery of information-processing capabilities. Understanding a patient's strengths and exploiting them are important in the learning process in occupational therapy. Teaching strategies should be geared to the patient's learning strengths (see Chapter 5).[60]

Researchers are seeking greater understanding of motor learning. Recent research by Parasher and Gentile[61] addresses the efficacy of "show" versus "tell" in providing instructions to the learner. They emphasize that two types of instructions—visuospatial and visuowritten—involve different processing and working memory systems. Visuospatial instructions are associated with right hemispheric functions. Visuowritten instructions involve interhemispheric transfer from the left to right hemispheres to produce visual representations of desired action goals. Parasher and Gentile determined that elderly persons have "greater difficulty than the young with the interhemispheric transfer or recoding of speech-based input required to derive a central representation of the action-goal." That is, showing the elderly learner the way to perform the task is better than verbally describing it. As more therapists involve themselves directly in research of this kind, occupational therapists may begin to elucidate differences in learning capabilities across the life span in the presence of a disability and hence will be able to teach skills more effectively.

***Executive Functions.*** Executive functions include the many skills used in problem solving, including problem recognition, goal formulation, planning and organization, initiation, and self-regulation and monitoring. If a person is to engage in independent, purposeful, and self-serving behavior, intact executive functioning is essential. The frontal lobes are linked inextricably with executive functions. Patients with frontal lobe lesions have difficulties with (among other things) initiating behavior, switching from one strategy to another, using mistakes to alter performance, and dealing with distractions.

In functional mobility training, difficulties with executive functions may manifest as difficulties with problem solving in novel situations. For example, the strategy used to learn to roll on a mat is not applicable in a bed, in which sheets and pillows are present and the surface is often softer. A new strategy must be learned in this situation, which could prove difficult for patients with impaired executive functions.

***Language and Communication.*** The left hemisphere is responsible for propositional language (conveying meaning through actual word order, word choice, and specific combinations of words and phrases into sentences). *Aphasia* is defined as the loss of language abilities (which may be on a continuum of mild to severe) caused by brain injury, usually to the dominant left hemisphere. Aphasia can affect the individual's auditory comprehension, verbal expression, repetition, naming, oral reading, reading comprehension, and written expression.[52] The therapist must address aphasia in therapy for functional mobility skills and, depending on whether the patient has expressive or receptive impairments or both, must develop a unique plan of action to ensure success in treatment.

The right hemisphere is responsible for affective language (prosody, or melody of speech, and the conveying of meaning through emotional tone via changes in stress, tempo, rhythm, duration, and intonation of speech sounds). The right hemisphere also is said to process pragmatic language. Pragmatics refers to a rule system that delineates the appropriate use of language according to situational contexts and constraints. In other words, pragmatics involves the meaning conveyed by the words themselves through the use of gesture, body language, facial expression, and other nonverbal means.[62] With brain injury to the right hemisphere, deficits in communication can occur; however, they are frequently more subtle than those noted with dominant left hemisphere involvement. With right-sided brain injury, patients exhibit flattened affects. Their speech, though fluent, is characterized by aprosodia, verbosity, and tangentiality. Additionally, these patients may be unable to discern prosody or nonverbal cues in the communication attempts of others. This can have an enormous effect on the therapist-patient relationship, and attempts at training such patients in functional mobility skills may prove difficult unless the therapist understands that communication deficits are present. Only then can the therapist devise an individualized treatment plan with these specific problems in mind.

*Psychological Components.* The therapist must appreciate the psychiatric sequelae associated with CVA to facilitate the rehabilitation process (see Chapter 2). Cerebral ischemia is associated with two types of depressive disorders. One type is depression meeting symptom criteria for major depression given in the *Diagnostic and Statistical Manual of Mental Disorders*, fourth edition. The other type is minor depression meeting symptom criteria for dysthymic depression (excluding the 2-year duration criterion) given in the manual. An association between the location of left-side anterior lesions and major depression among patients with acute stroke has been reported by three different groups of investigators.[6,39,69] Patients with depression in the rehabilitation setting are challenges for staff members and require supportive psychotherapeutic interventions. Additionally, they may benefit from psychopharmacologic treatment. Professionals working with these patients must recognize the signs of depression early because depression can have a significant impact on the patient's ability to participate in the rehabilitation process, concentrate during therapy sessions, and learn new skills.

In *Descartes' Error: Emotion, Reason and the Human Brain*, Damasio, a renowned neurologist, argues persuasively if not controversially that an inextricable link exists between cognition and emotion.[24] Damasio's thesis suggests for the work of occupational therapists a truth they perhaps have known implicitly for years: a person cannot be separated into apportioned packages of cognitive characteristics distinct from emotional and physical characteristics. The whole being, which is more than the sum of biopsychosocial factors that interplay and are interdependent on each other, must be considered.

## STRATEGIES FOR SPECIFIC IMPAIRMENTS

### Language Impairments

Different types of strategies may be used when approaching the patient with communication difficulties sustained as a result of damage to the right and left hemispheres. The therapist should consider the following guidelines when working with patients with left hemisphere involvement resulting in aphasia[62]:

1. Avoid speaking in a loud voice. Although the temptation is great, no hearing loss has occurred, and loud speech often makes the patient feel like a child.
2. Give the patient ample time to respond so the patient has time to process the response for which the therapist is asking.
3. Observe the patient for signs of fatigue or anxiety; do not pressure the patient.

4. Encourage expression of thoughts or ideas through whatever means the patient has available (e.g., posturing and gesturing).
5. If comprehension is a problem, ask simple, short questions and deemphasize spoken interaction; use gesture, facial expression, and pantomime to provide the patient with clues as to the response desired.
6. For the patient with comprehension problems, cueing through the tactile medium is most beneficial. For example, if rolling is the desired activity, ensure that hand placement "tells" the patient the response needed.

### Pragmatic Impairments

Therapists should consider the following guidelines when working with patients with right hemisphere involvement[62]:

1. Minimize distractions because an attention deficit may be present and interfering in treatment.
2. Have the patient demonstrate the ability to do an activity rather than rely on a report of the way the activity is accomplished. Demonstration is crucial because patients with right-sided lesions have a tendency to minimize their deficits or simply not recognize them.
3. Ensure that the patient is focused on the task at hand.
4. Go through sequences with the patient, having the patient repeat the correct order in which to carry out the task. If the goal is sit-to-stand, have the patient describe with the therapist the necessary steps (i.e., come to the edge of the bed, bring the feet back, lean forward).
5. Provide feedback on statements irrelevant to the situation. Patients with right-sided lesions are verbose at times and may complicate simple directions in the process.
6. Try to promote awareness of facial gestures as communication. This awareness is important because patients have a tendency not only to be devoid of facial expression but also to be unable to perceive the expressions of others.
7. Increase awareness of the patient's current situation (e.g., the reason the patient requires assistance with bed mobility and transfers).
8. Help the patient relearn the rules of taking turns in conversation.

### Apraxia

Apraxia is a disorder of skilled movement in the absence of impaired motor functioning or paralysis.[38] The left hemisphere appears to be superior to the right in the control of certain types of complex, sequenced motor acts; if damage is sustained to the left hemisphere, the patient's ability to acquire and perform tasks involving skilled movements may be impaired. Many forms of apraxia have been identified; as with many of the other disturbances discussed, they may be attributable to a number of causes or anatomic lesions. The forms of apraxia, caused largely by damage to the left frontal and inferior parietal lobes, include ideational, ideomotor, and buccofacial apraxia.

According to Bonfils, Affolter has developed a treatment technique of nonverbal guiding to stimulate and facilitate the patient's perceptual systems, thereby influencing cognitive systems. The therapist manually guides the patient in an activity, allowing exploration of objects and supporting surfaces in the process. This form of manual guidance is a "hand-over-hand" approach, with the therapist maintaining light but direct contact with the patient's extremities as the patient goes through the motions of carrying out a functional activity. The goal of this therapeutic approach is not the output of the movement pattern but rather the problem-solving process believed to be taking place.[13]

Heavy emphasis on the tactile-kinesthetic approach, that is, the tactile-kinesthetic exploration of the environment by the patient with facilitation from the therapist, is the defining feature of this technique; additionally, the technique is nonverbal, making it useful for the patient with apraxia. Affolter contends that the patient with apraxia is dealing with a perceptual deficit and needs to be treated with a functional approach. The therapist can use this approach to assist the patient if motor movement breaks down; the therapist provides the intervention without the use of words, except perhaps after the movement in the form of feedback to the patient on performance. Thus the tactile-kinesthetic approach may be useful with patients with aphasia as well (see Chapter 19).[13]

The tactile-kinesthetic approach emphasizes the use of meaningful activities in the appropriate environmental context. In this approach, the singular use of therapy equipment such as the mat table is meaningless because the patient needs to learn to roll and sit up from a bed and must learn sit-to-stand from a variety of surfaces such as a bed, chair, wheelchair, couch, toilet, and tub. Mistakes are needed for learning to take place. Patients need to learn to adapt to different situations and modify movement and strategy accordingly. Gradually the patient must take control over the personal movement repertoire for any carryover to take place.

### Unilateral Inattention

Unilateral inattention is most commonly with right-hemisphere lesions and may exist with or without hemianopsia. Patients with unilateral inattention have symptoms that vary in specific sensory modality involvement and severity. The therapist should thoroughly assess sensory, motor, and visual manifestations, paying particular attention to assessing the patient's level of awareness of the problem. Often these patients experience a lack of recognition of the left side of the body; this may make

efforts at training in functional mobility tasks difficult because the ability to attempt to incorporate both sides of the body into the activity is neither automatic nor easy to facilitate by the therapist.

In her extensive work on the cognitive remediation of these patients, Toglia[81] describes specific treatment strategies that primarily focus on the need to heighten the patient's awareness of the problem. She recommends consistent use of self-monitoring strategies and error detection by the patient in the cognitive remediation process. Modification of the environment also may be necessary; for example, a patient particularly susceptible to environmental distractions may need to begin functional mobility training in a low-stimulus environment and gradually build to a higher-stimulus environment in therapy (see Chapter 19).

### Attentional Deficits

Depending on the nature of the patient's attention problem, the therapist may choose to focus on increasing sustained attention, shifting attention, and sustaining attention in the presence of auditory and visual distractors. Initially therapy may have to take place in a minimally distracting environment, but gradually the patient needs to develop tolerance to stimuli in the environment.

## FUNCTIONAL MOBILITY TASKS

Functional mobility tasks occur throughout the daily routine under varying circumstances within changeable environments. Each task requires the individual to stabilize the body in space or exhibit dynamic postural control. Das and McCollum[25] identified three major requirements for locomotion that can be applied to all functional mobility tasks:

1. Progression or movement in a desired direction
2. The ability to stabilize the body against the forces of gravity
3. The ability to make changes in movement in relation to specific tasks within different environments

This view of functional mobility is congruent to a systems approach for analyzing and explaining normal movement, an approach that emphasizes the interaction of the individual, task, and environment.[78]

## ACTIVITIES IN THE SUPINE POSITION

The performance of supine activities is often associated with the acute stages of the rehabilitation process. Bridging, rolling, and movement from sidelying-to-sit are basic functional mobility tasks that are necessary to the provision of nursing care and movement of the client from a bed to a wheelchair. However, these mobility sequences are also important to enabling the client to participate in a wide range of life areas. For example, consider the individual who chooses to lie on a beach to enjoy the sun and surf. The soft surface of the sand may require the individual to assume a bridge position to shift their position if rolling is inadequate. Supine activities require the individual to gain control of flexor and extensor patterns of the trunk, which can be viewed as a prerequisite for more advanced trunk positions.

## Bridging

***Analysis of Movement.*** In the functional mobility task of bridging, the back and hip extensors support the body against the forces of gravity. The arch formed when the upper back and feet are in contact with the supporting surface is maintained by the activation of muscles located on the underside of the arch. Use of the arms or legs increases the demands placed on the trunk musculature. When an arm or leg is raised (as in attempts to dress), the muscles located above the arch (the oblique abdominal muscles) must become active to support the limb.[26]

***Selected Problems.*** The mobility task of bridging is a challenge for patients with hemiplegia because of loss of activity in the extensors and the abdominal muscles. Combining this problem with early return of extensor activity results in ineffective and inefficient movement patterns.

Supine characteristics indicating decreased abdominal activity include the following:

- Upward and outward drawing of the ribcage (that is, the affected side rides higher in the cavity because the abdominal muscles do not tether the ribcage downward)
- Shortening of the neck resulting from unopposed elevation of the shoulder girdle
- Hypotonic appearance of the abdomen
- Shift of the umbilicus to the nonaffected side
- Reduced proximal stability effecting the lower extremities

Primitive extensor activity for all movements further diminishes flexor control because of reciprocal inhibition.[26]

***Treatment Strategies.*** Bridging is an important position that the patient should be instructed to assume early in the intervention process. Bridging is a mobility function necessary for the use of a bedpan, reduction of pressure on the buttocks, and movement within the bed (bed scooting).[45] In addition, the position of the low back and hips approximates the alignment required for the normal stance position.[45,79] Movement within this position can simulate further the movement required of the pelvis and lower extremities during ambulation, specifically forward motion of the pelvis, lateral and rotational pelvic shift, and advanced movement combinations of hip extension with knee flexion.[26]

The patient with hemiplegia may experience difficulty in assuming the crook-lying position and forming a bridge because of a variety of underlying causes. The lack of selective muscle activity on the affected side, caused by the use of mass patterns, prevents the patient from combining the necessary hip components of flexion and adduction.[11] Patient attempts to place the affected leg usually result in a mass pattern of movement characterized by hip flexion and external rotation and supination of the foot. The patient's inability to stabilize the pelvis while attempting this movement results in increased extension of the lumbar spine combined with forced extension of the nonaffected side into the supporting surface. Another possible reason for the increase in the extension of the lumbar spine is tightness of the hip flexors,[79] although this is unlikely in the early stages after stroke unless the patient exhibited tightness before sustaining the stroke.

The therapist can assist the patient to assume the crook-lying position. The therapist encourages the patient to assist with active flexion of the unaffected leg and may be required to assist and hold the required crook-lying position. Active flexion on the affected leg helps position the pelvis forward and may promote active holding of the affected leg in a flexed position.[45] The therapist may provide downward pressure on the flexed knee of the affected side to ensure appropriate foot placement.[11]

Active bridging can be used to improve selective extension of the hip and abdominal muscle activity. As the patient lifts the buttocks from the supporting surface, the therapist should make sure the patient does not use excessive extensor activity, which is characterized by extension of the hips, overarching of the back, and pushing of the head into the supporting surface. To improve selective movement, the therapist encourages the patient to initiate the movement by actively tilting the pelvis upward. The therapist may need to prepare the patient for this movement (Figure 14-1). After tilting the pelvis forward, the patient lifts the buttocks off the surface while holding the pelvis level. The therapist may assist this movement by placing one hand under the hemiplegic hip and one hand on the abdominals. If the feet are positioned close to the body, the therapist also may guide the femoral condyles forward toward the feet while applying downward pressure (Figure 14-2).

After the patient can maintain this position, the next step is to lift the unaffected foot off the surface while maintaining the pelvis level. The therapist should observe any asymmetries or rotation of the pelvis. The therapist must not permit the patient to drop the unaffected side to gain more stability. This task is difficult for the patient with hemiplegia because it places demands on the oblique abdominal muscles.[20,27,79] Bridging can be graded according to the patient's ability to control movements selectively. Placement of the feet further away from the buttocks

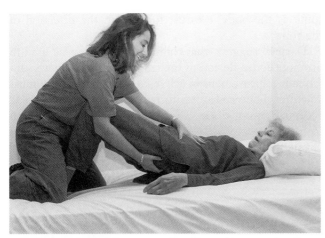

**Figure 14-1** In bridging, one should avoid increased extensor activity that results in arching of the back. To assist with selective movement of the pelvis, the therapist cues the gluteal region and the lower abdominals. This sequence may be applied first to the unaffected side and then to the hemiplegic side.

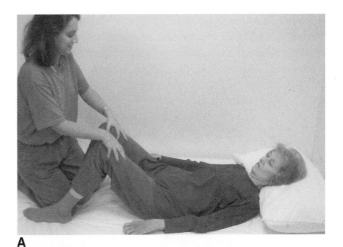

**A**

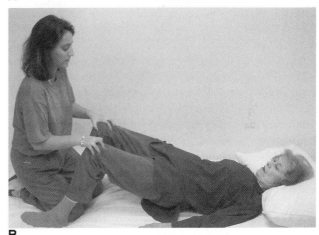

**B**

**Figure 14-2** **A,** As the patient gains selective control over the pelvis, the therapist can provide downward pressure through the knees and guide the femoral condyles forward toward the feet. **B,** The therapist asks the patient to lift the buttocks off the bed. Physical assistance can be diminished as the patient gains control.

requires a greater degree of selective activity to maintain knee flexion with hip extension.[27] Alternate lifting of the feet off the supporting surface while maintaining the level of the pelvis requires increased muscular activity and greater coordination (Figures 14-3 and 14-4).[79]

Bridging can be used to move up in bed and don pants while in a supine position. Therapists should instruct caregivers in the appropriate techniques to ensure that these movements are transferred into the patient's daily life routine. The occupational therapist can incorporate these movement strategies while training the patient in self-care activities.

## Rolling

*Analysis of Movement.* Rolling is an important part of bed mobility and an essential part of many other tasks. Research has demonstrated that normal adults use a variety of movement strategies to roll from supine to prone.[68]

One of the most common movement strategies used by young adults in rolling from supine to prone includes a lift-and-reach arm pattern. Movement of the head and trunk is initiated by the shoulder girdle; a unilateral lift of the leg also occurs. Rotation of the spine, which results in dissociation of the shoulder and pelvic girdles, is not observed (Figure 14-5).[68] This rotation was once assumed to be a prerequisite to attaining the ability to roll in a normal pattern of movement.[11]

The most important finding of this study is that normal adults have a repertoire of movements available to them, unlike patients after stroke, who are limited to stereotypical patterns of movement.[23] The environmental conditions of this study were limited to rolling on an exercise mat, and the subjects were asked to roll "as fast as you can." Thus the variety of patterns observed may relate to the temporal demands and implied goal of the task. The strategies used to roll for speed may differ significantly from the strategies used to target a particular object in the environment. Therapists who work with patients with hemiplegia must consider the rolling surface (environment), the goal of changing the position of the body while supine, and future mobility goals such as attaining supine-to-sit. Thus therapists must determine movement sequences most suitable to ensuring safety and maintaining essential components of movement that are nevertheless necessary for subsequent skills. Rotation of the spine during rolling is just one strategy that may be useful in providing a greater variety of movement possibilities for the patient with hemiplegia.[20,26,27]

***Rolling to the Hemiplegic Side: Selected Problems and Treatment Strategies.*** The patient with hemiplegia frequently rolls over using an extensor pattern to initiate the movement sequence because of lack of flexor control of the trunk and the early return of extensor activity. The patient relies on the unaffected side to push against the supporting surface, resulting in an arching of the axial spine as the body is thrust forward in the direction of the roll.

Davies[26] suggests that rolling activities can be used to promote active flexion of the trunk and thus achieve subsequent improvement in active control of the trunk musculature. The need exists to balance the concentric and eccentric contractions of the trunk muscles in proportion to the change in force exerted by gravity as the patient changes position.

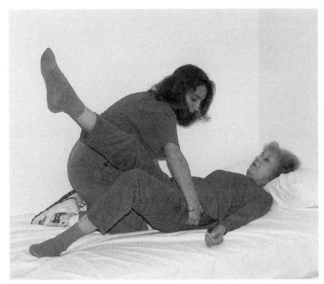

**Figure 14-3**    Lifting a leg off the supporting surface places increased demands on the abdominal muscles because the pelvis must be held up. The therapist asks the patient to lift the unaffected foot off the bed so that all the patient's weight is placed on the affected side. The patient must maintain the pelvis in a level position. This patient is experiencing difficulty maintaining the optimal pelvic position (left hemiplegia).

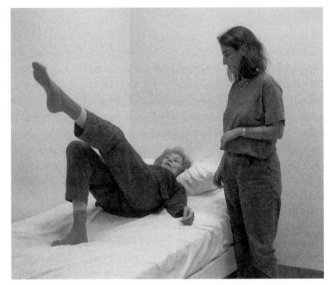

**Figure 14-4**    This patient has less difficulty in lifting the hemiplegic side (left hemiplegia).

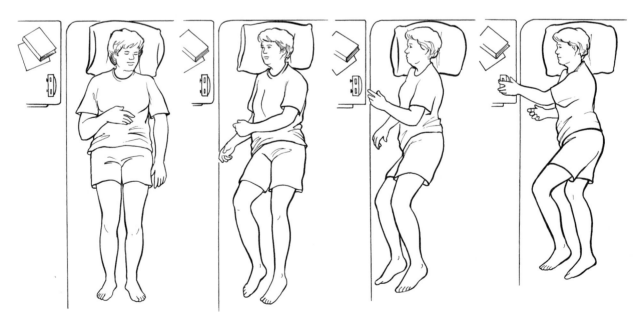

**Figure 14-5**    Research has determined that a common form of rolling observed in adults is initiated by a lift and reach above shoulder level; the shoulder girdle leads the movement, and a unilateral lift of the lower extremity follows. Many subjects also use a unilateral push of the lower extremity. A great variety of patterns is observed because of individual differences in build and strength and in the support surface.

The hemiplegic arm requires protection before rolling to the affected side is practiced. The therapist can provide this protection by prepositioning the arm, assisting the patient in bringing the shoulder and arm forward, and giving physical support to the hemiplegic arm while standing on the affected side.

The patient is encouraged to lift the unaffected arm and leg up and forward across the body; this movement is consistent with the pattern identified by Richter, Van Sant, and Newton.[68] This movement should occur without the patient pushing against the supporting surface with the unaffected foot (Figure 14-6). The patient may repeat this movement by returning to the supine position. A part of or the whole leg should be held in abduction and slowly lowered to the surface as the patient returns to the supine position.

As the patient gains control of this movement sequence, the next step is to lift the head from the surface to assist with initiation of movement. As the patient turns, the head is rotated toward the direction of the movement. Throughout the sequence, physical assistance should decrease as changes in the patient's ability to control movement occur.

***Rolling to the Unaffected Side: Selected Problems and Treatment Strategies.*** Rolling to the unaffected side may be more difficult for the patient with hemiplegia. The movement frequently is initiated by an extensor pattern that includes extension of the head, neck, and back. The patient relies on extension of the back to bring the hemiplegic leg over the trunk in a pattern of extension

that may be viewed as an inefficient compensatory strategy. The affected arm may be left behind as the patient rolls (Figure 14-7).[27]

When teaching patients to roll to the unaffected side, the therapist's goals are to decrease maladaptive compensatory strategies contributing to inefficient movement and enhance more effective and efficient patterns of movement. The patient may be instructed to use the stronger arm (Figure 14-8) to bring the hemiplegic arm up and forward while the therapist attempts verbally or physically to cue the movement of the pelvis and lower extremity. The

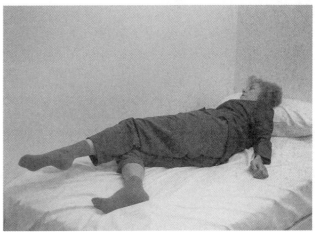

**Figure 14-7** Rolling toward the unaffected side. The patient should avoid using the back extensors to bring the lower extremity forward while neglecting the hemiplegic arm (left hemiplegia).

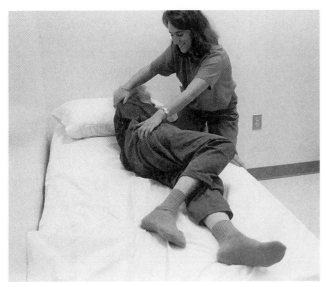

**Figure 14-6** Rolling toward the hemiplegic side (left hemiplegia) is accomplished by lifting the unaffected leg over the hemiplegic side without pushing off the bed surface. The therapist assists with movement of the shoulder and pelvic girdles.

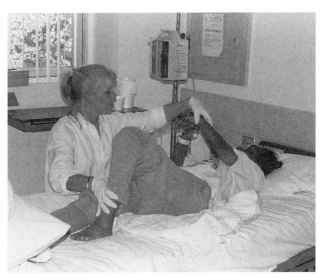

**Figure 14-8** Early in the rehabilitation process the therapists instructs the patient with left hemiplegia to use the stronger hand to assist in bringing the shoulder forward; the therapist positions the hemiplegic leg in hip and knee flexion to avoid an extensor pattern.

therapist supports the affected leg while assisting with anterior movement of the pelvis (Figure 14-9).

Repetition of this sequence may assist with learning. The therapist encourages the patient to lift the affected leg off the supporting surface and lower it slowly after returning to the supine position. This strategy is used to assist the patient in maintaining a slight degree of hip and knee flexion, which decreases reliance on the extensor compensatory pattern. An alternative method is to flex both legs to roll.[11,27]

## Supine-to-Sit

***Analysis of Movement.*** The transitional movement from supine-to-sit may be achieved through a variety of movement strategies. Adults have a tendency to use a momentum strategy to achieve the goal (Figure 14-10). Their movements are smooth and efficient as they "bound" out of bed, off the couch, or out of a chair. A momentum strategy requires forces within the trunk to be generated and transferred to the lower extremities to initiate the rolling sequence. Trunk muscles must contract concentrically to initiate and propel the movement; eccentric muscle contractions provide control. The reciprocal shortening and lengthening of muscle contractions provide maintained stability.

Many older adults demonstrate a tendency to use a force control strategy (Figure 14-11). The individual transfers forces from one body part to another as graduated changes in position occur. Rolling to side lying, then pushing up with the upper extremities, and swinging the lower extremities over the side of the bed is an example of this strategy. This method provides increased stability because concentric and eccentric forces are required in increments. Increased effort (force) must be used if momentum is lacking.[18,20,27,68,75]

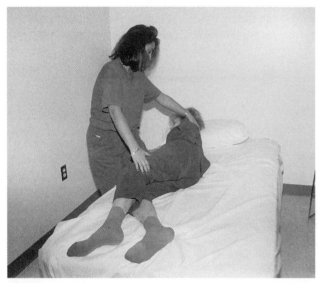

**Figure 14-9**    Assistance can be decreased as the patient gains control of the movement. The therapist is assisting with knee flexion and protraction of the shoulder (left hemiplegia).

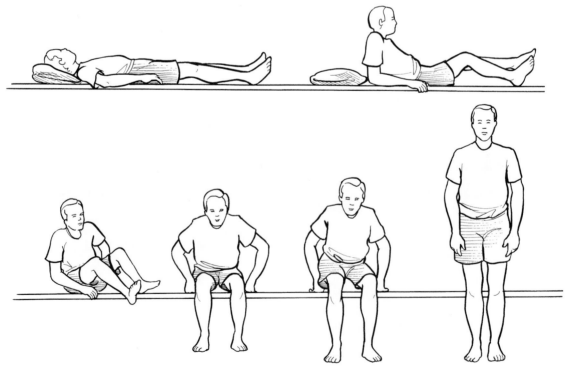

**Figure 14-10**    The most common movement strategy used by adults to get out of bed relies on momentum. Strategies vary greatly.

Evidence exists to support that older adults use their upper limbs to assist the trunk musculature when moving from supine-to-sit.[3] Thus therapists need to consider the movement strategies and positioning of the arms when retraining the supine-to-sit sequence. A great variety of movement possibilities to achieve a supine-to-sit sequence remains. The described sequence often is used spontaneously by patients after CVA and by the therapists as a method of instruction.[20] This sequence is referred to as *sidelying-to-sit* for the remainder of this chapter.

***Selected Problems.*** Movement from the side lying to seated position becomes a challenge for the patient after CVA because of the combined effects of limited muscular activity and maladaptive compensatory strategies. Patients lack appropriate postural alignment and stability.[20,26] The lack of flexor control of the trunk and early return of extensor activity interfere with the patient's ability to grade concentric and eccentric muscle activity effectively relative to the changing forces of gravity.[26] If inadequate control of the trunk musculature is evident, the patient must rely on compensatory strategies that may include overuse of the unaffected arm or leg or exaggerated use of head movements. The patient uses these compensatory strategies instead of effective lateral movements of the neck and trunk. When side lying, the patient flexes the head forward instead of laterally and uses the unaffected arm to move the body away from the supporting surface. The forward movement of the head may be a compensatory strategy to shift the center of gravity forward. The patient may be unable to combine lateral flexion and extension of the trunk because of lack of selective muscle activity. Hooking of the unaffected leg under the affected leg to lift and lower the leg over the side of the bed is yet another compensatory strategy many patients are instructed to perform. This strategy prevents selective movement of the pelvis in an anterior and lateral direction.[20,26] The patient with hemiplegia experiences difficulty whether rising from the hemiplegic or the unaffected side because of the problems presented.

Additionally, while changing positions, the patient may not exhibit appropriate head-righting responses; this deficit requires the patient to flex the neck laterally while controlling eccentric muscle activity on the opposite side. Furthermore, the patient also may be unable to move or place the affected limbs appropriately in preparation for transitional movement or may neglect the affected limbs entirely.

***Treatment Strategies.*** Many methods are suggested to retrain the patient in the supine-to-sit movement sequence. One method suggests that patients with hemiplegia be taught initially to roll toward the affected side to decrease the amount of effort required and reduce maladaptive strategies such as pulling and pushing to achieve the seated position.[20] Others suggest that the patient with hemiplegia be instructed to rise from both sides early in treatment to prevent associated reactions.[10,26,27] Another option is for the patient to start the movement sitting upright and learn to lie down first. This method may decrease the force gravity exerts on the trunk musculature as the patient first learns to control movement into gravity using eccentric muscle activity.[26] The physical environment and the patient's premorbid preferences for movement sequences also may influence the methods selected. Patients may benefit from learning more than one method to move more effectively in different environments.

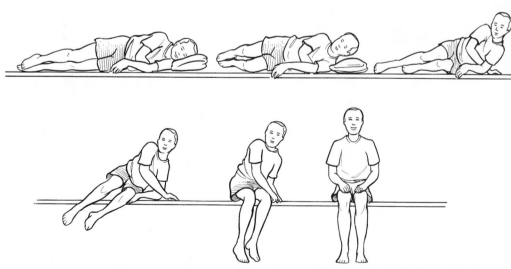

**Figure 14-11** A force control strategy for getting out of bed has the individual performing the task in two parts: the patient moves from supine to side lying and then pushes to a seated position. This strategy is useful for patients who exhibit reduced stability functions.

***Sidelying-to-Sit Toward the Affected Side.*** The therapist assists the patient in lifting the hemiplegic leg over the side of the bed; the head, neck, and upper thorax are brought forward, requiring the neck to flex laterally. Concurrently the nonaffected arm must be brought across the body and placed on the bed. The unaffected leg also must be lifted over the side of the bed as the patient pushes down with the hand. The movement of the unaffected leg as the patient simultaneously pushes with the hand adds a momentum strategy to this movement sequence; the weight of the leg assists the patient in attaining a seated posture. The therapist may be required to assist with bringing the unaffected shoulder forward over the base of support of the body. The therapist may place hands on the shoulder and pelvic girdle to give support and assist with movement of the unaffected leg (Figure 14-12). As the patient gains some control over this movement, the therapist may provide support to just the unaffected shoulder and pelvis (Figure 14-13). The therapist can use verbal cues or downward pressure on the shoulder physically to cue lateral flexion of the trunk and appropriate head righting. To reverse this sequence, the patient may require assistance with lifting the hemiplegic leg onto the bed. Care should be directed toward maintaining the hemiplegic shoulder in a forward position as the patient turns and lowers the body to the bed surface.[26]

When assuming a sitting position from the affected side, the patient is active in the trunk, particularly while bearing weight on the affected upper extremity; therapists should be mindful of this. Furthermore, the therapist may have to cue movement of the trunk on both sides to promote the correct sequence of lateral flexion and extension responses (Figure 14-14).

***Sidelying-to-Sit Toward the Unaffected Side.*** The sequence of movement in sidelying-to-sit toward the unaffected side remains the same as that in the previous example; however, the placement of the therapist's hands to assist movement changes. The therapist should

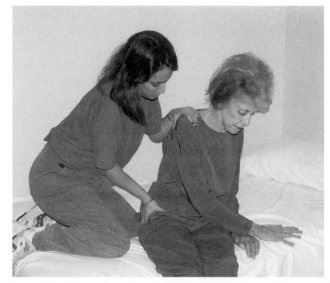

**Figure 14-13**    When the patient is able to control the trunk muscles actively, the therapist can decrease assistance. The therapist may cue lateral flexion of the head and trunk by providing downward pressure to the shoulder and pelvic girdles of the unaffected side.

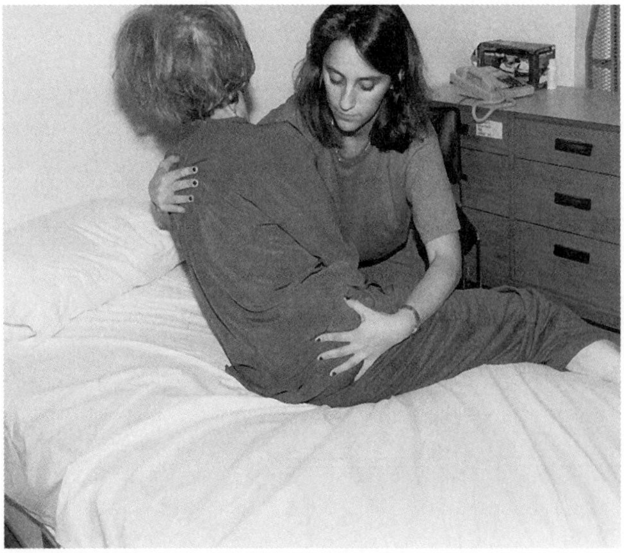

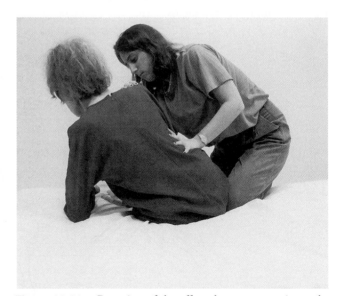

**Figure 14-12**    The therapist uses one arm around the patient's shoulders while the other hand provides downward pressure to the pelvis to assist with weight transfer in movement to a seated position (left hemiplegia).

**Figure 14-14**    Propping of the affected upper extremity as the patient prepares to assume the seated position. The therapist is assisting with lateral flexion of the unaffected side while observing for appropriate head and trunk alignment on the affected side.

instruct the patient to lift the affected arm while lifting the unaffected leg over the side of the bed. The therapist assists with movement of the affected leg forward and over the edge of the bed as the patient lifts the head, neck, and upper thorax over the sound arm (Figure 14-15). The therapist needs to ensure that the hemiplegic shoulder remains in a forward position as the patient begins to push down with the unaffected side. A movement sequence that begins as a force control strategy can

with increased motor control of the head, neck, and trunk become a momentum strategy.

Patients demonstrating a lack of lateral flexion of the neck require preparatory interventions. The patient should be positioned side lying on the unaffected side with the head on the bed (Figure 14-16, *A*). The patient lifts the head with the therapist's assistance as needed (Figure 14-16, *B*). The therapist then asks the patient to lower the head to the bed; this movement requires eccentric contraction of the lateral flexors. This maneuver is followed by active lifting of the head, which requires concentric muscle contractions. The therapist should not permit the patient to rotate or flex forward while performing this task. A visual target such as an alarm clock, television, or family picture may assist in establishing this task-related goal.[20]

Additional interventions to promote lateral flexion and extension of the trunk, which are necessary to perform sidelying-to-sit, are described in the section on sitting.

## ACTIVITIES IN SITTING

The ability to maintain a seated position and perform activities of daily living safely and efficiently is a goal many occupational therapists seek with their patients (see Chapter 7). In the acute stages after CVA (if the patient is medically stable), the therapist should begin to work on control of sitting and standing with the patient as soon as possible to promote the ability to manage the upright position and increase overall visual input in functional positions.[20]

### Analysis of Movement

For controlled movement in sitting the ability to bear and shift weight anteriorly, posteriorly, laterally, and in a

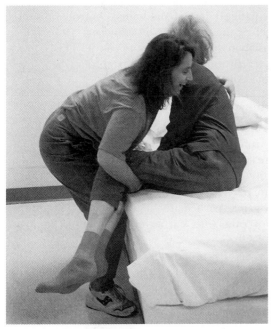

**Figure 14-15**   Rising from the unaffected side. For patients who require significant support, the therapist places one hand on the scapula while assisting with movement of the legs.

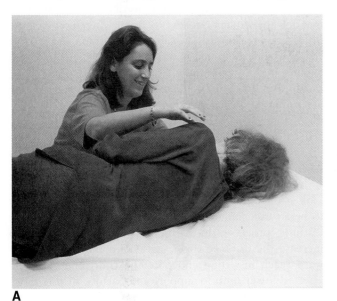

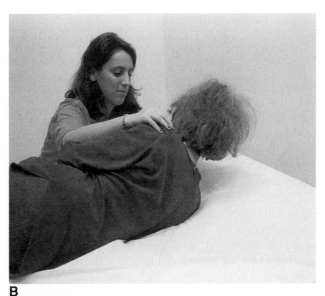

**A**                                           **B**

**Figure 14-16**   **A,** To encourage active control of the lateral neck muscles, the patient first learns to control eccentric contraction while lowering the head to the bed. **B,** This is followed by active lateral neck flexion while raising the head.

rotary pattern must be present. This suggests that the concentric and eccentric abilities of the trunk flexors and extensors and the ability to activate these muscle groups selectively relative to the task demand must be present. For example, for controlled anterior weight shift through the pelvis the need for concentric contraction of the low back extensors and an associated eccentric contraction of the trunk flexors (abdominals) is evident. In a posterior weight shift through the pelvis, the need for concentric contraction of the trunk flexors and an associated eccentric contraction of the trunk extensors is evident. With lateral weight shift through the pelvis the trunk extensors and flexors work together concentrically (shortening) on the non–weight-bearing side and eccentrically (lengthening) on the weight-bearing side.[11] During trunk rotation the primary muscles involved are the oblique muscles.

## Selected Problems

The trunk is crucial in postural control. The therapist must begin an assessment on functional capabilities in this area by close examination of the patient's ability to control movements in sitting. A full appreciation of the normal ranges of motion within the spine is useful when comparing patients with hemiplegia and the patterns they use with the normal population. The therapist must be cognizant that these ranges decrease with age; ascertaining the baseline from which these patients were operating before the onset of hemiparesis is important. Mohr[56] emphasizes the importance of establishing a patient's range of motion in spinal extension and flexion, lateral flexion, and rotation before treatment is implemented. This provides the therapist with information needed to decide whether interventions should include increasing ranges in these areas with the goal of promoting activation by the patient in these patterns for function. Davies[26] also recommends this approach. For example, passive mobilization of the lumbar spine for lateral flexion may be an important preparatory treatment to working on increased trunk control in activities requiring a lateral weight shift such as sidelying-to-sit. The therapist, having encouraged increased mobility in this plane, can progress to facilitation of the appropriate muscle contractions needed to hold and move into this position by placing the hand in the patient's axilla and assisting the side to lengthen while placing the other hand on the patient's opposite trunk to guide shortening on that side.

A deeper look at the location of movement and the way it is initiated is necessary before proceeding in evaluation. Ryerson and Levit[70] help categorize trunk movements in sitting by dividing them into movements initiated from the upper trunk versus the lower trunk. They further break anterior, lateral and posterior weight shifts in each of these categories and then provide functional examples for each movement pattern.

Davies[26] indicates that the abdominal muscles tend to be neglected in treatment. Appropriate recruitment of the abdominals is not possible because of the presence of hypotonicity in the trunk and changes in biomechanical alignment that keep the abdominals from working optimally. Davies goes further and points out that a number of patients with hemiplegia from CVA appear to have a bilateral loss of abdominal muscle activity and tone. This seems to be a function of the attachment of the abdominal muscles through a central aponeurosis connected to the linea alba; each side depends on the other for skilled movement to take place. Davies maintains that as a result of the patient's loss of abdominal control and subsequent neglect of these muscles by clinicians, patients begin to use compensatory strategies to move. This is evidenced by overactivation of the back extensors when attempting to move (see Chapter 7).

### Functional Activities in Sitting

Task-oriented functional practice must follow all "preparatory" trunk activity such as mobilization. Following hands-on treatment, one hopefully will see gains in passive mobility or the patient's ability to "find" the muscle and activate it. However, the patients themselves must use these gains, particularly in the context of a functional activity; otherwise, carryover is doubtful (Figures 14-17 and 14-18).

Gentile[31] has proposed two distinct processes that mediate skill learning: an explicit process and an implicit process. In the explicit process, patients consciously involve themselves with shaping the movements to achieve a specific goal. In the implicit process, the main concern is the dynamics of force generation, which is not under the conscious control of the patient. Implicit processes rely on the interplay of muscle contractions against the passive components affected by gravity and joint torques. Gentile suggests that for the explicit process to occur, therapists can use information consciously available to the patient and provide coaching such as around how a movement is organized and features in the environment. For implicit learning to occur, therapists must challenge themselves creatively to set up the environment to elicit a response from the patient that produces force generation as a by-product of the functional activity in which they are engaged. Clearly the therapist must set up opportunities for practice for the greatest benefit to occur to the learner.

Dean and Shepherd[28] designed a study specifically to look at the efficacy of task-related training, which proves to be an excellent example of using explicit and implicit learning processes in treatment. Their intent was to increase the distance stroke patients could perform forward reach in sitting and note the contribution of the affected lower limb to support and balance in this activity. Twenty subjects were used in this study. They had to be a minimum of 1 year past stroke. They were randomized into two groups—an experimental group that received treatment involving reaching forward for natural objects

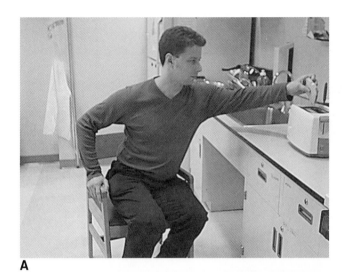

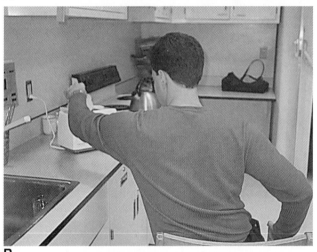

**Figure 14-17** **A,** Reaching for toast combines patterns of trunk lateral flexion and extension. **B,** Using the left affected arm to bear weight on the armrest results in scapula depression, which contributes to the shortening of the trunk muscles on the right side.

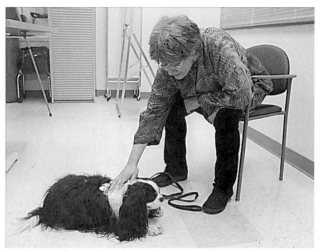

**Figure 14-18** A pet therapy dog is used to encourage trunk flexion and weight-bearing on the affected left arm and leg.

beyond arm's length (in a gradual progression) and a control group that received sham training with cognitive tasks within arm's length. Electromyography, videotaping, and two force plates (to evaluate the amount of lower extremity force generated during the activity and sit-to-stand) were used before and after training to gain objective measures. After training, subjects were capable of reaching farther and faster, suggesting that the affected lower limb was assisting more in support. Furthermore, the researchers noted that subjects demonstrated improved force generation of the affected lower limb in sit-to-stand. The explicit learning process subjects were engaged in was demonstrated by the problem solving and practicing of forward reaching farther and farther. The implicit learning process was activating the lower extremity in the process.[28,31]

## Scooting

*Analysis of Movement.* Scooting, or "butt walking," involves the transfer of weight over first one buttock and then the other, creating overall movement of the body anteriorly in a seated position.[10] Appropriate elongation of the trunk on the weight-bearing side and shortening on the non–weight-bearing side is required. This movement pattern is useful for a number of functional activities such as donning and doffing pants in a seated position. From a mobility perspective it allows the individual to approach the edge of a supporting surface to transfer.

*Selected Problems.* As indicated previously, problems with passive restriction in the trunk and the inability to activate trunk muscles selectively are of primary concern with this activity and may preclude the appropriate balance reactions needed for success and safety. The patient must have intact skin on the buttocks to practice scooting.

*Treatment Strategies.* Verbal or physical cueing to assist patients with scooting can be accomplished in a variety of ways, depending on the level of involvement of the individual. The therapist may elicit the desired movement pattern through a series of contacts in which the therapist first cues a lateral weight shift and then places the hand on the patient's pelvis to cue forward advancing of the hip on the non–weight-bearing side.[10] The therapist then changes hands to cue forward movement of the opposite buttock (Figure 14-19). Patients with more profound physical involvement may require added assistance by the therapist, particularly in advancing the buttock (Figure 14-20).

## Transfers

*Analysis of Movement.* The ability to move from a given surface to an adjacent surface safely and efficiently is a

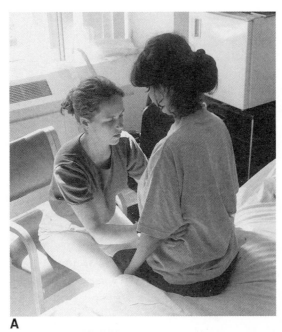

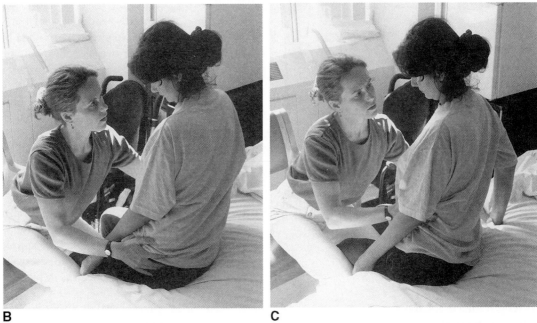

**Figure 14-19**    Scooting is an important skill for moving to the edge of a bed or seat and can be a useful movement pattern in activity of daily living tasks such as donning pants in a seated position. **A,** The patient begins in symmetrical sitting. **B,** The therapist can encourage scooting by first cueing a lateral weight shift and then advancing the non–weight-bearing buttock to move anteriorly **(C).**

primary goal in treatment for many of the patients with whom occupational therapists work. This maneuver requires enough forward flexion of the trunk over the feet to allow the individual to pivot about the feet and sit on the nearby surface.

***Selected Problems.*** Patients with neglect who attempt to transfer often succeed in transporting only half the body onto the supporting surface. Additionally, the left foot may be neglected, and the patient may be oblivious to proper left foot placement before transferring.

Many patients require considerable help to maintain a flat foot on the floor. This may be because of unilateral inattention, poor sensation on the affected side, shortened trunk muscles resulting in asymmetrical sitting, and shortening of the calf muscles on the affected side.

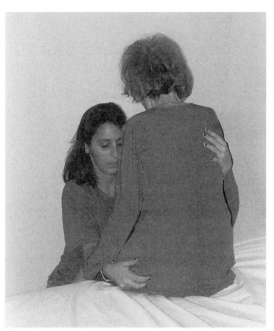

**Figure 14-20** Patients requiring a more direct contact to scoot can be guided first by the therapist to advance the buttock.

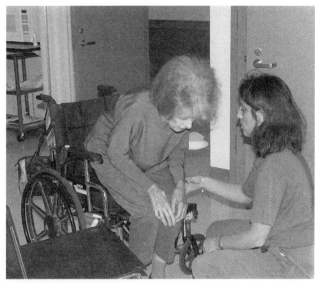

**Figure 14-21** To teach a patient to perform a squat-pivot transfer, the therapist should encourage the appropriate amount of anterior weight shift by instructing the patient to move the shoulders forward.

*Treatment Strategies.* Bobath[10] and Davies[27] describe the anterior weight shift that can be facilitated through contact on the patient's pelvis or scapulae. Carr and Shepherd[20] recognize the same forward weight shift and encourage patients to move the shoulders forward during active participation in transfers (Figure 14-21). All four therapists describe ways the therapist may use manual contact to the knee to draw the knee forward and encourage weight bearing on the hemiplegic side.

Patients have varying degrees of motor control for this activity. The therapist needs to create an environment in which the patient has enough guarding by the therapist to make training safe and enough "room" to try to make the transfer with as little assistance as possible. This is not always easy to do, and some patients inevitably require much assistance to transfer. However, the more the patient can be encouraged to do, the more the patient learns during the session. Consistent grading of the level of assistance a patient requires (i.e., minimal, moderate, or maximal) is important in measuring progress and communicating to other staff members the amount of help required by the patient to carry out the task.

In the initial stages of transfer training a patient may require maximal assistance, and the therapist may need to clasp both hands around the pelvis to pivot the patient from one surface to another. As the patient gains greater strength and control over balance, the therapist may reduce this level of assistance to a lighter hold around the pelvis and then the scapula.

Patients tend to be taught stand-pivot or modified stand-pivot (squat-pivot) transfers. Many therapists train stand-pivot transfers for the presumed benefits they afford in getting the patient into an upright position and putting full weight on the involved lower extremity. However, these transfers do not in any way resemble the maneuvers performed by normal subjects in moving from one surface to the other (i.e., coming to a full stand or turning and sitting down on an adjacent surface). As Shumway-Cook and Woollacott[78] point out, stand-pivot transfers may be more difficult because they do not allow the patient to use a momentum strategy; the need to come to a stand instead of pivoting blocks the benefits the momentum strategy provides.

Promoting weight shift onto the affected lower extremity is important during transfers and sit-to-stand activities. The therapist may position both knees around the patient's affected knee physically to assist a forward weight shift onto the lower extremity and guard against buckling at the patient's knee. For patients requiring less cueing and guarding, the therapist may assist the knee by placing a hand on the patient's distal femur and gently pulling anteriorly and then down toward the floor as the patient takes weight on the leg.

The role of the arms in this training process has become controversial. Bobath[10] and Davies[27] support using clasped hands in front of the body to facilitate a forward weight shift, placing the arms on a stool, chair, or other supporting surface. However, a study by Carr and Gentile[17] examined the role of the upper extremities in sit-to-stand and determined that "fixing" the arms (by holding a rod as subjects in the study did) had a tendency to cause an increase in what was described as *extension force* (the force needed by the lower extremities to extend the body into an upright position) and a decrease in momentum of the body during sit-to-stand; this determination may have implications for transfers. The authors advocate that patients work on increasing strength in the lower extremities (particularly in extension) to enhance functioning in sit-to-stand. They contend that although patients tend to use the hands to push down on the arm-rests of a chair to stand or alternatively swing the arms forward to assist horizontal and vertical propulsion of the body mass, these strategies cannot be used in varying environmental conditions[17] (Figures 14-22 to 14-25).

### Sit-to-Stand

*Analysis of Movement.* Sit to stand can be divided into different phases, depending on the description of the

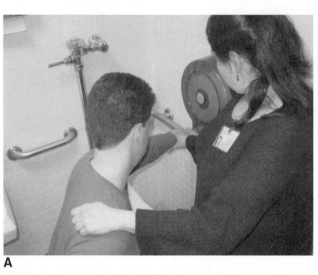

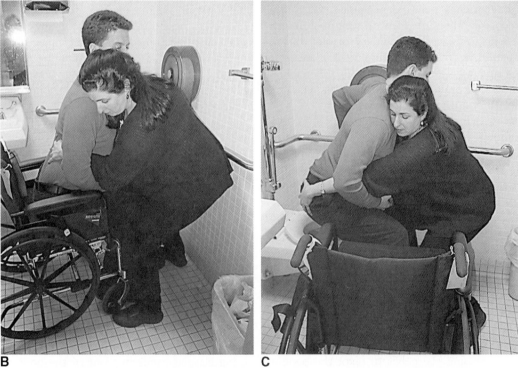

**Figure 14-22**    **A,** Use of a grab bar can encourage a forward weight shift in a transfer requiring greater physical assistance. **B,** Positioning and proper handling can be difficult with space constraints. This requires problem solving for the therapist, patient, and caregiver. **C,** While this patient may require moderate physical assistance to perform the transfer, he is actively encouraged to use the movements he is capable of in the transfer, in this case, thoracic extension.

researcher (Figure 14-26). Shepherd and Gentile[76] describe sit-to-stand using the terms *preextension phase*, a phase characterized by the beginning of the movement to the position in which the thighs are off the surface, and *extension phase*, the phase from the thighs-off position through the end of movement (full stand). Shenkman et al[75] describe four phases in sit-to-stand (Figure 14-27).

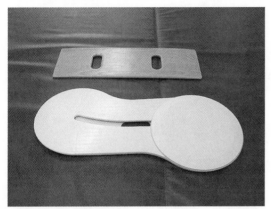

**Figure 14-23** A typical short sliding board and a Beasy board. These devices can be used to assist patients who have greater physical needs.

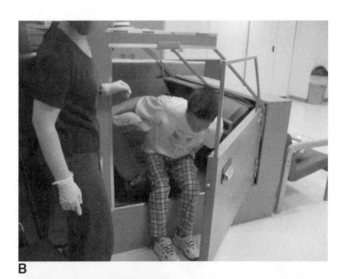

**B**

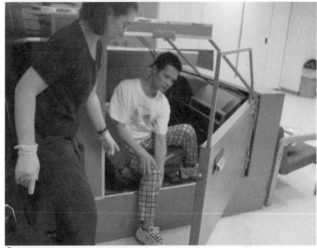

**C**

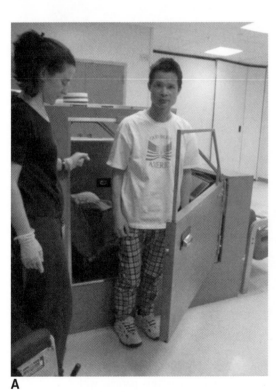

**A**

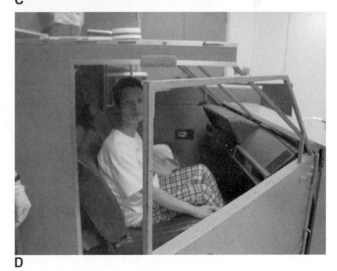

**D**

**Figure 14-24** **A,** Early practice with car transfers may take place using a simulated car in the clinic and where possible should progress to an actual vehicle. **B,** Controlled descent into gravity requires coactivation of the abdominal muscles (flexors) and back extensors to avoid injury in a constrained space. **C,** The patient is shown how to manage the affected leg during the transfer. **D,** Completion of the car transfer.

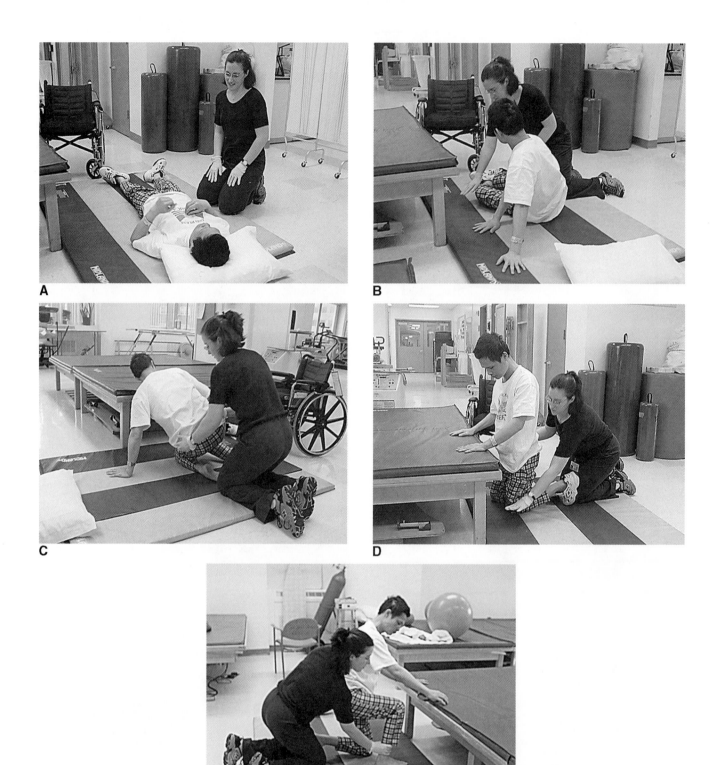

**Figure 14-25** **A,** Teaching the patient and caregiver how to get up safely from the floor is important before discharge to the community. **B,** The therapist instructs this patient with right-sided weakness to assume a side-sitting position on the left arm and hip. **C,** The therapist or caregiver assists the patient at the pelvis to assume weight on his knees. She uses a surface immediately in front of the patient to allow for arm support. **D,** The patient now is supported fully on his hands and knees. She prepares him for the next stage by asking him to shift his weight to his left. **E,** When the patient shifts weight over to the left knee, he is able to move his weaker right leg into a half-kneeling position.

*Continued*

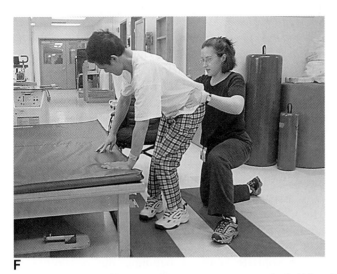
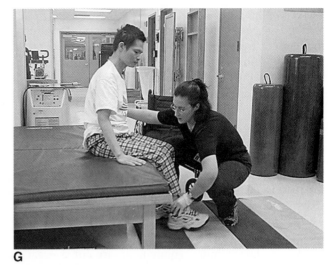

F                                    G

**Figure 14-25 cont'd**    **F,** From the half-kneeling position the patient assumes a standing position and begins to shift his weight to sit on the adjacent surface. **G,** The patient is seated safely.

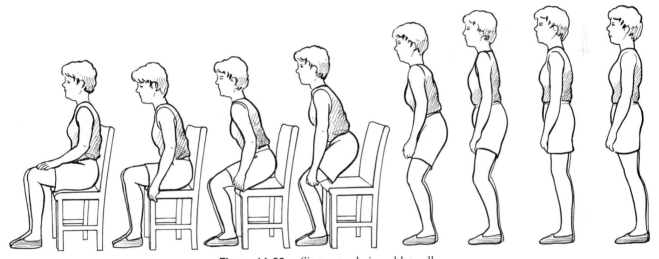

**Figure 14-26**    Sit-to-stand viewed laterally.

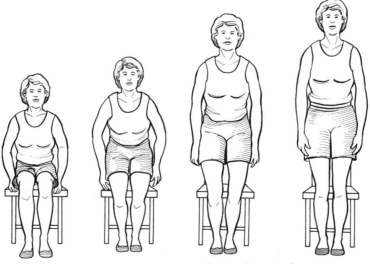

**Figure 14-27**    Sit-to-stand viewed anteriorly.

Phase 1 (Figure 14-28, *A*) is referred to as the *flexion momentum phase* and is used to generate the initial momentum for rising. During this phase, the center of mass is within the base of support, and eccentric contractions of the erector spinae are required to control forward motion of the trunk. Phase 2 (Figure 14-28, *B*) begins as the individual leaves the chair seat and ends at maximal ankle dorsiflexion. Forward momentum of the upper body is transferred to forward and upward momentum of the total body. The center of mass is now moving from within the base of support of the chair to the feet. By definition the phase is unstable and requires coactivation of hip and knee extensors. Phase 3 (Figure 14-28, *C*) is an extension phase during which the body rises to its full upright position by extension of the hips and knees. The stability requirements are not as great as in phase 2 because the center of mass is well within the base of support of the feet. Phase 4 (Figure 14-28, *D*) is a stabilization phase in which complete extension of the hips and knees occurs. Regardless of the way researchers divide the task, an appreciation of the biomechanics of this movement pattern is crucial in training and in understanding potential problems that occur in hemiplegia.

Carr and Shepherd[18] have outlined key factors that influence the way sit-to-stand is executed in normal individuals. The therapist must consider the role of foot position, the starting position of the trunk, the speed of movement, and the role of the upper limbs in balance and propulsion. Carr and Shepherd stated that:

1. Sit-to-stand is accomplished most easily when the initial starting position of the foot is in a somewhat posterior position (with the ankle in approximately 75 degrees of dorsiflexion).
2. Initiating active trunk flexion from the erect position and encouraging the individual to swing the trunk forward at a reasonable speed allows for the greatest generation of extension force in the lower limbs to raise the body vertically.
3. Increased velocity of trunk flexion facilitates extensor force in the lower limbs.
4. Constraint of the arms (as in holding the hemiplegic arm forward while attempting sit-to-stand) results in increased time producing sufficient lower limb extensor forces to stand.

Janssen, Bussman, and Stam[43] reviewed key factors affecting sit-to-stand by searching the literature for the most frequently mentioned determinants, and they found that chair height, use of armrests, and foot position significantly influence the ability to carry out sit-to-stand. Use of a higher chair resulted in lower moments needed at the knee and hip, using armrests lowered the moments needed at the hip, and repositioning feet from anterior to posterior allowed for lowering the maximum mean extension moments at the hip.

***Selected Problems.*** As mentioned in the previous section, patients may have difficulty maintaining their feet flat on the floor because of poor sensation, unilateral inattention, or shortening of the trunk and calf muscles.

Difficulties with spatial relations and praxis have been noted during transfer training, regardless of whether the therapist is training the patient for pivot transfers or sit-to-stand. Certain patients lean backward instead of forward while the therapist is attempting to transfer. These patients' actions are unpredictable and often run counter to those expected after instruction from the therapist.

As Arnadottir[5] has noted, transfers also reveal problems with organizing and sequencing and conditions such as ideational apraxia. These problems may become evident when a patient attempting to rise from bed omits the appropriate steps of handling the bedclothes in preparation to transfer (see Chapter 18).

*Motor impersistence,* a term first introduced by Fisher[29] to describe failure to persist at various tasks such as eye closure, breath holding, conjugate gaze, and tongue protrusion may explain some patients' inabilities to persevere with certain tasks such as transfers, sit-to-stand, and ambulation. These patients tend to collapse midway through the task, sometimes without warning, and reduced muscle strength, per se, does not appear to be the cause. Impersistence, in most studies, has been found to correlate more with right-hemisphere lesions than with left-hemisphere lesions.[29,49]

The manner in which the sit-to-stand movement pattern is executed may reveal who is at risk for falls. Cheng et al[21] found that when comparing stroke patients who had a history of falls against stroke patients who had no history of falls, the differences were clear in measurable parameters such as body weight distribution. Stroke patients with a history of falls executed the task of sit-to-stand asymmetrically, taking much more weight on their sound side.[21] This suggests that, certainly from the point of view of safety concerns, stroke patients need as many opportunities as possible to develop better control of their affected lower limbs in sit-to-stand.

***Treatment Strategies.*** Bobath[10] describes the need to begin training patients in sit-to-stand from a fairly high seat (Figure 14-29, *A*), progressing gradually to lower seats or a plinth (Figure 14-29, *B*). Other studies have substantiated her assertion such as the one concluding that high-surface chairs can decrease significantly the joint ranges of motion needed at the hip and knee, making rising from a higher chair much less stressful than rising from a lower chair.[16]

Stretching the arms forward also is recommended by Bobath[10] and Davies[27] in practicing sit-to-stand. As mentioned previously, Carr and Gentile[17] maintain that normal trunk flexion is accompanied by some arm flexion; fixing the arms in specific positions during the activity may actually prove detrimental to the typical movement pattern. Encouraging weight bearing on the affected leg

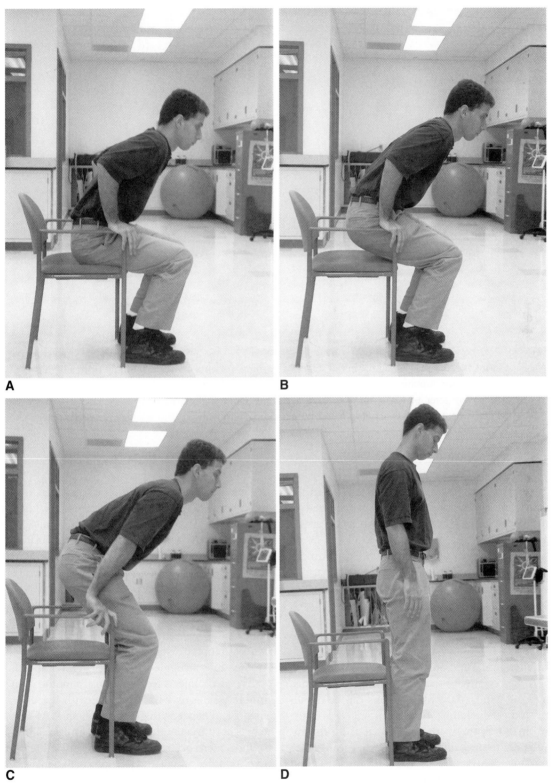

**Figure 14-28**    **A,** Phase 1 of sit-to-stand. **B,** Phase 2 of sit-to-stand. **C,** Phase 3 of sit-to-stand. **D,** Phase 4 of sit-to-stand.

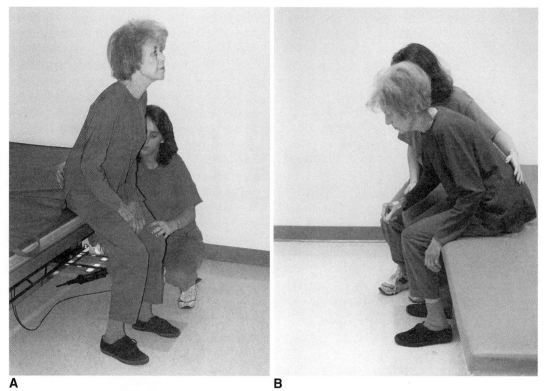

**Figure 14-29    A,** During the initial stages of learning, patients may find standing from a high surface easier. Among other things this provides the patient with a feeling of success. **B,** The patient can attempt lower surfaces after becoming more skillful. Varying the surfaces from which patients practice standing is important to promote learning and enables the patient to cope with varying situations that arise in the real world.

by pulling the knee forward also is emphasized. Bobath,[10] Davies,[27] and Carr and Shepherd[19] agree on the need to practice intermediate stages and sitting down by reversing the sequence.

Verbal or physical cues may be required to promote appropriate weight bearing on the affected lower extremity are recommended as for transfer training. In Figure 14-30, the therapist's assistance provides much stability for the patient. In Figure 14-31, the therapist needs only to cue the patient through the distal femur to get the desired response.

Carr and Shepherd[17] and Shepherd and Gentile[76] have conducted studies clarifying the role of the trunk, arms, and feet in sit-to-stand. Many implications can be drawn from these studies, including the importance of training patients to go from sit-to-stand by actively flexing the trunk, using momentum to swing the trunk forward, decreasing contracture of the calf muscles, and practicing from a higher-than-normal seat initially. Carr and Shepherd,[19] through their extensive study of motor learning and control, have emphasized the importance of task-specific training, structured practice outside therapy sessions, correct feedback about performance, and a way

to quantify and challenge performance. A system for training sit-to-stand in which a gradual lowering of the seat occurs is considered beneficial because it provides a form of progressive resistive exercise that improves muscle strength and control in a task-specific activity.[17]

Because getting the feet back and under in sit-to-stand is so important, training patients to move to the edge of the supporting surface to allow for this is necessary. Afterward, forward flexion of the trunk to bring the center of mass over the base of support can occur. A patient who attempts to stand without doing this is set up for a tremendous struggle or failure (Figure 14-32).

Normal subjects frequently use a momentum strategy in mobility skills as a way to move with less energy requirements and hence with greater efficiency. Momentum strategy is used frequently in rising from bed, and no cessation of movement occurs. The momentum strategy can be used in a modified way with appropriate patients who have sustained CVA because it allows them to use the force generated by forward flexion to take them into an upright position. They then need adequate stability when their thighs are off the supporting surface to prevent them from falling forward. Momentum provides the patient with an

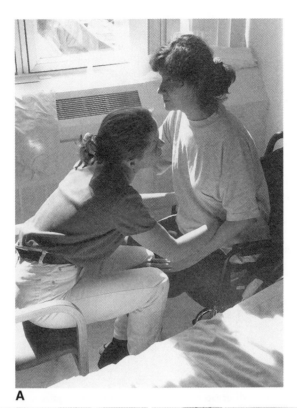

A

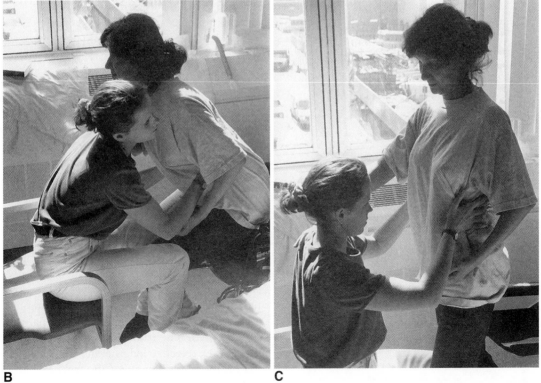

B                                    C

**Figure 14-30**  **A,** The therapist promotes weight bearing on the patient's affected lower extremity in sit-to-stand by placing the knees around the patient's affected knee, drawing the patient forward **(B),** and discouraging "buckling" when the patient achieves the standing position **(C).**

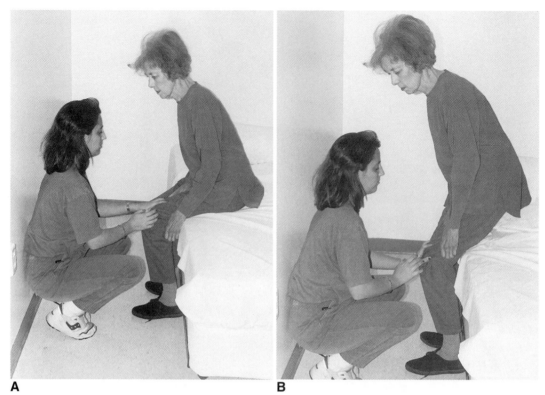

**A**    **B**

**Figure 14-31**    Patients with greater motor control still may require some cueing to equalize the weight bearing between the lower extremities if they have a tendency to stand up using their unaffected side more than the other. **A,** The therapist places a hand on the distal femur of the affected lower extremity, draws the knee anteriorly, and then applies downward pressure as the patient comes to stand **(B).**

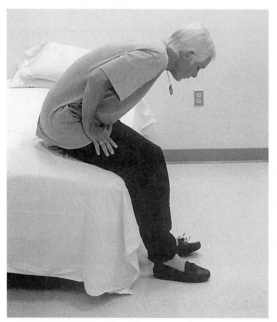

**Figure 14-32**    Foot placement is important in sit-to-stand. Note how far forward this individual's feet are as he attempts to stand.

efficient ability to move but by definition requires an ability to control for stability in its execution; patients with poor trunk control or significant cognitive impairments are not candidates for using such a strategy. When introducing the momentum strategy in therapy, the therapist must adequately guard the patient from falling.

## ACTIVITIES IN STANDING

### Analysis of Movement

The ability to stand is a goal many patients with hemiplegia want to achieve because the drive to be upright is strong. Patients should be provided the opportunity to practice standing and shifting their centers of gravity in all directions and reaching for functional objects in the environment. The trunk responses needed for controlled sitting (i.e., selective lengthening and shortening depending on the requirements of the task) also are needed for controlled standing; however, these trunk responses are carried out over a much narrower base of support.

### Selected Problems

Standing may prove challenging for patients with severe hemiplegia who have only one side of the body available to use for movement; moving with one half of the body is stressful work. The slow, laborious effort of standing and attempting to move in this position causes an increase in posturing and skeletal muscle activity. Movements often are lacking in spontaneity and must occur at a conscious level for the patient. Postural deviations noted in sitting in these patients become even more exaggerated in standing. The patient who "fixes" the upper limb must stay upright while sitting because the patient fixes even more in the struggle to stay upright on two feet.

### Treatment Strategies

As stated previously, standing as early as possible if medical clearance is permitted is ideal for patients. Standing helps increase the patient's level of arousal and can be motivating. Bobath,[10] Davies,[27] and Carr and Shepherd[20] emphasize the need to help the patient stand so that body segments are aligned properly and weight is accepted through the affected lower extremity. For some patients, accomplishing this requires all of their attention and energy. Therefore the therapist should be mindful of the need (at least initially) to train the patient to stand and take weight on the affected lower extremity in a quiet, minimally distracting environment. This may be even more critical for patients with attention disorders manifesting as distractibility, impulsivity, and irritability with increased stimulation. As noted earlier, the therapist must consider the need to incorporate competing stimuli into therapy gradually; otherwise, the therapist cannot assert that functional balance has been achieved.

Achieving weight shift in standing requires a substantial amount of cueing by the therapist because patients often are fearful of standing on the affected leg because of reduced muscle strength, postural control, and sensation. Visual disturbances also may make standing a frightening activity for the patient.

Initially, the use of a wall (Figure 14-33) may be desirable to offer the patient substantial support; however, this should not be used to train functional reach in standing because postural muscle activity in the legs is reduced (with the help of the wall) when the patient makes an arm movement. A manually guided approach is useful to help the patient learn the desired end point of the movement pattern. Contact by the therapist directly on the pelvis (with one hand on each side) offers optimal control to guide the weight shift, and the therapist gradually can taper the amount of guidance required as the patient begins to activate more.

Free-standing balance should be attempted as soon as possible (see Chapter 8). Standing while simultaneously scanning the environment or having a conversation with the therapist is challenging and meaningful (Figure 14-34).

A progression to standing and reaching prepares the patient to be able to perform personal self-care and instrumental activities of daily living safely and efficiently in a standing position. The patient needs to practice reaching in all directions in functional environments (Figure 14-35). As Carr and Shepherd[20] have outlined, this should include reaching overhead, to the side, backward, and down, progressing to unilateral and bilateral reaching to the floor. Recent research has demonstrated that the pattern of postural muscle activity in response to postural adjustments can be modified by training. This finding suggests the need for task-specific training to ensure the patient has a broad repertoire at hand when confronted with solving a movement problem in standing.

A commonly held view about asymmetrical hemiparetic gait is that it may be subject to amelioration by balance training emphasizing weight bearing on the paretic lower extremity. However, a study by Winstein et al[87] in which hemiparetic subjects received specific balance training with a specially designed feedback device revealed that balance in standing may be improved, but no carryover into a more symmetrical gait pattern occurs. This suggests that skill acquisition has a task-specific

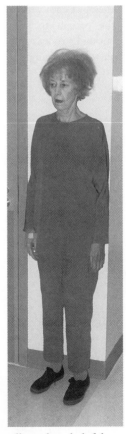

**Figure 14-33** A wall can be a helpful starting place in teaching a patient to maintain a standing position. The wall can assist the patient to achieve alignment of body parts in what can be a frightening position to assume. However, the wall does not substitute for the need to learn to stand and function in open space.

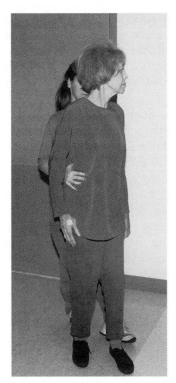

**Figure 14-34**    The therapist cues weight shifting in standing while encouraging the patient to scan the environment. Standing and looking around a room can prove challenging for patients in the initial stages of learning to stand.

nature, and therapists cannot assume progress achieved in one skill area can be carried over or transferred to another. This finding calls into question many commonly held beliefs about the use of developmental progression to increase functional capabilities in upright positions. The effect of the environment on postural control has been explored increasingly in the motor learning literature, but research typically has been done on the able-bodied population. A study conducted by Abreu[1] examined the effect of environmental predictability on postural control after stroke. This study was conducted with subjects in a seated position; findings revealed that an unpredictable environmental model facilitated a more stable response from patients than the response seen with a predictable environment. These findings challenge the assumption that therapy is best conducted in an undemanding environment. Abreu hypothesizes that the interaction between postural control systems and information processing systems is complex and requires significant exploration if therapists are to be successful in matching patients and tasks.

Shumway-Cook and Woollacott[78] also note that although researchers have been painstakingly studying the biomechanical aspects of transfers, a paucity of information on the perceptual strategies used for these activities is available. Mulder, Pauwels, and Neinhaus[59] describe human beings as "biological problem-solving

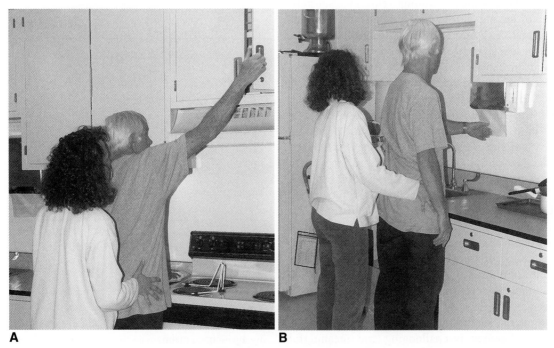

**A**                                                          **B**

**Figure 14-35**    Training for weight shifting and reaching in standing should occur within a functional context because task-specific training is most beneficial to the learner. Reaching up **(A),** forward **(B),** . . .

machines." They see no separation among motor, perceptual, and cognitive systems in the performance of movement problem solving. They describe the nervous system as a flexible, plastic, self-organizing entity. After injury, the spontaneity under which it functions is lost. The authors carried out a series of experiments with amputees in which they studied balance by measuring postural sway. They noted that these subjects, when given the STROOP test while trying to maintain balance, displayed an increase in postural sway. They concluded that

a dual-task world is the environment in which rehabilitation must take place, not the structured, unidimensional laboratory. The authors also assert that human movement studies should include more than isolated motor output and must examine the interaction between cognitive and sensory aspects of a task.

The body of research regarding the relationship between attention and postural control, as a function of age, has been increasing. Rankin et al[67] looked at the effect of a cognitive task on the neuromuscular responses involved

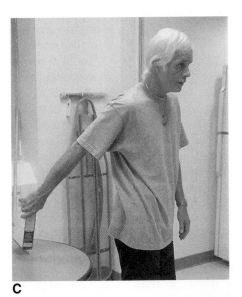

C

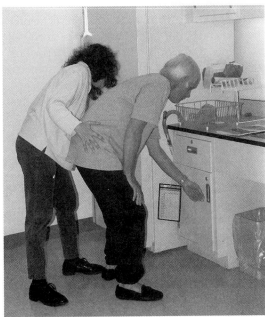

D

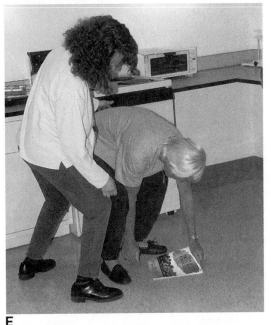

E

**Figure 14-35 cont'd**    backward (**C**), reaching down (**D**), and toward the floor (**E**). These patterns are among the many patterns of movement the patient should practice within functional activities. Occupational therapists are uniquely qualified with their expertise in task analysis to train patients to perform basic and instrumental activities of daily living.

in reactive balance control in normal young versus older adults. Subjects were analyzed on a standing platform while undergoing perturbations. Electromyographic activity was measured and compared when subjects underwent the balance activity alone and then with the addition of the cognitive task (in this case, a math task). Indeed, for both groups, muscle activity declined when the secondary task was performed; however, the results also indicated that the dual-task activity had a greater impact on balance control in older adults than the younger adults. Therapists need to be mindful of how dual tasks may contribute to the risk for falls in the elderly.

Brauer, Woollacott, and Shumway-Cook[15] looked further, exploring the attentional demands of balance recovery for balance-impaired elderly persons and, additionally, how cognitive demand affected postural stability in these individuals. Fifteen healthy older adults were compared with 13 older adults with clinical balance impairment. Each group was exposed to balance disturbances while standing on a platform. The dual-task used to assess attentional demand involved responding to the balance perturbations while giving a verbal reaction to auditory tones presented to the subjects. The results from this study led the researchers to conclude that recovery of balance for balance-impaired individuals was more attentionally demanding, and additionally, recovery of balance was slower and less efficient when simultaneously performed with a cognitive task.

Their conclusions have far-reaching implications for occupational therapists, whose primary role is to train patients in functional activities, which, by definition, include dual tasks. The dual task paradigm is a useful guide in standing activities because the patient is challenged to develop skill and not merely stand and think only of maintaining balance. This behavior is hardly functional and must be borne in mind as therapists label patients independent in these activities (see Chapter 8). However, while therapists must set up real-life situations to evaluate and treat their patients, they must be mindful of what the literature is indicating to determine the appropriate approach with patients who have standing balance impairments.

Sit-to-stand and stand-to-sit may be the same in certain basic ways. However, the key differences have implications for treatment. First, movement duration has been found to be longer in stand-to-sit than in sit-to-stand.[50,77] In stand-to-sit, lower limb extensors are working in a flexed position and execute the task by lengthening rather than shortening the way they do in sit-to-stand. Controlling the descent is a difficult task for muscles with compromised strength, and certainly in the initial stages following stroke, many patients with hemiplegia sit by letting go and almost collapsing into a seated position, rather than executing a smooth, controlled descent into a seat. Practicing stand-to-sit with patients is important

and should get greater practice time than it probably currently does. Gaining control in sit-to-stand does not translate to stand-to-sit.

## ADJUNCT TECHNIQUES TO ENHANCE SKILL ACQUISITION

### Feedback

Although encouragement of patients is important in the rehabilitation process and should not be eliminated, therapists must consider the relevance of feedback to the learning process and not confuse the two. Therapists are often too liberal in their use of feedback with patients, using the guiding principle of "more feedback is better" and that feedback facilitates learning.

In her review of this topic, Winstein[86] provides research findings indicating that less information feedback creates a better learning environment and probably forces the learner to develop problem-solving strategies. A great deal of research is being conducted on normal, healthy individuals in this area, and although the findings may prove applicable to the areas in which occupational therapists work, they have yet to be tested on patient populations that have sustained CVA and should be approached with some caution on the part of the therapist.

Gentile[32] describes two kinds of augmented feedback an instructor can provide to learners:

1. Knowledge of performance, defined as knowledge of information about movement
2. Knowledge of results, defined as knowledge of information about the performer-environment interaction

She goes on to suggest that the demands of the task best dictate the most efficacious form of feedback. Activities that can be characterized according to the taxonomy of tasks as closed and consistent motion tasks require information about the movement to be transmitted from the instructor to the learner. For example, when training a patient in rolling over in bed or achieving sit-to-stand from a wheelchair, the provision of feedback about placement of the extremities and maintenance of alignment is useful. Tasks that can be categorized as open and variable motionless tasks according to the taxonomy of tasks by definition are subject to changing environmental conditions, and therefore feedback to the learner should focus on incorporation of environmental factors into the approach used and selection of movement strategy and pattern. For example, standing up while on a bus requires anticipation of the motion of the bus, movement of persons in the immediate environment, and consideration of changing space constraints.

Many therapists videotape patients to provide information on performance and show and measure improvement in skill. This can prove useful, particularly with patients who may lack awareness about their performance (see Chapter 4).

## Modeling

Recently, some research in motor learning has been dedicated to the effects of modeling in teaching motor skill. A substantial review can be found in the sports coaching literature.[41] However, the physical rehabilitation literature contains scant published research studies examining the use of modeling and its effects on physically disabled adults during training in activities of daily living and mobility skills. Nevertheless, modeling is used frequently in rehabilitation settings to promote skill acquisition is self-care, transfers, walking, and wheelchair mobility. Therapists often use themselves and other patients as models. In addition, they use drawings, photographs, and videotapes to enhance motor performance. However, the most efficacious forms of modeling have yet to be explored with this population.

The viability of modeling as a topic for motor behavior researchers has been well documented in the literature, however. Much of this research has been based on Bandura's social learning theory of modeling.[7] Bandura claims that modeling not only is a fundamental means of modifying existing behavior patterns but also is important to the acquisition of new modes of behavior. McCullagh, Weiss, and Ross[55] note that Bandura's original theory actually was designed for the acquisition and modification of social skills and behaviors, and motor learning researchers originally did not adopt this model, speculating that theories of motor skill acquisition would not be congruent with it. However, a shift in thinking in this area occurred in the 1980s, and many researchers are now examining the role visual demonstrations play in providing information to the observer before the action.[55] An integral component of Bandura's model is the concept of the formation of a cognitive representation by the observer viewing the model.[7] Understanding the nature of this cognitive representation is important in conceptualizing the way the modeling process aids or hinders the observer.

## Mental Imagery

Mental imagery has been used as a research treatment modality to enhance the rate of motor skill acquisition and improve skill accuracy. A substantial body of research exists that suggests that mental practice can improve learning of new motor skills in healthy individuals, and indications point to the concept that mental practice should be considered a complement to physical rehabilitation and not a substitute for physical practice.[42] Regarding individuals with stroke, the literature suggests that mental imagery, as measured by electroencephalogram activity, may produce activation of the sensorimotor cortex in individuals with left-sided hemiplegia. Occupational therapists should consider increasing the use of this clearly potent modality to improve their patients' performance in functional mobility tasks.

## Manual Guidance

Manual guidance is a controversial subject because therapists often feel they cannot possibly begin to teach patients new movement skills without helping them to "feel" the appropriate movement pattern or assisting the patient into the desired position. Too much handling encourages the patient not to be active and obviously runs counter to expectations desired in therapy. Selective use of hands-on support is obviously the more expedient approach to take, and therapists must become aware when their hands interfere with the active learning process that needs to take place for patients to develop skills.

## EVALUATION TOOLS

Bobath[10] devised an evaluation tool for use with the adult hemiplegic patient that progressed from simple to more selective movement patterns with an emphasis on the quality of movement patterns executed by the patient. This assessment strictly looks at the quality of movement and balance reactions and does not address the way a patient carries out specific functional mobility activities. Rather the assessment targets the places where movements may contribute to difficulty with the normal execution of mobility tasks. The assessment is thorough in this regard but takes a long time to administer and is not standardized.

Currently the only standardized evaluation for mobility skills is Carr and Shepherd's Motor Assessment Scale for Stroke Patients.[18] This test assesses the following eight areas:
1. Supine to side lying
2. Supine to sitting over side of bed
3. Balanced sitting
4. Sitting to standing
5. Walking
6. Upper arm function
7. Hand movements
8. Advanced hand activities

The advantages of the Motor Assessment Scale include the following:
1. It tests recovery specific for the patient recovering from CVA.
2. It takes less time to administer and infringes little on treatment time.
3. It is simple to administer and has objective and clear descriptions of criteria for rating patients.
4. It is sensitive to changes in patients' motor recovery status and therefore is useful in describing patient progress over time.

The Functional Independence Measure was developed by the Uniform Data System at the State University of New York at Buffalo as a standardized way for professionals to evaluate patient progress regarding levels of assistance needed to perform personal self-care, functional mobility, communication, cognition, and social interaction. Each area is graded on a scale of 1 to 7, with a score of 1 indicating total dependence and 7 indicating complete independence. The areas of functional mobility covered in this test include transfers to bed, chair, and toilet and tub and locomotion and stairs. This test is used in rehabilitation centers across the United States and has been found to have good to excellent reliability.[34,35]

The Assessment of Motor and Process Skills is a standardized test created by occupational therapists that simultaneously evaluates motor and process skills to predict effect on the ability to perform instrumental activities of daily living. Such an evaluation tool, if developed for personal self-care and functional mobility skills, would prove invaluable for occupational therapists (see Chapter 20).

## ANTICIPATING CHANGING ENVIRONMENTS

The ultimate goal of functional mobility retraining is to have the patient resume the roles and activities associated with the lifestyle before the CVA. This goal presumes that patients need to transfer reacquired mobility skills to environments unique to the individual lifestyle and participation patterns. The treatment setting presents a predictable environment in which the physical aspects of therapeutic equipment and furnishings remain unchanged from one treatment session to another. The patient's home environment also may be viewed as fairly predictable because of the patient's familiarity with the surroundings. The physical layout and home furnishings change little over time, even if home modifications are introduced. Nevertheless, therapists frequently observe problems as the patient attempts to make the transition from the treatment setting to the home environment. Unexpected problems occur within the closed home environment, and community-based activities challenge the individual's ability to solve newly encountered problems. The occupational therapist is well qualified to address these dilemmas through task analysis of occupations and careful consideration of the environmental contexts in which each task is performed.[71] The patient recovering from CVA is required to generalize and adapt mobility skills learned in the clinic setting to meet the changing environmental demands encountered on discharge. This generalization and adaptation occurs through the interaction among multiple systems: perceptual, cognitive, sensory, and motor. This chapter previously presented specific strategies for ameliorating performance impairments influencing functional mobility. These strategies should be incorporated throughout the intervention process as a means to attain generalization and encourage participation in life situations or instrumental activities of daily living on discharge.

### Strategy Development

The research examining normal movement sequences has found great variety in the movement patterns used to perform each mobility task. A single pattern may be identified as occurring more frequently during rolling, although many subjects use alternative patterns that are equally effective. Similarly the methods described to retrain patients to roll over also vary. No single correct strategy is available to achieve this mobility task. Strategy development is more than learning to use a normal pattern of movement; it results from the patient's exploration of movement possibilities in relation to tasks occurring in different environments.[78] Thus the occupational therapist may use several methods of instruction while assisting the patient in learning movement limitations and determining future mobility potentials.[71,78] The two primary strategies for functional mobility include a force control strategy and a momentum strategy.[23] Early in the intervention process, patients may benefit from instruction in a force control strategy to prevent secondary impairments of fixations and resultant development of inappropriate compensatory strategies.[10,18,20,26,27] This method of instruction also is preferred for patients who do not have adequate stability of the trunk musculature because it may facilitate independent performance.[20] A momentum strategy or a combination of momentum and force control may be introduced if stability of the trunk is evident. Momentum is more efficient, requires less muscular activity, and approximates more normal-looking movement.

Not all patients are able to achieve a momentum strategy, but many patients may attempt to do so on their own in the home environment, particularly if it was their preferred method of movement before the stroke. Therapists need to anticipate this possibility and explore momentum as an alternative before discharge. Transition from a force control to a momentum strategy requires simple, concise instruction to move quickly without stopping the movement. The therapist may use manual cues at the shoulder girdle to ensure safety. Demonstration by the therapist also is helpful. The practice of momentum strategies also may prepare the patient to control movement during stressful life situations that occur unexpectedly and require quick transitional movements.

### Practice Conditions

To prepare the patient to resume the previous lifestyle, the occupational therapist must consider carefully the conditions under which practice takes place. The goal of intervention is to maximize retention and transfer of acquired skills to everyday life situations the patient will encounter.[37] The therapist must increase the demands of the learning context during practice to prepare the patient to respond to unpredictable events. Chapter 5 presented an overview of factors the therapist considers when structuring the practice conditions in stroke rehabilitation. The following are considerations specific to functional mobility retraining.

***Blocked and Random Practice.*** Blocked practice in functional mobility retraining is the rote practice of mobility functions in sequence. For example, the patient initially practices rolling to the unaffected side, then to the affected side, then to the seated position. Repetition of experiences and a degree of mastery must occur at each level before the patient proceeds to the next level of skill. This method of structuring practice initially may assist the patient in gaining proficiency during the practice session but is not effective in preparing the patient to engage in self-care tasks in which changes in the position of the body occur randomly in response to task requirements. For example, the patient rolls to the left to reach for a brush on the table; it is just beyond reach. The patient rolls back to supine and assumes a bridge position, pushing upward in bed. The patient then rolls again and is able to grasp the brush. Random practice of mobility tasks improves learning, retention, and the ability to solve motor problems encountered in life situations.[74] Schmidt[72] recommends that randomized practice be incorporated throughout the intervention process. Mobility tasks should be interspersed with other tasks such as activities of daily living training in which the patient must make transitional movements in a natural context. The trial-and-error exploration of functional mobility in this context initially may prove difficult for the patient. Progress may be slow, and the therapist may be tempted to instruct the patient in a single movement strategy to speed progress. Varying the practice conditions increases the contextual interference, facilitating generalization as the patient relies on multiple processes and promoting the development of versatile motor strategies.[44,81]

Schmidt notes one exception in which a part-to-whole method of practice may be beneficial. Early in the intervention process, when the patient is acquiring foundational skills, practicing of component movements may be necessary. For example, the patient initially may need to gain control of lateral flexion of neck and trunk muscles before these movements can be incorporated into the sidelying-to-sit sequence. Schmidt suggests that as soon as patients are able to perform these component movements, they should be integrated immediately into programs emphasizing random practice.[72] This method of practice can be used only with mobility functions that are readily divided into natural component parts.[73,86]

***Varying the Practice Conditions for Specific Tasks.***
Gentile's taxonomy of motor tasks[32,33] is useful for determining the most appropriate practice conditions for each mobility task. Objects, persons, and the spatial temporal characteristics of each task influence the motor strategies selected. Sabari[71] suggests that the occupational therapy process inherently considers the importance of the regu-

latory conditions to task performance. Occupational therapists frequently adapt and regulate the environment to facilitate mobility functions, as in adjusting the height of a bed in preparation for a transfer (Figures 14-36 and 14-37). Similarly, the amount of verbal cues and physical assistance is adjusted to foster independent performance and skill development. Sabari also directs attention to the crucial role occupational therapists assume as regulators throughout mobility retraining.

### Closed Tasks

Early in the treatment process, most functional mobility tasks may be considered closed, and the environmental features are regulated easily to improve performance. Rolling over and coming to a seated position in a hospital bed occurs on a stationary surface. The therapist can regulate the environment further by positioning pillows and bed linens appropriately, raising the bed guard rails, adjusting the height of the bed, limiting the number of persons moving around the patient's bed, and positioning the body in a fairly static position to assist the patient if needed. Another important characteristic of a closed task is that movement is self-paced and no temporal constraints are placed.

The therapist's role as a regulator can be equated with the degree of assistance or handling provided. The therapist initially may give significant physical assistance and use a variety of adjunct techniques to promote perceptual, cognitive, and sensory processing. As the patient regains control of movements in desired sequences, physical assistance and the amount of cueing is reduced gradually or eliminated.[71]

### Variable Motionless Tasks

Bed mobility becomes a variable motionless task if the therapist is not present to regulate certain features of the environment. Patients preparing to get out of bed

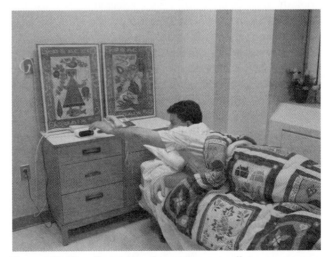

**Figure 14-36** Requiring the patient to roll in response to the buzzer of an alarm clock while under a heavy quilt is an example of how a therapist regulates the spatial and temporal characteristics of the environment.

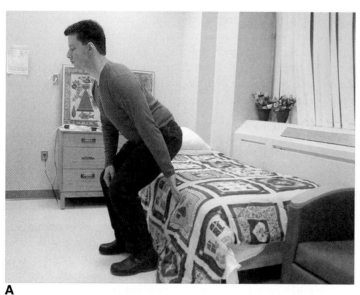
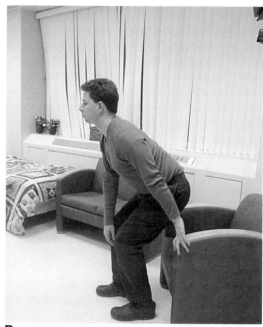

**A**    **B**

**Figure 14-37** **A** and **B,** Varying the sitting surface when practicing sit-to-stand and stand-to-sit assists the patient to learn flexible strategies.

independently may find the pillows and bed linens in disarray, making movement difficult; the bed guard rails are lowered, the top of the bed remains slightly elevated, and the height of the bed may be too high. Simultaneously the patient may be receiving verbal encouragement to "hurry up." Without the therapist present to structure the environment, the patient may experience difficulty and may use compensatory strategies incompatible with the restoration of performance component deficits. The patient may hook the unaffected leg under the affected leg and use the hands to pull up to a seated position.

This comparison illustrates the way overstructuring the environment does not prepare the patient recovering from stroke to develop flexible motor strategies. The patient needs to have opportunities to process information and acquire the ability to solve future problems.[2,72] Abreu[1] studied the effects of environmental regulation on postural control and found that unpredictable environments elicited improved control. These findings are contrary to beliefs occupational therapists have held concerning the grading of tasks from simple to complex and the structuring of environments from predictable to unpredictable. Abreu[1] postulates that the results of this study indicate that both types of environments should be incorporated concurrently in the intervention process. The therapist may regulate the environment but not on all trials. Perhaps the height of the bed is adjusted and the guard rails are elevated on one trial, whereas the next session may require the patient to instruct the therapist verbally in the arrangement of the immediate surroundings in preparation for the mobility task.

### Consistent Motion Tasks

During consistent motion tasks, the pace of the environment remains the same and the environment moves. These tasks are associated with mechanical devices such as conveyor belts. Most functional mobility tasks do not meet this criterion.

### Open Tasks

Many advanced mobility skills meet the criterion of an open task in which the spatial and temporal parameters of movement are determined by events occurring in the environment. Open tasks require more precise timing of movement, and the patient is challenged to anticipate and react to unexpected events. Sit-to-stand on a moving train, plane, or bus are examples of open tasks. Practice of these tasks should occur in the actual environment whenever possible.[40,71] Patients who are physically capable of attempting these advanced skills should be engaged in them while in the rehabilitation setting whenever possible.

Patients who do not have adequate foundational skills while hospitalized can benefit from interventions to improve future potential for the acquisition of advanced mobility skills. Patients need to be introduced to unpredictable environments in which they have the opportunity to explore movement strategies and develop problem-solving abilities. Early in the intervention process the therapist's handling techniques to prepare and assist the patient can be modulated using different degrees of tactile, proprioceptive, and kinesthetic input as the patient engages in functional mobility tasks. For example, as the patient learns to transfer, the therapist can vary the sensory cues and amount of assistance.[9] Responding to changes in sensory input may be helpful in the development of anticipatory postural adjustments.[78]

## SUMMARY

The performance of functional mobility tasks should not occur in isolation, as in a gross mobility mat program. Practice of mobility skills while the patient is engaged in life tasks presents opportunities to solve unexpected problems that arise as the patient manipulates different objects and encounters changing support surfaces and changing temporal demands. The following are some suggestions for altering the regulatory features in the clinical environment.

### Rolling

- Practice rolling on a narrow surface such as a sofa.
- Encourage abrupt change in direction, as in reversing the movement in midstream.
- Practice rolling under a heavy quilt.
- Try rolling with an object such as a newspaper in the hand.
- Attempt propping to side lying to adjust pillows.
- Practice rolling in a darkened room.
- Ask the patient to roll quickly.

### Sidelying-to-Sit

- Attempt sidelying-to-sit with an immediate reach pattern.
- Practice sidelying-to-sit on a narrow surface.
- Try modifying the sequence to get out of a chaise longue chair.
- Practice sidelying-to-sit on a soft surface such as a sofa.
- Ask the patient to come to sitting as "fast as they can."

### Sit-to-Stand

- Use varying seat surfaces:
  Chair with arms
  Chair without arms
  Reclining chair with a significant seat depth
  Aluminum patio chair
  Side of the sofa
  Middle of the sofa
  Chair with wheels such as a desk chair
  Stool
  Swivel chair
  Dentist's chair
  Chair in theater or stadium
  Seat on public transportation (such as a bus or subway)

- Incorporate varying standing surfaces:
  Different textures of carpet
  Linoleum
  Tile floor
  Grass
  Concrete
- Include varying speed of movement.
- Account for varying objects and pets in the environment.
- Incorporate changing lighting.
- Attempt holding of various objects:
  Coat
  Briefcase
  Shopping bag
- Relearn turning right and left.

## REVIEW QUESTIONS

1. What effect does the patient's place in the life cycle have on planning relevant treatment in functional mobility retraining?
2. What effect does damage to the right hemisphere have on functional mobility skills?
3. How does a lack of awareness of disability differ from denial, and what are the implications of lack of awareness for functional mobility retraining?
4. How can the tactile-kinesthetic approach (such as the Affolter approach) be incorporated into treatment with a patient with apraxia?
5. What is the force control strategy?
6. What are the three major task requirements for locomotion that can be applied to all functional mobility tasks?
7. What three possible interventions can be used to maximize a patient's ability to achieve lateral trunk flexion?
8. What is the pusher syndrome?
9. What implications for treatment may be derived from the research done by Carr, Shepherd, and Gentile on sit-to-stand?
10. What current information about a dual-task paradigm can be incorporated into occupational therapy interventions?
11. How can the therapist structure the practice of functional mobility tasks, considering the venue of care?

## REFERENCES

1. Abreu BC: The effect of environmental regulations on postural control after stroke, *Am J Occup Ther* 49(6):517-525, 1995.
2. Abreu BC, Toglia JP: Cognitive rehabilitation: a model for occupational therapy, *Am J Occup Ther* 45(7):439-448, 1987.
3. Alexander NB, Grunawalt JC, Carles S, et al: Bed mobility task performance in older adults, *J Rehabil Res Dev* 37(5):633-638, 2000.
4. American Occupational Therapy Association: Practice framework: domain and process, *Am J Occup Ther* 56:609, 2002
5. Arnadottir G: Neurobehavioral deficits related to cortical dysfunction. In Arnadottir G: *The brain and behavior: assessing cortical dysfunction through activities of daily living*, St Louis, 1990, Mosby.

6. Astrom M, Adolfsson R, Asplund K: Major depression in stroke patients: a 3-year longitudinal study, *Stroke* 24(7):976-982, 1993.

7. Bandura A: *Principles of behavior modification*, New York, 1969, Holt, Rinehart, Winston.

8. Bernstein N: *The coordination and regulation of movement*, Elmsford, NY, 1967, Pergamon.

9. Bly L: What is the role of sensation in motor learning? What is the role of feedback and feedforward? *NDTA Network* 5:5, 1996.

10. Bobath B: *Adult hemiplegia: evaluation and treatment*, ed 3, Oxford, 1990, Butterworth-Heinemann.

11. Bobath B: *Adult hemiplegia: evaluation and treatment*, ed 2, London, 1978, Heineman.

12. Bogousslavsky J, Van Melle G, Regli F: The Lausanne stroke registry: analysis of 1,000 consecutive stroke patients, *Stroke* 19(9): 1083-1092, 1988.

13. Bonfils KB: The Affolter approach to treatment: a perceptual-cognitive perspective of function. In Pedretti LW, editor: *Occupational therapy practice skills for physical dysfunction*, ed 4, St Louis, 1996, Mosby.

14. Bourbonnais D, Noven SV: Weakness in patients with hemiparesis, *Am J Occup Ther* 43:313, 1989.

15. Brauer SG, Woollacott MH, Shumway-Cook A: The interacting effects of cognitive demand and recovery of postural stability in balance-impaired older adults, *J Geronotol A Biol Sci Med Sci* 56(8):M489-M496, 2001.

16. Burdett RG, Habasevich R, Pisciotta J, et al: Biomechanical comparison of rising from two types of chairs, *Phys Ther* 65(8): 1177-1183, 1985.

17. Carr JH, Gentile AM: The effect of arm movements on the biomechanics of standing up, *Hum Mov Sci* 13:175, 1994.

18. Carr JH, Shepherd RB: *Neurologic rehabilitation: optimizing motor performance*, Oxford, 1998, Butterworth-Heinemann.

19. Carr JH, Shepherd RB: A motor learning model for rehabilitation. In Carr JH, Gordon J, Gentile AM, et al: *Movement science: foundations for physical therapy in rehabilitation*, Rockville, Md, 1987, Aspen.

20. Carr JH, Shepherd RB: *A motor relearning programme for stroke*, Oxford, 1987, Butterworth-Heinemann.

21. Cheng PT, Wu SH, Liaw MY, et al: Symmetrical body weight distribution training in stroke patients and its effect on fall prevention, *Arch Phys Med Rehabil* 82(12):1650-1654, 2001.

22. Crosson C, Crosson BA, Barco, PP, et al: Awareness and compensation in postacute head injury rehabilitation, *J Head Trauma Rehabil* 4:46, 1989.

23. Crutchfield CA, Barnes MR: *Motor control and motor learning in rehabilitation*, Atlanta, 1993, Stokesville.

24. Damasio AR: *Descartes' error: emotion, reason, and the human brain*, New York, 1994, GP Putnam's Sons.

25. Das P, McCollum G: Invariant structure in locomotion, *Neuroscience* 25(3):1023-1034, 1988.

26. Davies PM: *Right in the middle: selective trunk activity in the treatment of adult hemiplegia*, New York, 1990, Springer-Verlag.

27. Davies PM: *Steps to follow: a guide to treatment of adult hemiplegia*, New York, 1985, Springer-Verlag.

28. Dean CM, Shepherd RB: Task-related training improves performance of seated reaching tasks after stroke: a randomized controlled trial, *Stroke* 28(4):722-728, 1997.

29. Fisher CM: Left hemiplegia and motor impersistence, *J Nerv Ment Dis* 123:201, 1956.

30. Ford-Smith CD, Van Sant AF: Age differences in movement patterns used to rise from a bed in the third through fifth decades of age, *Phys Ther* 73:305, 1992.

31. Gentile AM: Implicit and explicit processes during acquisition of functional skills, *Scand J Occup Ther* 5:7-16, 1998.

32. Gentile AM: Skill acquisition: action, movement and neuromotor processes. In Carr JH, Gordon J, Gentile AM, et al: *Movement science: foundations for physical therapy in rehabilitation*, Rockville, Md, 1987, Aspen.

33. Gentile AM: A working model of skill acquisition with application to teaching, *Quest* 17:3, 1972.

34. Granger CV, Hamilton BB: The Uniform Data System for medical rehabilitation report of first admissions for 1990, *Am J Phys Med Rehabil* 71(2):108-113, 1992.

35. Granger CV, Hamilton BB, Linacre JM, et al: Performance profiles of the Functional Independence Measure, *Am J Phys Med Rehabil* 72(2):84-89, 1993.

36. Hall ET: *The hidden dimension*, New York, 1966, Doubleday.

37. Hartman-Maeir A, Soroker N, Oman SD, et al: Awareness of disabilities in stroke rehabilitation: a clinical trial, *Disabil Rehabil* 25(1):35-44, 2003.

38. Heilman KM: Neglect and related disorders. In Heilman KM, Valenstein E, editors: *Clinical neuropsychology*, New York, 1979, Oxford University.

39. Herrmann M, Bartles C, Wallesch CW: Depression in acute and chronic aphasias: symptoms, pathoanatomical-clinical correlations and functional implications, *J Neurol Neurosurg Psychiatry* 56(6):672-678, 1993.

40. Higgins JR, Spaeth RK: Relationship between consistency of movement and environmental condition, *Quest* 17:61, 1972.

41. Hodges NJ, Franks IM: Modeling coaching practice: the role of instruction and demonstration, *J Sports Sci* 20(10):793-811, 2002.

42. Jackson PL, Lafleur MF, Malouin F, et al: Potential role of mental practice using motor imagery in neurologic rehabilitation, *Arch Phys Med Rehabil* 82(8):1133-1141, 2001.

43. Janssen WG, Bussman HB, Stam HJ: Determinants of the sit-to-stand movement: a review, *Phys Ther* 82(9):866-879, 2002.

44. Jarus T: Motor learning and occupational therapy: the organization of practice, *Am J Occup Ther* 48(9):810-816, 1994.

45. Johnstone M: *Restoration of motor function in the stroke patient*, ed 2, New York, 1983, Churchill Livingstone.

46. Joseph R: Parietal lobes. In Joseph R, editor: *Neuropsychology, neuropsychiatry and behavioral neurology*, New York, 1990, Plenum.

47. Joseph R: The right brain. In Joseph R, editor: *Neuropsychology, neuropsychiatry and behavioral neurology*, New York, 1990, Plenum.

48. Joseph R: Confabulation and delusional denial: frontal lobe and lateralized influences, *J Clin Psychol* 42(3):507-520, 1986.

49. Joynt RL, Benton AL, Fogel ML: Behavioral and pathological correlates of motor impersistence, *Neurology* 12:876, 1964.

50. Kralj A, Jaeger RJ, Munih M: Analysis of standing up and sitting down in humans: definitions and normative data presentation, *J Biomech* 23(11):1123-1138, 1990.

51. Krefting LH, Krefting D: Cultural influences on performance. In Christiansen C, Baum C, editors: *Occupational therapy: overcoming human performance deficits*, Thorofare, NJ, 1991, Slack.

52. Lapointe LL: Neurogenic disorders of communication. In Minifie FD, editor: *Introduction to communication sciences and disorders*, San Diego, 1994, Singular.

53. Levine RE: Culture: a factor influencing the outcomes of occupational therapy, *Occup Ther Health Care* 4:1,3, 1987.

54. Marsden CD, Rothwell JC, Day BL: The use of peripheral feedback in the control of movement. In Evarts EV, Wise SP, Bousfield D, editors: *The motor system in neurology*, Amsterdam, 1985, Elsevier Biomedical.

55. McCullagh P, Weiss MR, Ross D: Modeling considerations in motor skill acquisition and performance: an integrated approach. In Pandolf KB, editor: *Exercise and sport sciences reviews*, Baltimore, 1979, Williams & Wilkins.

56. Mohr JD: Management of the trunk in adult hemiplegia: the Bobath concept, *Topics in neurology*, 1990, American Physical Therapy Association.

57. Mohr JP, Foulkes MA, Polis AT, et al: Infarct topography and hemiparesis profiles with cerebral convexity infarction : Stroke Data Bank, *J Neurol Neurosurg Psychiatry* 56:344-351, 1993.

58. Mosey AC: *Psychosocial components of occupational therapy*, New York, 1986, Raven.

59. Mulder T, Pauwels J, Neinhaus B: Motor recovery following stroke: towards a disability-orientated assessment of motor dysfunctions. In Harrison AH, editor: *Physiotherapy in stroke management*, Edinburgh, 1995, Churchill Livingstone.

60. Neistadt ME: The neurobiology of learning: implications for treatment of adults with brain injury, *Am J Occup Ther* 48:421, 1993.

61. Parasher RK, Gentile AM: Translating instructions into spatially-directed limb movements, *Abstr Soc Neurosci* 21:422, 1995.

62. Pimental PA: Alterations in communication, *Nurs Clin North Am* 21(2):321-337, 1986.

63. Poole JI: Application of motor learning principles in occupational therapy, *Am J Occup Ther* 45(6):531-537, 1991.

64. Posner MI, Inhoff AW, Friedrich FJ: Isolating attentional systems: a cognitive-anatomical analysis, *Psychobiology* 15:107, 1987.

65. Posner MI, Rafal RD: Cognitive theories of attention and the rehabilitation of attentional deficits. In Meier MJ, Benton A, Diller L, editors: *Neuropsychological rehabilitation*, New York, 1987, Churchill Livingstone.

66. Rafal RD, Posner MI, Friedman JH, et al: Orienting of visual attention in progressive supranuclear palsy, *Brain* 111(pt 2):267-280, 1988.

67. Rankin JK, Woolacott MH, Shumway-Cook A, et al: Cognitive influence on postural stability: a neuromuscular analysis in young and older adults, *J Gerontol A Biol Sci Med Sci* 55(3):M112-M119, 2000.

68. Richter RR, Van Sant AF, Newton RA: Description of adult rolling movements and hypothesis of developmental sequences, *Phys Ther* 69(1):63-71, 1989.

69. Robinson RG, Kubos KL, Starr LB, et al: Mood disorders in stroke patients: importance of location of lesion, *Brain* 107(pt 1):81-93, 1984.

70. Ryerson S, Levit K: *Functional movements reeducation*, New York, 1997, Churchill Livingstone.

71. Sabari JS: Motor learning concepts applied to activity-based interventions with adults with hemiplegia, *Am J Occup Ther* 45(6):523-530, 1991.

72. Schmidt RA: Motor learning principles for physical therapy. In Lister MJ, editor: *Contemporary management of motor control problems: proceedings of the Second STEP Conference*, Alexandria, Va, 1991, Foundation for Physical Therapy.

73. Schmidt RA, Lee TD: *Motor control and learning: a behavioral emphasis*, ed 2, Champaign, Ill, 1999, Human Kinetics.

74. Shea JB, Morgan RL: Contextual interference effects on the acquisition, retention, and transfer of a motor skill, *J Exp Psychol Learn Mem Cogn* 5:179, 1979.

75. Shenkman M, Berger RA, Riley PO, et al: Whole-body movements during rising to standing from sitting, *Phys Ther* 70(10):638-648, 1990.

76. Shepherd RB, Gentile AM: Sit-to-stand: functional relationship between upper body and lower limb segments, *Hum Move Stud* 13:817, 1994.

77. Shepherd RB, Hirschorn AD: Standing up and sitting down at two different seat heights. Proceedings of the sixteenth International Society of Biomechanics Congress, 1997, Tokyo.

78. Shumway-Cook A, Woollacott MH: *Motor control: theory and practical applications*, ed 2, Baltimore, 2001, Lippincott Williams and Wilkins.

79. Sullivan PE, Markos PD, Minor MD: *An integrated approach to therapeutic exercise: theory and clinical application*, Reston, Va, 1982, Reston.

80. Taub E: Somatosensory deafferentation research with monkeys: implications for rehabilitation medicine. In Ince LP, editor: *Behavioral psychology in rehabilitation medicine: clinical implications*, Baltimore, 1980, Williams & Wilkins.

81. Toglia J: Generalization of treatment: a multicontext approach to cognitive perceptual impairment in adults with brain injury, *Am J Occup Ther* 45(6):505-516, 1991.

82. VanSant A: Life-span development in functional tasks, *Phys Ther* 70(12):788-798, 1990.

83. Van Zomeren AH, Brouwer WH: *Clinical neuropsychology of attention*, Oxford, 1994, Oxford University Press.

84. Warren M: A hierarchical model for evaluation and treatment of visual perceptual dysfunction in adult acquired brain injury, part 1, *Am J Occup Ther* 47(1):42-54, 1993.

85. Weintraub S, Mesulam NM: Visual hemispatial inattention: stimulus parameters and exploratory strategies, *J Neurol Neurosurg Psychiatry* 51(12):1481-1488, 1988.

86. Winstein CJ: Knowledge of results and motor learning-implications for physical therapy, *Phys Ther* 71(2):140-149, 1991.

87. Winstein CJ, Gardner ER, McNeal DR, et al: Standing balance training: effect on balance and locomotion in hemiparetic adults, *Arch Phys Med Rehabil* 70(10):755-762, 1989.

88. World Health Organization: *International classification of functioning, disability and health* (short version), Geneva, 2001, The Organization.

89. Zola-Morgan S, Squire LR: Neuroanatomy of memory, *Ann Rev Neurosci* 16:547-563, 1993.

sheila m. hayes

**chapter 15**

# Gait Awareness

**key terms**

| | | |
|---|---|---|
| assistive devices | hemiplegic gaits | orthotic devices |
| cerebellar strokes | ipsilateral pushing | proprioceptive deficits |
| gait analysis | perceptual deficits | visual deficits |
| gait patterns | | |

**chapter objectives**

After completing this chapter, the reader will be able to accomplish the following:

1. Understand normal gait components.
2. Identify common gait deviations after a cerebrovascular accident.
3. Understand the basics of gait retraining.
4. Identify and describe commonly used orthoses and assistive devices.

In the management of a stroke patient, gait analysis and gait training traditionally have been the responsibility of physical therapists. Because of the interdisciplinary approach used to rehabilitate the stroke patient, much sharing of information occurs between team members regarding the patient's functional and mobility status. Occupational and physical therapists often "cotreat" to enhance problem solving regarding specific barriers to independence in activities of daily living.

Just as physical therapists have much to gain by familiarizing themselves with terminology and treatments used by occupational therapists (e.g., in the area of perceptual motor deficits), occupational therapists should find it beneficial to have a basic understanding of normal gait components, common gait deviations after a stroke, and gait retraining. An integrated approach to treatment of the stroke patient necessitates a working knowledge of the terminology, evaluation techniques, and rationale for treatment of other disciplines.

The physical therapist should perform a thorough examination before gait analysis and retraining. This examination includes factors such as range of motion, posture and bony alignment, strength, motor control, coordination, sensation, and balance. The therapist notes any deficits in these areas. The therapist is then ready to observe and analyze gait and to speculate on which of the deficits may be contributing to a specific gait deviation. The therapist can address specific deficits with appropriate treatment interventions and modalities.

Gait analysis is the objective documentation of gait[61] and ranges in complexity from observational assessment to quantitative analysis using instrumented gait analysis systems. These systems can include tools such as videotaping, three-dimensional motion analysis, dynamic electromyograms, and force plates. A variety of such quantitative systems are available and vary widely in sophistication and price.[12,52]

Kinematic analysis evaluates movement patterns, including the movement of the body, and specific angles between body segments (joint angles) as the body moves through the gait cycle. Observational gait analysis is a qualitative method of kinematic analysis. When kinematics is measured by instrumented analysis, it is considered a quantitative gait analysis.[52] Observational gait analysis is the visual inspection of walking.[71] Although not as reliable as quantitative gait analysis, observational gait analysis is the method most often used by practitioners. Most physical therapists do not have access to highly technical evaluation equipment, although videotaping is now more commonly available. Perry developed a systematic method for observational gait analysis that helps standardize this evaluation.[64]

Observational gait analysis is an acquired skill that requires much practice and repetition. The physical therapist must learn how to look at nine different points on the body (head, shoulders, arms, trunk, pelvis, hips, knees, ankles, feet) while simultaneously comparing the observed gait with normal gait features, in three body planes. When one is first learning gait analysis, observation of as many normal gaits as possible is necessary. When one is first performing observational gait analysis in the clinic, the recommendation is that the physical therapist choose patients who can tolerate walking for several minutes. This allows the therapist to apply Perry's approach to viewing trunk and limb excursions during the gait cycle.

Observational gait analysis should take place in the sagittal and frontal planes. The frontal or coronal view must include anterior and posterior vantage points. Certain motions such as leg rotation and foot abduction and adduction take place in the transverse or horizontal plane, although the therapist usually is not in a position to observe motion specifically in this plane. In normal gait, most movement occurs in the *sagittal* plane, whereas in abnormal gait, many of the deviations are observed as compensations in the *frontal* (coronal) and *transverse* (horizontal) planes[61] (Figure 15-1).

## TERMINOLOGY

Physical therapists must first familiarize themselves with the components of the normal gait cycle and with the terminology used to describe these components before they can analyze the gait of a person who has had a stroke. A cycle begins when the heel of one foot touches the ground and ends after the leg and body have advanced through space and time and the heel of that *same* foot hits the ground again.

The cycle includes a period when the leg is in contact with the ground, which is followed by a period when it is advancing through space. Thus the gait cycle of one leg can be divided into two phases: the stance phase (in which the leg is in contact with the ground) and the swing phase

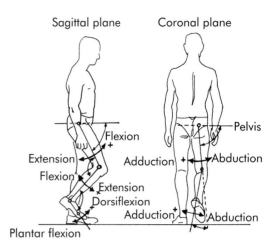

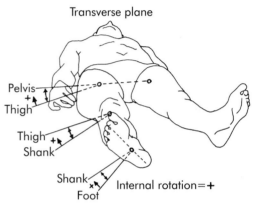

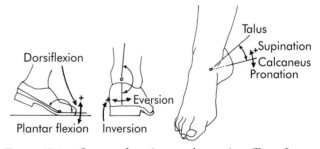

**Figure 15-1** System of naming angular motion. (From Inman VT, Ralston HJ: *Human walking,* Philadelphia, 1981, Williams & Wilkins.)

(in which the leg is off the ground). The stance phase makes up 60% of the gait cycle, and the swing phase makes up 40% (Figure 15-2). In a normal gait, the opposite leg also is going through a gait cycle simultaneously (i.e., has a stance phase and a swing phase). Each leg has two periods at the beginning and end of stance when the opposite leg is also in contact with the ground. These are called the periods of *double support.* Together they account for 10% of the initial stance phase and 10% of the end of stance for both legs.

The phases of swing and stance are further divided into substages. The language used to describe these subdivisions uses the traditional terms or the terms developed at

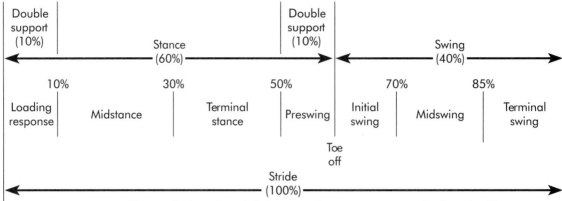

**Figure 15-2** Phases of gait cycle and their proportions as percentages of gait cycle. (From Ounpuu S: *Evaluation and management of gait disorders*, New York, 1995, Marcel Dekker.)

**Table 15-1**

**Gait Terminology**

| TRADITIONAL | RANCHO LOS AMIGOS |
|---|---|
| **Stance Phase** | |
| *Heel strike:* The beginning of the stance phase when the heel contacts the ground; the same as initial contact | *Initial contact:* The beginning of the stance phase when the heel or another part of the foot contacts the ground |
| *Foot flat:* Occurs immediately following heel strike when the sole of the foot contacts the floor; occurs during loading response | *Loading response:* The portion of the first double support period of the stance phase from initial contact until the contralateral extremity leaves the ground |
| *Midstance:* The point at which the body passes directly over the reference extremity | *Midstance:* The portion of the single limb support stance phase that begins when the contralateral extremity leaves the ground and ends when the body is directly over the supporting limb |
| *Heel off:* The point following midstance when the heel of the reference extremity leaves the ground; occurs prior to terminal stance | *Terminal stance:* The last portion of the single limb support stance phase that begins with heel rise and continues until the contralateral extremity contacts the ground |
| *Toe off:* The point following heel off when only the toe of the reference extremity is in contact with the ground | *Preswing:* The portion of stance that begins the second double support period from the initial contact of the contralateral extremity to lift off of the reference extremity |
| **Swing Phase** | |
| *Acceleration:* The portion of beginning swing from the moment the toe of the reference extremity leaves the ground to the point when the reference extremity is directly under the body | *Initial swing:* The portion of swing from the point when the reference extremity leaves the ground to maximum knee flexion of the same extremity |
| *Midswing:* The portion of the swing phase when the reference extremity passes directly below the body: extends from the end of acceleration to the beginning of deceleration | *Midswing:* The portion of the swing phase from maximum knee flexion of the reference extremity to a vertical tibial position |
| *Deceleration:* The swing portion of the swing phase when the reference extremity is decelerating in preparation for the heel strike | *Terminal swing:* The portion of the swing phase from a vertical position of the tibia of the reference extremity to just before initial contact |

From O'Sullivan SB, Schmitz TJ, editors: *Physical rehabilitation assessment and treatment*, Philadelphia, 1994, FA Davis.

Rancho Los Amigos Medical Center in Los Angeles (Table 15-1). Because the terms are similar, physical therapists often use a mixture of old and new terms unless the facility in which they work advocates strict adherence to one terminology. Most physical therapists are familiar with the Rancho Los Amigos terminology because of the abundance of research, literature, and gait assessment forms that have been produced by the pathokinesiology service and physical therapy department at that facility.[62]

The Rancho Los Amigos definition of swing phase is divided into the substages of initial swing, midswing, and terminal swing. The stance phase is divided into initial contact, loading response, midstance, terminal stance, and preswing (Figure 15-3). Within these substages, the physical therapist observes the joint displacements and movements occurring at the trunk, pelvis, hip, knee, ankle, and toes. Figure15-4 illustrates the phases of the gait cycle and the corresponding normal joint displacements that occur as the body moves through the sagittal plane.

Other terms used in describing gait cycles are stride, step, cadence, and velocity. A *stride* is equal to a gait cycle (i.e., from heel strike of one leg to the next heel strike of the same leg). Stride can refer to distance (stride length) or time (stride time) in the gait cycle of one leg. A *step* is described as the distance (step length) or time (step time) from the heel strike of one leg to the heel strike of the opposite leg (Figure 15-5).

## RELIABLE GAIT PARAMETERS

*Cadence* is the number of steps or strides per unit of time. Walking velocity equals speed: the distance walked divided by time. Because time-distance variables are the components of gait that can be measured most reliably, therapists can use them in assessing improvement in stroke patients.[36,66,68] For example, persons who have had

a stroke with a resulting hemiparesis typically walk with a slower than normal gait.[48,57] Routine recording of the cadence and velocity of these patients is an objective way of documenting change over time. The measure is valid to show improvement for physical therapists that do not have access to the instrumented gait analysis systems mentioned previously.

Improvements in cadence and velocity also can be an indication of functional improvement and limb recovery. A study of hemiplegic patients by Harro and Giuliani[40] showed positive correlations between high scores (greater than 90) on the motor portion of the Fugl-Meyer motor assessment scale and the ability to increase walking speeds. Richards et al[66] studied 18 hemiplegic subjects divided into three subgroups: slow, intermediate, and fast walkers. They found that the fast walkers had movements and muscle activations more like those of able-bodied subjects than the slow or intermediate speed walkers.

## HEMIPLEGIC GAITS

The type of gait of a person who has had a stroke depends on where in the brain the insult has occurred and which systems are affected, such as motor, sensory, balance, coordination, perceptual, and visual systems. If a motor area in the cortex or a motor track is involved, hemiplegia or hemiparesis is manifested in the contralateral limbs. The location of the infarction within these areas determines whether the arm or the leg is more impaired. Not all stroke patients are hemiplegic or hemiparetic, nor do all hemiparetic patients have the same degree of motor deficits. Unfortunately, the term *hemiplegic gait* frequently is applied to all individuals with hemiparesis, although many varieties and degrees of deficits exist.[36] Individuals who have suffered ischemia in areas of the brain supplied by the anterior cerebral artery

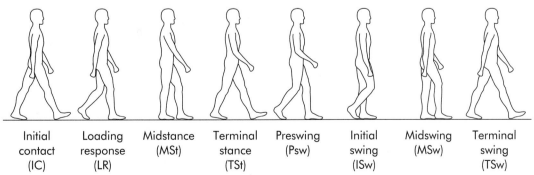

| Initial contact (IC) | Loading response (LR) | Midstance (MSt) | Terminal stance (TSt) | Preswing (Psw) | Initial swing (ISw) | Midswing (MSw) | Terminal swing (TSw) |

**Figure 15-3** Phases of gait cycle shown with corresponding body position for sagittal plane motion. (From Ounpuu S: *Evaluation and management of gait disorders*, New York, 1995, Marcel Dekker.)

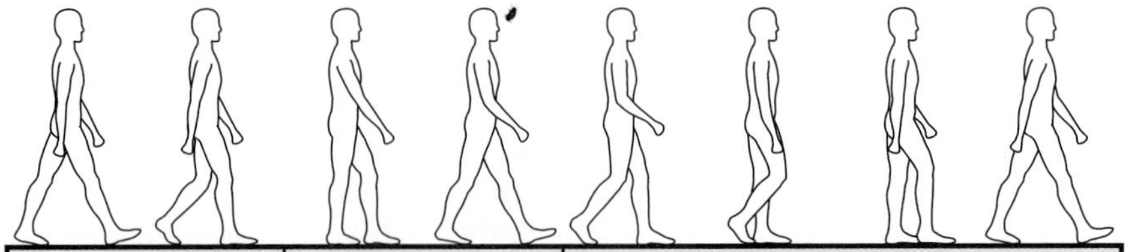

| | Weight acceptance | | Single limb support | | Swing limb advancement | | | |
|---|---|---|---|---|---|---|---|---|
| **Reference limb** | IC | LR | MSt | TSt | PSw | ISw | MSw | TSw |
| **Opposite limb** | PSw | PSw | ISw/MSw | TSw | IC/LR | MSt | MSt | TSt |
| **Trunk** | Erect ————————————————————————→ | | | | | | | |
| **Pelvis** | 5° Forward rotation | 5° Forward rotation | 0° | 5° Backward rotation | 5° Backward rotation | 5° Backward rotation | 0° | 5° Forward rotation |
| **Hip** | 25° Flex | 25° Flex | 0° | 20° Apparent hyperext | 0° | 15° Flex | 25° Flex | 25° Flex |
| **Knee** | 0° | 15° Flex | 0° | 0° | 40° Flex | 60° Flex | 25° Flex | 0° |
| **Ankle** | 0° | 10° Plantar flex | 5° Dorsiflex | 10° Dorsiflex | 20° Plantar flex | 10° Plantar flex | 0° | 0° |
| **Toes** | 0° | 0° | 0° | 30° MTP Ext | 60° MTP Ext | 0° | 0° | 0° |

**Figure 15-4**   Range of motion summary. (Courtesy Rancho Los Amigos Medical Center Physical Therapy Department and Pathokinesiology Laboratory, Downey, Calif.)

usually have greater deficits in the leg. Those with ischemic lesions in areas supplied by the middle cerebral artery have greater arm involvement, although leg weakness is usually also present in varying degrees. Middle cerebral artery infarctions are the most common type of stroke.[16] The gait deviations seen with these lesions are those most often described by the generic term *hemiplegic gait*. Following are descriptions of some of the more common alterations.

During the stance phase of the hemiparetic leg, a patient may exhibit "foot flat" or even a "forefoot first" at the initial contact instead of a heel strike with adequate ankle dorsiflexion. The patient also may exhibit plantar flexion (forefoot first) *and* supination (in the frontal plane) at initial contact and then begin to bear weight precariously on the lateral border of the foot.[17,35,52,60]

During the loading response, while the patient is still in double limb support, weight is being "loaded," or accepted,

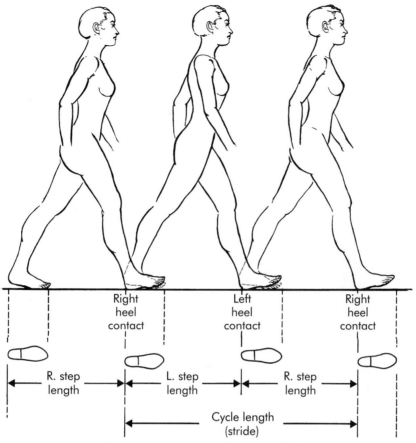

**Figure 15-5** Distance dimensions in a gait cycle. *R.*, Right, *L.*, left. (From Inman VT, Ralston HJ: *Human walking*, Philadelphia, 1981, Williams & Wilkins.)

onto the leg. Normally, 10 to 15 degrees of knee flexion is needed to absorb the forces of momentum and body weight. This flexion may be absent, in which case the knee remains extended or even hyperextends (genu recurvatum) during midstance, as the body moves forward. In this instance, no tibial advancement occurs over the foot because no dorsiflexion is occurring at the ankle (Figure 15-6).

Midstance begins the period of single limb support. In addition to knee hyperextension, the therapist also may observe trunk and hip flexion as the body attempts to move its center of mass forward over a stiff knee. The problem may be compounded by pelvic retraction. Other patients may display the opposite scenario during midstance on the paretic leg; knee flexion may be excessive in the sagittal plane, with concurrent excessive dorsiflexion and hip flexion.[2,17,52,60]

In the *frontal* plane, lateral trunk lean may be excessive over the ipsilateral leg during midstance or a positive Trendelenburg's sign may be evident, both of which indicate weak hip abductors of the stance leg. A positive Trendelenburg's sign is present when excessive lateral displacement of the pelvis occurs over the stance leg, with

an excessive lowering of the pelvis on the contralateral swing leg.[54,61]

During the terminal stance phase, which is still a period of single limb support, normal hip extension may be absent along with the ability to transfer weight onto the forefoot in preparation for push off. Dorsiflexion at the ankle joint may continue to be excessive or diminished. Lack of heel rise can occur in the *sagittal* plane, combined with excessive dorsiflexion, and the contralateral leg makes initial contact early.[2,36,52,61]

The preswing phase is the final stance stage and the second double support period. A lack of knee flexion (normally between 30 and 40 degrees) often occurs in the paretic leg, accompanied by a lack of ankle joint plantar flexion at the end of preswing.[2,17,60,62]

Many of the deviations observed in the hemiparetic limb during stance can contribute to a *decreased step length* by the *opposite* leg. The body is not able to complete its normal excursion forward because of lack of movement, or ineffective movement, of the pelvis, hip, knee, or ankle of the hemiparetic limb. The opposite limb may "step to" instead of stepping *past* the paretic limb. Step length also can be reduced in the hemiparetic leg.

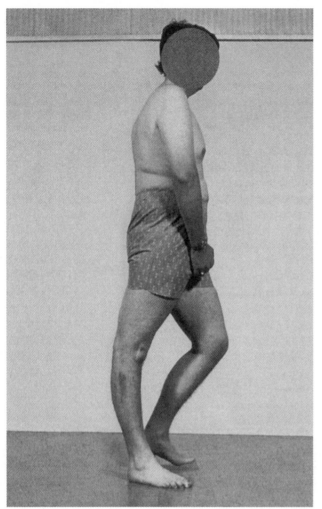

**Figure 15-6**    Genu recurvatum in midstance caused by a rigid plantar flexion contracture (greater than 15 degrees). Tibia is prevented from advancing forward, driving the knee posteriorly into recurvatum, impeding progression, and reducing momentum. (From Adams J, Perry J: *Human walking*, Philadelphia, 1994, Williams & Wilkins.)

The therapist sometimes can see the swing phase of the paretic limb as a mass flexion movement instead of a series of sequential flexion movements.[36,48] More often the swing phase is characterized by a stiff-legged swing, with a decrease in hip flexion and in the velocity and amount of reciprocal knee flexion and extension. The velocity of the entire paretic limb is often decreased.[36,56] The decrease in hip flexion, together with the lack of knee flexion and dorsiflexion, often results in *circumduction* to advance the stiff limb.* *Circumduction* occurs when the patient swings the leg through in a semicircle and is most noticeable when looking at the patient in the frontal plane (Figure 15-7). The patient combines external rotation and abduction at the hip to lift the leg out to the side

*References 2, 36, 49, 54, 60, 62.

**Figure 15-7**    Supination of foot during swing phase resulting from uninhibited activity in the tibialis anterior. Circumduction of hip is also present during this swing phase. (From Davies P: *Steps to follow: the comprehensive treatment of patients with hemiplegia*, New York, 2000, Springer-Verlag.)

and then adducts and often internally rotates the leg to bring it back in.[54] In a normal gait pattern, no abduction, adduction, or external or internal rotation occurs in the frontal plane during the swing phase.[62]

The limited knee flexion in the preswing phase persists into the initial swing phase and often throughout the entire swing phase. The toe drag first seen in the initial swing phase may continue because of the decreased knee swing but also may be a consequence of decreased hip flexion and decreased ankle dorsiflexion. The patient can initiate compensatory hip hiking at this stage to assist with clearing the toes as the leg advances.[2,36,52,56,60] Other compensations used to counteract toe drag are increased hip and knee flexion or vaulting by the opposite (stance) leg. Vaulting occurs when the person rises up on the toes of the stance foot for better clearance of the swing leg.[2]

In the midswing phase the pelvis may remain retracted instead of rotating forward to neutral. Hip hiking and leg circumduction may continue, especially if knee flexion and dorsiflexion remain limited. Dorsiflexion may be decreased or absent, with the ankle assuming a plantar-flexed (foot-drop) position. The foot may supinate during midswing because of an imbalance in ankle dorsiflexor muscle function[17,23,52,62] (see Figure 15-7). Normally, the anterior tibialis and long toe extensors dorsiflex the foot symmetrically. Some stroke patients have overactive anterior tibialis muscles and weak long toe extensors, causing the medially placed anterior tibialis tendon to pull the foot into supination.[23]

As the limb progresses toward the terminal swing phase, many patients are unable to extend the knee while simultaneously flexing the hip and ankle. Instead, knee extension is decreased, and the foot initially contacts the ground with the knee flexed.[52,56] The pelvis still may be retracted or may not have rotated forward past neutral. This, in addition to the decrease in knee extension, results in a decreased step length by the paretic leg. Other subjects may exhibit knee extension with plantar flexion during the terminal swing phase, instead of the normal dorsiflexion seen in preparation for upcoming heel strike.[36,62] In still other persons, adduction of the hip with knee extension can be so pronounced as to cause the swing leg to cross in front of the stance foot. Patients literally end up tripping over themselves.

## CAUSES OF GAIT DEVIATIONS

One cannot overemphasize that the causes of the aforementioned *observed* gait deviations may vary from patient to patient. For example, a common deviation at initial contact is foot flat or forefoot first instead of heel strike. This abnormality could result from weak dorsiflexor muscles,[26,27,49,51,62] excessive activity of the plantar flexors,[2,48,49,62] a decreased ability to perform fast reciprocal movements,[36,46,49] disruption in the central generation of preprogrammed muscle activation,[44] noncontractile soft tissue tightness in the plantar flexors,[2,21,26,62] or a pathologic condition of the ankle joint. Even when soft tissue tightness and joint contractures are ruled out, hypotheses vary and often conflict about the precipitating factor. This is especially true when the issue of voluntary versus reflex skeletal muscle activation is addressed. A number of recent papers and publications provide an abbreviated review of the literature on this topic.*

## TREATMENT INTERVENTIONS

The physical therapist first addresses deficits identified during the physical assessment that are contributing to the abnormal gait, such as decreased range of motion and strength. Interventions can include basic modalities and therapeutic exercise and a variety of approaches to address the lack of movement and voluntary control. Many interventions are based on theories that advocate facilitation of normal movement and sensory stimulation of the patient by the therapist. In this context, the patient is a passive recipient of the therapist's efforts. However, during the past 20 years, therapists gradually have shifted away from using these more traditional therapeutic approaches to using the motor control perspective. The

motor control approach also is based on a theoretical model, but it does not advocate specific treatment techniques that are done by the therapist to the patient. In the motor control model the main task of the therapist is not to facilitate normal movement but to structure the environment in such a way that the patient actively will relearn to use the affected limbs functionally. The motor control relearning theory is based on research from a variety of fields: neurophysiology, muscle physiology, biomechanics, and psychology.[20,39] Patients are believed to learn by actively trying to solve problems (see Chapter 6). Therefore, therapists should structure tasks to promote acquisition of the movements needed to solve specific motor control problems in a variety of situations (see Chapters 4 and 5). This pertains not only to patients with a hemiplegic gait but also to patients with motor control deficits described in the following sections.

Disordered motor control most likely has many causes. Individual therapists have the responsibility to keep abreast of the latest research in this area and in the area of recovery of function after stroke. By doing so, gait training becomes an ever-changing and challenging task for therapist and patient. Although this chapter focuses on deficits that impair gait, other deficits exist (and are noted). Recent publications provide comprehensive reviews of all the impairments that accompany specific stroke syndromes.[11,13,35,78]

## OTHER ABNORMAL GAIT PATTERNS

The list of abnormal gait patterns that can appear after stroke is too extensive to be covered completely in a single chapter. Therefore, what follows are examples of abnormal gaits that are particularly challenging to the physical therapist. Each deficit results from damage in the particular part of the brain described.

### Cerebellar Strokes

A person who has an infarct in the cerebellum caused by occlusion or hemorrhage of a vertebral or a cerebellar artery may exhibit completely different gait deviations than a hemiparetic patient. The cerebellum is composed of three parts or lobes: the flocculonodular lobe, the anterior lobe, and the posterior lobe. The *flocculonodular* lobe also is called the *vestibulocerebellum* because most of its input is from the vestibular nuclei in the pons. The *anterior* lobe also is known as the *spinocerebellum* because most of its input is from the spinocerebellar tracts via the inferior cerebellar peduncle and the superior cerebellar peduncle. The *posterior* lobe also is known as the *neocerebellum* and contains most of the cerebellar hemispheres. The hemispheres receive their major input from the cortex via the middle cerebellar peduncle.

In addition, the cerebellum can be divided longitudinally into functional zones perpendicular to the horizontal

---

*References 21, 26, 31, 36, 40, 41, 45, 46, 48.

fissures dividing the lobes. The most medial structure is the vermis. Adjacent to the vermis, on either side, is the pars intermedia (intermediate section) of the cerebellar hemisphere. Lateral to this is the bulk of the cerebellar hemisphere.

Gait is influenced most by the flocculonodular and anterior lobes. Consequently, infarcts in these areas lead to difficulty maintaining a proper stance and walking.[55] Damage to the flocculonodular lobe (vestibulocerebellum) causes head and neck ataxia. Truncal tremor is often severe. The patient often uses a wide-based stance with the feet apart to increase stability. Any attempt to bring the feet together or walk with one foot directly in front of the other causes loss of balance. Ataxia or dysmetria of the limbs is not common.

Damage to the anterior lobe, especially the medial aspect, causes a disruption in the sensory input (via the spinocerebellar tracts) that is related to agonist-antagonist muscle activity. Lower limb ataxia or dysmetria is also present, but upper limb ataxia is usually absent. Lesions in a cerebellar hemisphere result in ipsilateral limb dysmetria or hypotonia, in addition to other deficits. Although the damage does not affect postural stability, the gait appears ataxic and staggering because of the limb dysmetria.[52]

The cerebellum is supplied by three main arteries: the posterior inferior cerebellar artery, the anterior inferior cerebellar artery, and the superior cerebellar artery. These arteries are part of the posterior circulation—the vertebrobasilar system. The posterior inferior cerebellar artery is a branch of the vertebral artery, whereas the anterior inferior cerebellar artery and superior cerebellar artery are branches of the basilar artery. Chapter 1 describes in detail the territories supplied by these arteries and their associated areas.[3,4] In general, these arteries supply the areas of the cerebellum that their names imply, in addition to parts of the brainstem. Some areas of vascularization in the cerebellum overlap because of the many free cortical anastomoses[4] (Figure 15-8). Although one artery may supply one particular lobe predominantly, this overlapping may result in additional blood coming from the distal branches of another artery. However, as a rule, the superior cerebellar artery supplies the superior cerebellar peduncle, the anterior inferior cerebellar artery supplies the middle cerebellar peduncle, and the posterior inferior cerebellar artery supplies the inferior cerebellar peduncle.[4]

A cerebellar stroke resulting from occlusion of the posterior inferior cerebellar artery usually is referred to in the literature as a *lateral medullary syndrome* (Wallenberg's syndrome)[13,35,78] because it was believed that the posterior inferior cerebellar artery supplied the lateral medulla and parts of the cerebellum. Recently this term has been disputed, based on evidence that the lateral medulla is supplied less frequently by the posterior inferior cerebellar

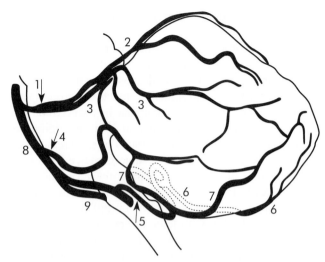

**Figure 15-8** Lateral view of cerebellar arteries. *1*, Superior cerebellar artery; *2*, medial branch of superior cerebellar artery; *3*, lateral branch of superior cerebellar artery; *4*, anterior inferior cerebellar artery; *5*, posterior inferior cerebellar artery; *6*, medial branch of posterior inferior cerebellar artery; *7*, lateral branch of posterior inferior cerebellar artery; *8*, basilar artery; *9*, vertebral artery. (From Bogousslavsky J, Caplan L, editors: *Stroke syndromes*, Cambridge, England, 1995, Cambridge University Press.)

artery than previously thought.[3] If the lateral medulla is spared, an infarct of the posterior inferior cerebellar artery territory is apparent as a headache on the ipsilateral side, vertigo, nausea and vomiting, nystagmus, and limb and gait ataxia. If the lateral medulla is involved, the foregoing signs and symptoms are present. In addition, interruption of the sympathetic nerve fibers can cause Horner's syndrome. Cranial nerves V, IX, and X also are affected.[3,77]

Involvement of cranial nerves V, IX, and X results in ipsilateral loss of pain and temperature in the face (V), dysphagia (IX), and dysphonia (X). Pain and temperature may be decreased on the opposite side of the body because of the interruption of the ascending spinothalamic tracts. This combination of cerebellar and medullary signs constitutes Wallenberg's lateral medullary syndrome. In either type of posterior inferior cerebellar artery infarct, the inferior cerebellar peduncle and the inferior aspect of the cerebellum are affected. The result is ipsilateral limb ataxia and gait ataxia.[3,77] In addition, the patient tends to fall to the side of the lesion (ipsilateral axial lateropulsion) and has difficulty shifting weight toward the contralateral leg.[3]

Earlier texts reported that posterior inferior cerebellar artery infarcts are the most common,[13] but recent findings have shown that superior cerebellar artery infarcts occur as frequently.[3,4] Superior cerebellar artery infarcts have several different clinical manifestations. Dysarthria is one of the most frequent. Limb dysmetria and gait ataxia, as well as ipsilateral axial lateropulsion, are also common symptoms.[3] Anterior inferior cerebellar artery infarcts are the least common. In addition to vertigo and ataxia, tinnitus and deafness are present. Auditory involvement, along with peripheral facial palsy, are classic signs of anterior inferior cerebellar artery infarcts, and differentiate them from superior cerebellar artery or posterior inferior cerebellar artery infarcts.[3,77]

Gait retraining after a cerebellar stroke is focused on relearning the way to correct balance losses. Patients first must learn the point in space where their center of gravity is positioned optimally over their base of support for stability. Then they must relearn the way to realign their center of gravity constantly with their base of support. This task is most difficult during ambulation when the center of gravity is shifted anterior to the base of support as the body moves forward.[76]

Balance retraining should encourage active problem-solving by the patient (see Chapter 8). Being held upright by the therapist while walking does not promote functional independence. Likewise, assistive devices that require upper extremity weight bearing (e.g., walkers) may prevent loss of balance but do not promote functional improvement because they do not challenge the patient to relearn balance control.[5,14] The patient merely is stabilized externally and is not required to use or integrate postural reflexes.

Activities that require active weight shifting and goal-oriented reaching are encouraged and practiced while the patient is standing (see Chapter 14). The therapist can introduce progressively more challenging exercises and activities as the patient becomes more adept.[5] Initially, some patients find it beneficial to walk with their nonaffected side next to a high mat. The hand of the nonaffected side is placed on the surface of the mat for support. The patient can advance the dysmetric limb more easily if the opposite (sound side) hip maintains contact with the high mat during stance. Later, the patient uses a cane only to prevent loss of balance or as a cue to shift weight to the less affected side, not as a maximal assistive device.

## Ipsilateral Pushing

An unusual motor behavior that hemiplegic patients sometimes display in the clinic is ipsilateral pushing. The patients tend to push away from the unaffected side in any position. Davies[23] described the syndrome in 1985 and called it the *pusher syndrome*. The syndrome is not medically recognized, and the literature is scant on this subject. A study by Pedersen, Wandell, and Jorgensen[63] examined whether the syndrome was localized to a specific right parietal lobe lesion, but they found no association. The same study also found no significant association between ipsilateral pushing and two perceptual deficits, hemineglect and anosognosia. Further research is needed to investigate the role of other deficits. For instance,

Pedersen, Wandell, and Jorgensen[63] suggested investigating the role of subcortical sensory pathways and relay stations and the effects of exaggerated sensory feedback from the affected side. Damage to any area involved in processing sensory information can cause impairments when that input is needed to coordinate spatial movement.[10] Posterior parietal lobe infarcts can cause a variety of visual perceptual disorders besides hemineglect and anosognosia.[78] The hippocampus also is believed to play a role in spatial orientation,[10,22] and if it does, the result of damage to that area needs to be examined.

The original description of the pusher syndrome was based solely on a practitioner's observation. The syndrome was thought most often to be associated with left hemiplegia and perceptual deficits (especially left neglect), left visual field neglect with or without homonymous hemianopsia, impaired body scheme and body image, and visuospatial deficits.[23]

Although research has not confirmed the existence of a pusher syndrome, ipsilateral pushing does exist. The cause may not be identifiable, but the behavior still occurs and was seen in as many as 10% of the 327 stroke patients in the study by Pedersen, Wandell, and Jorgensen.[63] Gait training for patients with ipsilateral pushing is a definite challenge, as is transfer training. During sit-to-stand activities, some patients project themselves quickly out of a chair toward their hemiparetic side. If left unguarded, they fall. Transferring toward the stronger side is difficult because they are always pushing away from that side. Although easier, transfers toward the hemiparetic side are dangerous because of the lack of motor control on that side. Standing requires assistance to prevent falling to the weak side.

Walking with an assistive device, such as a cane in the stronger hand, is initially unproductive, because these patients tend to use the cane to push themselves toward the hemiparetic leg. They appear unable actively to shift weight onto the strong leg. The more these patients are supported (to prevent falling to the paretic side), the more they push into the helper.

Gait retraining is based on the same principles discussed in the ataxic gaits section. Patients must relearn the way to adjust their center of gravity over their base of support while standing. This implies a need for conscious awareness of their loss of balance. Although Pedersen, Wandell, and Jorgensen[63] found no significant correlation between anosognosia and ipsilateral pushing, patients were questioned only about limb weakness and visual field deficits, not about balance deficits. Patient self-assessments of the location of their center of gravity in relation to their base of support have yet to be investigated. This author has observed that these patients can relearn to balance themselves, and this was confirmed by the Pedersen study. Of interest is that data collected by Pedersen, Wandell, and Jorgensen[63] demonstrated that at discharge, patients with ipsilateral pushing had lower scores on the Barthel index than those *without* ipsilateral pushing had *on admission* to the hospital. In addition, patients with ipsilateral pushing had significantly increased length of hospital stays and recovery periods. Relearning to maintain balance while walking is a formidable task indeed for patients with ipsilateral pushing.

Trial and error is encouraged to promote active problem solving. The degree of difficulty in relearning to maintain balance while walking is compounded by changes in sensation, strength, motor control, and feedback circuits following the infarction. Visual and tactile goals can be most helpful. Having patients walk around a high mat or table cues patients where to shift their weight to avoid falling. The use of parallel bars is discouraged; patients must learn to weight shift with the trunk to correct balance losses and not merely to pull on a bar to remain upright. Patients can advance to using a cane once they have mastered trunk control. Hands-on techniques used by the therapist to facilitate movement are discouraged. The patients simply will push into the hands of the therapist.

At times, leg weakness interferes with a pusher syndrome patient's ability to relearn postural control and weight shifting. Davies[23] advocated splinting the hemiparetic knee in extension while having the patient work on active weight shifting during functional standing activities. Splinting the knee this way reduces the amount of pushing by the patient while standing. One can assume that the added stability somehow reassures patients and gives them time to assess accurately whether they are balanced. Perhaps the degrees of freedom have been limited, allowing patients to concentrate on one task—weight shifting—to achieve a functional goal without having to concern themselves with an unstable knee. At this time, only speculations can be made about what reduces the pushing tendency and why. Although treatment techniques were suggested for gait training patients with ipsilateral pushing, no controlled studies have been done to verify their efficacy, and they are based solely on this and other practitioners' clinical experiences.

## Proprioceptive Deficits

Loss of sensation after a stroke can compound motor deficits. In particular, loss of proprioception can greatly impede motor recovery after stoke.[28] Proprioception is conveyed to the cerebellum and to the cerebral cortex. Information about joint position and muscle activity is sent to both, but the information projected to the cerebellum is not recorded as conscious perception. The information is used to ensure coordinated limb movements. In contrast, the information sent to the cortex can be perceived consciously and provides awareness of limb position and movement.[35]

Proprioceptive input from muscle spindles, joint receptors, and cutaneous touch receptors reaches the cerebellum through the inferior cerebellar peduncle via the ipsilateral dorsal spinocerebellar tracts. The same information reaches the somatosensory area of the cerebral cortex via the ipsilateral posterior columns of the spinal cord, which cross in the medulla and ascend in the medial lemniscus to the thalamus and then to the cortex.

Middle cerebral artery strokes can impair awareness of proprioception at the cortical level. Although all sensations can be affected, proprioception and two-point discrimination are usually more impaired than pain and temperature perception.[13] The deficits are manifested in the contralateral arm and leg. Cerebellar artery strokes cause loss of the unconscious, rapid proprioceptive input required for the smooth, automatic movements of gait. Loss of sensory input regarding agonist-antagonist muscle activity disrupts the continuous modulation of these muscles that is required for coordinated gait movements.

A study by Kusoffsky, Wadell, Nilsson[47] found that patients with proprioceptive loss after cortical stroke were able to regain a greater amount of function in the leg than in the arm. One explanation they gave for this was that gait greatly depends on centrally generated activation patterns, and these patterns in turn do not depend on peripheral sensory mechanisms. These central pattern generators originate in the spinal cord and are controlled by locomotor centers in the brainstem. These centers are influenced by the cerebellum, the basal ganglia, and the cerebral cortex.[37] The physical therapist can take advantage of this phenomenon by emphasizing functional gait as much as possible.

Along with vestibular and visual input, proprioceptive information contributes to a patient's ability to maintain a stable upright position. Input from muscle spindles and joint receptors provides valuable information not only about the position of a limb in space but also about the environment.[44,76] The ability to react to uneven surfaces or changes in ground texture depends on this input, and its impairment puts a patient at higher risk of falling. Coordinated limb movements may be decreased, and the person may be unable to judge the step length or limb joint excursions needed for maneuvering in the environment.

Vision can help to compensate for the proprioceptive loss.[35,44,59,76] As with other deficits, the physical therapist should encourage a problem-solving approach. The patient must learn consciously to use visual input, which was not necessary before. Occasionally mirrors are useful, although the therapist should evaluate these aids individually for each patient. Mirrors can hinder as often as they help patients, especially those with visuospatial deficits.

The therapist's role is to provide a variety of settings in which the person can practice using visual cues. In addition, biofeedback can be used to provide auditory cues. One type of biofeedback unit is a limb load monitor that can signal a person when the foot contacts the ground. Standard biofeedback units provide information about the force of muscle contraction during strengthening exercises (see Chapter 10).

## Visual Deficits

Visual impairments from strokes also can affect gait. The most common visual deficit in hemiplegic patients is homonymous hemianopsia,[77] which occurs when an infarction involves the optic tract, the lateral geniculate body, or the optic radiation to one occipital cortex. A branch of the internal carotid artery, the anterior choroidal artery, supplies most of the optic tract and the optic radiation, with some coverage by branches of the middle cerebral artery and the posterior cerebral artery.[78] The visual cortex is supplied mainly by the posterior cerebral artery but also is supplied by some middle cerebral artery collaterals.[9,18] Homonymous hemianopsia also can result from an isolated occlusion of the calcarine branch of the posterior cerebral artery, but in this case no concurrent hemiplegia or hemisensory loss occurs.[33]

When homonymous hemianopsia is present, visual information about one half of a person's environment is missing. The temporal half of the visual field of one eye and the nasal half of the visual field of the other eye are absent. Loss of the left half of the visual field accompanies left hemiplegia, and loss of right visual field accompanies right hemiplegia. As mentioned previously, balance is maintained by an intricate communication network between the visual, vestibular, and proprioceptive systems. If vision is impaired, one aspect of this network is functioning abnormally. The ability to maintain balance is at risk if the patient does not learn to use other systems for feedback about the environment.[22]

Self-awareness of the visual deficit is crucial for patients. They must test this new awareness in a variety of situations and environments to ensure safety on discharge from the hospital and maximize functional independence (see Chapter 16).

## Perceptual Deficits

Perceptual deficits such as left neglect or visual neglect are neurobehavioral deficits that can affect gait. These phenomena and their manifestations, causes, and clinical implications are discussed elsewhere (see Chapters 18 and 19).[10,33] Ipsilateral pushing also may be classified as a neurobehavioral deficit.

Hemineglect and hemianopsia are separate entities that can often coexist.[8] Likewise, neglect and sensory loss can develop together or independently. Communication between the occupational and physical therapists concerning a patient's perceptual status is a necessity and helps determine the best treatment approach to maximize function and ensure consistency of treatment interventions. Information obtained from formal testing by the occupational therapist can provide valuable insights for the physical therapist formulating the gait retraining program.

## Orthotic Interventions

An orthosis (from the Greek adjective *orthos*, meaning "straight") is an external device that improves a person's function when applied to a body part.[50] The more commonly used term for an orthosis is a *brace*. Orthoses now are named according to the joints they encompass. Short leg braces are known as *ankle-foot orthoses* (AFOs). A long leg brace is known as a *knee-ankle-foot orthosis* (KAFO) or a *hip-knee-ankle-foot orthosis* if it contains a hip joint and a knee joint. The newer terminology is more descriptive and specific and avoids confusion.

Orthotic devices are prescribed by a physician and fabricated by an orthotist. The physical therapist provides input to the physician and orthotist about which temporary devices have been assessed in the clinic before a permanent orthosis is prescribed. The physical therapist is also responsible for gait training the individual with the orthotic device. Training includes donning and doffing instructions, skin inspections, and patient education as well as the actual gait training.

Orthotic devices are classified in four categories: stabilizing (supportive), functional (assistive), corrective, and protective. All orthoses are used to increase function.

Stabilizing and functional orthoses are the two type most often used with stroke patients. Stabilizing orthoses are used to prevent unwanted motion such as plantar flexion at the ankle or knee buckling. Functional orthoses have an element that compensates for lost muscle strength by assisting with movement. Stabilizing orthoses are not intended as a way to correct a fixed deformity in an adult; they only can stabilize and accommodate a deformity. Corrective orthoses are used to correct or realign parts of a limb. They are used for infants and young children to help correct flexible skeletal deformities. These orthoses should not be used to correct a fixed deformity in an adult. A stabilization orthosis can be used, but only to support the fixed deformity. Protective orthoses protect a portion of a limb from weight-bearing forces (e.g., a limb with a fracture).[32]

The orthotist adheres to basic physical principles when fabricating an orthosis to control a weak joint. An orthosis that provides three points of pressure is the most common type.[73] One of the three forces is directed toward the joint itself, and the other two end forces are directed opposite to the main force (Figure 15-9). This principle is important for the occupational therapist to learn because of its relevance to adaptive shoe equipment. Figure 15-9, *B*, illustrates the three points of pressure used with an AFO that is providing a dorsiflexion assist. The main point of pressure is on the dorsum of the foot. The two counter pressures are at the posterior calf and

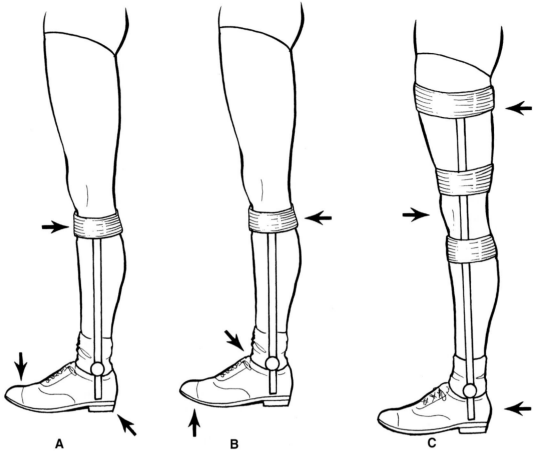

**Figure 15-9**    **A,** Three points of pressure of an ankle-foot orthosis with dorsiflexion stop. **B,** Three points of pressure of a dorsiflexion assist ankle-foot orthosis. **C,** Three points of pressure of a locked knee-ankle-foot orthosis. (These illustrations are diagrammatic only.)

the distal plantar surface of the foot. Elastic laces, often used to facilitate donning a shoe with stroke patients, eliminate the main point of pressure and result in loss of orthotic effectiveness. Therefore, elastic laces should not be used with dorsiflexion-assist braces. Elastic laces should be used cautiously with solid ankle AFOs that prevent dorsiflexion (see Figure 15-9, *A*) because the foot needs to be held snugly in the AFO and shoe. This is especially true if plantar flexion spasticity is present.

Another orthotic principle states that the longer the lever arms, the less force needs to be applied at the three points of pressure. Therapists need to consider bony landmarks and superficial nerves when implementing these principles.[73] The orthotic joint axis of motion should be aligned with the skeletal joint; otherwise, abnormal pressures can be applied in the wrong areas, such as under calf bands, with movement or positioning.[32,73]

Orthotic devices can be made of a variety of materials, the most common of which are metal and plastic. Plastic orthoses are in total contact with a limb and are worn inside the shoe. Metal orthoses are attached to a shoe and held in place on the limb with straps or bands.

An AFO is the most commonly used orthosis for patients with a hemiplegic gait and is the most appropriate.[52,64,84] An AFO can affect knee motion and ankle motion. Knee buckling can be reduced, in stance, by adjusting the amount of dorsiflexion at the ankle joint. Similarly, knee hyperextension (genu recurvatum) can be avoided by controlling the amount of plantar flexion. Therefore the therapist can avoid using a heavier KAFO to control the knee.

Plastic orthoses usually are made from high-temperature thermoplastic materials such as polypropylene. They require high temperatures for molding and therefore are shaped over a model, such as a plaster cast impression of the patient's leg. They are more resistant to continued stress than the low-temperature thermoplastics used for upper limb orthoses.

The simplest and most commonly used plastic AFO is the posterior leaf splint or spring[32] (Figure 15-10, *A*). The leaf spring is used when the main gait deviation is "foot drop" during the swing phase. The orthosis functions as a dorsiflexion assist device because of its flexibility. The plastic of the calf portion is displaced in stance

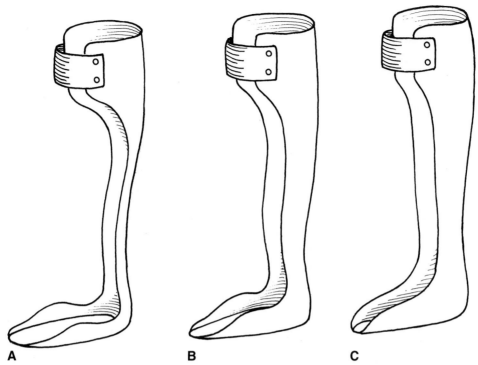

**Figure 15-10** **A,** Posterior leaf splint or posterior leaf orthosis. **B,** Modified ankle-foot orthosis. **C,** Solid ankle-foot orthosis.

and then springs back to a 90-degree angle during swing. The ankle joint is held at this 90-degree angle during swing. Foot drop and toe drag are avoided. This orthosis, however, does not afford any mediolateral stability at the ankle joint. If this is of concern, then the therapist can try a more substantial orthosis.

A modified AFO has a wide calf upright with lateral trimline borders that are just posterior to the malleoli (Figure 15-10, *B*). Usually the foot plate encompasses more of the lateral and medial borders of the foot. This results in more control of calcaneal and forefoot inversion and eversion. The increased width of the calf portion offers somewhat more resistance to plantar flexion in swing and stance.

The most supportive AFO is the solid ankle AFO (Figure 15-10, *C*). The lateral trim lines extend even farther forward, anterior to the malleoli. Because of its construction, the solid ankle AFO is designed to prevent ankle motion and foot motion in any plane. The device controls dorsiflexion, plantar flexion, inversion, and eversion.

A variety of hinged plastic AFOs are now available to allow certain motions and to block others. The ankle joint components are too numerous to mention, and newer components are being designed continuously. The orthotist can use different combinations of joints and stops to allow, limit, or prevent movement. For example, the therapist may wish to allow dorsiflexion past neutral (90 degrees) in stance to allow normal tibial advancement over the foot but block plantar flexion at neutral to prevent foot drop in swing and knee hyperextension in stance.

Another group of plastic AFOs is referred to as *tone-inhibiting AFOs*. Most of these AFOs initially were designed for use with children with cerebral palsy.[25] Several types have been designed more specifically for use with adult hemiplegics.[53] The common denominator is the flexibility allowed by these orthoses, in the foot and in the ankle. In theory, this flexibility allows more normal weight-bearing contacts on the plantar surface of the foot throughout stance, which promotes normal mobility in the foot during stance rather than having the foot held in one position. Mueller et al[53] documented the foot-loading patterns obtained when using two different tone-inhibiting AFOs. They assessed biomechanical alignment and foot stability, and one orthosis—the dynamic ankle-foot orthosis—was found to have had significant effects at the lateral forefoot with respect to force. The authors concluded that this effect might support the medial longitudinal arch of the foot and increase the stability of the forefoot as it is loaded. They theorized that this in turn might allow the forefoot to be loaded at a faster velocity. They did not investigate the effects of correct biomechanical alignment on muscle electromyographic activity.

The use of this type of AFO is based on the same principles that underlie the use of serial casting.[19,25] Both were believed, by some practitioners, to reduce abnormal muscle activity. However, the scientific literature so far does not confirm that the prolonged stretch afforded by serial casting has a central inhibitory effect.[1,15,19,24,83] Changes in sarcomere number and connective tissue caused by immobilization, positioning, and stretch can influence muscle contraction force.[1,15,21,38] In addition, muscle length also can influence the manifestation of hyperreflexia.[1,20,21] Perhaps these mechanical properties of muscle are influenced by tone-inhibiting orthoses. By promoting better biomechanical alignment and normal muscle length, these AFOs may exert an effect on peripheral rather than central factors that, over time, could otherwise augment stretch reflexes. Further research is needed—especially long-term, controlled studies—to investigate the many variables that influence motor control and muscle function. The term *tone inhibiting* may have to be reconsidered until a more complete and universally accepted definition of tone exists along with what contributes to normal and abnormal tone.

Metal orthoses were the main type of orthotic devices used before the 1970s.[32] Metal AFOs still are used for certain stroke patients who cannot tolerate the total contact of a plastic AFO for whatever reason. The components usually consist of two metal uprights attached to an ankle joint. The metal is usually aluminum, but sometimes heavier steel is needed for control. The ankle joint is attached to a stirrup that is fastened beneath the heel of the shoe. The proximal ends of the upright are attached to a calf band.

The metal ankle joint is usually a single- or double-channel (chamber) type (Figure 15-11). Other types of ankle joints are described in detail elsewhere.[21,32,49] A single-channel ankle joint can assist dorsiflexion with a spring placed in the channel. Plantar flexion also can be limited to prevent genu recurvatum by placing a pin in the channel. A double-channel ankle joint can prevent dorsiflexion and plantar flexion by using pins in both channels. Small screws hold the pins in the chambers. The degree of dorsiflexion or plantar flexion (i.e., the ankle joint angle) can be determined by the degree to which the pins are driven into the channels by tightening the screws. Springs and pins can be used in combination to stop one movement and assist another.

The metal uprights attached to the ankle joint and stirrup offer a certain amount of foot and ankle mediolateral control. However, if additional support is needed (e.g., to prevent severe foot inversion), a strap can be added that applies pressure to the lateral malleolus in a medial direction and is secured around the medial upright. Because it prevents varus positioning of the ankle, the strap is called a *varus correction strap*. Force can be applied in the opposite direction with a strap to prevent foot eversion and a valgus foot position. This strap then is called a *valgus correction strap*. A varus correction strap is more common.

The simplest type of metal AFO is the Veterans Administration Prosthetic Center shoe clasp orthosis, which consists of a single narrow metal upright that attaches to the heel counter of a shoe with a metal clasp and a calf strap (Figure 15-12). The orthosis offers dorsiflexion assist only, with no mediolateral or plantar flexion control.

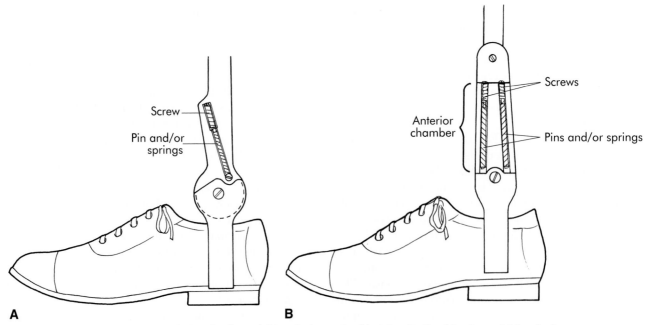

**Figure 15-11**   **A,** Single-channel (chamber) metal ankle joint. **B,** Double-channel (chamber) metal ankle joint.

Occasionally a KAFO with knee locks may be prescribed for a patient who requires additional knee control. However, the additional weight, the prevention of normal knee joint excursions during swing, and increased energy cost caused by these factors greatly limit the potential for functional ambulation.[52,64,84] In addition, donning and doffing a KAFO are difficult for hemiplegic patients (see Figure 15-9, C).[84]

A KAFO combines the features of an AFO with a knee joint and (in the case of a metal orthosis) metal uprights that extend proximally up the thigh. Thigh bands secure the KAFO on the upper leg. The simplest knee joint is a hinge, and the most common locks to maintain knee extension are drop ring locks.[32] The thigh component of plastic KAFOs usually is made of the same thermoplastic material as the AFO component. Metal and plastic combinations also can be used.[29,32,49]

As previously mentioned, KAFOs are seldom used for hemiparetic patients. Occasionally, a preexisting knee joint deformity or ligamentous laxity is exacerbated by walking because of the now weak muscular support. In such instances, no alternative may be available to using a KAFO to allow minimal household ambulation. A KAFO or a knee extension splint sometimes is used as an initial training device to enhance stability. These are used only as temporary measures and not as long-term orthotic devices.[20,52,84]

The physical therapist has the responsibility of reevaluating the orthotic device on an ongoing basis, especially

in the outpatient or home therapy setting. In this era of decreased length of hospital stays, patients sometimes are prescribed an orthotic device while still in the early stages of recovery. As motor control improves, the orthotic device may need to be modified or discontinued to allow more active movement by the patient.

## ASSISTIVE DEVICES

The assistive devices most commonly used with stroke patients are canes, walkers, and occasionally two crutches. Hemiparetic patients whose balance is impaired minimally and who have functional strength in the opposite upper extremity may use a cane. Two crutches or a walker require at least some functional use of both upper extremities. Both devices provide more external stability, with the walker providing more stability than the crutches. The main function of a cane is to increase the base of support and thereby improve balance.[70] The base of support is increased by providing another contact with the floor. Canes also decrease the need for abductor muscle tension to stabilize the pelvis in stance on the paretic side.[58,70] This in turn helps to prevent dropping of the contralateral pelvis (a positive Trendelenburg's sign) in stance when the cane is used in the hand opposite the hemiparetic leg. Using the opposite hand also helps simulate the reciprocal arm and leg movements of a normal gait.

A variety of canes are on the market, ranging from a simple wooden straight cane to a tripod "walk cane" (also called a *hemiwalker*). At a level in between these two canes are the narrow- and wide-based quadruped canes (quad canes) (Figures 15-13 to 15-16). Widening the base of support provides more stability. Physical therapists may begin training with a fairly wide-based cane because of hemiparesis and impaired balance. They should advance patients as quickly as possible to the least amount of assistance required to ensure a safe, stable gait. Patients often are kept inadvertently on a maximally wide base of support cane when it is no longer needed. This prevents the patient from maximizing functional ambulation for two reasons: (1) normal weight shifting to the hemiparetic leg is limited, and (2) cadence is slower than it is with a smaller device[70] or no device. The key word is *safety*. Maximum use of the involved leg should be encouraged along with normal trunk and pelvic movement, provided that patient safety is not compromised.

Two crutches occasionally are used: axillary or (more often) forearm (Lofstrand) crutches (Figure 15-17). Certain cerebellar stroke patients or others who have impaired balance but functional use of both arms and hands may be trained with these devices. These patients require the extra postural support afforded by the second crutch but have enough motor control to be able to advance the crutches reciprocally.

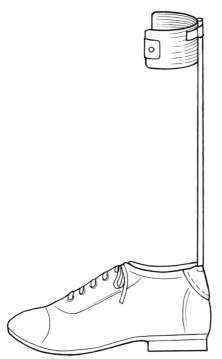

**Figure 15-12** Veterans Administration Prosthetic Center orthosis for dorsiflexion assist.

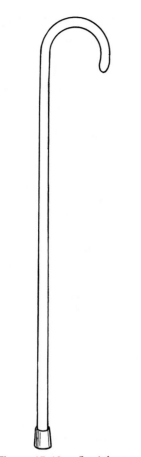

**Figure 15-13**   Straight cane.

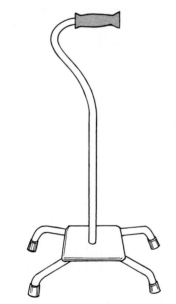

**Figure 15-14**   Wide-based quad cane.

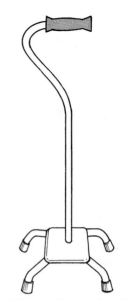

**Figure 15-15**   Narrow-based quad cane.

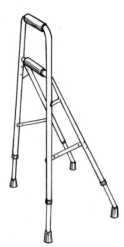

**Figure 15-16**   Hemiwalker or walk cane.

Therapists may use walkers for training stroke patients who have functional use of both arms and hands but need greater outside support than that afforded by two crutches. Occasionally a walker may allow functional use of a hemiparetic arm even though balance is sufficient with a cane. In this case, the patient also should practice gait training with a cane to promote optimum postural control. If patients have sufficient control of the paretic arms, they also may use walkers when it is necessary for them to transport objects around the house (e.g., in the kitchen).

Standard walkers are the most stable assistive devices because they provide four points of contact with the ground. The base of support is greatly increased. A variety of walkers are available as well. In addition to standard walkers with four legs, rolling walkers with front wheels only, with four wheels, and platform attachments are also available. Rolling walkers allow a more normal reciprocal gait, but the therapist must take care to prevent the walker from "running away" with the patient. A stroke patient with insufficient arm and hand strength to lift a walker may have the ability to maintain a grip on

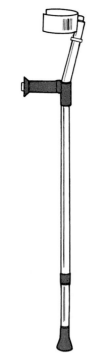

**Figure 15-17** Lofstrand crutch.

| | ← Progression | | | |
|---|---|---|---|---|
| **Begin new cycle** | | **Begin cycle** | **Start** | |
| | ② | | ○ | Two point contralateral **A** |
| ① | | ① | Ⓡ | (two devices) |
| | ② | | Ⓛ | |
| ① | | ① | ○ | |
| | | | | |
| ① | | ① | Ⓡ | Two point contralateral **B** |
| | ② | | Ⓛ | (left hand, right foot) |
| ① | | ① | ○ | |
| | | | | |
| | ② | | Ⓡ | Two point ipsilateral **C** |
| ① | | ① | Ⓛ | (left hand, left foot) |
| ① | | ① | ○ | |
| | | | | |
| ① | | ① | ○ | |
| | ② | | Ⓡ | Three point—left **D** |
| ① | | ① | Ⓛ | |
| ① | | ① | ○ | |

**Figure 15-18** **A** to **D**, Diagrammatic view of assisted gaits. (From Smidt G, Mommens MA: Gait patterns, *Phys Ther* 60:553, 1980.)

the rolling walker and push it forward. Some walkers have pressure-sensitive brakes that prevent forward movement when the patient pushes down on the walker.

As mentioned in the cerebellar stroke section, postural control sometimes is sacrificed for stability when a walker is used. The patient has no need to relearn balance and control if the walker provides needed support. As mentioned, safety is the ultimate concern. If safe, functional ambulation is not possible without a walker, then safe, independent ambulation with a walker is the preferred choice.

The type of gait pattern taught to the stroke patient depends on a number of factors, including balance, strength, and coordination.[58,70] The therapist also should consider cognitive and perceptual deficits, including apraxias.

Smidt and Mommens[72] suggested terminology for describing walking patterns. *Point* refers to the number of contacts made with the floor, including with feet and assistive devices, during the forward progression of the gait cycle (Figures 15-18 and 15-19). For example, a four-point contralateral gait indicates that two feet and two assistive devices (such as canes being advanced one at a time) are being used (see Figure 15-19, *A*). The more contacts on the floor at any given moment, the more stable the person is while walking. In addition, the pattern can be called a *delayed pattern* if the assistive device is advanced before the limbs. Delayed patterns provide more stability than moving a limb concurrently with an assistive device. Following are the most common gait patterns taught to stroke patients.

## GAIT PATTERNS

### Two-Point Contralateral Gait Pattern Using One Device

Hemiparetic patients with a nonfunctional arm often are taught a two-point contralateral gait pattern using one assistive device. A device, such as a cane, is held in the unaffected hand. The cane and the paretic leg are advanced together (one point), and then the unaffected leg is advanced alone (second point) (see Figure 15-18, *B*). The cane may be advanced first and then the paretic limb followed by the unaffected limb for a more stable pattern. This pattern is a delayed contralateral two-point gait pattern (see Figure 15-19, *B*). In Figures 15-18, *B*, and 15-19, *B*, the right leg is the hemiparetic leg.

### Four-Point Contralateral Gait Pattern Using Two Devices

The devices used in a four-point contralateral gait pattern could be canes or crutches. The therapist might choose this type of gait for stroke patients who have functional

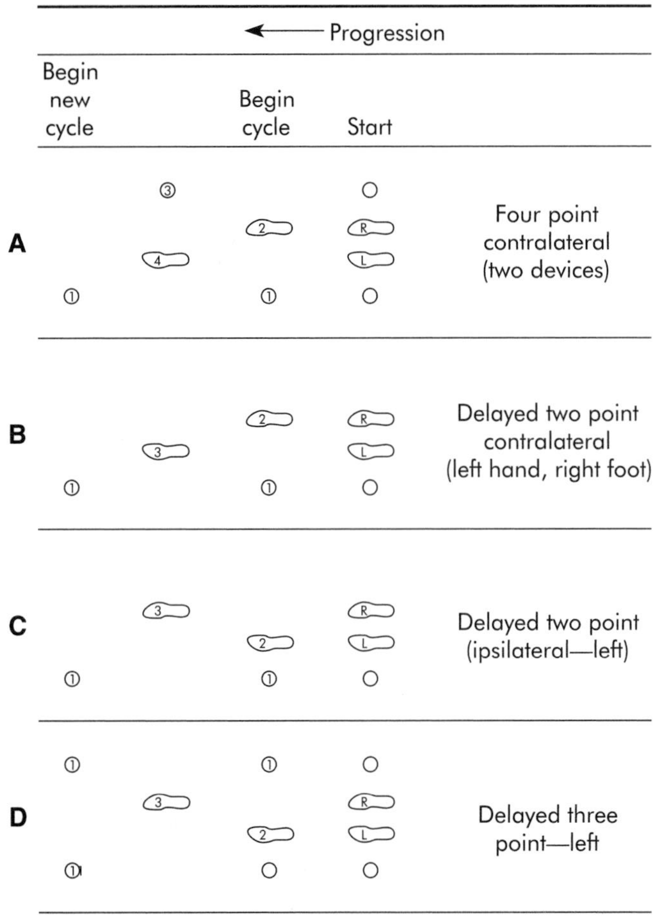

**Figure 15-19**  A to D, Diagrammatic view of assisted gaits. (From Smidt G, Mommens MA: Gait patterns, *Phys Ther* 60:553, 1980.)

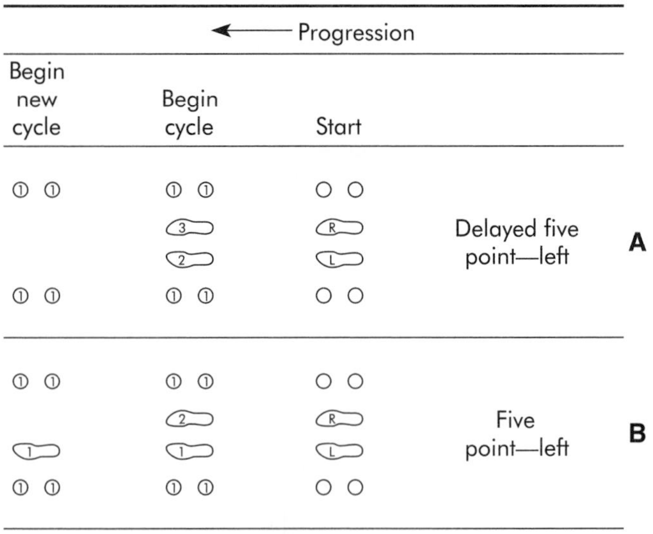

**Figure 15-20**  A and B, Diagrammatic view of assisted gaits. (From Smidt G, Mommens MA: Gait patterns, *Phys Ther* 60:554, 1980.)

use of all four limbs but have impaired balance. They require bilateral support but are able to advance each device (two points) and each leg (two points) individually and reciprocally. Although this is a stable gait pattern, it is not used often with hemiparetic patients. Sometimes a patient recovering from a cerebellar stroke will be taught this pattern to encourage coordinated reciprocal arm and leg movements and postural control.

### Two-Point Contralateral Gait Pattern Using Two Devices

If the previously mentioned patients regain sufficient postural control, they might be advanced to using a two-point contralateral pattern (see Figure 15-18, *A*). They still would be using two crutches or canes but would be moving one device and the opposite leg simultaneously (one point) followed by the other device and opposite leg (second point).

### Five-Point Gait Pattern Using One Device

Therapists may train patients with a walker if they have functional control of all four extremities but require

greater trunk control than that afforded by a cane. For example, certain patients who have had cerebellar strokes may never recover adequate postural stability to be able to use two canes. A walker allows the patient to use five points of contact: the four legs of the walker and one of the patient's legs. The patient advances the walker simultaneously with one leg and then places all four of the walker legs firmly on the floor at the same time as the patient's foot. This pattern is called a *five-point gait pattern* (Figure 15-20, *B*). If the patient moves the walker first, followed by the patient's leg, the pattern is called a *five-point delayed gait pattern* (Figure 15-20, *A*). Other authors refer to this gait pattern as a "3-1-point" or "modified 3-point" pattern.[65] The basic sequence is the same, however.

Therapists may train previously mentioned patients with a rolling walker. They may choose this device for two reasons: (1) the walker is in constant contact with the floor while being advanced, therefore affording maximum postural control, and (2) the walker is in constant motion, therefore the patient is able to take equal step lengths and to increase speed. With the standard walker, the patient is forced to use a "step-to" type of gait pattern (the walker is advanced, then the foot, then the other foot) that prevents a normal stride and limits velocity.[72] In making the decision to use a rolling walker, the physical therapist also must consider the patient's ability to control the continuous forward motion of the walker, as mentioned previously.

### Three-Point Gait Pattern Using Two Devices

Three-point gait patterns seldom are used with stroke patients and are used more often with patients who have orthopedic conditions requiring weight relief on one leg (see Figures 15-18, *D*, and 15-19, *D*).

## GUARDING TECHNIQUES

The goal of gait training after stroke is to have the patient walk as efficiently, safely, and independently as possible. To promote optimum functional ambulation, for the patient to experience postural instability to relearn the way to correct these imbalances is important.

With this in mind, the therapist must be as close to patients as necessary to prevent them from falling or injuring themselves and yet not inhibit them from learning the way to right themselves. Therapists must allow patients to take some risks without jeopardizing the patients' safety or their own safety. This is not an easy task, especially for new therapists. The ultimate horror for any therapist is having a patient fall. Obviously, until therapists are comfortable with patients and know how much, if any, outside support they need, guarding too much is better than guarding too little. Regardless, the goal always should be safe, optimum function, and the therapist needs to reevaluate on an ongoing basis how much guarding is needed and in what type of setting and on what type of surface activities should be performed.

Hemiparetic patients walking with a cane most often are guarded on the weaker side. The therapist stands slightly posterior and lateral to the affected side.[65,70] The therapist is then in the best position to assist the patient. Should patients lose their balance or stumble, they may have difficulty preventing a fall to the weaker side because of decreased sensation and decreased strength and control of the paretic leg. The therapist can control patients with the hand closest to them at the hip or pelvis and can control patients' shoulder and trunk with the other hand if necessary.

The use of gait belts or guarding belts varies from therapist to therapist and from institution to institution, but most facilities advocate their use in the initial stages of gait training and on stairs. The patient's safety is of the utmost concern. At times, a patient is uncontrollable without a gait belt. Other times, the belt can be a hindrance to patients relearning postural control if the therapist is inadvertently tugging on the belt with every step. Therapists must evaluate each patient individually. The size of the patient in comparison to the therapist also may need to be considered. The therapist should decide which anticipatory actions need to be taken to protect the patient from harm based on clinical assessment and sound judgment.

When guarding a patient who is ascending stairs, the therapist is positioned posterior and to the weaker side. The patient should be trained using a railing at the stronger side. Initially, the therapist may teach the patient to ascend one step at a time, leading with the stronger leg. When the patient is descending, the therapist stands in front of and lateral to the affected side so as to provide assistance if the patient's knee buckles. Using the railing, the patient steps down one step at a time, leading with the paretic leg. A patient who regains functional strength of the paretic leg may advance to the step-over-step method of stair climbing, with close guarding by the therapist. Ascending and descending stairs with only a cane or two canes is difficult and requires excellent balance. Some home environments may necessitate such training, but it should be undertaken with sufficient guarding, and the therapist carefully should weigh the safety risks.

Guarding techniques need to be taught to family members as soon as possible during inpatient rehabilitation. Family participation in gait training provides the opportunity for practice and repetition of newly learned techniques.

## BODY WEIGHT SUPPORT SYSTEMS

Gait training with body weight support involves the use of an overhead suspension system and a harness that supports a percentage of the patient's weight as he or she walks on a treadmill (Figure 15-21). The amount of weight supported can be decreased as the person's gait pattern improves. This new approach to gait training is based on studies of adult "spinal cats." These animals underwent low thoracic spinal transection and then were trained on treadmills with their hindquarters supported.[7,69,74] Later investigators found that pools of spinal locomotor cells show evidence of "learning" during step training.[30]

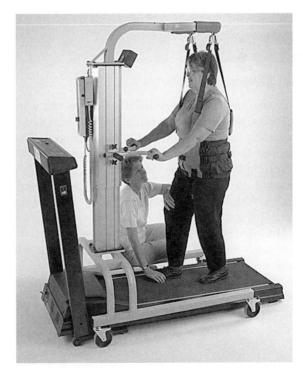

**Figure 15-21** LiteGait System. (From Mobility Research, LiteGait, PO Box 3141, Tempe, AZ 85280; 1-800-332-WALK; www.litegait.com.)

Even before body weight support treadmill training (BWSTT), gait training on a treadmill was known to encourage task-specific motor relearning.[67] This agrees with motor control/motor learning principles mentioned earlier. Proponents of these theories believe that gait training improves recovery of walking more effectively than working on isolated limb control or on a single component of the gait cycle (see Chapter 6).[9,85]

The use of a suspension system for patients with stroke and spinal cord injuries was suggested first by Finch, Barbeau, and Arsenault[34] and Barbeau and Blunt.[6] Early studies suggested that BWSTT leads to a better recovery of walking, including speed over ground, endurance, and amount and type of assistance needed, than conventional therapy.[42,43,82] A later study showed that BWSTT is superior to treadmill training without body weight suspension. In this study, Visintin et al[81] randomized 100 subjects into a BWSTT protocol or treadmill training without body weight support. At the end of 6 weeks of training, the BWSTT group showed significantly greater improvements in every outcome measure, including functional balance, motor recovery, gait velocity, and endurance. These higher scores persisted 3 months after training.

Training with BWSTT at velocities that approach normal walking velocities has been shown to improve a person's "self-selected overground walking velocity."[75] As mentioned previously, higher velocities of walking correlate with an improved gait pattern.[66] The long-term benefits of BWSTT over conventional therapy (i.e., longer than 3 months) now are being investigated.

## Case Study

### GAIT TRAINING AFTER STROKE

This case study in no way reflects the patient's whole treatment program because emphasis also is placed on increasing strength and function in the trunk and left arm and in the leg. In addition, frequent sessions of cotreating by the occupational and physical therapists occurred to enhance communication about specific treatment concerns (e.g., the subluxated shoulder) and functional goals.

H.C. is a 54-year-old male who was admitted to the emergency room of a university medical center with sudden onset of left-sided weakness. Two weeks earlier he had undergone a mitral valve repair and a single coronary artery bypass with a left saphenous vein graft. He had had an uneventful postoperative recovery course and was discharged to his home and prescribed a β-blocker.

On admission, the neurologic workup and results included (1) a computed tomography scan of the head showing early lucency in the right subcortical area;

(2) noninvasive flow studies (on the second day) showing accelerated flow velocities in the right middle cerebral artery suggestive of stenosis and normal flows in the anterior cerebral arteries, posterior cerebral arteries, and basal artery; and (3) a transesophageal echocardiogram revealing trace mitral regurgitation, normal left ventricular function, and no intracardiac or aortic mass or thrombus.

The attending neurologist concluded that H.C. had suffered an infarct in the right corona radiata and putamen in the territory supplied by the lenticulostriate branches of the right middle cerebral artery. The cause of the infarct was most probably an embolus of cardiac origin that developed after the mitral valve repair. H.C. was prescribed anticoagulant medication and was stabilized medically. Twelve days later he was transferred to the rehabilitation unit of the same medical center.

On admission to the rehabilitation unit, H.C. had symptoms of a pure motor syndrome with left upper extremity weakness that was greater than the left leg weakness, minimal left lower facial droop, and no sensory loss. He was alert and oriented and most cooperative although somewhat deconditioned because of the previous cardiac surgery.

Physical assessment revealed normal passive range of motion of the left arm and leg, although both legs manifested tight hamstrings and could perform only a straight leg raise to barely 60 degrees. A finger-width subluxation was present in the left shoulder. Strength testing revealed that the left arm was grossly 2 to 3 out of 5 throughout. He was able to extend the left knee completely while sitting (3 out of 5), but the hip flexors were weaker (2 out of 5). He exhibited no isolated voluntary ankle movement, although dorsiflexion was 2 out of 5 with simultaneous flexion of the hip and knee, and plantar flexion was 2 out of 5 during simultaneous extension of these proximal joints. He did not at that time (or ever) exhibit any spasticity in the limbs during passive testing by the therapist, with the exception of mild, unsustained ankle clonus. He exhibited no ankle edema despite the leg weakness and previous vein graft for the coronary artery bypass graft surgery.

His gait was evaluated initially while he was walking around a high mat with his right side next to the mat, using his right arm and the mat to "unload" the left leg. During static standing, he required contact guarding and verbal cues to extend the left hip and knee actively. He had a tendency to bear most of his weight on the stronger right leg. When cued to stand with equal weight on both legs, he was unable to maintain an upright posture and would fall to the left because the knee would buckle. He required minimal assistance to maintain the hip and knee in extension when bearing weight symmetrically.

Initially he was able to take 10 steps around the mat with minimal assistance. His gait analysis was as follows: Uneven step lengths were observed; the left was greater although less controlled than the right. The shorter step with the right leg resulted in a "step-to" type of gait pattern—the right leg stepping to meet, instead of pass, the left leg. He exhibited a decrease in single-limb stance time on the left leg. His cadence was slow—approximately 40 steps per minute.

During the left leg stance, the heel did not strike at initial contact; the foot was flat. The loading response resulted in excessive knee flexion that was greater than the normal 10 to 15 degrees. To prevent buckling in midstance, the knee snapped back into hyperextension (genu recurvatum). Instead of bringing his body forward by allowing the tibia to advance over the foot (dorsiflexion), he kept the ankle angle fixed and flexed the hip and trunk over the foot. He did not push off at the end of stance. Instead, he quickly took a short step with the right leg to unload the left one as soon as possible.

Because the resulting right leg position was next to the left leg instead of beyond it, the left leg was unable to assume the normal preswing position of hip extension and 40-degree knee flexion (see Figure 15-4). Instead, the left hip and knee were in full extension, and he was forced to initiate swing on the left from this position.

During the swing phase of the left leg, H.C. exhibited decreased hip and knee flexion and a foot drop because of the weak dorsiflexors. This resulted in his toes scraping the floor. He displayed mild lateral trunk flexion to the right in an attempt first to initiate swing from the previously mentioned abnormal preswing position and then to clear the toes throughout the swing phase.

H.C. was put on a program of active assistive range of motion and strengthening exercises for the left arm and leg. Treatment of the leg emphasized functional strengthening in weight-bearing positions (e.g., sit-to-stand exercises for hip and knee strengthening).

During the initial stage of gait training, a posterior leaf splint orthosis was used to assist with dorsiflexion during the swing phase on the left side. This splint was chosen to encourage a more efficient swing phase and to discourage the patient from leaning to the right to clear the left leg during swing. Because of its flexibility, the posterior leaf splint did not restrict activity at the left ankle or knee during stance. Although the knee was unstable, H.C. was still in the early stages of recovery. Sacrificing mobility for stability (i.e., blocking any ankle dorsiflexion and knee flexion in stance) was not beneficial. Doing so would have forced him to move compensatorily because it is normal to dorsiflex up to 10 degrees at the ankle during midstance and terminal stance. The therapist offered close supervision to contact guarding at the knee because of possible knee buckling resulting from excessive dorsiflexion. H.C. was taught to be aware of the difference between excessive knee flexion and recurvatum. He was soon able to identify correctly when he was in either of these abnormal positions even if he could not always prevent them.

H.C. quickly advanced from ambulation around the high mat to ambulation with a narrow-based quad cane and then a straight cane. He had the advantage of recovering much of his hip extension and abduction strength, which meant he did not require a large degree of outside support from an assistive device for these muscles.

Functional training included standing balance retraining in single-limb and double-limb weight-bearing positions. Modified versions of activities that the patient previously had enjoyed (soccer) and a few new ones (golf putting and baseball) were introduced. H.C. practiced ambulation in a variety of environments and on both even and uneven terrains in preparation for discharge. H.C. even practiced getting through busy revolving doors.

After 6 weeks of inpatient rehabilitation, H.C. was evaluated for a permanent ankle-foot orthosis (AFO). His left leg strength had improved enough to allow him to isolate dorsiflexion and plantar flexion in any position grossly in the 2 out of 5 range, ankle inversion and eversion in the 2 out of 5 range, and toe flexion and extension in the 1+ out of 5 range. His hip flexors improved minimally to 2+ out of 5, and knee extension also improved minimally to 3+ out of 5.

During ambulation, H.C. continued to manifest knee recurvatum in stance and did not push off at the end of stance because of weak plantar flexors. During swing, he continued to exhibit a foot drop and toe drag. The physiatrist, physical therapist, and orthotist performed a joint observational gait analysis. Because of the continued plantar flexor and dorsiflexor weakness during the swing and stance phases and less than

## Case Study

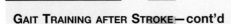

### GAIT TRAINING AFTER STROKE—cont'd

normal knee extension strength, they decided that H.C. required minimal knee control and ankle control from an AFO. In addition, the weak ankle invertors and evertors necessitated mediolateral control by an orthosis. Therefore a posterior leaf splint was deemed insufficient. However, because H.C. was continuing to progress and did not require maximum support at the knee, a solid ankle AFO was also inappropriate. The general consensus was that H.C. should be allowed to have as much movement at the ankle as possible without jeopardizing his safety to promote development of a normal gait pattern.

For this reason the team decided to order a hinged polypropylene AFO with free dorsiflexion at the ankle and a plantar flexion stop at 90 degrees. The hinged ankle with free dorsiflexion allowed him to move the tibia normally over the foot (dorsiflexion) in midstance and terminal stance. The plantar flexion stop at 90 degrees prevented foot drop in swing and recurvatum in stance. The orthosis improved his gait by allowing the normal joint excursions at the knee and ankle in stance while preventing abnormal movements in stance and swing. The promotion of normal joint excursions at the ankle in stance allowed him to take equal step lengths with both legs.

On discharge to his home, H.C. was able to ambulate independently indoors with a straight cane and the hinged AFO, but he required supervision outdoors. He was able to ascend and descend stairs step-over-step using a railing and ascend and descend curbs and ramps with the straight cane, all with distant supervision. He could perform simple home exercises independently for left leg and arm strengthening. He returned to work full-time as a university professor and continued with outpatient physical therapy 3 times a week for 6 months after discharge. He regained full functional use of the left upper extremity including finger function (albeit with decreased coordination), fine motor control, and strength. He also continued to receive occupational therapy for several months as an outpatient.

## SUMMARY

The aim of this chapter is to familiarize the occupational therapist with processes used by physical therapists during gait evaluation and training of patients who have had a stroke. The most common type of gait disorders are those resulting from a middle cerebral artery infarction.

The application of orthotic devices is not an exact science. To assume that a particular abnormal gait always requires one specific type of orthotic device is not accurate. Therapists must evaluate devices on an individual trial basis. Use of a specific device or pattern requires individualized attention.

Those well-versed and experienced in motor control research[20,36,39,41,85] believe that the trend in physical therapy is moving away from earlier theoretical models of treatment techniques and toward a motor control model. The emphasis is no longer on specific treatment techniques to "facilitate" movement but on active problem solving by the patient to promote skilled movement and motor relearning. Treatment programs need to be based on specific motor control deficits, varied, and meaningful to the patient and must take place in numerous environments.

One can no longer assume that certain treatment techniques are effective. Effectiveness needs to be validated by research. Weinstein et al[85] examined the effect that balance-training and weight-shifting activities during standing have on the hemiplegic gait. Although patients who received training improved their standing symmetry significantly, training did not translate into improved weight shifting during ambulation. This study clearly demonstrates the hazards of assuming that transfer of training occurs from one functional task to another. For example, it would be convenient to assume that the techniques used to improve the standing balance of a patient with ipsilateral pushing will improve the ability to walk. However, no evidence supports this theory. Further research such as that of Weinstein et al[85] is imperative for therapists to validate the rationales for their treatment procedures for stroke patients. To do otherwise denies the patient the most beneficial treatment approach.

The case study was unusual because the patient exhibited no spasticity and had voluntary, isolated control of all muscles but had decreased strength. However, several authors questioned the role of spasticity in preventing normal movement[1,20,21,41] and pointed to weakness as the more limiting factor. Spasticity is well known to increase the incidence of muscle contracture and thereby alter the biomechanical efficiency of a muscle.* In this respect, only the ankle joint was at risk and minimally so. The patient was a model patient for other reasons. He was not cognitively impaired, and he was motivated to return to work. He was aware (although grudgingly at times) of the need for faithful adherence to a regular exercise program of repeated practice of newly learned motor skills.

Therapists always should be aware of the need for careful physical assessment, individualized treatment programs that are based on research findings, and ongoing reevaluation of the effectiveness of the treatment program in promoting optimum function.

---

*References 1, 20, 21, 26, 38, 41.

# REVIEW QUESTIONS

1. What constitutes a gait cycle?
2. What are the phases and subphases of the gait cycle?
3. What are step, stride, and cadence?
4. What type of cerebral infarct is associated with the typical "hemiplegic gait"?
5. What are some of the variables that can cause a deviation from the normal joint excursions during a gait cycle?
6. In what way does the motor control model differ from the more traditional theoretical models underlying the different therapeutic techniques?
7. What are some of the manifestations of a posterior inferior cerebellar stroke?
8. What makes treatment of patients demonstrating ipsilateral pushing so challenging?
9. What helps compensate for proprioceptive loss after stroke?
10. What are the main differences between metal and plastic orthotic devices?
11. What orthotic device is used most commonly with stroke patients?
12. What assistive devices are used most commonly with stroke patients?
13. What determines the type of gait pattern that will be taught to a stroke patient?

# REFERENCES

1. Ada L, Canning C: Anticipating and avoiding muscle shortening. In Ada L, Canning C, editors: *Key issues in neurological physiotherapy*, Boston, 1990, Butterworth-Heinemann.
2. Adams JM, Perry J: Gait analysis: clinical application. In Rose J, Gamble JG, editors: *Human walking*, Baltimore, 1994, Williams & Wilkins.
3. Amarenco P: Cerebellar stroke syndromes. In Bogousslavsky J, Caplan L, editors: *Stroke syndromes*, Cambridge, England, 2001, Cambridge University Press.
4. Amarenco P: The spectrum of cerebellar infarcts, *Neurology* 41:973, 1991.
5. Balliet R, Harbst KB, Kim D, et al: Retraining of functional gait through the reduction of upper extremity weight bearing in chronic cerebellar ataxia, *Int Rehabil Med* 8(4):148-153, 1987.
6. Barbeau H, Blunt R: A novel interactive locomotion approach using body weight support to retrain gait in spastic paretic patients. In Wernig A, editor: *Plasticity of motoneuronal connections*, Amsterdam, 1991, Elsevier.
7. Barbeau H, Rossignol S: Recovery of locomotion after chronic spinalization in the adult cat, *Brain Res* 412:84, 1987.
8. Barton JJS, Caplan LR: Cerebral visual dysfunction. In Bogousslavsky J, Caplan L, editors: *Stroke syndromes*, Cambridge, England, 2001, Cambridge University Press.
9. Bassile CC, Bock C: Gait retraining. In Craik RL, Oatis CA, editors: *Gait analysis: theory and practice*, St Louis, 1995, Mosby.
10. Bingman VP, Zucchi M: Spatial orientation. In Cohen H, editor: *Neuroscience for rehabilitation*, Philadelphia, 1993, JB Lippincott.
11. Bogousslavsky J, Caplan L, editors: *Stroke syndromes*, Cambridge, England, 2001, Cambridge University Press.
12. Bontrager E: Instrumented gait analysis. In DeLisa JA, editor: *Gait analysis in the science of rehabilitation*, monograph 002, Baltimore, 1998,

Department of Veterans Affairs, Veterans Health Administration, Rehabilitation Research and Development Service, Scientific and Technical Section.
13. Branch EF: The neuropathology of stroke. In Duncan P, Badke MB, editors: *Stroke rehabilitation*, Chicago, 1987, Mosby.
14. Brandt T, Krafczyk S, Malsbenden I: Postural imbalance with head extension: improvement by training as a model for ataxia therapy, *Ann N Y Acad Sci* 374:636, 1981.
15. Brower B, Davidson LK, Olney SJ: Serial casting in idiopathic toe walkers, *J Pediatr Orthop* 20(2):221-225, 2000.
16. Brust JB: Circulation of the brain. In Kandel ER, Schwartz JH, editors: *Principles of neural science*, ed 4, New York, 2000, McGraw-Hill.
17. Burdett RG, Borello-France D, Blatchly C et al: Gait comparison of subjects with hemiplegia walking unbraced, with ankle-foot orthosis, and AIR-Stirrup® brace, *Phys Ther* 68:1197, 1998.
18. Caplan LR: Visual perceptual abnormalities. In Bogousslavsky J, Caplan L, editors: *Stroke syndromes*, Cambridge, England, 2001, Cambridge University Press.
19. Carlson SJ: A neurophysiological analysis of inhibitive casting, *Phys Occup Ther Pediatr* 4:31, 1984.
20. Carr JH, Shepherd RB: A motor learning model for rehabilitation. In Carr JH, Shepherd RB, editors: *Movement science foundations for physical therapy in rehabilitation*, Gaithersburg, Md, 2000, Aspen.
21. Carr JH, Shepherd RB, Ada L: Spasticity: research findings and implications for intervention, *Physiotherapy* 81:421, 1995.
22. Cohen H: Special senses 2: the vestibular system. In Cohen H, editor: *Neuroscience for rehabilitation*, Philadelphia, 1999, JB Lippincott.
23. Davies PM: *Steps to follow*, Berlin, 1985, Springer-Verlag.
24. De Deyne PG: Application of passive stretch and its implications for muscle fibers, *Phys Ther* 81(2):819-827, 2001.
25. Diamond M, Ottenbacher K: Effect of tone-inhibiting DAFO on stride characteristics of an adult with hemiparesis, *Phys Ther* 70:423, 1981.
26. Dietz V, Quintern J, Berger W: Electrophysiological studies of gait in spasticity and rigidity: evidence that altered mechanical properties of muscle contribute to hypertonia, *Brain* 104(3):431-449, 1981.
27. Dimitrijevic MR, Faganel J, Sherwood AM et al: Activation of paralyzed leg flexors and extensors during gait in patients after stroke, *Scand J Rehabil Med* 13:109, 1981.
28. Duncan PW, Badke MB: Determinants of abnormal motor control. In Duncan PW, Badke MB, editors: *Stroke rehabilitation*, Chicago, 1987, Mosby.
29. Edelstein J: Orthotic management and assessment. In O'Sullivan S, Schmitz TJ, editors: *Physical rehabilitation: assessment and treatment*, ed 4, Philadelphia, 2001, FA Davis.
30. Edgerton VR, Roy RR, de Leon RD et al: Does motor learning occur in the spinal cord? *Neuroscientist* 3:287, 1997.
31. Engardt M, Knutsson E, Jonsson M, et al: Dynamic muscle strength training in stroke patients: effect on knee extension torque, EMG activity, and motor function, *Arch Phys Med Rehabil* 76(5):419-425, 1995.
32. Faculty of Prosthetics and Orthotics, New York University School of Medicine and Post Graduate Medical School: *Lower limb orthotics*, New York, 1986, New York University School of Medicine and Post Graduate Medical School.
33. Ferro JM: Neurobehavioral aspects of deep hemispheric stroke. In Bogousslavsky J, Caplan L, editors: *Stroke syndromes*, Cambridge, England, 2001, Cambridge University Press.
34. Finch L, Barbeau H, Arsenault B: Influences of body weight support on normal human gait: development of a gait training strategy, *Phys Ther* 71:842, 1991.
35. Gilman S, Newman SW: *Clinical neuroanatomy*, ed 8, Philadelphia, 1992, FA Davis.
36. Giuliani CA: Adult hemiplegic gait. In Smidt GL, editors: *Gait in rehabilitation*, New York, 1990, Churchill Livingstone.

37. Glatt SL, Koller WS: Gait apraxia. In Spivack BS, editor: *Evaluation and management of gait disorders*, New York, 1995, Marcel Dekker.

38. Goldspink G, Williams P: Muscle fiber and connective tissue changes associated with use and disuse. In Ada L, Canning C, editors: *Key issues in neurological physiotherapy*, Boston, 1990, Butterworth-Heinemann.

39. Gordon J: Assumptions underlying physical therapy intervention. In Carr JH, Shepherd RB, editors: *Movement science foundations for physical therapy in rehabilitation*, Gaithersburg, Md, 2000, Aspen.

40. Harro CC, Giuliani CA: Kinematic and EMG analysis of hemiplegic gait patterns during free and fast walking speeds, *Neurol Rep* 11:57, 1987.

41. Held JM: Recovery of function after brain damage: theoretical implications for therapeutic intervention. In Carr JH, Shepherd RB, editors: *Movement science foundations for physical therapy in rehabilitation*, Gaithersburg, Md, 2000, Aspen.

42. Hesse SA, Bertelt C, Jahnke MT, et al: Treadmill training with partial body weight support compared with physiotherapy in non-ambulatory hemiparetic patients, *Stroke* 26(6):976-981, 1995.

43. Hesse SA, Bertelt C, Schaffrin A, et al: Restoration of gait in non-ambulatory hemiparetic patients by treadmill training with partial body weight support, *Arch Phys Med Rehabil* 75(10):1087-1093, 1994.

44. Jones LA: Somatic senses 3: proprioception. In Cohen H, editor: *Neuroscience for rehabilitation*, Philadelphia, 1999, JB Lippincott.

45. Knutsson E: Gait control in hemiparesis, *Scand J Rehabil Med* 13 (2-3):101-108, 1981.

46. Knutsson E, Martensson A: Dynamic motor capacity in spastic paresis and its relation to prime mover dysfunction, spastic reflexes, and antagonist co-activation, *Scand J Rehabil Med* 12:93, 1980.

47. Kusoffsky A, Wadell I, Nilsson BY: The relationship between sensory impairment and motor recovery in patients with hemiplegia, *Scand J Rehabil Med* 14(1):27-32, 1982.

48. Lehmann JF: Lower limb orthotics. In Redford JB, editor: *Orthotics etc*, ed 3, Baltimore, 1986, Williams & Wilkins.

49. Lehmann JF, Condon SM, Price R, et al: Gait abnormalities in hemiplegia, *Arch Phys Med* 68(11):763-771, 1987.

50. Licht S: Preface to the first edition. In Redford JB, editor: *Orthotics etc*, ed 3, Baltimore, 1986, Williams & Wilkins.

51. McComas AJ, Sica RE, Upton AR, et al: Functional changes in motor neurons of hemiparetic patients, *J Neurol Neurosurg Psychiatry* 36(2):183-193, 1973.

52. Montgomery J: Assessment and treatment of locomotor deficits in stroke. In Duncan PW, Badke MB, editors: *Stroke rehabilitation: recovery of motor control*, Chicago, 1987, Mosby.

53. Mueller K, Cornwall MW, McPoil TG et al: Effect of two contemporary tone-inhibiting AFOs on foot-loading patterns in adult hemiplegics: a small group study, *Top Stroke Rehabil* 1:1, 1995.

54. Norkin C: Gait analysis. In O'Sullivan S, Schmitz TJ, editors: *Physical rehabilitation: assessment and treatment*, ed 4, Philadelphia, 2001, FA Davis.

55. Oestreich L, Troost BT: Cerebellar dysfunction and disorders of posture and gait. In Spivack BS, editor: *Evaluation and management of gait disorders*, New York, 1995, Marcel Dekker

56. Olney SJ, Griffin MP, Monga TN, et al: Work and power in gait of stroke patients, *Arch Phys Med Rehabil* 72(5):309-314, 1991.

57. Olney SJ, Richardes CL: Hemiplegic gait following stroke, *Gait Posture* 4:136, 1996.

58. Olsson EC, Smidt GL: Assistive devices. In Smidt GL, editor: *Gait in rehabilitation*, New York, 1990, Churchill Livingstone.

59. O'Sullivan SB: Motor control assessment. In O'Sullivan SB, Schmitz TJ, editors: *Physical rehabilitation: assessment and treatment*, ed 4, Philadelphia, 2001, FA Davis.

60. O'Sullivan SB: Stroke. In O'Sullivan SB, Schmitz TJ, editors: *Physical rehabilitation: assessment and treatment*, ed 4, Philadelphia, 2001, FA Davis.

61. Ounpuu S: Clinical gait analysis. In Spivack BS, editor: *Evaluation and management of gait disorders*, New York, 1995, Marcel Dekker.

62. Pathokinesiology Service and Physical Therapy Department: *Observational gait analysis handbook*, Downey, Calif, 1991, Professional Staff Association of Rancho Los Amigos Medical Center.

63. Pedersen PM, Wandell A, Jorgensen HS: Ipsilateral pushing in stroke: incidence, relation to neuropsychological symptoms, and impact on rehabilitation—the Copenhagen stroke study, *Arch Phys Med* 77(1):25-28, 1996.

64. Perry J: The mechanics of walking. In Perry J, Hislop H, editors: *Principles of lower extremity bracing*, Washington, DC, 1977, American Physical Therapy Association.

65. Pierson FM: Ambulation aids, patterns and activities. In *Principles and techniques of patients care*, ed 2, Philadelphia, 1999, Saunders.

66. Richards CL, Malouin F, Dumas F, et al: Gait velocity as an outcome measure of locomotor recovery after stroke. In Craik RL, Oatis C, editors: *Gait analysis: theory and application*, St Louis, 1995, Mosby.

67. Richards CL, Malouin F, Wood-Dauphinee S, et al: Task-specific physical therapy for optimization of gait recovery in acute stroke, *Arch Phys Med Rehabil* 74(6):612-620, 1993.

68. Richards CL, Olney SJ: Hemiparetic gait following stroke. II. Recovery and physical therapy, *Gait Posture* 4:149, 1996.

69. Rossignol S, Barbeau H, Julien C: Locomotion of the adult chronic spinal cat and its modification of monoaminergic agonists and antagonists. In Goldberger ME, Gorio A, Murray M, editors: *Development of plasticity of mammalian spinal cord*, Spoleto, Italy, 1986, Springer-Verlag.

70. Schmitz TJ: Preambulation and gait training. In O'Sullivan S, Schmitz TJ, editors: *Physical rehabilitation: assessment and treatment*, ed 4, Philadelphia, 2001, FA Davis.

71. Sisto SA: An overview of the value of information resulting from instrumented gait analysis for the physical therapist. In DeLisa JA, editor: *Gait analysis in the science of rehabilitation*, monograph 002, Baltimore, 1998, Department of Veterans Affairs, Veterans Health Administration, Rehabilitation Research and Development Service, Scientific and Technical Section.

72. Smidt GL, Mommens MA: System of reporting and comparing influence of ambulatory aids on gait, *Phys Ther* 60(5):551-558, 1980.

73. Smith E, Juvinall RC: Mechanics of orthotics. In Redford JB, editor: *Orthotics etc*, ed 3, Baltimore, 1986, Williams & Wilkins.

74. Smith JL, Smith LA, Zernicke RF et al: Locomotion in exercised and non-exercised cats cordotomized at 2 and 12 weeks of age, *Exp Neurol* 16:393, 1982.

75. Sullivan KJ, Knowlton BJ, Dobkin BH: Step training with body weight support: effect of treadmill speed and practice paradigms on post-stroke locomotor recovery, *Arch Phys Med Rehabil* 83:683, 2002.

76. Tiderksaar R: Falls in older persons. In Spivack BS, editor: *Evaluation and management of gait disorders*, New York, 1995, Marcel Dekker.

77. Timmann D, Ciener HC: Cerebellar ataxia. In Bogousslavsky J, Caplan L, editors: *Stroke syndromes*, Cambridge, England, 2001, Cambridge University Press.

78. Toole JF: *Cerebrovascular disorders*, ed 5, Philadelphia, 1999, Lippincott Williams & Wilkins.

79. Unsworth C, Warburg CL: Assessment and intervention strategies for cognitive and perceptual dysfunction. In O'Sullivan S, Schmitz TJ, editors: *Physical rehabilitation: assessment and treatment*, ed 4, Philadelphia, 2001, FA Davis.

80. Viradens P, Bogousslavsky J: Anterior choroidal artery territory infarcts. In Bogousslavsky J, Caplan L, editors: *Stroke syndromes*, Cambridge, England, 2001, Cambridge University Press.

81. Visintin M, Barbeau H, Korner-Bitensky N, et al: A new approach to retrain gait in stroke patients through body weight support and treadmill stimulation, *Stroke* 29(6):1122-1128, 1998.

82. Visintin M, Finch L, Barbeau H: Progressive weight bearing and treadmill stimulation during gait retraining of hemiplegics: a case study, *Phys Ther* 68:807, 1987.

83. Walsh EG, Wright GW, Brown K, et al: Biodynamics of the ankle in spastic children: effect of chronic stretching on the calf musculature, *Exp Physiol* 75(3):423-425, 1990.

84. Walters RL, Garland DE, Montgomery J: Orthotic prescription for stroke and head injury. In American Academy of Orthopedic Surgeons: *Atlas of orthotics*, ed 2, St Louis, 1985, Mosby.

85. Weinstein CJ, Gardner ER, McNeal DR, et al: Standing balance training: effects on balance and locomotion in hemiparetic adults, *Arch Phys Med* 70(10):755-762, 1989.

lorraine aloisio*

**chapter 16**

# Visual Dysfunction

**key terms**

| | | |
|---|---|---|
| accommodation | scanning | visual acuity |
| anatomy of the eye | stereopsis | visual field |
| functional optometrist | strabismus | visual pathways |
| pursuits | treatment | visual perception |
| saccades | vergence | visual screening |

**chapter objectives**

After completing this chapter, the reader will be able to accomplish the following:

1. Present an overview of visual processing, including anatomy of the eye, neuronal processing, and pathophysiology in relation to stroke.
2. Outline procedures for vision screening and visual perception evaluation.
3. Outline treatment procedures as they pertain to functional abilities.

Occupational therapy has made great strides in the screening and treatment of visual disorders in the past 2 decades. This chapter integrates the occupational therapy literature with various other disciplines. The goal of this chapter is to provide therapists with a comprehensive evaluation and treatment framework for patients who experience visual dysfunction after stroke. A comprehensive understanding of the visual system and the way function is affected after an individual experiences a physical trauma (e.g., a cerebrovascular accident [CVA]) is emphasized.

## A TEAM APPROACH

The processing of visual information is a complex act that usually is screened and evaluated by one or more mem-

bers of the rehabilitation team. These members may include the neurologist, ophthalmologist, neuroophthalmologist, occupational therapist, and others. One highly important member often missing from this team is the rehabilitative optometrist, more commonly known as the *functional optometrist* (Box 16-1). The functional optometrist works with the occupational therapist to assess and manage the functional aspects of vision. These aspects include the ability to use binocular vision, fixate, scan and locate objects, and use accommodation skills successfully.[9,13,14,31] The occupational therapist relies heavily on the results of the functional optometrist's assessment to provide appropriate treatment and enhance the patient's quality of life.

Many occupational therapists must go outside the rehabilitation program or clinic to use the services of the functional optometrist. Only a few rehabilitation facilities currently use a functional optometrist's services regularly.[21,31] With the high prevalence of visual system

---

*I wish to dedicate my effort in writing this chapter to my father, Fred R. Aloisio.

**Box 16-1**

## Suggestions for Collaboration and Development of a Vision Team

Begin with an occupational therapist who has either some visual experience or a strong interest in the area of visual function. The reason for this clearly is to foster respect and understanding of the differences of the two professions (i.e., occupational therapy and functional optometry) and of how they overlap.

### IN-HOUSE FACILITY

- The occupational therapist should contact the appropriate department to speak with the functional optometrist or similar vision professional. The therapist should explain his or her interest in this profession and how one believes these areas of expertise overlap.
- The therapist should ask this professional to provide an in-service to the occupational therapy department to discuss the types of patients whom occupational therapists treat and why information from the functional optometrist is important to one's profession and patient treatment.
- The occupational therapist should also provide an in-service to the optometric department so that they can further understand what role occupational therapists play in enhancing functional vision skills.
- The therapist should invite potential team members to rounds and discuss the occupational therapy aspects of the patients afterward.
- The therapist should have the functional optometrist tour the occupational therapy department and ask the other occupational therapists to be involved in vision-related treatment during that visit. If that is not possible, the therapist might suggest meeting in a patient's room and collaborating on the vision problems of that patient.
- Case studies can be completed by either profession or can be reported as a collaborative effort. The Optometric Extension Program provides numerous outlets for lectures and case study collaboration between out two professions (see Box 16-3).

### OFF-SITE GENERATED

- The steps are generally the same if the therapist's facility does not have a functional optometrist or similar member on staff.
- The informed or interested occupational therapist first can contact the universities in the area that provide education for functional optometrists and other potential team members and request a meeting with the professors or residents to explain one's intentions.
- The therapist may be able to receive a list of the functional optometrists in the area by calling the Optometric Extension Program as indicated in Box 16-3.

For both on-site facility and off-site generation, the therapist's department probably will require permission from the director of rehabilitation, if not from the director of the facility. The therapist should be prepared to state the case in detail regarding goals and objectives and should include the ability for publishing future case studies, holding lectures regarding vision in that facility, and improving patient progress, which is the most important reason for this entire effort.

dysfunctions after stroke, a great need exists to have these professionals as part of the rehabilitation team. For example, an apparent deficit in a visual cognitive skill such as figure-ground (i.e., finding an article of clothing in a drawer) actually may be caused by refractive, binocular, accommodative, ocular motility, or pattern recognition problems. Therefore, to help patients regain complex functions, treatment must start at the basic processing level and proceed through a hierarchy of skills, according to Hellerstein and Fishman.[12] Warren's hierarchy of visual perceptual skill development[29] is similar. This framework states that higher-level skills (visuocognition, visual memory, pattern recognition) evolve from the integration of lower-level skills (oculomotor control, visual fields, visual acuity) and subsequently are affected by disruption of lower-level skills.

The functional optometrist's assessment, management, and collaboration with other team members is essential for the success of the individual. The functional optometrist's role does not replace the need for ophthalmologic and neuroophthalmologic intervention. If damage has occurred to ocular structures or to the ocular motor system, one should call an ophthalmologist or neuroophthalmologist to provide diagnostic and therapeutic care. Surgical or medical treatment may be necessary to minimize loss of sight. However, after the patient is stable, evaluation and treatment of the functional aspects of vision is essential.[5,9,30]

## ANATOMY OF THE EYE

The eye includes the cornea, iris, lens, vitreous chamber, and retina (Figure 16-1).

### Cornea

The cornea is the first structure light hits after it is reflected from an image.[6] Corneal tissue is completely transparent. Light is refracted, or bent, to a great degree by the cornea. Efferson[6] describes the refraction of light by discussing the way a stick placed into water appears bent at the point where it enters the water (Figure 16-2).

Damage to the cornea from abrasions, burns, congenital conditions, and disease-related processes can alter the spherical shape of the cornea and disturb the quality of the image that falls on the retina. In keratoconus the cornea slowly becomes steeper and more cone-shaped, distorting the image and causing reduced vision.[6,28]

### Iris

Behind the cornea is the iris, the colored portion consisting of fibers that control the opening of the pupil, the dark circular opening in the center of the eye. Constriction and dilation of the pupil control the amount of light entering the eye in a fashion similar to the way the f-stop on a camera changes the size of the aperture to control the amount of light and depth of field. In bright light the opening constricts, and in dim light it dilates, allowing light in to stimulate the photoreceptor cells of the retina. This constriction and dilation are under auto-nomic nervous system control with sympathetic and parasympathetic components. Under sympathetic stimulation (fight-or-flight reactions) the pupils dilate, perhaps giving rise to the expression "eyes wide with fear." Under parasympathetic stimulation the pupils constrict.[6]

### Lens

Behind the iris is the lens. The lens is involved in focusing and accommodation and is a biconvex, circular, semirigid, crystalline structure that focuses the image on the retina. The lens of the eye is analogous to the external optical lens system of a camera. A camera is focused by turning the lens to change the distance of the lens from the film, effectively increasing or decreasing the power of the lens and allowing near or distant objects to be seen more clearly.[6,8] The eye achieves the same effect (a change in the power of the lens) by the action of tiny ciliary muscles that act on suspensory ligaments, changing the thickness and curvature of the lens. A thicker lens with a greater curvature produces higher power and the ability to see clearly at near distances. A thinner lens and flatter curvature produce less optical power and the ability to see distant objects clearly (Figure 16-3). Accommodation is the process of lens thickening and thinning.[6,17]

Ideally the lens brings an image into perfect focus so that it lands on the fovea, the area of central vision. If the focused image falls in front of the retina, however, a blurred circle falls on the fovea (Figure 16-4). In this case the lens is too thick and has too much optical power. This can be one of the causes of myopia (nearsightedness). One simple remedy is to place a negative (concave) lens externally in front of the eye in glasses to reduce the power of the internal lens and allow the image to fall directly on the fovea. A similar type of problem occurs in hyperopia (farsightedness), in which the image falls in the back of the retina. In presbyopia ("old eyes") the flexibility of the lens fibers decreases and the lens becomes more rigid. Accommodation becomes weaker until the image

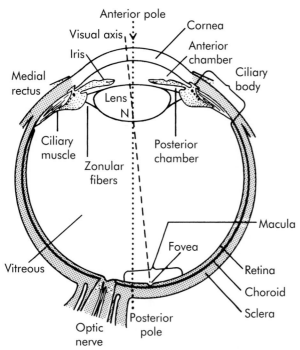

**Figure 16-1**    Horizontal section of the eye. (From Wolff E: *Anatomy of the eye and orbit*, ed 7, London, 1976, HK Lewis.)

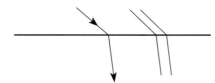

**Figure 16-2**    Refraction—the bending of light at the air-water interface. (From Umphred DA, editor: *Neurological rehabilitation*, ed 3, St Louis, 1995, Mosby.)

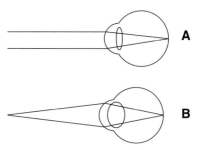

**Figure 16-3**    Focusing and accommodation. **A,** Thinner lens and flatter curvature produce less optical power and ability to see distant objects clearly. **B,** Thicker lens and greater curvature produce higher power and ability to see clearly at near point. (From Umphred DA, editor: *Neurological rehabilitation*, ed 3, St Louis, 1995, Mosby.)

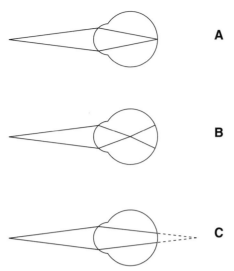

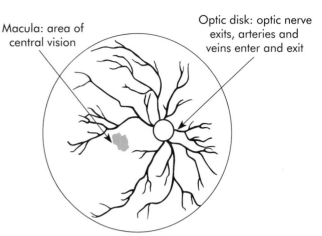

**Figure 16-5** Retinal topography.

**Figure 16-4** **A,** Perfect focusing as the lens brings the image directly onto the fovea. **B,** Focused image falling in front of retina with a blurred circle on fovea, producing myopia (near-sightedness). **C,** Focused image falling in back of retina producing hyperopia (farsightedness). (From Umphred DA, editor: *Neurological rehabilitation*, ed 3, St Louis, 1995, Mosby.)

can no longer be focused on the retina. When this occurs, a person may wear a positive lens externally to aid in vision.[6,21]

Cataracts also can affect the lens, impairing the general clarity of vision because of a loss of transparency in the crystalline lens. Incoming light tends to scatter inside the eye, causing glare problems.

### Vitreous Chamber

The vitreous chamber, the space behind the lens, is filled with a gelatinous substance.[17]

### Retina

The retina, located at the back of the eye, is the photosensitive layer that receives the pattern of light reflected from objects, similar to the film in a camera. Efferson's topography of the retina[6] (Figure 16-5) includes the optic disk, where the optic nerve exits and arteries and veins emerge. The optic disk also is called the *blind spot*, because it contains no photoreceptor cells. The macula is temporal to the optic disk and contains the fovea, which is essential for central vision. The surrounding retina is vital for peripheral vision and defines a 180-degree half sphere.[6,17]

## NEURONAL PROCESSING: VISUAL PATHWAYS

### Retina

According to Kelly,[15] the visual fields are "the way in which the visual world is projected onto the retina."[1] The

left and right hemivisual fields project to the temporal and nasal hemiretinal fields. Figure 16-6 shows the visual pathways.[1] Based on the work of Mason and Kandel,[16] the visual field is the view seen by the two eyes without movement of the head. If the foveae of both eyes are fixed on a single point in space, a left and right half of the visual field can be defined. The left half of the visual field projects on the nasal retina of the left eye and the temporal retina of the right eye. The right field projects on the nasal retina of the right eye and the temporal retina of the left eye. Light originating in the center of the visual field enters both eyes; this area is called the *binocular zone*. In either half of the visual field a monocular zone also may be defined: light from the temporal portion of the hemifield projects only onto the nasal hemiretina of the eye on the same side because the nose blocks light from reaching the opposite eye (Figure 16-7).[16] This monocular portion of the visual field also is called the *temporal crescent* because it constitutes the crescent-shaped temporal extreme of each visual field. Because no binocular overlap occurs in this region, vision is lost in the entire temporal crescent if this region of the retina is damaged severely. Árnadóttir[1] explains that fibers from the retina form the optic nerves on each side. The optic nerves meet in the optic chiasma, where fibers from the nasal hemiretina cross to the opposite side. The optic tract is continuous with the optic chiasma and carries fibers from the ipsilateral temporal hemiretina (the inner visual field) and contralateral nasal hemiretina (the outer visual field) (see Figure 16-6). The optic tract on each side projects to the lateral geniculate body of the thalamus. The optic radiation then carries visual information from the lateral geniculate body to the calcarine cortex in the occipital lobe. During the radiation, the fibers fan out from the upper part of the bundle carrying information from the lower visual field that runs posteriorly in the parietal lobe. The lower part of the bundle, with information from the upper visual field, loops around the temporal

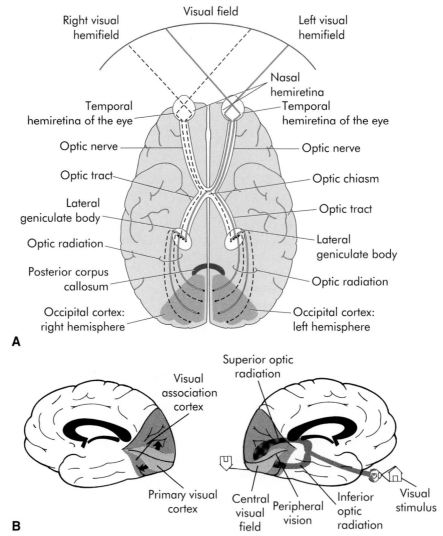

**Figure 16-6**    The visual pathways. **A,** Inferior view depicting flow of information from the visual fields to the visual cortex (visual fields = 180 degrees). **B,** Medial view of components of the visual cortex and visual processing. (**B** from Árnadóttir G: *The brain and behavior: assessing cortical dysfunction through activities of daily living,* St Louis, 1990, Mosby.)

horn of the ventricles in the temporal lobe on its way to the visual cortex. A stimulus in the superior visual field is projected to the inferior retina, resulting in an inverted image (see Figure 16-7).[1,16] Because of this inversion, information from the superior visual field is carried by the inferior optic radiation. The inverted image then is carried to the cortex. In the primary visual cortex around the calcarine fissure (Brodmann's area 17), the occipital pole is essential in vision from the central or middle visual field, whereas peripheral vision is facilitated by a more anterior part of the medial occipital cortex. The association areas (Brodmann's areas 18 and 19) receive information from the primary visual cortex. They integrate this information with previous experiences and information from other sensory modalities and form visual memory

traces.[12] The different processes can occur at the same time, a phenomenon termed *parallel processing*.[1,4,11]

## Photoreceptors

Photoreceptors on the retina convert light energy falling on them into electrical impulses that the brain can analyze. Cohen and Fox[4] state that the photoreceptor layer includes two classes of photoreceptors: rods and cones. Efferson[6] explains that the cone or rod shape is the dendrite of the cell. Variations in shape and slight variations in pigment give each cell different sensitivities. The rod cell has greater sensitivity to dim light but less sensitivity to color. The cone cell has greater sensitivity to color and high-intensity light but less to reduced-light conditions. The greatest concentration of cone cells occurs in the

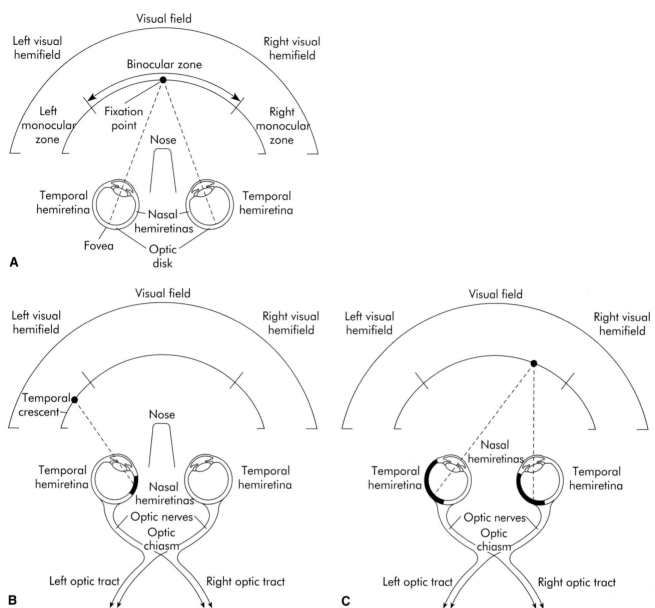

**Figure 16-7**  The visual field has binocular and monocular zones. **A,** Light from the binocular zone strikes both eyes, whereas light from the monocular zone strikes only the eye on the same side. The hemiretinas are defined with respect to the fovea, the region in the center of the retina with the highest acuity. The optic disk, the region where the ganglion cell axons leave the retina, is free of photoreceptors and therefore creates a gap, or blind spot, in the visual field for each eye. **B,** Light from a monocular zone (temporal crescent) falls only on the ipsilateral nasal hemiretina and does not project on the contralateral retina because it is blocked by the nose. **C,** Each optic tract carries a complete representation of one half of the binocular zone in the visual field. Fibers from the nasal hemiretina of each eye cross to the opposite side at the optic chiasm, whereas fibers from the temporal hemiretina do not cross. In the illustration, light from the right half of the binocular zone falls on the left temporal hemiretina and right nasal hemiretina. Axons from these hemiretinas thus contain a complete representation of the right hemifield of vision. (From Mason C, Kandel ER: Central visual pathways. In Kanel ER, Schwartz TH, Tessel TM, editors: *Principles of neural science*, ed 3, Norwalk, Conn, 1991, Appleton & Lange.)

fovea and macula; the concentration of cone cells decreases and the concentration of rod cells increases with increased distance from the macula.

Efferson[6] describes the phenomenon responsible for the high degree of neural representation in the foveal region that accounts for the tremendous conscious awareness of the central view, called *convergence*. The degree of convergence is greatest at the periphery of the retina; many photoreceptor cells synapse on each ganglion cell. This accounts for poor acuity but high light sensitivity. The closer to the macula, the smaller the degree of convergence; at the fovea, no convergence occurs. One photoreceptor cell synapses with one bipolar cell and one ganglion cell. The visual pathway begins a three-neuron chain exiting through the optic nerve; this chain consists of rods and cones synapsing with bipolar and ganglion cells. This one-to-one correspondence between photoreceptor and ganglion cells in the fovea means that a significant degree of neural representation of the foveal image occurs in the brain. This representation accounts for the individual's primary awareness of objects in the foveal field and secondary awareness of objects in the peripheral field. Conscious visual awareness of the environment is influenced primarily by objects in the foveal field. However, continuous information about the environment is flowing through the peripheral retina, usually subconsciously. Attention quickly shifts from foveal to nonfoveal stimulation if changes in light intensity and rapid movement occur. For example, an individual who is reading is using the fovea. If a familiar person enters the room, the peripheral field becomes stimulated and the individual becomes aware of the other person's presence, clothing, and ambulation pattern.

### Five Neuronal Control Systems

Five separate movement systems maintain the fovea on a target, and each of these systems shares the same effector pathway, that is, the three bilateral groups of ocular motor neurons in the brainstem, according to Goldberg, Eggers, and Gouras.[11] These systems include the following:

- Vestibuloocular movement uses vestibular input to hold images stably on the retina during brief or rapid head rotation. This movement stabilizes the eye as the head moves.
- Optokinetic movements use visual input to hold images stably on the retina during sustained or slow head rotation. These eye movements are used while driving a car and reading street signs, recognizing persons while walking down a hall, and window shopping.
- Saccadic eye movements keep the fovea on a visual target by keeping objects of interest on the fovea; these movements help the eye shift rapidly from target to target.[11] Saccadic movements resemble the quick phase of vestibular nystagmus. Accurate saccadic eye move-

ments also can occur in response to sounds, tactile stimuli, memories of locations in space, and even verbal commands (e.g., look left).

- Smooth pursuit movements hold the image of a moving target on the fovea. The smooth pursuit system moves the eyes in space to keep a single target on the fovea by calculating the speed at which the target is moving and then moving the eyes accordingly. Smooth pursuit requires the individual to attend to an object and voluntarily pursue it, unlike optokinetic movements, which are involuntary.
- Vergence movements move the eyes in opposite directions so that the image is positioned on both foveae. When a person views a moving object, each eye moves differently to keep the image of the object aligned precisely on each fovea. If the object moves closer, the eyes must converge. If the object moves away, the eyes diverge.[11]

### Eye Movement System

Six muscles attach to each eye: the superior rectus, inferior rectus, medial rectus, lateral rectus, superior oblique, and inferior oblique. The recti originate at the apex of the orbit and insert on the sclera (the outer coat of the eyeball) anterior to the equator of the eye. The obliques approach the eye from the anteromedial aspect and insert posterior to the equator (Figure 16-8).[11]

The medial rectus adducts and rotates the eyes inward, whereas the lateral rectus abducts and rotates the eyes outward. The superior rectus uses elevation and intorsion to move the eyes upward; it is assisted by the inferior rectus, which uses depression and extorsion to move the eyes downward. The superior oblique uses depression and intorsion to rotate the eye downward and outward, whereas the inferior oblique uses elevation and extorsion to rotate the eye upward and outward.[6-8]

In coordinated eye movement, a muscle of one eye is paired with a muscle of the opposite eye to produce movement in the six cardinal directions of gaze. These paired primary muscles are termed *yoke muscles*. In any conjugate movement (both eyes moving the same amount in the same direction), the yoke muscles receive equal innervation.[28] To follow a moving target upward and to the left, the left eye moves upward and away from the nose and the right eye moves upward and toward the nose. This demonstrates that each pair of muscles in one eye has a functional complement in the other orbit that can rotate the eye in the same place but in the opposite direction.[11]

Extraocular muscles are innervated by three groups of motor neurons the cell bodies of which form nuclei in the brainstem. The lateral rectus is innervated by the motor neurons of the nervus abducens (cranial nerve VI) in the pons. The medial inferior and superior recti and the inferior oblique muscles are innervated by the ocular motor

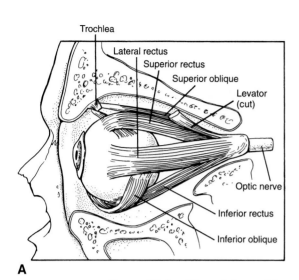
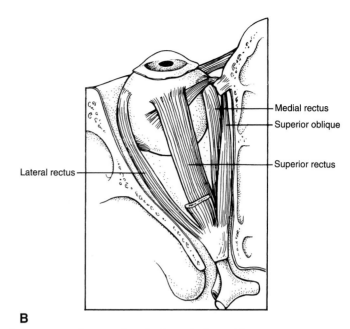

**Figure 16-8** The origins and insertions of the extraocular muscles. **A,** Lateral view with orbital wall cut away. The recti insert in front of the equator of the globe, and contraction rotates the cornea toward the insertion. The obliques insert behind the equator, and contraction rotates the cornea away from the insertion. The superior oblique muscle passes through a pulley of bone, the trochlea, before it inserts. **B,** Superior view with roof of orbit cut away. (From Goldberg ME, Eggers HM, Gouras P: Ocular motor system. In Kandell ER, Schwartz TH, Tessel TM, editors: *Principles of neural science,* ed 3, Norwalk, Conn, 1991, Appleton & Lange.)

neurons that form the nervus oculomotorius (cranial nerve III) in the midbrain. The superior oblique muscle is innervated by the nervus trochlearis (cranial nerve IV) in the midbrain. Cranial nerve III is located at the level of the superior colliculus, whereas cranial nerve IV is located at the level of the inferior colliculus; both are located in the midbrain.[7,11,26]

One should note the existence of the epicanthus, which is a fold of skin extending from the root of the nose to the median end of the eyebrow, covering the inner canthus (the angle at either end of the slit between the eyelids) and caruncle (the small fleshy growth). The epicanthus is a characteristic of certain races and may occur as an anomaly in white persons. This anatomic structure does not impair vision yet is similar to what an individual experiencing esotropia may present when visually screened during oculomotor performance.

## PATHOPHYSIOLOGY REGARDING CEREBROVASCULAR ACCIDENT

Individuals who sustain brain damage (cerebrovascular accident, traumatic head injury, tumor) often exhibit visual system dysfunctions that may occur within the primary visual pathway (sensory or motor), associative visual pathway (perceptual), or within both pathways.[2]

Dysfunction in the visual pathways leads to primary visual deficits, including decreases in near and distant acuity; accommodation; visual fields; oculomotor range of motion; convergence; quality of saccadic, pursuit, fixation, and functional scanning; color perception; stereopsis; symptoms of central blindness; and strabismus.[2,26] At times the terminology may be confusing. Bouska, Kauffman, and Marcus[3] refer to the aforementioned skills as *primary visual skills,* Hellerstein and Fishman[13] refer to them as the *basic processing level,* Warren[29] describes them as the *lower level skills* in her hierarchic framework, and Scheiman[22] calls them *visual information processing skills.* Whatever the term, they are the most basic and functional visual skills necessary for the development and management of all visual perception and visual motor activities, and they must be intact for a person to receive, process, interpret, and respond appropriately to input from the environment (Table 16-1).

Occupational therapists must be aware of the primary functional visual skills and the ways deficits in one or more of these areas affect the quality of life of patients with whom they work. A comprehensive understanding of the visual system is necessary because the occupational therapist is often in the best position to observe functional vision problems, administer visual screening appraisals, and observe functional skills. The functional

**Table 16-1**

**Visual Skills and Their Associated Functions and Resulting Dysfunctions after Cerebrovascular Accident**

| VISUAL SKILL | VISUAL FUNCTION | VISUAL AND PERCEPTUAL DYSFUNCTIONS |
|---|---|---|
| Visual acuity | Clarity of vision at near point and distance; 20/20 refraction | Vision blurred in one or both eyes consistently or inconsistently; visual fatigue; task incompletion |
| Accommodation | Process of focusing whereby the lens changes curvature so that various viewing distances remain clear | Blurred vision; inattention; poor concentration; eyestrain; visual fatigue |
| Visual fields | The peripheral area of vision up, down, in, and out when both eyes are positioned straight forward | Inability to read or starting to read in the middle of the page; ignoring of food on one half of the plate; difficulty orienting to stimuli in specific areas of space |
| Oculomotor range of motion; fixation; saccades and pursuits | Ability of both eyes to move within the six cardinal positions of gaze (right, left, inferior, superior, inferior oblique, superior oblique); maintenance of gaze for 10 seconds; small precise eye jumps; following a moving stimulus | Excessive head movement; frequent loss of place; skipping of lines; poor attention span; slow copying; difficulty when driving, reading, writing; difficulty tracking in all planes |
| Vergence | The ability to bring the eyes together smoothly and automatically along the midline to observe objects singly at near distance (convergence) or to move the eyes outward for single vision of distant objects (divergence) | Difficulty focusing; decreased depth perception; difficulty and confusion in interpreting space; decreased eye-hand coordination in self-care and hygiene; difficulty in driving, sports, communication, and ambulation |
| Strabismus | Deviation of one eye or one eye at a time from the object of regard, where the eye not in use is turned | Esotropia (inward turn); exotropia (outward turn); hyperopia (upward turn); hypopia (downward turn); double vision or suppression; decreased eye-hand coordination during mobility tasks; overreaching or underreaching; difficulty with reading and near tasks |
| Functional scanning | Ability to read or write from left to right precisely and smoothly without errors | Omitting letters, words, numbers; losing place when returning to next line; exaggerated head movement; using finger as pointer; abnormal working distance |
| Color perception | Ability to perceive colors | Muddy or impure color; color may fade out; difficulty finding items by color |
| Stereopsis | Depth perception and its relationship to spatial judgment | Problematic binocular system; deficits in three-dimensional perception; decreased spatial judgment especially in fine motor areas |

optometrist is the most qualified professional to assess and rehabilitate visual efficiency and the visual perceptual system. Vision, the dominant sense for gathering information, should be evaluated by a functional optometrist who has extensive experience in vision rehabilitation and functional vision care. Consultation with a functional optometrist by the rehabilitation team is crucial so that all health care providers have a good understanding of the patient's visual deficits and functional results. The team then can establish treatment strategies using a multidisciplinary approach. Improved visual processing often helps speed progress in other rehabilitative areas, including occupational therapy, speech therapy, therapeutic recreation, and physical therapy.[13]

**Functional Visual Skills**

The following sections describe primary functional visual skills; Table 16-1 lists the skill, function, and dysfunction associated with each.

*Visual Acuity.* Clarity of vision, or visual acuity, is essential in each eye at near and far points.[8] Near vision acuity is the ability to see, inspect, identify, and understand objects clearly at near distances, within an arm's length. Distance acuity is the ability to see, inspect, identify, and understand objects clearly at a distance.[18] Refraction is the process used to evaluate the optical system of the eye. Refraction is used to determine whether an individual suffers from myopia (nearsightedness), hyperopia (farsightedness), and/or astigmatism (the lens is not spherical but oval and causes light rays to focus at two different points). Refraction also is used to determine whether an individual will benefit from glasses and the appropriate prescription.[8,21] If visual acuity is decreased for near or distance tasks, vision is blurry and visual fatigue or eyestrain may be present. Corrective lenses focus the angle of light through the lens so the angle of reflection of the light on the retina is equal to the refraction, and the environment is focused. The therapist must be aware that changes in the individual's visual acuity occur often. Therefore the lens prescription that was correct before the incident more than likely has changed and vision has become worse. Adding to this deficit may be the inability of patients to express verbally that they cannot see clearly. Evaluation of the lense prescription by the optometric or ophthalmologic team is imperative.

Another important determination is whether the individual is suffering from low vision, other visual deficits that follow, or low vision with a complexity of visual deficits. Not all patients benefit from low-vision devices. Magnifiers, darker backgrounds, and greater illumination help only so much. The therapist must be aware of the other visual deficits that have occurred and treat them accordingly. Treating visual deficits is much more than treating low-vision issues.

*Accommodation.* Accommodation is the ability to change the focus of the eye to see objects at different distances clearly.[18] The normal human visual system is physiologically focused for objects at distances of 20 feet and greater. If an object is brought closer than 20 feet, the eye must make a focusing adjustment or the object appears blurred. The accommodative system of the human eye works so well that most people are totally unaware that they even have a focusing system.[22] When an individual reads the mail and then looks up at the clock on the wall to determine the time, that person uses the accommodative system. If accommodative disorders are diagnosed, one or more of the following may be present: discomfort and eyestrain for all visual tasks, blurred vision, inattention during occupational therapy sessions, poor concentration, visual fatigue, rubbing of the eyes, or difficulty with activities of daily living that require sustained close work.

*Visual Fields.* The visual fields extend approximately 65 degrees upward, 75 degrees downward, 60 degrees inward, and 95 degrees outward when the eye is in the straight forward position. The total field of vision is approximately 180 degrees.[17] Visual fields are essential areas of the visual system that allow the individual to orient effectively to stimuli in specific areas of space. One uses visual fields when driving, walking, reading, and eating and in all daily living skills. Inferior field loss causes

difficulty with mobility, including poor balance, tendency to trail behind others when walking, walking next to walls and touching them for balance, trouble seeing steps or curbs, shortened and uncertain stride while walking, and trouble identifying visual landmarks. Superior field deficit causes difficulty in seeing signs, reading and writing; misreading of words, poor accuracy, slow reading rate, inability to follow lines of text, and inaccurate check writing are additional difficulties.[1,9,21]

*Oculomotor Range of Motion.* Oculomotor range of motion is the ability to move the eyes in the six cardinal positions of gaze (right, left, inferior, superior, superior oblique, inferior oblique) using smooth and even motion without stress. For the eyes to move within these quadrants, three areas must be intact: fixation/stability, saccadic function, and pursuit function. Fixation is the ability to locate and inspect a series of stationary objects with both eyes quickly and accurately. Most individuals are able to sustain precise fixation with no observable movement of the eyes for 10 seconds.[21] Saccadic functions include eye movements enabling the individual to redirect the line of sight rapidly so that the point of interest stimulates the fovea. Saccadic function consists of a jump from one fixation point to the next with a slight pause to process the information (as in reading). Pursuit function is the ability to follow a moving object such as a ball in flight or moving vehicle in traffic smoothly and accurately with both eyes. Difficulty with fixation results in off-task behavior and may give the impression that the person is inattentive or impulsive. Saccadic dysfunction usually manifests itself through undershooting of the target of interest; at times, overshooting of the target may be observed. Pursuit dysfunction is a condition in which the individual is unable to follow a moving target accurately. Pursuit problems play a significant role in activities of daily living such as driving and sports and any other activities in which the individual or the object of regard is moving.[28]

*Vergence.* Vergence includes convergence and divergence. Vergence is the ability to bring the eyes together smoothly and automatically to observe objects singly at near distance (convergence), or to move the eyes outward for single vision of distant objects (divergence). Vergence is associated reflexively with accommodation and divergence with relaxation of accommodation. The function of this reflex is to allow near or far objects to be single and clear. Problems in vergence can occur if the eye movement system is out of coordination with accommodation or damage to cranial nerves III, IV, or VI has occurred. Problems can be slight, with merely a tendency for the eyes to converge in or out too far, or they can be greater in magnitude. Tendencies to underconverge or overconverge are called *phorias* and are not visible to the observer. Some phorias may worsen to the extent that binocularity (the ability of both eyes to act as a single unit to obtain a three-dimensional scene viewed with depth and meaning) breaks down, at which point the individual displays strabismus. Vergence ability is needed for singular binocular vision and is basic to all activities. At near distances an individual may have difficulty finding objects; eye-hand coordination may be decreased, affecting self-care and hygiene tasks; and reading may be difficult. Distance tasks that may be affected include driving, sports, movies, communication, wheelchair mobility, and ambulation.[6]

*Strabismus.* Strabismus, or tropia, is a visible turn of one eye that may be constant, intermittent, or alternating between eyes. Strabismus may result in double vision; long-term strabismus may suppress or turn off the vision in the wandering eye.[6] Suppression is a neurologic function that is an adaptation to the intolerable situation of double images. Suppression is exhibited only in long-term strabismus because apparently the brain cannot learn to suppress past the time of peak plasticity (until approximately 7 years).

The developing brain must choose which eye has the visual direction by using motor and tactile inputs. The other foveal image then is suppressed neurologically. The peripheral vision in the suppressing eye is still normal, and the eye is not by any means blind.[6,24] In strabismus one eye may turn outward (exotropia), inward (esotropia), upward (hypertropia), or downward (hypotropia). These are the most common forms of strabismus. Strabismus may be intermittent, occurring occasionally and alternating switching use to the right or left eye or suppressing just the right eye or left eye. Strabismus may be constant (the same eye is always in or out) or comitant (the amount of turn is always the same regardless of whether the person is looking up, down, right, left, or straight ahead). Newly acquired strabismus (from stroke or head injury) is usually noncomitant; eye turn changes depend on the direction in which the eyes are looking. Any strabismic disorder may result in an inability to judge distance, underreaching or overreaching for objects, covering or closure of one eye, double vision, head tilt or turn, "spaced out" appearance, difficulty reading, and avoidance of near tasks. Strabismus may also affect posture and the patient's perception of position in space.

*Functional Scanning.* Functional scanning refers to the ability to scan a page of print from left to right without skipping letters, words, or lines. A person should be able to scan with precise and smooth eye saccades. Functional scanning also relates to writing tasks and the ability to maintain print appropriately on each line. Problems with functional scanning result in poor speed and numerous errors, losing of place on a line of print, incorrect stating of letters or words while reading, inability to read or write from left to right, skipping around the page, and using the finger as a pointer.[2]

*Color Perception.* Color perception may be impaired in individuals who experience right hemisphere or bilateral lesions.[24] This symptom is different from color agnosia in which the patient is unable to name colors correctly as a result of an inability to interpret sensory information. Individuals with defective color perception may see colors as "muddy" or "impure" in hue, or the color of a small target may fade into the background, decreasing the ability to differentiate it from the background. Total loss of ability to discern color (achromatopsia) is rare but can occur.[3]

*Stereopsis and Depth Perception.* Stereopsis is binocular visual perception of three-dimensional space or depth. Depth perception is used during all activities involving spatial judgments, in particular fine motor and eye-hand coordination tasks in which judgment of relative depth is required (threading a needle, placing toothpaste on a toothbrush, hammering). Walking over curbs and up and down stairs requires depth perception.

## Corneal Diseases

As previously stated, corneal diseases and abrasions usually have occurred before CVA and not because of it. The Boston Scleral Lens currently exists, invented by The Boston Foundation for Sight founder Dr. Perry Rosenthal. This lens allows the cornea to breathe while covered by the lens. The lens rests on the sclera and creates a space over the cornea that is filled with artificial tears. By filling the surface irregularities of the cornea to restore vision, protecting it from exposure to air and the rubbing effect of blinking, and providing a reservoir of oxygen that allows the eye to heal, this cushion of fluid is responsible for restoring vision. The lens received Food and Drug Administration approval in 1994 and has achieved an 80% success rate in more than 300 patients.[19,20]

*Cortical Blindness.* Cortical blindness refers to a significant decrease in visual acuity with severe blurring that is uncorrectable by lenses. Such blindness can be a total or almost total loss of vision resulting from bilateral cerebral destruction of the visual projection cortex (area 17). Deficits include blurred vision and decrease in acuity.

## Age-Related Changes

Although CVAs affect many age groups, a much higher incidence occurs among elderly persons. The most common condition affecting the vision of elderly persons is cataracts. General clarity of vision is impaired because of a loss of transparency of the crystalline lens of the eye. The lens slowly loses its ability to prevent oxidation, and liquidation of the outer layer begins. The normally soluble proteins adhere, causing light to scatter; vision slowly declines.[6,7]

Age-related macular degeneration is the leading cause of blindness in the Western world. Loss of central vision occurs from fluid that leaks from the deeper layers of the retina, pushing the retina up and detaching it from the nourishing layer. New vessel growth, hemorrhage, and atrophy further destroy central vision. All near-point activities of daily living (reading, sewing, cooking) are affected, and safety is compromised.[6]

In arteriosclerosis, vision may or may not be affected. Hardening of the retinal arteries may occur, eventually leading to ischemia in the areas of the retina dying from oxygen deprivation. Hypertension usually is accompanied by arteriosclerosis. Retinal bleeding and edema may occur, which can affect central vision if the macula is involved.

Diabetes can affect the lens. In the "sugar cataract," sorbitol collects within the lens, causing an osmotic gradient of fluid into the lens, which leads to disruption of the lens matrix and loss of transparency. As the fluid increases and decreases within the lens, the person's vision also fluctuates, depending on the sugar level. Retinal effects include microvascular damage and microaneurysms. Retinal ischemia may reduce central vision. Ischemia leads to the growth of new vessels that are weak and frequently leak and cause hemorrhage. The hemorrhage attracts fibrotic development, which puts traction on the retina, pulling it off and leading to retinal detachment and blindness.[6] (Laser treatment may prevent retinal detachment.)

Glaucoma is caused by an increase in intraocular pressure. This pressure interferes with the flow of blood and nutrients at the optic disk. Severe glaucoma can cause field loss and eventually complete blindness.

Ptosis is a dropping or drooping of the upper eyelid from paralysis. Ptosis should not be confused with blepharoptosis, which is a drooping of the upper eyelid because of aging and is usually genetic. However, both conditions interfere with the ability to see, and both cause visual fatigue. Blepharoptosis can be corrected with surgery, with restored vision.

The occupational therapist should obtain the patient's visual history. Visual impairments may have existed previously and may not be a result of a stroke; however, previous impairments may have a greater impact with newly acquired deficits.

## EVALUATION: VISION SCREENING

Much discussion currently is taking place regarding visual acuity and whether occupational therapists should screen for it. As long as the therapist has a comprehensive understanding of vision and the correct administration of screening procedures, the therapist can perform screening. However, all the visual assessment tools used by occupational therapists are used for screening only. One must address visual acuity skills before making any other visual determination. The therapist then refers the patient being screened for a comprehensive visual evaluation by an experienced functional optometrist. When screening for visual acuity, Snellen's chart generally is used. This is the chart seen in optometrists' and ophthalmologists' offices. These professionals are trained extensively in this area. By no means does the author suggest that occupational therapists are as capable in a procedure such as this. However, this screening acts as a baseline and should be given and discussed with either of the previously mentioned optometric professionals within or outside the facility, as the case may be, again stressing the importance of collaboration in both professions.

The following is a comprehensive list of screening procedures that therapists can use within the facility. The visual screening should not be time consuming. As the therapist becomes familiar with the screening and patient responses, the screening techniques will be easier to complete.

Numerous visual screening assessments currently on the market have the occupational therapist in mind. Some state the word "pediatric" but are appropriate for adults, since the procedures are exactly the same and only the treatment varies. Some screening assessments include the following:

- *Understanding Vision Deficits: A Guide for Occupational Therapists* by Mitchell Scheiman, OD
- *The Aspects of Functional Vision and Screening* by Raquel M. de Benabib, MS (video and booklets)
- *The Visual Skills Appraisal* by Regina Edwards, MA
- *The Brain Injury Assessment Battery for Adults* (biVaBa) by Mary Warren, MS, OTR

Before screening, the head, neck, trunk, and pelvis should be aligned appropriately to the midline orientation. If the patient being screened wears glasses, they should be used during the screening. If the patient states that the glasses do not improve vision, or if the patient is unable to verify improved vision, the screening should be performed initially with glasses on and then with glasses off.

The occupational therapist should observe the patient during screening. The therapist should note the head position, eye alignment, eye-head dissociation, presence of excessive head movement, and the use of the upper extremities to stabilize the head (i.e., hand under chin).

The following is a description of vision screening processes, which should be administered in a well-illuminated room free of glare and reflection[3,6,23]:

1. Distance Visual Acuity
*Equipment:* Distance acuity chart (Snellen's chart), occluder or eye patch, and 20-foot measure
*Setup:* Fixate distance acuity chart on a well-lighted wall at patient's eye level 20 feet away.

*Procedure:* Cover the patient's left eye with occluder or patch. Ask the patient to identify letters on the 20/40 line. If the patient appears confused by the lines and letters, cover all other lines on the chart and expose only the line being used. If necessary, expose only one letter at a time. If the patient continues to have problems, attempt to test visual acuity using the Lea Symbols Test.[31] Continue until the individual misses more than 50% of the letters on a line. Cover the patient's right eye with occluder or patch and repeat the steps. Record acuity as last line in which the individual can identify successfully more than 50% of the letters.

*Functional implications:* If visual acuity is poorer than 20/40 or if a two-line difference or more is evident between the two eyes, a referral is necessary and corrective lenses may need to be prescribed.[31]

2. Ocular Mobility

*Equipment:* Penlight

*Setup:* Have patient sit facing therapist. Penlight should be approximately 12 inches from the eyes. Do not shine the light directly into the eyes; instead direct the light so that it is pointing slightly above eye level at the brow.

*Procedure:* Ask the patient to follow the penlight and move it in a large H pattern to the extremes of gaze. Then move the penlight in a large O pattern. Allow the patient to fixate on the light for 10 seconds before moving it.

*Functional implications:* Observation of pursuits should be smooth and precise without anticipating responses. Note visual fatigue or stress and whether the patient reports diplopia (double vision). Observe whether the patient looks away, loses the target, or squints or blinks excessively. The patient may display inability to attend to visual tasks, difficulty reading or completing writing tasks, and problems with spatial orientation during walking.[15]

3. Near Point of Convergence

*Equipment:* Penlight and ruler

*Setup:* Practice this procedure on a partner to determine when the penlight is positioned at 2, 4, and 6 inches from an individual's eyes.

*Procedure:* Slowly move the penlight toward the patient at eye level and between the eyes, making sure not to shine the light in the eyes. Ask the patient to keep the eyes on the light and state when two lights are seen. After this occurs, move the light another inch or two closer and then begin to move it away from the patient. Ask the patient to state when one light only is seen. Watch the eyes carefully and observe whether they stop working together as a team; one eye may drift outward. Record the distance at which the patient reports double vision and the recovery to single vision.

*Functional implications:* Double vision should occur within 2 to 4 inches of the eyes. A recovery to single vision should occur within 4 to 6 inches. A patient with a binocular vision problem may not report double vision because the eye that turns out is suppressed. Thus all eye movements should be observed before screening.

4. Stereopsis

*Equipment:* Viewer-free random dot test

*Setup:* Individual's head position should be vertical. If any head tilt occurs, it negates this screening.

*Procedure:* Hold the viewer-free random dot test 16 inches from the patient's eyes and ask the patient to describe what is seen. A patient with stereopsis should report seeing a square box in the upper left, an E on the upper right, a circle on the lower left, and a blank box on the lower right. Give the patient about 20 to 30 seconds to observe the targets. If the patient has difficulty, try tilting the target slightly to the left or right.

*Functional implications:* The patient should be able to identify all three symbols correctly. A patient with constant strabismus is unable to identify any of the shapes. Patients with less severe strabismus or phoria may have normal responses. Some patients may report double vision on this task, which suggests that strabismus is present.

5. Accommodation

*Equipment:* Isolated letters and occluder or eye patch

*Setup:* Make a target by photocopying the near visual acuity chart, cutting out the 20/30 targets, and taping them to a tongue depressor. Place one target on each side of the tongue depressor so as to make two screening targets.

*Procedure:* Patch the left eye. Hold the tongue depressor with the 20/30 target about 1 inch in front of the right eye. The patient should be unable to identify the stimulus on the tongue depressor at this distance. Slowly move the target away and ask the patient to report as soon as the target is identifiable. Using a ruler, measure and record the distance at which the patient is able to identify the stimulus. Divide 40 by the measurement to determine the amplitude of accommodation. If the patient is able to identify the target at 8 inches, divide 40 by 8, which equals 5 D. To compare the patient's amplitude of accommodation to the expected amplitude for the patient's age, use the following formula: expected amplitude = 18 − one third of the patient's age.[21] The following are examples of the way to use this equation:

A 9-year-old child: Expected amplitude = 18 − ($\frac{1}{3}$ × 9)
Expected amplitude = 18 − 3 = 15 D

A 45-year-old adult: Expected amplitude = 18 − ($\frac{1}{3}$ × 45)
Expected amplitude = 18 − 15 = 3 D

*Functional implications:* The amplitude of accommodation should be 2 D of the expected finding for the patient to pass the screening test. Observe all eye movements. Problems include blurred vision, poor concentration, inattention, visual fatigue, and eyestrain.

6. Saccades

*Equipment:* Two fixators with red and green targets and scanning chart

*Setup:* Have the patient keep the head erect and vertical.

*Procedure:* Hold two tongue depressors (one with a red target and one with a green target) 16 inches from the patient's face and about 4 inches from the midline. Give the patient the following instructions: "When I say red, look at the red target. When I say green, look at the green target. Do not look until I tell you." Have the patient look from one target to the other five round trips or a total of 10 fixations. Determine whether the patient can maintain attention to complete five round trips (ability). Score 1 to 5. Observe accuracy using one eye movement or multiple eye movements. Score 1 to 5. Observe head and body movement and assign a score of 1 to 5.

*Functional implications:* Adults without visual impairment should receive a perfect score.[3] Any score less than that denotes problems with saccadic function; the patient requires further evaluation. Poor saccades result in poor concentration and attention and difficulty reading and writing.

7. Visual Field

*Equipment:* Occluder or eye patch, black dowels with white pins on the ends or a wiggling finger

*Setup:* Make sure the patient is seated facing the examiner.

*Procedure:*

1. One-examiner presentation: The patient holds the occluder over the left eye. The therapist wiggles a finger out to the side and asks the patient to say "now" on first detecting the movement of the wiggling finger. The patient should look at the therapist's nose the entire time and ignore any arm movement. Begin with the hand slightly behind the patient about 16 inches away from the head. Slowly bring the hand forward while wiggling a finger. Continue randomly testing different sections of the visual field in 45-degree intervals around the visual field. Proceed to the left eye, asking the patient to occlude the right eye. If using the dowel technique, slowly bring the dowel in from the side until the patient reports seeing the small pin at the end of the dowel.

2. Two-examiner presentation: Examiner 1 stands behind the seated patient and examiner 2 sits facing the patient about 30 inches in front so that the face of the examiner and patient are at the same level.[10] Test each eye individually, being careful to patch the other eye. Examiner 2 closes one eye and instructs the patient to "fixate and keep looking at my open eye. Examiner 1 will be showing you one or more fingers very quickly. Don't try to look at the fingers. Keep looking at my open eye and when you see a finger or fingers, tell me how many you see."[10] Examiner 1 presents one or two fingers randomly for a 1-second duration to each quadrant of the visual field of the patient's unpatched eye. The fingers in the upper quadrant point down, and those in the lower quadrant point up. The fingers are presented 18 inches from the patient and at approximately 20 degrees from the line of fixation.[10]

3. Two-examiner left-right field simultaneous presentation: No patch is used during this screening. The patient looks at examiner 1 while examiner 2 stimulates both hemifields simultaneously. This screening looks for visuospatial hemiimperception, which usually is referred to as *extinction, hemiinattention,* or *unilateral spatial neglect.* When both hemifields are stimulated simultaneously, all or part of one hemifield is less responsive to stimulation; the patient responds to single stimuli and not to the affected side when both sides are stimulated.[10]

*Functional implications:* Visual field impairments have significant implications for the safe performance of many functional activities, including driving and mobility. Visually guided movement through space becomes impaired, as does efficient eye movement. Reading and near activities can be affected if central field loss is present.[6] Persons with visuospatial hemiimperception leave out parts of the text when reading or fail to perceive traffic to the left when driving or crossing the street.[10]

NOTE: These confrontation fields are considered a gross test as compared with a visual field perimeter test. Many patients cannot perform the perimeter test because it requires a higher cognitive level. These tests usually are not performed by occupational therapists. Observations are important and give the occupational therapist much information about the way in which patients move about the environment and the way they move their bodies and use spatial orientation.[6]

## VISUAL PERCEPTUAL EVALUATIONS

Tsurumi and Todd[27] state that much of the research on visual perception evaluation has been done using representations rather than real objects and real space. Visual perception testing uses two-dimensional representations of inverted forms as the stimulus material. The authors suggest that these two-dimensional figures, although useful measures of certain cognitive analysis skills, should not be correlated with the ability to perceive the three-dimensional world of objects and space.

Occupational therapists obtain more helpful information using more functional assessments. These assessments usually are in the form of checklists and observations of patients within the clinic or home setting.

### Hemianopsia

Hemianopsia is a visual field defect that results in loss of vision on the contralateral half of the visual field (Figure 16-9). The therapist can evaluate this defect

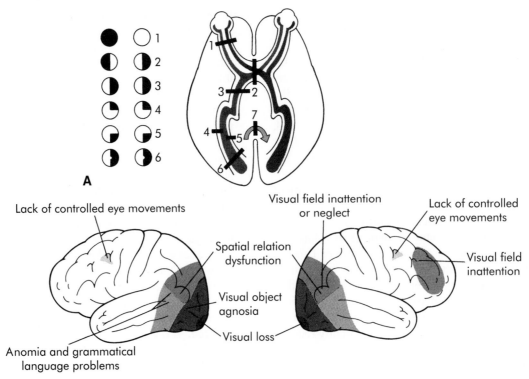

**Figure 16-9**    Visual processing deficits. **A,** The visual pathway viewed from the base of the brain (inferior view). The dark bars indicate lesions at different sites in the pathway. The numbers refer to visual-field disturbances according to location of the lesion: *1,* lesion of the optic nerve, leading to blindness in the corresponding eye; *2,* lesion of the optic chiasma, leading to bilateral temporal field defect; *3,* lesion of the optic tract, resulting in complete loss of visual field on the contralateral half of the visual field, or homonymous hemianopsia; *4,* lesion of the optic tract in the temporal lobe, resulting in loss of vision in the upper quadrant of the contralateral visual field in both eyes; *5,* lesion of the optic track in the parietal lobe, resulting in loss of vision in the lower quadrant of the contralateral visual field in both eyes; *6,* lesion in the occipital cortex, leading to visual loss in the contralateral visual hemifield with macular sparing; *7,* lesion in the posterior corpus callosum, resulting in a disrupted route, causing pure word blindness, or alexia without agraphia. **B,** Lesion sites that can produce visuospatial relation problems, or anomia and grammatical language problems related to spatial relations. Unilateral visual neglect is related to dysfunction of the inferior parietal lobe, cingulate gyrus, and dorsolateral frontal lobe, especially on the right side. (From Árnadóttir G: *The brain and behavior: assessing cortical dysfunction through activities of daily living,* St Louis, 1990, Mosby.)

using confrontation testing, as described previously. Patients with pure hemianopsias are aware of their visual losses and spontaneously learn to compensate by moving their eyes (foveae) toward their lost visual fields to expand their visual spaces to gather information right and left of midline.

## Unilateral Visual Inattention

Unilateral visual inattention is a condition in which a patient with normal sensory and motor systems fails to orient toward, respond to, or report stimuli on the side contralateral to the cerebral lesion. Efferson[6] states that this condition has been documented in patients who demonstrate no accompanying visual field defects or limb sensory or motor losses. The condition usually is not seen alone but is associated with accompanying sensory and motor defects such as hemianopsia, decreased tactile proprioceptive and stereognostic perception, and paresis or upper limb paralysis. LeDoux and Smylie[15a] report that inattention is a hemisphere defect. They described a patient shown bilateral hemispheric visual perceptual slides who made visuospatial errors in left space. The patient suffered from a right-sided lesion. When the same slides were directed only to the right visual field (left hemisphere), performance improved. Efferson hypothesized that the deficient hemisphere failed to receive or orient toward incoming information, whereas the intact receiving hemisphere remains oblivious and goes about its own business. Efferson suggests assessing using confrontation testing. If visual field loss is ruled out, then the stimuli should be applied using auditory, tactile, and visual modalities. The therapist should assess the patient's eyes, neck, head, and trunk position at rest and during activities. Persistent deviation toward the side of the lesion may indicate inattention. The therapist may rule out unilateral visual inattention if the patient is capable of tracking visual targets from ipsilateral to contralateral space, maintaining fixation, and fixating on visual targets right and left of midline on command. Slow searching or failure to search may be considered inattention. The therapist should note and carefully observe asymmetries in performance and during functional activities such as eating, filling out a form, reading, dressing, and maneuvering through the environment. The occupational therapist should note unawareness regarding doorways and hallways and turns made only in one direction (see Chapters 18 and 19).

Cancellation, crossing out, line bisection, and drawing and copying tasks may aid in indicating patient's impairment but may not result in information regarding how the impairment affects daily living tasks. Toglia[25] developed a unilateral inattention functional rating scale, including shaving both sides of the face, combing both sides of the hair, and eating from both sides of the tray.

### Cortical Blindness

A vision specialist or functional optometrist should assess cortical blindness and variations of it. Cortical blindness is a total or almost total loss of vision resulting from bilateral cerebral destruction of the visual projection cortex (area 17).

### Color Imperception

Color imperception may be measured by using Ishihara's color plates or color-sorting or color-matching tasks. Patients with defective color perception have difficulty with some visual perceptual tasks because contextual cues related to color and shading are unavailable to them.[6]

### Visual Agnosia

*Visual agnosia* is defined by Efferson[6] as a failure to recognize visual stimuli (objects, faces, letters) even though visual sensory processing, language, and general intellectual functions are preserved at sufficiently high levels. Three types of agnosia exist: visual, tactile, and auditory. Agnosia is tested by placing common objects in front of the patient and asking the patient to name them. Normal responses include the name of the item and its described or functional use. Abnormal responses are confabulatory and perseverative. The therapist must rule out anomia before evaluation. A person with visual agnosia is able to name the object if another sensory modality (e.g., tactile) is used to obtain information about the object.

### Spatial Relations

Spatial relations are discussed in Chapters 18 and 19 of this text but are mentioned here briefly. All visuospatial disabilities involve some problem with the apprehension of the spatial relationships between and within objects.[28] These problems include an inability to localize objects in space, estimate their size, and judge their distance and impaired memory for the location of objects and places. Further difficulties include the inability to trace a path or follow a route from one place to another and problems with reading and counting. Assessments to judge spatial relations include the following:

- Touching a number of targets in all parts of the visual field while fixating on a central point
- Determining which objects are closest and farthest in proximity to the patient
- Describing the position of objects in the patient's room from memory
- Describing a floor plan of the room arrangement in the patient's house

The therapist may assess reading and counting by asking the patient to read and observing performance and documenting errors. Pages of scanning materials (letters and numbers) often give additional information about spatial planning during reading. The therapist should control the size and density of the print.

## TREATMENT CONSIDERATIONS

Patients with visual field losses who are evaluated by a functional optometrist may be prescribed prism systems or yoked prisms to expand their viewing fields. They also may use oculomotor techniques emphasizing calisthenics, pursuit, saccades, and scanning techniques.

The occupational therapist should encourage the use of appropriate glasses or prisms during treatment sessions and use awareness techniques to help the patient understand the way visual defects interfere with various activities. The occupational therapist should emphasize conscious attention to detail while teaching organized scanning techniques for the deficient field. Increased speed and accuracy of eye movement during recognition tasks are essential aspects of therapy. Walking or another movement modality is necessary to integrate vision, movement, and perception. Planning routes verbally and visually assists the patient in thinking about and "going into" the deficit area. Use of markers when reading may be helpful. An L-shaped marker assists the patient in going over to that area before beginning to read each line.[10,12]

Treatment for unilateral visual inattention includes various techniques (see Chapter 19). Again, increasing the patient's cognitive awareness of inattention is a primary factor. The patient should be aware of the nature of the field loss and the way it affects vision. The patient with normal visual fields but with visual extinction should be treated the same as the patient with an actual field loss; the visual experience is similar. The therapist should provide performance examples in the environment to demonstrate the biased view.

The therapist should emphasize visual scanning and awareness of the way eye and eye-head movements may be used to compensate. Training then should continue to the next level in which larger and quicker pursuits and saccades are made with longer fixations into unattended space. Training may be accomplished with interesting targets held by the therapist (small colored lights, bright objects of interest to the patient, pictures of family or friends taped to pencils). Pursuit and tracking of the target from attended to unattended space should be stressed first. Use of saccades in unattended space comes next. Initially, eye-head movements are acceptable, but eventually eye movements should dissociate from head movements. The visual field remains the same if the head moves into the unattended space but the eyes remain on a target in the attended space. Daily right-left scanning should be done independently and move farther into the unattended space each day.[6,17,29]

As treatment progresses, increased awareness and scanning abilities should be incorporated in increasingly complex visual perceptual and visuomotor tasks. However, inattention often increases with task complexity; the therapist must monitor the patient and tasks carefully. Useful tasks for assessment include the following:

- Surveying a room repetitively
- Using scanning techniques to observe and name objects
- Moving toward and touching objects right and left of midline
- Assembling objects from pieces on the floor and table
- Completing an obstacle course
- Bringing a chart back to the therapist who left it on a counter

Scanning always should be stressed, especially during functional activities: dressing, shaving, and moving through the environment. The patient must learn to monitor the influence of inattention on functional performance and heed the admonition that "When something doesn't make sense, look into the unattended space and it usually will."[6] Using markers when reading, slowing the pace by reading aloud, and following text using a finger as a pointer are helpful adaptations.

Patients cannot feed or dress themselves unless they have been taught to scan and locate objects in the affected field. Computer use may be difficult, especially if the patient did not use one before the impairment. If the patient did use a computer before the impairment, the therapist should

screen and evaluate acuity and glare factors and scanning and pursuit abilities. Scanning and depth perception are not intact in patients wearing eye patches. Some patients may suffer from vestibular disorders and depend more on their visual skills to compensate for balance reactions (see Chapter 9).

Efferson[6] reports that no reliable studies are available regarding treatment of cortical blindness, color imperception, and visual agnosia. She instead presents the principles of Bouska, Kauffman, and Marcus.[3] If cortical blindness or simultanagnosia is suspected, the therapist must first attempt to increase the patient's knowledge of foveal and peripheral vision—where the patient is fixating. The therapist may use a small headlamp under subdued lighting to teach the patient to position the eyes in midline of the head. The therapist asks the patient to move the light (and thus the head and eyes) to locate fairly large, bright stimuli placed on a plain background. As acuity and localization skills improve, stimuli and background become smaller and more complex (e.g., from a box to a paper clip). The patient should point accurately to and manipulate targets after locating them with the light or keep the light on the target while moving the target with one hand. With color imperception, treatment should involve materials and tasks using sharp color contrasts with minimal detail and progress to less contrast (more hues) with more detail.[1]

The treatment of patients with agnosia should progress according to the abilities that return in spontaneous recovery from agnosia. Common objects should be used in treatment. Presentations should occur in front of the patient, not off to either side. Tactile input with or without visual input should be encouraged and can be used as a compensatory mechanisms; however, tactile input may not be helpful in every case.

Color and facial agnosia may be treated by continually drilling the patient regarding two or three personally important names or colors. The patient may be helped to pick out or memorize cues for associating names with faces.

Efferson points out that treatment for visuospatial deficits should follow basic developmental considerations and progress from simple to more complex tasks. (If the evaluation suggests disorders in body scheme, tactile or vestibular input, or right-left discrimination, these areas should be dealt with first.)

Patients who do not know their location in space must internalize spatial understanding before they can make judgments regarding the space around them. Gross motor spatial training should encourage movement in all planes wherever possible. Patients should look at or fixate on a target and move their bodies near it by rolling, crawling, using a wheelchair, or ambulating. Auditory stimuli should be used, including alternative sounds and playing music, and should be presented constantly to the patient. Patients should be able to state where the stimulus is, point to it, and move toward it. Vision should be occluded before movement activity but made available during movement. The next level after this training segment incorporates retrieving items from the occupational therapy kitchen. The therapist can ask the patient to retrieve items from "behind you in the drawer on the right," "the table next to you," or "the bottom cabinet below your waist." Patients also can place items in various positions within a room. They then should stand when able or sit, if necessary, in the middle of the room, close their eyes and try to visualize, verbalize, and point to where the objects are in relation to themselves from memory. Having located the objects, the patients then should move through the area and pick up each item they put down in sequence. Functional carryover always should be used (e.g., having patients remember through visualization where they put their glasses in the living room before they begin searching) (Box 16-2).[6]

## PERCEPTUAL RETRAINING WITH COMPUTERS

Numerous computer programs have been developed for rehabilitation of brain damage sequelae such as impaired cognition, attention, sequencing, memory, and perception. Because the computer is a highly visual medium, it has become an obvious tool for treatment of visual perceptual dysfunction. Treatment with computers has been termed *computer-assisted therapy*. No large or conclusive treatment studies have yet defined the outcome of computer-assisted therapy compared with conventional therapy. Some reports indicate that computer-assisted therapy helps to motivate patients with poor attention and motivation. The therapy provides perceptual variables (number, size, speed) and immediate feedback and is an automatic control for learning. Visual perceptual training with computers should be viewed as one part of select patients' treatment programs. Some patients, especially elderly patients, have no interest in working on or learning the computer and are not motivated to use it. The computer does not require perceptual, vestibular, and motor responses that typically are required for daily living activities. Low-vision aids are available for individuals suffering from macular degeneration, cataracts, diabetic retinopathy, glaucoma, detached retina, or retinitis pigmentosa. Low-vision aids include magnification and enhancement for most software programs. These aids are helpful when used with the appropriate population. Low-vision aids should not be suggested unless a primary visual assessment, or at least a visual screening, has been administered. Use should be justified and not just based on trial and error. Use of the computer should be limited

---

**Box 16-2**

### Suggested Functional Activities to Treat Visual System Dysfunction after Cerebrovascular Accident

The following functional activities address visual fixation, scanning, and saccades. Some activities also address accommodation, eye-hand coordination, and figure-ground skills. Postural control and upper extremity performance play primary roles in these activities.

A vestibular component may be added as the patient progresses by placing items behind him or her so that he or she must rotate to retrieve them or by placing items lower than the patient so a change in head position must occur. During activities the patient always should maintain as much visual fixation as possible, especially if using vestibular responses.

1. Sorting activities are necessary adjuncts to activities of daily living and are performed every day. The more meaningful the task is to an individual, the greater the result in completion.
   a. Sorting of items on the shelf in a medicine cabinet. Sequence can be written by the therapist or demonstrated.
   b. Sorting of silverware from caddies or dishwasher bin into silverware receptacle in a drawer. If this task is too difficult, the therapist can color code sets of spoons, forks, and butter knives and then remove coding one set at a time.
   c. Sorting of dinnerware by pattern, color, and size; removing it from the dishwasher, dish drainer, or table; and placing it on another surface. After sorting, the patient may set the table or put the dinnerware away in a high or low cabinet.
   d. Sorting of coins in a coin holder.
   e. Sorting of laundry by color, pattern, or size as stated on labels. The therapist may ask the patient to hang pants in one section of a closet and sweaters in another. Pants and sweaters may be placed on hangers in a different manner, which addresses spatial orientation.
2. Placing toothpaste on a toothbrush or a gel cleanser on a small brush to clean jewelry, small vases, or bowls is a useful task. So too is placing mustard from squeeze containers onto small cheese and bread wedges (cut out from cookie cutters or cut with a knife following a straight path distinguished with food coloring or mustard).
3. The therapist may place colored spots on a large mirror; the patient then cleans the spots off of the mirror.
4. The therapist may use baking activities. The patient then should place ingredients in all quadrants, including high, low, and rotary positions.
5. Hanging birthday cards or artwork created in the therapy room—either by color coordination, alphabetical order of artist, or written or verbal cues from therapist.

**Box 16-3**

**Computer Programs for Visual Perceptual Training**

Optometric Extension Program
2912 S. Daimler St.
Santa Ana, CA 92705
(714) 250-8070

Bernell Corporation
750 Lincolnway East
P.O. Box 4637
South Bend, IN 46634
(800) 348-2225

Psychological Software Services Programs
Odie Bracey
Psychological Software Services
6555 Carollton Ave.
Indianapolis, IN 46229

Life Science Associates Programs
R. Gianutsos
Life Science Associates
1 Fenemore Road
Bayport, NY 11705
(diagnosis and training)

to those who have previous knowledge of computers, who have a stated goal to return to using a computer for work or leisure, and who enjoy computer work (Box 16-3).

## REVIEW QUESTIONS

1. What is the role of the functional optometrist in the evaluation and treatment of vision dysfunction after CVA?
2. Which deficits are considered primary visual deficits?
3. What are the norms for visual fields?
4. What are examples of age-related visual dysfunctions that may complicate the evaluation of a stroke patient?
5. For which patient population are computers a useful treatment modality?

## REFERENCES

1. Árnadóttir G: *The brain and behavior: assessing cortical function through activities of daily living*, St Louis, 1990, Mosby.
2. Bouska MJ, Gallaway M: Primary visual deficits in adults with brain damage: management in occupational therapy, *Occup Ther Pract* 3:1, 1991.
3. Bouska MJ, Kauffman NA, Marcus SE: Disorders of the visual perception system. In Umphred DA, editor: *Neurological rehabilitation*, ed 2, St Louis, 1990, Mosby.
4. Cohen H, Fox CR: The visual and vestibular systems. In Cohen H, editor: *Neuroscience for rehabilitation*, Philadelphia, 1993, JB Lippincott.
5. Cohen AH, Rein LD: The effect of head trauma on the visual system: the doctor of optometry as a member of the rehabilitative team, *J Am Optom Assoc* 63:530, 1992.
6. Efferson L: Disorders of vision and visual perceptual dysfunction. In Umphred, editor: *Neurological rehabilitation*, ed 3, St Louis, 1995, Mosby.
7. Farber S: *Neurorehabilitation: a multisensory approach*, Philadelphia, 1992, Saunders.
8. Gianutsos R, Matheson P: The rehabilitation of visual perceptual disorders attributable to brain injury. In Meier M, Diller L, Benton A, editors: *Neuropsychological rehabilitation*, London, 1986 Churchill Livingstone.
9. Gianutsos R, Ramsey G, Perlin RR: Rehabilitation optometric services for survivors of acquired brain injury, *Arch Phys Med Rehabil* 69(8):573-578, 1988.
10. Gianutsos R, Suchoff IB: Visual fields after brain injury: management issues for the occupational therapist. In Scheiman M, editor: *Understanding and managing vision deficits: a guide for occupational therapists*, Thorofare, NJ, 1997, Slack.
11. Goldberg ME, Eggers HM, Gouras P: Ocular motor system. In Kandel ER, Schwartz TH, Tessel TM, editors: *Principles of neural science*, ed 3, Norwalk, Conn, 1991, Appleton & Lange.
12. Hellerstein LF, Fishman B: Visual rehabilitation for patients with brain injury. In Scheiman M, editor: *Understanding and managing vision deficits: a guide for occupational therapists*, Thorofare, NJ, 1997, Slack.
13. Hellerstein LF, Fishman B: Vision therapy and occupational therapy: an integrated approach, *J Behav Optom* 5:122, 1990.
14. Kalb L, Warshowsky TH: Occupational therapy and optometry: principles of diagnosis and collaborative treatment of learning disabilities in children, *Occup Ther Pract* 3:77, 1991.
15. Kelly DD: Sexual differentiation of the nervous system. In Kandel ER, Schwartz TH, editors: *Principles of neural science*, New York, 1985, Elsevier.
15a. LeDoux JE, Smylie C: Left hemisphere visual process in a case of right hemisphere symptomatology: implications for theories of cerebral lateralization, *Arch Neurol* 37:157, 1980.
16. Mason C, Kandel ER: Central visual pathways. In Kandel ER, Schwartz TH, Tessel TM, editors: *Principles of neural science*, ed 3, Norwalk, Conn, 1991, Appleton & Lange.
17. Moses R, Hart W: *Adler's physiology of the eye: clinical application*, St Louis, 1987, Mosby.
18. Richards RG, Oppenheim GS: *Visual skill appraisal*, Novato, Calif, 1984, Academic Therapy.
19. Romero-Rangel T, Stavrou P, Cotter J, et al: Gas-permeable scleral contact lens therapy in ocular surface disease, *Am J Ophthalmol* 130(1):25-32, 2000.
20. Rosenthal P, Cotter JM, Baum J: Treatment of persistent corneal epithelial defect with extended wear of a fluid-ventilated gas-permeable scleral contact lens, *Am J Ophthalmol* 130(1):33-41, 2000.
21. Scheiman M: Optometric model of vision, part one. In Scheiman M, editor: *Understanding and managing vision deficits: a guide for occupational therapists*, Thorofare, NJ, 1997, Slack.
22. Scheiman M: Optometric model of vision, part two. In Scheiman M, editor: *Understanding and managing vision deficits: a guide for occupational therapists*, Thorofare, NJ, 1997, Slack.
23. Scheiman M: Screening for visual acuity, visual efficiency and visual information processing problems. In Scheiman M, editor: *Understanding and managing vision deficits: a guide for occupational therapists*, Thorofare, NJ, 1997, Slack.
24. Scotti G, Spinnler H: Color imperception in unilateral hemisphere-damaged patients, *J Neurol Neurosurg Psychiatry* 33:22, 1970.
25. Toglia J: Unilateral visual inattention: multi-dimensional components, *Occup Ther Pract* 3:18, 1991.

26. Toglia J: *Cognition and perception: principles and practice workshop*, New York 1990 (oral presentation).
27. Tsurumi K, Todd V: Theory and guidelines for visual task analysis and synthesis. In Scheiman M, editor: *Understanding and managing vision deficits: a guide for occupational therapists*, Thorofare, NJ, 1997, Slack.
28. Vaughan D, Asbury J: *General ophthalmology*, Los Altos, Calif, 1974, Lange Medical.
29. Warren M: A hierarchal model for evaluation and treatment of visual perceptual dysfunction in adult acquired brain injury, Part I and Part II, *Am J Occup Ther* 47:42, 1993.
30. Warshowsky TH: Principles of optometric rehabilitation, *Pract Optom* 4:4, 1993.
31. Zoltan B, Siev E, Freishtat B: *The adult stroke patient: a manual for evaluation and treatment of perceptual and cognitive dysfunction*, Thorofare, NJ, 1986, Slack.

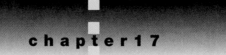

carolyn a. unsworth

**chapter 17**

# How Therapists Think: Exploring Therapists' Reasoning When Working with Patients Who Have Cognitive and Perceptual Problems Following Stroke

### key terms

clinical reasoning

conditional reasoning

expert therapist

interactive reasoning

narrative reasoning

novice therapist

phenomenological

pragmatic reasoning

procedural reasoning

tacit knowledge

generalization reasoning

worldview

### chapter objectives

After completing this chapter, the reader will be able to accomplish the following:

- Define clinical reasoning, and identify and define the main forms of clinical reasoning.
- Describe the differences between a more phenomenological approach versus a more biomedical approach to patient care.
- Describe how an understanding of clinical reasoning can enhance practice in the area of cognitive and perceptual dysfunction with patients following stroke.
- Provide examples of situations in which a therapist might use procedural, interactive, conditional, and pragmatic reasoning.
- List the five stages in the development of expertise and the key features of each phase.
- Successfully work through the Review Questions at the conclusion of this chapter.

This chapter reviews how a therapist uses clinical reasoning in the context of practice with patients who have cognitive and perceptual problems following stroke. Because this chapter provides an overview of research literature in the field of clinical reasoning, the content relates to therapists working with all patient groups. However, the case example that illustrates the text is specific to patients with cognitive and perceptual problems following stroke. The chapter examines the different forms of clinical thinking such as scientific versus the phenomenological approaches to patient care and then explores in detail the kinds of reasoning popularly identified in occupational therapy literature, including narrative, procedural, interactive, conditional, and pragmatic reasoning. Influences on clinical reasoning also are explored, such as the therapist's worldview. Because many academics and therapists agree that the use of case studies that demonstrate expert reasoning provides excellent opportunities for students to develop their own reasoning skills, the reasoning processes of an expert therapist obtained during my research in this field are used to illustrate the text. The final section of the chapter examines how clinical reasoning skills develop as students or new graduates progress over time from novice to expert. Occupational therapists can use this information to make expert clinical reasoning more explicit and therefore easier for students and novice therapists to learn and incorporate in their practice.

## WHAT IS CLINICAL REASONING?

### Definition of Clinical Reasoning

To put it simply, *clinical reasoning* may be defined as the thinking processes of therapists when undertaking a therapeutic practice. Although occupational therapists have written extensively about clinical reasoning over the past 20 years, they are still just beginning to understand what clinical reasoning is and its importance to practice. Mattingly and Fleming[43] describe clinical reasoning as being a practical know-how that puts theoretical knowledge into practice and a complex (yet often common-sense) way of thinking to find what is best for each patient.

Unsworth[68] states, "To me, clinical reasoning is how I think and make decisions when I'm planning to be with a client; when I'm with a client; and afterwards, when I reflect on therapy. It involves intuition, judgment, empathy, and common sense . . .

"It's how I think about what the client is telling me and what I observe . . .

"It's what I pay attention to and ignore . . .

"It's what I respond to immediately or note for future reference . . .

"It's the way I try to understand my client as a human being . . .

"It's how I draw on my knowledge of previous clients, their difficulties and successful and unsuccessful solutions, . . .

"It's the way I draw on my theoretical knowledge and apply this in practice . . .

"It's the stories I share with other therapists about our clients, the therapy we provide and how we feel about it . . .

"It's the way I consider the total picture including how much therapy time I can spend with the client, financial reimbursement issues, and the support available from the client's family . . .

"It's the process of deciding what course of action to take with the client, and how I modify or change this over time.

"The way I reason has changed over time, due to greater experience and mentoring from expert occupational therapists and other health professionals. The way I reason in my OT practice makes me different from other health professionals."*

### Development of Clinical Reasoning in Occupational Therapy

Rogers and Masagatani[53] conducted the first empirical study of clinical reasoning in occupational therapy in 1982. The following year, Rogers[51] delivered an Eleanor Clarke Slagle lecture that focused on clinical reasoning. This lecture, coupled with a presentation by Donald Schön (an expert in the analysis of professional practice) to the American Occupational Therapy Association Commission on Education, stimulated the American Occupational Therapy Research Foundation to set up the Clinical Reasoning Study. The study was designed by an anthropologist (Mattingly) and several occupational therapists including Fleming, Gillette, and Cohen and was influenced greatly by Schön as the consultant on the project.[44] The study ran between 1986 and 1990 and was reported extensively in the special issue on clinical reasoning of the *American Journal of Occupational Therapy* in November 1991. In 1994, Mattingly and Fleming[43] published this work in a book. The content of this chapter draws on the foundation laid by Mattingly and Fleming in the Clinical Reasoning Study and extends these ideas using research and theoretical literature from the past 10 years from Sweden, the United Kingdom, Australia, and North America.

### Clinical Reasoning and Theory

The first consideration is the use of clinical reasoning to explore the practical theories of the profession. One of the aims of the Clinical Reasoning Study was to make

---

*Reprinted with permission from Unsworth CA: *Cognitive and perceptual disorders: a clinical reasoning approach to evaluation and intervention*, Philadelphia, 1999, FA Davis.

explicit the tacit knowledge contained in the practical theories used by the therapists studied. The study argued that this tacit knowledge could be shared if a language to describe therapists' reasoning could be developed. Hence the study aimed to examine the types of reasoning processes used by therapists to use their many practical theories.

Mattingly and Fleming[43] made the distinction between espoused theories and theories-in-use. Espoused theories are those held true by the discipline. These theories are intelligent speculations about the workings of a particular phenomenon, which then usually are tested out and refined through research. Theories-in-use, or practical theories, are those generated by practice. Although many scientists do not support the notion that theory can arise from practice, researchers such as Mattingly and Fleming[43] and Schön[56] believe this is possible. Many of these practical theories are passed verbally among therapists when working together, and they often guide therapists in their day-to-day practice. Theories-in-use generally are accompanied by a large fund of tacit knowledge. Often therapists cannot describe what they are doing or why; in other words, their expert knowledge is tacit. While this knowledge remains undocumented, it cannot be used to contribute to the fund of knowledge for the profession. Hence a language to describe how and why therapists use certain techniques or communicate in particular ways is needed.

In addition to the way clinical reasoning can be used to explore the practical theories of the profession, one also must consider that the construct of clinical reasoning is itself developing into a theory. Knowledge of clinical reasoning has been growing steadily over the past 20 years and is evolving slowly into a theory derived from practice. If clinical reasoning is evolving into a theory, what is the relationship between this and other theories or frameworks that guide occupational therapy practice? Kielhofner[34] described conceptual practice models as bodies of knowledge developed in occupational therapy for its practice. However, whereas some models can be applied to many patient groups, some are more targeted for patients with particular problems. Hence Stanton, Thompson-Franson, and Kramer[58] described some conceptual practice models as generic and others as specific to the patients problem areas. To think about these generic models as umbrella models, such as the Canadian Model of Occupational Performance[13,37] or the Model of Human Occupation,[33] is useful. In the field of cognitive and perceptual dysfunction, an umbrella conceptual practice model is used with a specific practice model such as the Cognitive Disabilities Model,[3] the dynamic interaction approach,[62] the quadraphonic approach,[1] the retraining approach,[6] the neurofunctional approach,[28] or the compensatory or rehabilitation approach.[23,63] The evolving theory of clinical reasoning seems to interface smoothly with all of these conceptual practice models. A clinical reasoning approach cannot replace any model, and yet such an approach can be used to complement these models and add a different perspective to clinical work. Using a clinical reasoning approach with an umbrella and specific practice model ensures that the therapist acknowledges and can describe scientific and phenomenological approaches to patient care (as are described next) and has a language to describe the kinds of thinking that guides practice, including why one chooses a particular practice model. Figure 17-1 depicts this relationship between a generic occupational therapy (umbrella) conceptual practice model, specific conceptual practice models, and clinical reasoning.

## CLINICAL REASONING WITH PATIENTS WHO HAVE COGNITIVE AND PERCEPTUAL PROBLEMS FOLLOWING STROKE

At some point in their careers most occupational therapists work with patients who have cognitive and perceptual problems. One of the largest groups of patients with such problems is the group of stroke survivors. The American Heart Association[5] estimates that each year approximately 700,000 Americans will have a stroke. Documented evidence indicates that at any one time approximately 3 million persons in the United States have a stroke-related disability that requires ongoing management and care.[2] Global estimates of incidence of cognitive and perceptual problems following stroke vary enormously because of differences in assessments used, populations studied, and time since stroke onset. However,

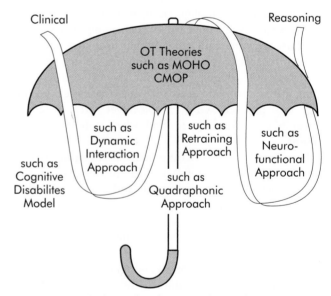

**Figure 17-1** Relationship between the evolving theory of clinical reasoning and other conceptual practice models. *OT,* Occupational therapy; *MOHO,* Model of Human Occupation; *CMOP,* Canadian Model of Occupational Performance.

Kong, Chua, and Tow[35] estimate that approximately 41.5% of persons who experience stroke and are more than 75 years old experience some deficit in this area. Closer examination of specific impairments shows that 82% of patients who are 2 to 3 days past a stroke experience some unilateral neglect[59] and that 23% of patients have more lasting experience of this problem.[49] The incidence of apraxia is reported to be lower, with estimates of up to 30% of patients with left hemisphere damage experiencing problems.[19] When working with patients after stroke, the language of clinical reasoning can aid occupational therapists in describing their practical and espoused theories (and how these translate into day-to-day therapy) to colleagues, students, and the patient and patient's family. Descriptions of the key types of reasoning that form this language are described in the next section.

The conceptual practice model that the therapist adopts guides the kinds of evaluations and interventions that the therapist will undertake,[67,68] and the section Procedural Reasoning describes this in more detail. For example, a therapist who uses a remedial or bottom-up approach such as the retraining approach[6] assumes that remediation of function is possible, and this fundamental belief helps shape all the reasoning that follows. Such therapists believe that reorganization of brain activity is possible following stroke. Reorganization refers to the ability of the central nervous system to reconfigure and adapt itself in various biologic and functional ways to perform an activity. In contrast, a therapist who uses an adaptive, or top-down, framework such as the compensatory or rehabilitation approach[23,63] to patient care believes that the therapist needs to work with patients in the everyday occupations the patients want and need to do and that the environment can be modified or that compensatory strategies can be used to assist patients to complete tasks. In other words, the therapist starts at the top, which is the desired occupation rather than working with the patient on the underlying performance components. When using a top-down approach, the therapist does not assume generalization of compensation strategies taught from one activity to another.[68]

Theoretical information provides only the starting point for therapy. Many writers suggest that only through clinical practice can clinical practice develop and creative solutions be found for problems that are not mentioned in texts.[14,55] When problems or obstacles arise in therapy, occupational therapists need to be able to reason to reach a solution. For example, theoretically, therapists know to assess the patient's sensation to exclude these problems before the assessment of complex perceptual problems. But what if the patient has insufficient or unreliable language, making sensory testing impossible? What if the patient is depressed and refuses to undergo sensory testing? Only through learning about clinical reasoning and developing a language to help therapists reason through these problems and seek answers with colleagues can practice develop.

## CASE STUDY: SALLY AND SAM

The next section deals specifically with the different types of clinical reasoning therapists use. To illustrate these different types of thinking, clinical reasoning examples from Sally are provided. Sally is an expert occupational therapist working with a 28-year-old male patient, Sam, who experienced cognitive and perceptual problems along with motor weakness on his right side following a left-sided anterior communicating artery stroke. Sally is the senior therapist in a team of eight therapists at a rehabilitation facility with 60 beds. She manages a caseload of patients with neurologic problems following stroke, head injury, or disease processes such as Parkinson's. The examples of Sally's reasoning are based on research transcripts in which Sally retrospectively described her therapy sessions with Sam.[67] Three transcripts were recorded, one following an initial outpatient evaluation session with Sam, another following a typical treatment session, and a third when Sam was being discharged from regular outpatient services. Hence transcript excerpts are headed with Evaluation, Intervention, or Discharge Session. These transcripts have been modified (and pseudonyms used) to protect the identity of the patient and therapist or more clearly to illustrate a particular form of reasoning. Sally's description of Sam together with details of his impairments, therapy goals, and the occupational issues he faces are outlined in the following section, which examines the difference between chart talk and narrative reasoning.

## A LANGUAGE TO DESCRIBE THE TYPES OF CLINICAL REASONING

This section explores the different types or modes of clinical reasoning. Although several different types of reasoning are described, these types basically fit into a more biomedical or a more phenomenological approach to patient care. As described by Mattingly,[40] the profession of occupational therapy deals in two practice spheres, the biomedical sphere that focuses on the mechanical body and the social, cultural, and psychological sphere that concerns the meaning of the illness to the person. Hence, Mattingly refers to occupational therapy as the two-body practice. Usually, these more scientific versus more phenomenological approaches to patient care coexist uneasily. However, Mattingly notes that many occupational therapists seem to be able to shift rapidly and easily between thinking about the patient's disease processes (body as a machine or the physical body) and the patient's illness experience (the lived body). Mattingly describes how some therapists can integrate these two approaches so seamlessly that "biomechanical means may be used to achieve phenomenological ends or the reverse." The synthesis of these two perspectives into what is called best practice in occupational therapy also reflects the paradigm shifts the professions has undergone over the past 40 years.

Therapists require different types of reasoning when working in these two different spheres and need different ways of communicating this reasoning. When occupational therapists are talking about the patient's medical problem, they are more likely to use a kind of language that Mattingly and Fleming[43] described as chart talk. In contrast, when the therapist is thinking about the patient as a person who also has a medical problem, the therapist is more likely to reason in what Mattingly and Fleming describes as the narrative form. Mattingly[41] describes occupational therapy clinical reasoning as being "largely tacit, highly imagistic, and deeply phenomenological mode of thinking." Mattingly therefore suggests that narrative reasoning is the best basis for most clinical reasoning in occupational therapy. Narrative reasoning means that stories are told or created to assist the therapist to make sense of what is happening with the patient. When thinking about the patient as a person, their illness experience, and what therapy will mean for the patient's present life and future, therapists commonly think and talk in the narrative form. These two ways of communicating clinical reasoning are described next.

## Narrative Reasoning and Chart Talk

Therapists use narratives or stories to convey their thinking to other professionals, students and novice therapists, and patients. Viewed in this light, narrative reasoning is a way of reporting or giving words to the other forms of clinical reasoning, which are discussed later in this section.[60] Narrative reasoning is also a form of phenomenological understanding. Narratives can take the form of storytelling or story creation. Storytelling can reveal how the therapist treated and interacted with the patient and also can be used to explain how the therapist perceives the patient to be managing the disability. Storytelling is most predominant when therapists are carrying out the day-to-day procedures of evaluating and treating patients, trying to understand the patient as a person, and what is happening in therapy.[4] Story creation, however, involves creating a picture of the future with the patient that includes setting goals to work toward in therapy. Story creation is more common when therapists envision a future for the patient, or engage in conditional reasoning (described in detail later). However, the story created for therapy usually does not proceed without the need for revision, and experienced therapists are adept in changing the therapeutic story midstream.[39] In the following example, Sally tells the story of Sam to the researcher. The emphasis of this narrative is on Sam as a person rather than the medical aspects of Sam's stroke.

*Evaluation Session, Part 1.* "Basically the idea behind this initial outpatient session is just looking at basic home independence for Sam. He was discharged home a couple of days ago, so he is back here every day at the moment as an outpatient. It was actually a self-discharge. We were heading toward that anyway, and the plan was for Sam to live in a bungalow or trailer on his family's property. He used to live in a trailer at the back of their property, but this has rotted out and they've pulled it down. They [his family] actually have a very small house, and it's just not really appropriate for him to be living there since he has teenage stepsiblings, and he is a very independent young man, he wants to have his own space, which you can really understand for a young man, so the idea for him is either to get a bungalow at the back of his family property again or go to a community-based group home. However, that hasn't worked out yet, and so Sam is in the family home for the moment. Sam had his stroke 6 weeks ago. He was in intensive care for 3 days, indicating the severity of the infarct, which was in the left anterior communicating artery. The CT [computed tomography] scan revealed a reasonably large lesion area, and consistent with his lesion, Sam experiences difficulties with walking, and he is using a 3-point stick. He also has reduced movement in his right arm, and particularly, he has difficulty using his hand since the movements are slowed and his grasp is reduced. He's also got some moderately severe cognitive problems.

"Sam, prior to his stroke, was unemployed, was a drug user, and didn't have a lot that interested him in his life other than playing the guitar, so in terms of finding activities that are meaningful for him, it's been quite hard, and we spent some really worthwhile time in therapy using the Interest Checklist and found that cooking is one activity he loves. He is really motivated, he is a terrific guy, he's really cooperative and tries really hard and seems to always understand the rationale, even though I always explain to him why we are doing what we are doing. So I suppose the two reasons why we chose this cooking activity for today are one, looking toward him in the long term developing a repertoire of basic meals he can prepare in his own place, and also because it specifically works on improving his planning and problem-solving skills, attention, and also his standing tolerance."

In contrast to narrative reasoning is the kind of language therapists use when speaking with colleagues about a patient's biomedical problems. Although the foregoing example is largely in the narrative form, Sally does slip into another kind or more factual description when she talks about Sam's medical problems. Mattingly and Fleming[43] reported that when therapists discussed procedural aspects of the patient's physical condition, shared treatment goals, and planned evaluations and interventions, they were more likely to use chart talk and scientific forms of reasoning. During these discussions, therapists tended to use a biomechanical way of understanding the patient's problems. For example, in the following excerpt Sally discusses aspects of Sam's splinting regimen using chart talk.

***Intervention Session, Part 1.*** "A lot of the focus with Sam in the past few weeks has been on him getting functional use of his right hand, which is his dominant hand. He's actually got quite increased muscle tone as you can see there. He has a night splinting regimen, and going back a few weeks ago, he basically forgot he had a right hand, he just wasn't initiating using it, and he quickly taught himself to be left dominant. So we're really pleased with the progress he's making in extending his wrist and MCP [metacarpophalangeal] and PIP [proximal interphalangeal] finger joints. We are talking about his splint at the moment because I did quite a radical change to the splint last Friday, and I was asking him if it was giving him any pain because it does give him a little bit of pain as we have been gradually increasing the extension of his wrist and of his fingers. He told me he took it off midway through the first night, but that he has been able to wear it through the last couple of nights."

Although therapists usually write case notes in the brief and factual language of chart talk, chart talk and narrative reasoning possibly may be interwoven when therapists are describing the patient. This idea was suggested previously when noting that occupational therapists seem to be able to weave between a biomedical and phenomenological understanding of the patient. In the first transcripts from Sally, one can see how she slips between discussing Sam as a person and describing the facts of his stroke. Research evidence also supports that therapists interweave these forms of reasoning when discussing and describing their patients.[64-66]

### The Therapist with the Three-Track Mind

Mattingly and Fleming[43] suggested that when describing the patient's biomedical problems, therapists tended to use chart talk. The kind of reasoning that supports this sphere of patient care draws on scientific reasoning. More specifically, Fleming[25] referred to this kind of thinking in occupational therapy as *procedural reasoning*. When reasoning in the narrative form and considering the meaning of the illness for the patient (in other words, when using a phenomenological perspective to patient care), occupational therapists use two other types of reasoning, which Fleming labeled *interactive* and *conditional reasoning*.

Fleming[25] also suggested that therapists seem to be able to think in these reasoning tracks simultaneously. Hence the phrase, "the therapist with the three-track mind" was coined. Therapists seem to monitor the procedural aspects of the treatment, such as the evaluations and interventions to be used with the patient and how the patient is performing, while being able to elicit the patient's cooperation and understand the person's response to the treatment using interactive reasoning.[24] Therapists also seem to be engaged in considering the patient's condition and how this could alter over time and to imagine how the patient's past, present, and future could be facilitated by occupational therapy intervention. Fleming and Mattingly[27] argued that experienced therapists were able to use these forms of reasoning in rapid succession or use different forms almost simultaneously. Fleming[24] suggested that "Reasoning styles changed as the therapist's attention was drawn from the clinical condition to another feature of the problem, and to how the person feels about the problem, almost simultaneously, using different thinking styles; and they did not 'lose track of' their thoughts about aspects of a problem as those components were temporarily shifted to be the background while another aspect was brought into the foreground."

Although Mattingly and Fleming[43] identified these three modes of reasoning together with narrative reasoning, subsequent theoretical and empirical publications have suggested that these might not be the only forms of reasoning used. In fact, occupational therapists and other allied health scientists have now documented multiple types of clinical reasoning including scientific, diagnostic, pragmatic, management, collaborative, predictive, ethical, intuitive, propositional, and patient-centered.[31,38,52,54] In this chapter, only the most commonly described forms of reasoning are presented, together with comments on their interrelationship. Hence, this chapter explores narrative, scientific, procedural, interactive, conditional, pragmatic reasoning, and a newly identified form of reasoning termed *generalization reasoning*.

***Procedural Reasoning.*** Therapists use procedural reasoning when thinking about the patient's problems and the kinds of evaluation, intervention, and outcome measurement procedures to use. Whereas interactive and conditional reasoning are based more in the phenomenological sphere and therefore are narrative forms of reasoning, procedural reasoning is based more in the biomedical sphere and therefore draws on scientific reasoning. Scientific reasoning almost exclusively forms the basis for medical reasoning and decision making. Scientific reasoning is the process of hypothesis generation and testing that generally is referred to as hypothetico-deductive reasoning. This form of reasoning most often is used to make a diagnosis of the patient's medical condition. Although occupational therapists are more concerned with identifying the patient's occupational problems rather than the medical diagnosis, therapists do draw on the ideas of scientific reasoning when reasoning procedurally.

In the medical decision-making literature, terms such as *diagnosis, prognosis and prescription, cue identification, hypothesis generation, cue interpretation,* and *hypothesis evaluation* are used commonly.[22] However, in the occupational therapy literature, terms such as *problem identification* and *goal setting* are more common. When determining what the patient's problems might be and selecting appropriate interventions, Fleming[24] identified that therapists were involved in a variety of procedural reasoning strategies and methods of thinking. These methods of thinking include the four-stage model of problem solving, which is based on the hypothetico-deductive reasoning, goal-oriented problem solving, task environment, and pattern recognition of the medical model. Each of these methods of thinking is described briefly.

Procedural reasoning generally begins with problem identification, and Elstein, Shulman, and Sprafka[22] developed a four-stage model of problem solving that focuses on problem identification. Fleming suggests that therapists may use this model when determining what the patient's occupational problems are.

The four stages in this model are as follows:
1. Cue acquisition: The therapist gathers cues or pieces of information about the patient and the patient's difficulties.
2. Hypothesis generation: The therapist generates several plausible explanations for the observed cues.
3. Cue interpretation: The therapist compares each hypothesis with the cue set and selects the most logical or best hypotheses to explain the cues.
4. Hypothesis evaluation: Finally, the therapist asks which is the best hypothesis by evaluating which cues generally are thought to be necessary for selecting each hypothesis and for the presence of critical cues for selecting each hypothesis. In this way, one hypothesis should be identified as the best.

All problem solving in occupational therapy is goal directed so that therapists and patients work together to ensure the patient can participate in desired and needed occupations. Although therapy is conducted mostly in clinical environments, therapists are thinking constantly about translating what is being accomplished into the patient's home environments. Hence procedural reasoning also is concerned with considering the environment in which the task is being conducted. Pattern recognition refers to a therapist's ability to identify the kinds of patient cues and features that occur together. For example, a therapist who observes a patient go several times to get the necessary toiletries for the morning bathroom routine may question whether the patient has a planning and organization problem or difficulties with memory. However, adding this information to many other observations of difficulties with planning, judgment, and problem solving prompts the therapist to consider difficulties with executive functions. The ability to recognize patterns of cues and behaviors becomes part of the therapist's tacit knowledge.[24] In other words, the therapist recognizes these patterns without needing actually to think through or articulate the emerging trend. Finally, current practice culture is driven by providing evidence to support the evaluations and interventions therapists select to use with patients. Therefore an occupational therapist is reasoning procedurally when asking, "What evidence is there to support the treatments I offer?"

In the following example that illustrates procedural reasoning, Sally describes setting up a cooking task with Sam.

*Intervention Session, Part 2*

INTERVIEWER: I notice you just set up the fry pan, so tell me about that.

SALLY: Yes. I basically set it up due to the timeframe for this session and the demands on Sam. We've been gradually upgrading the task demands on Sam, but today I said to Sam that I would set the fry pan up and also because reaching that would be extremely hard for him. He would have to lean right over the table, and also I was planning to put the rice on to cook, just to let him focus on the one task today.

INTERVIEWER: So, you would do the rice, and he would do the stir-fry vegetables in the pan?

SALLY: Yes and that's sort of been from past experience because when he has to attend to two things, he will forget one of them, like the rice. So once we sort of feel that he's managing cooking one dish well, then we'll upgrade it and include the second dish, the rice, and we would probably have something like a prompt sign on the table for him to remind him to check the rice and also the timer which we always use.

In the example of procedural reasoning, Sally talks about some of the difficulties that Sam has with the cooking task because of his memory and planning difficulties. However, more that just looking at Sam's problems, in this transcript excerpt, Sally goes on to incorporate into the activity her understanding of how Sam learns. This kind of reasoning is referred to as interactive reasoning and is described in the next section.

*Intervention Session, Part 3*

SALLY: I think with Sam, he's the sort of guy that learns from repetition. So, by letting him go in and make mistakes—you will see later, he comes back to the table and I've actually let him come back without the can opener and all those things—so that's a way for him to stop and think what he needs.

***Interactive Reasoning.*** Therapists use interactive reasoning to consider the best approach to communicate with the patient and also to understand the patient as a person. In the Clinical Reasoning Study, Mattingly and Fleming[43] found that although therapists reported their procedural practices, they did not report their interactions with the patient. Hence, they referred to interactive reasoning as the underground practice. Therapists often see patients at times in their lives that are difficult; their health or well being is challenged, and they may be experiencing their body in a new way. This can be frightening for the patient, who may respond with confusion or anger. The skilled therapist needs to be able to communicate effectively with the patient so as to share information about the patient's progress and prognosis, and the therapist can gain an understanding of how the patient perceives the disability and views the future.[43] However, because many patients who experience stroke also have a clinical lack of insight to their problems, the therapist faces the additional difficulty of collaborating with patients who may not have any understanding of their problems. Therapists need to take extra care with these patients to establish meaningful and realistic goals.

In its most simple form, interactive reasoning is concerned with how the therapist communicates with the patient. In the following example, Sally reasons about the way she interacts with Sam to make sure he can follow through with what she wants him to do.

*Evaluation Session, Part 2.* "I'm just sort of basically explaining to Sam the actual movement I want him to do. Often, if I can, I try to decrease the verbal cues and actually look at giving some physical cues as well. That carries right over to all of his program. So, for example, when we do personal care, I really have to use a combination of both physical cues and verbal prompting. I'm trying to certainly decrease that. I think with Sam and a lot of patients with stroke or brain injuries, it just takes much longer for them to respond. It just doesn't go in as quickly as it does with us. My strategy with Sam at the moment is give him the instruction or prompt him and then give him some time to respond, and then go on to give him some physical guidance as well."

More than just basic communication, interactive reasoning is also about understanding the patient as a person who has interests, needs, and values, as well as problems, so that the therapist can understand the disability from the patient's perspective. Interactive reasoning stems from the way therapists value the patient as an individual, and the therapist's deeply held humanistic beliefs. In the following example, Sally indicates that she understands Sam as an easygoing person who might want to take the easy way, even though he often can achieve more than he thinks.

### Intervention Session, Part 4

SALLY: That's another one of the jokes we have. He's been asking me for months about having elastic shoelaces, and I just said, 'No way, you're not having elastic shoelaces. You don't need them.'

INTERVIEWER: How does he know about them?

SALLY: I don't know. He just came out of the blue one day, and I said, "Who told you about those?" And he is the kind of guy that will say to you, "Anything to make my life easier, I will do." He will say, "I'm a bit slack," and that's his personality. I was having a joke with him before saying, "At least I believed in you," because now he's doing his shoelaces independently. I just said to him, "Imagine if we got you elastic shoelaces. You would look a bit silly out there with these big elastic shoelaces." So joking around with him has worked really well.

In this example, Sally also talks about joking around with Sam as a way of building a shared language between them and also gaining his cooperation in therapy. In the following example, Sally elaborates further on this use of humor in therapy.

*Intervention Session, Part 5.* "Yes, and I use humor as well. That's the approach I often take with people but especially with people like Sam, who are really laid back and low key, that really works well. Sam responds much better to a friendship sort of approach, just encouragement rather than the dictator sort of approach. That's not something Sam goes for. In fact, he bumps up against that approach, and I think that's been a pattern throughout his life. . . . With Sam in particular, like I said, sort of having our own private joke, like I say, I'm the hand police, and so if I see him not using his hand I only have to say 'hand police,' and we can have a bit of a laugh. And we can also laugh a bit at some of the failures he's had, and you obviously have to pick the people you do that with. You wouldn't do that with someone who has got poor insight, but Sam has excellent insight. But, like I said, that's my approach with a lot of people, but with other people you just don't use it because it's not appropriate, and they get very upset if you sort of stir them up a little bit, but with Sam, no, he's not problem at all."

From a variety of authors, Mattingly and Fleming[43] put together a list of purposes for which interactive reasoning is used:

1. Engage the patient in therapy.[42]
2. Know the patient as a person.[15]
3. Understand the patient's disability from the patient's point of view.[42]
4. Individualize the therapy for the patient to match the treatment goals with the person, disability, and experience of the disability.[26]
5. Convey a sense of acceptance/trust/hope to the patient.[36]
6. Break tension through the use of humor.[57]
7. Build a shared language of actions and meanings.[17]
8. Monitor how the treatment session is going[26] and demonstrate interest in the patient and the patient's concerns without indicating disapproval or distaste of the condition.[12]

Hence, interactive reasoning is concerned with collaborating with the patient as a partner in the therapy process. Together the therapist and patient must devise goals that are meaningful to the patient and also serve to promote the patient's occupational functioning. Humor seems to be one way to facilitate patients to collaborate in the therapy process, and Mattingly and Fleming[43] discussed several other strategies that therapists use to engage patients in this collaboration. These strategies include the following:

"1. Creating choices. Therapists try to engage clients in therapy by providing choices in relation to problem areas the client wants to work on, and the specific occupations or activities they might use in therapy.

"2. Individualizing treatment. A therapy program that is uniquely tailored for the client, through both the ingenuity of the therapist and the involvement of the client, generally keeps the client engaged in therapy. While the goals of therapy for a client with a memory problem may be quite similar, the way the therapy program is structured, and the activities that the client and therapist choose are usually different for each client.

"3. Structuring success. Therapists often structure, or manipulate therapy to provide the client with opportunities for success, and thus promote their alliance. Therapists are often in the business of revealing problems, and then working with the client to reduce their impact. Unless the client has some successes along the way, it is very hard to keep the client motivated, or to maintain a positive relationship with the client. Therapists often talk about keeping the client optimally challenged. This includes pushing the client to achieve, but not so far that he fails. This has been described as the 'just right challenge.'[11,18]

"4. Joint problem solving. Another approach therapists use to facilitate client engagement in therapy is to ask the client to help them in the problem solving process. For example, if the therapist has difficulty in using a piece of equipment, or in devising a strategy for a transfer, calling on the client for his input enables him to take a strong and active role in therapy if only for a short time.

"5. Gift exchange. The final two strategies that Mattingly and Fleming[43] found [that] therapists use to build an alliance with their clients were more personal in nature. The researchers found that therapists would go out of their way, or their formal roles to do something nice for the client such as bake a cake for a client's birthday. In this way the therapist shows a willingness to care for the client in a more personal way. In exchange, clients often feel more committed to co-operate in therapy. Clients may also give gifts to the therapist. These may be as simple as a flower, a few words of thanks or a hug, all of which demonstrate their personal thanks for the therapists' involvement in their treatment.

"6. Exchanging personal stories. Exchanging personal experiences is another powerful way to develop a bond with a client. Mattingly and Fleming[43] found this was commonly used by clinicians to engage the clients in therapy, and that clinicians were usually aware of the value of this strategy."*

Sally talks about the importance of patients choosing their own therapy activity. This illustrates the point made before about creating choices for the patient and also supports the idea of a patient-centered practice.

*Intervention Session, Part 6.* "Now we're upgrading his program, and we have a hand function group that Sam will start coming to. In this group we are looking at a lot of active wrist and finger extension because that's what he really needs to work on, and a lot of gross grasp because he really has trouble extending his third, fourth, and fifth fingers at this stage. Even in the hand function group, although I don't actually run it, two of the other OTs [occupational therapists] do, it's actually fantastic, and the therapists find out what it is the person who wants to do. We have had people in the group eating using chopsticks in their other hand or practicing putting CDs in and out of their player. We really try and keep people motivated by choosing their own therapy activities, and it's a really great fun group that people get a lot out of, I think, more than doing therapy on a one-to-one basis. A lot of my patients, from my experience working here, if they can't see or understand why they are doing a stupid exercise, you just lose them. As I said, we really try to emphasize here that patients choose meaningful activities."

Finally, the following transcript excerpt shows an example of how Sally structures the therapy session to ensure that Sam has some success. The motivating effect of this success pushes patients forward in their therapy programs.

*Evaluation Session, Part 3.* "We've just finished making toasted cheese sandwiches with Sam, and he did so well. And I made sure that Sam could do nearly all of this activity, since I'm challenging him with the stir-fried vegetables, so its good to balance this a bit with a cooking task that he can complete successfully. I was telling him how well his right hand is working now, and he was like so many other patients who say. 'Gosh, couldn't I use my hand at the start?' and we'll say, 'No,' and they'll just be amazed, so yes, having this success in an activity just keeps them going, I think."

---

*Reprinted with permission from Unsworth CA: *Cognitive and perceptual disorders: a clinical reasoning approach to evaluation and intervention,* Philadelphia, 1999, FA Davis.

*Conditional Reasoning.* Conditional reasoning was the last mode to be identified in the Clinical Reasoning Study. In describing the emergence of this mode, Fleming[24] wrote, "Later we realized that there was a third type of reasoning that therapists employed when they thought of the whole problem within the context of the person's past, present, and future; and within personal, social and cultural contexts. This was an especially useful form of reasoning, which therapists used when they wanted to, as they say, 'individualize' the treatment for the particular person. We called this 'conditional reasoning' because it took the whole condition into account."

Conditional reasoning takes the whole of the patient's condition into account as the therapist considers the patient's temporal contexts (past, present, and future), and his personal, cultural, and social contexts. Fleming[24] proposed that this form of reasoning is based in the cultural and social processes of understanding one's self and others and is used when the therapist wishes to understand the patient from a phenomenological perspective. In other words, a therapist uses this form of reasoning in trying to understand what is meaningful to patients in their world by imagining what their life was like before the illness or disability, what it is like now, and what it could be like in the future. In the following transcript excerpt, Sally is thinking through the issues surrounding Sam's life at home and what the future holds. This example not only illustrates conditional reasoning (e.g., discussing how Sam's condition has changed and on what his residential care situation is conditioned) but also shows aspects of what some authors describe as ethical reasoning,[7] where Sally imagines how Sam might behave in different residential settings and how his drug use may affect other residents.

*Discharge Session, Part 1.* "Now, we're talking about a big issue for Sam at the moment, it's the breakdown of his residential situation at home. He's still in his parents' house, but he can't stay there much longer, and they want him out. It's really hard because a lot of the residential settings [supervised housing such as nursing homes] are too low level for him, or the ones that he could live in and have day-to-day contact with someone in attending care support, there's no vacancies or he doesn't like them, and the other issue with him is if he goes into a group home, other people are at risk. He actually, unfortunately, shares his drugs around, and most of these houses have young men with brain injuries, and so we have a responsibility to ensure, you know—they can't obviously make an informed decision about whether to take the drugs Sam offers them. With Sam it's a premorbid thing, and essentially we have come to the realization he is not going to change. He's tried drug counseling, then we had a consultant, then social workers have tried, his mum has tried, and she is tearing her hair out, but he just—it's

something he likes to do no matter what we say. He acknowledges there is a high risk of psychotic incidences and all these things, but he just doesn't really budge from that. You know, when it comes down to the crunch, he just can't resist the temptation.

"So, essentially the two things we are trying to do at the moment is one, structure all of his time, since its when he's bored that he starts smoking drugs and things. Secondly, looking into attendant care so that he has someone helping him to live in a shared house, because if we look at him coming to our transitional living house, which is just across the road here, and I was also, at the end of the session, discussing with him the increased responsibilities that would be on him, and he is a very capable young man. He can make basic meals for himself now. Like, you didn't see him walk in, but he is now mobile with a stick, which he is hardly using. He has really well exceeded all of our expectations for someone with such a serious stroke. He still has ongoing cognitive impairments with things like memory and problem solving and planning, but with repetition and things, he can really learn to do things himself. It's really hard at the moment until we find out whether there's a bed available in one of the nearby group share houses. He is quite keen about that idea, but still his favored option is for himself to get a trailer or a bungalow on his family block."

Fleming[24] described the third form of reasoning as the most elusive. Conditional reasoning is not always conscious and therefore is more difficult to get at, understand, and describe. Conditional reasoning requires more than a simple knowledge of the patient's condition; it also calls for an understanding of how the condition has affected the individual's work, social situation and leisure, and view of self. Fleming[24] reported that therapists who were more interested in patients' medical conditions or occupational therapy treatment procedures than the patients themselves did not seem to use conditional reasoning. This is often the case with less experienced therapists who are still grappling with the patients' medical conditions and are still learning about putting an occupational therapy treatment program together. Hence conditional reasoning seems to be more pervasive in the thinking of experts rather than novice therapists.[29,66]

To convey a sense of the patient's past, present, and future and to map out how therapy is progressing, the therapist may remind the patient (and self) of a time when the patient could not do a task or activity. This may be particularly useful when therapy is progressing slowly or some of the routine aspects have become boring. Importantly, these reminders show the patient and therapist how the condition is progressing and that together they may yet reach their shared vision of the future.[24] For example, to encourage Sam, Sally talks about how much improvement he has made and how this helps him toward his goal of independent living.

*Intervention Session, Part 7.* "I'm just saying to him, 'Sam, you've made such great progress.' I remind him of when he first started in the kitchen and his endurance really limited how long he could work, and we used to make really simple meals like toasted sandwiches. And now he can make a stir-fry, and he can use his right hand to stabilize very effectively when he chops vegetables, and how he can concentrate for much longer on the job. I find Sam responds really well to reminders of how far he's come and how far this will get him in the future in terms of living in a more independent home environment, and that's a real motivator to keep going in therapy."

To summarize, Mattingly and Fleming[43] use the term *conditional* in three different ways. In its most simple form, the therapist thinks about the patient's whole condition and the meaning attached to this. The therapist also thinks about how the patient's condition could change and what this would mean for the patient, and finally the therapist thinks about whether the imagined life will be achieved and realizes that this is conditioned on the patient's participation in the therapy program and the shared image of the future.

## Pragmatic Reasoning

Schell and Cervero[54] reviewed Fleming's[25] conceptualization of the three tracks of clinical reasoning and postulated theoretically that this account of reasoning neglected the reasoning surrounding the environmental influences that affect thinking and the therapist's personal context. They referred to these kinds of reasoning as pragmatic reasoning. They suggested that organizational, political, and economic constraints and opportunities affect a therapist's ability to provide an occupational therapy service, as do personal motivation, values, and beliefs. In the following example, Sally describes how at the facility in which she works, she must use the Functional Independence Measure (Adult FIM[SM], 1995) as an outcome measure.[28a]

*Evaluation Session, Part 4.* "Last week just before Sam's discharge from inpatient care, I rescored his FIM and discussed that with the team as well. We use FIM as one of our outcome measures here. I don't really mind doing it, but like I have no choice anyway since that's what management has said we'll do."

Therapy often is constrained or promoted by issues over which the therapist may have little control, such as reimbursement for service, the kinds of services and equipment that can be provided given the patient's length of stay, whether the patient can afford to purchase equipment, and the kinds of services available in the community for the patient on discharge.[64] Another important note is that pragmatic reasoning as influenced by the environmental/practice context appears to interface directly with therapists' procedural, interactive, and con-

ditional reasoning. In the earlier example, when reasoning conditionally, Sally also reasoned pragmatically about how Sam's residential options were constrained by the number of supported community housing places that were available.

Time pressures are another common source of pragmatic reasoning. Therapists must consider what can be achieved in one session or across the patient's admission. Therapists feel the pressure of patients waiting for them and having to treat more than one patient at a time. Sally also talks about having to share therapy time when the patient is at his or her best.

*Evaluation Session, Part 5.* "We are trying to gradually increase his endurance, but you get to the stage where his face is going to fall into his cereal, [and] there's no point. You just have to sort of respect that fatigue and also respect the role of the other therapists, because if I see him first, it's not fair if I exhaust the guy, and everyone else gets nothing out of him, either in physical therapy or neuropsych. assessment or whatever it may be."

My empirical research has shown that although many instances of pragmatic reasoning were found in the transcripts relating to the therapist's practice context, few related to the therapist's personal context.[64] Hence one really must question whether pragmatic reasoning is in fact only concerned with the practice context and whether the therapist's personal context is not related to clinical reasoning but to something else.

## Worldview

*Worldview* is a useful term to describe the influence of the therapists' personal views about life on their thinking and reasoning. Although Schell and Cervero[54] proposed that these personal belief and values form the personal context component of pragmatic reasoning, one has difficulty imagining that therapists could reason actively with their deeply held sociocultural beliefs.[64] Rather, personal context seems to be something that influences clinical reasoning. The term *worldview* seems to be the best way to describe the factors that make up one's personal context.[70,73] Worldview commonly is understood as an individual's underlying assumptions about life and reality.[32] Hence worldview encompasses the therapist's ethics, values, and beliefs, faith and spirituality, and motivation. If the therapist's worldview influences reasoning, then therapists also must acknowledge that this may be a positive or negative influence. Therapists also must acknowledge that they have varying degrees of insight to the influence of their worldviews on reasoning and therefore varying ability to modulate this influence if desired. The most popular method of researching clinical reasoning is for the researcher to ask the therapist to tell what he or she is thinking about after a therapy session has ended.[67] As mentioned previously, in my research, I found that therapists rarely if ever revealed any information about their world-views or how this influenced their reasoning. This is not surprising given that worldview beliefs are deeply held and that individuals find that they cannot, or may not want to, articulate these beliefs. Hence to research and gain an understanding of the influence of worldview on clinical reasoning is difficult.[64] However, in some brief glimpses to her worldview, Sally's transcripts did reveal the personal satisfaction she gains from working with patients who have neurologic problems.

*Evaluation Session, Part 6.* "I think OTs [occupational therapists] are really great at empowering people and help them to feel they are in control and they have some say. I think OTs do that better than a lot of other professions. . . . I love to work with people with disabilities, so I think if you actually enjoy the contact and seeing people achieve things, it's such a rewarding job. That comes across in your approach."

The transcripts also revealed Sally's disappointment that Sam cannot achieve what she considers to be his potential because of drug use.

*Discharge Session, Part 2.* "Even though he's motivated and you can say, 'Sam, you've just made such amazing gains,' when he does use drugs, he just loses all his cognition basically. He sits there, and his mother reports he spaces out for 24 hours at a time, and it's a real shame. I have seen this fellow going from being full assistance in absolutely every activity of daily living to being fully independent in personal care, basic domestic activities, and basic community activities, so he really has done remarkably well, so it's a bit disappointing. You try not to dwell on it too much, but it is disappointing from a therapist's point of view because you think he could just keep on improving, but the drug use is holding him back, but at the same time that's his life."

Although Mattingly and Fleming[43] did not describe worldview specifically or its relationship to clinical reasoning, their text is rich with descriptions of how the therapist's personal qualities, abilities, or style influences therapy. Further research is required, perhaps using interview techniques, to explore the relationship of therapists' worldview to clinical reasoning.[65]

### Generalizing Form of Reasoning

Finally, in each of the forms of reasoning discussed before (procedural, interactive, conditional, and pragmatic), research has shown that therapists seem to draw on their experiences to enrich the kind of reasoning in which they are engaged.[65] Rather than being described as a separate form of reasoning, this form of reasoning seems to be an extension of the other forms. I call this *generalization reasoning*. Although generalization reasoning has similarities to simple pattern recognition (as described in relation to

pragmatic reasoning), it seems to go beyond simple pattern recognition of a set of cues. Therapists seem to reason initially about a particular issue or scenario with a patient, then reflect on their general experiences related to the situation (i.e., making generalizations), and then refocus the reasoning on the patient. This seems to occur in rapid succession, as in the following excerpt in which Sally reasons interactively about how she is communicating with the patient.

*Intervention Session, Part 8.* "Often, if I can, I try to decrease the verbal cues and actually look at giving some physical cues as well. That carries right over to all of his program. Physically, even though he has significant problems in all areas in terms of transfers and bed mobility and everything. So, for example, when we do personal care, I really have to use a combination of both physical cues and verbal prompting. I'm trying to certainly decrease that. I think with Sam and a lot of patients with stroke or brain injuries, it just takes much longer for them to respond. It just doesn't go in as quickly as it does with us. My strategy with Sam at the moment is give him the instruction or prompt him and then give him some time to respond, and then go on to give him some physical guidance as well."

In summary, this generalization form of reasoning seems to enrich the other reasoning modes and also seems to be used more frequently by expert rather than novice therapists.[65]

### Putting It All Together: A Summary of the Different Modes of Reasoning

Before summarizing the different kinds of clinical reasoning and influences on reasoning such as worldview, exploration of the interaction of the three tracks of clinical reasoning is important. Although some researchers examine procedural, interactive, and conditional reasoning in isolation from each other,[29] it seems that these forms of reasoning can occur in rapid succession or even simultaneously. As described earlier, Fleming[24] described how therapists can think in "many tracks simultaneously." For example, Fleming[25] writes that "in using conditional reasoning, the therapist appears to reflect on the success or failure of the clinical encounter from both the procedural and interactive standpoints and attempts to integrate the two." Although the notion of the simultaneous use of the three tracks should not be taken too literally, therapists certainly can see evidence in their clinical reasoning transcripts of the rapid blending of different modes of reasoning. For example, Sally uses all three forms of reasoning in the following brief explanation of one aspect of her therapy session. Procedural reasoning is underlined, conditional reasoning is in bold, and interactive reasoning is italicized.

*Intervention Session, Part 9.* "Another thing I'm working on with Sam is his speed. He's very slow to process information and therefore slow in executing tasks, *and I find that he also tends to self-distract a fair bit by chatting.* But at the same time that's hard because I'm Sam's case manager, which means that I monitor his whole program, and since he's just gone home, *we have been having long chats about how he was coping at home since I want to find out how he's doing and what he's having difficulty with, whether he's following through by making his own breakfast and using his dressing aids and things like that,* so in a way I'm distracting him a little bit, *but he has to learn to cope with distractions in his environment.*"

The relationship between the three main modes of reasoning can be illustrated by the use of a Venn diagram in which the three circles each represent a different mode of reasoning and yet show that each mode does not occur in isolation from the others.[65] These three forms of reasoning are related to the other modes described in this chapter, as illustrated in Figure 17-2.[64] Figure 17-2 presents the relationships between the different forms of reasoning, or influences on clinical reasoning, using the analogy of the basic structures of the brain. Starting at the top of this figure is worldview. This was described previously in the chapter as an influence on reasoning rather than a form of reasoning. Worldview is at the top of the diagram because it influences all the modes of reasoning, and like the idea of higher cortical function, worldview represents fairly sophisticated thinking that includes one's morals, ethics, and sociocultural perspective. The next level of the brain can be described crudely as the engine or working areas. Hence, this is where the main forms of reasoning (procedural, interactive, and conditional) occur, as illustrated using a Venn diagram. These forms of reasoning are more scientific (such as procedural reasoning) or draw more on phenomenological forms of thinking and therefore can be described as narrative forms of reasoning (such as interactive and conditional reasoning). At this level, the therapist's reasoning basically is driven by the patient (such as the patient's strengths and weaknesses, goals, and desires). Finally, at the most basic level of operation, which is similar to the brainstem, is pragmatic reasoning. Similar to fundamental brain functions such as breathing, pragmatic reasoning involves thinking related to things over which therapists often do not have much control. For example, the therapist reasons pragmatically about what might be achieved with a particular patient given the patient's maximum length of stay, which often is dictated by the payment or reimbursement system. In contrast to the patient-driven forms of reasoning described previously, pragmatic reasoning is context driven. Generalized reasoning can occur in connection with procedural, interactive, conditional, and pragmatic reasoning. The arrows that flow around Figure 17-2 indicate that each influence on reasoning or form of reasoning influences the others to a greater or lesser extent. Finally, one must acknowledge that this representation of clinical reasoning operates within the patient-centered practice of occupational therapy. In other words, this diagram assumes that therapists practice within a patient-centered framework.

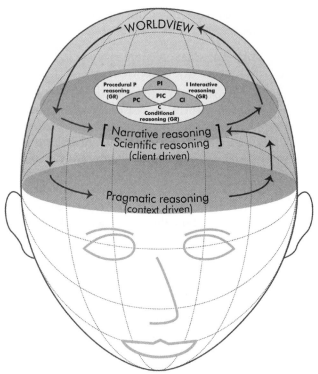

**Figure 17-2**    The relationship between the different forms of clinical reasoning within the patient-centered practice of occupational therapy. *GR,* Generalized reasoning. (From Unsworth CA: Clinical reasoning: how do pragmatic reasoning, worldview and client-centredness fit? *Br J Occup Ther* 67[1], 10-19, 2004.)

## CLINICAL REASONING AND EXPERTISE

### Differences Between the Clinical Reasoning of Novice and Expert Therapists

Over the past 15 years, research in health sciences has shown consistently that experts have better general problem solving and clinical reasoning skills than novice therapists.[61] The occupational therapy literature contains a wealth of information about the differences in the clinical reasoning of novice and expert therapists[16,29,50,60] and how students can improve their reasoning skills.[14,45-48] The purpose of this section is to review what is known about the clinical reasoning of expert therapists and strategies to enhance clinical reasoning so that students and novice therapist can hasten their own journey to expert status.

Like most skills, clinical reasoning can be graded along a continuum. Different points along the continuum are marked by certain characteristics that indicate an individual's skill level. Dreyfus and Dreyfus[20,21] presented a five-stage model of skill acquisition based on their study of chess players and airline pilots. They suggested that as students develop a skill, they pass through five stages of proficiency: novice, advanced beginner, competent, proficient, and expert. Benner[8] and Benner and Tanner[10] incorporated this model in their studies of the acquisition of skill in nursing, and since that time, most health science research regarding clinical reasoning incorporates the Dreyfus and Dreyfus model. Benner[8] suggested that as a therapist passes through the five stages of proficiency, changes in three aspects of skilled performance occur.

A shift in reliance from abstract principles to past experiences occurs, a change in perception of the situation occurs (i.e., a shift from perceiving all parts of the picture equally to viewing the whole situation in which only parts are relevant), and a change from detached observer to involved performer occurs. Based on the work of Dreyfus and Dreyfus,[20] Benner,[8] and Benner and Tanner,[10] Table 17-1 outlines the stages in the development of expertise and some of the characteristics of therapists at each stage.

Research with occupational therapists and other allied health professions has revealed a variety of aspects of clinical reasoning processes that differ between novices and experts. For example, Collins and Affeldt[16] suggest

**Table 17-1**

**Stages and Characteristics in the Development of Expertise**

| STAGE | THERAPIST CHARACTERISTICS |
| --- | --- |
| 1. Novice | Novices do not have experience of the situations in which they will be involved. To enter the clinic and gain experience in these areas, students are taught about theories, principles, and specific patient attributes.<br><br>A novice is usually rigid in the application of these rules, principles, and theories. However, rules cannot guide the therapist to do all the things that need to be done in the multitude of situations and contexts in which the therapist works.[8] A clinician can acquire only "context-dependent judgment" through participation in real situations.[48] |
| 2. Advanced Beginner | Advanced beginners have been involved in enough clinical situations to realize, or to have had pointed out to them, the recurring themes and information on which reasoning is based. An advanced beginner may begin to modify rules, principles, and theories to adapt them to the specific situation.<br><br>Advanced beginners do what they are told or what the text dictates as the correct procedure but may have difficulty prioritizing in more unusual circumstances those parts of the procedure that are least important or those aspects that are vital.<br><br>Advanced beginners have to concentrate on remembering the rules and therefore have less ability to apply them flexibly.<br><br>Dreyfus and Dreyfus[20] suggest that an awareness of the client as a person beyond the technical concerns does not usually develop until the student has advanced to this stage. |
| 3. Competent | Competent therapists are able to adjust the therapy to the specific needs of the patient and the situation but may have difficulty altering initial treatment plans. Benner[8] suggests that a therapists are competent once they are consciously aware of the outcome of their actions. This is typical of a therapist who has been in the job for 2 to 3 years. However, a competent therapist is said to lack the speed and flexibility of the proficient therapist. Efficiency and organization are achieved at this stage through conscious or deliberate planning. |
| 4. Proficient | Proficient therapists are flexible and are able to alter treatment plans as needed. Proficient therapists have a clear understanding of the patient's whole situation rather than an understanding of the components alone. Proficient practitioners have a perception of the situation based on experience rather than deliberation. Given that the proficient therapist has a perspective of the overall situation, components that are more and less important stand out, and the therapist can focus on the problem areas. |
| 5. Expert | Expert therapists approach therapy from patient-generated cues rather than preconceived therapeutic plans. Experts anticipate and quickly recognize patient strengths and weaknesses based on their experience with other patients. The expert therapist does not need to rely on rules and guidelines to take appropriate action but rather has an intuitive grasp of the situation. Experts often find it difficult to explain this intuition.[48] |

From Unsworth CA: *Cognitive and perceptual disorders: a clinical reasoning approach to evaluation and intervention,* Philadelphia, 1999, FA Davis.

that whereas novices tend to focus on one aspect of a situation and one observation triggers one association, experts can focus on many aspects of a situation and a single observation can trigger multiple associations. Although a more experienced therapist may reason holistically and react quickly to a problem with a total solution, a novice may reason step by step and react more slowly to a problem with only a partial solution. Robertson[50] supported this empirically through research that found that more experienced therapists had more integrated problem representations (that is, a well-organized body of knowledge). In addition, because occupational therapists reason in narratives, therapy is like telling or creating a story.[43] Mattingly and Fleming[43] suggest that expert therapists have a greater capacity than novices to make revisions to the story as therapy progresses.

Other differences between novices and experts include the way experts reason intuitively and have more tacit knowledge. This contrasts to the reasoning of a new practitioner, which seems to require conscious effort. Strong et al[60] reported that experts viewed gaining an understanding of their patients in terms of their illness and disability and of patients' perceptions of the effect of these on their lives as more important than did student therapists. Students placed a higher value on knowledge and understanding of the patient's problems, whereas expert therapists placed more emphasis on good communication skills. Hallin and Sviden[29] also found that expert therapists seemed to have an excellent understanding of the patient.

Finally, my research on the differences between the clinical reasoning of novices and experts[69] found that experts make complex skills look simple. The experts in this study were articulate and able to present the clinical reasoning that supported their therapy with confidence. Similar to the findings of Mattingly and Fleming,[43] Hallin and Sviden,[29] and Benner, Hooper-Kyriakidis, and Stanard,[9] experts seem to draw on their past experiences when planning and executing therapy and use this knowledge to anticipate patient performance and modify or change the therapy plan as needed. In addition, although the students in this study had had recent exposure to literature on patient-centered practice, the expert therapists appeared to have embraced this concept and were incorporating this approach in their work. Robertson[50] also noted this trend. Finally, expert therapists seemed to have a greater capacity to undertake an activity that met several patient goals or were more likely to be doing several things with the patient at once. Rather than suggesting that they were impatient or pressured by time, this finding indicated an efficiency of time use that novices had not yet developed.

### Enhancing the Student's Clinical Reasoning Skills

The progression of a therapist from novice to expertise is not assured. Although some therapists reach competent or proficient practice levels of expertise, they may never attain expert status. In addition, as can be understood from the foregoing examples, expertise is not necessarily reflected in the depth or breadth of experience nor years of practice. Therefore a relatively young therapist might possibly possess an intuitive grasp of the situation, generate therapy from patient-generated cues, recognize patient strengths and weaknesses based on past experience, and thus be considered an expert. This section presents a summary of ideas from occupational therapy literature that examines how students and novice therapists can improve their clinical reasoning and thus hasten their journey from novice to expert. More specific details of teaching strategies to enhance student's development of clinical reasoning skills may be found in Higgs[30] and Neistadt.[45]

The following list provides example strategies for novice and student therapists to try that will assist them better in honing clinical reasoning skills.

- Learn what clinical reasoning is and the different modes of reasoning. When undertaking cognitive and perceptual dysfunction coursework, try to integrate this with knowledge of clinical reasoning techniques.[45,68] In these courses, scientific and procedural forms of reasoning can dominate to the extent that insufficient attention is paid to the patient's experience of the disability, priorities, and life story.[48]
- Spend time reflecting on the patient's experience of the illness and disability and the patient's perceptions of how these affect his or her life. One might achieve this after a patient interview in which the student/therapist asks the patient about what the disability means to him or her and its effect on life.[60]
- Use case scenarios from experts to make expert therapist reasoning and hypothesis generation more explicit. In this way, students can learn to model their practice on an expert's.[50] Students can generate their own case studies and work in pairs to describe evaluation and treatment processes and thus facilitate self-evaluation and critical reflection.[45] As Mattingly and Fleming's study[43] revealed, mentoring from an expert therapist is just as influential as formal education is on a novice's practice.
- Note significant similarities and differences between patients and reflect on how these differences can influence treatment.[16]
- Develop relationships among data so that treatment planning is guided by a thorough understanding of the problem situation.[50]
- Explore probable consequences of treatments before enactment.[16]

Finally, an important way to enhance student development of clinical reasoning skills is to provide them with structured ways to reflect on their clinical encounters. A key aspect of clinical reasoning is the ability to reflect on what has been experienced in therapy and to go forward in response to this reflection. Having told stories, novice therapists need time to reflect on their meaning and significance. Expert reasoning relies on the ability to reflect on, and learn from, therapeutic encounters as an individual and from sharing experiences with other therapists. Much has been written in the medical[56] and education literature[71,72] regarding the training of doctors and teachers to be reflective. Teaching occupational therapy students and novice therapists to become more reflective by writing diary entries following therapy sessions and providing opportunities to reflect on their therapy encounters with more experienced occupational therapists also is important.

## SUMMARY

Occupational therapists who work with patients who have cognitive and perceptual problems following stroke often find themselves working in environments that are dominated by the medical model. This means that in subtle or more obvious ways occupational therapist do not always fit in with the approach taken by the rest of the team. Although most occupational therapists seem to marry scientific and phenomenological approaches to patient care successfully in practice, explaining this practice to others may prove more difficult. These explanations are hindered by the tacit nature of much of this knowledge. This chapter has explored the ways that therapists think and reason. Using Mattingly and Fleming's foundation work[43] in this field, the chapter has presented a language to describe the clinical reasoning that supports the more scientific and phenomenological approaches to patient care. Using this language helps novice and expert therapists to explain practice to colleagues and patients and helps therapists to articulate more clearly their goals and the methods used to reach them. In the challenging area of treating patients with cognitive and perceptual problems following stroke, the ability to communicate the clinical reasoning that supports practice is particularly important. The chapter concluded by presenting an overview of what we know about the differences between novice and expert practice and the role of clinical reasoning in expert practice and highlighted techniques that novice therapists can use to hasten their journey from novice to expert therapist status.

## ACKNOWLEDGMENT

I would like to thank Sheridan Vines (BAppSc.[Occ.Ther], AccOT) for sharing her rich knowledge and intuitions during a clinical reasoning research program conducted through the School of Occupational Therapy, La Trobe University. Thanks also to Geoffrey Campbell (graphic designer at Amanda Roach Designs, Windsor, Melbourne), who patiently translated my drawings of the relationship between the different modes of clinical reasoning into Figure 17-2.

## REVIEW QUESTIONS

1. What is clinical reasoning in occupational therapy?
2. Describe the difference between narrative and scientific forms of reasoning. How do Fleming's three tracks of reasoning relate to narrative and scientific forms?
3. Using first-person writing style, write a short narrative about one of your clinical encounters with a patient. Reflect on this encounter and identify in the margins what kinds of reasoning you were using at different times during the session.
4. The case study used to illustrate the chapter described Sally and Sam. Sam recently had discharged himself to home. Imagine that Sam was married with a child rather than single and that he had returned home to this environment. Also consider that Sam was working as a printer before his stroke and that he is keen to get back to this and does not use drugs. Write a chart report of your outpatient goals for Sam (i.e., a one paragraph summary that could be placed in Sam's medical record). Then write a short narrative indicating your therapy aspirations for what you and Sam hope to achieve over the next 2 months. Indicate the kind of future you predict for Sam and what kind of treatment activities you might use.
5. What are some of the hallmarks of clinical expertise?
6. What are three approaches novice therapists can use to hasten their journey from novice to expert therapist status?

## REFERENCES

1. Abreu BC: *The quadraphonic approach: management of cognitive and postural dysfunction*, New York, 1990, Therapeutic Service Systems.
2. Agency for Health Care Policy and Research: *Post stroke rehabilitation guidelines*, No 95-0662, Washington, DC, 1995, The Agency.
3. Allen CK: *Occupational therapy for psychiatric diseases: measurement and management of cognitive disabilities*, Boston, 1985, Little, Brown.
4. Alnervik A, Sviden G: On clinical reasoning: patterns of reflection on practice, *Occup Ther J Res* 16:98-110, 1996.
5. American Heart Association: *2002 heart and stroke statistics supplement*. Retrieved April 14, 2003, from www.Americanheart.org.
6. Averbuch S, Katz N: Cognitive rehabilitation: a retraining approach for brain-injured adults. In Katz N, editor: *Cognitive rehabilitation: models for intervention in occupational therapy*, Boston, 1992, Andover Medical.
7. Barnitt R, Partridge C: Ethical reasoning in physical therapy and occupational therapy, *Physiother Res Int* 2:178-194, 1997.
8. Benner P: *From novice to expert: excellence and power in clinical nursing practice*, Menlo Park, Calif, 1984, Addison-Wesley.
9. Benner P, Hooper-Kyriakidis P, Stanard D: *Clinical wisdom and interventions in critical care: a thinking-in-action approach*, Philadelphia, 1999, Saunders.
10. Benner P, Tanner C: Clinical judgment: how expert nurses use intuition, *Am J Nurs* 87(1):23-31, 1987.

11. Berlyne DE: Laughter, humor, and play. In Lindzert G, Aronson E, editors: *The handbook of social psychology*, Reading, Mass, 1969, Addison-Wesley.

12. Bradburn SL: Psychiatric occupational therapists' strategies for engaging patients in treatment during the initial interview, Unpublished master's thesis, Medford, Mass, 1992, Tufts University.

13. Canadian Association of Occupational Therapists: *Enabling occupation: an occupational therapy perspective*, Ottawa, 1997, The Association.

14. Cohn ES: Clinical reasoning: explicating complexity, *Am J Occup Ther* 45:969-971, 1991.

15. Cohn ES: Fieldwork education: shaping a foundation for clinical reasoning, *Am J Occup Ther* 43(4):240-244, 1989.

16. Collins LF, Affeldt J: Bridging the clinical reasoning gap, *Occup Ther Pract* 1:33-35, 1996.

17. Crepeau EB: Achieving intersubjective understanding: examples from an occupational therapy treatment session, *Am J Occup Ther* 45(11):1016-1025, 1991.

18. Csikszentmihalyi M: Play and intrinsic rewards, *Humanistic Psychol* 15:41-63, 1975.

19. de Renzi E: Apraxia. In Boller F, Grafman J, editor: *Handbook of neuropsychology*, vol 2, Amsterdam, 1989, Elsevier.

20. Dreyfus HL, Dreyfus SE: *Mind over machine: the power of human intuition and expertise in the era of the computer*, New York, 1986, Free Press.

21. Dreyfus SE, Dreyfus HL: A five-stage model of the mental activities involved in directed skill acquisition, Unpublished report supported by the Air Force Office of Scientific Research, USAF (Contract F49620-79-C-0063), Berkeley, 1980, University of California.

22. Elstein AS, Shulman LS, Sprafka SA: *Medical problem solving: an analysis of clinical reasoning*, Cambridge, Mass, 1978, Harvard University Press.

23. Fisher AG: An expanded rehabilitative model of practice. In Fisher AG, editor: *Assessment of motor and process skills*, ed 2, Fort Collins, Colo, 1997, Three Star Press.

24. Fleming MH: The therapist with the three track mind. In Mattingly C, Fleming MH: *Clinical reasoning: forms of inquiry in a therapeutic practice*, Philadelphia, 1994, FA Davis.

25. Fleming MH: The therapist with the three-track mind, *Am J Occup Ther* 45(11):1007-1014, 1991.

26. Fleming MH: Proceedings of the institute on clinical reasoning for occupational therapy. In *Educators*, Medford, Mass, 1990, Clinical Reasoning Institute, Tufts University.

27. Fleming MH, Mattingly C: Giving language to practice. In Mattingly C, Fleming MH: *Clinical reasoning: forms of inquiry in a therapeutic practice*, Philadelphia, 1994, FA Davis.

28. Giles GM, Wilson JC: *Occupational therapy for the brain injured adult: a neurofunctional approach*, London, 1992, Chapman & Hall.

28a. Guide for the Uniform Data Set for Medical Rehabilitation (Adult FIMSM), (1995). Version 5.0. Buffalo, NY: State University of New York at Buffalo.

29. Hallin M, Sviden G: On expert occupational therapists' reflection—on practice, *Scand J Occup Ther* 2:69-75, 1995.

30. Higgs J: Developing clinical reasoning competencies, *Physiotherapy* 78:575-581, 1992.

31. Higgs J, Jones M: *Clinical reasoning in the health professions*, ed 2, Melbourne, 2000, Butterworth-Heinemann.

32. Hooper B: The relationship between pretheoretical assumptions and clinical reasoning, *Am J Occup Ther* 51(5):328-338, 1997.

33. Kielhofner G: *The model of human occupation: theory and application*, ed 3, Philadelphia, 2002, Lippincott Williams & Wilkins.

34. Kielhofner G: *Conceptual foundations of occupational therapy*, ed 2, Philadelphia, 1997, FA Davis.

35. Kong KH, Chua KS, Tow AP: Clinical characteristics and functional outcome of stroke patients 75 years and older, *Arch Phys Med Rehabil* 79(12):1535-1539, 1998.

36. Langthaler M: The components of a therapeutic relationship in occupational therapy, Unpublished master's thesis, Medford, Mass, 1990, Tufts University.

37. Law M, Baptiste S, Carswell A, et al: *Canadian Occupational Performance Measure*, ed 2, Toronto, 1994, CAOT Publications Ace.

38. Lyons KD, Crepeau EB: The clinical reasoning of an occupational therapy assistant, *Am J Occup Ther* 55:577-581, 2001.

39. Mattingly C: The narrative nature of clinical reasoning. In Mattingly C, Fleming MH: *Clinical reasoning: forms of inquiry in a therapeutic practice*, Philadelphia, 1994, FA Davis.

40. Mattingly C: Occupational therapy as a two-body practice: the body as machine. In Mattingly C, Fleming MH: *Clinical reasoning: forms of inquiry in a therapeutic practice*, Philadelphia, 1994, FA Davis.

41. Mattingly C: What is clinical reasoning? *Am J Occup Ther* 45:979-986, 1991.

42. Mattingly C: Thinking with stories: stories and experience in a clinical practice, Unpublished doctoral dissertation, Cambridge, 1989, Massachusetts Institute of Technology.

43. Mattingly C, Fleming MH: *Clinical reasoning: forms of inquiry in a therapeutic practice*, Philadelphia, 1994, FA Davis.

44. Mattingly C, Gillette N: Anthropology, occupational therapy, and action research, *Am J Occup Ther* 45:972-978, 1991.

45. Neistadt ME: Teaching strategies for the development of clinical reasoning, *Am J Occup Ther* 50(8):676-684, 1996.

46. Neistadt ME: The classroom as clinic: applications for a method of teaching clinical reasoning, *Am J Occup Ther* 46:814-819, 1992.

47. Neistadt ME: Classroom as clinic: a model of teaching clinical reasoning in occupational therapy education, *Am J Occup Ther* 41:631-637, 1987.

48. Neistadt ME, Atkins A: Analysis of the orthopedic content in an occupational therapy curriculum from a clinical reasoning perspective, *Am J Occup Ther* 50:669-675, 1996.

49. Pedersen PM, Jorgensen HS, Nakayama H, et al: Hemineglect in acute stroke-incidence and prognostic implications: the Copenhagen stroke study, *Am J Phys Med Rehabil* 76(2):122-127, 1997.

50. Robertson LJ: Clinical reasoning, part 2: novice/expert differences, *Br J Occup Ther* 59:212-216, 1996.

51. Rogers JC: Eleanor Clarke Slagle Lectureship—1983; Clinical reasoning: the ethics, science, and art, *Am J Occup Ther* 37:601-616, 1983.

52. Rogers JC, Holm MB: Occupational therapy diagnostic reasoning: a component of clinical reasoning, *Am J Occup Ther* 45:1045-1053, 1991.

53. Rogers JC, Masagatani G: Clinical reasoning of occupational therapists during the initial assessment of physically disabled adults, *Occup Ther J Res* 2:195-219, 1982.

54. Schell BA, Cervero RM: Clinical reasoning in occupational therapy: an integrative review, *Am J Occup Ther* 47:605-610, 1993.

55. Schön DA: *Educating the reflective practitioner*, San Francisco, 1988, Jossey-Bass.

56. Schön DA: *The reflective practitioner: how professionals think in action*, New York, 1983, Basic Books.

57. Siegler CC: Functions of humor in occupational therapy, Unpublished master's thesis, Medford, Mass, 1987, Tufts University.

58. Stanton S, Thompson-Franson T, Kramer C: Linking concepts to a process for working with clients. In Townsend E, editor: *Enabling occupation: an occupational therapy perspective*, Ottawa, 1997, Canadian Association of Occupational Therapists.

59. Stone SP, Halligan PW, Greenwood RJ: The incidence of neglect phenomena and related disorders in patients with an acute right or left hemisphere stroke, *Age Ageing* 22(1):46-52, 1993.

60. Strong J, Gilbert J, Cassidy S, et al: Expert clinicians' and students' views on clinical reasoning in occupational therapy, *Br J Occup Ther* 58:119-123, 1995.

61. Thomas SA, Wearing AJ, Bennett M: *Clinical decision making for nurses and health care professionals*, Sydney, Australia, 1991, Harcourt Brace Jovanovich.

62. Toglia JP: A dynamic interactional approach to cognitive retraining. In Katz N, editor: *Cognitive rehabilitation: models for intervention in occupational therapy*, Boston, 1992, Andover Medical.

63. Trombly CA: Theoretical foundations for practice. In Trombly CA, editor: *Occupational therapy for physical dysfunction*, ed 4, Baltimore, 1995, Williams & Wilkins.

64. Unsworth CA: A new conceptualisation of clinical reasoning in occupational therapy, *Br J Occup Ther* 2004 (in press).

65. Unsworth CA: Using head-mounted video camera to explore current conceptualizations of clinical reasoning in occupational therapy, *Am J Occup Ther* 2004 (in press).

66. Unsworth CA: Clinical reasoning of novice and expert occupational therapists, *Scand J Occup Ther* 8:163-173, 2001.

67. Unsworth CA: Using a head-mounted video camera to study clinical reasoning, *Am J Occup Ther* 55:582-588, 2001.

68. Unsworth CA: *Cognitive and perceptual disorders: a clinical reasoning approach to evaluation and intervention*, Philadelphia, 1999, FA Davis.

69. Unsworth CA, Warburg CL: Assessment and treatment planning strategies for cognitive and perceptual dysfunction. In O'Sullivan SB, Schmitz TJ, editors: *Physical rehabilitation: assessment and treatment*, ed 4, Philadelphia, 2001, FA Davis.

70. Van Belle HA: *Basic intent and therapeutic approach of Carl Rogers*, Burnaby, British Columbia, 1980, Academy Press, Wedge Publishing Foundation.

71. Valli L: *Reflective teacher education: cases and critiques*, Albany, NY, 1992, State University of New York Press.

72. Witherell C, Noddings N: *Stories lives tell: narratives and dialogue in education*, New York, 1991, Teachers College Press.

73. Wolters AM: On the idea of worldview and its relationship to philosophy. In Marshall PA, Griffioen S, Mouw R, editors: *Stained glass: worldviews and social science*, New York, 1989, University Press of America.

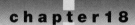

# Impact of Neurobehavioral Deficits on Activities of Daily Living

## key terms

| | | |
|---|---|---|
| activities and participation | body neglect | neurobehavior |
| activities of daily living | client factors | occupational performance |
| activity analysis | clinical reasoning | perseveration |
| agnosia | context | praxis |
| A-ONE | deficit-specific approach | spatial neglect |
| aphasia | executive control functions | spatial relations |
| areas of occupation | ideational apraxia | top-down approach |
| assessment methods | motor apraxia | |

## chapter objectives

After completing this chapter, the reader will be able to accomplish the following:

1. Establish a relationship between neurobehavioral concepts and activity performance.
2. Apply the theory on which the Árnadóttir OT-ADL Neurobehavioral Evaluation (A-ONE) is based as a structure for clinical observations of stroke patients.
3. Provide conceptual and operational definitions for neurobehavioral impairments and disability.
4. Apply clinical reasoning skills based on the A-ONE theory for hypothesis testing.
5. Relate the *International Classification of Functioning, Disability and Health* and the Occupational Therapy Practice Framework to the A-ONE theory and neurobehavioral concepts.
6. Provide examples of how strokes can cause different patterns of impairments affecting task performance.

Referrals to occupational therapy for patients who have had cerebrovascular accidents (CVAs) usually are made when the resulting impairments are suspected to affect activity performance. In the United States, 4.7 million persons with varying degrees of neurologic impairment are reported to be stroke survivors.[5] When neurobehavioral impairments result from a CVA, they can affect the performance of daily activities. This chapter contains discussions on the effect of neurobehavioral deficits on activity performance. Topics such as occupational performance, neurobehavior, function of the cerebral cortex, activity limitation, patterns of impairment resulting from different types of CVA, and application of clinical reasoning during assessment are discussed. However, before considering these issues, the following questions might be useful to consider: What are activities of daily living? What is neurobehavior? What is neurobehavioral deficit? How is neurobehavior related to activity performance? and How is the effect of neurobehavioral deficits on activity performance detected?

## ACTIVITIES OF DAILY LIVING

Activities of daily living (ADL) are defined by the U.S. Department of Health and Human Services[68] as basic daily activities such as eating, grooming, toileting, and dressing. The "Occupational Therapy Practice Framework: Domain and Process" (Framework),[50] which is an official document of the American Occupational Therapy Association, defines ADL, sometimes referred to as basic or personal activities of daily living, as activities "that are oriented toward taking care of one's own body." These activities include bathing or showering, bowel and bladder management, dressing, eating, feeding, functional mobility, personal device care, personal hygiene and grooming, sexual activity, sleep/rest, and toilet hygiene. These ADL can be classified as one of seven areas of occupational performance according to the Framework. The other six areas of occupation are instrumental activities of daily living, education, work, play, leisure, and social participation. Furthermore, five aspects of the domain of occupational therapy to which occupational therapists attend during the process of providing services in addition to areas of occupation are defined: client factors, performance skills, performance patterns, context, and activity demands.

The previously listed areas of occupation are human activities that are typically part of daily life. These areas can be broken down into specific tasks. For example, the area of dressing includes tasks such as putting on a shirt, trousers, socks, and shoes and manipulating different types of fasteners. Client factors, including body functions and structures, are the foundation of human performance. These fundamental factors residing from within the individual are required for successful performance of different tasks. The eight main groups of body

functions in the Framework based on the *International Classification of Functioning, Disability and Health* (ICF),[73] a document developed by the World Health Organization, include a group of mental functions (affect, cognition, perception) divided into global functions such as consciousness, orientation, sleep, temperament and personality, and energy and drive as well as into specific functions such as attention, memory, perceptual functions, thought, higher-level cognition, mental functions of language, calculation, motor planning, psychomotor functions, emotional functions, and functions related to experience of self and time; a group of sensory functions and pain; neuromusculoskeletal and movement-related functions; cardiovascular, hematologic, immunologic, and respiratory functions; voice and speech functions; digestive, metabolic, and endocrine functions; genitourinary and reproductive functions; and functions of skin and related structures. Each of these groups can be subdivided into smaller units or factors. For example, the group of neuromusculoskeletal and movement-related functions can be subdivided into functions of muscles and bones, muscle functions, and movement functions. Muscle functions can be divided further into muscle power, tone, and endurance. These subunits are required for task performance. The client factors or functional elements of task performance are used in different combinations and to varying degrees depending on the particular task.

The performance contexts of the Framework include cultural, physical, social, personal, spiritual, temporal, and virtual conditions that influence the engagement of the individual in performance areas.[50] The performance context therefore can provide environmental support or produce barriers. Because the occupational therapist views the individual as an occupational being,[21] the occupational therapist's center of attention is the parameter of performance areas that include different tasks. The client factors and context are viewed subsequently in relation to those tasks. Table 18-1 shows important aspects of the domain of occupation as given in the Framework, in view of the main themes of this chapter—that is, neurobehavior and ADL—and relates the Frameworks terminology to the classification systems of the ICF and the Árnadóttir OT-ADL Neurobehavioral Evaluation (A-ONE). The ICF describes three components: body structures and functions that can become impaired, activities and participation referring to capacity and performance that can become limited or restricted, and environmental factors that can act as facilitators and barriers of performance.[73]

In summary, ADL are one type of occupation or activity according to the Framework. Furthermore, *occupational performance* is the ability of an individual to accomplish activities by interaction of client factors, performance skills, performance patterns, and context of that individual.

**Table 18-1**

**Comparison of Terminologies Used in Different Classifications Systems**

| FRAMEWORK | ICF | A-ONE | |
|---|---|---|---|
| **Areas of occupation** | **Activities and participation** | **Activity performance; activities of daily living (ADL)*** | **Activity limitation: errors in task performance and possible limitation/restriction of independence resulting in required assistance** |
| Activities of daily living* | Self-care* | Dressing | Supervision needed during task performance |
| dressing* | dressing* | shirt/upper body garments | Verbal assistance needed during task performance |
| personal hygiene and grooming* | washing* | pants | Physical assistance needed during task performance |
| personal device care | caring for body parts* | socks | |
| toilet hygiene* | toileting* | shoes | |
| bathing, showering* | eating* | fastenings | |
| bowel and bladder management | drinking* | Grooming and hygiene | |
| functional mobility* | looking after one's health | wash face and upper body | |
| eating* | Communication* | comb hair | |
| feeding* | Mobility | shave/apply cosmetics | |
| sexual activity | Domestic life areas | brush teeth | |
| sleep/rest | acquisition of life necessities | toilet hygiene | |
| Instrumental activities of daily living | household tasks | bath or shower | |
| care of others | caring for household objects and assisting others | Transfers and mobility | |
| care of pets | Interpersonal interactions and relationships | sitting up in bed | |
| child rearing | Major life areas | transfers to standing or chair | |
| communication device use | education | maneuver around | |
| community mobility | work and employment | toilet transfers | |
| financial management | economic life | tub transfers | |
| health management/maintenance | Community, social, and civic life | Feeding | |
| home establishment/management | General tasks and demands | drink from mug/glass | |
| meal preparation and clean up | Learning and applying knowledge | feed with fingers | |
| safety procedures/emergency responses | purposeful sensory experiences | use fork or spoon | |
| shopping | *Activity limitation* | use knife | |
| Education | *Participation restriction* | Communication | |
| Work | | comprehension | |
| Play | | expression | |
| Leisure | | | |
| Social participation | | | |
| **Performance patterns** | **Activities, participation and personal contextual factors** | **Habits and routines are noted and used in reasoning about client factors but are not specifically addressed** | **Not addressed; related to ADL** |
| Routines | Task demands (routines) | | |
| Roles | Habits (personal context) | | |
| Habits | Limited participation | | |

| Context | Contextual factors | Contextual factors | Contextual restrictions |
|---|---|---|---|
| Cultural<br>Physical<br>Social<br>Personal<br>Spiritual<br>Temporal<br>Virtual | Environmental factors<br>physical environment<br>social environment<br>attitudinal environment<br>Personal factors<br>gender<br>race<br>lifestyle<br>habits<br>social background<br>education<br>profession | Environmental factors: Their influence on activity performance is considered and helping aids used are listed.<br>Personal factors considered for ADL.<br>gender<br>social background<br>profession | Environmental factors and possible restrictions are considered and listed.<br>Personal factors considered and listed during ADL performance:<br>gender<br>profession<br>social background |
| **Client factors (based on ICF; see next column)**<br>Body functions*<br>Body structures | **Body functions***<br>Neuromusculoskeletal and movement-related functions:<br>Functions of joints and bones<br>Muscle functions*<br>  power (strength)<br>  tone (flaccid/spastic)<br>  endurance<br>Movement functions*<br>  motor reflex<br>  involuntary movement reaction (righting and supporting reactions)<br>  control of voluntary movement (eye-hand coordination, bilateral integration, eye-foot coordination)<br>  involuntary movement functions (tremors, ticks, motor perseveration)<br>  gait pattern functions<br>Sensory functions* and pain<br>  proprioception<br>  touch/temperature/pressure/discrimination<br>  seeing (visual acuity, visual fields)<br>  hearing<br>  vestibular<br>  taste<br>  smell<br>  pain | **Central nervous system function**<br>Motor function<br><br>Sensory reception and simple gnosis<br>tactile<br>proprioceptive/kinesthetic<br>visual<br>auditory | **Neurobehavioral dysfunction/impairments**<br>Motor dysfunction<br>diminished strength<br>altered tone:<br>spasticity/rigidity/flaccidity<br>athetosis, tremor, or involuntary movements<br>motor perseverations<br>motor impersistence<br>dysarthria<br><br>Agnosia<br>astereognosis<br>visual agnosia<br>auditory agnosia related to comprehension |

Continued

**Table 18-1**

## Comparison of Terminologies Used in Different Classifications Systems—cont'd

| FRAMEWORK | ICF | | A-ONE | |
|---|---|---|---|---|
| | Mental functions (affective, cognitive, perceptual) | General performance | Impaired general performance | |
| | Global: | | | |
| | consciousness* | Alertness | impaired alertness | |
| | orientation (to person, place, time, self, and others)* | Orientation is considered under memory and topographical disorientation | | |
| | sleep | | | |
| | | initiative | impaired initiative | |
| | | motivation | impaired motivation | |
| | temperament and personality* energy and drive (motivation,* impulse control,* interests,* values) | temperament and personality are considered in relation to emotional functions | | |
| | Specific: | | | |
| | attention* | Attention | Attention and arousal dysfunctions | |
| | | | impaired alertness | |
| | | | altered attention | |
| | | | distractibility | |
| | | | performance latency | |
| | memory* | Memory | Memory dysfunction | |
| | | | working and short-term memory | |
| | | | long-term memory | |
| | | | orientation | |
| | | | confabulation | |
| | mental functions of sequencing complex movement (praxis)* | Praxis | Apraxia | |
| | | ideation | ideational apraxia | |
| | | sequencing and timing of activity steps | motor apraxia | |
| | | programming of motor movement | impaired organization and sequencing of activity steps | |
| | perception* | Spatial relations | Spatial relations dysfunction | |
| | | foreground/background | spatial relations impairment | |
| | | depth/distances | topographic disorientation | |
| | | Body scheme | Body scheme dysfunction | |
| | | | anosognosia | |
| | | | somatoagnosia | |
| | thought* (recognition, categorization, generalization, awareness of reality, logical/ coherent thought, appropriate thought content) | Higher cognitive and executive functions | Cognitive disturbances | |
| | | judgment | lack of judgment | |
| | | insight | decreased insight | |
| | | abstract thinking | concrete thinking | |
| | | | confusion | |

| | | |
|---|---|---|
| higher-level cognition* (judgment, concept formation, time management, problem solving, decision making) calculation | | |
| psychomotor functions | | |
| experience of self and time functions | | |
| emotional functions | Emotional functions | Emotional disturbances<br>apathy<br>depression<br>lability<br>euphoria<br>irritability<br>aggression<br>frustrations<br>restlessness |
| mental functions of language* (reception and expression) | Language functions<br>comprehension<br>expression | Language dysfunction<br>Sensory (Wernicke's) aphasia<br>jargon aphasia<br>anomia<br>paraphasia<br>expressive (Broca's) aphasia<br>dysarthria |
| Voice and speech functions<br>articulation functions<br>fluency and rhythm of language functions<br>alternative vocalization functions | | |
| *Impairments*<br>Body structures<br>Nervous system* | | |

From Árnadóttir G: *A-ONE training course: lecture notes*, Reykjavík, Iceland, 2003, Guðrún Árnadóttir. Material drawn from Occupational therapy practice framework: domain and process, *Am J Occap Ther* 56(6):609-639, 2002; World Health Organization: *The international classification of impairments, of functioning, disability and health—ICF,* Geneva, 2001, The Organization; and *The brain and behavior: assessing cortical dysfunction through activities of daily living,* St Louis, 1990, Mosby. Selected samples related to occupational performance with a specific focus on activities of daily living and neurology.
*Item relates to A-ONE terminology.

## NEUROBEHAVIOR: THE PROCESS OF LINKING OCCUPATION TO NEURONAL ACTIVITY

*Neurobehavior* is, according to Árnadóttir,[7,9] defined as "behavior based on neurological function, in particular occupational behavior, also referred to as occupational performance. Elements of neurobehavior include different types of sensory stimuli provided by different tasks. These stimuli are processed by different mechanisms of the central nervous system (CNS) and result in different types of behavioral responses. Feedback from the responses affects new sensory stimuli."[9] Neurobehavior therefore includes the different types of pertinent neurologic client factors, also referred to as *body functions*, necessary for performing different aspects of occupation. "All tasks provide sensory stimuli. Some factors relate to the reception of sensory stimuli, others to CNS processing of that information including for example different factors associated with perception, cognition, emotion, and praxis. Additional factors or functions relate to different behavioral responses, such as affect and movement. The mechanism of nervous-system processing and neurobehavior leading to occupational performance is a complex interaction where different combinations of factors are involved depending on the task."[7,9,12] Figure 18-1 illustrates the elements of neurobehavior. A *neurobehavioral deficit* is defined by Árnadóttir[7,12] as a functional impairment of an individual manifested as defective task performance resulting from a neurologic processing dysfunction that affects client factors such as affect, body scheme, cognition, emotion, gnosis, language, memory, motor movement, perception, personality, praxis, sensory awareness, spatial relations, and visuospatial skills.

## THEORETICAL RELATIONSHIP BETWEEN OCCUPATIONAL PERFORMANCE AND NEUROBEHAVIOR

The relationship between neurobehavior and ADL may be best described from a theoretical perspective. The theory behind the A-ONE[12] explains how neurobehavior is related to ADL. This is a factor-relating theory, according to the conceptual framework described by Dickoff, James, and Wiedenbach,[27] because following the development of terminology including definitions, the theory relates factors of neurobehavioral body functions to ADL task performance. The A-ONE theory proposes a relationship between different factors: the ability to perform daily activities, neurobehavioral impairments, and the CNS origin of the neurobehavioral dysfunction. In other words, a relationship between daily activities and neuronal processing is proposed. Research studies that support these statements have been conducted, and some of them indicate that impairments cause activity limitation, thus raising the theory to the situation-producing or third level of theory development.[8,12,31,32,60]

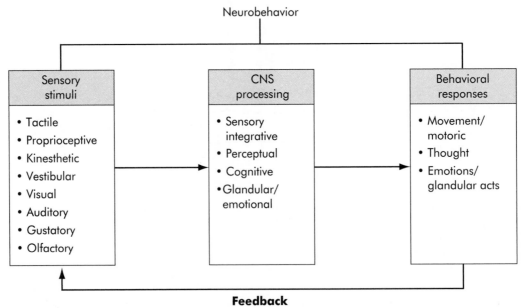

**Figure 18-1**    Elements of neurobehavior include different types of sensory stimuli. These stimuli are processed by different mechanisms in the central nervous system (CNS) and result in different types of behavioral responses. Feedback from the responses affects new sensory stimuli. (Adapted from Llorens LA: Activity analysis: agreement among factors in a sensory processing model, *Am J Occup Ther* 40:103, 1986.)

## DETECTING THE EFFECT OF NEUROBEHAVIORAL DEFICITS ON ACTIVITY PERFORMANCE

The therapist can detect the effect of neurobehavioral deficits through observation of occupational performance. Because neurobehavioral deficits often interfere with independence, therapists can benefit from detecting these impairments while observing ADL and can gain an understanding of the factors affecting the patient's activity limitation. Subsequently, therapists could begin determining the most pertinent intervention method.[12] Therapists can use a systematic analysis of occupational performance as a structure for clinical reasoning to help them assess functional independence related to task performance and to detect dysfunctional neurologic client factors. Such information can be important when intervention methods are aimed at simultaneous activation of activity and impairment levels, deficit specific approaches or rehabilitation frame of reference in which emphasis is on educating the patient's social support system. This method allows the therapist to analyze the nature or cause of a functional problem that requires occupational therapy intervention, as recommended by Holm and Rogers,[37,57] and so make the analysis from the view of occupations.

Activity analysis has been referred to commonly as the process of examining activities in detail by breaking them into their components to understand and evaluate tasks. Therapists study client factors that are needed to perform specific skills or tasks and the effects impaired client factors have on task performance.[12,41] Blesedell Crepeau[17] describes three types of activity analysis: task-, theory-, and individual-focused analysis. In task-focused activity analysis the following aspects are considered: the range of skills and components needed to perform the activity, typical performance methods, performance context, cultural meaning of the activity, and the therapeutic potential of the activities. Theory-focused activity analysis is performed with intervention potential in mind. In this case, the therapist makes the analysis by focusing on performance problems based on definitions of function and dysfunction as related to a particular theory. Individual-focused activity analysis, however, focuses on the client as opposed to the activity. Activity knowledge as related to therapeutic principles is integrated with the client's goals. Other important aspects of this type of analysis are interests, strengths, and needs of the patient and the performance context.

In the A-ONE, the therapist uses activity analysis to identify different client factors and possible manifestations of CNS dysfunction during ADL performance. During the instrument development of the A-ONE, activity analysis was used to determine which client factors are necessary for performance of particular tasks and how dysfunction of specific factors is revealed by neurobehavioral responses during performance of activities. As during the A-ONE focused activity analysis, the therapist keeps in mind different possible neurologic factors and impairments and the theoretical definitions of functional and dysfunctional behavior, thus the analysis goes beyond traditional task focused activity analysis. The analysis could be classified as theory focused, however. Because "occupation" refers to activities of everyday life performed with the aim of occupying oneself and "occupational performance" is the ability to carry out the previously mentioned activities,[50] one could refer to a theory-focused analysis of occupational performance when applying the A-ONE. An example might explain this process better. A meaningful task, such as eating, calls for a goal-directed, purposeful response. Various factors are involved, such as food and cutlery, as well as client factors such as visuospatial relationships, muscle tone, and emotional state. Carrying out the behavior required to eat requires different client factors. When analyzed with the required factors in mind, the quality of the response reveals information not only about independence in ADL but also regarding neurobehavioral impairments—the problems that interfere with independence, such as misjudging distances when reaching out for a cup or not knowing how to use cutlery[12] (Figure 18-2). The focus is thus on activity or occupational performance and how it is limited by impairments in view of the A-ONE theory, not on impairments.

### Function of the Cerebral Cortex: The Foundation of Task Performance

Occupational therapists observe performance of daily activities regularly as they work with stroke patients. With the use of activity analysis, detection of components of occupational performance or client body factors is possible, including functions and structures, by applying the terminology used by the ICF and the Framework. These factors are necessary for activity performance. Subsequently, therapists can detect the type and degree of severity of neurobehavioral impairments that interfere with activity performance. The body functions then can be related to functional areas of the brain responsible for different neurologic processing functions. Many of the client body factors are based on neurologic function, which takes place at different levels of the CNS. According to Árnadóttir,[12] several CNS areas may contribute to a particular type of neurologic processing, resulting in simultaneous or parallel processing at different locations, which contributes to processing of the same body functions. During activity performance, different types of processing may be taking place simultaneously. Neuronal processing in the brain varies in complexity. Viewing three levels of functional complexity in the cortex based on Luria's theories[42,43] is common. These commonly are called *primary*, *secondary*, and *tertiary cortical zones* or *projection areas*.

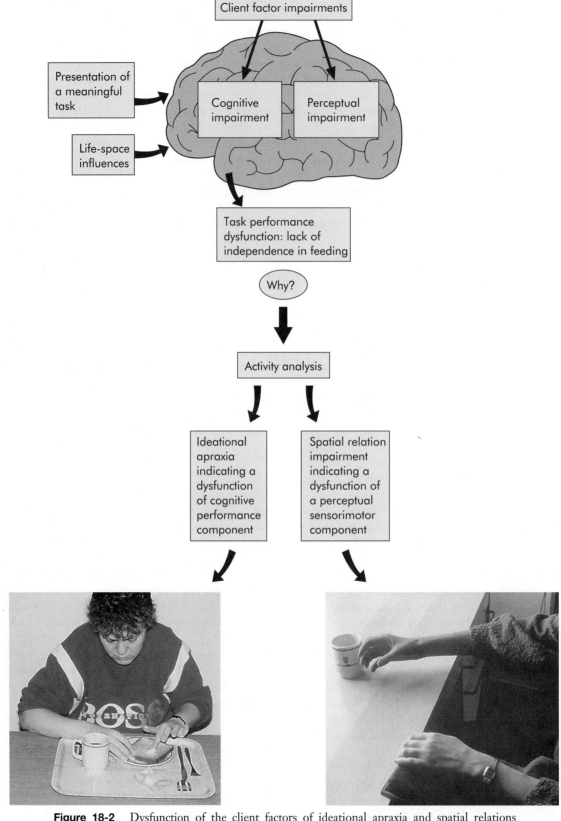

**Figure 18-2**   Dysfunction of the client factors of ideational apraxia and spatial relations impairment revealed by activity analysis during the observation of feeding performance. (Adapted from Árnadóttir G: *The brain and behavior: assessing cortical dysfunction through activities of daily living,* St Louis, 1990, Mosby.)

## Functional Localization for Neurologic Processing of Client Body Factors

Primary areas are concerned with direct processing of primary sensory and motor information. These areas include the primary somesthetic sensory cortex in the postcentral gyrus of the parietal lobe, the primary visual cortex around the calcarine fissure on the medial side of the occipital lobe, the primary auditory cortex in the superior temporal gyrus of the temporal lobe, and the primary motor cortex in the precentral gyrus of the frontal lobe.[12]

All cortical areas, other than the primary ones, are association areas that (except for the motor association cortex) receive information from the primary areas and integrate it with information from other areas. The secondary association areas are adjacent to and connected with primary cortical areas. They are involved in more complex processing aspects of a single sensory or motor function. These areas include the visual association cortex surrounding the primary visual cortex in the occipital lobe, the auditory association cortex in the temporal lobe, the somatosensory association area in the superior parietal lobule, and the premotor cortex in the frontal lobe.[12]

The tertiary, or higher-order, association areas are involved in complex integration of information from many different cortical areas. Three such higher-order cortical association areas exist: the prefrontal cortex, the limbic cortex, and the parietotemporaloccipital cortex, on the border of the three posterior lobes. The dorsolateral prefrontal cortex is involved in complex motor functions, concept formation, abstraction, intelligence, judgment, attention, intention, sequencing, and timing and organization of activity steps and behavior as well as emotional processing. The limbic association cortex includes the orbitofrontal part of the prefrontal cortex, the temporal pole, and the parahippocampal gyrus on the medial aspects of the temporal lobes and the cingulate gyrus of the cortex. The limbic association cortex is concerned with memory and with motivation and emotional aspects of behavior. The parietotemporo-occipital cortex is involved with processing of complex sensory functions based on information from two or more of the secondary association areas of the three posterior lobes. Figure 18-3 illustrates functional organization of the cerebral cortex.[12] Although function can be related to different anatomic areas, one must remember that plasticity permits deviations from the usual localization sites under certain conditions such as injury or developmental abnormality.

To summarize, the frontal lobes are responsible for motor functions, including motor speech; motor praxis; emotions; intelligence; cognition including attention and working memory; and executive control functions such as ideation, intention, judgment, and motivation. This refers to neuromusculoskeletal and movement-related factors, including muscle and movement functions, according to the ICF terminology; voice and speech functions; and global and specific mental functions. The parietal lobes are concerned with the processing of somesthetic information—and more complex sensory input from different sources, which includes sensory reception of somesthetic information—and specific mental functions related to memory and sequencing of complex movement as well as to perception and emotional functions, according to the ICF. The occipital lobes process visual information (i.e., visual sensory functions and specific mental functions related to visual perception), and the temporal lobes process auditory information and long-term memory, emotion, and motivation. These functions are classified by the ICF as sensory functions of hearing, voice, and speech functions, global mental functions of temperament and personality, and specific mental functions of memory, perception of hearing, and emotional functions. Table 18-2 summarizes the functions of the different cortical lobes of the brain and relates them to primary, secondary, and tertiary functional areas in these lobes. As indicated in the table, several functional areas in different lobes may contribute to a particular neurologic function. Therefore different cortical areas may be responsible for processing particular neurologic body functions or client factors.

When considering CNS localization of client factors necessary for task performance, the therapist must keep in mind that the cortex does not function in isolation. The cortex communicates by various pathways with other CNS areas that also contribute to neuronal processing, including the thalamus, which contains nuclei that relay information to and from the cortex. The thalamus is involved in sensory, motor, emotional, memory, and complex mental functions. The hypothalamus affects automatic functions, such as endocrine and emotional functions, and regulation of metabolism, temperature, and sleep. The basal ganglia and cerebellum affect coordination and tone of motor functions. The cerebellum also is involved in equilibrium. The brainstem houses fiber tracts that bring information to and from the cortex as well as different types of nuclei and the reticular formation. Reticular formation plays an important role in alertness and attention and contributes to cardiovascular and respiratory control.

## Processing of Praxis

Although certain neurologic functions can be assigned to specific cortical or subcortical locations within lobes, several CNS areas help process particular neurologic body functions.[12] Árnadóttir[12] summarized neurologic information resulting in several different processing models indicating processing sites of different functions in the cortex. One example is the processing model for praxis. Praxis takes place in two steps: ideation, referring to concept

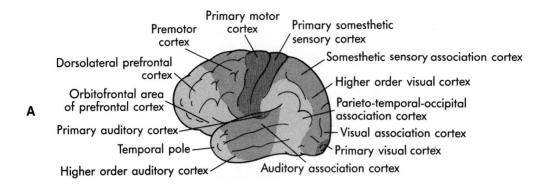

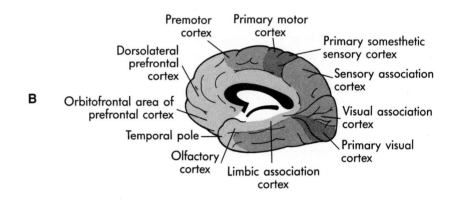

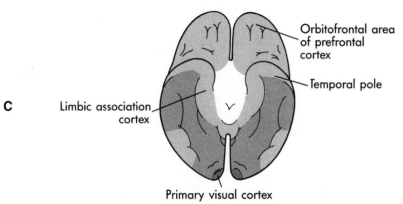

**Figure 18-3**    Functional organization of the cerebral cortex. **A,** Lateral surface. **B,** Medial surface. **C,** Inferior surface. The different shades refer to primary, secondary, and tertiary functional areas of the cortex. (From Árnadóttir G: *The brain and behavior: assessing cortical dysfunction through activities of daily living,* St Louis, 1990, Mosby.)

formation related to an activity, classified by the ICF and the Framework as the client factors of specific mental function related to thought and higher level cognition including sequencing of complex movement; and planning and programming of movement,[13] which can be related to the neuromusculoskeletal and movement-related functions of the ICF. The result of praxis is motor execution.[4] The ideation involved in praxis requires function of the frontal lobes (prefrontal and premotor areas) and of areas around the lateral fissure. The visuokinesthetic motor engrams or memory molecules for movement are stored in the left inferior part of the parietal

lobe,[35] the left hemisphere in general being superior in storing routinely used codes.[34] Access to the left inferior parietal lobe is needed for either side of the body to move. Information goes from this area to the premotor area, which programs movement before the information is conveyed to the primary motor cortex in the left hemisphere (which controls execution of movements of the right side of the body). The premotor cortex on the left side connects with the premotor cortex of the right side by way of the anterior fibers of the corpus callosum and in turn relays the visuokinesthetic motor information to the right hemisphere. The right premotor cortex pro-

**Table 18-2**

## Functions of the Cerebral Cortex

| FUNCTIONAL AREA | ANATOMIC AREA | CLIENT FACTORS: NEUROLOGIC BODY FUNCTIONS |
|---|---|---|
| **Frontal lobes** | | |
| Primary motor area | Precentral gyrus | Execution of movement |
| Secondary association area | Premotor cortex | Planning and programming of movement |
| | Frontal eye field | Sequencing, timing, and organization of movement |
| | Broca's area in the left inferior frontal gyrus | Voluntary eye movements |
| | Supplementary motor area | Programming of motor speech |
| | | Intention of movement |
| Tertiary association area | Orbitofrontal and dorsolateral prefrontal cortex | Ideation |
| | | Concept formation |
| | | Abstract thought |
| | | Intellectual functions |
| | | Sequencing, timing, and organization of action and behavior |
| | | Initiation and planning of action |
| | | Judgment |
| | | Insight |
| | | Intention |
| | | Attention |
| | | Alertness |
| | | Personality |
| | | Working memory |
| | | Emotion |
| **Parietal lobes** | | |
| Primary somesthetic sensory area | Postcentral gyrus | Fine touch sensation, proprioception, kinesthesia |
| Secondary somesthetic sensory association area | Superior parietal lobule | Coordination, integration, and refinement of sensory input |
| | | Tactile localization and discrimination |
| | | Stereognosis |
| Tertiary association area | Inferior parietal lobule | *Gnosis:* recognition of received tactile, visual, and auditory input |
| | | *Praxis:* storage of programs or visuokinesthetic motor engrams necessary for motor sequences |
| | | *Body scheme:* postural model of body, body parts, and their relation to the environment |
| | | *Spatial relations:* processing related to depth, distance, spatial concepts, position in space, and differentiation of foreground from background |
| **Occipital lobes** | | |
| Primary visual sensory area | Calcarine fissure | Visual reception (from the opposite visual field) |
| Visual association area | Brodmann's areas 18 and 19 | Synthesis and integration of visual information |
| | | Perception of visuospatial relationships |
| | | Formation of visual memory traces |
| | | Prepositional construction of language comprehension and speech |

*Continued*

**Table 18-2**

## Functions of the Cerebral Cortex—cont'd

| FUNCTIONAL AREA | ANATOMIC AREA | CLIENT FACTORS: NEUROLOGIC BODY FUNCTIONS |
|---|---|---|
| **Temporal lobes** | | |
| Primary auditory sensory area | Superior temporal gyrus | Auditory reception |
| Secondary association area | Superior and middle temporal gyri (Wernicke's area) | Language comprehension |
| | | Sound modulation |
| | | Perception of music |
| | | Auditory memory |
| Tertiary association area | Temporal pole, parahippocampus | Long-term memory |
| | | Learning of higher-order visual tasks and auditory patterns |
| | | Emotion |
| | | Motivation |
| | | Personality |
| **Limbic lobes** | | |
| Tertiary association area | Orbitofrontal cortex in frontal lobe, temporal pole, and parahippocampus in the temporal lobe | Attention |
| | | Motivation |
| | | Emotions |
| | Cingulate gyrus in frontal and parietal lobes | Long-term memory |

Adapted from Árnadóttir G: *The brain and behavior: assessing cortical dysfunction through activities of daily living*, St Louis, 1990, Mosby.

grams movements and instructs the adjacent primary motor cortex on the execution of movement of the left side of the body (Figure 18-4).

## PROCESSING DURING TASK PERFORMANCE

Motor praxis (as described previously) is only one type of neurologic body function related to neurobehavior. The type of client factor and the degree of involvement depend on the task to be performed. As mentioned, several processing mechanisms may be involved simultaneously in the performance of a particular activity. Árnadóttir has demonstrated this through analysis of activity such as brushing hair.[12] A person sitting in front of a mirror by a sink where the brush is located has three routes by which sensory information related to this particular task will reach the cortex. The person notes the brush visually, and this information travels through the visual pathway to the primary visual cortex where it is synthesized and further analyzed by the association areas. Memories and ideational processes are brought into play; as a result, the person gets the idea to want to brush the hair. Similarly, when the person is instructed verbally to brush the hair, this auditory input travels over the auditory pathway to the primary auditory area of the cortex in the temporal lobe where it is processed by the association areas. Subsequently, the input is compared with informa-

tion in memory stores, yielding an idea based on the auditory information.

The third pathway is somesthetic. A person who grasps or is handed a brush receives tactile and proprioceptive information, which (after it reaches the primary sensory cortex in the parietal lobe) is analyzed by the association areas and integrated with prior experiences.

Information from all three pathways travels from the pertinent primary receptive areas to secondary and tertiary areas where further processing takes place. Attention processes, memory processes, emotions, and higher-order thought are brought into play. The sensory information is integrated with previous experiences, and responses are planned. A response may be emotional or motoric, resulting in different processing mechanisms depending on the nature of the response. Simultaneous processing of information takes place as information from the different secondary association areas is fed into the limbic system, the tertiary association areas in the prefrontal lobe, and the temporal pole, where higher cognitive functions including emotion and memory take place. Different fiber connections in a hemisphere, between hemispheres, and between the cortex and other CNS structures play important roles in this processing.

During processing, ideation, intent to perform an action, and preparation of a sequenced plan of action occur; all result in flow of information to the primary

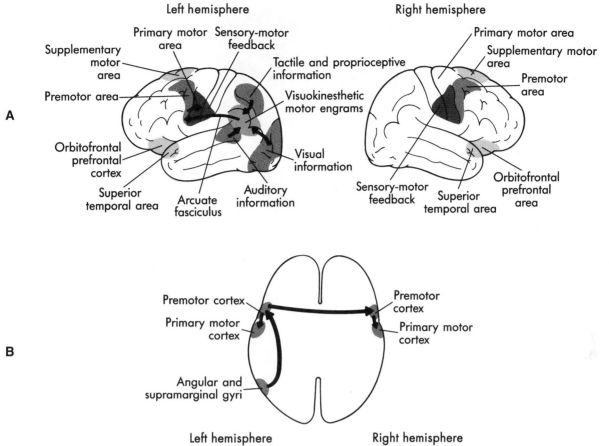

**Figure 18-4**    Processing of motor praxis. **A,** Active functional areas of the left and right hemispheres during praxis. **B,** Transverse view of the most commonly accepted sequential processing model of motor praxis.[35] (From Árnadóttir G: *The brain and behavior: assessing cortical dysfunction through activities of daily living,* St Louis, 1990, Mosby.)

motor cortex and ultimately in the functional response of picking up the brush. This process requires praxis. The intention to perform an action is relayed to the frontal lobes and supplementary motor areas. From the lower left parietal lobe (which houses visuokinesthetic motor engrams), information travels to the left premotor cortex (which is responsible for planning and sequencing of movement) on its way to the middle part of the primary motor cortex of the frontal lobe in the left hemisphere (which is responsible for movement performed by the right hand). A series of feedback movement interactions and readjustments follow. This series is based on continuous sensory information from the activity. During the complex process of performing "simple" activity, other responses (e.g., emotional and verbal) may be elicited. Such responses require function of processing areas different from the ones mentioned previously. Figure 18-5 illustrates some of the processing components that take place during the activity of brushing hair. The task performance that results from this kind of processing may reveal substantial information about function and subsequent dysfunction of the cerebral cortex.

## DYSFUNCTION OF THE ACTIVITIES OF DAILY LIVING AREA OF OCCUPATION AS A RESULT OF CERBROVASCULAR ACCIDENTS

Cerebrovascular accidents may affect neurologic client factors. Dysfunction of these factors may interfere subsequently with primary ADL. Neurobehavioral impairments may be related to dysfunction of neurologic body functions, which have been classified into four groups according to the ICF[73] on which the client factors of the *Framework*[50] are based. These groups are (1) neuromuscular functions, (2) sensory functions and pain, (3) mental functions, and (4) voice and speech functions. These functions have been related previously to concepts used in the A-ONE theory in Table 18-2. The terms may be defined in two ways. A concept traditionally is used for a general, abstract idea. Conceptual definitions are definitions of the concepts themselves, generalized and abstract. Conceptual definitions can be found in dictionaries. However, operational definitions refer to how particular concepts are measured and observed (e.g., test items with which particular concepts can be measured).

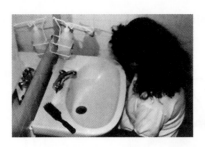

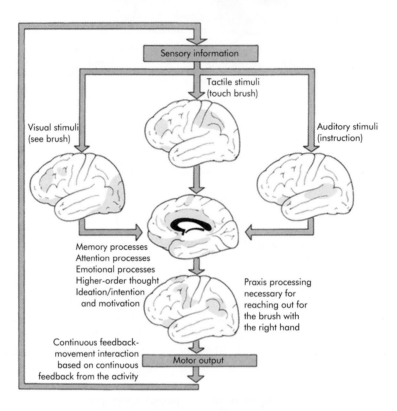

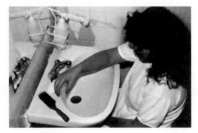

**Figure 18-5**    Different cortical areas involved in processing of various client factors during an activities of daily living task. A person sitting by a sink preparing for grooming is asked to brush her hair. Note that three types of sensory stimulation can lead to performance. (From Árnadóttir G: *The brain and behavior: assessing cortical dysfunction through activities of daily living,* St Louis, 1990, Mosby.)

The content of the following sections are based on concepts from the A-ONE.

### Conceptual Definitions of Terms

The frontal lobes process functions related to neuromusculoskeletal and movement-related client factor functions including muscle and movement functions, according to the ICF terminology; voice and speech functions; and global and specific mental functions.[7] Dysfunction of the frontal lobes, for example, may affect neuromusculoskeletal body functions processed in the primary motor and premotor areas. Subsequently, the therapist may observe impairments including paralysis of the contralateral body side, muscle weakness, and spasticity. The distribution of impairments is related to lesion localization in the primary motor cortex. Table 18-3 includes definitions of impairments or dysfunction of neurologic client factors and relates these to different cerebral lobes.[7,12]

The parietal lobes process somatosensory and complex sensory information from multimodal stimuli. When a dysfunction of the parietal lobes occurs, impairments related to different functional areas may develop, and these can be related to dysfunctions of client factors, in particular somesthetic sensory functions and specific mental functions.[12] Dysfunction of the inferior parietal lobe, which processes information from the secondary association areas of all three posterior lobes, for example, may lead to impairments related to perceptual and motor processing of client factors, in particular specific mental functions related to sequencing of complex movement, memory, and perception. These impairments include motor and ideational apraxia, if the left inferior parietal lobe is involved, because the visuokinesthetic motor engrams are stored in this area. Spatial relations disorders also may be present. These disorders have been defined conceptually as difficulties in relating objects to each other or to the self. Such difficulties may include difficulties with foreground and background perception, depth and distance perception, perception of form constancy, perception of position in space, or constructional apraxia.[12] See Table 18-3 for definitions of terms and different lesion sites.

The occipital lobe houses primary and secondary processing areas for visual information. The tertiary area for visual processing is located mainly in the inferior parietal lobe. If a dysfunction of the occipital lobe occurs, impairments are related to visual sensory functions and specific mental functions related to perception of visual information referring to the Framework classification of client factors.[7] Lesions of the association area, for example, cause visual agnosia. Different types of visual agnosias exist, including visual object agnosia; visuospatial agnosia, which is a spatial relations disorder of visual origin; prosopagnosia; color agnosia; and associative visual agnosia.[12] Visual object agnosia is defined conceptually as the inability of a patient to recognize, name, or demonstrate use of objects seen and results from distorted visual perception, regardless of visual acuity.[62] The affected person can see and describe the components of the object but cannot recognize the object itself (see Table 18-3 for additional definitions of terms and lesion sites).[12]

The temporal lobes are involved with two types of processing—auditory and limbic—that can be related to sensory functions of hearing, voice and speech functions, global mental functions of temperament and personality, and specific mental functions of memory, perception of hearing, and emotional functions. The lateral sides of the hemispheres house primary and secondary processing sites for auditory stimuli and perceptual processing of such information. The tertiary processing area for these functions is located in the inferior part of the parietal lobe.[7] A lesion of the auditory association cortex in the left hemisphere, for example, can cause anomia because the memory stores for nouns are located in this area. Anomia is loss of the ability to name objects or retrieve names of persons; the person does have fluent speech. As previously, Table 18-3 relates defined impairments to dysfunction of different cortical and subcortical areas.

## Manifestation of Neurobehavioral Impairments During Task Performance: Operational Definitions of Concepts

Operational definitions are how concepts are measured and observed. Following is a review based on Árnadóttir's operational definitions of terms[12] from the A-ONE regarding how one can detect neurobehavioral impairments during task performance in the areas of grooming and hygiene, dressing, functional mobility, eating, and functional communication. Each of these performance areas comprises several tasks. For successful completion of each of the tasks, involvement of several neurologic client factors is necessary. Dysfunction of client factors resulting in the previously defined impairments is manifested differently during performance. The following examples indicate the effect of different impairments on task performance in the various performance areas. This review refers to the terms used in the classification systems of the Framework and the ICF (see Table 18-3 for conceptual and operational definitions of terms). Some impairments affect specific ADL areas. Other impairments are more pervasive and may appear in any ADL performance area or may need to be addressed specifically. One must keep in mind that behavior is flexible and neurobehavioral impairments are complex. Some have similar factors—such as the impairments of unilateral body neglect and unilateral spatial neglect, which both include attention to stimuli—and may be manifested similarly. For others the anatomic neuronal networks lie close together. The following behavioral examples are guidelines for detecting impairments. However, they cannot be taken for granted without knowledge of neurobehavior, cortical function, activity analysis, and clinical reasoning because similar behaviors may result from different impairments at times. Thus the behavior of not washing one arm during the task of washing the upper part of the body may be caused by unilateral body neglect when it occurs in an individual with right hemisphere dysfunction. However, an individual with left hemisphere dysfunction may need assistance to wash the affected arm, partly because of motor paralysis, and also may need guidance to wash the other arm and body parts because of ideation problems and difficulty in organizing and

*Text continued on p. 400*

**Table 18-3**

## Cortical Impairments as Related to Anatomic Location and Definitions of Terms*

| IMPAIRMENT AND CORTICAL LOCATION | CONCEPTUAL DEFINITION | OPERATIONAL DEFINITION |
|---|---|---|
| **Aggression** | | |
| Prefrontal cortex, hypothalamus, medial forebrain bundle | Angry, destructive ideas or behaviors intended to be physically or emotionally injurious and aimed at domination; may be manifested as hostility and attacking and destructive behavior | Shows hostility or aggression toward activity or persons; may throw things at therapist when therapist tries to encourage performance |
| **Impaired alertness** | | |
| Prefrontal cortex, particularly orbitofrontal area; reticular formation | A basic arousal process "in which the awake person is unable to respond to any stimulus in the environment"[62] | Is more or less unaware of what is going on in surrounding environment |
| **Anomia** | | |
| Auditory association cortex on the lateral side of the left temporal lobe | Loss of the ability to name objects or retrieve names of persons; fluent speech | Has difficulty finding names of objects |
| **Anosognosia** | | |
| Right inferior parietal lobule; specific sensory thalamic nuclei, reticular formation, basal ganglia; prefrontal and premotor frontal lobe[59] | Denial or lack of awareness of a paretic extremity accompanied by lack of insight regarding the paralysis; paralyzed extremities may be referred to as objects or perceived out of proportion to other body parts | Does not identify a paralyzed body part as own; may deny it completely as a separate object or recognize it and reject it (e.g., patient may complain about "somebody's" arm and not recognize it as own) |
| **Apathy** | | |
| Prefrontal cortex; posterior internal capsule, basal ganglia[59], medial forebrain bundle and reticular formation | Shallow affect, psychomotor slowing, blunted emotional responses, lack of interest in the environment and inaction | Has a lack of emotion or feeling during activity performance and communication, lack of interest in things that generally are found exciting, and indifference during performance |
| **Astereognosis** | | |
| Superior parietal lobule | Sometimes referred to as *tactile agnosia*; failure to recognize objects, forms, size, and shape of objects by touch alone; includes failure of shape discrimination, texture, size, and weight. Refers to a failure of somesthetic recognition (tactile and proprioceptive), although somesthetic reception of tactile and proprioceptive stimuli is still intact | Needs to observe performance to accomplish dressing activity; unable to button shirt unless compensating by observing performance; if in doubt, should be checked by having patient recognize objects of different shapes, size, and texture with eyes closed (e.g., coins, ring, and pen) |

| | | |
|---|---|---|
| **Impaired attention** | | |
| Prefrontal cortex, thalamus, reticular formation | Inability to attend to or focus on a specific stimulus; possible distraction from presence of other irrelevant environmental stimuli; inability to screen out irrelevant stimuli | Does not continue an activity; does not attend to instruction or activity; does not attend to mistakes; may focus attention on irrelevant details and not on global environment |
| **Broca's aphasia/expressive aphasia** | | |
| Premotor area of left frontal lobe | Dysfunction of Broca's motor speech area, resulting in expressive aphasia indicated by a loss of speech production; used in the A-ONE as a synonym for expressive aphasia | Has total expressive aphasia or nonfluent speech; is unable to express self verbally |
| **Concrete thinking (lack of abstract thinking)** | | |
| Prefrontal cortex | Inflexible thinking; cannot use internal speech to generalize from similarities among situations; opposite of abstract thinking on a linear continuum of thinking | Is unable to generalize from one situation to another; may ask what time it is while eating breakfast; cannot think of simple solutions that require some thought (e.g., calculations); unable to gain abstract meaning of proverbs |
| **Confabulations** | | |
| Prefrontal cortex | Unconscious fabrication of stories or excuses to fill in memory gaps; may be within limits of reality or patient may not consider rules of reality and then will be identified easily; associated with lack of inhibitions and lack of judgment, as well as memory problems | Does not remember what happened during weekend and comes up with an explanation not grounded in reality |
| **Confusion** | | |
| Prefrontal and diffuse dysfunction—bilateral; thalamus and reticular formation | Lack of ability to think clearly, resulting in disturbed awareness and orientation regarding time, place, and person; impaired interpretation of external environment and slowed responses to verbal stimuli[24]; cognitive disturbance | Talks about past as present; is not oriented to time and place |
| **Depression** | | |
| Left frontal lobe and left basal ganglia, right frontal and right parietal lobes[39] | Affective disorder manifested as sadness, hopelessness, or loss of general interest in usual performance; may be accompanied by loss of appetite, loss of energy, sleeping disorders, and feelings of worthlessness | Has sad affect or expression during activity performance |
| **Disorientation** | | |
| Limbic system and limbic cortex in medial temporal lobe and prefrontal cortex | Inability to give personal information regarding self, disability, hospital stay, or time of day without language problems; relates to specific memory problems | Has an inability to give exact information regarding date (day, month, year) and time of day; may not be able to name institution but knows context of situation (i.e., that current environment is an institution); may not be able to name therapist but knows that therapist belongs to staff |

*Continued*

**Table 18-3**

## Cortical Impairments as Related to Anatomic Location and Definitions of Terms*—cont'd

| IMPAIRMENT AND CORTICAL LOCATION | CONCEPTUAL DEFINITION | OPERATIONAL DEFINITION |
|---|---|---|
| **Distractibility** | | |
| Prefrontal cortex, reticular formation | Diversion of attention | Becomes distracted by environmental stimuli such as conversation in next room or somebody entering the room (note two components of field dependency: distraction and perseveration) |
| **Dysarthria** | | |
| Primary motor cortex in frontal lobe, primary sensory cortex in parietal lobe and cerebellum | Weakness or altered neuronal control of muscles responsible for speech production or defective sensory feedback about movement of those muscles | Has problems with articulation of speech musculature; has slurred speech |
| **Echolalia** | | |
| Prefrontal cortex | A form of perseveration; echoing what is heard | Repeats what is heard. Patient is asked, "Can you comb your hair?" Patient replies, "Can you comb your hair?" |
| **Field dependency** | | |
| Prefrontal cortex | Uninhibited, inadequate, and irrelevant stereotypic actions that replace selective goal-directed actions corresponding to specific tasks; impulsiveness related to elementary orienting reflex[42]; field dependency thus has a dysfunction of an attention component and perseverative component | Becomes distracted from particular task performance by specific stimuli (e.g., is washing hands, suddenly sees denture brush, and incorporates it into the hand-washing activity by scrubbing the hands with the denture brush) |
| **Frustration** | | |
| Prefrontal cortex, hypothalamus | An appearance of agitation and intolerance in behavior that may be manifested emotionally, verbally, or physically | Becomes excited or intolerant when trying hard to perform or unable to perform (may be manifested emotionally, verbally, or physically) |
| **Homonymous hemianopsia** | | |
| Primary visual cortex around calcarine fissure in either hemisphere | Loss of a visual hemifield contralateral to a cerebral lesion | Has visual field defect to visual field that is contralateral to a cerebral lesion; is aware of deficit and tries to compensate for it by using head movements to scan both visual fields |

| | | |
|---|---|---|
| **Ideational apraxia**<br>Prefrontal and premotor cortex in either hemisphere, left inferior parietal lobule, and corpus callosum | A breakdown of knowledge of knowing what is to be done to perform that results from loss of a neuronal model or a mental representation about the concept required for performance; lack of knowledge regarding object use; also refers to sequencing of activity steps or use of objects in relation to each other (NOTE: Therapist should rule out comprehension difficulties) | Does not know what to do with toothbrush, toothpaste, or shaving cream; uses tools inappropriately (e.g., smears the toothpaste on face); sequences activity steps incorrectly so that there are errors in end result of tasks (e.g., puts socks on top of shoes) |
| **Impaired initiative**<br>Prefrontal cortex and supplementary motor cortex[23]—predominantly right hemisphere | Inability to initiate performance of an activity when need to perform is present | Sits without initiating an activity; can describe activity performance but displays inertia in initiating it |
| **Decreased insight**<br>Prefrontal cortex | Insight—a discovery stage, with increasing awareness of the whole self; decreased insight—lack of insight into personal condition and disability | Does not have insight into disease or disability; does not make realistic statement regarding future plans; makes unrealistic comments regarding disability |
| **Irritability**<br>Prefrontal cortex—particularly orbitofrontal cortex and hypothalamus | Excessive sensitivity to stimulation; includes quick excitability manifested as annoyance, impatience, or anger | Appears annoyed; may verbally indicate dislike or be physically agitated out of proportion to stimulus that evoked behavior |
| **Jargon aphasia**<br>Left auditory association cortex in left temporal lobe | Language disorder manifested as fluent speech output that cannot be understood by others because the sequences necessary for intelligible speech phonemes are not available; results from a failure of comprehension because person receives no feedback about own speech performance | Has fluent but unintelligible speech |
| **Impaired judgment**<br>Prefrontal cortex | Inability to make realistic decisions based on environmental information; unable to make use of feedback from own errors | Does not turn off water taps after washing; does not put brakes on wheelchair and makes unsafe transfers; goes to dining room without dressing or combing hair; does not care whether clothes are turned inside out or back to front, even when those facts have been pointed out |

*Continued*

**Table 18-3**

## Cortical Impairments as Related to Anatomic Location and Definitions of Terms*—cont'd

| IMPAIRMENT AND CORTICAL LOCATION | CONCEPTUAL DEFINITION | OPERATIONAL DEFINITION |
|---|---|---|
| **Lability** | | |
| Prefrontal cortex | Pathologic emotional instability; alternating states of gladness and sadness, including inappropriate crying | Has mood swings; cries or laughs inappropriately |
| **Long-term memory loss** | | |
| Hippocampus of limbic system connected to parahippocampus of medial sides of temporal lobes by dentate gyrus; thalamus and corpus callosum | Lack of storage, consolidation, and retention of information that has passed through working memory by way of different sensory networks in a permanent form; lack of ability to retrieve this information | Demonstrates failure in retrieving information that was processed before onset of disability and information that should have been mobilized from working to long-term memory after disability occurred |
| **Impaired motivation** | | |
| Prefrontal cortex, particularly orbitofrontal cortex, medial forebrain bundle, and hypothalamus | Lack of willingness to perform, with or without a perceived need | Does not initiate or continue an activity unless really accepting the need, although physical ability to perform is present (e.g., does not attempt to eat at mealtimes and may refuse to participate in activity); refuses to get up in morning or perform activities, although physically able to perform and has been motivated previously to perform by same activities |
| **Motor apraxia** | | |
| Premotor frontal cortex of either hemisphere, left inferior parietal lobe, corpus callosum, basal ganglia, and thalamus | Loss of access to kinesthetic memory patterns so that purposeful movement cannot be achieved because of defective planning and sequencing of movements, even though idea and the purpose of task are understood; used as a synonym for *ideomotor apraxia* | Has difficulties related to motor planning (e.g., cannot sequence and plan movements necessary to adjust grasp on a hairbrush when moving it from one side of head to other to turn the bristles toward hair) |
| **Impaired motor function** | | |
| Primary motor cortex, anterior internal capsule, basal ganglia, thalamus, and cerebellum | Flaccidity, decreased strength, rigidity, spasticity, ataxia, athetosis, tremor | Has difficulty stabilizing objects such as containers that must be opened; has difficulty reaching unaffected axilla when washing; has difficulty dressing because of a paralyzed arm or inability to button because of tremor |
| **Mutism** | | |
| Supplementary frontal cortex, cingulate gyrus, reticular formation | Impaired initiation of speech; lack of speech, although speech function is present | Does not attempt to speak or communicate |

| Impaired organization and sequencing | | |
|---|---|---|
| Prefrontal cortex | Inability to organize thoughts with activity steps properly sequenced (component of ideational apraxia but can occur separately as the first indication of impairment in a progressive disease process or last step of regressing ideational problems) | Has difficulties sequencing and timing steps of an activity; does not complete one activity step before starting another (e.g., does not take off glasses before taking off a T-shirt with a tight neck hole; puts on shoes before putting on the trousers; washes too quickly, resulting in poor performance) |
| **Paraphasia** | | |
| Prefrontal cortex or left lateral temporal lobe | Expressive speech defect characterized by misuse or replacement of words or phonemes during active speech | Replaces words with incorrect similar or dissimilar words (e.g., may identify an apple as an orange because both are fruits) |
| **Perseveration** | | |
| Premotor and/or prefrontal cortex | Repeated movements or acts during functional performance as a result of difficulty in shifting from one response pattern to another; refers inertia on initiation or termination of performance[22,42,43]; *prefrontal* perseveration—repetition of whole actions or action components; *premotor* perseveration—compulsive repetition of the same movement | Repeats movements or acts and cannot stop them once initiated (e.g., attempts to put on shirt without any progress—nay pull a long sleeve up arm past wrist [premotor perseveration]; moves comb toward mouth instead of hair after having brushed teeth [prefrontal perseveration]) |
| **Restlessness** | | |
| Prefrontal cortex | Uneasiness, impatience, inability to relax | May be impatient (e.g., cannot wait for therapist to start an activity); may have trouble staying in one place during activity |
| **Right-left discrimination impairment** | | |
| Right inferior parietal lobule; also could be left temporal or parietal lobe dysfunction | Inability to discriminate between right and left body sides or to apply the concepts of left and right to the external environment; includes an inability to understand and use concepts of left and right; comprises several factors, including a verbal component, a nonverbal component of tactile sensory discrimination and stimuli location, and spatial relations and visuospatial components[75] | Does not discriminate between left and right side of body on verbal command |
| **Short-term memory loss** | | |
| Limbic system and limbic association cortex in orbitofrontal areas or temporal lobes | Lack of registration and temporary storing of information received by different sensory memory modalities, be it somatosensory, auditory, or visual; refers to working memory in that a person must keep different aspects in mind while working on different memory tasks such as reasoning, comprehension, and learning; length of working or short-term memory depends on nature of assignments | Does not remember instructions throughout evaluation; may have to be reminded to comb hair several times |

*Continued*

**Table 18-3**

## Cortical Impairments as Related to Anatomic Location and Definitions of Terms*—cont'd

| IMPAIRMENT AND CORTICAL LOCATION | CONCEPTUAL DEFINITION | OPERATIONAL DEFINITION |
|---|---|---|
| **Somatoagnosia** | | |
| Right inferior parietal lobule | Disorder of body scheme; diminished awareness of body structure and failure to recognize own body parts and their relationship to each other[75]; difficulty relating own body to objects in external environment | Puts legs into armholes or arms into legholes; brushes mirror image of teeth instead of own teeth or washes mirror image of face instead of own face |
| **Somesthetic sensory loss** | | |
| Postcentral gyrus in either parietal lobe, posterior internal capsule, specific thalamic sensory nuclei | Loss of tactile sensation, proprioception, or kinesthesia | Has difficulty manipulating objects because of lack of sensation; is aware of sensory loss and tries to compensate (e.g., using visual clues) |
| **Spatial relations impairment** | | |
| Usually right inferior parietal lobule | Difficulty relating objects to each other or to self; synonymous with *visuospatial agnosia* when such difficulties are due to visuospatial impairment | Is unable to find armholes, legholes, or bottom of shirt; pulls sleeve in wrong direction; overestimates or underestimates distances when reaching for objects |
| **Topographic disorientation** | | |
| Inferior parietal lobule or occipital association cortex | Difficulty finding way in space as a result of amnestic or agnostic problems; manifested as problems finding way in familiar surroundings or learning new routes | Does not know way to bedroom or bathroom |
| **Unilateral body neglect** | | |
| Inferior parietal lobule, right cingulate gyrus, prefrontal cortex, reticular formation, specific sensory thalamic nuclei, posterior internal capsule | Failure to report, respond, or orient to a unilateral stimulus presented to body side contralateral to a cerebral lesion; can result from defective sensory processing or attention deficit, resulting in ignorance or impaired use of extremities; (used as a synonym for unilateral body inattention); usually affects left side of body | Does not dress affected body side; does not pull shirt all the way down on affected side; gets shirt stuck on affected shoulder and does not try to correct it or does not realize what is wrong |

**Unilateral spatial neglect**

Inferior parietal lobule, right cingulate gyrus, prefrontal cortex, reticular formation, specific sensory thalamic nuclei, posterior internal capsule

Inattention to or neglect of visual stimuli presented in extrapersonal space of side contralateral to a cerebral lesion as a result of visual perceptual deficits or impaired attention[36]; it may occur independently of visual deficits or with hemianopsia[75] (synonymous with unilateral visual neglect)

Does not account for objects in visual field on affected side—usually left side; when moving, runs into furniture, doorways, or walls located in affected visual field

**Visual object agnosia**

Visual association cortex, left or bilateral and posterior corpus callosum

Inability to recognize, name, or demonstrate use of objects seen, resulting from distorted visual perception regardless of visual acuity[65,75]; can see and describe components of object but cannot recognize object itself

Does not identify objects in either visual field on verbal command but can if allowed to touch them; may not be able to recognize a razor but can describe it as a T shape; is not able to explain an object's use but recognizes it when to allowed touch it

**Wernicke's aphasia/sensory aphasia/receptive aphasia**

Auditory association cortex in left lateral temporal lobe

Deficit in auditory comprehension of language; may affect semantic speech performance (manifested as paraphasia or nonsensical syllables because auditory feedback is impaired)[15,33]; impaired repetitions

Has difficulty comprehending spoken language; does not understand one- or two-word commands; does not perform according to verbal instruction; may have problems obtaining meaning from complex language (e.g., prepositions)

Courtesy G. Árnadóttir, Reykjavík, Iceland.
*Conceptual definitions of some common impairments seen in individuals with cerebrovascular accidents and examples of operational definitions from the A-ONE instrument.zRelation of impairments to dysfunctional central nervous system areas is simplified.
†A-ONE, Árnadóttir OT-ADL Neurobehavioral Evaluation.

sequencing the activity steps of the task. The patient also may have comprehension difficulties, which complicates the situation. The behavior of not washing an arm therefore may result from unilateral body neglect or ideational apraxia, depending on the situation. Therefore the following examples are to be used only as guidelines. Clinical reasoning and knowledge of neurobehavioral impairments and how the impairments group together in different diagnostic categories are crucial for effective differentiation and classification of impairments.

***Personal Hygiene and Grooming Performance Area.***
Three areas of occupation in the Framework are included in the grooming and hygiene domain of the A-ONE: personal hygiene and grooming, toilet hygiene, and bathing or showering. The performance of grooming and hygiene activities comprises several tasks; for example, washing the face and body and bathing or showering; performing oral hygiene (including brushing teeth); combing hair; shaving; applying cosmetics, deodorants, or perfumes; and performing toilet hygiene. These tasks may be affected by dysfunction of different client factors, resulting in various behavioral outcomes. Dysfunction of neuromusculoskeletal and movement-related functions can result in paralysis, muscle weakness, and spasticity. Paralysis or muscle weakness may be manifested as difficulty in washing the affected arm or axilla (Figure 18-6, *A*). The individual may need to learn to use one-handed techniques to overcome the impairment. Adapted equipment also may be needed for the individual to reach body parts such as the

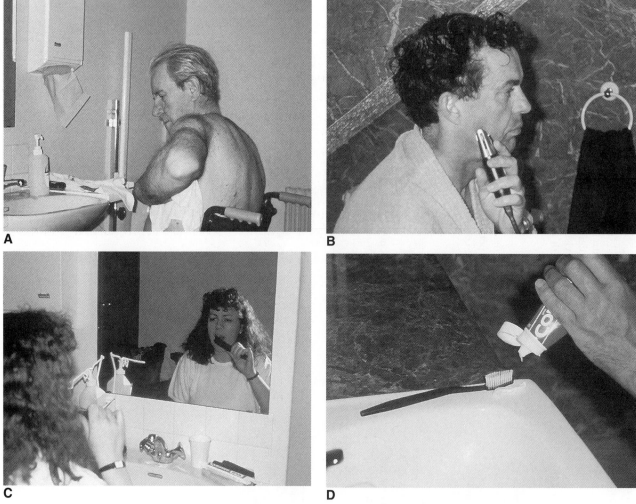

**Figure 18-6** Dysfunction of neurologic client factors manifested during grooming and hygiene tasks. **A,** Paralysis results in difficulty washing the affected axilla. **B,** Motor apraxia makes manipulation of razor difficult. **C,** Prefrontal perseveration, a part from the previous task of brushing the teeth, is perseverated during combing so that the comb is moved toward the mouth instead of the hair. **D,** Spatial relations impairment results in underestimation of distances when the individual attempts to place toothpaste on a toothbrush.

back or, if balance is poor, the feet. Stabilizing objects may be a problem; the individual may need a nonslip pad under the soap. While brushing teeth, the person may have problems opening the tube of toothpaste and may need to learn to compensate by stabilizing it between the knees or teeth. The same applies to other containers and the opening of lids. If the individual uses dentures, an adapted toothbrush or a suction brush for stabilization may be necessary (see Chapter 27).

Dysfunction of sensory functions can result in impaired tactile and proprioceptive sensation, astereognosis, or hemianopsia with a loss of a visual field, or a loss of part of a visual field may be present. Problems with tactile sensation, proprioception, or stereognosis affect object manipulation. An individual with such problems who does not suffer from inattention or neglect will be aware of the impairment and attempt to compensate for it (e.g., by using vision for sensory feedback). If a part of a visual field is defective or hemianopsia is present, an individual may have to compensate by turning the head. If an individual only has this impairment and not neglect, the individual will be aware of the problem and will be able to describe it, with insight into the dysfunction, and compensate for it.

Dysfunction of the client factor of sequencing complex movement, classified as specific mental functions, can lead to motor apraxia and motor perseveration. Individuals with motor apraxia have difficulty with motor planning; they may have difficulty adjusting the grasp of a razor when moving from one side of the face to another

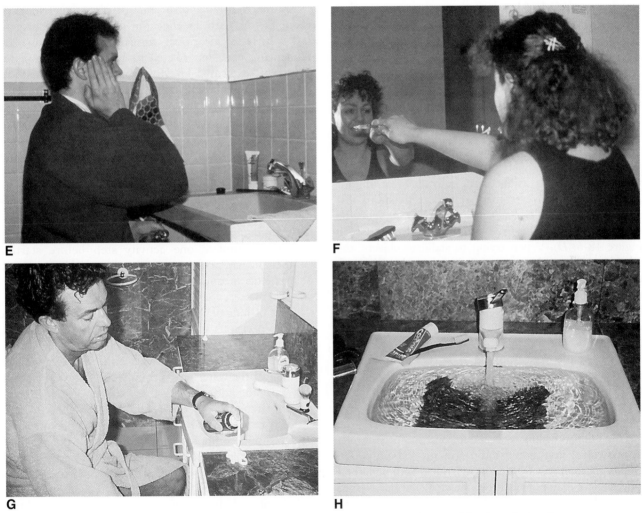

**Figure 18-6, cont'd**  **E,** Unilateral body inattention during shaving. Aftershave lotion is spilled from a bottle held in left hand while individual is reaching with right hand to face and looking into mirror. **F,** Somatoagnosia. Woman cannot differentiate between a mirror image and her own body when brushing her teeth. **G,** Ideational apraxia. Man does not know what to do with shaving cream. **H,** Lack of judgment. Water has been left running with the washcloth in the sink, producing a safety hazard.

or when moving the razor to the chin. This requires sequencing and planning of fine finger and wrist movements so that the razor is turned toward the face for effective use (Figure 18-6, *B*). Similarly, motor apraxia may influence the ability to comb or brush hair. The performance may be adequate on the side where the individual starts brushing but when moving the brush to the other side of the head or to the back, the individual has difficulty adjusting the hand movements required to turn the brush toward the hair. Manipulating a toothbrush and other items may be similarly difficult and manifested as "clumsiness."

Premotor perseveration may be manifested as repetition of the movements of washing the face; the individual cannot stop the movements and take the washcloth to other body parts. Prefrontal perseveration is perseveration of whole acts. The affected individual, having completed one task such as brushing the teeth, begins another activity such as combing but perseverates a part of the previous action program. As a result, the individual approaches the mouth with the comb (Figure 18-6, *C*).

If a dysfunction of the perceptual processing aspect of the specific mental functions client factor is present, a spatial relation disorder, difficulty with left-right discrimination, unilateral body inattention or neglect, unilateral visual inattention or neglect, anosognosia, or somatoagnosia may be expected. Spatial relation disorder may be manifested during hygiene and grooming tasks as difficulty in determining distances. An individual reaching for a toothbrush may overestimate or underestimate its distance. When the individual squeezes toothpaste onto the toothbrush, the paste may end up beside the brush (Figure 18-6, *D*). When trying to stabilize objects, the individual may reach next to the object, resulting in ineffective performance. For example, an individual may reach with the washcloth into the space next to the water faucet instead of under the faucet. When manipulating objects such as dentures, the individual may have problems determining the top from the bottom part of the dentures and the front from the back and left from right.

Impairments related to neglect or inattention can result from dysfunction of the specific mental function factor of perception or attention. In unilateral body neglect, or inattention, the individual does not use the affected limb according to available control. For example, the individual may not use the arm for stability while attempting to open a bottle. An individual with unilateral body neglect may not wash the affected side but washes other body parts systematically. The same may apply to other tasks as well, such as shaving and combing, in that the individual only attends to one side of the face or hair. A man holding an aftershave bottle in the left hand while looking at his own face in the mirror and reaching with the right hand to the face may tilt the bottle without noticing it and spill the liquid (Figure 18-6, *E*).

In unilateral spatial inattention or neglect, the individual randomly may locate all items in the affected visual field only when accidentally seeing them or may not notice an object at all in the affected visual field and does not systematically compensate for the impairment by rotating the head as required.

An individual with somatoagnosia cannot differentiate between the mirror image and self. An individual thus affected may attempt to wash the mirror image of the face instead of the actual face (Figure 18-6, *F*). These individuals may not be able to differentiate between their own body parts and those of others. For example, an individual may grab another person's arm and attempt to use it to hold onto objects. *Somatoagnosia* is defined in the A-ONE as a severe dysfunction that usually is accompanied by ideational apraxia and often by spatial relation disorders.

Dysfunctions of global and specific mental function client factors with an effect on grooming and hygiene tasks include ideational apraxia, organization and sequencing problems related to activity steps, impaired judgment, decreased level of arousal, lack of attention, distraction, field dependency, impaired memory, and impaired intention. Ideational apraxia may appear during grooming and hygiene activities; an individual may not know what to do with the toothbrush, toothpaste, or shaving cream or may use these items inappropriately (e.g., smear toothpaste over the face or spray the shaving cream over the sink (Figure 18-6, *G*). An individual with organization and sequencing difficulties only may have the general idea of how to perform but may have problems timing and sequencing activity steps. Such a patient may not complete one activity step before starting another or may perform activities too quickly as a result of problems in timing activity steps, resulting in a poor performance.

Lack of judgment may appear as an inability to make realistic decisions based on environmental information, providing that perception of those impulses is adequate. An individual so affected may leave the sink area without turning off the water taps or may leave the wash cloth in the sink, not noticing that the water level is increasing and threatening to overflow (Figure 18-6, *H*).

Field dependency has an attention component and a perseveration component. Individuals with this dysfunction may be distracted from performing a particular task by specific stimuli that they are compelled to act on or incorporate into the previous activity. For example, if an individual with field dependency sees a denture brush while washing the hands, that person may incorporate the brush into the activity and scrub the hands with the denture brush.

An individual with short-term memory problems may not remember the sequence of activity steps or instructions throughout activity performance. The therapist may have to remind an individual several times to comb the hair, even though the individual does not have comprehension problems.

Lack of initiation may occur during performance of grooming and hygiene tasks; the individual may sit by the sink without performing, even after being asked to wash. With repeated instructions to begin, the individual may indicate that the activity is about to start, yet nothing happens. After several such incidents and if the therapist asks for a plan, the individual may state a detailed plan of action in which the water will be turned on, the washcloth will be picked up and put under the running water, soap will be put on the cloth, and washing will begin. The individual has a plan of action but cannot start the plan. This impairment may be associated with ideational problems as well.

***Dressing Performance Area.*** The dressing performance includes the tasks of dressing the upper part of the body, including putting on items such as underwear, T-shirts, pullovers, sweaters, shirts, bras, cardigans, or dresses; put-

ting on pants, socks, pantyhose, and shoes; and manipulating fasteners, such as zippers, buckles, laces, or Velcro. Following are some examples of the effect of neurobehavioral impairments on task performance in this area. Dysfunction of neuromusculoskeletal and movement-related client factors affecting this performance area can result in paralysis of a body side. Individuals with one-sided paralysis must learn one-handed dressing techniques (Figure 18-7, *A*).

Dysfunction of the mental factor of sequencing complex movement can manifest as perseveration. Premotor perseveration may appear during dressing; the individual is unable to stop movements that have been initiated. For example, when the individual is placing an arm in a sleeve, the individual may keep pulling the arm into the sleeve until the end of the sleeve is up to the elbow or shoulder (Figure 18-7, *B*).

Defective specific mental function factor of perception may result in spatial relation disorders such as difficulty figuring out the front and back, the inside and outside, and the top and bottom of an article of clothing.

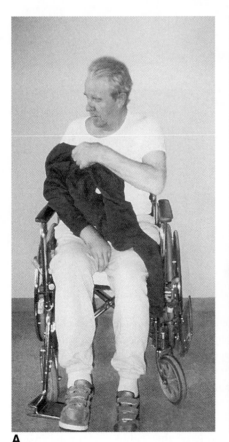

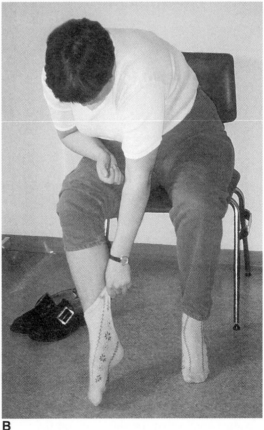

**A**                                                **B**

**Figure 18-7**   Dysfunction of neurologic client factors manifested during dressing tasks. **A,** Paralysis requires use of one-handed dressing techniques. **B,** Premotor perseveration results in repetitions of movements so that the leghole may be pulled up to the knee; the patient pulls the sock repeatedly, although it is already in place.

*Continued*

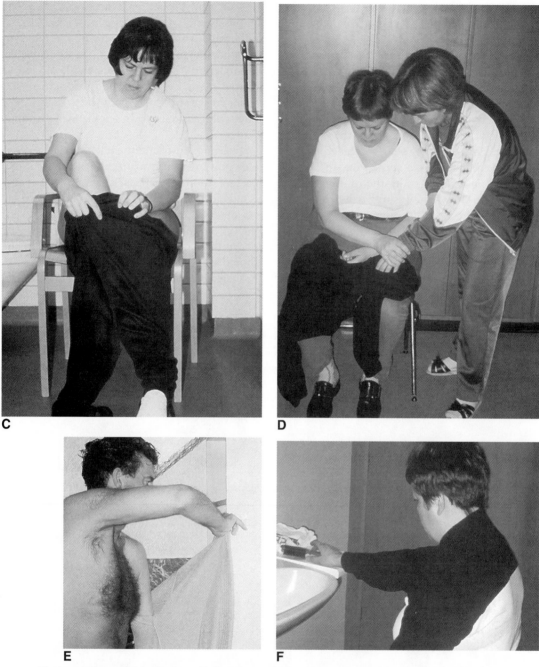

**Figure 18-7, cont'd**    **C,** Spatial relations impairment, in which the patient places both legs in the same leghole. **D,** Somatoagnosia. Woman attempts to dress the therapist's arm instead of her own. **E,** Unilateral body neglect. Man attempts to hang up his gown without having undressed his left arm. **F,** Field dependency. The sight of a comb distracts a woman in the middle of a dressing task. Woman discontinues dressing and begins combing.

Although the individual knows that the shirt goes on the upper part of the body and is trying to get the arm through the sleeve, the arm may be put through the neckhole instead of the sleeve or in the right sleeve instead of the left. An individual may place both legs in the same leghole (Figure 18-7, *C*) or may not perceive that one of the legholes is turned inside out. Right-left disorientation can be related to visuospatial problems; for example, an individual may put the right shoe on the left foot. An individual with spatial relation disorder may pull the sleeve in the wrong direction when attempting to put on a shirt. The individual may be unable to tie shoelaces

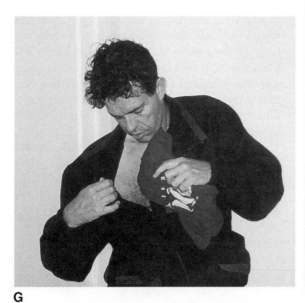

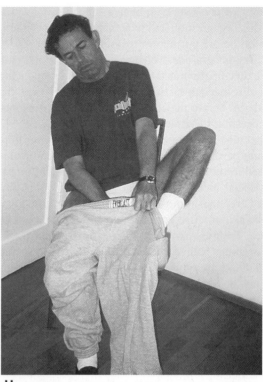

**G**

**H**

**Figure 18-7, cont'd  G,** Ideational apraxia. Man knows that the T-shirt should go under the sweater but does not know how to accomplish the goal. **H,** Organization and sequencing impairment. Man puts on socks and shoes before trousers, resulting in difficulties donning trousers.

because of difficulty handling the spatial relations aspects of manipulating shoestrings. Velcro fastenings on shoes may be folded back on themselves instead of being passed through the D-loop before being folded backward. Somatoagnosia may manifest as a patient attempting to dress a therapist's arm instead of their own (Figure 18-7, *D*) or when they attempt to place their legs into the armholes of a shirt. Thus they have problems with differentiating their own body from the therapist's body and relating objects to corresponding body parts. This is not only a spatial relation problem but also a defect in body image. An individual with only a visuospatial problem cannot find the correct armhole but realizes that a shirt is related to the upper body. This realization is not evident in individuals with somatoagnosia because of their body scheme dysfunction.

Unilateral body neglect may be severe, or less severe unilateral body inattention may be present. In severe cases an individual may not dress or undress the affected arm. The individual may even leave the arm in the armhole when undressing and attempt to hang the shirt on a clothes peg on the wall, not cognizant that the arm is still in the armhole (Figure 18-7, *E*). However, the problem is not always this severe or apparent. At times the shirt may get stuck on an affected shoulder without the individual notic-

ing it, or the shirt may not be pulled properly down on the affected side. An individual with unilateral visual neglect or inattention may not put on clothes that are placed in the left visual field because they remain unnoticed.

Dysfunction of global and specific mental function client factors may be seen as field dependency, ideational problems, or impaired judgment. Field dependency is illustrated by an individual in the middle of the activity of putting on a sweater. Having placed both arms through the correct armholes and the neck through the neckhole, the patient is distracted by the sight of a comb. The activity of dressing subsequently is discontinued immediately as the individual grabs the comb and starts combing his or her hair. After combing, the individual may or may not go back to the task of putting on the shirt (Figure 18-7, *F*). A person might not know what to do with the clothes or how to put them on. A person with ideational apraxia may be able to perform certain activities automatically, such as putting on a sweater. Difficulty arises when the person realizes the T-shirt or undershirt has not been put on under the sweater. The individual may not be able to plan the necessary activity steps to correct the mistake. The T-shirt may get tucked down the neckhole instead of the sweater being removed and the activity started over (Figure 18-7, *G*). An individual with ideational apraxia also may attempt to put a sock on over a shoe. An individual who only has organization and sequencing problems might put shoes on before putting on trousers (Figure 18-7, *H*). However, the general ideas of how to put the clothes on and where they fit are intact. Organization and sequencing problems also may appear when an individual dresses the unaffected arm before the affected one and then runs into difficulty dressing the affected arm.

The therapist also may detect impaired judgment during dressing performance. An individual may be improperly dressed in the hallways or the dining area, indicating a lack of social judgment. Spatial relation disorder also may affect dressing performance. An affected individual may not be able to differentiate the front and the back of the clothes. Trousers may be put on with the front pockets and fastenings turned backward. Because these spatial relations deficits are of visual origin, the affected individual may not be able to identify the mistakes. However, when a therapist points out that the trousers are backwards, an individual with a lack of judgment might comment that it does not matter how the trousers are worn.

A subject with intact judgment would attempt to make corrections, ask for assistance, or otherwise indicate a desire to have the performance corrected.

***Functional Mobility Performance Area.*** The performance area of functional mobility includes the tasks of rolling over and sitting up in a bed, transferring to and from a bed, transferring to and from a chair, transferring to and from a toilet, transferring to and from a bathtub or a shower, and moving from one room to another. The previously defined impairments or defective client factors may interfere with the tasks of this performance area (see Chapter 14). Following are some examples of how these dysfunctions may be manifested.

If a dysfunction of the neuromusculoskeletal and movement-related functions, such as paralysis is present, it affects strength and control of one body side and thus affects mobility and balance. An individual therefore may need assistance with transfers, require a wheelchair or walking aids, or require supervision or personal assistance for mobility (Figure 18-8, *A*).

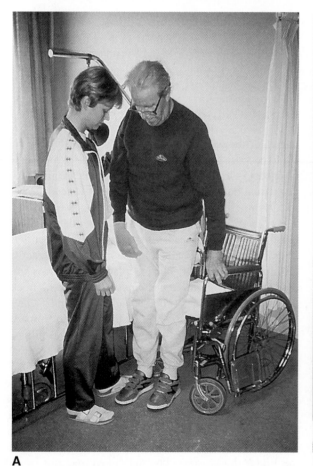

**A**

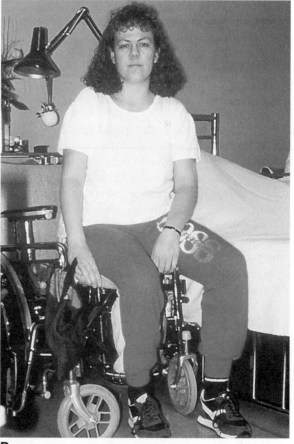

**B**

**Figure 18-8**   Dysfunction of neurologic client factors manifested during functional mobility tasks. **A,** Paralysis affects strength and balance. Individuals require assistance when transferring from bed. A wheelchair is needed for mobility. **B,** Unilateral body neglect. Woman only moves intact body side over to wheelchair and leaves affected side in bed.

Dysfunction of the client factor of specific mental functions of sequencing complex movement may lead to perseveration and motor apraxia as previously mentioned. Individuals with premotor perseveration may not be able to stop the movements of wheeling a wheelchair; as a result, they continue wheeling and moving after reaching the desired destination.

Dysfunctions of the specific mental functions perceptual factor may result in spatial relation disorders in which the affected individual may misjudge distances. The individual may park a wheelchair too far from a bed or chair for a transfer. An individual with unilateral body neglect or inattention may not account for the affected body side when moving. Such an individual may hit furniture with the affected arm or walk into obstacles such as doorways. When transferring from the bed to a chair, an individual may only move the unaffected side to the chair, leaving the affected side in bed or off the chair (Figure 18-8, *B*). An individual with severe neglect also may have the impairment of anosognosia. These individuals may deny that their affected arm or side is a part of themselves. The affected limb may be referred to as an

object, or these individuals may claim that someone else's arm is lying in bed with them. One man with anosognosia was heard to comment that he was going to occupational therapy and that he would "need to bring the arm along," because the occupational therapist "always works on the arm." Unilateral spatial neglect or inattention refers to the phenomenon in which the individual does not account for visual stimuli from the affected visual field. The individual may walk or wheel into obstacles such as garbage cans, furniture, doorways, or other individuals (Figure 18-8, *C*). Topographic disorientation, in which the person has visuospatial problems or memory problems regarding spatial locations also may be present. The individual does not know the way to different, familiar locations such as the bathroom, dining room, bedroom, or therapy department.

If a dysfunction of the global and specific mental factors is present, ideational apraxia or organization and sequencing problems may occur during transfers and mobility tasks. Individuals with ideational apraxia may not know how to get into bed. They literally may throw themselves into the bed. An individual may not know how to wheel

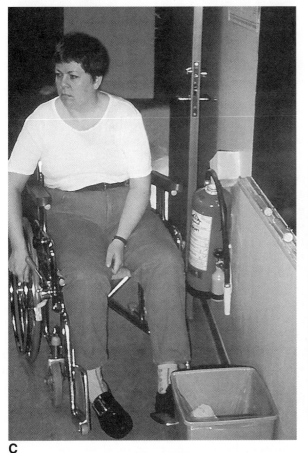

**C**

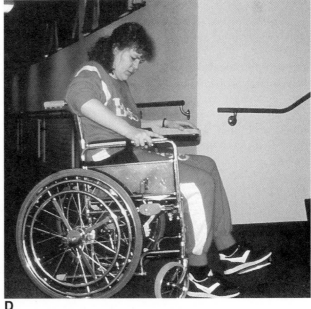

**D**

**Figure 18-8, cont'd**    **C,** Unilateral spatial neglect. Woman wheels into a garbage can in a neglected left visual field. **D,** Ideational apraxia. Woman does not know how to propel the wheelchair and pushes down on the armrest instead of the wheel.

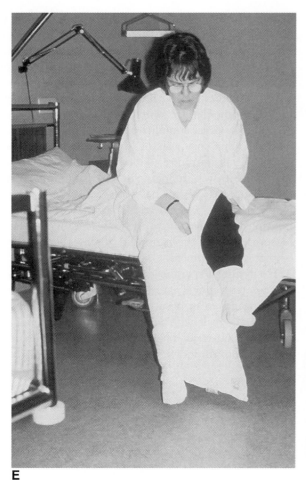
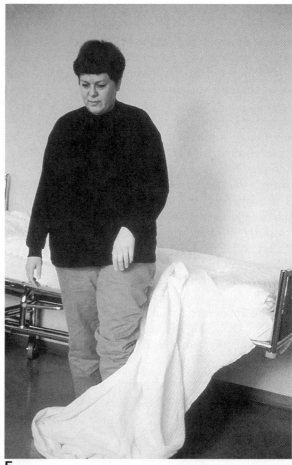

**E**                    **F**

**Figure 18-8, cont'd**    **E,** Organization and sequencing impairment. Woman does not lift off the blanket before sitting up in bed. **F,** Organization and sequencing impairment and ideational apraxia. Woman attempts to walk away from bed without having moved the blanket.

a wheelchair and may push down repeatedly on the armrest (Figure 18-8, *D*). (However, the therapist should rule out attention problems.) An individual with organization and sequencing problems may sit up in bed without taking off the blanket but will remove the blanket before standing up (Figure 18-8, *E*). However, an individual with additional ideational apraxia may sit up without lifting the blanket off and then attempt to stand up and walk away without moving the blanket, thus producing a safety hazard (Figure 18-8, *F*). An individual with organization and sequencing problems only may not put on wheelchair brakes before transferring or take them off before moving. This particular performance difficulty might occur when memory problems are present as well. If memory problems without impaired judgment are present, the results of the unsafe transfers (e.g., instability) may remind these individuals to lock the brakes.

***Eating Performance Area.*** Neurobehavioral impairments or dysfunction of the previously mentioned client factors may affect dysfunction of eating performance,

such as chewing and swallowing, drinking from a glass or a cup, eating without utensils (only using the fingers), eating with a fork or a spoon, and using a knife to cut or spread. Many of these tasks are accomplished earlier in the developmental sequence than some of the tasks mentioned previously.

A dysfunction of the neuromusculoskeletal and movement-related factors may result in paralysis of one side of the body, resulting in poor sitting balance and use of only one arm. Tactile and proprioceptive sensation in the affected hand and arm may be impaired because of defective sensory functions. All these impairments may affect eating tasks that require sitting balance and bilateral integration of the arms (e.g., stabilizing a slice of bread while buttering it or a slice of meat while cutting it, eating an egg, or peeling an orange). Because of the impairments, these eating tasks may require different performance techniques, helping aids, or personal assistance.

An individual with motor apraxia classified as dysfunction of the specific mental factor of sequencing complex movement according to the ICF classification system may

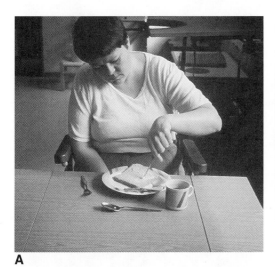

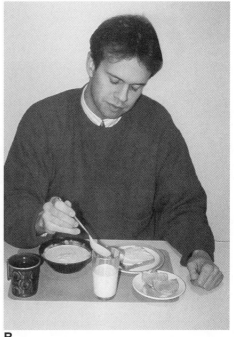

**A**                                         **B**

**Figure 18-9**   Dysfunction of neurologic client factors manifested during feeding and eating tasks. **A,** Motor apraxia makes manipulation of a knife difficult when buttering bread. **B,** Prefrontal perseveration. Man continues to move the spoon toward the glass instead of drinking from it, after having used the spoon to eat yogurt.

*Continued*

spill soup when moving the spoon from the bowl to the mouth, a task that requires much significant adjustment of fine finger and wrist movements to keep the spoon level. Motor apraxia may result in "clumsy movements" when spreading butter, resulting in problems manipulating the knife (Figure 18-9, *A*). Premotor perseveration is demonstrated when an individual cannot stop the movements of bringing the spoon to the mouth from the bowl after having finished the soup. Another example is the continuation of chewing movements after the food has dissolved in the mouth. Prefrontal perseveration, or perseveration of actions rather than movements (a cognitive factor), may manifest when an individual who has finished eating yogurt with a spoon reaches out for the spoon again to use it to get a sip of milk from a glass rather than drink directly from the glass (Figure 18-9, *B*).

Dysfunction of specific mental perceptual factors affecting eating behavior may result in spatial relation disorders; an individual trying to stabilize a slice of bread to butter it may misjudge distance and grab the plate instead of the bread (Figure 18-9, *C*). The individual may also overestimate or underestimate distances and reach beside the cup instead of grabbing the cup. Unilateral body neglect may occur during eating when the individual does not use the hand in a natural relation to its available function. Individuals may start eating bread using the left hand, "forget" that the bread is in the hand, and

proceed to eat other items as the hand holding the bread slides off the table (Figure 18-9, *D*). Unilateral spatial neglect may manifest in that the individual may not attend to objects or food in the affected visual field. For example, an individual may not notice a fork in the left visual field and attempts to solve the problem by grabbing the next person's fork located by a plate in the right visual field (Figure 18-9, *E*). Individuals may not eat food located in the affected visual field although they enjoy that particular type of food.

Dysfunction of global and specific mental function factors may result in ideational apraxia in which the affected individual does not know which utensils to use or how to use them. The individual may simplify the activity by using the fingers to eat meat instead of a fork. The person also may misuse objects. An individual may attempt to eat the soup with a knife. Activity steps may be left out of the sequence, resulting in defective performance. An affected individual may not take the shell off an egg before eating it or may not peel an orange before biting it. An individual may have the proper object in hand but may not know how to use it for the situation at hand: the individual may open a teabag, remove the tea leaves, and place them in the cup instead of placing the bag in the cup. Individuals may misuse objects; for example, they may sprinkle salt on the butter container (Figure 18-9, *F*). Field dependency may be manifested during feeding

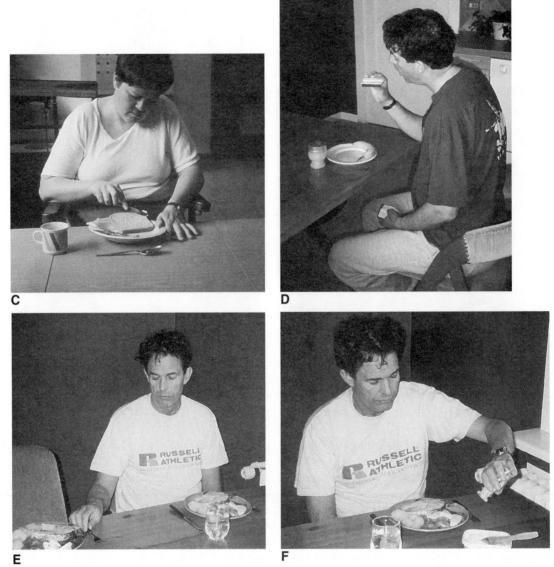

**Figure 18-9, cont'd    C,** Spatial relations impairment. Woman attempts to stabilize a piece of bread but misjudges distances and grabs the side of the plate instead. **D,** Unilateral body neglect. Man does not attend to a piece of bread in left hand; hand slides unnoticed off the table, and man grabs another slice with right hand. **E,** Unilateral spatial neglect. Man does not notice fork in his left visual field but solves problem by borrowing a fork from the next plate in the right visual field. **F,** Ideational apraxia. Man does not know what salt is used for and shakes it over butter container.

activities. Individuals may start grabbing food items before having positioned themselves properly at the table. Individuals also may grab items as they are seen, although the items are inappropriate for the activity at hand.

***Communication.*** *Communication* refers to how the individual expresses needs and understands others in the social environmental context. According to the A-ONE classification, such expression and understanding are important aspects of daily activities, often closely intertwined with other activities, and so are included in the communication domain. Communication includes, among other things, the ability to talk, comprehend, read, and write. The ICF[73] classifies communication referring to reception and production of messages and to carrying on conversation under activities and participation. Dysfunction of any of the following factors can affect communication: neuromusculoskeletal and movement-related functions, sensory functions, specific mental functions of sequencing complex movement, memory, perception, and thought, and voice and speech functions. This may result in Broca's or expressive aphasia, in which the individual is not capable of verbal expression or has nonfluent speech. Dysarthria is a problem with articulation of speech musculature and can be due to primary motor or sensory involvement, resulting in slurred speech. Premotor perseverations of speech occur when an individual repeats the same words or syllables over and over, unable to shift to other words or syllables. A prefrontal perseveration may be at work when an individual repeats a concept from a previous question; for example, when the individual is asked about numbers, such as the length of the hospital stay, followed by a question regarding which month it is, the answer may be "the thirteenth," indicating a perseveration of the concept of numbers. An individual with auditory processing dysfunction resulting in sensory aphasia or Wernicke's aphasia, also termed *receptive aphasia*, may have difficulty comprehending spoken language; for example, the individual may not understand one- or two-step instructions, may not perform according to verbal instruction, or may have difficulty obtaining meaning from complex language. When this impairment is accompanied by jargon aphasia, the individual has fluent but unintelligible speech because the individual does not receive auditory feedback about personal performance.

Dysfunction of the specific mental function factors may present as the memory impairment anomia, in which the individual has fluent speech but has difficulty remembering names. An affected individual may present with paraphasia, in which words are misused or misplaced; this can be a problem with classification of concepts. An individual with paraphasia may use a word from the same group of concepts as the intended term but not the correct word. The individual may call apples oranges or claim to be going to school instead of the clinic. Mutism may occur if intention is affected and manifests as lack of an attempt to speak or communicate.

***Pervasive Impairments.*** According to the A-ONE classification,[7,11,12] impairments can be classified as specific or pervasive in relation to activity performance. The impairments described in the previous sections and affecting specific tasks of an ADL domain are classified as specific because they are observed in relation to the particular task, whereas other impairments are not task specific. Thus some impairments are not necessarily tied to a particular performance area but can occur in relation to any performance area. Emotional and affective disturbance, such as apathy, depression, frustration, irritability, aggression, and lack of motivation, are examples of this because they may affect task performance in different areas of occupation.

As stated earlier, different impairments have different effects on task performance. The behavioral examples described in this chapter are intended as guidelines to assist therapists in detecting impairments during activity analysis for assessment purposes. This information, used with the appropriate theoretical background and clinical reasoning, is important in determining intervention strategies. Occasionally, differentiation between impairments with similar behavioral manifestations may be difficult, particularly for less experienced therapists. Knowledge of neurologic function and of how impairments are grouped in different diagnostic categories may be valuable for clinical reasoning in such instances.

## PATTERNS OF IMPAIRMENTS RESULTING FROM CEREBROVASCULAR ACCIDENTS

In a preceding section, neurobehavioral impairments were defined and related to different cortical areas. Involvement of dysfunction affecting client factors depends on various pathologic conditions resulting in CVA and the different anatomic areas involved. The cerebral blood supply depends mainly on three arteries in each hemisphere: the middle and anterior cerebral arteries, which are branches of the internal carotid artery, and the posterior cerebral artery, which is a branch of the basilar artery, formed by the union of the vertebral arteries.[40] Two major types of cerebrovascular dysfunction cause neurologic lesions: (1) ischemia, or insufficient blood supply to the brain, which is responsible for 70% to 80% of all strokes, and (2) hemorrhage, or bleeding, caused by a ruptured blood vessel, which accounts for the remaining 15% to 20% of strokes.* Hemorrhage results in swelling and compression of brain tissue. Different subtypes of CVA occur. Ischemia is subdivided into thrombosis, or blood flow obstruction caused by a local process in one or more blood vessels; embolism, in which blood flow obstruction is caused by materials from distant parts of the vascular system; and decreased systemic perfusion, or hypoperfusion, in which low systemic perfusion pressure results in reduced blood flow.[3,5,12,20,68]

Hemorrhage is subdivided into subarachnoid hemorrhage, which occurs at the surface of the brain and intracerebrally; and intraparenchymal hemorrhage, or bleeding in the cerebral tissue.[2,3,12,20] Each type of CVA results in different patterns of impairment. The type of impairment and severity depend mainly on the anatomic location of the lesion.[4,5,20] These further depend on the rate of arterial occlusion, adequacy of the collateral circulation, resistance of brain structures to ischemia,[20] duration and severity of ischemia, hematoma size, and underlying mechanism of hypoperfusion[74] and on edema.

If the middle cerebral artery is occluded, affecting blood supply to the lateral aspect of the hemisphere, the impairments vary depending on which branches of

---

*References 2, 3, 5, 12, 20, 68.

the artery and which hemisphere is affected. If the insult affects the upper trunk of the middle cerebral artery, which supplies the lateral aspects of the frontal and parietal lobes, hemiplegia is to be expected on the contralateral body side, especially of the face and arm, along with hemisensory loss, including tactile and proprioceptive information. This type of insult also may cause impairment of a visual field to the opposite site of the lesion. If the right hemisphere is impaired, unilateral neglect of space and body may result, as well as attention deficits, including unilateral body inattention and unilateral spatial inattention, anosognosia, spatial relation dysfunction, unilateral motor apraxia of the left side (if not paralyzed), lack of judgment, lack of insight, field dependency, and organization of behavior and activity steps. Emotional disturbances such as apathy, lability, and depression also may be present. If the left hemisphere is involved, speech and language functions may be impaired, and bilateral motor apraxia may be present. Ideational apraxia and perseverations also may be present. Emotional disturbances such as depression and frustration may be present. If the lower trunk of the middle cerebral artery is affected, visual field defect of the contralateral visual field, Wernicke's aphasia caused by involvement of the left hemisphere, and emotional disturbances may be present.[12,20]

If the anterior cerebral artery, which supplies the medial and superior aspects of the frontal and parietal lobes, is occluded, the paralysis and sensory loss will be greatest in the foot. Unilateral apraxia may result from dysfunction of the anterior part of the corpus callosum. Speech disturbance, or inertia of speech in a form of mutism, can be related to dysfunction of the supplementary motor area. Bilateral involvement of the anterior cerebral artery—or ruptured aneurysm of the anterior cerebral arteries or the anterior communicating artery, resulting in hemorrhage—may lead to behavioral disturbances related to dysfunction of limbic structures and the medial aspects of the frontal lobe.[12,20]

Occlusion of the posterior cerebral artery, which supplies the medial and inferior aspects of the temporal and occipital lobes, may result in homonymous hemianopsia or loss of a visual field. This loss results because of dysfunction of the visual cortex in the occipital lobe. Visual agnosia may be present (e.g., prosopagnosia, color agnosia, or visual object agnosia). Left-sided lesions may cause alexia and associative visual agnosia or naming difficulties. Bilateral lesions cause cortical blindness. Problems with spatial relations may be present, as well as right-left discrimination, alexia, agraphia, acalculia, and memory.[12,20]

Dysfunctions affecting other arterial branches that supply structures adjacent to the cortex can cause lesions in the cerebellum, basal ganglia, caudate nuclei, thalamus, and the internal capsule. These lesions can result in various combinations of impairments.

Systemic hypoperfusion results in a diffuse cerebral dysfunction affecting the watershed regions or the border zones in the periphery of the major cerebral arteries. The hippocampus and the adjacent temporal structures on the medial side of cortex also may be involved. The cerebellum and brainstem nuclei sometimes are involved as well. The resulting impairments include agitation; simultanagnosia, in which an object is seen as fragmented; brainstem reflexes; coma; confusion; memory disturbances with accompanying confabulations; restlessness; and occasional gait ataxia.[20] Tables 18-4 and 18-5 indicate patterns of impairments as they relate to dysfunction of different cerebral arteries and different CNS areas as a result of various vascular pathologic conditions (see Chapter 1).

## CLINICAL REASONING INVOLVED IN USING THE A-ONE

When applying the A-ONE principles to evaluate simultaneously occupational performance and dysfunctional client factors that limit the performance, the therapist applies different types of clinical reasoning, according to Árnadóttir.[7,9] These are interactive reasoning, as interaction between the client and therapist takes place, and procedural reasoning,[45] also termed *diagnostic*[37,57] or *scientific reasoning*,[18] referring to hypothesis formation following interpretation of cues about the nature of problems that interfere with occupational performance. Further exploration is necessary in relation to the A-ONE. When observing dressing performance, the therapist may not detect a critical cue such as not dressing one arm. The therapist interprets this cue, and other cues, by using previously described conceptual and operational definitions from the theory behind the A-ONE instrument and forms hypotheses. Possible hypotheses might be (1) lack of somesthetic sensory input from the arm, (2) unilateral body neglect—in which the person does not attend, usually to the left arm—that may or may not be paralyzed, (3) organization and sequencing problems in which the person is leaving an activity step out of the performance, or (4) ideational apraxia, in which the person does not have an idea of what to do with the shirt or how to put it on. In addition to considering definitions of terms when choosing the appropriate hypotheses, or determining which impairment is most likely to cause the particular activity limitation, the therapist keeps in mind indications of impairments during other activities because these might support a particular hypothesis. The neurologic information on functional localization and patterns of impairments as related to different diagnoses or different cerebral arteries described in the previous section also would be included in the reasoning and hypothesis formation. Thus, if the patient (1) knows in general how to use objects, not to mention if the patient can state a plan of action for the activity performance, but does not use

**Table 18-4**

## Cerebral Artery Dysfunction: Cortical Involvement and Patterns of Impairment

| ARTERY | LOCATION | POSSIBLE IMPAIRMENTS |
|---|---|---|
| | | **Dysfunction of either hemisphere** |
| Middle cerebral artery: upper trunk | Lateral aspect of frontal and parietal lobe | Contralateral hemiplegia, especially of the face and the upper extremity<br>Contralateral hemisensory loss<br>Visual field impairment<br>Poor contralateral conjugate gaze<br>Ideational apraxia<br>Lack of judgment<br>Perseveration<br>Field dependency<br>Impaired organization of behavior<br>Depression<br>Lability<br>Apathy |
| | | **Right hemisphere dysfunction** |
| | | Left unilateral body neglect<br>Left unilateral visual neglect<br>Anosognosia<br>Visuospatial impairment<br>Left unilateral motor apraxia |
| | | **Left hemisphere dysfunction** |
| | | Bilateral motor apraxia<br>Broca's aphasia<br>Frustration |
| Middle cerebral artery: lower trunk | Lateral aspect of right temporal and occipital lobes | **Dysfunction of either hemisphere**<br>Contralateral visual field defect<br>Behavioral abnormalities |
| | | **Right hemisphere dysfunction**<br>Visuospatial dysfunction |
| | | **Left hemisphere dysfunction**<br>Wernicke's aphasia |
| Middle cerebral artery: both upper and lower trunks | Lateral aspect of the involved hemisphere | Impairments related to both upper and lower trunk dysfunction as listed in previous two sections |

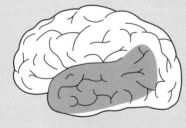

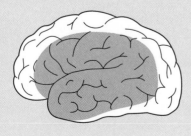

*Continued*

**Table 18-4**

## Cerebral Artery Dysfunction: Cortical Involvement and Patterns of Impairment—cont'd

| ARTERY | LOCATION | POSSIBLE IMPAIRMENTS |
|---|---|---|
| Anterior cerebral artery | Medial and superior aspects of frontal and parietal lobes | Contralateral hemiparesis, greatest in foot<br>Contralateral hemisensory loss, greatest in foot<br>Left unilateral apraxia<br>Inertia of speech or mutism<br>Behavioral disturbances |
| Internal carotid artery | Combination of middle cerebral artery distribution and anterior cerebral artery | Impairments related to dysfunction of middle and anterior cerebral arteries as listed above |
| Anterior choroidal artery, a branch of the internal carotid artery | Globus pallidus, lateral geniculate body, posterior limb of the internal capsule, medial temporal lobe | Hemiparesis of face, arm, and leg<br>Hemisensory loss<br>Hemianopsia[20] |
| Posterior cerebral artery | Medial and inferior aspects of right temporal and occipital lobes, posterior corpus callosum and penetrating arteries to midbrain and thalamus | **Dysfunction of either side**<br>Homonymous hemianopsia<br>Visual agnosia (visual object agnosia, prosopagnosia, color agnosia)<br>Memory impairment<br>Occasional contralateral numbness<br><br>**Right side dysfunction**<br>Cortical blindness<br>Visuospatial impairment<br>Impaired left-right discrimination<br><br>**Left side dysfunction**<br>Finger agnosia<br>Anomia<br>Agraphia<br>Acalculia<br>Alexia |
| Basilar artery proximal | Pons | Quadriparesis<br>Bilateral asymmetric weakness<br>Bulbar or pseudobulbar paralysis (bilateral paralysis of face, palate, pharynx, neck, or tongue)<br>Paralysis of eye abductors<br>Nystagmus<br>Ptosis<br>Cranial nerve abnormalities<br>Diplopia<br>Dizziness<br>Occipital headache<br>Coma[20] |

**Table 18-4**

**Cerebral Artery Dysfunction: Cortical Involvement and Patterns of Impairment—cont'd**

| ARTERY | LOCATION | POSSIBLE IMPAIRMENTS |
|---|---|---|
| Basilar artery distal | Midbrain, thalamus, and caudate nucleus | Papillary abnormalities<br>Abnormal eye movements<br>Altered level of alertness<br>Coma<br>Memory loss<br>Agitation<br>Hallucination[20] |
| Vertebral artery | Lateral medulla and cerebellum | Dizziness<br>Vomiting<br>Nystagmus<br>Pain in ipsilateral eye and face<br>Numbness in face<br>Clumsiness of ipsilateral limbs<br>Hypotonia of ipsilateral limbs<br>Tachycardia<br>Gait ataxia[20] |
| Systemic hypoperfusion | Watershed region on lateral side of hemisphere, hippocampus and surrounding structures in medial temporal lobe | Coma<br>Dizziness<br>Confusion<br>Decreased concentration<br>Agitation<br>Memory impairment<br>Visual abnormalities caused by disconnection from frontal eye fields<br>Simultanognosia<br>Impaired eye movements<br>Weakness of shoulder and arm<br>Gait ataxia[20] |

the left hand according to muscle strength, or (2) has other impairments that fit with the picture of right hemisphere dysfunction such as spatial relations impairment, one would probably suspect unilateral body neglect or inattention to body side as a result of right hemisphere dysfunction. The therapist would consider sensation in the arm because this may or may not be defective if neglect or inattention exists and could affect arm use. The therapist also would check insight into activity limitations and occupational errors by using the pervasive scale. If sensory loss exists, the patient is aware of the problem and how it affects performance. If neglect or inattention exists, the patient will not be aware consistently of the impairment and its effect on activity performance. If, however, cues indicate the client is having difficulties with object use in other activities as well, cannot state a plan of action, or has language problems that might indicate a defect in inner language, as well as problems forming a plan of action, one might come to the conclusion that the impairment of ideational apraxia limits the dressing performance. Thus the therapist might hypothesize that ideational apraxia caused by left hemisphere dysfunction might be the nature of the problem that interferes with task performance.[7] This information may be useful combined with other types of reasoning such as conditional reasoning[45] (see Chapter 17) when making decisions regarding intervention methods, as discussed later.[7]

## ASSESSMENT METHODS

Occupational therapists use basically two evaluation and intervention approaches when working with patients with neurologic conditions: deficit-specific approach, also termed *micro level, bottom-up, restorative,* or *remedial approach* and functional adaptation or compensation approach, also referred to as *macro level, top-down,* or *adaptive approach.*[47,48,66] Evaluation tools used when applying the deficit-specific approach are aimed at the impaired body structures and functions, using the ICF terminology or dysfunctional client factors, referring to

**Table 18-5**

## Cerebrovascular Dysfunction in Noncortical Areas: Patterns of Impairment

| LOCATION | POSSIBLE IMPAIRMENTS |
|---|---|
| Anterolateral thalamus, either side | ■ Minor contralateral motor abnormalities<br>■ Long latency period<br>■ Slowness<br><br>**Right side**<br>■ Visual neglect<br><br>**Left side**<br>■ Aphasia[20] |
| Lateral thalamus | ■ Contralateral hemisensory symptoms<br>■ Contralateral limb ataxia[20] |
| Bilateral thalamus | ■ Memory impairment<br>■ Behavioral abnormalities<br>■ Hypersomnolence[20] |
| Internal capsule or basis pontis | ■ Pure motor stroke[20] |
| Posterior thalamus | ■ Numbness or decreased sensibility of face and arm<br>■ Choreic movements<br>■ Impaired eye movements<br>■ Hypersomnolence<br>■ Decreased consciousness<br>■ Decreased alertness<br><br>**Right side**<br>■ Visual neglect<br>■ Anosognosia<br>■ Visuospatial abnormalities<br><br>**Left side**<br>■ Aphasia<br>■ Jargon aphasia<br>■ Good comprehension of speech<br>■ Paraphasia<br>■ Anomia[20] |
| Caudate | ■ Dysarthria<br>■ Apathy<br>■ Restlessness<br>■ Agitation<br>■ Confusion<br>■ Delirium<br>■ Lack of initiative<br>■ Poor memory<br>■ Contralateral hemiparesis<br>■ Ipsilateral conjugate deviation of the eyes[20] |
| Putamen | ■ Contralateral hemiparesis<br>■ Contralateral hemisensory loss<br>■ Decreased consciousness<br>■ Ipsilateral conjugate gaze<br>■ Motor impersistence<br><br>**Right side**<br>■ Visuospatial impairment<br><br>**Left side**<br>■ Aphasia[20] |

**Table 18-5**

## Cerebrovascular Dysfunction in Noncortical Areas: Patterns of Impairment—cont'd

| LOCATION | POSSIBLE IMPAIRMENTS |
|---|---|
| Pons | ■ Quadriplegia<br>■ Coma<br>■ Impaired eye movement[20] |
| Cerebellum | ■ Ipsilateral limb ataxia<br>■ Gait ataxia<br>■ Vomiting<br>■ Impaired eye movements[20] |

the terminology of the Framework. The evaluation tools of the functional approach are aimed at the activity level or occupational performance. During the last decade or so, different authors within occupational therapy have emphasized the importance of focusing on task performance or occupational functioning when assessing patients rather than focusing on impairments. They also have emphasized the importance of developing standardized tests that relate occupational performance to client factors or performance skills.* The A-ONE provides information on performance task dysfunction in different ADL domains and the dysfunctional neurobehavioral client factor functions that might affect ADL performance, as is evident by exploring the case studies that follow this review.

The case studies illustrated in Figures 18-10 and 18-11 describe two patients who sustained CVAs that resulted in different patterns of impairments based on involvement of different cerebral arteries. The A-ONE assessment was used to evaluate ADL performance and the type of severity of neurobehavioral impairments that interfered with task performance. The studies demonstrate how neurobehavioral impairment interferes with ADL performance and how the two types of dysfunction—dysfunction of client factors and their effect on performance tasks—may be evaluated simultaneously as recommended by several authors.* The case studies show two individuals who need physical assistance with all items in the dressing domain of the Functional Independence Scale of the A-ONE. The lack of functional independence is caused by different neurobehavioral impairments in each of the cases, resulting from different diagnoses. In Figure 18-10, *A*, Ms. Wilson has sustained a CVA on the right side; unilateral body neglect, spatial relations impairment, unilateral spatial neglect, organization and sequencing problems, and left hemiplegia interfere with the dressing performance (as indicated by scores on the Neurobehavioral Specific

Impairment Subscale of the A-ONE). In Figure 18-11, *A*, Mr. Johnson has sustained CVA on the left side; the impairments of ideational apraxia, motor apraxia, perseveration, organization and sequencing, and right hemiplegia interfere with dressing performance. The dressing domain is one of five domains on the Functional Independence Scale of the A-ONE. Summary sheets from the A-ONE indicating scores in the other functional domains and different neurobehavioral impairments are also shown for both individuals (see Figure 18-10, *B* and *C*, and Figure 18-11, *B* and *C*).

A therapist interested in applying a deficit-specific approach to evaluate dysfunction of client factors (e.g., muscle strength and tone, motor apraxia, spatial relations, neglect, and memory) has a choice of applying test batteries or evaluations aimed at specific impairments. Examples of test batteries used by occupational therapists to evaluate a range of impairments in patients with CVA are the Lowenstein Occupational Therapy Cognitive Assessment (LOTCA)[39] and the Rivermead Perceptual Assessment Battery (RPAB).[69] Examples of standardized deficit-specific tests available in occupational therapy departments for evaluating some of the impairments mentioned in the cases presented in Figure 18-10 and 18-11 are the Behavioral Inattention Test (BIT)[72] for unilateral neglect or inattention; the Motor-Free Visual Perception Test—Vertical (MVPT—V),[46] a deficit-specific evaluation that could be used to examine presence of spatial relations impairments, the Test of Every Day Attention (TEA)[56]; for attention deficits, the Behavioral Assessment of the Dysexecutive Syndrome (BADS)[70] for evaluating prefrontal dysfunction; Rivermead Behavioral Memory Test (RBMT)[71] for everyday memory functions; the Self-Reporting Awareness Test[1] and the Assessment of Awareness of Disability[63] for evaluating insight; a test for imitating gestures[25] used to evaluate ideomotor apraxia; and a test for ideational apraxia.[26]

Use of deficit-specific tests as a follow-up of the functional evaluation has been suggested by some authors under specific conditions. These conditions include circumstances in which the therapist has difficulties defining

---

*References 8, 12, 16, 30, 37, 44, 64.

# Functional Independence Scale and
# Neurobehavioral Specific Impairment Subscale

**Name** Ms. Wilson        **Date** 6/13/03

## Independence Score (IP):

4 = Independent and able to transfer activity to other environmental situations.
3 = Independent with supervision.
2 = Needs verbal assistance.
1 = Needs demonstration or physical assistance.
0 = Unable to perform. Totally dependent on assistance.

## Neurobehavioral Score (NB):

0 = No neurobehavioral impairments observed.
1 = Able to perform without additional information, but some neurobehavioral impairment is observed.
2 = Able to perform with additional verbal assistance, but neurobehavioral impairment can be observed during performance.
3 = Able to perform with demonstration or minimal to considerable physical assistance.
4 = Unable to perform due to neurobehavioral impairment. Needs maximum physical assistance.

## List helping aids used:

• Wheelchair
• Nonslip for soap and plate
• Adapted toothbrush
• Velcro fastening on shoes

PRIMARY ADL ACTIVITY      SCORING      COMMENTS AND REASONING

| DRESSING | IP SCORE | | | | | COMMENTS |
|---|---|---|---|---|---|---|
| Shirt (or Dress) | 4 | 3 | 2 | ① | 0 | Include one armhole, fix shoulder |
| Pants | 4 | 3 | 2 | ① | 0 | Find correct leghole |
| Socks | 4 | 3 | 2 | ① | 0 | One-handed technique, balance |
| Shoes | 4 | 3 | 2 | ① | 0 | Balance |
| Fastenings | 4 | 3 | 2 | ① | 0 | Match buttonholes, Velcro through loop |
| Other | | | | | | |

| NB IMPAIRMENT | NB SCORE | | | | | COMMENTS |
|---|---|---|---|---|---|---|
| Motor Apraxia | ⓪ | 1 | 2 | 3 | 4 | |
| Ideational Apraxia | ⓪ | 1 | 2 | 3 | 4 | |
| Unilateral Body Neglect | 0 | 1 | 2 | ③ | 4 | Leaves out left body side |
| Somatoagnosia | ⓪ | 1 | 2 | 3 | 4 | |
| Spatial Relations | 0 | 1 | 2 | ③ | 4 | Finding correct holes, front/back |
| Unilateral Spatial Neglect | 0 | 1 | ② | 3 | 4 | Leaves out items in left visual field |
| Abnormal Tone: Right | ⓪ | 1 | 2 | 3 | 4 | |
| Abnormal Tone: Left | 0 | 1 | 2 | ③ | 4 | Sitting balance/bilateral manipulation |
| Perseveration | ⓪ | 1 | 2 | 3 | 4 | |
| Organization/Sequencing | 0 | 1 | ② | 3 | 4 | For activity steps |
| Other | | | | | | |

Note: All definitions and scoring criteria for each deficit are in the Evaluation Manual.

**Figure 18-10** **A,** Árnadóttir OT-ADL Neurobehavioral Evaluation (A-ONE): sample from the dressing domain of the Functional Independence Scale and the Neurobehavioral Specific Impairment Subscale for Ms. Wilson.

# Árnadóttir OT-ADL
# Neurobehavioral Evaluation
# (A-ONE)

**Name**    Ms. Wilson

**Date**    6-13-03

**Birthdate**    4-15-1943

**Age**    60

**Gender**    Female

**Ethnicity**    Caucasian

**Dominance**    Right

**Profession**    Dressmaker

**Medical Diagnosis:**
Right CVA 6/20/03. Ischemia.

**Medications:**

**Social Situation:**
Lives alone in an apartment building on third floor
Has two adult daughters

**Summary of Independence:**
Needs physical assistance with dressing, grooming, hygiene, transfer, and mobility tasks because of left-sided paralysis and perceptual and cognitive impairments. Is more or less able to feed herself if meals have been prepared. No problems with personal communication, although perceptual impairments will affect reading and writing skills. Also has lack of judgment and memory impairment, which affect task performance. Is not able to live alone at this stage. If personal home support becomes available, will need a home evaluation because of physical limitation and wheelchair use. Needs recommendations regarding removal of architectural barriers or suggestions for alternative housing. Unable to return to previous job as a dressmaker.

FUNCTIONAL INDEPENDENCE SCORE (optional)

| FUNCTION | TOTAL SCORE | % SCORE |
|---|---|---|
| Dressing | 1,1,1,1,1= 5/20 | |
| Grooming and Hygiene | 1,2,1,1,3,0= 8/24 | |
| Transfer and Mobility | 1,1,1,1,1= 5/20 | |
| Feeding | 4,4,4,3= 15/16 | |
| Communication | 4,4= 8/8 | |

**Figure 18-10, cont'd**    **B,** A-ONE summary sheet for the case of Ms. Wilson.

deficits, when a new therapist needs to refine observation skills,[51,52] when therapists require an aid in quantification of the severity of the deficit,[52] and or when the therapist needs to report efficacy of treatment in research studies.[44]

The previous sections have described how the therapist can detect neurobehavioral impairments during observation of task performance by the use of activity analysis based on the A-ONE theoretical framework. Functional assessments may include nonstandardized and standardized observations. According to Burke,[19] non-

standardized assessments "do not require adherence to specific instructions for administration. They are appropriate for a wide range of settings, situations, materials, and individuals. Their usefulness for generalizing results from one individual to another is limited, however, because the materials, time allotments, and assistance may all vary." Nonstandardized tests may be useful for measuring progress in one individual, if the therapist is able to replicate the same situation at a later time.[19,54] According to Unsworth,[67] a nonstandardized hypothesis

## LIST OF NEUROBEHAVIORAL IMPAIRMENTS OBSERVED:

| SPECIFIC IMPAIRMENT | D | G | T | F | C |
|---|---|---|---|---|---|
| Motor Apraxia | | | | | |
| Ideational Apraxia | | | | | |
| Unilateral Body Neglect | 3 | 3 | 3 | 1 | |
| Somatoagnosia | | | | | |
| Spatial Relations | 3 | 3 | 3 | 1 | |
| Unilateral Spatial Neglect | 2 | 2 | 3 | 1 | |
| Abnormal Tone: Right | | | | | |
| Abnormal Tone: Left | 3 | 3 | 3 | 1 | |
| Perseveration | | | | | |
| Organization | 2 | 2 | 2 | 1 | |
| Topographic Disorientation | | | 3 | | |
| Other | | | | | |
| Sensory Aphasia | | | | | |
| Jargon Aphasia | | | | | |
| Anomia | | | | | |
| Paraphasia | | | | | |
| Expressive Aphasia | | | | | |

| PERVASIVE IMPAIRMENT | ADL |
|---|---|
| Astereognosis | ✓ |
| Visual Object Agnosia | |
| Visual Spatial Agnosia | ✓ |
| Associative Visual Agnosia | |
| Anosognosia | |
| R/L Discrimination | ✓ |
| Short-Term Memory | ✓ |
| Long-Term Memory | |
| Disorientation | ✓ |
| Confabulation | |
| Lability | ✓ |
| Euphoria | |
| Apathy | |
| Depression | ✓ |
| Aggressiveness | |
| Irritability | |
| Frustration | |

| PERVASIVE IMPAIRMENT | ADL |
|---|---|
| Restlessness | |
| Concrete Thinking | ✓ |
| Decreased Insight | ✓ |
| Impaired Judgment | ✓ |
| Confusion | |
| Impaired Alertness | |
| Impaired Attention | ✓ |
| Distractibility | ✓ |
| Impaired Initiative | |
| Impaired Motivation | |
| Performance Latency | |
| Absent Mindedness | |
| Other | |
| Field Dependency | ✓ |
| | |
| | |
| | |

Use (✓) for presence of specific impairments in different ADL domains (D = dressing, G = grooming, T =transfers, F = feeding, C = communication) and for presence of pervasive impairments detected during the ADL evaluation.

### Summary of Neurobehavioral Impairments:

Needs physical assistance for most dressing, grooming, hygiene, transfer, and mobility tasks because of left-sided paralysis, spatial relations impairments (e.g., problems differentiating back from front of clothes and finding armholes and legholes), and unilateral body neglect (i.e., does not wash or dress affected side)finding. Does not attend to objects in the left visual field and needs verbal cues for performance. Also needs verbal cues for organizing activity steps. Does not know her way around the hospital. Does not have insight into how the CVA affects her ADL and is thus unrealistic in day-to-day planning. Has impaired judgment resulting in unsafe transfer attempts. Leaves the water running after hygiene and grooming activities if not reminded to turn it off. Is emotionally labile and appears depressed at times. Is not oriented regarding time and date. Presents with impaired attention, distraction, and defective short-term memory requiring repeated verbal instructions.

### Treatment Considerations:

### Occupational Therapist:

### A-ONE Certification Number:

**Figure 18-10, cont'd**  **C,** A-ONE summary sheet for the case of Ms. Wilson. (Courtesy G. Árnadóttir, Reykjavík, Iceland.)

# Functional Independence Scale and
# Neurobehavioral Specific Impairment Subscale

**Name**  Mr. A. Johnson                                         **Date**  7/5/03

**Independence Score (IP):**

4 = Independent and able to transfer activity to other environmental situations.
3 = Independent with supervision.
2 = Needs verbal assistance.
1 = Needs demonstration or physical assistance.
0 = Unable to perform. Totally dependent on assistance.

**Neurobehavioral Score (NB):**

0 = No neurobehavioral impairments observed.
1 = Able to perform without additional information, but some neurobehavioral impairment is observed.
2 = Able to perform with additional verbal assistance, but neurobehavioral impairment can be observed during performance.
3 = Able to perform with demonstration or minimal to considerable physical assistance.
4 = Unable to perform due to neurobehavioral impairment. Needs maximum physical assistance.

**List Helping Aids Used:**

• Wheelchair

PRIMARY ADL ACTIVITY   SCORING   COMMENTS AND REASONING

| DRESSING | IP SCORE | | | | | COMMENTS |
|---|---|---|---|---|---|---|
| Shirt(or Dress) | 4 | 3 | 2 | ①| 0 | Assistance with right arm |
| Pant | 4 | 3 | 2 | ① | 0 | Stuck because of friction from shoe |
| Socks | 4 | 3 | 2 | ① | 0 | One-handed technique, balance |
| Shoes | 4 | 3 | 2 | ① | 0 | Attempts without opening sock |
| Fastenings | 4 | 3 | 2 | ① | 0 | Does not know how to handle buckle |
| Other | | | | | | |

| NB IMPAIRMENT | NB SCORE | | | | | |
|---|---|---|---|---|---|---|
| Motor Apraxia | 0 | ① | 2 | 3 | 4 | Left hand |
| Ideational Apraxia | 0 | 1 | 2 | ③ | 4 | Problems with belt, shoes before trousers |
| Unilateral Body Neglect | ⓪ | 1 | 2 | 3 | 4 | Stuck because of friction |
| Somatoagnosia | ⓪ | 1 | 2 | 3 | 4 | |
| Spatial Relations | ⓪ | 1 | 2 | 3 | 4 | |
| Unilateral Spatial Neglect | ⓪ | 1 | 2 | 3 | 4 | |
| Abnormal Tone: Right | 0 | 1 | 2 | ③ | 4 | Sitting balance/bilateral manipulation |
| Abnormal Tone: Left | ⓪ | 1 | 2 | 3 | 4 | |
| Perseveration | 0 | 1 | 2 | ③ | 4 | Repeats pulling sleeve, sock |
| Organization/Sequencing | 0 | 1 | 2 | ③ | 4 | Assistance with activity steps |
| Other | | | | | | Shoes before trousers |

Note: All definitions and scoring criteria for each deficit are in the Evaluation Manual.

**Figure 18-11**  **A,** Árnadóttir OT-ADL Neurobehavioral Evaluation (A-ONE): sample from the dressing domain of the Functional Independence Scale and the Neurobehavioral Specific Impairment Subscale for Mr. Johnson.

# Árnadóttir OT-ADL
# Neurobehavioral Evaluation
# (A-ONE)

**Name** ___Mr. A. Johnson___    **Date** ___7-5-03___

**Birthdate** ___4-17-62___    **Age** ___41___

**Gender** ___Male___    **Ethnicity** ___Caucasian___

**Dominance** ___Right___    **Profession** ___Carpenter___

**Medical Diagnosis:**

Left CVA due to ruptured aneurysm and cerebral hemorrhage

**Medications:**

**Social Situation:**

Married with two sons, 3 and 5 years old. Lives in own house in a village, a 1-hour drive from the hospital. Worked as a carpenter. Wife works full time in office. Children in day care. Wife is supportive but under a lot of strain because of the present situation.

**Summary of Independence:**

Needs physical assistance with all dressing, grooming, and hygiene tasks because of right-sided paralysis, ideational apraxia, organization and sequencing impairment, motor apraxia, and perseverations. Slow performance. Has receptive aphasia so verbal instructions not sufficient. Uses pantomime to indicate needs because of inability to use verbal expression. Is able to maneuver in a wheelchair but needs physical assistance with all transfers. Is able to drink and feed himself if food has been prepared, cut, and buttered. Unable to use knife (to peel, etc.) by using one-handed techniques, partially because of ideational apraxia, clumsy movements of left hand, and paralysis of right hand. Needs considerable assistance in most ADL tasks. Will need examination re architectural barriers at home and personal assistance before discharge. Unable to assume previous job and role of family provider.

FUNCTIONAL INDEPENDENCE SCORE (optional)

| FUNCTION | TOTAL SCORE | % SCORE |
|---|---|---|
| Dressing | 1,1,1,1,1 = 5/20 | |
| Grooming and Hygiene | 1,2,1,1,1,0 = 6/24 | |
| Transfer and Mobility | 1,1,3,1,1 = 7/20 | |
| Feeding | 4,4,4,1 = 13/16 | |
| Communication | 1,1 = 2/8 | |

**Figure 18-11, cont'd    B,** A-ONE summary sheet for Mr. Johnson.

testing approach for evaluation could be useful for therapists who have not had the chance to complete the required training for standardized assessments such as the A-ONE and the Assessment of Motor and Process Skills[29] (see Chapter 20). Most authors agree that standardized assessments have established, during their developmental process, uniform standards regarding assessment conditions, materials, and instructions for collecting and analyzing information that must be followed precisely. Furthermore, particular assessments may require specific training programs.* Thus the development of conceptual and operational definitions can be considered an important aspect of providing uniform standards. Some authors[6,14,55] additionally request that norms be established to complete the standardization process, referring to collecting information about the typical performance of an average person.

---

*References 6, 14, 15, 19, 53, 55, 58, 67.

## LIST OF NEUROBEHAVIORAL IMPAIRMENTS OBSERVED:

| SPECIFIC IMPAIRMENT | D | G | T | F | C |
|---|---|---|---|---|---|
| Motor Apraxia | 1 | 3 | | 3 | |
| Ideational Apraxia | 3 | 3 | 3 | 3 | |
| Unilateral Body Neglect | | | | | |
| Somatoagnosia | | | | | |
| Spatial Relations | | | | | |
| Unilateral Spatial Neglect | | | | | |
| Abnormal Tone: Right | 3 | 3 | 3 | 3 | |
| Abnormal Tone: Left | | | | | |
| Perseveration | 3 | 3 | | 1 | |
| Organization | 3 | 3 | 3 | 1 | |
| Topographic Disorientation | | ? | | | |
| Other | | | | | |
| Sensory Aphasia | | | | | ✓ |
| Jargon Aphasia | | | | | |
| Anomia | | | | | |
| Paraphasia | | | | | |
| Expressive Aphasia | | | | | ✓ |

| PERVASIVE IMPAIRMENT | ADL |
|---|---|
| Astereognosis | NT |
| Visual Object Agnosia | |
| Visual Spatial Agnosia | |
| Associative Visual Agnosia | |
| Anosognosia | |
| R/L Discrimination | |
| Short-Term Memory | NT |
| Long-Term Memory | NT |
| Disorientation | NT |
| Confabulation | |
| Lability | |
| Euphoria | |
| Apathy | |
| Depression | ✓ |
| Aggressiveness | |
| Irritability | |
| Frustration | ✓ |

| PERVASIVE IMPAIRMENT | ADL |
|---|---|
| Restlessness | |
| Concrete Thinking | ✓ |
| Decreased Insight | NT |
| Impaired Judgment | ✓ |
| Confusion | |
| Impaired Alertness | |
| Impaired Attention | ✓ |
| Distractibility | |
| Impaired Initiative | |
| Impaired Motivation | |
| Performance Latency | ✓ |
| Absent Mindedness | |
| Other | |

Use (✓) for presence of specific impairments in different ADL domains (D = dressing, G = grooming, T = transfers, F = feeding, C = communication) and for presence of pervasive impairments detected during the ADL evaluation.

### Summary of Neurobehavioral Impairments:

Has considerable ideational apraxia, sensory and expressive aphasia, and paralysis of right side, so requires extensive physical assistance in many ADL tasks. Limited use of left upper extremity for fine object manipulation due to motor apraxia. Takes long time to learn new skills because of ideational problems and comprehension. Incomplete testing of memory items because of communication problems. Appears depressed and frustrated at times, especially when unable to express self. Impaired judgment relating to inadequate organization and sequencing, as well as ideational apraxia. Brings electric razor toward running water. Attempts transfers without wheelchair brakes on.

### Treatment Considerations:

### Occupational Therapist:

### A-ONE Certification Number:

**Figure 18-11, cont'd**   **C,** A-ONE summary sheet for Mr. Johnson. (Courtesy G. Árnadóttir, Reykjavík, Iceland.)

## SUMMARY

The information in this chapter has provided guidelines for the observation of stroke patients during task performance with the purpose of detecting impairments that interfere with independent performance. The conceptual and operational definitions provided in this text, based on the A-ONE theory, are important to ensure consistency of the method. The review allows therapists to interpret cues and to form hypotheses regarding impairments and activity limitation. However, this information has limitations and as presented in this text is not standardized. In contrast, the A-ONE evaluation is standardized; that is, it includes detailed administration and scoring instructions and provides normative data and criterion references. Several studies of validity and reliability have been conducted to ensure the A-ONE does what its developer claims it does and that it measures the traits consistently.[10-12,31,32,49,60] The instrument requires a training seminar for therapists to ensure reliability. Thus the evaluation itself permits comparison across patients in addition to monitoring of progress, regardless of which trained therapist administers and interprets the evaluation. The results provide useful information for choice of treatment based on strengths and weaknesses of the patient, from the perspective of client factors and activity performance. Occupational therapists must gather valid, reliable information that can be used to build treatment guidelines. Therefore consistent terminology must be developed and, as suggested by Holm and Rogers,[37] data collection must be made by use of valid, reliable instruments to ensure usefulness and integrity of the information.

In short, the A-ONE instrument allows the therapist to detect impairments that interfere with task performance to understand factors underlying functional dependence. Such information aids therapists in understanding the reasons for the activity limitations. In other words, the instrument aids the therapist in analyzing the nature or cause of a functional problem requiring occupational therapy intervention. Subsequently, therapists can speculate about the best intervention for activity limitation and impairments (see Chapter 19). Therapists can base the decision on information from the evaluation and the therapist's knowledge of different intervention methods, whether they are focused on the level of activity performance or the CNS level of the client factors. This could be within a deficit-specific intervention approach in which, for example, different sensory stimuli can be provided with the aim of affecting neuronal processing (e.g., at the cortical level) based on different theories. Furthermore, assessment could be done by using a combination of the two major approaches, keeping neuronal factors in mind during activity performance, as is being recommended in the quadraphonic approach[1] or when applying adaptive frameworks such as the rehabilitation frame of reference[28] in which the information is used to develop adaptive techniques or inform the client's support system about the suggested techniques or about what to expect in terms of impairments and activity limitations in the client's performance. However, one must keep in mind that at present no functional assessment prescribes treatment, and therefore clinical reasoning is necessary to combine evaluation results with available treatment choices, as well as patient's specific conditions such as conceptual factors. Furthermore, research studies are needed to test the efficacy of intervention and theories.[38,61,65] For such testing, valid and reliable instruments are mandatory.

## REVIEW QUESTIONS

1. Which kind of lesions may produce unilateral motor apraxia of the left side of the body?
2. What is the difference between the impairments of disorientation and confusion?
3. Which impairment(s) might cause an individual to place both legs in the same leghole of a pair of pants?
4. If an individual does not wash both sides of the body spontaneously, impairments such as unilateral body neglect, organization and sequencing problems, or ideational apraxia might be suspected. Can clinical reasoning be used to differentiate between the different possible impairments, and if so how?
5. What is the difference between expected impairments in the presence of a right middle cerebral artery dysfunction compared with expected impairments of a left middle cerebral artery dysfunction?

## REFERENCES

1. Abreu BC: Evaluation and intervention with memory and learning impairments. In Unsworth C, editor: *Cognitive and perceptual dysfunction: a clinical reasoning approach to evaluation and intervention*, Philadelphia, 1999, FA Davis.
2. American Heart Association: *American Stroke Association: impact of stroke*, 2002. Retrieved February, 24, 2003, from www.strokeassociation.org/presenter.jhtml?identifier=1014
3. American Heart Association: *American Stroke Association: impact of stroke*, 2002. Retrieved February, 24, 2003, from www.strokeassociation.org/presenter.jhtml?identifier=1033
4. American Heart Association: *American Stroke Association: impact of stroke*, 2002. Retrieved February, 24, 2003, from www.strokeassociation.org/presenter.jhtml?identifier=1052
5. American Heart Association: *American Stroke Association: impact of stroke*, 2002. Retrieved February, 24, 2003, from www.americanheart.org/presenter.jhtml?identifier=2762
6. Anastasi A, Urbina S: *Psychological testing*, ed 7, Upper Saddle River, NJ, 1997, Prentice Hall.
7. Árnadóttir G: *A-ONE training course: lecture notes*, Reykjavík, Iceland, 2003, Gudrún Árnadóttir.
8. Árnadóttir G: The A-ONE instrument: sensitivity to activity limitation and impairment in dementia. Poster presentation at the thirteenth World Congress of Occupational Therapists, World Federation of Occupational Therapists, Stockholm, Sweden, 2002.
9. Árnadóttir G: Neurobehavior: the key to occupation. Poster presentation at the thirteenth World Congress of Occupational

Therapists, World Federation of Occupational Therapists, Stockholm, Sweden, 2002.

10. Árnadóttir G: Review of instrument development: Árnadóttir OT-ADL Neurobehavioral Evaluation (A-ONE). Poster presentation at the thirteenth World Congress of Occupational Therapists, World Federation of Occupational Therapists, Stockholm, Sweden, 2002.

11. Árnadóttir G: Evaluation and intervention with complex perceptual impairment. In Unsworth C, editor: *Cognitive and perceptual dysfunction: a clinical reasoning approach to evaluation and intervention*, Philadelphia, 1999, FA Davis.

12. Árnadóttir G: *The brain and behavior: assessing cortical dysfunction through activities of daily living*, St Louis, 1990, Mosby.

13. Ayres AJ: *Developmental dyspraxia and adult onset apraxia*, Torrance, Calif, 1985, Sensory Integration International.

14. Bailay DM: *Research for the health professional: a practical guide*, ed 2, Philadelphia, 1997, FA Davis.

15. Benson J, Schell BA: Measurement theory: application to occupational and physical therapy. In Deusen JV, Brundt D, editors: *Assessment in occupational and physical therapy*, Philadelphia, 1997, Saunders.

16. Bernspång B, Fisher AG: Differences between persons with right or left cerebral vascular accident on the assessment of motor and process skills, *Arch Phys Med Rehabil* 76(12):1144-1151, 1995.

17. Blesedell Crepeau E: Activity analysis: a way of thinking about occupational performance. In Neistadt ME, Blesedell Crepeau E, editors: *Willard and Spackman's occupational therapy*, ed 9, Philadelphia,1998, Lippincott-Raven.

18. Boyt Schell B: *Clinical reasoning: the basis of practice*. In Neistadt ME, Blesedell Crepeau E, editors: *Willard and Spackman's occupational therapy*, ed 9, Philadelphia,1998, Lippincott-Raven.

19. Burke JP: Selecting evaluation tools I. In Royeen CB, editors: *AOTA self study series: assessing function*, Rockville, Md, 1989, American Occupational Therapy Association.

20. Caplan LR: *Stroke: a clinical approach*, ed 2, Boston, 1993, Butterworth-Heinemann.

21. Clark FA, Parham D, Carlson ME, et al: Occupational science: academic innovation in the service of occupational therapy's future, *Am J Occup Ther* 45:300, 1991.

22. Damasio AR: The frontal lobes. In Heilman KM, Valenstein E, editors: *Clinical neuropsychology*, ed 2, New York, 1985, Oxford University Press.

23. Damasio AR, Anderson SW: The frontal lobes. In Heilman KM, Valenstein E, editors: *Clinical neuropsychology*, ed 3, New York, 1993, Oxford University Press.

24. Daube JR, Sandok BA: *Medical neurosciences: an approach to anatomy, pathology and physiology by systems and levels*, Boston, 1978, Little, Brown.

25. De Renzi E, Fabrizia M, Nichelli P: Imitating gestures: a quantitative approach to motor apraxia, *Arch Neurol* 37(1):6-10, 1980.

26. De Renzi E, Lucchelli F: Ideational apraxia, *Brain* 111(pt 5):1173-1185, 1988.

27. Dickoff J, James P, Wiedenbach E: Theory in a practice discipline. I. Practice oriented discipline, *Nurs Res* 17(5):415-435, 1968.

28. Duran L, Fisher AG: Evaluation and intervention with executive functions impairment. In Unsworth C, editor: *Cognitive and perceptual dysfunction: a clinical reasoning approach to evaluation and intervention*, Philadelphia, 1999, FA Davis.

29. Fisher AG: *Assessment of motor and process skills*, vol 1, *Development, standardization, and administration manual*, ed 4, Fort Collins, Colo, 1999, Three Star Press.

30. Fisher AG, Short-DeGraff M: Improving functional assessment in occupational therapy: recommendations and philosophy for change, *Am J Occup Ther* 47(3):199-201, 1993.

31. Garðarsdóttir S: Tengsl milli færni við, athafnir daglegs lífs (ADL) og taugaatferlis hjá sjúklingum sem fengið hafa heilablóð fall, *Iðjupjálfinn* 22:10, 2000.

32. Gardarsdóttir S, Kaplan S: Validity of the Árnadóttir OT-ADL neurobehavioral evaluation (A-ONE): performance in activities of daily living in persons with left and right hemisphere damage, *Am J Occup Ther* 56(5):499-508, 2002.

33. Geschwind N: Specialization of the human brain, *Sci Am* 241:80, 1979.

34. Goldberg E, Costa LD: Hemisphere differences in the acquisition and use of descriptive system, *Brain Lang* 14:144, 1981.

35. Heilman KM, Gonzalez Rothi LJ: Apraxia. In Heilman KM, Valenstein E, editors: *Clinical neuropsychology*, ed 3, New York, 1993, Oxford University Press.

36. Heilman KM, Watson RJ, Valenstein E: Neglect and related disorders. In Heilman KM, Valenstein E, editors: *Clinical neuropsychology*, ed 3, New York, 1993, Oxford University Press.

37. Holm MB, Rogers JC: The therapists thinking behind functional assessment II. In Royeen CB, editor: *AOTA self study series: assessing function*, Rockville, Md, 1989, American Occupational Therapy Association.

38. Huin-ing Ma, Trombly CA: A synthesis of effects of occupational therapy for persons with stroke. I. Restoration of roles, tasks and activities, *Am J Occup Ther* 56:260, 2002.

39. Itzkovich M, Elazar B, Averbuch S, et al: *Lowenstein occupational therapy cognitive assessment: LOTCA™ Manual*, Pequannock, NJ, 1990, Maddack Inc.

40. Kiernan, JA: *Barr's the human nervous system: an anatomical viewpoint*, ed 7, Philadelphia, 1998, Lippincott-Raven.

41. Llorens LA: Activity analysis: agreement among factors in a sensory processing model, *Am J Occup Ther* 40(2):103-110, 1986.

42. Luria AR: *Higher cortical functions in man*, ed 2, New York, 1980, Basic Books.

43. Luria AR: *The working brain: an introduction to neuropsychology*, New York, 1973, Basic Books.

44. Mathiowetz V: Role of physical performance component evaluations in occupational therapy functional assessment, *Am J Occup Ther* 47(3):225-230, 1993.

45. Mattingly C, Fleming MH: *Clinical reasoning: forms of enquiry in a therapeutic practice*, Philadelphia, 1994, FA Davis.

46. Mercier L, Hebert J, Colarusso RP, et al: *MVPT-V Motor free visual perception test—vertical format—manual*, Novato, Calif, 1997, Academic Therapy Publications.

47. Neistadt ME: The neurobiology of learning: implications for treatment of adults with brain injury, *Am J Occup Ther* 48(5):421-430, 1994.

48. Neistadt ME: Occupational therapy for adults with perceptual deficits, *Am J Occup Ther* 42(7):434-440, 1988.

49. Newer MR, Árnadóttir G, Martin AA, et al: A comparison of quantitative electroencephalography, computed tomography, and behavioral evaluations to localize impairment in patients with stroke and transient ischemic attacks, *J Neuroimaging* 4:82, 1994.

50. Occupational therapy practice framework: domain and process, *Am J Occup Ther* 56(6):609-639, 2002.

51. Okkema K: *Cognition and perception in the stroke patient: a guide to functional outcomes in occupational therapy*, Gaithersburg, Md, 1993, Aspen.

52. Phillips ME, Wolters S: Assessment in practice: common tools and methods. In Royeen CB, editor: *AOTA self study series: stroke—strategies, treatment, rehabilitation, outcomes, knowledge and evaluation*, Bethesda, Md, 1996, American Occupational Therapy Association.

53. Polgar JM: Critiquing assessments. In Neistadt ME, Blesedell Crepeau E, editors: *Willard & Spackman's occupational therapy*, ed 9, Philadelphia, 1998, Lippincott-Raven.

54. Reed KL, Sanderson SN: *Concepts of occupational therapy*, ed 4, Philadelphia, 1999, Lippincott Williams & Wilkins.

55. Richardson PK: Use of standardized tests in pediatric practice. In Case-Smith J, Allen AJ, Pratt PN, editors: *Occupational therapy for children*, ed 4, St Louis, 2001, Mosby.

56. Robertson I, Ward T, Ridgeway Y, et al: *The test of everyday attention (TEA)*, Bury St Edmunds, England, 1994, Thames Valley Test Company.

57. Rogers JC, Holm MB: The therapists thinking behind functional assessment I. In Royeen CB, editor: *AOTA self study series: assessing function*, Rockville, Md, 1989, American Occupational Therapy Association.

58. Royeen CB: *A research primer in occupational and physical therapy*, Bethesda, Md, 1997, American Occupational Therapy Association.

59. Starkstein SE, Robinson RG: Neuropsychiatric aspects of stroke. In Coffey CE, Cummings JL, editors: *Textbook of geriatric neuropsychiatry*, Washington, DC, 1994, American Psychiatric Press.

60. Steultjens EM: A-ONE: De Nederlandse Versie, *Ned Tidskrift Ergoterapie* 26:100, 1998.

61. Steultjens EM, Dekker J, Bouter LM, et al: Occupational therapy for stroke patients: a systematic review, *Stroke* 34:676-687, 2003

62. Strub RL, Black FW: *The mental status examination in neurology*, ed 2, Philadelphia, 1985, FA Davis.

63. Tham K, Bernspång B, Fisher A: Development of the assessment of awareness of disability, *Scand J Occup Ther* 55:46, 1999.

64. Trombly CA: Anticipating the future: assessment of occupational function, *Am J Occup Ther* 47(3):253-257, 1993.

65. Trombly CA, Hui-ing Ma: A synthesis of effects of occupational therapy for persons with stroke. II. Remediation of impairments, *Am J Occup Ther* 56:250, 2002.

66. Unsworth C: Introduction to cognitive and perceptual dysfunction: theoretical approaches to therapy. In Unsworth C, editor: *Cognitive and perceptual dysfunction: a clinical reasoning approach to evaluation and intervention*, Philadelphia, 1999, FA Davis.

67. Unsworth C: Reflections on the process of therapy in cognitive and perceptual dysfunction. In Unsworth C, editor: *Cognitive and perceptual dysfunction: a clinical reasoning approach to evaluation and intervention*, Philadelphia, 1999, FA Davis.

68. US Department of Health and Human Services: *Clinical practice guideline number 16: post-stroke rehabilitation*, Rockville, Md, 1995, US Department of Health and Human Services.

69. Whiting S, Lincoln N, Bhavnani G, et al: *RPAB: The Rivermead behavioural memory test*, Windsor, 1985, NFER-NELSON.

70. Wilson BA, Alderman P, Burgess H, et al: *Behavioral assessment of the dysexecutive syndrome (BADS)*, Bury St Edmunds, England, 1996, Thames Valley Test Company.

71. Wilson BA, Cockburn J, Baddely A: *RBMT: The Rivermead behavioural memory test*, Suffolk, England, 1989, Thames Valley Test Company.

72. Wilson BA, Cockburn J, Halligan P: *Behavioral inattention test: manual*, Suffolk, England, 1987, Thames Valley Test Company.

73. World Health Organization: *The international classification of impairments, of functioning, disability and health—ICF*, Geneva, 2001, The Organization.

74. Yatsu FM, Grotta JC, Pettigrew LC, et al: *Stroke: 100 maxims*, St Louis, 1995, Mosby.

75. Zoltan B: *Vision, perception, and cognition: a manual for the evaluation and treatment of the neurologically impaired adult*, ed 3, Thorofare, NJ, 1996, Slack.

kerry brockmann rubio
and glen gillen

**chapter 19**

# Treatment of Cognitive-Perceptual Deficits: A Function-Based Approach

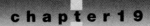

## key terms

| | | |
|---|---|---|
| Affolter approach | insight | perception |
| aphasia | integrated functional approach | perseveration |
| apraxia | memory | problem solving |
| attention | multicontextual approach | spatial relations |
| cognition | neurobehavior | unilateral neglect |
| concrete thinking | organization/sequencing | |

## chapter objectives

After completing this chapter, the reader will be able to accomplish the following:

1. Understand the different approaches to treatment of cognitive and perceptual (processing) impairments and be aware of research conducted on each approach.
2. Recognize the importance of context, psychosocial issues, and meaningful activity in treatment planning for this population.
3. Apply the multicontextual and Affolter approaches to treatment of processing impairments.
4. Discuss different treatment approaches to individual neurobehavioral impairments.
5. Realize the relevance and importance of occupation-based activities in the treatment of cognitive and perceptual impairments.

Few things are more interesting or frustrating to a therapist than observing a stroke survivor with severe neglect or apraxia attempting unsuccessfully to perform an activity. Cognitive and perceptual (processing) impairments can severely impair a person's ability to participate in everyday activities. Frequently, the priority for occupational therapists is to determine what can be done to improve the performance in activities for stroke patients with processing impairments.

This chapter reviews studies and other literature on treatment approaches and discusses suggestions for treating processing impairments that frequently are found in persons who have sustained a stroke. The reader should review Chapters 17 and 18 for a full overview of this topic.

## NEUROBEHAVIOR

*Neurobehavior* has been defined as any behavioral response resulting from central nervous system processing. Neurobehavior is considered the basis of performance in activities of daily living (ADL).[4] In this chapter the term *neurobehavior* refers to cognitive and perceptual components of behavior, including praxis, attention, memory, spatial relations, sequencing, and problem solving.

## TREATMENT APPROACHES

Approaches to stroke rehabilitation can be directed at the level of impairment, activity limitations, or participation restrictions. *Impairment* refers to body dysfunction; *activity limitation*, to task performance dysfunction; and *participation restriction*, to problems in life situations. Approaches aimed at the level of participation restrictions have the greatest impact on the stroke survivor's quality of life.[42] Unfortunately, many times in current practice, participation restrictions are deemphasized, whereas impairment or activity limitation is emphasized. Therapists must strive to provide service in all three areas of need while promoting issues relevant to the patient's quality of life. See Chapter 3.

Processing impairments commonly are described in the literature, but the focus often is placed on assessment of these impairments. Controlled studies relating to treatment effectiveness in the stroke population are few,[64] and studies supporting specific treatment approaches for cognitive and perceptual impairments are even rarer. In a survey on cognitive and perceptual rehabilitation, most occupational therapists said they perceived a need for treatment guidelines and more treatment techniques and materials for this population.[68]

Treatment approaches to perceptual or cognitive impairments generally are classified in one of two categories: (1) the functional or adaptive approach or (2) the remediation or restoration approach. The functional or adaptive approach emphasizes techniques to assist the patient in adapting to deficits, changing the environmental parameters of a task to facilitate function, and using a person's strengths to compensate for loss of function. Remediation, or restoration, emphasizes the use of techniques to facilitate recovery of the actual cognitive or perceptual skills affected by the stroke. Each approach has strengths and limitations, and therapists often use both approaches during stroke rehabilitation (Table 19-1).

### Functional Approach

The functional approach uses repetitive practice in particular activities, usually daily living tasks, to help the patient become more independent. This approach is designed to treat symptoms rather than the cause of the dysfunction.[21] Some occupational therapists believe their role in cognitive and perceptual rehabilitation lies solely in the realm of a functional approach, involving training in compensatory techniques and only with tasks directly related to functional performance.[55] This approach appears most compatible with research indicating that family members and financial providers rank independence in ADL as the highest priority for rehabilitation.[15,51]

Therapists use the functional approach to train patients to function by compensating. An example of compensation is the use of an alarm watch to remind someone with poor memory to take medication. Compensation circumvents the problem. Some therapists believe the use of compensation should be limited to patients who have accepted the permanence of the perceptual or cognitive deficit.[56] Only persons who can benefit from compensation should be taught these strategies; that is, they must have a basic understanding of their skills and the permanence of their limitations because the use of compensa-

**Table 19-1**

| Comparison of Functional and Remedial Approaches | |
| --- | --- |
| **FUNCTIONAL/ADAPTIVE** | **REMEDIAL/RESTORATIVE** |
| Emphasizes occupational skills | Emphasizes component skills |
| Targets symptoms of dysfunction | Targets cause of dysfunction |
| Uses compensatory techniques and environmental adaptation | Uses tabletop activities (pegboard, computer) to improve underlying cognitive and perceptual skills |
| Uses repetitive practice of daily living activities to improve performance | Assumes improved performance in pegboard or tabletop activity will translate into improved performance in everyday activities |
| Usually uses task-specific strategies that are not generalizable | Shows little generalizability to improved performance in functional tasks |

tion for disability requires that the individual recognize the need to compensate. The patient must be a self-starter, must be goal directed, and must want to learn new strategies. Successful compensation requires practice, repetition, and overlearning of the strategies.[71]

Environmental adaptation is more appropriate for those who cannot use compensatory strategies as a result of poor insight of disability. Adaptation involves changing the characteristics of the task or environment. This technique is used in patients with poor learning potential. An example of adaptation is the use of contrasting colors for a plate and placemat for someone with figure-ground difficulties. Establishing a routine and constant environment with repeated participation in familiar activities is often the most successful strategy for these individuals. The adaptive approach relies on caregivers to implement treatment strategies.[71]

A significant limitation of the functional approach is the task specificity of the strategies and lack of generalizability to other tasks.[13] For example, the use of an alarm timer to take medications on time does not help the patient remember a repertoire of other activities, such as to take a shower, start meal preparation, or get to a doctor's appointment, unless the patient specifically has been trained to do so.

## Remedial Approach

Remediation (or restoration or transfer of training) emphasizes restoration of the function or skill lost as a result of the stroke. Remedial treatment relies on several assumptions: the cerebral cortex is malleable and can adapt, and the brain can repair and reorganize itself after injury. Practice and repetition are assumed to result in learning. In turn, learning results in a more organized, functional system. Another assumption is that tabletop activities, such as pegboard tasks or computer activities, directly affect the underlying processing skills required for the patient to perform those activities. The most important assumption is that improved task performance of tabletop activities will be carried over to improved performance in functional activities.[13,21,47]

Although this approach has been successful when used in the initial stages of treatment,[21] most studies show only short-term results, generalization only to similar tasks,[64] or little effectiveness from remedial training for neurobehavioral impairments.[21,28] For this approach to be successful, treatment sessions must be frequent and lengthy.

Neistadt[46] believes that only those patients who show transfer of learning to tasks that are different in multiple characteristics are appropriate candidates for the remedial approach to processing impairments. Therapists widely agree that practice of a subcomponent skill, such as problem solving or attention to task, must occur in multiple contexts for successful transfer of learning.[71] According to Neistadt,[45] therapists always should train

for transfer of skills because the patient's home environment is always different from the clinic setting. Those who can transfer learning only to similar tasks should be restricted to a functional/adaptive approach to maximize their training potential.[46]

## Recommended Approach

Determination of the appropriate treatment approach for the stroke patient with processing impairments relies on the results of the assessment. Important questions include the following: Does the patient have the potential to learn? Is the patient aware of errors during task performance; and if so, does the patient have the potential to seek solutions to those errors? If the patient has poor learning potential and is unlikely to benefit from the use of cues or task modification, a strictly functional approach involving domain-specific training would be recommended.[61] Domain-specific training requires little or no transfer of learning (generalizability) and involves repetitive performance of a specific functional task using a system of vanishing cues. (*Vanishing cues* are cues that are provided at every step of task performance but then gradually are removed. The goal is to establish a program in which the patient can successfully perform the task with a minimum number of cues.) This type of training is hyperspecific, and the learning associated with it persists only if the task and environmental characteristics remain unchanged.

The remedial and functional approaches involve teaching the patient new behaviors. The difference is in whether emphasis is placed on performance skills or areas of occupation. Research indicates that the use of one approach exclusively always has some disadvantages; therefore consideration of the patient's learning potential and ability to generalize information, the severity of the injury, and the overall health, age, and support systems is important.[46] Research supports the use of the functional training approach[48,57] or a combination of a functional approach with a cognitive or perceptual remedial approach.[20,41,63] In a study by Edmans, Webster, and Lincoln,[22] stroke patients with perceptual impairments (as assessed by the Rivermead Perceptual Assessment Battery) received the transfer of training or functional approach to treatment of perceptual impairments. Improvement was noted in perceptual skills and ADL skills with both approaches, with no significant difference found between either approach in perceptual or ADL skill acquisition.

Traditionally the therapist has used a restorative or functional approach; however, Abreu et al[1] have proposed an integrated functional approach to treatment using principles from both approaches simultaneously. In this approach, areas of occupation and context are used to challenge processing skills. Because individuals engage in occupations as integrated wholes—not as separate attention machines, categorizers, or memory coders—treatments

**Box 19-1**

### Tooth-Brushing Task: Treatment of Neurobehavioral Impairments

**SPATIAL RELATIONS/SPATIAL POSITIONING**

Positioning of toothbrush and toothpaste while applying paste to toothbrush
Placement of toothbrush in mouth
Positioning of bristles in mouth
Placement of toothbrush under faucet

**SPATIAL NEGLECT**

Visual search for and use of toothbrush, toothpaste, and cup in affected hemisphere
Visual search and use of faucet handle in affected hemisphere

**BODY NEGLECT**

Brushing of affected side of mouth

**MOTOR APRAXIA**

Manipulation of toothbrush during task performance
Manipulation of cap from toothpaste
Squeezing of toothpaste onto toothbrush

**IDEATIONAL APRAXIA**

Appropriate use of objects (toothbrush, toothpaste, cup) during task

**ORGANIZATION/SEQUENCING**

Sequencing of task (removal of cap, application of toothpaste to toothbrush, turning on water, and putting toothbrush in mouth)
Continuation of task to completion

**ATTENTION**

Attention to task (for greater difficulty, distractions such as conversation, flushing toilet, or running water may be added)
Refocus on task after distraction

**FIGURE-GROUND**

Distinguishing white toothbrush and toothpaste from sink

**INITIATION/PERSEVERANCE**

Initiation of task on command
Cleaning parts of mouth for appropriate period of time and then moving bristles to another part of mouth
Discontinuation of task when complete

**VISUAL AGNOSIA**

Use of touch to identify objects

**PROBLEM SOLVING**

Search for alternatives if toothpaste or toothbrush is missing

---

that are not aimed at real-life contexts are irrelevant to real life. With this integrated functional approach, treatment may be focused on a subcomponent skill such as sustained attention, but daily occupations are used as the modality. For example, a self-feeding task can be used to improve sustained attention to task. Mealtime is often distracting. Eating can be a difficult task if attention deficits are present. A system of vanishing cues and a gradual increase in the amount of environmental distraction can be used to address inattention to task and activity participation.

The use of a functional approach is supported by today's health care industry, which seeks documentation of patient's functional competence in ADL. Only cost-effective interventions that directly affect functional status are embraced in today's health care environment.

Any functional task can be used to address a myriad of neurobehavioral impairments. For occupational therapists to use their skills in activity analysis to evaluate an activity for its effectiveness in addressing particular cognitive or perceptual deficits is imperative. Box 19-1 contains an example of using everyday function to address neurobehavioral performance skills.

## TREATMENT CONSIDERATIONS

Therapists must consider many factors while preparing a treatment plan. A stroke survivor may not have the same needs as a person with a closed-head injury, encephalitis, or a gunshot wound to the head. All have brain injury, but they have different patterns of behavior and recovery. Likewise, one must remember that no two stroke patients are alike. Each person with a stroke is a unique individual with special needs, goals, and problems.

### Population

The therapist should consider the patient's age; studies have found a functional decline with familiar and practiced tasks as adults age.[18] Expectations for functional level vary for different age ranges. A young stroke victim surely has different goals and aspirations than one who is older than 65 years. The therapist also must consider the person's previous level of function when establishing goals. A person who was not independent before a stroke probably will not achieve independence after the stroke. Cultural differences often emerge during evaluation and should be supported during treatment planning. The importance placed on occupations varies among cultures, so one should take care to ensure that goals and activities are culturally relevant to each patient.

### Environment

The importance of the environment or setting in which treatment takes place cannot be underestimated. Patients plan and perform ADL differently and with greater independence[52] at home than in the clinic setting.[49] Exposure to different environments and contexts requires patients to adapt strategies and solve problems,[35] leading to greater independence in a variety of situations.

The adaptation of purposeful activities to ensure success is of primary importance in occupational therapy. Success depends on the therapist's ability to analyze the activities and the patients' strengths, weaknesses, and needs to present the most relevant and challenging activity.

### Psychosocial and Emotional Issues

Many factors influence quality of life after a stroke. Occupational therapists frequently measure quality by examining physical recovery and performance of self-care as the primary indicators.[54] However, research indicates that even with good physical and functional recovery, persons show decreased socialization and leisure activity after a stroke.[3] Many patients sustain not only significant loss in functional ability after a stroke but also difficulty adjusting emotionally to the new lifestyle. Occupational therapists must address all factors relating to quality of life. Enhanced quality of life should be the ultimate priority in the planning of treatment (see Chapters 2 and 3).

Group treatment has been suggested as a way to facilitate socialization and communication by patients.[19] Groups provide reinforcement for socially acceptable behaviors. In addition, a stroke survivor may be more inclined to share feelings and concerns with a group of other stroke survivors because they are more likely to understand those feelings. Many occupational therapists have established support groups for stroke victims and their families.[23,26]

### Meaningful Activity

Although the underlying theory of occupational therapy revolves around the use of meaningful activity in treatment, addressing the use of meaningful activity in the treatment of processing impairments is still important. Activities used in treatment not only should address the impairment but also should be meaningful and relevant to each patient.

In the early 1990s, greater emphasis was placed on the participation of patient and family in goal setting. The health professions are recognizing that quality health care requires the patient and family to help establish a plan of care. The Joint Commission on Accreditation of Healthcare Organizations and the Commission on Accreditation of Rehabilitation Facilities require documentation of patient and family involvement in treatment planning, discharge planning, and education. Who knows better what activities and goals are meaningful and relevant than the patient and family?

## NEUROBEHAVIORAL IMPAIRMENTS IN THE STROKE POPULATION

Processing impairments in the stroke population are part of an interactive process involving the patient, the activity at hand, and the context in which the task is being performed.[61] Cognition and perception are a dynamic process, constantly changing and reacting to internal and external stimuli. Therapists must address neurobehavioral impairments in the context of the situation, according to the person's needs and goals. This is why a generic, general approach does not work for the patients included in this population.

Neurobehavioral impairments often are noted in stroke survivors. Lesions from a stroke may cause localized loss of function such as language comprehension. More often, strokes cause a variety of neurobehavioral impairments associated with the severity of the infarct. General treatment strategies for persons with cognitive and perceptual impairments after stroke are addressed next. Commonly noted neurobehavioral impairments are discussed individually later in the chapter.

## INTERVENTION STRATEGIES

Treatment strategies for cognitive and perceptual impairments are common in the literature; however, little research is available regarding the efficacy of these approaches. The need for research studies to support the many approaches being used in this population is great. Until much of this research is conducted, therapists must rely on techniques and approaches that appear successful (but perhaps are not yet proven).

### Activity Processing

Activity processing is especially helpful in cognitive rehabilitation because the therapist discusses the purpose and results of the activity with the patient. The therapists can discern awareness by the patient from feedback provided during and after activity participation. Activity processing enhances the patient's metacognition (knowledge of one's own cognitive ability and ability to monitor one's own performance) and general knowledge. Activity processing emphasizes the purpose of the activity in the rehabilitation process.[12] For example, when practicing spatial positioning during a dressing task, the therapists should instruct the patient on the spatial requirements for each step of the activity and the purpose of using the dressing task to improve spatial skills. As the patient performs the task, the patient and the therapist should discuss performance and strategies to perform the activity.

### Behavior Modification

Use of behavior modification techniques such as prompting, shaping (reinforcing responses that increasingly resemble the sought-after behavior), and contingent reinforcement (reward contingent on an appropriate response) are common in the stroke and/or brain injury population. Behavior modification techniques with intermittent praise and reinforcement to improve independence in daily activity have been successful.[27,39]

Use of prompts and cues is key to successful cognitive and perceptual rehabilitation. Cues can be faded by reducing the number, frequency, or specificity of the prompts.[71] For example, a therapist initially may provide detailed cues at every step of task performance, such as "Look to the left to find the soap." Cues should be tapered and should become less detailed as the patient progresses (e.g., "Have you remembered all the steps?"). Therapists should provide prompts and cues in a calculated and graded fashion. The use of cues and prompts is part of cognitive and perceptual rehabilitation and is an essential way of facilitating patient insight, error detection, and strategy development (Table 19-2).

### Group Treatment

Group treatment in the stroke population is often effective. Group treatment can yield situations more like real life, because they are less structured and can generate unpredictable events and provide distractions. In a group, patients can get feedback from their peers (which is often more meaningful), share similar experiences, and exchange problem-solving and coping strategies. Group treatment allows patients to learn from others' mistakes, practice monitoring their own behavior, and see that their problems are not unique.

Two approaches to treatment of neurobehavioral impairments that are particularly relevant to occupational therapy are the multicontextual and Affolter approaches. Although many approaches specific to cognitive and perceptual intervention are described in the literature, these two approaches have broad potential for stroke patients with neurobehavioral impairments.

### Multicontext Approach

The multicontext approach was developed by Joan P. Toglia, an occupational therapist, and is based on the dynamic interactional model of cognition.[61] This model views cognition as a product of constant interaction among the individual, the task, and the environment. In the multicontext approach the patient's processing abilities and self-monitoring techniques are used to facilitate learning for different tasks or environments (Box 19-2).

The ability to transfer information from one situation to another is an essential component of the multicontext approach. Toglia[62] believes transfer of skills must be taught throughout the learning process and during treatment sessions, not at the time of discharge. The ability to transfer learning across tasks can be facilitated by varying treatment environments or altering the nature of a task. Varying degrees of similarity between activities and having the patient practice a targeted strategy in different environments and with varying activities also can aid skills transfer. A near-transfer task is one that differs from the original task by only one or two surface characteristics (Box 19-3). If the original task is donning *shorts* in bed, a near-transfer task is donning a pair of *pants* in bed.

### Table 19-2

### Prompting Procedures

| PROMPTS | RATIONALE |
|---|---|
| "How do you know this is the right answer/procedure?" or "Tell me why you chose this answer/procedure." | Refocuses patient's attention to task performance and error detection. Can patient self-correct with a general cue? |
| "That is not correct. Can you see why?" | Provides general feedback about error but is not specific. Can patient find error and initiate correction? |
| "It is not correct because ..." | Provides specific feedback about error. Can patient correct error when it is pointed out? |
| "Try this [strategy]" (e.g., going slower, saying each step out loud, verbalizing a plan before starting, or using a checklist). | Provides patient with a specific, alternate approach. Can patient use strategy given? |
| Task is altered. "Try it another way." | Modifies task by one parameter. Can patient perform task? Begin again with grading of prompting described previously. |

Adapted from Toglia JP: Attention and memory. In Royen CB, editor: *AOTA self-study series: cognitive rehabilitation*, Rockville, Md, 1993, American Occupational Therapy Association; and Toglia JP: Generalization of treatment: a multicontext approach to cognitive perceptual impairment in adults with brain injury, *Am J Occup Ther* 45:505, 1991.

Intermediate-transfer tasks change three to six surface characteristics and are not as readily identified with the original task. An example is donning underwear from a sitting position (type of clothing, type of material, positioning, and sequence of task have changed). Far-transfer tasks share just one, if any, surface characteristics but are still conceptually similar to the original task. The use of one-handed principles taught for lower body dressing applied to upper body dressing is an example of a far transfer. Very far transfer is the generalization or application of previously learned information in novel or spontaneous situations.

Initially, the number of stimuli and complexity of tasks remain unchanged throughout the process of exposure to tasks with changing surface characteristics. As the patient shows consistent ability to use targeted strategies in a variety of situations, the number of stimuli and the complexity of tasks are increased.

The multicontext approach emphasizes the use of functional activities and a variety of gross motor, computer, and tabletop tasks. Therapists should vary treatment activities. Explicit teaching of the transfer from remedial to functional activities is essential.[47] A patient must understand that scanning for coins on a tabletop promotes the use of visual scanning in everyday activities.

Awareness during task performance is a focal point of this approach. Emphasis is on teaching the patient to be more aware of cognitive or perceptual strengths and weaknesses and ways to compensate.[47] The therapist should use awareness questions, estimation of performance, and strategy investigation before and after task performance. The therapist questions the patient about the difficulty of the task, the accuracy of task performance, and the amount of assistance needed. The patient should be given immediate feedback on the accuracy of responses to awareness questioning. Initially, the therapist asks the patient these questions during or after task performance. As accuracy of responses improves, the therapist asks the patient to predict task performance before engaging in the activity. The therapist also teaches the patient to ask questions such as "How am I doing?" "Am I implementing that strategy?" and "Am I forgetting anything?" The therapist also should give the patient questions about the strategy used to complete the task, such as "How did you keep track of what to do next?"[58] The use of these techniques helps the patient detect errors, estimate task difficulty and performance, increase self-awareness, and use self-monitoring skills. Teaching processing strategies such as prioritizing, clustering related information, planning ahead, time management, and awareness questioning yields deeper and more organized processing of information.[62]

Transfer of training is more likely to occur in patients with localized lesions such as a stroke than in those with diffuse injury such as anoxia or closed-head injury. Persons with diffuse injury tend to have poorer information-processing skills. Someone with a localized pattern of injury is expected to retain better learning capacity than is one with diffuse injury.[47] Neistadt[47] believes that transfer of learning between tasks that are different in more than three to six characteristics is difficult for brain-injured subjects and that the likelihood of generalization of learning to different tasks is greater when greater emphasis is placed on explicit teaching for transfer.

The therapist may use the multicontext approach when the patient shows potential for improvement through the use of environmental modification, assistance, or cues. This approach facilitates training techniques in a variety of task situations and environments to place increasingly difficult demands on the patient. The goal of this approach is to train the patient to use self-monitoring and

## Box 19-2

### Principles of the Multicontext Approach

- Transfer of skills must be taught, not just presumed to occur.
- Strategies taught to patients must be practiced in a variety of environments with many different tasks.
- Metacognitive skills are critical components of learning and the ability to generalize.
- Training of metacognitive skills and self-awareness is incorporated throughout treatment.
- Transfer of learning occurs through a graded series of tasks that decrease in similarity.
- Awareness questioning is used to help the patient detect errors, estimate task difficulty and performance, and predict outcomes.

Adapted from Toglia JP: Generalization of treatment: a multicontext approach to cognitive perceptual impairment in adults with brain injury, *Am J Occup Ther* 49:711, 1995.

## Box 19-3

### Examples of Task Surface Characteristics

- Color
- Shape
- Size
- Positioning
- Number of steps required
- Physical surroundings
- Spatial arrangement
- Familiarity of object/task
- Sequence of steps

Adapted from Toglia JP: Generalization of treatment: a multicontext approach to cognitive perceptual impairment in adults with brain injury, *Am J Occup Ther* 45:505, 1991.

compensation strategies to handle task performance in a variety of situations.[61]

## Affolter Approach

The Affolter approach is a treatment approach based on tactile-kinesthetic input provided to patients with cognitive and perceptual impairments. This approach was developed by Felicie Affolter, who holds degrees in child psychology, audiology, and language pathology. Affolter has noted that the tactile-kinesthetic sensory system is essential for interaction with the environment and that interaction with the environment results in increasingly complex skills.[9] Through tactile-kinesthetic input, connections between movement and its effect on objects lead to information regarding cause-and-effect relationships. Cause and effect assists in the development of cognitive connections in daily activities.[17] Emphasis is placed on providing appropriate input to facilitate a problem-solving process rather than a focus on the end product or specific skills.[9,17] According to Affolter, therapists must be sure to teach problem solving and not merely splinter skills, which rarely are carried over.[17]

*Guiding* is the main principle of the Affolter approach[9] (Box 19-4). The therapist places a hand over the patient's hand and guides the manipulation of objects as the patient performs the task.[17] The patient may respond with initial increased skeletal muscle activity, which often relaxes as the activity continues. Guiding often results in increased attention and sustained focus on the task at hand. Patients who previously were unable to brush their hair may begin to take over the purposeful movement and start to brush their hair while being guided by the therapist (Figure 19-1). The amount of guiding fluctuates with the patients' change in muscle activity and active participation in the task. Guiding initially should be performed on a supported surface rather than through air.

The surface provides tactile feedback, allows patients to explore the environment, and provides feedback on distance and spatial relationships. For example, when assisting patients to reach for their shoes, the occupational therapist should guide the patients' hand along the surface of the leg to the foot (Figure 19-2). During a hygiene task, the occupational therapist can guide the patients' hand along the edge of the sink to reach for the faucet.[9]

When assisting the patient in solving problems, the therapist or caretaker must offer the patient possibilities, not solutions.[9] The therapist must create an environment that facilitates cognitive-perceptual learning by providing problems to be solved.[17] The patient must be allowed to make mistakes during treatment to use problem-solving skills. Therapists often correct mistakes too quickly. The patient may not even realize a mistake has been made or take the opportunity to address the problem (such as spilled milk on a tray or a washcloth dropped on the floor). Guiding the patient through the process of cleaning up the milk or picking up the washcloth may be the most meaningful part of the treatment session.

A good activity is one that does not rely on outside feedback but provides its own through its success or completion.[17] The change of resistance of the knife against the cutting board and the aroma of a freshly cut orange are cues that tell the patient the task is complete. Use of functional and purposeful activities is essential to keep patients motivated. The environment also should be appropriate to the task: dressing in a bedroom, hygiene

---

**Box 19-4**

### GUIDING PRINCIPLES[9]

While guiding the patient, the therapist should do the following:

- Place his or her hand over the patient's whole hand, down to the fingertips.
- Keep talking to a minimum.
- Guide both sides of the body when possible.
- Move along a supported surface to give the patient maximum tactile feedback.
- Involve the whole body in the task to challenge posture.
- Provide changes in resistance during the activity.
- Allow the patient to make mistakes to give opportunities to solve problems.

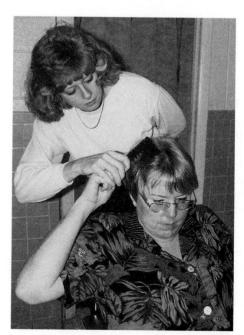

**Figure 19-1**    Patient is guided through a hair-brushing task.

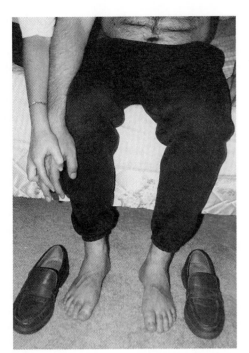

**Figure 19-2**    Guiding of the patient's hand along a supported surface (leg) as he reaches for a shoe.

activity in a bathroom. Wiping a countertop that is not dirty or stacking cones is not purposeful because there is no problem to be solved.[9]

The Affolter approach deemphasizes talking because most or all of the feedback should come from the activity.[17] Communication is nonverbal, provided through the tactile-kinesthetic sense. Instructions are not necessary to initiate guiding. It may be helpful for the therapist to say, "I'm going to guide your body/hands with my hands. My hands will tell you what I want you to do." Instead of telling the patient to grab the toothbrush, the therapist physically guides the patient through the process of reaching for the toothbrush and toothpaste.[9] As the patient begins to understand the purpose of the task through the tactile-kinesthetic input, participation in the task increases. Refraining from speaking allows the patient to process information without excess stimulation.

Patients perceive the environment by being guided physically through task performance. Because the therapist is in direct contact with the patient, the therapist gains direct feedback about the patient's attention to task, sequencing, problem solving, and muscle tone.[9]

Cognitive-perceptual training occurs regularly throughout the patient's day. Collaboration with other members of the health care team and education of families and caregivers on Affolter principles (Box 19-5) are vital because if the treatment plan is not supported and continued at home and in the clinical setting, the patient may

**Box 19-5**

**AFFOLTER PRINCIPLES[9]**

■ Physically guiding the patient's hands/body in functional activities
■ Emphasis on input rather than on output
■ Less focus on skills; more focus on facilitation of problem solving
■ Purposeful, meaningful tasks; must be a problem to be solved

experience conflict and confusion. Families often feel overwhelmed and helpless; training them to provide tactile-kinesthetic input during task performance allows them to participate in the recovery of their loved one.[9]

## TREATMENT APPROACHES FOR SPECIFIC NEUROBEHAVIORAL IMPAIRMENTS

Therapists rarely observe perceptual or cognitive deficits in isolation. Usually these deficits overlap and are difficult to interpret because of their complexity. Little research has been conducted or published on outcomes of specific treatment approaches for isolated perceptual and cognitive deficits, with the possible exceptions of memory impairments and unilateral neglect. However, therapists continue to assess these impairments individually, and using a combination of general and specific treatment approaches to neurobehavioral impairments does help sometimes. With this thought in mind, information on distinct treatment approaches related to specific impairments follows.

### Apraxia

According to Ayres,[5] praxis is one of the most important connections between brain and behavior; it is what allows persons to interact with the physical world. Apraxia is a dysfunction of purposeful movement that does not result primarily from motor, sensory, or comprehension impairments.[4] Although many different types of apraxia have been named and defined, the labels used to classify them are not universally accepted.[6] For relevance in this chapter, however, they fit into two general categories: motor and ideational apraxia.

Patients with apraxia are often unaware of their deficits, creating a dilemma for planning therapeutic interventions. However, one study concluded that patients with more severe cognitive (and motor) impairments showed the most significant improvement in ADL.[32] The study demonstrated the obvious potential for improvement with severely apraxic patients using compensatory strategy training for ADL skills and therefore negates the idea that severely apraxic patients have poor potential for improvement. Box 19-6 lists general treatment guidelines for patients with apraxia.

***Motor Apraxia.*** Motor apraxia is a defect in symbolic or expressive gestures. Motor apraxia is the inability to produce the individual elements in a sequence of tasks even as the patient retains the concept or idea of the task. Árnadóttir[4] has described movements in patients with motor apraxia as clumsy and inflexible. Someone with motor apraxia has difficulty imitating a motor command and difficulty sequencing and orienting elements of a task together. It may be helpful for the therapist to give only general information about the activity goal and leave out the specific instructions.[6] For example, when working on morning ADL with the patient, the therapist should use a general statement of "Let's get ready" instead of step-by-step instructions for each task. Having the patient visualize task movements and sequences before carrying out the task may be helpful. This visualization gives the patient a visual model to which to refer in performing the task.

***Ideational Apraxia.*** Ideational apraxia involves a disruption in the concept formation of action planning. The ability to select and organize movements to execute an action is impaired. This impairment often is seen in a person's attempt to use objects: faulty or inappropriate tool use is the hallmark of ideational apraxia. Often the patient with ideational apraxia seems confused, stubborn, or uncooperative. Treatment considerations for this dysfunction include step-by-step commands for each task[6] because patients with this disorder cannot grasp the general concept or idea of the activity but may be able to perform individual components of the task on command.

Use of Affolter's guiding techniques for patients with apraxia can promote task continuation through the tactile-kinesthetic sensation of smooth, rhythmic movement. Physical guiding provides the patient who has ideational apraxia with possibilities (not solutions). For example, as one guides a patient during a tooth-brushing task, one should guide the patient's hand toward objects at the sink but not directly at the appropriate object. The therapist should give the patient opportunity to plan and execute the appropriate movements.

A noncontrolled study of apraxic patients by van Heugten and other[33] viewed ADL tasks as occurring in three stages: initiation of activity, execution of activity, and control and/or correction during the activity. Treatment emphasis then was placed on the stage(s) at which each patient predominantly had problems, with emphasis on compensatory strategies for intervention. Interventions were provided in hierarchical order for instructions, assistance, and feedback. Improvements in ADL function were significant, whereas improvements in motor planning and motor skills were small.

### Perseveration

Perseveration is demonstrated by the inability to shift from one concept to another or to change or cease a behavior pattern once having started it. Perseveration also refers to the inability to translate knowledge into action (initiation of a task). The person is "stuck in set"— unable to discard the previous set of behaviors—or is unable to "activate" for a new situation. The person stuck in set is attempting to solve another problem with information relevant to a previous problem.

Bringing perseveration to a conscious level and training the patient to inhibit the perseverative behavior has been successful.[31] Other strategies include redirecting attention, assisting the patient in initiating a new movement or task, and engaging the patient in tasks that involve repetitive action (e.g., washing the face or body, stirring food, or sanding wood) to promote successful task participation.

### Unilateral Neglect

Of all the neurobehavioral impairments discussed in this chapter, unilateral neglect has received the most attention in the health care literature (see Chapter 16 for information on visual field loss versus neglect). Neglect not only occurs in the horizontal plane but also is manifested in vertical and radial planes (*vertical* implying neglect of stimuli upward or downward, and *radial* implying close to or far from the body). The existence of these phenomena requires therapists to check for the presence of this disorder and implement a treatment program to include all neglected spaces.[30,37] The most widely supported theories explaining unilateral neglect involve the attention and arousal mechanisms of the brain. The attentional theories speculate that neglect results from impaired attention abilities. The theory is that the right hemisphere is usually dominant for attentional skills and that left-side neglect resulting from a stroke in the right hemisphere therefore is seen more frequently than right-side neglect

---

**Box 19-6**

### GENERAL TREATMENT APPROACHES FOR PERSONS WITH APRAXIA

- Provide tactile, kinesthetic, and proprioceptive input before and during the activity to help guide movements.
- Keep commands simple, with minimal wordiness.
- Make frequent use of spontaneous situations, keeping activity on a subcortical level.
- Perform activities in their usual environments.
- Work in a relaxed environment with few distractions.
- Use goal-directed activities to decrease confusion.
- Provide contextual and environmental cues.

from a stroke in the left hemisphere, depending on hemispheric lateralization. Arousal theories state that left-side neglect occurs as a result of decreased stimulation to the injured hemisphere and overarousal in the noninjured hemisphere. According to this theory, the hyperaroused hemisphere pays greater attention to the contralateral space and body, and the unaroused hemisphere pays little attention to space and body contralateral to it. Research has not supported the arousal theory[14]; many therapists support, at least in part, the attentional theories.

General treatment principles that have been recommended in the literature include use of visual markers, visual scanning training, cueing for visual anchoring, increased stimulation to the affected side, movement or activation of the affected extremity in the affected hemispace, and training awareness of neglect to facilitate compensation.[16,41,58]

Anosognosia, the impaired awareness of neglect or other deficits, is a fundamental problem in the rehabilitation of neglect. The ability to improve this lack of awareness by fostering understanding of the activity limitation and its effect on function is a key component of treatment.[29] Studies have shown, however, that patients with the most severe neglect have demonstrated greater improvement in neglect behaviors.[13,24] Persons who have severe impairments benefit from the use of external cues such as verbal reminders and colored anchors to improve function. Mildly impaired patients who show faulty scanning may be helped only if they can be trained to use internal cues to improve their scanning ability.[13] The ability to internalize strategies is the skill most pivotal and most difficult to achieve for the brain-injured population.

***Spatial Neglect.*** Neglect of the environment and space contralateral to the lesion site is referred to as *spatial neglect*. Visual scanning activities are the most common and successful treatment approaches for spatial neglect and visual field cuts. The focus of this approach is to train the patient continually to scan the environment for relevant stimuli and to attend to stimuli in the affected hemisphere. Principles guiding this approach include grading activities from simple to complex, providing consistent feedback, repeating activities, and using visual scanning in the context of functional activities.[34] Cognitive or perceptual training is generalized well to similar tasks; therefore continuous training with similar tasks in treatment will likely yield the greatest benefit with generalization. This principle was demonstrated in a group of studies involving a scanning machine and multiple wheelchair movement conditions to demonstrate improvement in wheelchair mobility and decreased contact with obstacles.[40,66,67] The ability to scan the environment decreases as the attention demands of the task increase[13]; therefore, task performance must be kept simple when accurate scanning of the environment is necessary. Anchoring

techniques are used to cue the patient and organize the scanning pattern. Warren[65] recommends combining scanning with manipulation of whatever is being scanned to increase success. Studies have found that an individual has a stronger mental representation of a visual image if the person has explored the image or object by touch.[65] Other studies[38,69] have demonstrated decreased neglect symptoms by combining trunk rotation with a scanning activity.

Activation or active use by the impaired (usually left) hand, paired with perceptual anchoring, has been found to reduce the signs of neglect. Whether the positive effect is a result of the actual movement of the impaired arm or by a spaciomotor cueing process is a matter of controversy.[29] Results from studies looking at passive movement of the affected extremity have been inconclusive, whereas activation of bilateral upper extremities has been shown not to improve neglect.[53]

Scanning training combined with a scanning machine for treatment of spatial neglect has had some success. The scanning machine has a moving light that the patient visually tracks from one point to another. A flashing stimulus light combined with verbal cues also has been successful in assisting patients to anchor the beginning and end of scanning movements.[13]

Prism lenses and hemispatial eye patching have been used to treat spatial neglect with some success. Prisms deviate the visual field to the right; although the subjects initially misreach to the right, most begin to compensate after repeated exposure (adaptation effect). The aftereffect is the tendency to point opposite the optical displacement of the prisms after they are removed. In studies by Rossi, Kheyfets, and Reding[60] and Rossetti, Rode, and Pisella,[59] short-term improvements in neglect were noted in experimental groups of persons who wore prisms compared with controls who received standard treatment. Frassinetti et al[25] noted similar improvements in their small experimental group and noted decreased neglect behaviors 5 weeks after treatment was discontinued. Interestingly, the decrease in neglect occurred only for those patients who showed the adaptation effect and the aftereffect during assessment. Another study[7] noted significantly improved attention to the left visual field in the experimental group of subjects who wore glasses with the right half field obscured by patches. Improvement in functional activities (Functional Independence Measure scores) also was noted with this group compared with controls; however, the significant disparity between control and experimental groups makes these findings difficulty to interpret.

Some examples of functional treatment activities focusing on visual scanning include scattering items for mealtime across both visual fields, using diminishing cues to help the patient find needed items during the meal, and strategically arranging items for grooming and hygiene so the patient must scan the neglected space for successful task performance. Again, the occupational therapist should provide diminishing verbal cues to teach the patient to scan visually and independently.[34]

Although popular some years ago, the use of computers to treat neglect has shown little promise.[57] Certainly the use of computers in the brain-injured population (as with any other neurobehavioral impairment) may be relevant if the patient uses computers for work or leisure activities. The use of computer games to treat spatial neglect, however, has not been validated (especially the use of widely available software made specifically for "cognitive retraining"). These computer activities do not provide realistic or meaningful challenge for most patients, and they have been reported to have no generalizing effect.[48] Overall, the remedial or transfer of training approach for unilateral neglect frequently has been unsuccessful.[24]

Although caloric stimulation with cold water in the left ear, optokinetic stimulation through induced nystagmus, and vibration of the neck muscles have been shown to cause improvement in spatial neglect, little evidence exists of these effects lasting after treatment termination.[30]

*Body Neglect.* Inattention or neglect of body parts contralateral to the lesion site is termed *body neglect*. Activities requiring bilateral integration or use of both sides of the body have been used to treat the disorder. Affolter's guiding techniques also may be useful. Guiding may allow a patient to perform a bilateral task with an otherwise nonfunctional extremity. Guiding the hemiparetic extremities can provide useful tactile-kinesthetic input because the patient's body is taken through familiar movement patterns. Guiding may help increase attention to the neglected side by "activating" the affected extremities. Tasks that provide increased sensory stimulation to the affected extremities (e.g., applying lotion or bathing with a washcloth) also may decrease neglect.

Compensatory strategies for body neglect include using a tactile stimulator (e.g., vibrating beeper) to draw attention to the unattended body side, a buzzer that sounds randomly to redirect attention to affected side, and auditory (verbal or nonverbal) stimulation through earphones to increase arousal to affected side. Attention to affected extremities during functional activities such as dressing or wheelchair transfers has not been shown to improve neglect (unless specifically set up for stimulation during those activities).

No strong evidence is available showing that rehabilitation focusing on neglect behaviors improves patient's ADL skills or independence.[11]

## Aphasia

Language-processing defects are referred to as *aphasia*. Although treatment of aphasia typically is addressed by the speech pathologist, an understanding of how to facilitate communication with aphasic patients is critical. Box 19-7 outlines helpful hints for use with aphasic patients and their caregivers.

Many of the techniques of awareness questioning described in the discussion of the multicontextual approach are not useful with aphasic patients. Approaches, especially cueing strategies, must be adjusted for the aphasic brain-injured population. Cues normally provided verbally may be more effective when provided by tactile or visual means for those with receptive aphasia. For example, instead of telling a patient to pay attention to the left arm, tapping the left arm or using gestures to indicate visual scanning to the left arm may be more successful. Therapists of patients with expressive aphasia may find it helpful to work closely with the speech therapist to establish a communication system that facilitates awareness questioning (e.g., use of writing, drawing, or gestures by patients to give the therapist information about their ability to estimate task difficulty, detect errors, or predict outcomes).

### Organization/Sequencing Deficits

The ability to organize thoughts requires the integration of multiple skills, including praxis, sequencing, and problem-solving. *Sequencing* refers to the ability to plan and carry out events in proper order, progression, and time.[4] Sequencing and organization deficits represent the breakdown of a complex integration of skills, including use of sensory feedback and organization. Patients with sequencing and organization deficits can be trained to use a daily planner, or tape recordings, or cue cards (depending on whether they perform better with auditory or visual cues) to help sequence the steps of daily tasks. Gradually increasing the number of steps in a task can increase a patient's tolerance and ability to perform more complex tasks (Box 19-8).

**Box 19-7**

### APHASIA: TIPS FOR FAMILY MEMBERS

- Persons with aphasia understand speech more easily when only one person talks to them at a time. Extra noise only creates confusion.
- Give the patient enough time to respond.
- Carefully phrase questions to make it easier for the patient to respond; for example, use yes/no and either/or questions.
- Use visual cues or gestures with speech to help the patient better understand.
- Never force the patient to respond.
- Use concise sentences.
- Do not rush communication. Rushed communication with a person who has aphasia can increase frustration and decrease the effectiveness of communication.

**Box 19-8**

### SEQUENCING DEFICITS: TIPS FOR FAMILY MEMBERS

- Frustration and error can be lessened by step-by-step directions written in a simple format (e.g., a checklist).
- Maps and diagrams may be useful.
- Visual aids often prove helpful, especially when combined with verbal instructions or physical guiding.
- Frequent, routine practice should help reinforce the sequencing of daily activities.

**Box 19-9**

### PERCEPTUAL PROBLEMS: TIPS FOR FAMILY MEMBERS

- Overstimulation from visual information may increase the problem.
- Getting rid of unnecessary objects and equipment lessens the demands on the patient and simplifies the task. For example, the tabletop should be cleared of objects that look alike so that the patient does not confuse them.
- Slowing down while reaching for an object or walking into a new area is usually helpful.

## Spatial Relations Syndrome

Spatial relations syndrome is the label given to disorders with impairment in the perception of spatial relationship of objects. These disorders include impairments with figure-ground, position in space, spatial relations, and form and space constancy skills. Topographic disorientation also is classified sometimes as part of spatial relations syndrome. Recommendations for spatial impairments include training patients to move slowly through their environments, encouraging patients to touch objects in the environment frequently, teaching patients to handle objects by the base, and using verbal cues or feedback instead of gestures.[50] Perceptual impairments are often difficult for families to understand. Educating the caregivers about these disorders and instructing them on how they can help their loved ones (Box 19-9) is especially important.

*Spatial Relation Dysfunction.* Spatial relation dysfunction is an impairment in relating objects to one another or to the self. Some examples of functional activities for patients with spatial deficits include identification and orientation of clothing during a dressing activity. This includes matching buttons and buttonholes together on a shirt or working on the ability to orient shoelaces during a one-handed tie. Wheelchair transfers require the ability to position the body in relation to a bed or other object and spatial orientation to maneuver wheelchair brakes and armrests in the correct direction. Simple meal preparation is another activity that requires spatial orientation and positioning because of tasks as locating and selecting needed items, stirring food, and setting the table.[34]

The use of the computer for visuospatial retraining has little or no effect on visuospatial skills and no carryover to functional activities.[28] Thus the use of computer programs aimed solely at addressing visuospatial skill retraining appears to be an ineffective remediation technique. A computer screen provides information as a two-dimensional image. Spatial relation impairment is a three-dimensional problem. For persons who use the computer for work or leisure, however, the use of the keyboard or mouse while working on the computer can be an effective, challenging, and meaningful modality.

*Spatial Positioning Impairment.* The concept of spatial positioning involves accurate placement or positioning of objects, including body parts. That impairment may be associated with impaired proprioception, however. This disorder is linked with language comprehension. Concepts such as *above*, *in*, and *under* are interpreted according to position in space and language skills.

Treatment for spatial positioning impairment should include increasing the patient's awareness of the impairment and teaching compensatory strategies. Matching colored markers for correct placement of objects can be helpful. Treatment ideas include having the patient practice placing a glass on top, in front, to the right, and to the left of a plate on command, placing certain objects (cups or utensils) in a row and having the patient identify which object is in a position different from those of the others. If language skills are impaired, the patient can be asked to create a place setting from a model. Repetition of specific spatial concepts, with emphasis on attention to detail and compensatory strategies (e.g., Velcro shoe strap goes toward the colored marker), may be helpful.

Treatment techniques for right-left discrimination problems include providing activities that stress right and left differences, such as dressing and grooming. In addition, therapists may use color or other markers to distinguish the right from the left side of items such as clothing and shoes.

*Figure-Ground Impairment.* Figure-ground deficits involve the inability to distinguish the foreground from the background. Treatment strategies for figure-ground deficits should include teaching the patient to be cognitively aware of the deficit and to slow down enough during task performance to identify all the relevant objects or stimuli before handling or manipulating them. The environment can be adapted to make it simple and uncluttered (e.g., organizing drawers or shelves). The use of stark contrast between objects (e.g., the plate and table during mealtime) is helpful for patients with this disorder. Sorting objects such as utensils from a kitchen drawer or nuts and bolts from a toolkit can be a good therapeutic activity; the sorting can be made more difficult with the addition of smaller and larger objects, thereby adding the element of size discrimination. The sorting should have a purpose, such as using the utensils for a cooking task.

***Topographic Disorientation.*** Topographic disorientation is difficulty finding direction in space.[4] The use of compensatory techniques and environmental adaptation, progressively reduced as the patient demonstrates learning, is often successful in the treatment of this disorder. Therapists can use markers such as colored dots to identify a route the patient must travel every day. The therapist gradually removes cues as the patient memorizes the route. One successful treatment program described by Borst and Peterson[10] used the patient's intact skills of right-left discrimination and language to assist with functional mobility. In this treatment program the patient practiced following directional instructions (e.g., "Go left at the next door"). The patient then was asked to draw the path from room to room on a map of the clinic area. Such an exercise would be especially helpful in the home setting. At first the therapist may need to assist the patient with correctly orientating the map with each turn. The therapist should withdraw verbal cues slowly. Next, the patient should attempt to go from room to room with only brief glances at the map. The last step is to withdraw the use of the map altogether. Generalization of this type of treatment is unlikely; therefore, treatment should take place only in the most meaningful environment.

## Agnosia

*Agnosia* typically is defined as the inability to recognize sensory stimuli. Agnosia presents as a defect of one particular sensory channel, such as visual, auditory, or tactile. Examples include finger agnosia, visual agnosia, somatoagnosia, simultanagnosia, and tactile agnosia. These disorders rarely are seen in isolation, and little data have been published regarding treatment techniques for agnosia. However, because the defining principle of agnosia is impairment of one specific sensory modality, treatment usually focuses on teaching the patient to use the intact sensory modalities. For example, in tactile agnosia—the inability to recognize objects by handling them—the patient is taught to use visual, olfactory, and auditory senses to recognize objects.

***Somatoagnosia.*** Somatoagnosia is the decreased awareness of body structure and inability to recognize or relate body parts to each other. Treatment includes having the patient imitate body movements, identify, and appropriately use body parts during task performance, and practice simple tasks that require two body parts working together (e.g., opening a jar).

***Visual Agnosia.*** Visual agnosia can be broken down into visual object agnosia and visuospatial agnosia. Visual object agnosia is the inability to recognize objects through the visual senses, whereas visuospatial agnosia includes deficits of spatial relations, topographic orientation, and depth perception. Educating patients to use other intact sensory systems and avoiding reliance on visual information is the most successful treatment plan for patients with visual agnosia. One socially isolating agnosia is prosopagnosia, the inability to recognize familiar faces. Therapists must educate patients and their families to seek and provide other sensory information (e.g., voice recognition or familiar scents) to help the patient identify others.

***Simultanagnosia.*** Simultanagnosia is the inability to grasp the association between multiple stimuli presented simultaneously, including interpretation or integration of elements into a meaningful theme. Persons with simultanagnosia may recognize individual items—such as shoes, socks, pants, and shirts—but have no understanding about how they are related. Therapy emphasizes the intact ability to recognize specific stimuli. Attempts to make persons with simultanagnosia understand the relationship between their shoe and their foot probably will be unsuccessful. For a successful outcome, therapists can teach patients to recognize the shoe and the foot and can instruct them regarding what to do. Step-by-step instructions for primary ADL are often necessary for such patients. Perhaps the use of tape-recorded instructions for morning routines would be successful (visual cues are not helpful because the patient cannot visually integrate or understand the cues).

## Memory Impairments

Although memory impairments are not as common in persons who have sustained strokes as they are in those with closed-head injuries, dementia, or encephalitis, difficulty retaining information is nonetheless common in the stroke population.

Fractionated memory loss, which is usually material specific or modality specific, is the most common memory impairment in stroke survivors. These types of memory impairments are found in patients with focal lesions such as localized strokes and (less commonly) with diffuse brain diseases (such as dementia) or closed-head injury. Material-specific memory loss involves the loss of verbal or nonverbal memory as a result of unilateral damage to the medial temporal lobe. A stroke in the left medial temporal lobe leads to verbal memory loss, whereas a right medial temporal lobe infarct would result in nonverbal memory loss. Examples of verbal memory loss are the inability to recall a previous conversation or instructions given by a therapist. Examples of nonverbal memory loss are the inability to remember the route from home to the grocery store (or from the bedroom to the therapy gym) or the tune of a favorite song. When patients have material-specific memory loss, the therapeutic approach must take advantage of their intact systems. If patients are not retaining verbal information, the use of more gestures and body language may be effective. If spatial relationships are difficult to recall, reliance on the intact language system and use of step-by-step verbal directions may be helpful.

Modality-specific memory loss is associated with focal lesions of the fibers that connect the sensory processing areas (e.g., visual, tactile, sensory, and auditory) to the medial temporal lobes. Therefore, memory loss would correspond only to the affected sensory processing area. Treatment for modality-specific memory loss also should focus on using intact sensory systems to compensate for memory loss. For example, if during evaluation, a patient was unable to recall any information that was given orally by the therapist, the treatment plan would be focused on training techniques involving frequent tactile and visual cues such as hand-over-hand techniques and drawings and written programs.

Short-term memory is tied closely to attention. Most persons can hold about seven units of information in short-term memory. Short-term memory capacity can be increased by grouping information into more meaningful units ("chunking"). Long-term memory is believed to be coded and organized semantically or by meaning; therefore attaching specific meaning to information may aid retention of memories.

One strategy-based approach to improving memory involves the use of temporal tags. The belief is that when a memory is formed, it is associated not only with a certain context but also with a temporal tag (information about when memory occurred). If emphasis is placed on recalling *when* an event occurred, it may help the person recall the actual event that occurred. However, one of the hallmarks of most persons with stroke-associated memory loss is their inability to form strategies to recall information; relying too heavily on rote memory is frequently the result.

Rehearsal (repeating information several times) refreshes or regenerates information. Use of visual imagery, first-letter mnemonics, and rehearsal has helped some patients remember things such as items on a shopping list and persons' names. However, these techniques could not be generalized into everyday activities. Patients should be trained to create their own personal prompts or reminders and taught the way to use them in everyday life. Spaced retrieval, a technique in which information is retrieved at progressively longer intervals, has been a successful memory technique; unfortunately, the technique is limited by the small amount of material that can be retained.[29]

Although little evidence has been found showing that cognitive training can improve memory function, the functional use of memory aids has been demonstrated repeatedly.[29,36] Aids include calendars, logbooks, notes, tape recorders, time buzzers or alarms, and written, step-by-step instructions.

A patient with functional metamemory is able to process memories and monitor their content. More generally, the patient can appreciate, recognize, and assess the status of memory abilities. Metamemory (which is related to insight) therefore involves being aware of deficits and is clearly important in predicting the way a patient will approach a task. Treatment for a patient with metamemory deficits involves increasing the patient's awareness of the deficit; a patient who is unaware of memory impairment will be unable to implement compensation techniques.

Persons remember better through recognition (e.g., remembering whether eggs or orange juice were on a grocery list) than cued recall (e.g., remembering whether breakfast foods were on a grocery list); they remember better through cued recall than free recall (e.g., remembering what was on a grocery list). Therefore, providing the particular environment and cues that facilitate successful recall for each individual is important.

Few controlled studies exist that analyze the effects of rehabilitation for memory problems after stroke, and no evidence is available to support cognitive rehabilitation for memory impairments to improve memory skills or functional abilities.[44]

## Attention Deficits

Attention is an essential element in successful task performance. Poor ability to attend to a task often is misinterpreted as a lack of motivation or neglect. Accurate assessment of an attention impairment is important to implementing appropriate treatment techniques. One method that may be helpful in managing attention problems is changing the way occupational therapists speak to patients. The goal is to couple the patient's attention with the intended action; instructions should be in the logical sequence of the action. Instead of instructing a patient to "Scoot forward," the therapist would say, "Your bottom [*pause*]. Move it forward to the edge of the chair." The wording should correspond with the order in which the steps are to be executed and should allow the patient to attend to each step. The pause is important to allow the patient enough time to shift focus and process the information.[13]

Use of systematic training incorporating a series of tasks with progressively increasing attentional demands has resulted in improvements in memory and attention to task,[8] although other studies have failed to demonstrate support for remedial training in attention.[61]

Family members often are frustrated when their loved ones are distracted easily or are unable to focus on a task. Family members must be informed that stroke survivors do not behave erratically on purpose. Teaching the family the way to create a supportive environment is important (Box 19-10).

Attention has been described as having four distinct domains: alertness, selective attention, sustained attention, and divided or alternating attention. Therapists must train patients in each domain skill individually, and generalization from one domain to another should not be expected after training.[43]

***Selective Attention Impairment.*** The ability to focus on relevant stimuli while screening out irrelevant stimuli is referred to as *selective attention.* Training patients to react to certain environmental cues and ignore distractions may improve selective attention. For example, the therapist can ask a patient to follow audio-recorded instructions for a hygiene task (or meal preparation, if a more complex task is desired). After the patient is able to complete the task successfully, the therapist can add elements of distraction, such as a radio or television, one by one.

***Sustained Attention Impairment.*** Sustained attention is the ability to maintain attention over a period of time. Focusing and sustaining attention is improved by gradually increasing the attentional demands of activities, through choosing activities with longer duration and additional distractions. For example, a task such as combing hair in a quiet bathroom without a mirror initially may require less than 30 seconds of focused attention to complete (and have few inherent distractions). As the patient successfully completes these types of tasks, the therapist should choose activities that require focused attention to detail and have more distractions (e.g., straight razor shaving task with the radio playing in the background). Some support exists for providing specific training for attention to improve alertness and sustained attention, but no evidence exists that attention training affects functional abilities.[43]

***Alternating Attention Impairment.*** Alternating attention is shifting focus from one stimulus to another. For the brain-injured population, the therapist should plan graded activities from simple to complex that initially require the patient to shift attention from one stimulus to another. For example, a simple activity may consist of participating in a ceramics painting project (in which the patient alternates attention from the paint to ceramic vase); a more complex task would be to have the patient perform a dressing task while watching the news on television and having the patient repeat important daily events after completing the task. Initially, tasks should require only attention shifts between two focal points. As the patient successfully completes these tasks, the therapist should use activities incorporating more focal points (e.g., a meal preparation task in which focus must alternate among planning, following directions, searching for supplies, monitoring other foods, timing, and place setting).

## Concrete Thinking

Inflexible thought processes characterize persons who use concrete thinking. They have difficulty generalizing information from one situation to another and rely heavily on available sensory information.

Persons with impaired abstraction skills usually have poor ability to recognize and learn the cognitive and perceptual skills needed for a specific task. Therefore they may benefit only from learning splinter (nongeneralizable) skills in treatment and may demonstrate training only in those tasks that are similar to those learned.[47] Box 19-11 reviews suggestions for family members to facilitate communication and task performance with this population.

## Insight Problems

A patient's lack of awareness may lead others to think the patient lacks motivation. Insight is related to knowledge of self, abilities, and skills. Judgment and insight frequently are associated. Lack of insight can result in impulsiveness or an inability to plan for the future. Treatment for decreased insight should focus on family education, use of feedback about skills, and self-awareness training.[12]

Lack of insight can be a significant limitation in the rehabilitation process. If someone cannot recognize the need for cognitive rehabilitation, that person likely will have no motivation to learn. Pressure from family members or loved ones and use of positive reinforcement may help in these situations. Family and caregivers must

---

**Box 19-10**

### DISTRACTIBILITY: TIPS FOR FAMILY MEMBERS

- Help unclutter the environment. Turn off the television and close doors to decrease excessive noise.
- Allow only one or two visitors at a time.
- Establish eye contact.

---

**Box 19-11**

### COGNITIVE INFLEXIBILITY: TIPS FOR FAMILY MEMBERS

- Make statements and questions as simple and uncomplicated as possible.
- Explain the reasons for certain procedures. The person may have difficulty understanding the long-term effects of therapy or medical procedures. Explain these with smaller goals that are easier to accomplish.
- If possible, structure tasks so they consist of a series of related tasks rather than many unrelated tasks.

understand the safety implications for those with impairments of insight, judgment, or abstraction skills. Frequently these patients need heavy supervision at home because of their lack of safety awareness. Providing a safe environment is the first priority, and instructing family members on home adaptations is essential (Boxes 19-12 and 19-13). Feedback for this population should be immediate, concrete, and objective. Use of multiple media (visual, verbal, tactile) for feedback is most beneficial for retention of information.[12]

### Impaired Problem-Solving Skills

Problem solving is not a single function but an integration of multiple skills. New or unique circumstances require problem-solving skills; novel or different tasks in multiple contexts require a patient to call on these skills. Games and puzzles often are used to enhance problem-solving skills and are enjoyable and challenging for the patient. The use of games to practice newly learned problem-solving strategies is often less threatening than practice of ADL. The patient should understand the purpose of using a game to improve problem-solving skills. Strategies to practice include chaining (breaking down the sequence of component parts), performing one step at a time, and writing down each step of sequences.[71]

A case study by Yuen[70] involved a patient's decreased compliance in taking medication because of problem-solving and other difficulties. Compliance improved by structuring the environment, using assistive devices (e.g., pillbox timer), and cognitive cueing. Box 19-14 describes ways the family can assist patients with this impairment.

## GOALS

The ability to document occupational therapy evaluation and treatment information appropriately is more important than ever. The insurance industry reimburses for occupational therapy services according to information provided to them through documentation; the goals that are set for a patient are critical to the support of the plan of care by the insurance company. Functional outcomes have gained increasing support and in many cases are required by insurance companies for reimbursement. Therefore goals should be meaningful and sustainable; they must be valued and carried out by the patient outside the clinical environment.[2] Allen[2] describes examples of goals and documentation criteria for use in the brain-injured population (Box 19-15).

Cognitive and perceptual rehabilitation has become a specialized area of practice for many occupational therapy practitioners. Specialization may result in decreased adherence to the roots of the profession and a focus on just one segment or function of the individual. One must remember that all cognitive and perceptual skills work together to produce an integrated and complex system of behaviors. The focus of occupational therapists should be on the way neurobehavioral impairments affect patients' lives. The overall intent should not be to increase patients' attention span but to improve their ability to perform meaningful, relevant activities.

---

**Box 19-12**

### DENIAL AND LACK OF INSIGHT: TIPS FOR FAMILY MEMBERS

- Provide frequent reality orientation (e.g., explain why patient is in the hospital and with what activities patient is having problems).
- Be honest (but not critical) about the patient's condition or disabilities.
- If it is not dangerous, allow or even encourage the patient to try a desired activity. When the patient is unable to complete the task, calmly draw attention to it. Do not badger or gloat.
- Be patient. Remember that denial is a result of neurologic damage; it is not an effort to be stubborn on the part of the patient.
- Once you believe the patient can handle confrontation, challenging the patient may be necessary. Show that you can easily accomplish a task that the patient says no one can do.

---

**Box 19-13**

### IMPULSIVITY: TIPS FOR FAMILY MEMBERS

- Reward the patient for brief periods of self-control.
- Redirect the patient's attention to appropriate behavior.
- Place the wheelchair (or other equipment) out of sight to prevent the patient from being tempted to sit in it when alone.
- Ignore verbal outbursts whenever possible, and try not to take them personally.
- When the patient has some capability for control, be direct about your feelings but not critical. You may want to say things such as "My feelings are hurt when you talk to me this way" or "It embarrasses me when you tell other people things I have said to you about them."
- Keep dangerous objects such as knives and scissors in a safe place.

---

**Box 19-14**

### PROBLEM-SOLVING IMPAIRMENTS: TIPS FOR FAMILY MEMBERS

- Remove time restraints from tasks if possible.
- Provide written or verbal step-by-step instructions for tasks.
- Keep directions and tasks as simple as possible.

A general approach that can be used for every stroke patient with cognitive or perceptual impairments will never be found. The approach taken to treat each person who has had a stroke must be an integration of the person's previous function, support system, severity of injury, and personal needs and goals. Cognitive and perceptual rehabilitation is a challenging and rewarding part of the rehabilitation process.

### Box 19-15

## SAMPLE GOALS FOR PATIENTS WITH NEUROBEHAVIORAL IMPAIRMENTS

- Patient will properly sequence dressing tasks involving the legs with fewer than two verbal cues in three out of three trials.
- Patient will use grab bars or other objects for stability and safety during dressing task in three out of three trials.
- Patient will demonstrate appropriate use of pillbox for medication schedule in three out of three trials.
- Patient will prepare a shopping list from a recipe with all needed ingredients in two out of three trials.
- Patient will use 75% of objects and eat 75% of food placed on left side of midline, without verbal cues, in three out of three trials.
- Patient will prepare a simple, familiar meal with 80% recognition of errors in three out of five trials.
- Patient will use objects appropriately in hygiene tasks without assistance in two out of three trials.
- Patient will attend to and perform all steps of audio-cued grooming task in three out of three trials.
- Patient will plan and participate in community activities once a week in three out of five trials.

### Case Study 1

#### NEUROBEHAVIORAL DEFICITS AFTER STROKE

G.W., a 49-year-old man, was working as a security guard at a prison when he sustained a massive right middle cerebral artery cerebrovascular accident. He was hospitalized for 7 days and subsequently received occupational therapy on an outpatient basis. G.W.'s neurobehavioral deficits initially included severe left-side spatial and body neglect, anosognosia, and difficulty with spatial relationships, along with hemiparesis resulting in total dependence in mobility and all activities of daily living except eating (for which he needed moderate assistance).

Initial treatment plans focused on setting up functional activities such as eating, grooming, hygiene, and dressing. G.W. was required visually to scan the left side of space to find needed objects or use both arms to practice use of the left side of the body. (This was achieved through use of guiding techniques because no independent movement of left arm was present.) Diminishing verbal cues were used for G.W. to learn to attend to the left side of his body and left side of space during functional task performance. G.W.'s greatest initial impediment was his steadfast denial that his left arm and leg belonged to him (known as *anosognosia*). Fortunately, this denial diminished and was no longer present 4 weeks after the stroke.

Techniques such as matching color markers were minimally successful in treating spatial deficits. However, adaptive devices, such as elastic shoelaces (to prevent the need spatially to execute one-handed shoelace tying), and compensatory strategies, such as slowing down movements and keeping hands on supported surfaces while reaching, were highly successful in increasing G.W.'s independence in daily task performance.

As G.W.'s awareness of his disability improved, use of awareness questioning was emphasized. G.W. initially was questioned after (and then before) each task; he later learned to ask himself questions such as, "What do I do before I start?" "Do I see everything I need?" "Is there anything I forgot?" and "Did I pay attention to my left side?" Awareness questioning was the most successful technique for improving G.W.'s ability to achieve independent performance of basic self-care and eventually perform instrumental ADL without assistance. Initially he lived with his mother and brother after the stroke, but he returned to independent living in his apartment and at the time of discharge was working with vocational rehabilitation services to explore employment options.

### Case Study 2

#### ROLE OF FAMILY IN OVERCOMING NEUROBEHAVIORAL DEFICITS AFTER STROKE

M.A., an 82-year-old man, sustained a stroke in the left hemisphere at the age of 80 years and subsequently underwent above-the-knee amputation of his right leg as a result of peripheral vascular disease. M.A. was placed in a skilled nursing facility, and soon thereafter occupational therapy services were initiated. Neurobehavioral impairments noted at the time of evaluation included global aphasia, motor and ideational apraxia, and severe attention deficits. M.A. depended on others for all mobility and ADL skills, including eating. M.A.'s family was supportive and visited him daily at lunch and dinnertime. Much of the occupational therapy was focused on patient, family, and staff education. The family was taught to use Affolter guiding techniques, which they implemented at mealtime and for grooming and hygiene tasks. The family and staff were taught ways to facilitate communication through tactile and visual cues and guiding techniques, ways to decrease environmental stimulation and distractions, and ways to approach M.A. to help him attend to tasks. M.A. responded well to guiding techniques, requiring only occasional tactile cues after initiating the task (through guiding) to eat, comb his hair, and wash his face in a low-stimulus environment. Occupational therapy continued for 7 weeks (because M.A. also was seen for contracture management), and eventually M.A. was discharged from the skilled nursing facility to his family's care.

## REVIEW QUESTIONS

1. How is the integrated functional approach different from traditional functional approaches, and why is it the recommended approach for cognitive and perceptual impairments?

2. What are the basic principles of the multicontextual and Affolter approaches, and why are they relevant to occupational therapy for cognitive and perceptual impairments?

3. What neurobehavioral components are required to perform a hair grooming task? How can this task be used in the treatment of motor apraxia?

4. How can caregivers adapt environments to assist loved ones with cognitive or perceptual impairments?

5. What do most research-based studies reveal about the use of computers for cognitive and perceptual impairments? When is the use of computers most relevant?

## REFERENCES

1. Abreu B, Duval M, Gerber D, et al: Occupational performance and the functional approach. In Royeen CB: *AOTA self-study series: cognitive rehabilitation*, Rockville, Md, 1994, American Occupational Therapy Association.
2. Allen CK: Reporting occupational therapy services. In Allen CK, Earhart CA, Blue T: *Occupational therapy treatment goals for the physically ill and cognitively disabled*, Rockville, Md, 1992, American Occupational Therapy Association.
3. Ángeleri F, Ángeleri VA, Foschi N, et al: The influence of depression, social activity, and family stress on functional outcome after stroke, *Stroke* 24:1478, 1993.
4. Árnadóttir G: *The brain and behavior: assessing cortical dysfunction through activities of daily living*, St Louis, 1990, Mosby.
5. Ayres AJ: *Development dyspraxia and adult onset apraxia*, Torrance, Calif, 1985, Sensory Integration International.
6. Baggerly J: Sensory perceptual problems following stroke, *Nurs Clin North Am* 26(4):997-1005, 1991.
7. Beis JM, Andre JM, Baumgarten A, et al: Eye patching in unilateral spatial neglect: efficacy of two methods, *Arch Phys Med Rehabil* 80(1):71-76, 1999.
8. Ben-Yishay Y, Piasetsky EB, Rattok J: *A systematic method for ameliorating disorders in basic attention*, New York, 1987, Guilford Press.
9. Bonfils KB: The Affolter approach to treatment: a perceptual-cognitive perspective of function. In Pedretti LW, editor: *Occupational therapy: practice skills for physical dysfunction*, St Louis, 1996, Mosby.
10. Borst MJ, Peterson CQ: Overcoming topographical orientation deficits in an elderly women with a right cerebrovascular accident, *Am J Occup Ther* 47:551, 1993.
11. Bowen A, Lincoln NB, Dewey M: Cognitive rehabilitation for spatial neglect following stroke (Cochrane review). In *The Cochrane library*, Issue 3, Oxford, UK, 2002, Update Software.
12. Bruce MA: Cognitive rehabilitation: intelligence, insight, and knowledge. In Royeen CB, editor: *AOTA self-study series: cognitive rehabilitation*, Rockville, Md, 1994, American Occupational Therapy Association.
13. Calvanio R, Levine D, Petrone P: Elements of cognitive rehabilitation after right hemisphere stroke, *Behav Neurol* 11(1):25-57, 1993.
14. Cermak SA, Trombly C, Hausser J, et al: Effects of lateralized tasks on unilateral neglect after right cerebral vascular accident, *Occup Ther J Res* 11:271, 1991.
15. Condeluci A, Ferris LL, Bogdan A: Outcome and value: the survivor perspective, *J Head Trauma Rehabil* 7:37, 1992.
16. Cooke D: Remediation of unilateral neglect: what do we know? *Aust Occup Ther J* 39:19, 1992.
17. Davis JZ: The Affolter method: a model for treating perceptual disturbances in the hemiplegic and brain-injured patient, *Occup Ther Pract* 3:30, 1992.
18. Dickerson AE, Fisher AG: Age differences in functional performance, *Am J Occup Ther* 47(8):686-692, 1993.
19. Duncombe LW, Howe MC: Group treatment: goals, tasks, and economic implications, *Am J Occup Ther* 49:199, 1995.
20. Edmans JA, Lincoln NB: Treatment of visual perceptual deficits after stroke: single case studies on four patients with right hemiplegia, *Br J Occup Ther* 54:139, 1991.
21. Edmans JA, Lincoln NB: Treatment of visual perceptual deficits after stroke, *Int Disabil Stud* 11(1):25-33, 1989.
22. Edmans JA, Webster J, Lincoln NB: A comparison of two approaches in the treatment of perceptual problems after stroke, *Clin Rehabil* 14(3):230-243, 2000.
23. Evans R: Family stroke education, *Occup Ther Health Care* 2:63, 1985.
24. Fanthome Y, Lincoln NB, Drummond A, et al: The treatment of visual neglect using the transfer of training approach, *Br J Occup Ther* 58:14, 1995.
25. Frassinetti F, Angeli V, Meneghello F, et al: Long-lasting amelioration of visuospatial neglect by prism adaptation, *Brain* 125 (pt 3):608-623, 2002.
26. Friedland J: Social support for stroke survivors: development and evaluation of an intervention program, *Phys Occup Ther Ger* 7:55, 1989.
27. Guiles GM, Clark-Wilson J: The use of behavioral techniques in functional skills training after severe brain injury, *Am J Occup Ther* 42(10):658-665, 1988.
28. Hajek VE: The effect of visuo-spatial training in patients with right hemisphere stroke, *Can J Rehabil* 6:175, 1993.

29. Halligan PW, Cockburn JM: Cognitive sequelae of stroke: visuospatial and memory disorders, *Crit Rev Phys Rehabil Med* 5:57, 1993.

30. Heilman K, Valenstein E, Watson R: Neglect and related disorders, *Semin Neurol* 20(4):463-470, 2000.

31. Helm-Estabrooks N, Emory P, Albert ML: Treatment of aphasic perseveration, *Arch Neurol* 44(12):1253-1255, 1987.

32. van Heugten CM, Dekker J, Deelman BG, et al: Rehabilitation of stroke patients with apraxia: the role of additional cognitive and motor impairments, *Disabil Rehabil* 22(12):547-554, 2000.

33. van Heugten CM, Dekker J, Deelman BG, et al: Outcome of strategy training in stroke patients with apraxia: a phase II study, *Clin Rehabil* 12(4):294-303, 1998.

34. Jabri J: Providing visuoperceptual remediation treatment for stroke patients in the home setting, *J Home Health Care Pract* 4:36, 1992.

35. Jarus T: Motor learning and occupational therapy: the organization of practice, *Am J Occup Ther* 48(9):810-816, 1994.

36. Jennett SM, Lincoln NB: An evaluation of the effectiveness of group therapy for memory problems, *Int Disabil Stud* 13(3):83-86, 1991.

37. Kageyama S, Imagase M, Okubo M, et al: Neglect in three dimensions, *Am J Occup Ther* 48(3):206-210, 1994.

38. Karnath HO, Christ K, Hartje W: Decrease of contralateral neglect by neck muscle vibration and spatial orientation of trunk midline, *Brain* 116(pt 2):383-396, 1993.

39. Katzmann S, Mix C: Improving functional independence in a patient with encephalitis through behavior modification shaping techniques, *Am J Occup Ther* 48(3):259-262, 1994.

40. King T: Treatment of visual inattention using computerized overhead projection, *J Cogn Rehabil* 11:32, 1993.

41. Lin K, Cermak SA: Cognitive perceptual intervention in poststroke patients with unilateral neglect: an annotated bibliography, *Phys Occup Ther Geriatr* 10:63, 1991.

42. Lincoln N: Stroke rehabilitation, *Curr Opin Neurol Neurosurg* 5(5):677-681, 1992.

43. Lincoln NB, Majid MJ, Weyman N: Cognitive rehabilitation for attention deficits following stroke (Cochrane review). In *The Cochrane library*, Issue 3, Oxford, UK, 2002, Update Software.

44. Majid MJ, Lincoln NB, Weyman N: Cognitive rehabilitation for memory deficits following stroke (Cochrane review). In *The Cochrane library*, Issue 3, Oxford, UK, 2002, Update Software.

45. Neistadt ME: A meal preparation treatment protocol for adults with brain injury, *Am J Occup Ther* 48(5):431-438, 1994.

46. Neistadt ME: The neurobiology of learning: implications for treatment of adults with brain injury, *Am J Occup Ther* 48(5):421-430, 1994.

47. Neistadt ME: Perceptual retraining for adults with diffuse brain injury, *Am J Occup Ther* 48(3):225-233, 1994.

48. Neistadt ME: Occupational therapy treatments for constructional deficits, *Am J Occup Ther* 46(2):141-148, 1992.

49. Nygard L, Bernspang B, Fisher AG, et al: Comparing motor and process ability of persons with suspected dementia in home and clinic settings, *Am J Occup Ther* 48(8):689-696, 1994.

50. Olson E: Perceptual deficits affecting the stroke patient, *Rehabil Nurs* 16(4):212-213, 1991.

51. Papstrat LA: Outcome and value following brain injury: a financial provider's perspective, *J Head Trauma Rehabil* 7:11, 1992.

52. Park S, Fisher AG, Velonzo C: Using the assessment of motor and process skills to compare occupational performance between home and clinic settings, *Am J Occup Ther* 48(8):697-709, 1994.

53. Pierce SR, Buxbaum LJ: Treatments of unilateral neglect: a review, *Arch Phys Med Rehabil* 83(2):256-268, 2002.

54. Radomski MV: There is more to life than putting on your pants, *Am J Occup Ther* 49(6):487-490, 1995.

55. Radomski MV: Cognitive rehabilitation: advancing the stature of occupational therapy, *Am J Occup Ther* 48(3):271-273, 1994.

56. Radomski MV, Dougherty PM, Fine S, et al: Case studies in cognitive rehabilitation. In Royeen CB, editor: *AOTA self-study series: cognitive rehabilitation*, Rockville, Md, 1994, American Occupational Therapy Association.

57. Robertson IH, Gray JM, Pentland B, et al: Microcomputer-based rehabilitation for unilateral left visual neglect: a randomized controlled trial, *Arch Phys Med Rehabil* 71(9):663-668, 1990.

58. Robertson IH, North NT, Geggie C: Spatiomotor cuing in unilateral left neglect: three case studies of its therapeutic effects, *J Neurol Neurosurg Psychiatry* 55:799, 1992.

59. Rossetti Y, Rode F, Pisella L: Prism adaptation to a rightward optical deviation rehabilitates left hemispatial neglect, *Nature* 395:166, 1998.

60. Rossi PW, Kheyfets S, Reding MJ: Fresnel prisms improve visual perception in stroke patients with homonymous hemianopia or unilateral neglect, *Neurology* 40(10):1597-1599, 1990.

61. Toglia JP: Attention and memory. In Royeen CB, editor: *AOTA self-studies series: cognitive rehabilitation*, Rockville, Md, 1993, American Occupational Therapy Association.

62. Toglia JP: A dynamic interactional approach to cognitive rehabilitation. In Katz N, editor: *Cognitive rehabilitation: models for intervention in occupational therapy*, Boston, 1992, Andover Medical.

63. Toglia JP: Generalization of treatment: a multicontext approach to cognitive perceptual impairment in adults with brain injury, *Am J Occup Ther* 45(6):505-516, 1991.

64. Trombly C: Clinical practice guidelines for post-stroke rehabilitation and occupational therapy practice, *Am J Occup Ther* 49(7):711-714, 1995.

65. Warren M: Visuospatial skills: assessment and intervention strategies. In Royeen CB, editor: *AOTA self-study series: cognitive rehabilitation*, Rockville, Md, 1994, American Occupational Therapy Association.

66. Webster JS, Cottam G, Gouvier WD, et al: Wheelchair obstacle course performance in right cerebral vascular accident victims, *J Clin Exp Neuropsychol* 11(2):295-310, 1989.

67. Webster J, Jones S, Blanton P, et al: Visual scanning training with stroke patients, *Behav Ther* 15:129, 1984.

68. Wheatley CJ: Cognitive rehabilitation service provision: results of a survey of practitioners, *Am J Occup Ther* 48(2):163-166, 1994.

69. Wiart L, Bon Saint Come A, Debelleix X, et al: Unilateral neglect syndrome rehabilitation by trunk rotation and scanning training, *Arch Phys Med Rehabil* 78(4):424-429, 1997.

70. Yuen HK: Increasing medication compliance in a women with anoxic brain damage and partial epilepsy, *Am J Occup Ther* 47(1):30-33, 1993.

71. Zemke R: Task skills, problem solving, and social interaction. In Royeen CB, editor: *AOTA self-study series: cognitive rehabilitation*, Rockville, Md, 1994, American Occupational Therapy Association.

## SUGGESTED READINGS

Abreu B: Perceptual motor skills: assessment and intervention strategies. In Royeen CB, editor: *AOTA self-study series: cognitive rehabilitation*, Rockville, Md, 1994, American Occupational Therapy Association.

Allen CK, Earhart CA, Blue T: *Occupational therapy treatment goals for the physically and cognitively disabled*, Rockville, Md, 1992, American Occupational Therapy Association.

*AOTA self-paced clinical course: STROKE—strategies, treatment, rehabilitation, outcomes, knowledge, and evaluation*, Rockville, Md, 1996, American Occupational Therapy Association.

Davies PM: *Starting again: early rehabilitation after traumatic brain injury or other severe brain lesion*, Berlin, 1994, Springer-Verlag.

Katz N: *Cognition and occupation in rehabilitation: cognitive models for intervention in occupational therapy*, Rockville, Md, 1998, American Occupational Therapy Association.

Unsworth C: *Cognitive and perceptual dysfunction: a clinical reasoning approach to evaluation and intervention*, Philadelphia, 1999, FA Davis.

# Enhancing Engagement in Instrumental Activities of Daily Living

## key terms

Assessment of Motor and Process Skills

Canadian Occupational Performance Measure

disability

instrumental activities of daily living

## chapter objectives

After completing this chapter, the reader will be able to accomplish the following:

1. Understand the concept of instrumental activities of daily living.
2. Recognize the effect of a stroke on a person's engagement in instrumental activities of daily living.
3. Understand the relationship between the degree of impairment and engagement in instrumental activities of daily living and implications for evaluation and intervention.
4. Discuss the occupational therapy evaluation process for enhancing engagement in instrumental activities of daily living.
5. Discuss the Canadian Occupational Performance Measure and the Assessment of Motor and Process Skills.
6. Understand the basics of goal writing for performance of instrumental activities of daily living.
7. Understand the adaptive approach to occupational therapy intervention for instrumental activities of daily living intervention.

Rehabilitation is a restorative and learning process that hastens and maximizes a patient's functional recovery after a cerebrovascular accident (CVA) by addressing the resulting impairments, disabilities, and handicaps.[25] The main objective of rehabilitation is to restore functioning so that a patient can return or continue to live in the community.

All rehabilitation professionals focus on a patient's functional status and the functional status of the patient's family.* Depending on a rehabilitation professional's

---

*The term *family* refers to all members of a patient's close-knit social group, which may include a spouse, a partner, relatives, and friends.

perspective, though, the term *function* may take on a different meaning. From an occupational therapist's perspective, *function* is defined as a person's occupation—his or her engagement in activities that are meaningful and purposeful, including personal self-care; vocational, educational, social, and play and leisure activities; and instrumental activities of daily living (IADL).[11,13,18,41] Thus the main role of occupational therapists working with patients who have had a stroke is to facilitate the restoration of the ability to engage in daily occupation successfully so that the patients can return or continue to live in the communities where they live, work, and play.[13,43]

## CEREBROVASCULAR ACCIDENT AND INSTRUMENTAL ACTIVITIES OF DAILY LIVING

Instrumental activities of daily living are the more complex daily tasks, such as domestic chores, household management, shopping, and transportation, that must be performed for a person to continue living in the community (Box 20-1).[10,21,25,32,47] *Instrumental activities of daily living* is the most common term used to identify these domestic and community tasks, although other terms also have been used, including extended activities of daily living or domestic activities of daily living.[58] Instrumental activities of daily living tasks typically are differentiated from play and leisure activities because the engagement in play and leisure, although important to a person's well-being, is not necessarily required for independent community living. For persons who have had a stroke, a return to living in the community requires the ability to engage in not only basic self-care tasks but also IADL tasks.[25]

Studies from Sweden and Spain indicate that persons who have had a stroke tend to attain independence with basic self-care tasks to a greater degree than with IADL tasks.[8,40] A United Kingdom study indicates that the frequency of engagement in IADL tasks was significantly less than that before the stroke.[28] This trend is similar to one found in a study in the United States in which 1 year after a stroke, persons were generally sedentary, not involved in the routine care of the home, and isolated

---

**Box 20-1**

### Examples of Instrumental Activities of Daily Living

**HOME ENVIRONMENT**

**Meal Preparation Tasks**

Planning snacks and meals
Gathering food and materials
Preparing food
Using tools and appliances
Restoring food and materials
Setting the table

**Household Chores**

Washing windows
Handling garbage and recycling
Performing minor repairs
Watering lawn and plants
Raking leaves

**Communication Activities**

Using the telephone
Handling mail
Writing letters
Using a computer

---

**Box 20-1**

### Examples of Instrumental Activities of Daily Living—cont'd

**Miscellaneous Tasks**

Operating light switches
Opening doors and using keys
Operating television and radio
Caring for animals
Watering houseplants

**House Cleaning Routines**

Vacuuming rugs
Dusting furniture
Sweeping floors
Mopping floors
Washing dishes

**Laundry Tasks**

Washing, drying, and folding
Making the bed
Changing bed linens
Ironing clothes

**Financial Responsibilities**

Paying bills
Balancing checkbook

**Emergency Procedures**

Responding to a fire
Communicating an emergency

**COMMUNITY ENVIRONMENT**

**Mobility**

Riding a bus or subway
Taking a taxi
Driving a car

**Shopping**

Buying groceries
Buying clothes
Handling monetary transactions

from friends and previous leisure activities.[53] Another U.S. study revealed that for males who have had a stroke, dissatisfaction with their diminished activity level was associated with lack of involvement in home maintenance, traveling, and helping others.[2] From an Australian study, the capacity to engage in a range of social and domestic activities was a prime determinant of satisfaction with recovery following a stroke.[12] Despite these discouraging results, many persons who have had a stroke continue to engage in IADL despite the residual effects of the stroke. One study from the United Kingdom indicated that many persons who have had a stroke achieve independence with the performance of various IADL tasks such as shopping, using public transportation, coping with money, ironing, hanging out the wash, making the bed, cleaning the house, and preparing a snack, hot drink, or meal.[16]

Instrumental activities of daily living require greater interaction with the physical and social environment and a greater degree of skill (e.g., problem-solving and social skills) than basic self-care tasks.[20,47,54] Therefore any underlying impairments in a person's sensorimotor, cognitive-perceptual, or psychosocial capacity that may result from a CVA tend to affect the performance of IADL tasks to a greater degree than they affect basic self-care (Box 20-2). The presence of an impairment, however, is not predictive of a patient's level of performance of daily life tasks.[19,52] A Canadian study of persons with

### Box 20-2

**Potential Effect of Impairments on Instrumental Activities of Daily Living Tasks Compared with Self-Care Tasks**

- Hemiplegia of the arm may create more difficulty in opening a can of soup than in buttoning a shirt.
- Weakness in the leg may severely limit bending down to secure tools on a lower shelf in the garage but may be adequate to don a pair of slacks.
- Postural insecurity may result in a greater risk for injury when sweeping the floor than when standing to perform grooming tasks.
- Aphasia may make shopping for groceries at the local store more difficult than eating a meal at home.
- Visual inattention to the environment may make locating needed items in a kitchen more difficult than locating meal items on a table.
- Poor tactile sensation in the hand may lead to safety concerns when using a knife to prepare vegetables for a meal but not when buttering toast for breakfast.
- Depression resulting from the stroke experience may decrease the patient's motivation and desire to engage in more complex instrumental activities of daily living tasks that may seem overwhelming in their performance demands and energy requirements compared with simpler basic self-care tasks

right- and left-side CVA[29] found that the ability to prepare a sandwich and cup of tea could not be predicted accurately from the extent of upper or lower extremity weakness, cognitive function, visuospatial abilities, somatosensory functioning, or motor planning dysfunction. A pilot study[49] investigated the meal preparation skills (e.g., tuna salad or an omelette) of 10 ambulatory women with aphasia. No relationship was found between severity of aphasia and degree of cognitive-perceptual impairment, and all the women had retained some degree of meal preparation skill. Indeed, 60% attained the highest rating for the meal preparation task, indicating near normal or independent performance. Furthermore, despite a tendency for persons with right-side CVA to have left inattention and visuospatial difficulties and for persons with left-side CVA to have apraxia and aphasia, the overall ability to perform daily living tasks may be similar for both types of patients.[3] Research revealed that IADL performance in patients with right- and left-side CVA did not differ significantly despite the hemisphere-specific differences of their impairments.

## OCCUPATIONAL THERAPY SERVICES

The critical issue regarding the presence of underlying impairments resulting from a CVA and the performance of IADL tasks is whether occupational therapy intervention for a disability in IADL performance should be focused directly on improving a patient's underlying impairments. If a patient's IADL performance cannot be predicted from the degree of the impairment, changing a person's degree of impairment may not automatically improve IADL performance. Furthermore, other rehabilitation professionals focus their expertise on underlying impairments to reduce the degree of impairment and enhance functional status.[43] For example, a neuropsychologist addresses cognitive-perceptual function to evaluate formally the degree of a patient's left visual inattention. The presence of an underlying impairment is of concern to an occupational therapist when considering intervention for IADL performance, but the effect of an underlying impairment on a patient's ability to perform IADL tasks directs evaluation and intervention strategies.

Self-care and functional mobility are the most common variables used as outcome measures in studies of persons with CVA.[29] These variables also reflect the intervention strategies commonly used by occupational therapists. In a survey of occupational therapy directors in adult physical rehabilitation facilities across the United States in the 1990s, the 10 most frequently used intervention activities, ranked in order of frequency, were the following[39]:
1. Self-care
2. Upper extremity exercise
3. Functional mobility

4. Neuromuscular function
5. Homemaking
6. Cognitive and perceptual training
7. Community living skills
8. Physical agent modalities
9. Sensory reeducation
10. Assistive technology

Because upper extremity exercise was ranked the second most common intervention strategy used by occupational therapists and homemaking and community living skills were ranked fifth and seventh, respectively, occupational therapists may not be doing enough to prepare their adult patients for successful reintegration to the community and should reorder their intervention priorities accordingly.[39] Meal preparation has been recommended for inclusion in rehabilitation intervention for stroke patients, particularly those with meal preparation responsibility, because engagement in meal preparation tasks may help foster a sense of usefulness and purpose, an important component of the rehabilitation process.[29,49]

In the inpatient rehabilitation setting, occupational therapists typically evaluate IADL tasks such as meal preparation at the end of a patient's rehabilitation stay (if at all)[29] and often after much emphasis and intervention has been directed at the performance of self-care tasks. Although the importance of enhancing a patient's level of performance in self-care tasks is not disputed, the amount of therapy time devoted to tasks that may involve only 1 or 2 hours of a patient's day is questionable, particularly because the patient has the rest of the day in which to occupy time meaningfully. Occupational therapists need to consider a patient's perceptions of what is important for quality of life and life satisfaction. An Australian study revealed that occupational therapists and older adults living in the community differed in their perceptions of which IADL activities were the most important.[21] The occupational therapists tended to consider "important" those tasks necessary to live independently, whereas the older adults interpreted "important" those activities that held meaning, not just independence. Some patients who have had a stroke and their families may find more benefit participating in IADL tasks that are more satisfying rather than just those required for independent living.

Another issue arises when a patient has concluded inpatient rehabilitation and proceeds to outpatient or home health services, for which only a limited number of occupational therapy appointments may be reimbursed by a third-party payer. The length of stay is limited for inpatient rehabilitation services, and follow-up appointments for home health or outpatient services are limited as well. The time frame under which the third-party payer will provide payment for services often affects the patient's desire and ability to reengage in desired daily life tasks. Patients who have had a CVA have commented that the stress of inpatient rehabilitation prevented them from

benefiting completely from rehabilitation and that a period of time at home provided them with an opportunity to experience directly the ways the CVA had affected their lives.[53] These patients experienced renewed interest in improving skills and achieving independence in daily life tasks after time at home. Thus, by the time stroke patients are ready to enhance their skills, they may not be eligible to receive additional occupational therapy services. A Swedish study, focusing on persons with CVA 2 years after inpatient rehabilitation revealed an increase in dependence in IADL tasks, suggested needs are unmet several years after the initial CVA.[26]

Although engagement in daily activities may be dramatically different after a CVA, patients who have had a stroke clearly want and continue to engage in a variety of activities of daily living (ADL) despite the effect of the CVA. The role of the occupational therapist is to facilitate the patient's continued participation in meaningful and purposeful daily activities and adaptation to the changed status.[14-17] Ultimately, however, the quality of the patient's life is of the utmost importance. Occupational therapists who work in rehabilitation settings should not limit evaluation and intervention strategies to a patient's proficiency with basic self-care tasks or upper extremity function. They must expand the possibilities and assist each patient in engaging in an array of meaningful and valued activities that will bring personal satisfaction.[46]

## REHABILITATION EVALUATION PROCESS

Depending on the area of expertise, each rehabilitation professional fulfills a unique role during the evaluation process for IADL. Physical therapists may focus on a patient's ability to walk safely during IADL tasks such as riding the bus and watering the lawn. Social workers may focus on securing services to carry out IADL tasks if a patient is limited in the ability to perform these tasks and family members cannot take over the responsibility for them.

Despite the need for all rehabilitation professionals to focus on IADL tasks, the evaluation of rehabilitation programs tends primarily to use physical and self-care assessments.[24] Though standardized assessments of IADL may be more sensitive indicators of the consequences of a stroke than assessments of self-care tasks,[35,58] standardized assessments for IADL have not been developed as extensively as those for self-care tasks. No agreement exists as to the exact categories or items to be included in IADL assessments (Table 20-1).[10] Furthermore, their content often reflects specific cultural concerns and overemphasizes activities customarily performed by women.[58] Of note is the fact that most IADL assessments were developed outside of North America, and the applicability of these assessments to a North American population is questionable.[10]

**Table 20-1**

**Instrumental Activities of Daily Living Standardized Assessments**

| | RIVERMEAD ADL ASSESSMENT | ADELAIDE ACTIVITIES PROFILE | FRENCHAY ACTIVITIES INDEX | NOTTINGHAM EXTENDED ADL SCALE | INSTRUMENTAL ACTIVITY MEASURE |
|---|---|---|---|---|---|
| Authors | Whiting and Lincoln (1980)[59] | Bond and Clark (1998)[5] | Holbrook and Skilbeck (1983)[28] | Nouri and Lincoln (1987)[42] | Grimby et al (1996)[27] |
| Rating scale | 3-level | 4-level | 4-level | 4-level | 7-level |
| Focus | Degree of assistance in performance activities | Degree of participation in activities | Degree of participation in activities | Degree of difficulty and assistance engaging in activities | Degree of assistance in performing activities |
| Format | Observation | Interview | Interview | Self-report | Observation |
| Country of origin | United Kingdom | Australia | United Kingdom | United Kingdom | Sweden |
| Assessment items: | | | | | |
| Meal preparation | Prepare a meal Prepare a hot drink Prepare a snack | Prepare main meal Wash dishes | Prepare main meal Wash dishes | Make a hot drink Make a hot snack Wash dishes Take hot drinks between rooms | Cook a main meal Prepare simple meal |
| Domestic activities | Heavy cleaning Light cleaning Hand wash clothes Iron clothes Hang out washing Make bed | Heavy housework Light housework Wash clothes Household or car maintenance | Heavy housework Light housework Wash clothes Household or car maintenance | Housework Wash small clothing items Full clothes wash | Cleaning house Washing clothes |
| Gardening | — | Light gardening Heavy gardening | Gardening | Manage own garden | — |
| Productive activities | — | Voluntary or paid employment Care for other family members | Gainful work | — | — |
| Shopping/ community activities | Carry shopping Cope with money | Household shopping Personal shopping | Local shopping | Shopping Manage own money | Large-scale shopping Small-scale shopping |

*Continued*

**Table 20-1**

## Instrumental Activities of Daily Living Standardized Assessments—cont'd

| | RIVERMEAD ADL ASSESSMENT | ADELAIDE ACTIVITIES PROFILE | FRENCHAY ACTIVITIES INDEX | NOTTINGHAM EXTENDED ADL SCALE | INSTRUMENTAL ACTIVITY MEASURE |
|---|---|---|---|---|---|
| Transportation | Use public transport—bus<br>Transport self to shop | Drive a car or organize transport | Drive car or go on bus<br>Travel outings or car rides | Travel on public transport<br>Drive a car | Use public transportation |
| Leisure/social activities | — | Community social activities<br>Outdoor social activity<br>Invite persons to home<br>Hobby<br>Telephone calls to family/ friends<br>Attend religious events<br>Outdoor recreation or sporting activity | Social occasions<br>Hobby<br>Reading books | Go out socially<br>Use the telephone<br>Read newspapers or books<br>Write letters | — |
| Mobility: outdoors | Outdoor mobility<br>Crossing roads<br>Get in and out of car | Walk outdoors | Walking outside | Walk outside<br>Cross roads<br>In/out of car<br>Walk on uneven ground | Locomotion outdoors |
| Mobility: indoors | Indoor mobility<br>Mobility to lavatory<br>Move bed to chair<br>Move floor to chair | — | — | Climb stairs | — |
| Basic self-care | Drink<br>Clean teeth<br>Comb hair<br>Wash face and hands<br>Put on makeup or shave<br>Eat<br>Undress<br>Dress<br>Wash in bath<br>Get in and out of bath<br>Overall wash | — | — | Feed self | — |

Most IADL assessment tools rely on a self-report format; that is, the patient or a family member is asked a series of questions about a variety of IADL tasks in which a patient may engage at home. Most patients, even those without cognitive difficulties, encounter some difficulty rating their capacity to engage in IADL tasks, often rating what they do on a daily basis but not necessarily accurately rating what they might be capable of doing.[57] Although the importance of understanding a patient's and family's perceptions cannot be overemphasized, differences do occur between self-report standardized assessments and assessments based on a professional's observation.[6,9,48]

## Occupational Therapy Evaluation

Although IADL assessment tools can be valuable during the rehabilitation process to assess general outcomes and determine a need for support services, their utility is limited for occupational therapists. An Australian study revealed that only 11% of occupational therapists working with patients with CVA frequently used standardized assessments,[22] and a U.S. study revealed that occupational therapists who worked in home health were more likely to use a standardized assessment for self-care activities, and none identified using a specific assessment tool for IADL.[36] Few self-care or IADL assessment tools were designed specifically for occupational therapists and were based on an occupational therapy frame of reference.[30]

In the absence of appropriate standardized assessments, occupational therapists should rely on their expertise and skills in observing IADL performance during the evaluation process and, when possible, use IADL assessment tools developed for use by occupational therapists. As occupational therapists bring their expertise in occupation to the rehabilitation team, they should focus the evaluation process on a patient's ability to resume daily life activities in the environments in which the patient lives, works, and plays.[43] Therefore the evaluation process should begin with a focus on the daily life activities of concern to the patient and family.[18] In addition, if occupational therapists use evaluation strategies reflective of their unique perspective on function—that is, occupation—patients, families, and other health care professionals more readily identify their expertise from that of other professionals.[17]

Occupational therapists also are committed to client-centered practice; that is, the patient's knowledge and experience of daily life after a CVA is of central concern in rehabilitation services. Occupational therapists are guided by an ethical commitment to listen and respond to a person's priorities regarding meaningful and purposeful occupation in daily life.[7,13,43] A client-centered approach to occupational therapy intervention requires an occupational therapist actively to seek information of concern to the patient and family.[7] The rehabilitation evaluation

process is best begun with an interview of the patient, family, or both to identify those specific concerns.

## Interview Process

Occupational therapists should initiate the interview process by soliciting information regarding the daily life activities of concern, including any IADL tasks in which a patient would like to engage. Many interview formats can be used to gather this information. An informal conversation is the most casual and is often effective. For a more in-depth analysis of a patient's perspective on ADL, an interview based on the model of human occupation can yield specific insight into the patient's values, interests, and sense of personal causation—and habits and roles—with respect to IADL tasks (Box 20-3).[31]

During the interview, an occupational therapist also should gather information regarding the environment in which a patient will be performing IADL tasks.[43] Such an interview entails soliciting information about the physical layout of the home. *A Consumer's Guide to Home Adaptation*[1] contains a framework with which to guide an interview focused on the patient's home environment. The information in this booklet details the types of daily

---

**Box 20-3**

### Questions Based on the Model of Human Occupation

These questions are intended to guide an occupational therapist's reasoning regarding the type of information desired about a person's engagement in instrumental activities of daily living (IADL) and are not intended to be asked of a patient.

**PARTICIPATION, PERFORMANCE, AND SKILL**

- Does this person currently engage in IADL tasks that are desired and contribute to his or her well-being?
- Can this person do the IADL tasks that make up (or should make up) this person's life?
- Does this person exhibit the necessary communication/interaction, motor, and process skills to perform the IADL tasks he or she needs and wants to do?

**VOLITION**

**Personal Causation**

- Is this person aware of his or her abilities and limitations to engage in IADL tasks?
- Does the person feel capable of performing IADL tasks or certain aspects?

**Values**

- What are the person's values with respect to the ways IADL tasks should be performed?
- Can this person prioritize those IADL tasks that he or she considers most important?

*Continued*

life activities in which persons with disabilities are likely to engage in their home and provides questions about activities that are likely to be difficult. The booklet also provides information about home modifications and adaptations (see Chapter 25).

### Canadian Occupational Performance Measure

One standardized interview format that is useful in the evaluation process is the Canadian Occupational Performance Measure (COPM).[33] The COPM was developed from a

---

**Box 20-3**

### Questions Based on the Model of Human Occupation—cont'd

**Interests**

- What IADL tasks does this person enjoy doing?
- What aspects of doing IADL tasks does this person enjoy most?

**HABITUATION**

**Habits**

- What is the person's daily routine, and which IADL tasks are a part of this routine?
- What quality of life is provided by a routine of IADL tasks for this person?

**Roles**

- What are the person's current roles, and do any of these roles include a responsibility for IADL tasks?
- How does the person meet the obligations of roles associated with desired IADL?

**Performance Capacity**

- What are the consequences of sensory, motor, or other capacities for this person's experience of engaging in IADL tasks?
- How do experiences (e.g., left neglect, hemiparesis, or diminished enthusiasm) influence this person's performance of IADL?

**ENVIRONMENT: PHYSICAL AND SOCIAL**

**Physical**

- Do the spaces and objects this person uses support engagement in IADL tasks?

**Social**

- Do interactions with others support or inhibit this person's engagement in IADL?
- Do the person's social groups support engagement in meaningful roles associated with IADL?

Adapted from Kielhofner G, Forsyth, K: Thinking with theory: a framework for therapeutic reasoning. In Kielhofner G, editor: *A model of human occupation: theory and application*, ed 3, Philadelphia, 2002, Lippincott Williams & Wilkins.

---

patient-centered perspective and can be used with persons experiencing difficulty with the performance of daily activities, regardless of diagnosis or impairment. The COPM guides the occupational therapist through a semistructured conversation to identify the activities that the person wants, needs, or is expected to do in daily life and to identify problems or difficulties with those activities. The COPM also focuses on the person's perception of the importance of, performance of, and satisfaction with the identified activities of concern.

The format of the COPM guides the occupational therapist to ask questions about the person's engagement in daily activities, soliciting information about the person's morning-to-afternoon-to-evening routine. The COPM comprises six topic areas: (1) personal care, (2) functional mobility, (3) community management, (4) paid/unpaid work, (5) active recreation, and (6) socialization. The COPM also assists the occupational therapist to focus intervention on the person's goals. Furthermore, research evidence is sufficient to support the use of the COPM with patients with strokes.[4,23,51,62]

---

### Case Study 1: Part A

#### LIVING AT HOME: EVALUATION OF IADL PERFORMANCE

Karen, a 54-year-old woman, experienced visual blurring and partial left-side paralysis at home one day. Her husband took her to the hospital, where she was admitted and subsequently diagnosed with right-side CVA with moderate left-side hemiparesis. During her 6-day stay in the hospital, Karen rapidly made progress, spontaneously regaining much physical and cognitive-perceptual function, although the residual effects from the CVA were still apparent at discharge on day 7. Starting on the fourth day of her hospitalization, she received physical therapy to evaluate her walking. The physical therapist identified that although Karen's gait pattern had some minor irregularities, she did not require a cane or walker. The physical therapist, however, was concerned with the continued paresis of her left arm, mild left visual inattention, and short-term memory deficits. He recommended that she walk with supervision when outdoors and that she undergo outpatient physical therapy to address her irregular gait and overall physical function. Although the initial impact of the CVA had resolved substantially and Karen was essentially independent in performing basic self-care tasks (the nursing staff having recommended supervision and adaptive equipment for bathing), her neurologist questioned her ability to engage safely in household tasks and community activities. Therefore, he recommended that Karen be supervised throughout the day and that she avoid more complex activities such as cooking and community outings. To further address the residual effects of the CVA, the neurologist recommended that she receive outpatient occupational therapy.

Karen went to her first outpatient occupational therapy appointment 16 days after the CVA. During a casual initial interview, her occupational therapist gathered information about Karen's role in the family and community and the effect of the stroke on Karen's life, particularly the recommendation that she be supervised throughout the day. During this first conversation, the therapist realized the importance of Karen's desire to resume her previous activities, particularly those associated with her role as a wife, mother, grandmother, homemaker, and hobbyist. The therapist also recognized that Karen was unhappy with the prospect of continued daytime supervision. To further explore these areas of concern and gather more specific information about Karen's perception of her ability to engage in self-care, work, and leisure activities, the occupational therapist chose to use the COPM to identify Karen's primary concerns with specific activities.

The occupational therapist explained the purpose of the COPM and began by asking Karen questions about her morning activities since her discharge from the hospital. She continued with questions about other activities that Karen wanted or needed to engage in during the afternoon and into the evening. Throughout the interview, the therapist asked Karen which activities she found difficult or was unable to do. By the end, Karen had identified the six activities most important to her: (1) changing the bed, (2) preparing meals, (3) setting and combing her hair, (4) assisting her younger children with their homework, (5) sewing, and (6) playing with her grandchildren (Figure 20-1).

Her occupational therapist learned that two of the identified activities—changing the bed and meal preparation—were activities in which Karen was not engaging, based on her neurologist's recommendation. Karen had said that she did not feel physically capable of playing with her grandchildren and feared she might drop them. As for helping her children with their homework, Karen believed she wasn't "smart enough now" because she occasionally became confused during conversations with her children. Finally, Karen said that she was frustrated with combing and

setting her hair because "it just doesn't turn out the way it did before the stroke." This information from the COPM set the stage for the occupational therapist to begin identifying skills that would support Karen's engagement in daily life tasks and which skills might be limiting or preventing her participation in desired activities.

## Observation of Instrumental Activities of Daily Living Performance

Whether using a formal or an informal interview procedure, the occupational therapist should continue the evaluation process with an observation of a patient performing some IADL tasks of concern. Observation of such performance (and performance of other ADL tasks) is an important component of every evaluation process, particularly because one valuable contribution occupational therapists provide for the rehabilitation team is an evaluation of the ability of a patient to perform safely daily life tasks they desire or are required to perform to return and live safely in the community.[43]

The occupational therapist should not proceed first with a direct evaluation of the degree of a patient's impairments such as muscle strength, mental status, and depression.[45] Patients with CVA initially may experience a multitude of underlying impairments such as hemiparesis, left visual inattention, aphasia, and hemianopsia. Direct measurement of the severity of these underlying impairments, however, does not provide the occupational therapist with the information necessary to determine the way in which the patient will perform a specific IADL task. The interplay of a patient's impairments in the context of IADL performance and the environment in which those tasks are performed is the main focus of occupational therapy intervention.[43] Therefore, impairments resulting from a CVA are observed and evaluated best in the context of a patient's task performance.[45,47] Occupational therapists should use evaluation procedures that capture the full spectrum of a patient's IADL performance ability and should limit evaluation procedures that address a patient's cognitive, sensorimotor, and psychosocial function.[43] This evaluation strategy reflects a top-down approach in which an occupational therapist begins with an evaluation of a patient's ability to perform daily life tasks (the top) rather than beginning with an evaluation of a patient's underlying impairments (the bottom).[55] The Assessment of Motor and Process Skills (AMPS)[17] is one assessment tool

| | | IMPORTANCE |
|---|---|:---:|

**STEP 1A: Self-Care**

**Personal Care**
(e.g., dressing, bathing,
feeding, hygiene)

STYLING & COMBING HAIR — 8

DRESSING IN A TIMELY MANNER — 6

**Functional Mobility**
(e.g., transfers,
indoor, outdoor)

GETTING UP SAFELY FROM BATHTUB — 8

**Community Management**
(e.g., transportation,
shopping, finances)

**STEP 1B: Productivity**

**Paid/Unpaid Work**
(e.g., finding/keeping
a job, volunteering)

ASSISTING KIDS WITH HOMEWORK — 10

**Household Management**
(e.g., cleaning, doing
laundry, cooking)

CHANGING SHEETS — 9

PREPARING MEALS FOR FAMILY — 10

FOLDING TOWELS — 2

**Play/School**
(e.g., play skills,
homework)

**STEP 1C: Leisure**

**Quiet Recreation**
(e.g., hobbies,
crafts, reading)

SEWING — 8

NEEDLEPOINT — 5

MAKING X-MAS WREATHS — 5

**Active Recreation**
(e.g., sports,
outings, travel)

PLAYING WITH GRANDKIDS ON THE FLOOR — 9

BOWLING — 4

**Socialization**
(e.g., visiting, phone calls,
parties, correspondence)

**Figure 20-1**    Results from Karen's interview using step 1 of the Canadian Occupational Performance Measure. (Modified from Law M, Baptiste S, Carswell A, et al: *Canadian occupational performance measure,* Toronto, 1994, CAOT Publications ACE.)

for occupational therapists that reflects a top-down approach to evaluation.

## Assessment of Motor and Process Skills

The AMPS is a client-centered, task-oriented performance assessment of the quality of a person's performance in personal (basic self-care) and instrumental ADL and not the person's underlying impairments.[3,17] Developed specifically for use in occupational therapy and currently standardized internationally and cross-culturally on more than 50,000 persons, the AMPS tests the ability of a person to perform personal and instrumental ADL tasks. Although the AMPS does not measure a person's underlying impairment directly, its use does help clarify whether underlying impairments are influencing the ability to perform ADL tasks effectively and at what point in the performance the impairment may have an effect.[3] The AMPS can be used with any person who (1) desires to perform, even if at a marginal level, simple daily living tasks and (2) is familiar with at least two of the AMPS tasks (Box 20-4).[17] Moreover, the AMPS is not restricted to any specific diagnosis and has been used extensively with persons with CVA.

The AMPS requires no specialized equipment and can be conducted in any ADL-relevant setting within 60 minutes. The occupational therapist who uses the AMPS must attend a 5-day AMPS training course to become certified in its use.* For the assessment, the person chooses to perform two or three ADL tasks (from choices offered by the occupational therapist) that are culturally appropriate, familiar, and relevant to daily life. The choices range from simple to complex ADL tasks and reflect various cultural backgrounds, including American, British, Hispanic, Scandinavian, and Asian. The AMPS-trained occupational therapist ensures that the tasks chosen by the person are sufficiently challenging so that the practitioner can observe the person's ability to perform ADL tasks and note any difficulties. The task is performed in the person's usual manner to discern the natural ability to perform such tasks.[17]

Because the AMPS is a standardized measurement tool, to evaluate a person's performance accurately, an AMPS-trained occupational therapist must compare the performance against the criteria for the specified task. For example, one task choice is to prepare scrambled eggs, toast, and a beverage. According to the criteria for this particular AMPS task, the person is requested to use one or two eggs to make the eggs, use two slices of bread with one spread to prepare the toast, and pour a glass of juice or milk or a cup of coffee. The person prepares the eggs in a skillet or frying pan on a stove and uses a standard toaster or toaster oven. Finally, the person serves the eggs, toast, and beverage in appropriate dishes at a counter or table and restores the work space to its original condition.[17] No restrictions are placed on the way the task should be performed. The person is free to choose any method that accomplishes

---

**Box 20-4**

## Examples of Task Choices in the Assessment of Motor and Process Skills

### MEAL PREPARATION TASKS

Beverage from the refrigerator
Toast and boiled or brewed coffee or tea
Cold cereal and beverage
Eggs, toast, and beverage
Luncheon meat or cheese sandwich
Cakes, muffins, or brownies
Tossed salad with dressing
Fried ripe bananas (*plátanos*)
Beans and toast
Fried rice
Pasta with meat, sauce, green salad, and beverage

### HOUSEHOLD CHORES

Sweeping the floor
Making a bed
Ironing a shirt
Repotting a plant
Changing sheets on a bed with a duvet
Hand washing dishes
Folding laundry
Vacuuming
Cleaning a bathroom
Setting a table

### OUTDOOR HOME MAINTENANCE

Sweeping outside
Raking grass or leaves
Weeding

### COMMUNITY TASKS

Shopping

### PERSONAL ACTIVITIES

Eating a meal
Putting on socks and shoes
Upper body dressing
Upper body grooming and total body dressing

---

From Fisher AG: *Assessment of motor and process skills*, vol 2: User manual (ed 5), Fort Collins, Colo, 2003, Three Star Press.

---

*Occupational therapists and occupational therapy assistants are eligible to become certified in the use of the AMPS.

the objectives of the specified AMPS task the person agreed to perform.

After observing the person perform each ADL task, the occupational therapist rates the person's performance on 16 motor and 20 process skill items (Box 20-5) for each task performed. Motor skills are observable actions a person uses to move the body or objects during performance of an ADL task. Process skills are observable actions a person uses to (1) select and interact with and use tools and materials, (2) carry out individual actions and steps, and (3) modify performance on encountering problems. Process skills should not be equated with a person's cognitive capacity, such as attentional, memory, motor planning, and problem-solving skills. Cognitive skills reflect the person's underlying capacity for performance (i.e., the mind-brain-body system in the model of human occupation) and support the way a person organizes and adapts actions during task performance. For example, the ability to gather tools and materials to a work space requires many underlying cognitive skills such as attentional, memory, and problem-solving skills. These specific cognitive skills, however, are not observed directly during ADL performance. What is observed while a person gathers tools and materials is the behavioral output (occupational performance) of the person's underlying capacity (cognitive skills). Similarly, motor skills (as defined in the AMPS) also reflect the behavioral output of a person's underlying motor capacity and should not be equated with traditional motor skills such as muscle strength, range of motion, postural control, and motor planning.[17]

Because motor and process skills are observable actions expressed in the context of performing chosen, familiar, and life-relevant ADL tasks, each skill item is evaluated in terms of the way it contributes to the logical progression and outcome of task performance. Thus, each motor and process skill item is rated on a 4-point scale, in which 4 is competent, 3 is questionable, 2 is ineffective, and 1 is deficit. During each task, the person is rated on the competency of performance in each skill item. For example, an inpatient rehabilitation patient is shown to have moderate hemiparesis of the right upper extremity and a mild motor planning deficit as on a standardized assessment of impairment. An AMPS-trained occupational therapy assistant observed the patient preparing a meat sandwich for an AMPS assessment and scored this performance according to the criteria and examples in the AMPS manual. During the task, the patient was able to readily and consistently locate the needed tools and materials in the familiar occupational therapy clinic kitchen and thus received a score of 4 (competent performance) on the skill item *search/locates*. The patient received a score of 3 (questionable performance) on the process skill item *chooses* because the occupational therapy assistant questioned the appropriateness of using a steak knife to spread butter on a piece of bread. The patient received a score of 2 (ineffective performance) on the motor skill item *manipulates* because of difficulty manipulating the twist tie for the bag of bread, which was dropped on the counter two times. Finally, the patient received a score of 1 (deficit performance) on the motor skill item *grips* because the package of meat being grasped in the patient's right hand fell to the floor. Well persons also are expected occasionally to receive a score of 2, or even 1,

## Box 20-5

### Motor and Process Skills

**MOTOR SKILLS**

Stabilizes
Walks
Coordinates
Moves
Calibrates
Paces*
Aligns
Reaches
Manipulates
Transports
Grips
Positions
Bends
Flows
Lifts
Endures

**PROCESS SKILLS**

*Paces*
Uses
Inquires
Sequences
Gathers
Navigates
Adjusts
Attends
Handles
Initiates
Terminates
Organizes
Notices/responds
Benefits
Chooses
Heeds
Continues
Searches/locates
Restores
Accommodates

From Fisher AG: *Assessment of motor and process skills*, vol 2: User manual (ed 5), Fort Collins, Colo, 2003, Three Star Press.

*Paces is considered a motor and a process skill.

on a few skill items. The AMPS does not have a ceiling for motor or process skill abilities. Thus the AMPS detects a change in ability even in persons with higher functional abilities who still experience some difficulty with ADL performance.[17]

Once the items are scored for each task, the results are entered in the AMPS computer scoring program.* The computer analysis of the motor and process skill scores results in ADL motor ability and ADL process ability measures. The ability measures represents the placement of the person on a continuum of motor or process ability. Persons with higher motor ability measures are more skilled in their ability to move themselves and objects during task performance, and persons with higher process ability measures are more skilled in their ability to organize and adapt the actions of task performance to achieve an effective outcome. Persons with less ADL motor or ADL process ability are placed lower along the continuum of ability. Because the AMPS is a sensitive measurement tool, any change in the ability of a person to perform ADL tasks results in a change in the person's process or motor ability measure, or both. Therefore the AMPS is suited ideally to evaluate a change in ADL performance resulting from occupational therapy intervention.[17]

The administration of the AMPS, however, does not conclude with the computer generation of the motor and process skill ability measures. The occupational therapist or occupational therapy assistant (in collaboration with an occupational therapist) must still interpret the results in light of other information the practitioner has gathered about the person to use the results of the AMPS to plan occupational therapy intervention.

---

*The AMPS computer scoring program is available only to occupational therapists who have completed the 5-day AMPS training course.

### Case Study 1: Part B

#### LIVING AT HOME: ADDRESSING PROBLEMS WITH IADL PERFORMANCE

At the conclusion of the COPM interview with Karen during her first outpatient appointment, her occupational therapist learned that the activities of primary concern to her were (1) changing the bed, (2) preparing meals, (3) setting and combing her hair, (4) assisting her younger children with their homework, (5) sewing, and (6) playing with her grandchildren. She learned that Karen was concerned with the recommendation that she not engage in complex household or community activities and with being supervised during the day. (Her sister-in-law was staying with Karen while Karen's husband worked.) The occupational therapist, however, needed more objective information to begin intervention planning. Rather than informally observe Karen using the stove in the occupational therapy clinic, her occupational therapist wanted to use the AMPS to evaluate Karen's ADL motor and ADL process ability and solicit objective evidence to determine whether Karen was indeed safe in staying home alone and engaging in more complex IADL tasks. She also wanted to determine how Karen's underlying impairments (partial paralysis of the left arm, mild left visual inattention, and mild short-term memory deficits) might be affecting Karen's performance of daily life activities. The occupational therapist asked Karen whether she would be willing to perform some ADL tasks during the second outpatient appointment so that she could observe Karen's performance, and Karen agreed.

To conclude Karen's first outpatient appointment, her occupational therapist conducted a 10-minute AMPS interview, per guidelines in the AMPS manual. At the conclusion of the interview, Karen chose two tasks to perform for the assessment: (1) changing standard sheets on a freestanding bed and (2) preparing scrambled eggs, toast, and a beverage. During the interview, the occupational therapist ensured that these tasks were familiar to Karen; that they would be of sufficient challenge to her, given the mild residual effects of her right-side CVA; and that they were appropriate for the occupational therapy clinic. The occupational therapist stressed that because this was a formal assessment, she and Karen needed to agree to specific criteria for each task. To prepare eggs, toast, and a beverage, Karen understood and agreed that she would use two eggs, adding some milk, salt, and pepper; two slices of whole wheat bread with margarine for the toast; and a glass of orange juice. She also understood that she was to serve the eggs, toast, and orange juice at the table and clean her work spaces but she did not have to wash dishes or utensils. For changing the sheets, Karen understood and agreed that she was to remove the blanket, bedspread, sheets, and pillowcases; replace the sheets and pillowcases with clean sheets from the closet; place the blanket and bedspread on the bed; and dispose of the soiled sheets and pillowcases in the laundry hamper. Although these were the agreed criteria, Karen's occupational therapist also

### LIVING AT HOME: ADDRESSING PROBLEMS WITH IADL PERFORMANCE—cont'd

stressed that Karen could perform the tasks in her usual manner, using the tools, materials, and methods she preferred. During the AMPS interview process, the occupational therapist also determined which tools and materials Karen would like to use during the assessment—particularly in preparing the eggs, toast, and beverage in the kitchen—to ensure that all needed tools and materials would be available during the second appointment when Karen would be performing both IADL tasks.

When Karen returned 2 days later for her second outpatient appointment, the occupational therapist explained the assessment procedures again and oriented Karen to the kitchen and bedroom. Although these tasks were familiar to Karen, she had not performed them in the outpatient clinic, and the occupational therapist wanted to ensure that Karen knew where all the needed tools and materials were in the kitchen and how the stove and toaster worked. She even asked Karen to place needed tools and materials in locations in the kitchen approximating their locations in Karen's home. To approximate Karen's home environment further, her occupational therapist ensured that extra tools and materials, such as various cookware items, dishes, utensils, and food items, were stocked in the kitchen. After ensuring that Karen was oriented fully to the kitchen, her occupational therapist began the assessment by stating, "For this assessment, you agreed to prepare scrambled eggs, using two eggs, milk, salt, and pepper; two pieces of toast, using whole wheat bread and margarine; and a glass of orange juice and to serve it at the counter. Please leave your work space as you found it; however, you do not need to wash the dishes. If you have any questions, please feel free to ask. When you are finished, just let me know."

Karen then proceeded to prepare the eggs, toast, and beverage while her occupational therapist observed her performance and took notes to refer to afterward when she would score Karen's performance (Figure 20-2). Karen finished the task in approximately 12 minutes, after which she took a 5-minute coffee break while her occupational therapist scored her task performance on the 16 motor and 20 process skill items. Then the occupational therapist gave her the instructions for the second task—changing the sheets—which Karen performed while her occupational therapist again observed her performance.

Karen took approximately 8 minutes to complete this task. Afterward, her occupational therapist scored Karen's second performance. After the completion of both tasks, Karen and her occupational therapist discussed Karen's perception of her performance, particularly with reference to awareness of safety issues. Karen reported that she felt she was safe in using the stove and that her performance was fairly good because the eggs and toast were edible. Karen did share her frustration at feeling slow and awkward while changing the sheets. The occupational therapist said she also believed Karen's use of the stove was safe but that she would have more information after the results of the AMPS were entered in the computer scoring program. She also promised Karen that she would share those results with her during the next appointment.

Because the occupational therapist did not have a formal assessment tool with which to observe the other activities of concern to Karen (sewing, setting and combing her hair, assisting with her children's homework, playing with her grandchildren), she asked Karen if she could observe her engaging in sewing and setting and combing her hair during the third appointment. Based on the information she gained by observing Karen perform the two AMPS tasks, however, the occupational therapist believed she had some good information regarding Karen's motor and process skill abilities and that she not only could conduct an informal evaluation of these activities but also begin intervention to address Karen's concerns.

Later that afternoon, the occupational therapist entered the scores from both task performances into the computer scoring program. The AMPS Graphic Report showed Karen's ADL motor ability measure was 0.9 and her ADL process ability measure was 1.2 (Figure 20-3). Karen's ADL motor ability measure reflected that she experienced some mild difficulty in (1) positioning her body appropriate to the task, (2) coordinating her arms to stabilize task objects, (3) manipulating and gripping task objects with her left hand, (4) executing smooth and fluid left arm and hand movements, (5) lifting heavy objects, and (6) calibrating the force and extent of her left arm movements. Karen's ADL motor ability score of 0.9 indicated she would need some physical assistance to live in the community; 83% of all persons with a motor ability measure of 2.0 or lower require some kind of assistance.[17] Despite Karen's diminished motor ability to move herself and objects, her actions did not place her at risk for injury or a fall, and she was successful in achieving the desired outcome—preparing a meal with the use of a stove and changing the sheets on a bed. The occupational therapist reasoned that given Karen's current motor abilities, Karen possessed the skills to engage in a variety of activities despite the effect of the CVA. In fact, the therapist reasoned that continual engagement in various activities throughout Karen's day would help improve her overall motor ability.

When the occupational therapist interpreted Karen's ADL process ability measure, she was encouraged by the results. This measure of 1.2 indicated that she possessed sufficient ability to manage most daily life tasks, for 93% of persons who require minimal to substantial assistance with managing daily life tasks score below 1.0.[17] During both AMPS tasks, Karen demonstrated good awareness about avoiding injury or damage, and her occupational therapist reasoned that given Karen's current ability to organize and adapt her actions over time, Karen would not be at great risk for an accident during household chores and meal preparation tasks. This did not mean Karen's task performance was flawless. She did experience some mild difficulty in (1) choosing the tools and materials needed for the tasks (e.g., she did not choose orange juice for eggs, toast, and beverage, and she chose extra pillows from the closet when changing the sheets) and (2) restoring tools and materials (e.g., the margarine was not returned to the refrigerator). These problems also suggested Karen was experiencing some mild difficulty accommodating her actions to overcome problems, although minor ones, as they arose while she engaged in ADL tasks. Her occupational therapist reasoned, however, that these issues were not so much related to an underlying impairment of Karen's judgment but more to her mild memory deficit. The occupational therapist also reasoned that although Karen had demonstrated mild left visual inattention during an examination performed by her neurologist, this residual impairment did not appear to affect her ADL task performance at this time.

Given the objective results of the AMPS and the information she gathered during the initial interview, from a review of Karen's medical chart, and from a discussion with Karen's physical therapist, the occupational therapist was confident that Karen could begin to initiate and independently perform some IADL tasks at home on a trial basis. The occupational therapist called Karen's neurologist, shared the results of her evaluation, and indicated that she would work with Karen and her husband to set up a trial program at home, gradually expanding Karen's repertoire of independent activities. When Karen returned for her third outpatient appointment, her occupational therapist shared the results of the AMPS and her professional opinion of Karen's ability to begin engaging independently in home and community activities. Although the issue of community activities remained to be explored, Karen and her occupational therapist developed a plan for reengagement in favorite home activities and set goals to mark Karen's progress toward a return to a safe, independent, and meaningful life in the community.

## GOAL SETTING FOR REHABILITATION INTERVENTION

Thorough, consistent, well-documented evaluation procedures at each stage of a patient's rehabilitation are critical in guiding a professional's reasoning to establish realistic rehabilitation goals, plan interventions, and monitor a patient's progress. After a rehabilitation professional has conducted a thorough evaluation that reflects the professional's area of expertise and focuses on the areas of concern to the patient and family, the patient, family, and rehabilitation team members should collaborate to establish goals for the current phase of the patient's rehabilitation. The goals should be agreed on by the patient, the family, and the rehabilitation professionals and should be understood clearly by the patient and family.[25] If a patient and family members do not understand the rehabilitation goal, the goal is probably not appropriate or should be defined in terms that the patient and family members understand and find meaningful.

One current concern in the rehabilitation setting is that professionals may not be considering the patient's personal goals when planning intervention.[37,41,52] Evidence suggests more effort could and should be made to promote more collaboration between patients and rehabilitation professionals in the development of goals. If rehabilitation professionals agree to realistic goals that are important and meaningful to the patient and they make a concerted effort to initiate intervention directly

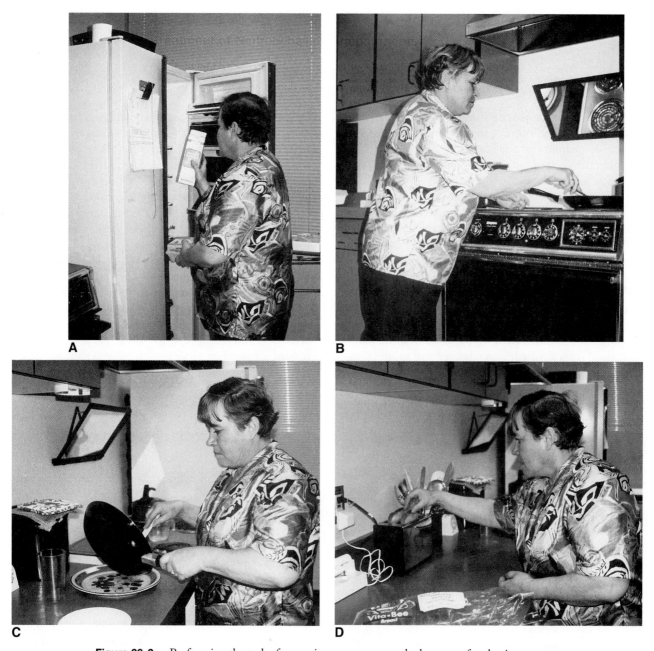

**Figure 20-2**    Performing the task of preparing eggs, toast, and a beverage for the Assessment of Motor and Process Skills. **A,** *Choosing* needed items for the task. **B,** Ineffective *positioning* of body; standing too far away to stir eggs. **C,** *Coordinating* two body parts toward the same action. **D,** *Initiating* a step of the task.

related to those goals, the professionals provide a purposeful experience that is immediately relevant to their patients' lives.[34] Rehabilitation goals should be realistic in terms of the patient's current level of ability (or disability) and potential for recovery from the CVA. Rehabilitation professionals should collaborate with the patient to develop goals for which the professionals can use their expertise to facilitate the accomplishment of those goals. Each rehabilitation professional possesses unique skills, and depending on the goals of the patient, a particular professional may be more suited to facilitate the accomplishment of a patient's goal. For example, if a patient with severe right leg hemiplegia decided the most important goal was to walk independently, a physical therapist would be the most qualified rehabilitation professional to collaborate with the patient and determine whether this goal was realistic. Finally, goals should be documented in explicit, measurable terms so that they serve as yardsticks by which to measure whether a patient is benefiting from rehabilitation services.[25]

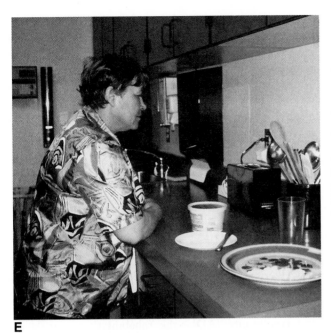

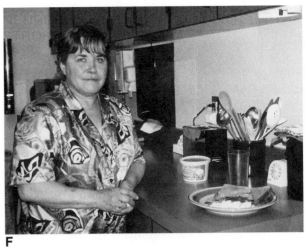

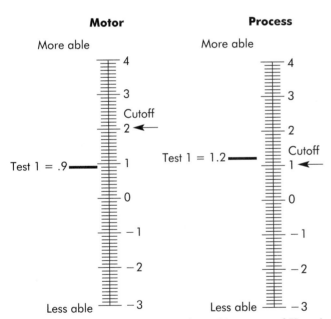

**Figure 20-2, cont'd**    **E,** Ineffective *sequencing* of steps for task results in a delay. **F,** Ineffective *heeding* of the task goal; no orange juice was served.

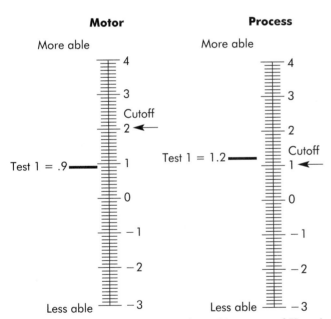

**Figure 20-3**    Computer-generated graphic report of Karen's Assessment of Motor and Process Skills results. AMPS ability measures indicate the degree of a person's motor and process skill ability to manage daily life tasks in the community.

## GOAL SETTING FOR OCCUPATIONAL THERAPY INTERVENTION

For occupational therapists, the process of establishing goals begins with the initial interview, which focuses on daily life activities of concern to the patient and family. No matter the stage of rehabilitation (inpatient, outpa-

tient, or home health), the initial interview always should address the daily life activities of concern to the patient, including IADL tasks when appropriate. The opportunity for any patient with a CVA to pursue desired engagement in IADL tasks always should be available.

To ensure that IADL goals are measurable and essential, occupational therapists should start with a clear description of a patient's initial status in relation to the potential goal. For example, a patient desires to prepare a simple lunch using the stove top. To monitor more effectively the patient's goal achievement, the occupational therapist first must identify and document where the patient started (that is, his or her initial status) in relation to the desired outcome. For example, an occupational therapist might document the following: "While preparing a simple lunch, patient is at risk for fall, requiring several cues to enhance her safety. She is at mild risk for injury when using a sharp knife as she frequently held the knife awkwardly and attempted to cut an apple without first stabilizing it on a cutting board." As this is where the patient starts, the occupational therapist then can write a goal for the patient to achieve. Thus a documented goal might be "During the preparation of simple lunches, patient will consistently perform in a safe manner that reduces her risk for injury." Following intervention, this goal then is compared with the patient's documented initial status to determine whether the patient is benefiting from rehabilitation intervention. For example, if the occupational therapist failed to document that the patient was initially at risk for a fall or an injury, no evidence would indicate that the patient needed to perform tasks in a safe manner to reduce the risk for injury. Even though the patient's risk for a fall or an injury might have been reduced substantially by discharge and the patient was now able to perform simple meal preparation tasks safely and without supervision, the patient's actual progress since admission could not be substantiated unless documentation was available to prove so (Table 20-2).

To establish that the goals are realistic, occupational therapists also should include information regarding a patient's current capacities and abilities. For example, to justify the goal "Patient will safely and independently prepare a simple lunch using the stove top," the occupational therapist should document that the patient demonstrates a capacity to learn new skills, is aware of his or her postural insecurity, and is cognitively capable of recognizing and responding to obvious safety hazards in the kitchen in his or her intact visual field. The inclusion of such information establishes that the patient is capable of benefiting from rehabilitation services and shows that goals are realistic and obtainable.

Goals specific to occupational therapy also should reflect the unique perspective of occupational therapy; that is, a patient's engagement in daily living activities. For example, a goal such as "Patient will achieve 120 degrees of shoulder flexion to place objects in upper kitchen cabinets" is not an appropriate occupational therapy goal. The statement "Patient will achieve 120 degrees of shoulder flexion" reflects a framework based on physical movement, not IADL performance. Goals also should not describe the type of intervention the occupational therapist intends to use to achieve the goal.[44] From the previous example, the statement "Patient will achieve 120 degrees of shoulder flexion to place objects on upper kitchen cabinets" reflects the occupational therapist's intervention strategy; that is, the plan to focus on improving the patient's underlying muscle strength to enhance the patient's active range of motion. If the goal is to place items on upper kitchen cabinets (a reflection of the patient's actual IADL performance), a variety of interventions are available with which to achieve this goal, not just to enhance the patient's active range of motion. An appropriate IADL goal in this example would be "Patient will place objects in upper kitchen cabinets safely and easily." Such goals reflect the daily life activities that patients need or want to perform, the expected outcome of occupational therapy intervention.

## REHABILITATION INTERVENTION

The patient and family members must be involved actively in all stages of recovery.[25] The intervention plan and goals should incorporate the role of the patient in the family. If a patient's prior responsibilities included home and community IADL, the rehabilitation team should encourage the family to involve the patient in the process of deciding to whom these responsibilities should be delegated. Many times a patient derives great satisfaction from engaging in an IADL with the assistance of family members or other individuals even though independent performance is not possible. For example, although a patient may not be able independently to prepare a batch of her grandson's favorite cookies because of an impairment in motor planning, she may be able to assist her son with parts of the task.

The rehabilitation team also should ensure that family members continue to maintain their roles in the family despite any new caregiving responsibilities that may be required. Assuming the role of a caregiver and taking over

**Table 20-2**

### Instrumental Activities of Daily Living Initial Status and Goals

| INITIAL STATUS | GOAL |
|---|---|
| Patient requires substantial physical assistance to retrieve and transport needed items within the kitchen. | Patient will prepare a light breakfast independently and safely. |
| Patient requires constant verbal cuing when setting the table. | Patient will set table correctly for dinner, requiring no verbal cuing. |
| Patient encounters great physical difficulty when attempting to vacuum and is unable to complete the task. | Patient will complete task of vacuuming a small room, experiencing an acceptable degree of difficulty. |
| Patient is unsafe when washing windows, requiring physical assistance to prevent a fall. | Patient will wash indoor windows safely and independently. |
| Patient displays very poor ability to use a computer keyboard and gives up in frustration. | Patient will be able to use a computer effectively to complete a one-page letter successfully. |
| Patient is unable to reach for and grasp light switches on the wall. | Patient will be able to operate light switches on the wall independently. |
| Patient requires many cues to ride the bus to the local shopping center. | Patient will ride the bus to the shopping center, requiring no verbal cues. |

household chores and responsibilities can be stressful, and the rehabilitation team should not assume that all family members are capable of performing the IADL tasks that the patient previously performed. Rehabilitation professionals must be aware of the shifting roles and responsibilities in the family and actively work with the family to manage their new roles and responsibilities (see Chapter 31).

## Occupational Therapy Approaches for Intervention

Intervention strategies occupational therapists use for patients with CVA tend to fall in two categories: (1) a remedial approach, in which a practitioner focuses intervention on the patient's underlying capacity (e.g., active range of motion, memory skills, motor planning, and visual attention) necessary to perform functional activities, and (2) an adaptive approach, in which a practitioner focuses intervention on the patient's ability to perform a specific activity.[38,39] The use of a remedial approach assumes that targeting a specific underlying impairment (e.g., visual inattention to the left environment) and focusing intervention on enhancing the patient's underlying capacity (e.g., attending and responding to visual stimuli in the left environment during visual training exercises) will be transferred to other activities in which the patient engages during the day and will result in overall improved performance of daily activities (see Chapter 19).

In contrast, the use of an adaptive approach assumes that patients have difficulty transferring learning across activities. For example, an adaptive approach for a patient with visual inattention of the left environment assumes that improving the patient's ability visually to locate a moving target on a computer screen will not transfer adequately and will not sufficiently improve the ability visually to locate a family member walking in a grocery store. Consequently, occupational therapists who follow an adaptive approach believe intervention should be focused on the skilled practice of the specific daily life activities of concern to the patient and that this promotes independent living.[38] Because the skills and knowledge being taught during rehabilitation should be meaningful to patients,[25] an adaptive approach directly relates the patients' goals to the intervention strategy and is particularly relevant as patients understand their disabilities in terms of the precipitating event and their ability to function.[39]

When implementing an adaptive approach, an occupational therapist may consider three aspects to promote a patient's IADL performance: (1) modifying the task, (2) modifying the method of accomplishing the task, and (3) modifying the environment (Table 20-3).[54] Modifying the task entails changing the performance requirements such that the overall objective of the task remains the same but the performance demands are better matched to the patient's abilities. For example, a home health patient with substantial right hemiparesis and low endurance wanted to shop for clothes but knew a trip to the local department store was not feasible. The occupational therapy assistant suggested that the patient consider sending away for some catalogs from which to shop. The occupational therapy assistant has modified the task of shopping such that the performance demands of shopping for clothes (in this case, by catalog rather than at the store) match the patient's current abilities. When modifying a task, an occupational therapist assists a patient in identifying those tasks that can be performed.

**Table 20-3**

### Adaptive Approaches to Intervention for Instrumental Activities of Daily Living Performance

| MODIFYING THE TASK | MODIFYING THE METHOD | MODIFYING THE ENVIRONMENT |
|---|---|---|
| **Problem: difficulty obtaining items in lower kitchen cabinets (because of diminished physical capacity)** | | |
| Ask for assistance when obtaining items or ask someone to obtain items before beginning the instrumental activities of daily living task. | Use a reacher to obtain needed items from lower shelves or sit on a footstool when reaching for items. | Install shelves that pull out on rollers or modify kitchen so that needed objects are on higher shelves. |
| **Problem: difficulty sequencing actions to prepare breakfast efficiently (because of diminished cognitive capacity)** | | |
| Prepare only simple breakfasts such as cold cereal or frozen breakfast entrees or ask that someone else prepare a portion of the meal. | Establish a routine to prepare breakfast, such as gathering needed items first and organizing on countertop before initiating food preparation. | Develop a manual that has written steps for each breakfast desired and keep on the countertop for reference. |

Adapted from Trombly CA: Retraining basic and instrumental activities of daily living. In Trombly C, editor: *Occupational therapy for physical dysfunction*, Baltimore, 1995, Williams & Wilkins.

In contrast, modifying the method of accomplishing the task requires that a patient learn new ways of performing the same task. In other words, the characteristics of the task remain the same, but the way the patient performs the task is adapted. For example, a 58-year-old patient receiving outpatient services was experiencing a memory impairment that affected his role as a father. He wanted to be able to call and talk with his three sons and two daughters, all of whom lived out of state, but he was embarrassed because he occasionally forgot to whom he was talking and often could not remember the significant events that he wanted to share with his children. The occupational therapist worked with him to develop a new routine in which he would write each of his children's names on a piece of paper and below each name those significant events he wanted to share. When he made a phone call, the name at the top of the page reminded him to whom he was talking and the notes below helped him remember what he wanted to say. In essence, the task of calling and carrying on a conversation remained the same, but the strategy required him to learn and implement a new method when making a telephone call. When considering modifying the method of the way a task is accomplished, an occupational therapist also considers a patient's capacity to learn and adapt actions to new performance demands.

Modifying the environment entails making some change in the physical or social environment to facilitate the patient's performance of the task. Suggesting modifications to the home for improved accessibility is an example of modifying the physical environment to enhance a patient's performance. The use of adaptive equipment, such as one-handed can openers and over-the-stove mirrors, is an aspect of modifying the environment; specifically, the tools and materials with which to perform the task. Modifying the social environment entails bringing another person into the environment whose presence can facilitate the person's performance. For example, a patient with moderate hemiparesis was receiving outpatient occupational therapy services in which she was focusing on preparing meals for her family. She reported to her occupational therapist that the one aspect of meal preparation she could not do at home was using the built-in microwave above the stove. The occupational therapist and patient discussed and tried various ideas, all of which were rejected by the patient as too costly (e.g., remodeling the kitchen) or too difficult (e.g., lifting the food items with a reacher adapted to hold microwave containers of food). In the end, the occupational therapist suggested that perhaps the patient needed to get assistance from one of her family members when she needed to use the microwave. Although the patient was initially reluctant, she also realized that of the suggestions, this was the most reasonable. Through further discussion with the occupational therapist, she recognized that she did not need to perform all tasks independently to retain her sense of competency and worth within the family.

Modifying the task, modifying the method of accomplishing the task, and modifying the environment are not mutually exclusive approaches. Using a long-handled duster (i.e., modifying the environment) when cleaning furniture also may entail a patient learning a new one-handed technique (i.e., modifying the method). Preparing cereal and juice for breakfast rather than eggs, toast, and coffee (i.e., modifying the task) also may require that needed items be placed on shelves within easy reach (i.e., modifying the environment). Taking a taxi rather than a bus to the local grocery store (i.e., modifying the task) also may entail a patient learning a new routine to pay the cabdriver, such as calling ahead, asking for the fare, and then placing the money in a shirt pocket for easy access (i.e., modifying the method). No matter which aspect of adaptation an occupational therapist considers, however, the capability of the patient is always the focus.

When suggesting adaptive approaches for IADL performance, occupational therapists should be aware that suggestions are made most effectively in a way that promotes discussion between the patient and the practitioner and that promotes the creation of a variety of options from which to choose. Of particular concern is the issue that learning new methods of performing tasks may compete with previous habits and preferences of performance.[60] For example, an occupational therapist working in home health suggested to a patient with significant right arm hemiparesis that she use a wheeled cart to transport dishes from the kitchen to the dining room table. This suggestion was met with considerable resistance by the patient because she insisted that the cart would be too complicated to use and that it would take up too much room in the kitchen. Considering the patient's preference for the way she believed the task should be performed, the patient and occupational therapist devised an alternative method whereby the patient was able to transport the dishes to the counter, then to a side table, and then to the dining room table.

Another issue to consider is that any new method of performing tasks must be reinforced in the patient's home environment, particularly if the tasks are learned in an inpatient rehabilitation setting. Without the assistance of family members to reinforce and assist with the new methods, the emotional and cognitive demands of changing performance, transferring new methods of performance from the clinic to the home, and developing new patterns of performance in the home may be more difficult. Finally, when occupational therapists make suggestions about adaptations to the home environment, these suggestions must incorporate not only the physical layout of the home but also the patient's current ability, personal feelings about the home adaptations, and the possible impact on family members of adapting the home.[60]

Occupational therapists should be cautious when extrapolating a patient's IADL performance in the rehabilitation setting to the home.[25] Intervention strategies that rely on adapted methods of performance only work if the patient also is taught the way to adapt performance in a variety of environments. If a patient is only taught the way to make meals using a microwave oven in the rehabilitation clinic and will be using a stove and oven at home to prepare meals, the patient may not be able to generalize the information unless the occupational therapist has focused on the patient's skill in adapting performance to different environments. Conversely, a patient may have difficulty mastering simple meal preparation in the outpatient occupational therapy clinic because of its unfamiliarity, but adaptive skills in performing the same meal preparation activities at home may be more apparent in the familiar environment.[61] Some objective evidence exists that older adults perform better at home regarding adaptive strategies when performing IADL tasks, although this has not been confirmed for persons with CVA.[45] The specific setting of the intervention also should be in as realistic a context as possible. For example, although practicing the component tasks of meal preparation such as cutting vegetables and opening cans of food is feasible in a dining room with just a table and the appropriate utensils, the same room would not be a realistic context in which to prepare a sandwich and a can of soup for lunch. Instrumental activities of daily living intervention, particularly when focusing on the patient's efficiency and safety during performance, should be conducted in as realistic a context as possible to recreate the rich complexity of options available when the patient is performing IADL tasks in a naturalistic environment.

A potential conflict may exist for occupational therapists who use an adaptive approach, particularly when providing services in inpatient settings for patients newly diagnosed with CVA. Some rehabilitation professionals recommend that adaptive devices be used only if other methods of performing the task are not available or cannot be learned.[25] They also assert that a patient mastering a method of performing the task without the use of adaptive devices will experience greater flexibility, satisfaction, and independence. From an occupational therapy perspective, the belief that adaptive devices should be a last resort is uncertain. Waiting to engage in certain activities until a patient's underlying impairments have improved or resolved can be discouraging for patients who want to begin engaging in specific activities. When adapting an activity to include the use of an adaptive device, an occupational therapist can facilitate a patient's ability to carry out an activity successfully, which may promote the patient's intrinsic recovery of underlying impairments.[14-16] For example, the use of a can opener designed for one-handed operation does not exclude the use of bilateral arm and hand movements. If movement is possible in the affected arm, a patient can and should use that movement when using the one-handed can opener. Thus the use of an adaptive device can help meet the goal of being able to open a can of food and promote a patient's intrinsic physical function at the same time. As such, occupational therapists should work closely with other rehabilitation professionals to explain their rationale for using an adaptive approach and should coordinate their intervention approach with other rehabilitation approaches.

Based on a review of rehabilitation outcome studies, evidence suggests that adaptive intervention approaches do improve a patient's performance of daily living tasks and level of independence and are more effective than remedial intervention approaches.[39] A U.S. survey of registered occupational therapists who worked primarily within home health care settings revealed that 84% reported being more concerned with using an adaptive approach rather than a remedial approach when working with patients who have had a stroke.[36] Furthermore, a recent synthesis of the best occupational therapy research evidence supports the provision of opportunities for patients to practice activities of their choosing within familiar contexts and training in the use of adaptations.[56]

Occupational therapists focus on purposeful activities that have value and meaning as their "modality" of intervention and actively seek the engagement of the patient rather than a passive response.[14-16] A patient's engagement in meaningful occupation requires more than just the ability to regain and control movement after a CVA; it also requires interest, motivation, cognitive and perceptual function, and support of the patient's family and community. The value of interventions for a patient's IADL performance that focus specifically on a patient's underlying motor impairments is questionable.[3] To limit the focus of intervention to a patient's motor performance limits the patient's chances of successfully engaging in desired IADL tasks on returning to the community. An adaptive approach that considers the sensorimotor, cognitive-perceptual, and psychosocial aspects of task performance and the physical and social environments in which the task performance occurs is more consistent with the philosophy of occupational therapy and more effective in assisting a patient in achieving desired goals in IADL performance.[39]

## Use of the Assessment of Motor and Process Skills to Guide Intervention

Assessment tools are valuable in assisting an occupational therapist in identifying the status of a patient's disability and can assist the practitioner in making decisions about intervention strategies. One distinct advantage of the

AMPS is the generation of an objective measure of a person's motor and process skill ability (see Figure 20-3). This information allows the occupational therapist to determine whether a person appears to be experiencing greater difficulty with motor or process skills and to plan intervention accordingly. For example, if a person has a low motor ability measure but a high process ability measure, an occupational therapist should consider whether the person could use these process skills to work around limitations of motor skills. Conversely, if a patient has a low process ability measure and the occupational therapist believes little improvement is possible with a patient's underlying impairments and the person's potential for learning new skills is limited, the practitioner can consider focusing intervention on training a person's family to assist with and support the patient's IADL performance.[44]

An assessment tool, however, should provide more information that just a number. According to Settle and Holm,[50] "To guide an intervention program, a tool should identify not only a patient's functional status, but also the specific factors that led to such a determination." The AMPS reflects this principle because it assists an occupational therapist in focusing on the specific actions of task performance (i.e., the specific motor or process skills) with which a person is experiencing difficulty and also the relative competencies a person possesses regarding performance.[44] To identify readily the motor and process skills that support or limit a person's IADL performance, the occupational therapist can examine the AMPS computer-generated report (Figure 20-4). Those motor or process skills that are effective for a person are identified as *adequate*, those skills that are ineffective are identified as *difficulty*, and those skills that are particularly problematic are identified as *markedly deficient*.

No "recipe" exists that an occupational therapist can follow to determine which intervention strategies will work best given the configuration of a person's motor and process skills. The occupational therapist's clinical reasoning guides the practitioner to decide which intervention strategies to use to assist a patient in achieving the stated IADL goals. The use of an adaptive approach, however, is highly recommended for use with the AMPS because the AMPS readily identifies those motor and process abilities that are intact and applicable to daily life tasks.[44] For example, from a computer-generated report, an occupational therapy assistant learns that a person is relatively able to initiate the steps of a task without hesitation (the process skill termed *initiates*). Using the AMPS as a framework by which to guide intervention, the occupational therapy assistant can develop intervention strategies that present a comfortable challenge to the person and that require competency in initiating the steps of a particular task. The recommendation is that the tasks to be mastered by the persons are tailored to their abilities to avoid stress.[25] The use of the AMPS supports this principle because it helps the occupational therapist identify performance skills that a person possesses and skills that are more problematic.

Because the AMPS readily identifies the motor and process abilities that are difficult or markedly deficient for the person, the occupational therapist can develop intervention strategies to assist the person in (1) enhancing ability with a specific motor or process skill and (2) adapting to the diminished skill ability by using other motor or process skills.[44] For example, a person with poor postural control has difficulty stabilizing her body while sitting in a wheelchair during IADL task performance (the skill item termed *stabilizes*). The occupational therapist may consider intervention strategies that enhance the person's ability to stabilize her body or adapt to the loss of stability by using other motor or process skills. To enhance the person's ability to stabilize her body while seated in the wheelchair, an occupational therapist may consider adapting the wheelchair (i.e., modifying the environment) with a seating system that promotes greater stability (see Chapter 24). To use the person's process skills to adapt to her diminished ability to stabilize her body, an occupational therapist might consider the implementation of a new strategy for the person to overcome her problem with instability (i.e., modifying the method of performance); that is, she may need to learn to place the affected arm on the wheelchair armrest to stabilize the trunk adequately when reaching for objects with the unaffected arm. In either scenario, the occupational therapist is using an adaptive approach for intervention.

The use of the AMPS during intervention also can assist an occupational therapist in modifying a task, particularly when examining the relative demand of IADL tasks and attempting to find tasks suited to the person's current abilities. The 56 IADL tasks included to date in the AMPS manual have been analyzed and placed on a hierarchical scale from easier to harder for motor and process abilities. An AMPS-trained occupational therapist can identify readily which IADL tasks are easier (or harder) with respect to motor or process skills and begin IADL intervention with the tasks that present an appropriate challenge to the person's motor or process skill ability. For example, folding a basket of laundry is an easier than average task with respect to process skill ability than the task of preparing a fruit salad, which is a harder than average task.[17] For a person with diminished process skills, a more appropriate challenge is to begin IADL intervention with easier than average tasks, such as folding laundry, and the other IADL tasks that are found at this end of the AMPS task hierarchy. As a person improves IADL task performance, more challenging tasks may be identified from the AMPS task hierarchy. Because rehabilitation intervention may be guided by the level of task difficulty with less complex or demanding tasks addressed first so that a patient experiences success,[25] the AMPS is suited ideally for use during rehabilitation intervention. This assumes, of course, that a patient is interested in pursuing a variety of IADL tasks for intervention and sees the relevancy of the intervention tasks to stated goals.

Repetition and practice between training sessions when the patient is on the unit or at home is also recommended for patients with CVA.[25] Because the AMPS motor and process skills are universal skills that are used in all IADL task performances,[17] the skill items may be emphasized in a variety of tasks and contexts. For example, the motor skill termed *positions* is the action of positioning

| **Client:** | Stuart | **Therapist:** | Steve Park |
|---|---|---|---|
| **ID:** | 3597-34 | **Gender:** | Male |
| **Age:** | 80 | **Evaluation Date:** | 05/23/03 |

The Assessment of Motor and Process Skills (AMPS) was used to determine how MR. STUART'S MOTOR and ORGANIZATIONAL/ ADAPTIVE (process) capabilities affect MR. STUART'S ability to perform fuctional DAILY LIVING TASKS necessary for COMMUNITY LIVING. The tasks were chosen from a list of standard functional activities rated according to their level of complexity. MR. STUART chose to perform the following tasks that MR. STUART considered to be meaningful and necessary for functional independence in the community:

Task 1: F-2 Luncheon meat or cheese sandwich
Task 2: L-1 Folding a basket of laundry

The level of complexity of the tasks chosen was easier than average or average. Overall performance in each skill area is summarized below using the following scale: ADEQUATE SKILL: no apparent disruption was observed, DIFFICULTY: ineffective skill was observed, MARKEDLY DEFICIENT SKILL: observed problems were severe enough to be unsafe or require therapist intervention.

The following strengths and problems were observed during the administration of the AMPS:

Adequate= A        Difficulty = D        Markedly Deficient = MD

## MOTOR SKILLS:

### Skills needed to move self and objects

| | A | D | MD |
|---|---|---|---|
| **Posture:** | | | |
| STABILIZING the body for balance | | X | |
| ALIGNING the body in a vertical position | X | | |
| POSITIONING the body or arms appropriate to the task | | X | |
| **Mobility:** | | | |
| WALKING around the task environment (level surface) | | X | |
| REACHING for task objects | | X | |
| BENDING or rotating the body appropriate to the task | | X | |
| **Coordination:** | | | |
| COORDINATING two body parts to securely stabilize task objects | | | X |
| MANIPULATING task objects | | X | |
| FLOWING by executing smooth and fluid arm and hand movements | | X | |
| **Strength and Effort:** | | | |
| MOVING by pushing and pulling task objects on level surfaces or opening and closing doors or drawers | X | | |
| TRANSPORTING task objects from one place to another | | | |
| LIFTING objects used during the task | | X | |
| CALIBRATING by regulating the force and extent of movements | | X | |
| GRIPPING by maintaining a secure grasp on task objects | | X | |
| | | X | |
| **Energy:** | | | |
| ENDURING for the duration of the task performance | | X | |
| Maintaining an even and appropriate PACE during task performance | | X | |

**Figure 20-4**    Computer-generated Assessment of Motor and Process Skills report.

*Continued*

**PROCESS SKILLS:**

**Skills needed to organize and adapt actions to complete a task**

| | A | D | MD |
|---|---|---|---|
| **Energy:** | | | |
| Maintaining an even and appropriate PACE during task performance | | X | |
| Maintaining focused ATTENTION throughout the task performance | X | | |
| **Using Knowledge:** | | | |
| CHOOSING appropriate tools and materials needed for task performance | | X | |
| USING task objects according to their intended purposes | X | | |
| Knowing when and how to stabilize and support or HANDLE task objects | | X | |
| HEEDING the goal of the specified task | | X | |
| INQUIRES: asking for needed information | X | | |
| **Temporal Organization:** | | | |
| INITIATING actions or steps of task without hesitation | | X | |
| CONTINUING actions through to completion | | X | |
| Logically SEQUENCING the steps of the task | X | | |
| TERMINATING actions or steps at the appropriate time | | X | |
| **Space and Objects:** | | | |
| SEARCHING for and LOCATING tools and materials | | X | |
| GATHERING tools and materials into the task workspace | | X | |
| ORGANIZING tools and materials in an orderly, logical, and spatially appropriate fashion | | | X |
| RESTORES: putting away tools and materials or straightening the workspace | | | X |
| NAVIGATES: maneuvering the hand and body around obstacles | X | | |
| **Adaptation:** | | | |
| NOTICING and RESPONDING appropriately to nonverbal, task-related environmental cues | | | X |
| ACCOMMODATES: modifying actions to overcome problems | | | X |
| ADJUSTS: changing the workspace to overcome problems | | X | |
| BENEFITS: preventing problems from reoccuring or persisting | | | X |

**Figure 20-4, cont'd**

the body or arms appropriately for the task, including the wheelchair relative to the task demands. The occupational therapist and other rehabilitation team members or family members may focus on this skill during a variety of tasks, facilitating a patient's ability to position the wheelchair while retrieving a carton of milk from the refrigerator, wiping the dinner table, or making the bed. The motor skill *positions* also is used during the performance of self-care tasks, and the occupational therapist may emphasize the repetition and practice of this skill during the morning self-care routine.

Finally, the AMPS may be given at any time during rehabilitation intervention and as often as warranted to determine whether a patient is making progress in IADL task performance. If a positive change occurs in a patient's motor or process ability measure, objective evidence is obtained that the patient is improving. The determination of a patient's progress, however, should not be based solely on the improvement in a patient's specific ability measure. The true benchmark by which progress should be judged is whether a patient is achieving the desired goals regarding daily life tasks.[44]

---

**Case Study 2**

**RETURNING HOME: IADL INTERVENTION DURING REHABILITATION**

One morning, Stuart, an 80-year-old retired railroad mechanic and watch repairman, awoke to discover that he could not move his left arm and leg to get out of bed. His wife called for an ambulance, and on his arrival at the local hospital, Stuart was found to have sustained a right CVA resulting in left hemiplegia. Initially, the impact of the right CVA was severe; Stuart experienced extensive left hemiplegia, including facial paralysis, visual inattention to the left environment, and tactile inattention to the left side of his body. Over the next 5 days, Stuart's condition improved somewhat. He started to regain some movement in his left hip and knee, and his attention to the left side of his body improved, although his left arm remained flaccid. Stuart's medical team believed a course of rehabilitation would be beneficial; however, given their knowledge of Stuart's health before the CVA (diabetes mellitus, hypertension, mild chronic obstructive pulmonary disease, and glaucoma) and his premorbid activity level (fairly sedentary), they decided a course of rehabilitation at a local skilled nursing facility (SNF) was the best option. Although Stuart expressed a strong desire to return home to live with his wife, the medical team was concerned that the couple had a limited community support system: a close friend who lived six blocks away and the manager of the assisted living complex where they lived. (Stuart and his wife had no children.) Although their friend and the manager volunteered to help out when Stuart returned home, the medical team was apprehensive about the success of this plan. They believed, however, that Stuart should be given the opportunity to return home and plans were made for admission to the skilled rehabilitation unit of a local nursing facility.

On Stuart's admission, the occupational therapist and occupational therapy assistant received a referral accompanied by Stuart's medical history. After deciding to initiate the evaluation process with an interview, they scheduled a half hour that afternoon for the occupational therapy assistant to interview Stuart. She planned to focus on Stuart's roles, routines, values, and interests regarding his daily occupation, the environments in which he typically occupied his time, and his concerns regarding the effect of the CVA on his daily life activities.

During the interview, the occupational therapy assistant discovered that Stuart lived in a small, rural town with his wife of 56 years. After his retirement from the railroad company in 1975, Stuart began a second career as a watch repairman. He and his wife managed a small repair shop for many years in the downtown shopping area of the town where they lived until his wife, because of frail health, could no longer assist with the business. Stuart reported that because his own health had been declining, they subsequently sold the business and moved to an assisted-living complex where they would no longer be responsible for the upkeep of a home. Their mornings consisted of rising around 7 AM, dressing, eating a breakfast that Stuart generally prepared, and watching a favorite television program at 10 AM. Two or three times a week, Stuart also took a shower in the morning. After their favorite program, Stuart and his wife enjoyed playing cards or taking short walks on the grounds of the complex. Together, Stuart and his wife prepared a light

lunch, generally followed by a short rest. During the afternoon, Stuart and his wife completed light household chores such as general cleaning and laundry or pursued more sedentary leisure activities such as listening to the radio or reading large-print books from the local library. For the more demanding household chores, such as cleaning the bathroom and vacuuming, they used the services of a cleaning agency. Because dinner was provided in the dining room of the complex, the evening was available for relaxation. Stuart and his wife often played cards again or watched television before retiring around 9 PM. Once a week, in the afternoon, the couple took a taxi to the local grocery store, although Stuart reported that this was becoming more difficult because his wife relied increasingly on the use of a wheelchair for community excursions. Finally, Stuart revealed that it was important for he and his wife to be together; although a neighbor and their close friend were looking in on his wife, Stuart believed her health would decline further if he was not at home with her.

The morning after the initial interview the occupational therapist continued the evaluation process with an informal observation of Stuart's self-care skills. She discovered Stuart required maximal assistance in donning his underwear, pants, shoes, and socks. With his T-shirt and button-down shirt, however, Stuart only required moderate assistance. When dressed and seated in a wheelchair, Stuart required minimal assistance with his grooming in front of a wheelchair-accessible sink, in addition to a few verbal cues to shave the left side of his face thoroughly and to comb the hair on the left side of his head. After Stuart's morning routine, his occupational therapist accompanied him to the dining hall, where she provided some physical assistance with Stuart's food preparation and a few verbal cues to draw Stuart's attention to food items located on the left side of his placemat.

Throughout the evaluation of Stuart's self-care skills, the occupational therapist noted that Stuart was able to sit independently in the wheelchair, although he had a tendency to lose his balance when reaching for items. He required moderate assistance to stand, but he was capable of following her instructions to enhance his stability. She noted that Stuart displayed no movement in his left arm, although she did not observe any gross neglect of his arm or other parts of his body that might result in an injury. Throughout his morning routine, she observed that Stuart initiated many of the required steps, indicating that he knew what needed to occur next, although he required some verbal cues to improve the quality of his performance because his techniques to perform tasks with one hand were awkward. He also needed occasional assistance to locate needed objects more quickly in his left visual field.

When the occupational therapist and occupational therapy assistant shared information from their sessions during their scheduled consultation time, they discovered that Stuart had voiced several concerns about going home. He believed it was important that he be able to help out around the house and not just sit all day long. Although he knew he and his wife would need assistance when he was discharged, he did not want to move from his current apartment to have someone live with them. Therefore Stuart and his wife needed to be able to manage on their own at night and at least during part of the day. (The social worker already had discussed with Stuart the possibility of someone assisting with Stuart's morning self-care routine if necessary and to perform other necessary tasks.) Both practitioners realized that Stuart was frustrated with his dependence on others and his lack of engagement in activities with his wife. Stuart obviously missed spending time with his wife, particularly because his wife was not able to make daily trips to the SNF because of her poor health. Stuart also had mentioned to the occupational therapy assistant that he was frustrated in not being able to call his wife on his own. When questioned further, Stuart said he often could not reach the telephone in his room, particularly from his bed, and he kept getting a wrong number or was disconnected.

After their discussion, the occupational therapist met briefly with Stuart in the afternoon to discuss potential goals. Stuart expressed an interest in being able to get ready in the morning with less assistance, to telephone his wife daily, to eat without anyone watching over him, and to play cards with his wife when she was able to make a trip to the SNF. To pursue additional information, the occupational therapist asked Stuart whether she could observe him while he telephoned his wife in his room. Stuart agreed, and he proceeded to dial his home telephone number. The occupational therapist realized that Stuart was unable to locate and press the correct buttons. She wondered whether this was due to a problem with Stuart's vision or visual attention and made a mental note to seek

more information from his medical chart. She also observed Stuart did not have much difficulty using only his right arm and hand, although she did note the placement of the telephone in the room was not accessible when Stuart was in bed. When someone answered the telephone and Stuart realized it was not his wife, he abruptly hung up the phone. Before additional frustration set in, Stuart's occupational therapist dialed the number for him and left the room for a few minutes to allow Stuart to talk privately with his wife.

After Stuart finished his telephone call, his occupational therapist returned and asked Stuart to play cards. She explained that she was curious as to whether Stuart was experiencing difficulty with his vision and the best way for her to explore this further was to again observe Stuart while he engaged in an activity. She further explained that she had an adapted card holder that would allow Stuart to hold his cards without the use of his hands. Because Stuart's favorite game was double solitaire, he said a card holder would not be necessary, although he said he might be interested in the device for other games. During the 5-minute game of solitaire, the occupational therapist observed that Stuart did not readily notice cards to be played on the left as frequently as he noticed cards on the right. She made a mental note to seek a referral to an optometrist to obtain more information.

With the information from Stuart's medical chart, the initial interview and observations of Stuart's morning self-care routine, use of the telephone, and playing of a card game, both occupational therapists had gathered enough information with which to complete the initial occupational therapy evaluation. From that evaluation, the following goals were set for the next week: (1) patient will readily locate food items when eating a meal without verbal cueing, (2) patient will don underwear and pants with moderate assistance, (3) patient will don shirt with minimal assistance, and (4) patient will independently, successfully, and to his satisfaction use the telephone in his room to call his wife daily. Both occupational therapists discussed the intervention plan for Stuart for the next week, which focused on the daily practice of the tasks Stuart valued, including a daily morning routine of dressing, grooming, and eating and practicing using the telephone in his room. They worked with Stuart twice a day and, as the week progressed, noted improvement with Stuart's self-care ability and his ability to use the telephone. This was due in part to the modifications made to

Stuart's physical environment; they obtained a telephone with enlarged buttons and rearranged the placement of the telephone in his room for easier access. Stuart was becoming more competent in using the phone, and by the end of the week he was pleased with successfully calling his wife with no assistance.

After 10 days his occupational therapy practitioners began to address the other concerns Stuart had expressed; namely, his desire to perform some IADL tasks so that he would not just sit around when he returned home. Stuart's physical capacity was improving; he now required only moderate to minimal assistance for dressing, and his visual attention to the left environment was improving. They decided that the occupational therapy assistant would administer the AMPS not only to gain some objective information regarding Stuart's ability to live independently in the community but also to clarify further Stuart's competencies and limitations regarding the performance of personal and instrumental ADL tasks.

After Stuart had spent 12 days in the SNF, his occupational therapy assistant conducted an AMPS interview in the morning. The AMPS interview focused on the IADL tasks that Stuart had performed before his CVA and that currently were of concern to him regarding living at home. Based on the types of IADL tasks that Stuart had performed in the past, was willing to perform for the assessment, and which would offer sufficient challenge, she offered five task choices to Stuart: (1) folding a basket of laundry, (2) getting a drink from the refrigerator, (3) preparing a meat sandwich, (4) polishing shoes, and (5) watering a plant. Because Stuart was concerned about meals at home, he chose to prepare a meat sandwich; because his wife hated to fold the laundry and "someone had to do it," folding a basket of laundry was his second choice.

That afternoon, Stuart's occupational therapy assistant initiated the first AMPS observation. The SNF did not have a laundry room similar to the one in Stuart's complex, but Stuart said he and his wife occasionally folded the laundry at the dining room table in their apartment when the laundry room was crowded. The occupational therapy assistant determined that the best place for the assessment was in a dining hall free from distractions. Before having Stuart start the task, she again explained the task criteria and observed Stuart as he folded approximately 20 items of laundry. Stuart took almost 20 minutes to fold the basket of laundry and was visibly fatigued on completing the

task. The occupational therapy assistant decided it would be better if Stuart waited until the next day to perform the second AMPS task. After Stuart returned to his room, she scored his performance.

The administration of the AMPS continued the next morning in a small kitchen on the rehabilitation unit, where Stuart prepared a bologna sandwich with mayonnaise and white bread. Before beginning the task, Stuart said he would use his wheelchair lap tray. Although the occupational therapy assistant was skeptical that Stuart would be able to maneuver his wheelchair and reach for objects in the kitchen, she allowed him to decide the way he would perform the task. She again observed Stuart; he took 17 minutes to prepare the sandwich. Although at times she was concerned about the risk for injury (e.g., Stuart used a paring knife to spread the mayonnaise), she did not intervene because she saw no obvious signs of imminent risk for injury and she wanted to evaluate Stuart's abilities regarding the way he would perform the task, not how she believed it should be performed. Again, Stuart was fatigued at the end of the task and returned to his room for a rest. She scored his performance and entered his scores from both tasks into the AMPS computer scoring program.[17]

The results of the computer analysis were not surprising to Stuart's occupational therapy assistant. Stuart's motor ability measure of −1.0 was substantially below 2.0; 84% of all individuals scoring 2.0 or below require some kind of assistance to manage daily life tasks in the community. Stuart's limited physical capacity as a result of the CVA was reflected in his low motor ability measure. Stuart's process ability measure of −0.4 was also below 1.0; 93% of individuals scoring 1.0 or below require some level of assistance to live in the community.[17] Stuart's underlying cognitive and perceptual capacity had been affected by the CVA but not to the same degree as his physical capacity. Although Stuart scored low on the process ability scale (relative to a process ability measure of 1.0 that reflected a greater ability to manage ADL tasks in the community), his occupational therapy assistant believed Stuart's significant motor skill difficulties also were affecting his ability to organize and adapt his actions effectively when engaging in personal and instrumental ADL tasks. She also believed Stuart demonstrated potential to learn new ways to adapt to his current motor skill difficulties.

### RETURNING HOME: IADL INTERVENTION DURING REHABILITATION—cont'd

Later that afternoon, before putting the computer-generated AMPS report in the medical chart (Figure 20-4), the occupational therapy assistant shared the results with the occupational therapist, and they spent a few minutes discussing the implications for Stuart's intervention plan. Based on their discussion, the occupational therapy assistant modified the intervention plan to include the practice of IADL tasks during her afternoon session with Stuart. They also included the following goals, in addition to Stuart's ongoing self-care goals, in the weekly progress note: (1) patient will transport needed items safely and effectively when setting a table, and (2) patient will organize his work space efficiently when folding laundry. Both goals were chosen because Stuart had indicated that he wanted to perform some household chores and meal preparation tasks when he returned home. Both goals reflected the performance of IADL tasks that were easier than average with respect to motor skills and within Stuart's current physical capacity, although both tasks still would present a challenge. Based on her observations of his performance, the occupational therapy assistant noted that Stuart's difficulty with transporting items appeared to limit his options as to where and how a task was performed and that his organizational skills as to where objects were placed in the work space made tasks more difficult. In the weekly note accompanying the goals, the occupational therapy assistant included this information and her evaluation that Stuart was demonstrating poor efficiency with both skills as a result of his limited physical capacity and his lack of experience performing tasks with one hand and from a wheelchair.

In modifying the intervention plan to include a focus on IADL performance, both practitioners realized Stuart would not make great gains with his motor skills or become independent with the performance of all IADL tasks. Yet they reasoned that if Stuart could perform some IADL tasks at home, he would rely less on outside services. Stuart would be pleased to remain at home, assisting with household chores and meal preparation tasks as much as he was able. (Stuart particularly enjoyed activities involving food.) Because the therapists were able to examine the AMPS hierarchy to determine which tasks were easier, they also could use an adaptive approach of modifying the tasks to present a comfortable challenge to Stuart in learning new skills. Finally, the motor and process skills that would be emphasized in the context of practicing IADL tasks also could be emphasized during Stuart's self-care activities.

To begin IADL intervention with Stuart, the occupational therapy assistant thoroughly examined the AMPS report. She began with Stuart's motor skills because these presented the greatest challenge to Stuart. She knew, however, that for Stuart to enhance his motor skills, he would have to rely on his process skills to change the way he performed IADL tasks.

Of the first three motor skills, *positions* presented the most difficulty for Stuart. To enhance Stuart's ability to position himself more effectively and reduce the need to stabilize his trunk while bending and reaching for objects, his occupational therapy assistant engaged Stuart in a variety of IADL tasks during their afternoon session and practiced positioning his wheelchair and his body relative to the demands of the task. In some cases a head-on approach with his wheelchair worked best; in others, a 45-degree angle was better. She provided feedback to Stuart regarding his performance and frequently solicited Stuart's opinion as to how he felt about the practice. She also asked Stuart to practice this skill when he attended his favorite weekly activities such as the gourmet tasting and popcorn party offered by the SNF activity program.

Although Stuart experienced some difficulty stabilizing his body—the motor skill termed *stabilizes*—the occupational therapist knew Stuart's physical therapy practitioners were focusing on Stuart's postural control, and she reported to them the difficulties Stuart was experiencing during the performance of IADL tasks. They also discussed some modifications to the seating of the wheelchair to help promote better stabilization of his trunk. His occupational therapy assistant also reasoned that if Stuart learned to position himself better relative to the demands of the task, the need for trunk stability would be less. Finally, because Stuart's ability to maintain an upright posture in the wheelchair—the motor skill termed *aligns*—was adequate, she did not need to address this area.

When looking at the next three motor skills—*walks, reaches,* and *bends* (Figure 20-5)—Stuart's occupational therapy assistant reasoned that these skills, although difficult for Stuart, were not of great hindrance to his performance. Stuart had received a score of 2 on *walks* for both tasks because he required a wheelchair for mobility, per the scoring criteria outlined in the AMPS manual.[17] His occupational therapy assistant reasoned that minor modifications could be made to Stuart's home environment, such as rearranging the kitchen cupboards and hall closets to reduce the demand for reaching and bending. She discussed these modifications with Stuart, and they made plans to meet with the manager of the complex because she had agreed to help out when Stuart returned home. Finally, regarding Stuart's ability to reach and bend, his physical therapy practitioners were focusing on enhancing his underlying physical capacity, which would help support his ability to reach and bend, although Stuart most likely would not regain full physical function during his 5-week rehabilitation stay.

Of all the motor skills, *coordinates* was the only one identified as markedly deficient on the report. This reflected the lack of functional use of the left arm, which made holding and stabilizing objects that typically required the use of two hands difficult. With this in mind, the occupational therapy assistant considered two adaptive approaches. First, she focused on modifying the method by which Stuart attempted to hold and stabilize objects. This entailed focusing on the use, whenever possible, of Stuart's left arm to serve as a "weight" or "block" to secure objects. During both IADL tasks for the assessment, Stuart made no attempt to use his left arm. This was due in part to Stuart's perception that his left arm was of no use. He had not yet learned that in some cases, his arm could be used as a weight to hold objects on his lap or a flat surface and as a block against which an object could be wedged. Because Stuart's left arm showed no signs of spasticity, this new method was feasible for him.

The second adaptive approach for the motor skill *coordinates* involved modifying the environment with the use of adaptive devices. Particularly for meal preparation tasks, Stuart and his occupational therapy assistant explored options for adaptive devices that would allow him to perform certain components of an IADL without struggling to stabilize objects during task performance. They explored the use of a modified cutting board and devices to stabilize dishes on the counter and pans on the stove, and those of interest to Stuart were used when he practiced preparing simple snacks and light meals during the afternoon. The occupational therapy assistant again recognized that the use of adaptive devices also entailed Stuart learning how to use them, reflecting a need to modify the method by which he accomplished a task. This relied on his process skill abilities to adapt and organize his actions despite the fact that the focus was on a motor skill.

Regarding the motor skill *manipulates* (Figure 20-6), Stuart's occupational therapy assistant chose an adaptive approach that again focused on modifying the environment. For example, Stuart had some difficulty manipulating objects with his right hand, such as when he was putting the fastener back on the bag of bread. This task typically requires the use of two hands, and Stuart's score of 2 reflected his difficulty in performing such a task with only one hand. For IADL tasks that relied more on his fine-motor capacity, Stuart and his occupational therapy assistant explored adaptive devices within his abilities, such as a clothespin to seal the bag of bread rather than the tiny fastener or twist

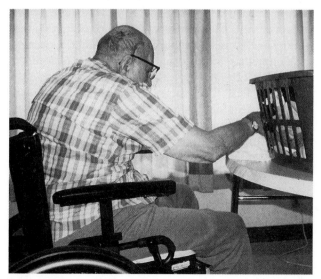

**Figure 20-5** Difficulty *bending* the body and *reaching* for task objects.

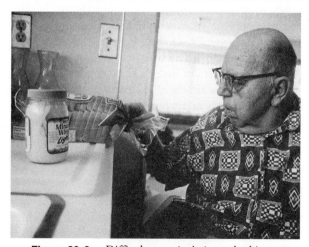

**Figure 20-6** Difficulty *manipulating* task objects.

### RETURNING HOME: IADL INTERVENTION DURING REHABILITATION—cont'd

tie that typically comes with a bag of bread. The motor skill *flows*, the ability to execute smooth and fluid arm movements, also presented some difficulty for Stuart. Because his CVA was fairly recent, more spontaneous recovery was likely, and this motor skill was not interfering greatly with Stuart's performance, it was decided not to emphasize this motor skill during intervention.

Of the next five motor skills—*moves*, *transports*, *lifts*, *calibrates*, and *grips*—only *transports* was chosen for particular emphasis during intervention. This reflected the occupational therapists' assumptions that Stuart's low scores on these motor skills reflected his underlying capacity (i.e., his diminished muscle strength) and that in the short time remaining for his inpatient rehabilitation, Stuart's overall strength probably would not increase significantly. Stuart's physical therapy practitioners developed an exercise program for Stuart, and he was engaging actively in many other activities at the SNF. These other opportunities to develop underlying physical capacity would support Stuart's ability to move, lift, and grip objects.

One significant issue, however, was Stuart's ability to transport objects from one place to another while moving his wheelchair. Although his wheelchair lap tray presented a stable platform on which to secure an object when moving it from one area of a room to another, it also presented some obstacles. Stuart's occupational therapy assistant recommended that he not use the lap tray while performing IADL tasks. Instead, she explored with Stuart different styles of wheelchair bags to hold the objects he needed to transport. Stuart also learned some new methods by which to transport objects, including sliding heavier objects along the countertop rather than transporting them in his wheelchair. The biggest issue, however, arose when Stuart attempted to transport food items after retrieving them from the refrigerator. Again, Stuart relied on practice to learn to retrieve food items, place them in a wheelchair bag or secure them in his lap, and safely transport them to a counter or table.

With the last of the motor skill items, *endures* and *paces*, Stuart's occupational therapy assistant recognized this would be an ongoing issue for Stuart. He became fatigued easily after 10 minutes of performing easier-than-average ADL tasks. Again, she reasoned that his underlying capacity (i.e., his cardiopulmonary endurance) was fairly compromised, particularly because of his history of mild chronic obstructive pulmonary disease, and that Stuart would need to adapt his daily routine to his limited capacity. Therefore she and Stuart explored the need to pace his activities throughout the day and not attempt to do too much at one time. This limitation presented a challenge to Stuart because he preferred to try as hard as he could during his therapy to get better faster and get home sooner. His occupational therapy assistant explained the need to temper his activity level so that he would not run out of energy by the end of the day, when his wife would need his assistance the most. Stuart reluctantly agreed, but from the occupational therapy assistant's perspective, he continued to push himself too hard while at the SNF.

The occupational therapy assistant next turned to the scores on Stuart's process skills and examined them regarding potential intervention strategies. One reason she surmised Stuart would be able to benefit from therapy was his ability to maintain focused attention throughout the task, the process skill *attends*. Although persons with right CVA have a greater tendency to distractibility, this was not the case with Stuart. In fact, during her discussion with the occupational therapist, Stuart's occupational therapy assistant learned that Stuart's tendency to delay his response to what was occurring in his left visual field (e.g., playing cards within his left visual field when playing solitaire) was probably reflective not of his ability to maintain his focused attention but his ability to notice and respond appropriately to nonverbal, environmental cues in his environment, the process skill *notices/responds*. As the optometrist had confirmed, his visual capacity also was diminished, which complicated his ability to notice environmental information to which he needed to respond.

Of the next five process skills, *chooses*, *heeds*, and *handles* presented some difficulty for Stuart. His occupational therapy assistant, however, was not concerned with the process skills *chooses* and *heeds* relative to the demands of the types of IADL tasks Stuart would engage in at home. On the AMPS report, *chooses* and *heeds* were identified as difficult (equivalent to a score of 2 [ineffective performance]) because he chose wheat bread to make the sandwich instead of white bread and did not sort the socks into pairs while folding the laundry, as specified in the task criteria to which he agreed before beginning each task. Yet these actions were not of major concern to the occupational therapy assistant because the consequences of his actions were minor. If Stuart ended up making a sandwich at home with mustard rather than the mayonnaise he originally considered, the consequences would not be of major concern. Stuart's occupational therapy assistant also believed that if Stuart were presented with more challenging situations in which he needed to remember information and act on it, the consequences might be of more concern.

Regarding Stuart's ability to know the way to stabilize and support task objects, the process skill *handles*, his occupational therapy assistant surmised that this resulted from Stuart's inexperience with performing tasks with one hand. As he practiced various methods of stabilizing and supporting task objects to adapt to his significantly diminished motor skill *coordinates*, Stuart learned more ways to stabilize and hold objects effectively. Because Stuart demonstrated an ability to use task objects according to their intended purpose—the process skill *uses* (Figure 20-7)—and an ability to ask effectively for needed information—the process skill *inquires*—the occupational therapy assistant did not need to address these skills.

Similar to the previous items, the process skills *initiates*, *continues*, *sequences*, and *terminates*, although presenting some difficulty for Stuart, were not of major concern. Stuart demonstrated the ability logically to sequence the steps of a task—the process skill *sequences*—and although he displayed some hesitation

when initiating some actions (the process skill *initiates*), his occupational therapy assistant surmised that this was Stuart trying to "figure out" the way he was going to perform a specific component of the task with his motor skill limitations. For example, the occupational therapy assistant had observed that Stuart hesitated for about 6 seconds before opening the refrigerator door. When she questioned Stuart after the assessment, he responded that he was trying to figure out how to get the door open with only one hand and also move his wheelchair. Similarly, Stuart would stop in the middle of an action, such as spreading the mayonnaise on a slice of bread, close the bag of bread, and then return to spreading the mayonnaise, a behavior reflecting the process skill *continues*. Stuart also spent a significant amount of time spreading the mayonnaise on the bread, reflecting ineffective performance in stopping actions at an appropriate time, the motor skill *terminates*. Although these skills were interfering with Stuart's overall efficiency in performing a task, they did not interfere greatly with the overall quality or outcome of the task. Consequently, the therapists did not emphasize these four process skills during Stuart's therapy.

The process skill *search/locates*, in contrast, was a skill that Stuart's occupational therapy practitioners believed should be emphasized during therapy. Both practitioners surmised that Stuart's diminished visual capacity (i.e., acuity, saccades, and pursuits) was affecting his ability to search for and locate needed items. They also believed Stuart's ability to attend visually to the environment, as observed on his admission to the SNF, still may be affecting his performance. For example, if Stuart initially did not see an item on a shelf, he quickly began looking on the next shelf down. To help Stuart develop a more effective search pattern, the occupational therapy assistant worked with Stuart to slow down when looking for items and to examine each area in his visual field carefully before moving on to the next area. She also made some recommendations—to Stuart for his home and to the SNF administrator for the facility—to modify the environment to ensure that adequate lighting was available.

The process skill *gathers* was also emphasized during intervention, in part as a way of adapting to Stuart's diminished motor skills (Figure 20-8). If Stuart were able to use more efficient strategies with which to gather items, he would rely less on his motor skills to transport items. The therapists applied the same reasoning to the

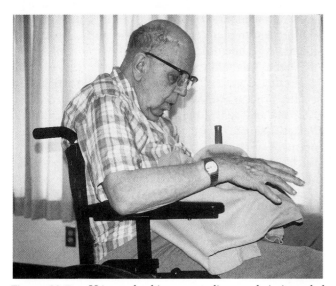

**Figure 20-7**    *Using* task objects according to their intended purpose.

## Case Study 2

### RETURNING HOME: IADL INTERVENTION DURING REHABILITATION—cont'd

process skill *organizes* (Figure 20-9). If Stuart were able to learn more efficient strategies with which to organize the tools and materials in his work space, these would reduce the demand on his motor skills. For example, when he folded the laundry for the assessment, Stuart had requested that the basket of laundry be placed on the table, where he proceeded to move it closer to him. This left a small space on which to fold

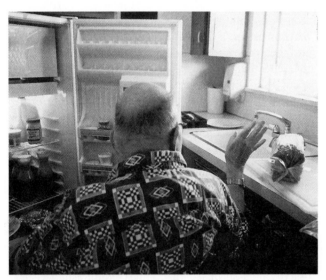

**Figure 20-8**    *Gathering* needed materials in the work space.

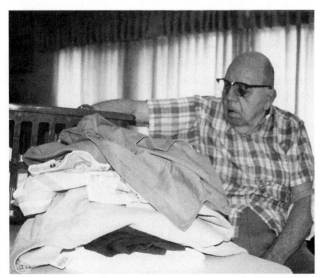

**Figure 20-9**    Ineffectively *organizing* materials in the work space results in limited work surface on which to fold clothes.

clothing. As Stuart folded more items, the space became crowded with the folded clothes, leaving him less space in which to fold clothes. By the end of the task, Stuart was folding the clothes on his lap because the table had no more space. Although this reflected Stuart's knowing that a lap could be used as a surface from which to fold clothes (see Figure 20-7), it created additional difficulty when performing the task. Focusing on this process skill, as reflected in his second IADL goal, required great patience on Stuart's part. He was not used to organizing his work space, and he reported to his occupational therapy assistant that he typically worked within the "mess" he created and did not pay much attention to having a "neat" work space. The OT assistant explained the reasoning for trying to organize his work space a bit better, referring to the example with the basket of laundry. She mentioned that had Stuart moved the basket of laundry to a different location, more space would have been available in which to fold the clothes. This challenging goal took considerable attention during their therapy sessions together because it was a challenging habit for Stuart to relearn.

As with the process skill *organizes*, the process skill *restores* had been identified as markedly deficient on the report. After discussion, Stuart's occupational therapy assistant realized that this too probably was related to Stuart's previous habits. He reported that he generally did not restore items right away and his wife frequently badgered him to clean up. Because this was a natural behavior of his, Stuart's occupational therapy assistant made little attempt to emphasize this process skill, except to point out to Stuart occasionally that he might save some time and energy if he restored items throughout the task.

To the surprise of both practitioners, Stuart's score on the process skill *navigates*, his ability to maneuver his hand and body around obstacles, had been identified as adequate on the report. They both believed the presence of visual inattention to the left environment might create some difficulty for Stuart during ADL tasks. They were correct, however, in their assumption that Stuart's underlying impairment with visual attention to the left environment did affect his ability to notice nonverbal environmental cues and respond appropriately; the process skill *notice/responds* was identified as markedly deficient on the report. To address this issue, the occupational therapy assistant again suggested modifying the environment to ensure adequate lighting. When she eventually spoke with Stuart and the manager of the assisted-living complex, she emphasized the need to simplify the visual environment to make it easier for Stuart to notice environmental cues. For example, Stuart mentioned that the tablecloth on the dining room table in his apartment was a bright floral print. Stuart's occupational therapy assistant explained that this might make it more difficult for Stuart visually to note items on the table and that a plain white tablecloth would be a better choice.

The last three process skills—*accommodates, adjusts,* and *benefits*—were the most important of the process skills because they reflected Stuart's ability to deal effectively with problems as they arose during task performance. Two of three process skills were identified as markedly deficient. Yet both occupational therapists needed to interpret this in light of Stuart's overall abilities. His low process scores on these items in part reflected his inability to overcome and adapt effectively to the many difficulties with motor skills. In other words, Stuart only recently had begun to practice new skills with his changed body since his CVA. Because this was the first time Stuart had attempted to perform IADL tasks, his difficulties were expected. For example, when preparing the sandwich, Stuart chose to keep the lap tray on his wheelchair while he worked in the kitchen. This presented additional problems because Stuart was not able to bend as far forward to reach objects, and the presence of the lap tray required additional maneuvering of the wheelchair to avoid hitting the countertop with the edge of the tray.

Stuart's underlying impairments were affecting his ability to adapt to problems as they arose. His occupational therapists surmised that Stuart's delay in turning over the knife he was using to cut the meat sandwich in half (i.e., not readily recognizing that he was using the knife incorrectly) may have resulted from his diminished visual capacity to see the knife blade (Figure 20-10). As such, this may have been affecting the process skill *accommodates.* Although Stuart's scores on *accommodates, adjusts,* and *benefits* were low, both occupational therapists believed Stuart still possessed the underlying cognitive capacity with which to learn to adapt and organize his actions more efficiently. They surmised that if Stuart concentrated on developing strategies with which to enhance his ability with specific motor or process skills or to adapt to his diminished motor skills by using his process skills, a greater repertoire of strategies with which to deal with problems would be available to Stuart.

During the final 3 weeks of inpatient rehabilitation, Stuart's goals for occupational therapy intervention focused on achieving greater independence with self-care skills and improved quality of performance with

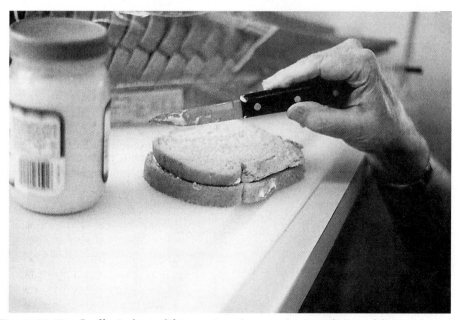

**Figure 20-10**    Ineffectively modifying actions (*accommodates*) results in a delay turning over the knife.

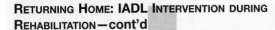

## Case Study 2

### RETURNING HOME: IADL INTERVENTION DURING REHABILITATION—cont'd

IADL tasks. He continued to practice performing IADL tasks, preparing simple snacks and light meals in the kitchen, watering houseplants, folding laundry, dusting, and cleaning countertops and tables. Throughout, Stuart's occupational therapy assistant focused on the way Stuart performed the task, working with him to develop strategies to accomplish the task more efficiently. Although this required Stuart to learn new methods, regaining movement was not the primary focus of the intervention. The focus was on Stuart's need to be able to engage in simple IADL tasks so that he and his wife could continue living in their home.

By the end of the Stuart's 5 weeks in the SNF rehabilitation unit, Stuart had made significant, although not outstanding, progress. As a result of a consistent morning self-care routine monitored by the occupational therapist, Stuart only required minimal assistance to get ready in the morning. (He did, however, require moderate assistance with showering.) Once Stuart was ready for the day, he was able to engage in simple IADL tasks such as washing a few dishes, getting a drink from the refrigerator, and setting the table without great difficulty. The rehabilitation team believed Stuart and his wife would be able to manage at home, with less assistance than they originally thought.

Just before Stuart's discharge, his occupational therapist used the AMPS to reevaluate him. This time, however, Stuart chose to set the table and iron a shirt as his two task choices. Neither the occupational therapist performing the AMPS (the occupational therapy assistant having performed the first assessment) nor Stuart's choosing different IADL tasks invalidated the results of the AMPS because the computer program accounted for both factors in the analysis. The results showed that his motor ability measure had improved from –1.0 to –0.7, a slight improvement. His process ability measure, however, improved significantly from –0.4 to 0.3, indicating that he was better able to organize and adapt his actions during task performance. Stuart demonstrated an enhanced ability to search more effectively for and locate items in his environment, handle and support objects, pace his performance, coordinate his body parts to hold and stabilize objects, transport and manipulate objects, and overcome problems as they arose during task performance. All these abilities supported Stuart's goal to return home and live in the community. Because his goal had been achieved, his rehabilitation was considered successful.

## ACKNOWLEDGMENTS

Leslie Duran is gratefully acknowledged for her feedback and assistance throughout the original preparation of this chapter. Appreciation for their assistance also is extended to Sally Huffman; Kathryn Kafalias; Stan Neiderhouse; Rehabilitation Institute of Oregon, Portland; and Eugene Good Samaritan Health Center, Eugene, Oregon.

## REVIEW QUESTIONS

1. Describe the perspective on function of occupational therapists compared with other rehabilitation professionals.
2. What do research studies reveal regarding the effect of a cerebrovascular accident on a person's engagement in IADL tasks?
3. What is the relationship between a person's degree of impairment resulting from a cerebrovascular accident and ability to perform IADL tasks?
4. Compare occupational therapy IADL assessments with those from other rehabilitation disciplines. What are the differences?
5. What are the advantages of using the Canadian Occupational Performance Measure with respect to a focus on IADL tasks?
6. Why is the use of IADL performance assessments recommended for use by occupational therapists?
7. What are the key elements that must be included in the documentation when writing goals for IADL performance?
8. Compare the adaptive and remedial approaches to occupational therapy intervention for IADL performance.
9. Describe the different aspects of adaptation that an occupational therapist considers when using an adaptive approach to IADL intervention.
10. What are the advantages of using the Assessment of Motor and Process Skills to guide intervention for IADL performance?

## REFERENCES

1. Adaptive Environments Center: *A consumer's guide to home adaptation*, Boston, 1993, The Center.
2. Atler KE, Gliner JA: Post stroke activity and psychosocial factors, *Phys Occup Ther Geriatr* 7:13, 1989.
3. Bernspang B, Fisher AG: Differences between persons with right or left CVA on the assessment of motor and process skills, *Arch Phys Med Rehabil* 76(12):1144-1151, 1995.
4. Bodium C: The use of the Canadian occupational performance measure for the assessment of outcome on a neurorehabilitation unit, *Br J Occup Ther* 1999:123, 1999.
5. Bond MJ, Clark MS: Clinical applications of the Adelaide activities profile, *Clin Rehabil* 12(3):228-237, 1998.
6. Branch LG, Meyers AR: Assessing physical function in the elderly, *Clin Geriatr Med* 3(1):29-51, 1987.
7. Canadian Association of Occupational Therapists: *Occupational therapy guidelines for patient-centered practice*, Toronto, 1991, The Association.

8. Carod-Artal FJ, González-Gutiérrez JL, Herrero JA, et al: Functional recovery and instrumental activities of daily living: follow-up 1 year after treatment in a stroke unit, *Brain Inj* 16(3): 202-216, 2002.

9. Carter J, Mant F, Mant J, et al: Comparison of postal version of the Frenchay activities index with interviewer-administered version for use in people with stroke, *Clin Rehabil* 11(2):131-138, 1997.

10. Chong, DK: Measurement of instrumental activities of daily living in stroke, *Stroke* 26(6):1119-1122, 1995.

11. Christensen C, Baum C: *Occupational therapy: overcoming human performance deficits*, Thorofare, NJ, 1991, Slack.

12. Clark MS, Smith DS: Factors contributing to patient satisfaction with rehabilitation following stroke, *Int J Rehabil Res* 21(2):143-154, 1998.

13. Commission on Practice, American Occupational Therapy Association: Occupational therapy practice framework: domain and process, *Am J Occup Ther* 56(6):609-639, 2002.

14. Eakin P: Occupational therapy in stroke rehabilitation: implications of research into therapy outcomes, *Br J Occup Ther* 54:326, 1991.

15. Eakin P: The outcome of therapy in stroke rehabilitation: do we know what we are doing? *Br J Occup Ther* 54:305, 1991.

16. Edmans JA, Towle D: Comparison of stroke unit and non-stroke unit inpatients on independence in ADL, *Br J Occup Ther* 53:415, 1990.

17. Fisher AG: *Assessment of motor and process skills*, ed 5, Fort Collins, Colo, 2003, Three Star Press.

18. Fisher AG: Functional measures. 1. What is function, what should we measure, and how should we measure it? *Am J Occup Ther* 46(2):183-185, 1992.

19. Fisher AG: Functional measures. 2. Selecting the right test, minimizing the limitation, *Am J Occup Ther* 46(3):278-281, 1992.

20. Foti D, Pedretti LW: Activities of daily living: section 1—self-care/home management. In Pedretti LW, editor: *Occupational therapy: practice skills for physical dysfunction*, St Louis, 1996, Mosby.

21. Fricke J, Unsworth C: Time use and importance of instrumental activities of daily living, *Aust J Occup Ther* 48:118, 2001.

22. Fricke J, Unsworth C: Occupational therapists' conceptions of instrumental activities of daily living in relation to evaluation and interventions with older clients, *Scand J Occup Ther* 5:180, 1998.

23. Gilbertson L, Langhorne P: Home-based occupational therapy: stroke patients' satisfaction with occupational performance and service provision, *Br J Occup Ther* 63:464, 2000.

24. Gompertz P, Pound P, Ebrahim S: The reliability of stroke outcome measures, *Clin Rehabil* 7, 290-296, 1993.

25. Gresham GE, Duncan PW, Stason WB, et al: *Post-stroke rehabilitation: clinical practice guideline*, No 16, AHCPR Pub No 95-0662, Rockville, Md, 1995, US Department of Health and Human Services, Public Health Service, Agency for Health Care Policy and Research.

26. Grimby G, Andrén E, Daving Y, et al: Dependence and perceived difficulty in daily activities in community-living stroke survivors 2 years after stroke: a study of instrumental structures, *Stroke* 29(9):1843-1849, 1998.

27. Grimby G, Andren E, Holmgren E, et al: Structure of a combination of functional independence measure and instrumental activity measure items in community-living persons: a study of individuals with cerebral palsy and spina bifida, *Arch Phys Med Rehabil* 77(11):1109-1114, 1996.

28. Holbrook M, Skilbeck CE: An activities index for use with stroke patients, *Age Ageing* 12(2):166-170, 1983.

29. Jongbloed L, Brighton C, Stacey S: Factors associated with independent meal preparation, self-care and mobility in CVA patients, *Can J Occup Ther* 55:259, 1988.

30. Kelly FA, Kawamoto TT, Rubenstein LZ: Assessment of the geriatric patient. In Kiernat JM, editor: *Occupational therapy and the older adult: a clinician manual*, Gaithersburg, Md, 1991, Aspen.

31. Kielhofner G, Forsyth, K: Thinking with theory: a framework for therapeutic reasoning. In Kielhofner G, editor: *A model of human occupation: theory and application*, ed 3, Philadelphia, 2002, Lippincott Williams & Wilkins.

32. Law M: Evaluation of occupational performance. In Trombly C, editor: *Occupational therapy for physical dysfunction*, Baltimore, 1995, Williams & Wilkins.

33. Law M, Baptiste S, Carswell A, et al: *Canadian occupational performance measure*, ed 3, Toronto, 1998, Canadian Association of Occupational Therapists.

34. Levine RE, Gitlin LN: A model to promote activity competence in elders, *Am J Occup Ther* 47(2):147-153, 1993.

35. Lindberg M, Fugl-Meyer AR: The long-term consequences of subarachnoid haemorrhage. 2. Prevalence of instrumental ADL disabilities, *Clin Rehabil* 10:69, 1996.

36. Moulton C: Current trends in the practice of home health care of occupational therapists treating patients who have had a stroke, *Occup Ther Int* 4:31, 1997.

37. Neistadt ME: Methods of assessing patients' priorities: a survey of adult physical dysfunction settings, *Am J Occup Ther* 49:428, 1995.

38. Neistadt ME: Occupational therapy treatment for constructional deficits, *Am J Occup Ther* 46(2):141-148, 1992.

39. Neistadt ME, Seymour SG: Treatment activity preferences of occupational therapists in adult physical dysfunction settings, *Am J Occup Ther* 49(5):437-443, 1995.

40. Nilsson AL, Aniansson A, Grimby G: Rehabilitation needs and disability in community living stroke survivors two years after stroke, *Top Stroke Rehabil* 6:30, 2000.

41. Northern JG, Rust DM, Nelson CE, et al: Involvement of adult rehabilitation patients in setting occupational therapy goals, *Am J Occup Ther* 49(3):214-220, 1995.

42. Nouri FM, Lincoln NB: An extended activities of daily living scale for stroke patients, *Clin Rehabil* 4:123, 1987.

43. Park S: Restoring occupational performance: rehabilitation services for older adults. In Larson KO, Pedretti LW, Stevens-Ratchford RG, editors: *ROTE: the role of occupational therapy with the elderly*, Bethesda, Md, 1996, American Occupational Therapy Association.

44. Park S: Treatment planning. In Fisher AG, editor: *Assessment of motor and process skills*, Fort Collins, Colo, 1995, Three Star Press.

45. Park S, Fisher AG, Velozo CA: Using the assessment of motor and process skills to compare occupational performance between clinic and home settings, *Am J Occup Ther* 48(8):697-709, 1994.

46. Radomski MV: There is more to life than putting on your pants, *Am J Occup Ther* 49(6):487-490, 1995.

47. Rogers JC, Holm MB: Assessment of self-care. In Bonder BR, Waner MB, editors: *Functional performance in older adults*, Philadelphia, 1994, FA Davis.

48. Rubenstein LZ, Schairer C, Wieland GD, Kane R: Systematic biases in functional status assessment of elderly adults: effects of different data sources, *J Gerontol* 39(6):686-91, 1986.

49. Sarno MT, Buonaguro A: Factors associated with independent meal preparation in aphasic females: a pilot study, *Occup Ther J Res* 3:23, 1984.

50. Settle C, Holm MB: Program planning: the clinical utility of three activities of daily living assessment tools, *Am J Occup Ther* 47(10):911-918, 1993.

51. Simmons DC, Crepeau EB, White BP: The predictive power of narrative data in occupational therapy evaluation, *Am J Occup Ther* 54(5):471-476, 2000.

52. Steinberg FU: Medical evaluation, assessment of function and potential, and rehabilitation plan. In Felsenthal G, Garrison SJ, Steinberg FU, editors: *Rehabilitation of the aging and elderly patient*, Baltimore, 1994, Williams & Wilkins.

53. Tangeman PT, Banaitis DA, Williams AK: Rehabilitation of chronic stroke patients: changes in functional performance, *Arch Phys Med Rehabil* 71(11):876-880, 1990.

54. Trombly CA: Retraining basic and instrumental activities of daily living. In Trombly C, editor: *Occupational therapy for physical dysfunction*, Baltimore, 1995, Williams & Wilkins.

55. Trombly C: The issue is—anticipating the future: assessment of occupational function, *Am J Occup Ther* 47:253, 1993.

56. Trombly CA, Ma H: A synthesis of the effects of occupational therapy for persons with stroke. I. Restoration of roles, tasks, and activities, *Am J Occup Ther* 56(3):250-259, 2002.

57. Van Herk IE, Arendzen JH: Measures to assess functional capacities of stroke patients living at home: a review of literature, *J Rehabil Sci* 8:66, 1995.

58. Ward G, Jagger C, Harper W: A review of instrumental ADL assessments for use with elderly people, *Rev Clin Gerontol* 8:65, 1998.

59. Whiting S, Lincoln NB: An ADL assessment for stroke patients, *Br J Occup Ther* 43:44, 1980.

60. Wilcock AA: *Occupational therapy approaches to stroke*, Melbourne, 1986, Churchill Livingstone.

61. Woodson AM: Stroke. In Trombly C, editor: *Occupational therapy for physical dysfunction*, Baltimore, 1995, Williams & Wilkins.

62. Wressle E, Samuelsson, Henriksson C: Responsiveness of the Swedish version of the Canadian occupational therapy measure, *Scand J Occup Ther* 6:84, 1999.

susan l. pierce

chapter 21

# Driving as an Instrumental Activity of Daily Living

## key terms

community mobility
driver rehabilitation therapist
ecological validity

independent transportation
on-the-road test

mobility prescription
predriving clinical screening

## chapter objectives

After completing this chapter, the reader will be able to accomplish the following:

1. Define *driving* as an instrumental activity of daily living.
2. Identify the role of occupational therapy in addressing driving issues at different stages of rehabilitation and recovery for the stroke survivor.
3. Understand the legal issues associated with involvement of driving issues and how to reduce liability exposure.
4. Identify performance deficits related to a cerebrovascular accident that can interfere with driving skills.
5. Understand the current accepted practice for a comprehensive driver assessment for the stroke survivor.
6. Identify resources for information, education, and referral.

In the continuum of activities of daily living (ADL), the occupational therapist must consider mobility in the rehabilitation process of the patient recovering from a cerebrovascular accident (CVA). Treatment planning for mobility issues should center on independent mobility for the patient in and around the house and community. With the accessibility offered by cars and federal mortgage assistance programs after World War II, studies of housing patterns of the elderly in 1970 and 1980 showed a dramatic move from rural to urban living. By 1980 the parents of today's baby boomers moved away from their parents' homes in the city and to the suburbs where they are now "graying in place." This movement pattern greatly changes the nature of the transportation needs of the elderly today and will continue to be a significant factor when the baby boomers become elderly.[31]

A century ago, individuals could walk to work, shops, friends' homes, churches, and most other destinations. Today, with the primary mode of transportation being the personal vehicle and with the distance separating homes and businesses in the suburbs, few destinations are now within walking distance. Impairments and activity limitations caused by a CVA or age further can shorten distances traversable on foot. Conference planners were surprised at the 1971 White House Conference on Aging when delegates ranked transportation third in importance, preceded only by income and health. Research confirms that in general older persons are not satisfied with their abilities to get around in the community.[5] Because persons must go into the community to meet almost all of their needs, the existence of facilities and services is meaningless without accessibility. Automobiles provide vital access to widely scattered services and facilities. Reduced mobility in the community by an individual can result in a lower self-esteem, depression, and feelings of uselessness, loneliness, and unhappiness.

The performance skills necessary for safe driving begin to deteriorate around the age of 55 and dramatically decline after age 75.[26] Approximately 72% of strokes occur in persons older than 65. In addition to normal aging conditions, the brain damage from a cerebral infarct and its clinical manifestations can affect the person's driving skills. The specific motor, sensory, and cognitive deficits depend on the location and severity of the cerebrovascular damage (see Chapters 1 and 18). This damage can cause one or more temporary or permanent impairments. Of the approximately 80% of persons who survive the initial period, 75% are left with residual perceptual-cognitive dysfunction.[19] Although these impairments may affect safe driving, the therapist must evaluate each patient recovering from a CVA individually because the location and nature of the stroke can produce different problems and deficits.

Independent transportation should be considered an instrumental activity of daily living (IADL). Achieving or not achieving independent transportation for a stroke survivor can impede or affect greatly all other instrumental activities of daily living. Frances Carp,[5] a California psychologist who has studied older drivers, uses the conceptual model in Figure 21-1 to detail the determinants of emotional and social well-being. Life maintenance needs include nourishment, clothing, medical care, banking, and

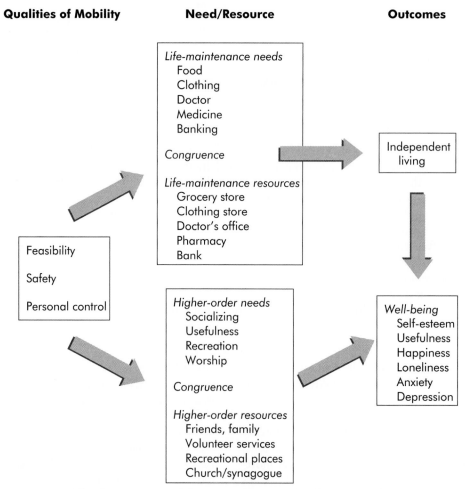

**Figure 21-1**   The determinants and dynamics of emotional and social well-being. (Modified from Transportation Research Board—National Research Council, Special Report 218, *Transportation in an aging society*, Washington, DC, 1988.)

pharmaceuticals. Community resources for meeting these needs include grocery and drug stores, department stores, physician's offices, and banks. If a person has no access to these resources, independent living becomes nearly impossible. Other needs, labeled *higher order*, include needs for social interaction, usefulness, recreation, and religious experience. Carp's research of investigative studies supports the idea that "if life is to have an acceptable quality, higher-order needs such as those expressed in trips for relaxation and enjoyment and religious activities are also essential."

The threat of losing a driver's license may have devastating effects on a stroke survivor's motivation to maintain independence in other areas of daily living. The primary fear of elderly persons is not death but losing their independence and becoming burdens to their loved ones.[3] Carp[5] states the following:

Loss of license is a serious fear among drivers, a threat to their autonomy, usefulness, and self-esteem. . . . A century ago people could walk to work, shops, others' homes, religious services, and most destinations. Few destinations [today] lie within walking distance for any person. . . . Mobility is a key influence on the congruence term in the model. . . . Satisfaction of life-maintenance and higher order needs require going out into the community. . . . The loss of a license would mean inability to go where they needed to go and therefore meet their needs independently. . . . Just as receipt of the first driver's license is an important rite of passage to adulthood and independence, license loss formally identifies one as "over the hill."

Driving is inseparable with being one's own person and taking care of oneself. The issue is more than just one of losing mobility. Rendering an opinion as to whether the patient recovering from a CVA is capable of driving is serious and demands careful attention by the rehabilitation team. Law enforcement officers or driver licensing personnel cannot address this issue effectively, which has potentially dangerous consequences to the stroke survivor or to pedestrians or other road users. Elderly drivers who do not self-regulate effectively are not detected easily with standard licensing procedures.[19] Furthermore, doubt exists as to whether most licensing staffs have the skills necessary to detect these problem drivers.[7]

## DRIVING AS AN ACTIVITY OF DAILY LIVING SKILL

Community mobility is paramount to the patient recovering from CVA and attempting to maintain a productive lifestyle in the work or social arenas. Being one of the most complex activities of daily living, driving certainly requires attention, careful consideration, and inclusion with other ADL issues. In other words, if the rehabilitation team addresses safety in mobility or safety in the kitchen for the stroke survivor, then certainly safety in

driving demands addressing. By including driving as an IADL, driving will be brought up and discussed early in the stroke survivor's rehabilitation and recovery. Such discussion will lead to patient and family education and acceptance early to reinforce their responsibility and requirements in the process of the patient's regaining independent driving or their need to investigate alternative transportation options. The discussion also will lessen the family's stress and anxiety over the issue of driving for their family member, for they will not have to shoulder the burden of telling the person that he or she cannot drive and then dealing with an angry family member.

Driving is an activity of daily living listed under community mobility in the Practice Framework of the American Occupational Therapy Association (AOTA).[23] Pierce[28] writes, "Each area of mobility requires a certain skill level in occupational performance. A hierarchy of skills dictates the order in which each area is addressed. Mobility in basic activities of daily living (BADL) is first, followed by mobility in instrumental activities of daily living (IADL). Some occupational therapy (OT) goals for motor, sensory, perceptual, and cognitive functioning must be achieved prior to ADL training and specifically mobility training."

The AOTA recently identified driver rehabilitation and training as one of the top 10 emerging practice areas for occupational therapists in the twenty-first century.[24] "As an activity that contributes to independence and quality of life, driving falls squarely within the province of occupational therapy practice," according to Johansson.[16] The discipline of occupational therapy has been given the role of evaluating patients regarding their ability to drive a motor vehicle primarily because of the wide spectrum of physical, cognitive, and perceptual skills that fall under the realm of occupational therapy.[17] In addition, occupational therapists have a background in psychosocial dysfunction that can be key in giving the therapist the necessary therapeutic attitude and approach to this sensitive issue to understand how it can affect the psychosocial and emotional well-being of the patient. The AOTA has identified older driver evaluation and retraining as an important specialty area for practitioners to consider because of the broad approach of the profession to evaluation and treatment.[20] John Eberhard, a senior research psychologist at the National Highway and Traffic Safety Administration has said that he "envisions a key role for the OT profession in maintaining elders' automotive proficiency. OT practitioners have clear insights into the need for mobility. They have the skills to assess functional mobility and the skills to enhance it."[25]

In all settings the occupational therapist is concerned with the performance level of ADL, with mobility being at the top of the pyramid (Figure 21-2). The daily living task of mobility may involve bed and wheelchair mobility,

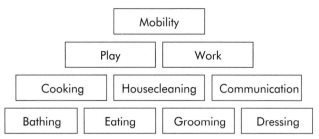

**Figure 21-2** Pyramid model for rehabilitation of activities of daily living.

transfers, walking, and driving. These tasks allow an individual to function independently by moving from one place to another. Successful community mobility may depend on the patient's ability to drive or use alternative transportation. Because persons of all ages can suffer a CVA, it is important that driving or transportation as a community mobility issue is on the ADL repertoire for the occupational therapist to explore, evaluate, and treat as necessary. The occupational therapist must understand the significance of community mobility for the total well-being of the patient. A holistic view presents driving as a vital link between the patient and the outside world.

## REHABILITATION TEAM'S RESPONSIBILITY

The entire rehabilitation team must address the issue of driving or transportation for the stroke survivor, with members addressing the issue within their own professional expertise (Figure 21-3). The rehabilitation team must get involved with this issue because they are concerned with the overall functioning of the patient and his or her resulting quality of life after a stroke. They are in the best position to identify any existing or potential contributors to driving risk. In addition, families need assistance and guidance with this highly sensitive issue before they take the family member home. The rehabilitation team must define a course of action that is fair and reasonable. They must weigh the patient-doctor or patient-therapist confidentiality versus public safety. The social and ethical dilemma faced by medical professionals and the department of driver licensing is to strike a balance between protecting the person's privilege to drive and the safety of other road users, including pedestrians, other drivers, and vehicle passengers.

Each team member has a role and responsibility and should be ready to address related issues as they arise. For example, the physician, as the head of the rehabilitation team and medical authority, must take a leading role with this issue. The physician should be the first to inform the patient and family of the need for a formal driving assessment. Without hesitation the physician should inform the stroke survivor and the family that the patient will not be able to drive until the road test has been completed.

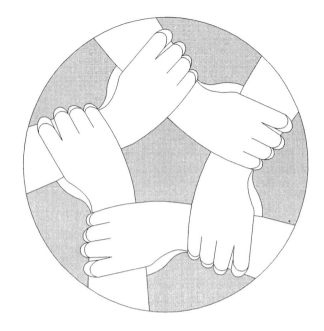

- Physician
- Social worker
- Occupational therapist
- Physical therapist
- Rehabilitation nurse
- Speech therapist
- Neuropsychologist

**Figure 21-3** Driving should be addressed as appropriate by each member of the rehabilitation team, following the same policies and procedures. The process depends on good communication between the team members.

The nurse can provide a list of medications with which the patient will be discharged home and note any side effects that could affect safe driving. The speech therapist may address the need for a patient with aphasia to begin carrying a personal identification card; if he or she is involved in an accident or is stopped by a police officer, the card would explain the speech difficulties. The speech therapist also may inform the occupational therapist of any language deficits that might be contraindicated for safe driving. For example, if the stroke survivor has global aphasia and needs to be evaluated for driving using driving aids, they may have difficulty with verbal instructions on a new task or with directions. The physical therapist can reinforce the reality that the person with dense right hemiplegia will not be able to use the right foot for driving because of lack of necessary motor and sensory function and can work on the goal of the patient's entering and exiting a vehicle with or without an orthotic device. The social worker can counsel the family to reinforce the team's discharge recommendations related to referral for a formal driving assessment after discharge and assist other members in identifying alternative transportation options.

The occupational therapist's role would be the most directly involved with the driving task. The occupational therapist would provide initial information for the patient and family, perform a predriving clinical screening, and eventually complete the equipment/vehicle assessment and the in-traffic assessment and make final recommendations to the physician, team, patient, family, and department of driver licensing, if necessary. The facility and or employer and the occupational therapy staff must decide whether one or more therapists will address driving issues throughout the entire process.

## OCCUPATIONAL THERAPIST'S CHANGING ROLE WITH THE STROKE SURVIVOR

The occupational therapist's background and training in evaluation and treatment in the performance areas of physical, visual, visual-perception, and cognition coupled with an understanding of diagnostic and age-related problem areas assists the therapist to understand the implications of driving. In addition, the occupational therapist's background and understanding of psychological and emotional issues assists the therapist greatly in handling the delicate issue of driving when just speaking of the issue can cause anxiety, defensiveness, and other psychological stress for not only the stroke survivor but also family members. The occupational therapist's role many times is to educate, listen, and counsel not only the patient but also family members. The occupational therapist's keen ability to look at the "whole person" is important to the process in considering all aspects of the issues of community mobility, including driving, and how all the different aspects are interrelated and depend upon one another.

The occupational therapist's role changes during different phases as the stroke survivor moves through acute care hospitalization, rehabilitation, discharge, and community follow-up. As the person moves through these phases, the occupational therapist addresses issues of driving relevant to each phase. The level of knowledge, skill, and training for the therapist varies during each phase. Driving or transportation should be an established ADL goal early on with all other ADL goals and have a well-defined course of action toward this goal.

### Acute Care Phase

During the initial hospital phase, the role for the occupational therapist is primarily one of inquiry and fact finding. One of the most common questions initially asked by a person in this phase is "Can I drive again?" or "When will I be able to drive again?" The therapist must be able to answer the question when asked and speak with confidence about how the rehabilitation team will address the concern. The therapist can inquire whether the stroke survivor had been a licensed driver before the CVA and

what was the frequency and circumstances of driving. For example, did the person drive to work or drive his or her children to school? Does the person live in a rural area or city? Was the person the primary driver in the family? Did the person drive intrastate, interstate, or just locally? Is the person at a stage at which he or she already had begun to limit driving to daylight only or within short distances of home? Is driving a goal for the person now? If the patient has memory, cognitive, or speech deficits, the family may need to be consulted to obtain or verify the information given by the patient. If the stroke survivor passes through the hospital phase quickly, then these questions may need to be explored by the therapist in the next phase. The point is that driving should be addressed early and as commonly as dressing, grooming, and other mobility issues. Whether the appropriate time is in the acute care phase or the rehabilitation phase, the therapist should be equipped to address driving in an appropriate way.

### Rehabilitation Phase

As the stroke survivor moves into the rehabilitation phase, the foregoing information would be passed on to the rehabilitation unit therapist. The primary occupational therapist would pick up the issue by addressing driving as an IADL in the initial evaluation for planning an intervention program with the stroke survivor as for other ADL such as dressing, bathing, and cooking. To address driving as an IADL and assess factors that may affect safe driving, the occupational therapist requires an understanding of all patient factors and skills involved in driving. With an understanding of the level of skill performance demanded in the driving task, the occupational therapist can include treatment of deficits, with driving in mind, much as the therapist would for other ADL tasks.

Driving an automobile is a complex task involving a hierarchy of skills. Adequate motor response and physical control of the vehicle are essential skills but are secondary to accurate perception and understanding of ever-changing traffic environments and unpredictable situations. A driver processes information and makes conscious or unconscious decisions using (1) environmental information such as traffic lights, road markings, road signs, and other road users; (2) attention and perceptual mechanisms using visual search, spatial relations, and time and space management; (3) reasoning, problem solving, and planning to analyze each situation and understand cause and effect; and (4) response by physical control, adjustment, and compromise. Table 21-1 gives an overview of occupational performance in driving.

### Preexisting or Progressive Age-Related Conditions

In addition to conditions or problems associated with the primary diagnosis, the therapist should explore other preexisting medical or aging conditions that require attention. Stressel[37] writes the following:

**Table 21-1**

## Occupational Performance in Driving for a Stroke Survivor

| BASIC SKILL AREAS | PERFORMANCE FACTORS |
|---|---|
| **Physical Demands** | |
| One functional upper extremity and left extremity | Operation of primary/secondary vehicle controls with or without adaptive equipment |
| **Visual Demands** | |
| Visual acuity: 20/40 in at least one eye | Reading/understanding road signs<br>Reading odometer and dash gauges<br>Can influence depth perception<br>Identification of stimuli seen in side vision |
| Peripheral vision: >130 degrees of total field of vision with both eyes | Awareness of stimuli in side vision<br>Visual scanning<br>More useful than visual acuity |
| Good eye function/quality of vision: disease or age-related problems | Cataracts: poor glare recovery, poor night vision<br>Diabetic retinopathy: blind spots, see incomplete driving scene<br>Glaucoma: blurriness, blindness |
| **Visual-Perceptual Demands** | |
| Spatial relations | Reading/responding to road signs/markings; perception of space around car |
| Figure-ground | Maneuvering through parking lot; finding road signs in a visually busy environment |
| Visual closure | Discrimination of high- and low-priority issues; seeing the whole picture with incomplete cues |
| Visual memory | Time and space management; delay response time |
| Form constancy | Visual analysis in busy and/or low-light environments |
| Visual discrimination | Analysis of road signs by shape and color |
| **Cognitive Demands** | |
| *Strategic skills* | Choice of route<br>Time of day to take trip<br>Planning a sequence of trips or stops<br>Evaluating general risks in traffic (under varying traffic, road, and weather conditions) |
| *Tactical skills* | Anticipatory driving behavior<br>Adjusting speed to varying traffic conditions<br>Quick decisions related to expected or unexpected situations<br>Judgment/reasoning to estimate risks |
| *Operational skills (combines physical, visual, and cognitive)* | |
| Attention: | |
| Focused | Responding to specific stimuli |
| Sustained | Maintaining focus during continuous driving |
| Selective | Maintaining focus in face of distractions |
| Alternating | Mental flexibility to focus between several tasks requiring attention |
| Divided | Responding simultaneously to multiple tasks or multiple task demands |
| Complex reaction time (appropriateness and timeliness of response) | |
| *Memory skills* | |
| Recent | Remembering destination, path to take, and event |
| Procedural | Subconscious operation of vehicle controls as old, learned behavior |

In general, aging results in the normal deterioration of the physical, cognitive, and visual functioning. People age at different rates, and age-related problems that are known to affect driver performance do not occur in all people at the same rate or to the same degree. The rate of decline is very individualized, and chronological age is not a good predictor of an individual's capabilities. As the prevalence of disease increases with age, it becomes more difficult to differentiate between functional losses due to the effects of disease versus functional loss associated with the aging process. . . . The process of aging is inescapable. Age-related changes are characteristically detrimental in nature, cumulative and irreversible over time, but often lack sharply defined points of transition. Changes begin at different chronological ages, progress at varying rates, and do not affect each body system in the same way. . . . Although some diseases and deterioration may present themselves suddenly, generally there is a slow accumulation of deficits.

Several examples to illustrate this point are the stroke survivor who has had insulin-dependent type 2 diabetes for 25 years. He was diagnosed with diabetic retinopathy and had two laser surgeries for treatment. Another stroke survivor has been on kidney dialysis for 2 years after having an allergic reaction to a medication that damaged the kidneys. Each of these preexisting conditions, separate from any deficits related to the CVA, could increase risk factors associated with safe driving and should be addressed separately in terms of the affect on the driving task. Box 21-1 lists other examples of non-CVA factors to consider. Communication with the family, rehabilitation physician, neurologist, and perhaps the primary care physician is important to synthesize the patient's entire medical history and consider all potential factors that may affect the stroke survivor returning to independent driving.

The second stage of involvement during the rehabilitation period is the crucial area of education of the stroke survivor and the family regarding individual responsibility in the whole process. In this phase the patient must be informed how, when, and by what process driving will be addressed. The therapist should be well spoken in the process, timing, referral procedures, and resources so as to speak with authority and confidence in the process. The stroke survivor and family should know at this point that the patient cannot drive until a driver rehabilitation therapist has completed a formal driving evaluation. By giving the patient the information at this stage, he or she will be prepared and cooperative in moving through the process and knowing what to expect along the way. The patient will understand that performance skill areas are being addressed that might affect driving skills so that he or she will be better prepared for the formal evaluation.

Driving is one area that scares many family members of stroke survivors. They need to be informed so they can provide the necessary assistance and support for the patient throughout the process. The family can begin dealing with this reality and plan for alternative transportation for the stroke survivor until the results of the formal driving evaluation are known. This should lessen their fears and anxiety and brings them into an active role in the process while allowing them to remain in the background regarding the decisions about driving. In other words, the family cannot be blamed for the stroke survivor's temporary or permanent loss of driving privileges. By addressing the driving issue in the medical setting, the family is relieved of having to address the issue themselves with the stroke survivor, which many times can cause frustration and emotional stress from the stroke survivor's anger, lack of insight, or poor judgment.

## Medical Reporting with Driver Licensing Authorities

Each state has licensing requirements and reporting laws. Many states do not require a driver to report a new medical episode resulting in disability between license renewals. Some states allow only a doctor to report a medical condition that may preclude safe driving. Other states may allow professionals such as a law enforcement officer or allied health professional, or even nonprofessionals such as a neighbor or family member to report a driver's medical condition or to raise a concern. Occupational therapists should investigate the requirements for the state in which they work so as to develop a procedure to use consistently with every patient to have a set policy approved by the administration and legal departments of the facility and understood by each team

### Box 21-1

#### Non–Cerebrovascular Accident Medical Factors That Potentially Can Affect Driving Safety

Previous history of cerebrovascular accident or transient ischemic attack

Diabetes

Visual problems such as cataracts, glaucoma, macular degeneration, or diabetic retinopathy

Arthritis and osteoarthritis

Surgeries that caused limitations such as hip/knee replacements or cervical laminectomy

Respiratory conditions such as emphysema or chronic obstructive pulmonary disease

Amputations

Other neuromuscular conditions such as polio, multiple sclerosis, or muscular dystrophy

Dementia

Polypharmacy: multiple medications with interacting effects; prescription and over-the-counter looked at separately and in synergistic combination

Psychological diagnoses such as bipolar disease, depression, or schizophrenia

Parkinson's disease

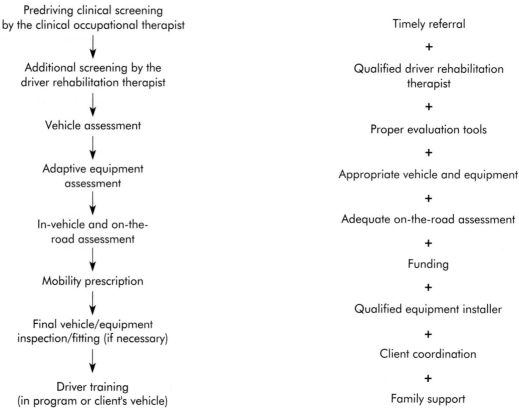

Predriving clinical screening
by the clinical occupational therapist

↓

Additional screening by the
driver rehabilitation therapist

↓

Vehicle assessment

↓

Adaptive equipment
assessment

↓

In-vehicle and on-the-
road assessment

↓

Mobility prescription

↓

Final vehicle/equipment
inspection/fitting (if necessary)

↓

Driver training
(in program or client's vehicle)

**Figure 21-4**    The driving assessment process for a stroke survivor.

Timely referral

+

Qualified driver rehabilitation
therapist

+

Proper evaluation tools

+

Appropriate vehicle and equipment

+

Adequate on-the-road assessment

+

Funding

+

Qualified equipment installer

+

Client coordination

+

Family support

**Figure 21-5**    Factors that influence the driving evaluation process.

member. Many states have medical advisory boards to their departments of driver licensing that are good resources for licensing requirements and the medical reporting process.

That testing procedures in driver examination offices do not evaluate fully all skills related to driving is common knowledge, particularly when the driver may have a medical condition or deficit that is not physically obvious. Examiners may not have knowledge of an applicant's diagnoses unless the person informs them or a physician provides written notification. They do not have an understanding of possible implications for driving. For example, a person with a complete right homonymous hemianopsia, which is a common vision deficit after a CVA, usually does not pass the visual requirements of most states for a minimum of 125 to 140 degrees of continuous field of vision. The typical methods of vision testing by driver licensing offices measure only visual acuity and not visual fields. A person can have 20/40 visual acuity, which is acceptable in most states; however, the driver examiner may never know the person has homonymous hemianopsia.

## Predriving Clinic Screening

A comprehensive driving assessment for a person who has had a stroke may include the steps illustrated in Figure

21-4. A successful completion of this process depends on many factors that can influence the outcome, as noted in Figure 21-5. The process should begin before the person is discharged from the inpatient stay with a discharge predriving clinic screening. The purpose of this step is threefold: (1) to assess any residual deficits in the areas of physical, visual, visual-perceptual, and cognitive performance skills; (2) to determine whether any of these deficits could or would interfere with driving performance; and (3) to determine whether a referral for the on-the-road test is appropriate now or should be delayed. Are there deficits related to primary or secondary diagnosis that still exist on discharge from the inpatient stay that could affect the stroke survivor's driving performance? At this step, the therapist should have knowledge of the appropriate state licensing laws and understand each skill performance area needed for safe driving so that the appropriate information can be passed on to the driver rehabilitation therapist. For example, if the patient has left neglect or serious visual-perceptual deficits, these conditions can be contraindicative of safe driving unless they resolve early. Another example is the field of vision requirement already discussed. If a stroke survivor has a complete homonymous hemianopsia, then the therapist should tell the patient that a return to driving may not be possible because of the requirements of the state unless

**Table 21-2**

**Examples of Cerebrovascular Accident–Related Deficits to Identify During Initial Assessment**

| DEFICIT | POTENTIAL ISSUES FOR FUTURE RETURN TO DRIVING |
|---|---|
| Left or right neglect | May not see or respond to road signs or markings; may ride to extreme right or left of lane; may miss turning lanes; will not look to affected side at intersections |
| Loss of field of vision | Will be surprised by unexpected stimuli or events that move into field of vision suddenly from blind area |
| Dense hemiplegia | May require adaptive devices to compensate for physical dysfunction in one or both affected extremities |
| Seizure | Most states have a required period of being seizure free with or without medication |
| Reflex sympathetic dystrophy | Pain or strong medications may affect mood and be a distracting factor |
| Visual-perceptual | See Table 21-1 |
| Aphasia | Misreads signs or other road user cues; becomes distracted when attempting to talk |
| Impulsivity, poor inhibition | Responds or reacts without thinking or seeing the consequences |
| Denial, poor insight | Does not see or understand his or her deficits; improvement difficult because he or she does not feel there is any need for improvement |
| Memory | May not remember where destination is or how to get there; becomes confused and anxious when cannot find street, misses a street, or is faced with a detour |

the condition resolves itself enough to meet the field of vision requirements. Table 21-2 has examples of problem areas to note.

When structuring the predriving clinical screening, the therapist should be guided by common sense to determine the specific clinical tests and techniques to use. Although much of the typical clinical tools and equipment can be used for this screening, the therapist may need additional specialized equipment for more relevance to driving.

Patients may be more cooperative with the clinical assessment if they appreciate its relevancy to the driving task. For example, the patient may feel frustrated and angry working on a puzzle or paper maze during predriving clinical screening but may understand the importance of a test that provides specific data related to driving such as reaction time, steering control, and divided attention. The therapist should describe the relevance of any test given so the patient will be motivated to perform well on the test. The physical and visual assessment is generally easy for the therapist to set up because the assessment and techniques used in these areas are similar to those used in other settings and with other disabilities.

The purpose of the predriving clinical screening is to identify problem areas and address these areas in relation to driving with minimal risk to the patient and therapist. The therapist should attempt to use clinical tools and tests during this phase that have the most significance to the driving task. Box 21-2 lists some of the more common clinical tests. Additional tools and devices are available on the market that can be used in the clinic with driver-related tasks and have a degree of face validity and statistical correlation (Box 21-3).

Engum et al[8] note the following: "Knowing the patient's diagnosis or pathology typically does not yield predictions about the patient's ability to drive. . . . Even

**Box 21-2**

**Examples of the Common Clinical Tests Used as Needed**

Trailsmaking Part A and B
Gardner Test of Visual Perceptual Skills
Motor-Free Visual Perceptual Test—3
Wechsler Adult Intelligence Scale (WAIS) Digit Symbol
WAIS Picture Completion
WAIS Digit Span
WAIS Block Design
Double letter cancellation task
Driver Performance Test
Cognitive Linguistic Quick Test
Mini-mental examination
Unilateral neglect test
Computerized reaction time
Road smart judgment test
Minnesota Rate of Manipulation
Gross Impairments Screening Battery of General Physical and Mental Abilities (GRIMPS)
Rey-Osterreith Complex Figure Test
Porteus Maze Test
Raven Progressive Matrices

loss of brain mass is not deemed to be an exact predictor of driving skills . . . neuropsychological tests which can detect gross organic impairment or provide useful catalogs of patients' impairments and abilities do not seem to assess driver potential."

Their 4-year research project with more than 230 brain-damaged patients led to the development of the Cognitive Behavioral Drivers Inventory (CBDI). This inventory is designed to assess aspects of cognitive functioning such as attention, concentration, rapid decision making, visual-motor speed and coordination, visual scanning and acuity,

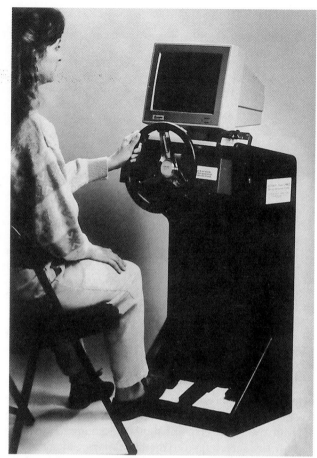

**Figure 21-6**   The Elemental Driving Simulator. (Courtesy Life Science Associates, Bayport, NY.)

and shifting attention from one task to another. Their results demonstrated that more than 95% of the patients receiving passing scores on the CBDI were judged independently by an on-the-road driving test as safe to operate a motor vehicle. Conversely, all patients who failed the CBDI were judged as unsafe drivers in the independently administered road test.[8] A subsequent study by some of the same authors in 1988 completed a double-blind test of the validity of the CBDI. Again, the authors found a high correlation between the results of the CBDI and the independent road test.[7] Although the CBDI is psychometrically strong, it has no face validity. Although the CBDI is useful, the Elemental Driver Simulator has face validity and may be better understood by patients as being relative to driving because it involves operating simulated primary car controls (Figure 21-6).

Gianutsos,[10] who assisted in developing the Elemental Driver Simulator, states, "road tests lack the basic psychometric requisites of tests—standardization, reliability and empirical validity." She describes the Elemental Driver Simulator as a "computer-based quasi-simulator that is based on objective, norm-referenced measures of the cognitive abilities regarded as critical for driving." These cognitive abilities include mental processing efficiency, simultaneous information processing, perceptual-motor skills, and impulse control. The Elemental Driver Simulator also attempts to measure insight and judgment by comparing self-appraisal with performance. Research by Gianutsos[10] and Engum et al[8] indicate a significant correlation in the Elemental Driving Simulator and CBDI. These researchers believe that their results confirm the reliability and validity of their clinical driving assessment programs. By using the Elemental Driver

Simulator or CBDI, the therapist obtains not only objective data but also recorded information relevant to the driving task. More importantly, data from these tests have demonstrated reliability and validity with published norms and standardized rules. The drawbacks to these tools are that they are expensive, time consuming to give, and require the use of a proper computer, which can be intimidating for an older person.

The predriving clinical screening can be organized similar to or along with a typical discharge evaluation of performance areas. The screening would be an obvious emphasis on driving skill requirements in an attempt to determine if the person is ready for referral for the on-the-road assessment or if the referral should be delayed to a better time. One should remember that if the person is referred too early, the results may produce negative consequences for the person's driving privileges. Discussion of the components of a predriving clinical screening follows.

**Physical Assessment**

The physical assessment should involve a brief functional look at the patient's active range of motion, muscle strength, sensory modalities, bilateral and unilateral gross and fine motor coordination, and any abnormalities such as spasticity, stereotypical patterns, and associated reactions. A slowing of physical functioning can affect reaction time in responding to stimuli in the environment. Slower reaction time among older drivers may be caused by strength and motor change or delayed visual processing. The loss of strength and range of motion can prevent the person from safely operating the primary or secondary controls of the vehicle. If the person has the necessary isolated control in the affected arm with appropriate sensation and smooth coordination, he or she may be able to continue using this arm for two-handed steering. In driving, an affected limb cannot be used at all if the necessary functional skills are not available since it could be unsafe and cause the driver to lose control of the vehicle. If the patient cannot use the affected arm safely, then various kinds of adaptive equipment and driving aids are available that can be used to aid one-handed steering or for reach of the turn signals (Figure 21-7). Some states require a spinner knob even if the person can palm the wheel and control it well with the remaining good arm. Compensatory techniques with special equipment can assist only with physically controlling a vehicle and do not resolve the person's other potential problem area with cognitive and visual skills.

Regarding lower extremity function, if the patient does not have isolated control in the right lower extremity, then the person will require a left foot gas pedal (see Figure 21-7). If the person has recovery in muscle strength, sensation, and coordination in the right leg, then the patient may be able to continue using this leg normally on the pedals. If the person wears a lightweight short leg brace and has some minimal movement in the ankle and all other factors—such as strength, sensation, and coordination—are good, then this person still may be able to use the right leg for gas and brake operation or just gas operation. If movement to the brake pedal is slow with or without a brace, or the hip or knee fatigues quickly, then teaching a two-footed driving method may be possible if this is allowed in the state of residence and the person has plantarflexion and dorsiflexion in the affected ankle. Proprioception is a must and should be evaluated carefully. The driver rehabilitation therapist will determine if the stroke survivor has good foot placement, good pedal regulation, and acceptable reaction time using the affected leg. The in-vehicle and on-the-road assessments will determine which method and what equipment, if any, is viable and necessary. After the moving assessment, the therapist may determine that the person requires equipment when initially it was thought they could use their affected upper or lower limb.

For secondary controls that are operated in a stationary position, the stroke survivor may be able to use compensatory methods for these controls; for example, using

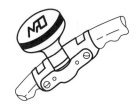

Spinner knob

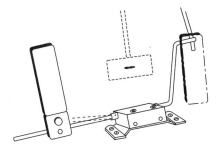

Left foot accelerator

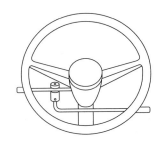

Turn signal crossover

**Figure 21-7**  Typical driving aids for a person recovering from cerebrovascular accident. (Courtesy Mobility Products and Design, Crow River Industries, Minneapolis, Minn.)

the left hand for inserting and turning the ignition key or operating the gearshift lever. If this is difficult, adaptive aids such as a gear selector crossover and key extension may be appropriate. Special panoramic mirrors can be beneficial when neck range of motion is limited or to increase visual awareness to the rear, sides, and blind spots (Figures 21-8 and 21-9). These mirrors do not compensate for loss of peripheral vision, so they are not useful for correction of homonymous hemianopsia.

## Visual Assessment

A visual assessment is crucial because driving depends so much on visual skills. A visual assessment is more than mere checking of a patient's visual acuity and depth perception. Scheiman,[32] a rehabilitation optometrist who works with patients with various diagnoses, states that good vision is more than clear vision: "the individual must have the ability to use his eyes for extended periods of time without discomfort, be able to analyze and interpret the incoming information, and respond to what is

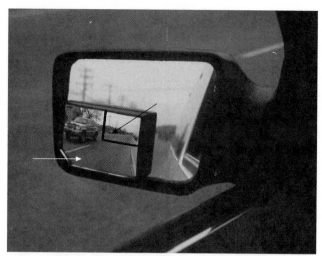

**Figure 21-8** SmartView Mirror by Interactive Driving Systems. This mirror eliminates the confusion noted in the typical spot convex mirror and increases rear vision by dividing the mirror into two areas. The outside half of the SmartView mirror *(white arrow)* shows objects in the blind spot of the vehicle, or Danger Zone. If a car is detected in the Danger Zone, the driver must not move in front of it. In this photograph the car shown is detected by the mirror to be in the driver's Danger Zone. The upper inside quadrant of the mirror *(black arrow)* is boxed and shows the Safe Zone. If a car is seen in the box—and stays in the box—the driver may move in front of it. (Courtesy Interactive Driving Systems, Cheshire, Conn.)

being seen." His experience indicates that nearly half of the patients admitted to a rehabilitation center with CVA or traumatic brain injury have visual system deficits, primarily in the area of binocular vision and accommodation. Other commonly reported vision problems include reduced visual acuity, decreased contrast sensitivity, visual field deficits, visual neglect, strabismus, oculomotor dysfunction, and accommodative and stereopsis dysfunction.

The stroke survivor should be evaluated visually according to the vision requirements for licensing of the state. This usually includes visual acuity of 20/40 in at least one eye and a total field of vision of at least 130 degrees. Eye test charts can be used to ascertain visual acuity. A commercially available stereoscopic vision tester that is self-contained and often used by driver licensing agencies may be applicable to a clinical setting. In addition to visual acuity, these machines also screen for depth perception or stereopsis, contrast sensitivity, road sign recognition, phoria, fusion, and horizontal perimeter vision. These machines have limitations that the therapist must take into consideration when using them and interpreting the results. For example, stereoscopic vision testers rely on binocular vision. If a patient does not possess binocular vision for whatever reason, this machine can be used only on a limited basis. Box 21-4 lists vision testing resources. If any suspicions of problem

areas arise, the stroke survivor should be referred to an eye care specialist. If the patient does not meet basic state requirements, an eye care specialist should see the patient before an on-the-road assessment.

Some states allow a loss of vision in the upper quadrant as long as the lateral median in the superior quadrant is normal (Figure 21-10). The exact degree of visual field available in each eye should be assessed quantitatively. Gianutsos and Suchoff[12] have suggested that perimetric and functional visual fields also are important to assess. A patient with complete homonymous hemianopsia may have only 90 degrees of total visual field. Whenever an occupational therapist suspects that a patient has any degree of peripheral vision loss, an objective test using machines such as the Goldman or Humphrey perimeter test should be used. An occupational therapy clinic generally cannot afford expensive, large objective perimeter machines that can quantitatively measure exact degrees of visual fields in all quadrants. The therapist can perform a finger confrontation test or use a horizontal perimeter tool and while this will confirm a complete hemianopsia, the test is not inclusive or objective. Before turning the patient down, the therapist must make a referral to a local eye care specialist that uses one of the machines noted previously to get an accurate report of the exact field of vision.

Aside from visual deficits that may occur because of the CVA, the occupational therapist also must consider the normal change in visual skills occurring as a result of the person's age. Testing eye range of motion, tracking, pursuits, and saccades can be done quickly with a few handheld sticks or other stimuli such as a tracking ball. As does any organ in the body, the eye loses some of its capability with age. The pupil of the eye becomes less elastic and restricts the amount of light let into the retina. Many elderly patients complain of difficulty driving at night or during weather conditions when the illumination is poor, such as in rain, fog, or snow. Cataracts, glaucoma, and macular degeneration are common among elderly persons. Cataracts, a clouding of the lenses, also can affect night driving and produce hazy vision during the day. Cataract surgery has a 90% success rate in a healthy older person who does not have comorbidities. Glaucoma, an increase in ocular pressure that damages the optic nerve and retinal nerve fibers, begins that to affect side vision first and then eventually compromises central vision. Glaucoma is a treatable condition, and a referral to the appropriate eye care specialist is important before performing the on-the-road assessment. The therapist should consider diabetic retinopathy for a person with a history of diabetes. When the degree of macular degeneration is so great that it affects the central vision to a point that the person cannot see anything in this visual area, then the patient needs to stop driving. Therapists can assess visual scanning, awareness, and attention in the clinic by using some of the subtests

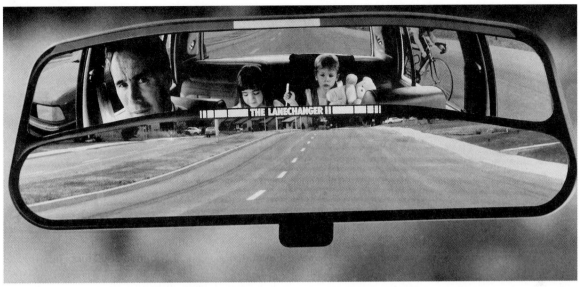

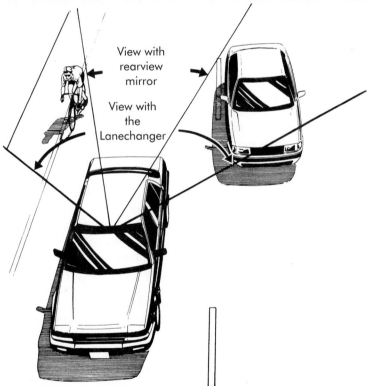

**Figure 21-9** **A,** The Lanechanger mirror combines a standard rearview mirror with a convex mirror. **B,** This convex mirror provides a wider angle of vision and increased safety. (Courtesy The Lanechanger, Quebec, Canada.)

**Box 21-4**

**Resources for Vision Testing Equipment**

Bernell Corporation
4016 North Home St.
Mishawaka, IN 46545
(800) 348-2225

Keystone View
Division of Mast Development
2212 East 12th St.
Davenport, IA 52803

Porto-Clinic
Driver Testing Equipment
1309 South Main Ave.
Scranton, PA 18504

Stereo Optical Company
3539 North Kenton Ave.
Chicago, IL 60641
(800) 344-9500

Visual Resource, Inc.
P.O. Box 51524
Bowling Green, KY 42102
(502) 842-5965

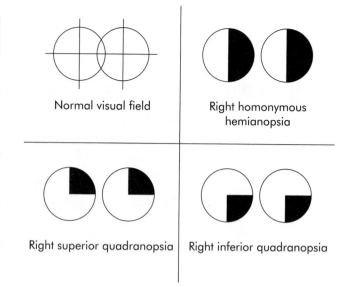

**Figure 21-10** Representation of normal visual field in the eyes and typical visual field defects.

in the visual-perceptual and cognitive tests discussed later in this chapter.

Because speed and movement can influence visual and visual-perceptual skills, the therapist must make the final determination of the proficiency and effectiveness of these areas for driving in the vehicle and in the dynamic moving traffic environment. For example, the speed of a vehicle decreases visual acuity and side vision. If a person has 200 degrees of visual field, at 20 miles per hour, the field is reduced to 104 degrees; at 40 miles per hour, to 70 degrees; and at 60 miles per hour, to 40 degrees. Speed also decreases visual acuity; the faster the speed, the less time available to react to visual stimuli in the environment.[34] The Visual Attention Analyzer Model 2000 (Visual Resources, Inc., Chicago, Ill.) assesses the size of the useful field of view and comprises three subtests to evaluate processing speed, divided attention, and selective attention (see Chapter 16).

### Visual-Perception and Cognitive Assessment

According to Toglia,[39] the limitation to the deficit-specific approach to perception is that "it equates difficulty in performance of a specific task with a deficit . . . [and] does not consider the underlying reasons for failure or the conditions that influence performance." For example, a patient may score low on a typical occupational therapy clinical test of visual-perceptual skills; nevertheless, the results may be a consequence of reduced visual acuity or accommodation and not necessarily a specific visual-perceptual deficit.

A stroke survivor who has serious visual-perceptual deficits will have difficulty throughout rehabilitation.[41] The occupational therapist will complete documentation and observations of deficits in these areas during routine evaluation and treatment. The stroke survivor probably should not be referred to the driver rehabilitation therapist until the deficit areas no longer interfere with basic ADL. If the therapist understands the definition of each visual-perceptual category and the way deficits in each area affect a person's basic self-care skills, a further analysis of driving tasks can show the way persistent problems in these areas can interfere with driving performance (see Chapter 18).

Driving requires a combination of perceptual skills in which cognitive performance plays a major role. Strong cognitive abilities are fundamental to attentiveness in the driving task, recognition of stimuli, and choice of the appropriate way to respond. A decline in cognitive abilities can significantly influence a person's ability to plan, judge, and act adequately. A cognitively impaired person may have difficulty maneuvering a vehicle through rapidly changing traffic with many unexpected actions and reactions from other drivers, passengers, pedestrians, and bicyclists. Cognitive impairment has been linked to higher motor vehicle crash rates in elderly individuals.[1] Problem areas may involve attention, orientation, concentration, learning (short-term memory), and problem solving. Diffuse cognitive deficits occur more frequently in patients with large frontal strokes, visuospatial deficits in right hemisphere strokes, and apraxia in left hemisphere strokes.[43] Unilateral neglect has been reported in half of the patients with right brain damage and in 20% to 25% with left brain damage.[37] Diller and Weinberg[6] report that "patients with left hemiparesis often experience accidents that are related to difficulties in dealing with space, while accidents in patients with right hemiparesis are often related to slowness in processing information."

Patients are generally more aware of motor problems than they are of cognitive problems.[14] Gresham et al[13] note that "unawareness of the stroke (or its manifestations) is often found in patients with lesions in the nondominant hemisphere. It can lead to impulsive, unsafe behavior in a patient who may otherwise appear relatively normal with respect to physical functioning." Patients' poor insight into their own problem areas can be dangerous because patients may not be aware of serious driver errors and the potentially fatal consequences of their actions.

The occupational therapist can use some common verbal and written tasks to assess the areas of visual perceptual functioning such as spatial relations, visual discrimination, form constancy, depth perception and visual memory, sequential memory, and visual closure. Two commonly used tests are the Gardner Test of Visual Perceptual Skills and the Motor-Free Visual Perception Test—3 that was standardized in 2003 for adults age 70 or older. The Motor-Free Visual Perception Test—Vertical is for those who have difficulty with horizontally presented stimuli such as stroke survivors.

Therapists can use a variety of cognitive tests to assess memory, language, orientation, attention, concentration, reasoning, and problem solving. The Helm-Estabrooks Cognitive Linguistic Quick Test can be administered in 20 to 30 minutes; is standardized for adults with acquired neurologic dysfunction, ages 18 to 89; and can be used to identify a person's cognitive strengths and weaknesses. This test gives a "snapshot" assessment of the status of these five cognitive domains: attention, memory, language, executive functions, and visuospatial skills. (see Chapter 18).

During the administration of these clinical tests, one must keep in mind that these tests are static and two dimensional and do not begin to simulate the dynamics of the driving task. French and Hanson[9] stated "controversy continues about which cognitive-perceptual assessments are the best predictors of behind-the-wheel performance." The authors summarize studies performed by Galski, Bruno, and Elhe in 1992 that found a significant correlation between seven tests: "Part A of the Trailsmaking Test, the Rey-Osterreith Complex Figure Test, the Porteus Maze Test, the Visual Form Discrimination, the Double Letter Cancellation, the Wechsler Adult Intelligence Scale—Revised Block Design Test, and Raven's Progressive Matrices and the behind-the-wheel evaluation. . . . the [continued] research suggests that a combination of neuropsychological testing, visual screening, physical functioning, and actual driving (simulators and on-the-road evaluations) is necessary to predict driving performance."

Engum et al[8] define basic operational and behavioral skills as "attention, concentration, rapid decision-making, stimulus discrimination/response differentiation, sequencing, visual-motor speed and coordination, visual scanning

**Table 21-3**

### Effects of Various Deficits in a Stroke Survivor on Driving Performance

| TYPE OF DEFICIT | EFFECT ON DRIVING PERFORMANCE |
|---|---|
| Higher cognitive functions, memory, ability to learn | Cannot remember route to take to location or loses way if makes wrong turn; may not remember road names but can remember the route; severe deficits in higher functions may impede safe driving; unless the patient recovering from cerebrovascular accident is a new driver, the inability to learn new tasks may not impede safe driving; may require directions to be repeated |
| Motor | Usually does not impede safe driving because compensatory driving techniques or adaptive driving aids can be used |
| Disturbances in balance and coordination | May impede car transfers or loading of mobility device (e.g., wheelchair or walker); steering device, left-foot accelerator, or turn signal adaptation may compensate for inability to use the upper or lower extremity |
| Somatosensory | Generally does not interfere with driving because a person does not use an extremity with lack of sensation or with limiting pain while driving |
| Vision disorders | Severe visual loss or ocular motility disturbances may impede safe driving; the deficit may lead to the patient not meeting driver licensing requirements; persons with homonymous hemianopsia are not allowed to drive in most states; other age-related deficits such as glaucoma, cataracts, and diabetic retinopathy may impede safe driving |
| Unilateral neglect | A contraindication for safe driving |
| Speech and language | Expressive aphasia, dysarthria, or apraxias of speech are usually not problems in driving, although attempting to carry on a conversation while driving may cause distraction; receptive aphasia may impede the driver from understanding directions or conversation |
| Pain | The unaffected extremities may be used to drive; does not impede driving unless it is so severe it causes a distraction |

and acuity and attention shifting." Table 21-3 describes several performance areas and the way deficits in these areas can affect driving performance.

An appropriate end to the predriving clinical screening may involve several tests to assess procedural memory for driving, knowledge of road rules, and road sign and/or situational problem solving, reasoning, and judgment. There are several formal tests that can be used. The Driver Performance Test, distributed by the Advanced Driving Skills Institute (Clearwater, Fla.), is a video of simulated real-world driving scenes and provides insight into the patient's perceptual capabilities, psychomotor responses, and decision-making strategies. Using a driver education defensive driving technique of identifying, predicting, deciding, and executing, the Driver Performance Test requires the patient to search for hazardous situations or conditions, identify potential and immediate hazards, predict the effect of the hazard, decide the way to evade the hazard, and execute evasive driving actions.[42] The drawback to this test is that it takes about 45 minutes to administer. Additional time is then necessary to review the answer video with the patient, an essential step for any learning or understanding to take place for the patient or the therapist.

Because the Driver Performance Test has no statistical validity, the therapist should decide whether to use valuable time administering it during this phase or letting the driver rehabilitation therapist use it in the next phase of the process. An important consideration is that this rapidly timed test may produce stress in the stroke survivor because it requires quick problem solving and decision making, marking on an answer sheet while having attention divided, and retaining information. The test taker has only a few seconds to choose an answer and then must go on to the next traffic scene because the test has no built-in delay or pause. If the test taker gets behind, he or she may become disorganized or distracted and not be able to respond to the next scene. Although quick thinking and reaction are important for driving, the Driver Performance Test may be a better tool to use after the patient has passed all clinical tests and road tests. In other words, the test may be a more effective tool to use when the therapist determines that the patient needs more practice, training, or review in the areas tested by the Driver Performance Test.

A unique Power Point–based driver education course is available from Drivers Edge (InterActive Enterprises Inc., Palatine, Ill.). that can be used to assess driving knowledge, road sign recognition, problem solving, and judgment. The course is designed to be worked through by the patient in the presence of the therapist, who can immediately assess the person's knowledge and judgment skills. The lessons covering all aspects of the driving environment use real traffic scenes, animations, graphics, short videos, and sound effects (Box 21-5). A computer is required.

## Box 21-5

### Resources for Assessment of Driving Knowledge and Judgment

Driver Performance Test and Safe Performance On Road Test:
Advanced Driving Skills Institute
19321 U.S. 19 North, Suite 401
Clearwater, FL 34624
1-800-327-6781
www.advdrivskills.com

Drivers Edge Rehabilitation Course:
InterActive Enterprises, Inc.
852 Martin Drive
Palatine, IL 60067
1-847-358-9508 (fax)
interactiveenterprises@comcast.net

## IMPORTANCE OF THE COMBINATION OF A PREDRIVING CLINIC SCREENING AND AN ON-THE-ROAD TEST

A comprehensive driver assessment should involve the two phases of a clinical assessment and an on-the-road assessment. In fairness to the stroke survivor, the therapist's decision regarding the patient's visual, perceptual, and cognitive abilities for driving should not be based solely on a clinical test or solely on an on-the-road test. In a 1994 review of driver assessment methods at the Jewish Rehabilitation Center in Montreal, Canada, the chief of research and her associates found that 95% of their patients were given on-the-road tests because no clear cutoff score based on typical clinical tests was reliable in predicting whether a person was unsafe to drive.[19] Earlier studies suggest that persons who pass tests for cognitive deficits do not require road tests.[23,33] Experienced certified driver rehabilitation specialists typically do not agree with this opinion, and other more recent studies have found that clinical testing alone is insufficient and recommend a mandatory driving test.[4,18,45]

A therapist should not deny a stroke survivor the opportunity to have the road test based on the clinical findings only unless the patient has obvious serious performance issues or does not meet the basic requirements given by the department of driver licensing. The therapist at this point can make only an assumption regarding significant deficits and the potential for them to interfere with driving performance. There is little correlation between typical clinical tests and real driving performance, so the therapist performing the formal driving test on the road should make the final conclusion regarding the stroke survivor's driving abilities. Occupational therapists who are experienced driver rehabilitation therapists say that some patients who do well on clinical tests perform poorly in the car. However, they agree that some patients who do poorly in the clinic perform well in the familiar environment of the car. Again, the decision lies in the occupational therapist's skill to combine clinical observations and analysis with clinical reasoning and judgment of in-car performance.

## DETERMINATION OF READINESS FOR THE ROAD TEST

Driving is one of the most complex activities a person may perform, requires integration of many performance areas, and should always be at the top of the ADL pyramid. Because of its complexity, driving should be one of the last ADL attempted following a stroke.[27] The stroke survivor must have reached all other ADL goals before being ready for the difficult ADL of driving. With abbreviated inpatient rehabilitation stays for stroke survivors becoming the norm, the driving evaluation should not take place until the patient has been discharged from the outpatient treatment program or has recovered to a maximal level of independence in the performance of other ADL. If the person is referred too early, he or she may not do well and may lose driving privileges. If the person is referred too late, then he or she may begin driving without an evaluation or the necessary medical approval and put other persons at risk.

Timeliness of the referral for the formal road test is important. Typically, the appropriate time for a referral to the driver rehabilitation therapist is not until 2 to 4 months after discharge from the inpatient facility. An exception to this timeline is if the person suffered a mild stroke or transient ischemic attack and recovered quickly with minimal residual deficits. This person may be evaluated as early as 2 to 4 weeks after discharge from the inpatient facility. The clinical occupational therapist is the best person to determine whether the stroke survivor is ready for the formal road test before discharge as an inpatient or to determine an estimation of time for readiness after discharge to include in the team's discharge planning and final recommendations to the patient and family. Input from all team members should be sought. The physician should provide only medical clearance when all parties agree that the stroke survivor is ready for the on-the-road assessment.

A timely referral by the physician or other team members may reduce the likelihood that the patient may begin driving with no supervision from a family member or friend. The physician should communicate effectively to the stroke survivor that he or she should abstain from all driving until an evaluation has been completed. This recommendation should be documented and verbally communicated to the person's caregivers. For liability protection of the rehabilitation facility and team members, the patient should be required to sign a form demonstrating understanding of the recommendations given and indicating willingness to comply. Each team member that has verbally given the same recommendations to the patient should document in the progress notes or discharge summary when and what instructions were given to the patient. If it appears that the person will not comply with the recommendations, the rehabilitation team (doctor or therapists) should advise the department of driver licensing.

The therapist should caution the patient and the family against practicing a week or so before the appointment with the driver rehabilitation therapist. This strategy is unsafe and needless and puts the patient at risk to be sued by parties for driving while impaired, which can cause personal and property damage. In addition, insurance companies may be able to claim fraud and violation of their regulations, so that they are not monetarily responsible for any damages ordered by a court. The potential consequences are not worth the risk and associated liability.

## OCCUPATIONAL THERAPIST AS A DRIVER REHABILITATION THERAPIST

The impact of persisting sensory, perceptual, motor, and cognitive deficits on driving risk levels must be addressed through an objective, formal evaluation on the road and in a specially adapted evaluation vehicle. The professional performing this part of the driving evaluation must have a medical background, knowledge of driver education principles, and special training and skill in in-vehicle techniques and methods. The allied health professional in this role is called the driver rehabilitation therapist to distinguish the therapist from a commercial driving school instructor.

According to the 2003 membership directory of the Association of Driver Rehabilitation Specialists, most therapists certified by this organization have an occupational therapy background. This organization offers a certification examination process leading to designation as a certified driver rehabilitation specialist. For education and knowledge of the field of driver rehabilitation, the Association of Driver Rehabilitation Specialists offers an annual conference. Adaptive Mobility Services, Inc., based in Orlando, Florida, offers progressive educational workshops for the allied health professional who needs didactic and practical learning in the field at various levels. They offer an annual symposium on Community Mobility that addresses all issues for the therapist, including driving. In 2002 the AOTA formed a driving network for therapists to use for networking. The AOTA now has a specialty section listserv for its members to communicate with one another through e-mail. They also have educational opportunities available at their annual conference, online courses, and planned specialized workshops. In 2004, AOTA will have a position paper and practice guidelines for driver rehabilitation. Box 21-6 has contact information.

After receiving a referral on a stroke survivor for the road test, the first step for the driver rehabilitation therapist

**Box 21-6**

**Resources for Professional Education, Driver Education Materials, and Networking**

AAA
Traffic Safety
1000 AAA Drive, Box 78
Heathrow, FL 32746-5080

Adaptive Mobility Services, Inc. (AMS)
Department of Continuing Education
1000 Delaney Ave.
Orlando, FL 32806
(407) 426-8020
www.adaptivemobility.com

American Occupational Therapy Association (AOTA)
4720 Montgomery Lane
Bethesda, MD 20814-1220
(800) 877-1383
www.aota.org/members/area3/index.asp

Association of Driver Rehabilitation Specialists (ADED;
   formerly called Association of Driver Educators for the
   Disabled)
711 South Vienna
Ruston, LA 71270
(800) 290-2344
www.aded.net or www.driver-ed.org

Safety Industries
P.O. Box 1137
McGill, NV 89318
1-775-235-7766

is to talk with the primary clinical occupational therapist in the inpatient or outpatient unit to obtain any pertinent information about the patient. If any questions arise about skill performance areas that the occupational therapist cannot answer, the driver rehabilitation therapist should talk with the person in the appropriate discipline, such as physical therapy, speech therapy, neuropsychology, or rehabilitation optometry.

Second, the driver rehabilitation therapist interviews the patient and the family. The therapist should review the medical history with the patient to assess any pertinent information that should be considered during the road test. The therapist should review the patient's progress in rehabilitation, discuss the unaccomplished goals in each discipline, and confirm all facts regarding the patient's driving history, driving circumstances, and other contextual information. Driving abilities may be impaired as a result of adverse drug effects or age-related factors such as physiologic changes and age-associated diseases and conditions including arthritis, cataracts, memory loss, and hearing loss. The therapist should explore the patient and family's knowledge and perspective of problems with other coexisting medical conditions in areas that may not necessarily be related to the CVA

diagnosis so as to understand the whole person. For example, if the stroke survivor has a history of diabetes and has had the right leg amputated, the driver rehabilitation therapist would be prudent to explore the potential problems that may occur in the patient's left leg. This may affect equipment recommendations in terms of a left foot gas pedal versus a set of hand controls.

The therapist should check the person's driver's license and ensure that it is still valid and should note any restrictions already placed on the license. A driver's license is considered public property, so the therapist can contact the appropriate office with the department of driver licensing to check on the status of the person's license. Most departments of driver licensing do not allow a person to drive if the license has been suspended or has expired. Most states have a medical advisory board that needs to become familiar with the driver rehabilitation therapist and the area that he or she covers. With the appropriate medical approval, the medical advisory board may issue a temporary driving permit for evaluation purposes only. The patient and family should be told that this permit is not to be used to practice before the road test appointment.

The on-the-road phase of the driver evaluation is crucial to the final decision about a person's driving abilities. The value of the in-vehicle and the in-traffic assessment cannot be underestimated. The professional performing this step must have knowledge of driver education principles, road rules, and state laws and must know how to assess all driving abilities in the car. This person must know the breakdown of performance components involved in specific driving tasks and must understand the purpose of planning a specific route for each person, what to look for, and the things that can be done to elicit underlying suspected behaviors. This professional is not a passive passenger sitting on the right side of the car simply giving directions. The person must have verbal, visual, and physical skills required to control the driver and the vehicle throughout the test.[30] The therapist must know how to approach the driver with constructive criticism and how to react and handle the emotional and psychological factors that come into play with this portion of the evaluation.

The occupational therapist's unique skill in analysis of activity and occupational performance is of great benefit in this role. The therapist's keen observation skills and knowledge of what to look for are also invaluable during the in-car work. Because the therapist understands the diagnosis and all implications so well, the therapist can plan a route specific to each patient. The therapist should strive for ecological validity, which simply means that the (evaluation and) training takes into consideration the actual environment from which the patient comes and to which the patient will return. The environment includes home, yard, neighborhood, and community: where the person works, plays, and/or goes to school.[28]

The driver rehabilitation therapist must have a working knowledge of deficits associated with a CVA, age-related issues, medication implications, and the relationship of all to the driving task. The driver rehabilitation therapist must appreciate the importance of driving to the stroke survivor and work in the patient's best interest while also considering the well-being of the public. Although only an allied health professional should be performing the predriving clinical screening based on professional licensure, ethical standards, and guidelines, many hospitals and rehabilitation centers consider using a commercial driving school instructor or a retired driver educator from a school to complete the on-the-road assessment so they do not have to invest in an evaluation car. They may consider the liability cost reduced by using a driving school, but this is not always the case.

## USE OF DRIVING SCHOOL INSTRUCTORS AND DRIVER EDUCATORS

The use of an individual without an allied health background in this role should be studied carefully and considered by the rehabilitation team, the employer, and legal counsel. This decision could result in an inadequate outcome if the person performing the road test does not understand diagnoses, disabilities, and the way to observe and assess each performance skill level in the car. The person's educational background, personal references, work history, and working knowledge of diagnoses should be considered carefully. State requirements for licensing as a commercial driving school instructor varies greatly, with no special training required to work with persons with disabilities. In many states a person can obtain a commercial driving instructor license by having a high school diploma, a good driving record with no criminal record, and proof of good health. Some states do require taking an in-depth driver education course to be licensed as a commercial driving instructor; however, other states require less. Many driving schools exist to teach new drivers to pass a road test so that they can obtain driver's licenses; the focus is not on analyzing driving behavior. In summary, a typical commercial driving school instructor is usually not a professional, has no understanding of disabilities, and tends to concentrate on teaching a person to pass a road test. The instructor's motivation is often to provide a revenue-generating service. A rehabilitation driving program would need to find a knowledgeable and experienced driving school instructor who has also obtained specialized training with disabilities. An instructor listed as a certified driving rehabilitation specialist (CDRS) with the Association of Driver Rehabilitation Specialists (formerly called Association of Driver Educators for the Disabled [ADED]) will have met these criteria but the credential does not speak to competency.

A driver educator may have a more professional approach. This individual has a professional college degree in education with special study in driver education and so is well equipped to educate a person regarding the driving task. This person, although having the professional background, would not have the medical background for understanding all medical implications of a stroke survivor. The biggest limiting factor today to finding a driver educator is that many high school driver education programs are being closed because of funding and liability issues; therefore fewer individuals opt for special study in this field, and consequently, fewer study programs exist for them. If a driver educator is used, the therapist must work with and advise this person about the patient's strengths and weaknesses and probable behaviors that may be observed or expected based on the predriving clinical screening. The therapist also can assist the driver educator in handling particular problem areas and provide recommendations for appropriate remedial training to see whether the driver can compensate for problems seen in the car. A Driver Educator can be similarly located by ADED as just noted.

If the driving instructor or driver educator has little or no experience working with stroke survivors, the therapist must remain closely involved with the road test to ensure proper and continued understanding of the driver's deficits and that the progress or lack of progress is observed correctly. The therapist may need to be in the evaluation vehicle only for the first and last session, but the therapist's concurrence with the recommendations and findings of the person performing the in-car assessment is important to document. The driver rehabilitation therapist should remain as the supervisor of the person performing the road test and can be held responsible for any decisions or actions made by this person. The members of the "driving team," comprised of the driver rehabilitation therapist and the driving school instructor or driver educator, always should keep in mind that they must follow a standard of care, show reasonable judgment, and avoid negligent action in their work and decisions. Any accidents or collisions in an evaluation car or wrongly clearing a person for driving can produce potential litigation against all parties associated with the driver evaluation process. The liability is not passed completely onto the person just performing the road test. The therapist and/or rehabilitation team that referred the stroke survivor to a particular person for the road test may share liability if wrong decisions are made or poor conclusions are drawn and incompetence is proved.

## VEHICLE AND EQUIPMENT ASSESSMENT

Before conducting the road test, the driver rehabilitation therapist must review the occupational therapist's predriving screening or perform one if the original screening is more than 6 months old. This information will assist the therapist in preparing for the potential deficit areas the patient may have and what adaptive equipment and driving route may need to be used. Determination of the vehicle and adaptive driving equipment appropriate for each patient depends largely on the physical and functional assessment results. The driver rehabilitation therapist and, if used, the driving school instructor or driver educator must objectively evaluate the equipment needs in the clinic and then in the evaluation vehicle. Final determination of equipment needs should be confirmed in a moving assessment in the evaluation vehicle; however, the patient's own vehicle must be considered at some point. The majority of adults, particularly elderly adults, typically own a vehicle with automatic transmission, which is required for the installation of most driving aids.

Usually the driving equipment needed by a person with left or right hemiplegia is minimal and not costly (between $75 and $450); but additional costs exist for special instruction and training on the devices in a dual-controlled vehicle. This training and practice should help prevent any accidents and allow the patient to become familiar with the devices. Proper use of the equipment also should be ascertained in a dynamic situation; however, the driver should be given sufficient learning time before being taken into complex traffic situations. A driving range or neighborhood with light traffic and speeds of 15 to 25 miles per hour is a safe, undemanding, and nonthreatening environment in which to start. Even if the patient has no equipment needs, this environment provides time for the patient to become familiar with the evaluation vehicle and the verbal directions of the therapist or instructor.

## ON-THE-ROAD DRIVING ASSESSMENT

A driver must make multiple decisions constantly and interpret information correctly and quickly for safe driving (Figure 21-11). Smith[35] states the following: "Driving

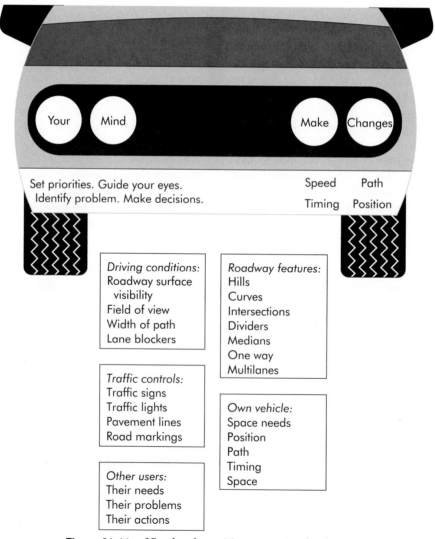

**Figure 21-11**    Visual and cognitive processing for driving.

a modern passenger vehicle on a clear day in light traffic does not overtax any dimension of performance (perceptual, cognitive, or physical). However, in heavy traffic at high speed, at night on poorly marked roads, at a complex intersection, or in a potential accident situation, the demands placed on drivers can exceed their abilities."

Smith[34] goes on to describe a step procedure necessary for safe driving:

"1. The driver must see or hear a situation developing (stimulus registered and sampled at the visual, auditory, or perceptual level).
2. The driver must recognize it (stimulus recognition at the cognitive level).
3. The driver must decide the way to respond (cognitive level).
4. The driver must execute the physical maneuver (motor level)."

Each individual should be given the opportunity for a behind-the-wheel evaluation with the exception of persons who do not meet state driver's licensing guidelines. Even if the evaluation consists only of driving range maneuvers, the mistakes observed on the range may demonstrate to the patient the potential danger in actual traffic. According to Gianutsos,[11] the New York State Vocational and Educational Services for Individuals with Disabilities committee that addressed this issue concluded in its report on August 13, 1993, that no candidate should be advanced to driving without a behind-the-wheel test. Numerous studies have investigated driving after a stroke or head injury. These patients can be most difficult to assess for driving because they may not only have physical disabilities that are readily visible but also may have more subtle visual, visuoperceptual, or cognitive problems not easily apparent by observation.

More than half of all stroke survivors who drove cars before their strokes stop driving afterward.[21] Factors that are associated most commonly with driving cessation are older age at the time of stroke and the presence of cognitive deficits.[13] Wilson and Smith[44] investigated the driving performance of patients after stroke using two control groups on a planned driving course. The results indicated that the patients recovering from stroke performed more poorly than did the control subjects. Specific problems identified included difficulties entering and leaving an interstate, lack of awareness of other potential interacting vehicles, and difficulty in reacting to emergency situations. Analyses of the more likely performance components causing the driving errors were concluded to be difficulty in visual scanning, lane positioning, appropriate speed, coordination of separate visual scans, interaction with same directional traffic, and maintaining a safe distance from other vehicles.

A simple 5- to 10-minute road test given by a state driver's license examiner is not adequate to assess fully all areas that must be considered in driving after a stroke.

The examiner primarily is evaluating physical control of the vehicle during basic skills tests such as perpendicular or parallel parking, backing up, three-point turns, and right and left turns. Many times drivers are not even tested in traffic, or if they are, traffic exposure is light and short. The panel of the U.S. Department of Health and Human Resources that determined poststroke rehabilitation guidelines reflected in their report that "stroke survivors may be able to pass a driving test despite having visuospatial deficits or problems with easy distractibility, impulsive behaviors, or slowed decision making that may impair their ability to drive safely under unpredictable road conditions."[13] In addition, the driver license examiner rarely has knowledge of all the adaptive equipment available for physical deficits to determine recommendations. The stroke survivor requires a medical-oriented evaluation and training in a dual-controlled vehicle, neither of which is available from driver license examiners. If adaptive equipment is required for continued safe driving, the stroke survivor generally requires a longer period of training because compensation or adaptation involves breaking old habits (e.g., using the left foot on a left side mounted gas pedal rather than the right foot).

Driving is an overlearned skill for the experienced elderly driver, so the on-the-road driving assessment phase generally does not require teaching the patient to drive. Many operational components come back naturally to the patient unless a residual memory problem associated with dementia, agnosia, or apraxia is evident. Patients' strategic skills may be impaired by any visual, visual-perceptual, or cognitive deficits that remain. Not to be overlooked is the increased anxiety and stress that this phase of the driver evaluation can invoke for the person being evaluated. The driver rehabilitation therapist in a supportive, therapeutic way can be a valuable asset during the first 15 minutes of the road test. The therapist should make every effort to relax the patient and to let the patient know what to expect and how the verbal directions will be given. The evaluation car may be different from the stroke survivor's, and this can affect his or her disposition. The evaluation vehicle may have many different types of adaptive equipment, and the therapist needs to know how to remove equipment that may get in the way of a driver. For example, if the brake or gas rod of a hand control is interfering with a driver who is using his or her right foot moving on and off the factory gas pedal and brake, the therapist should know how to remove these rods for this patient.[29] By allowing time to let the person become familiar with the evaluation vehicle, the driver may be more relaxed for the rest of the test. The driver rehabilitation therapist always should keep in mind how important driving is to each person and how crucial the final decision is on the rest of the person's life. This perspective aids the therapist in spending sufficient and quality time during the work in the car.

The therapist must understand and plan the goals, objectives, and structuring for the in-traffic assessment. Every mile of road the patient is requested to drive should have a purpose. Ramsey,[30] a driver educator from West Virginia who has more than 30 years of experience working with persons with diverse disabilities, states that if driver evaluators or educators go straight for more than a mile, they are "taking a joy ride" and are not assessing effectively a person's ability to drive. Driving straight is easier than making vehicle and speed adjustments for left and right turns and for merging. The visual and mental demands on the driver are greatly increased in executing multiple-step procedures with divided attention demands. The therapist can use a planned route by which to evaluate every patient. The route for a stroke survivor should focus on problem areas seen with the patient's particular deficit areas. Routes familiar and unfamiliar to the driver may have to be used to expose the person to many complex driving situations. If possible, the driver rehabilitation therapist should start or end the test in the driver's home environment, because the patient likely will perform better and be more relaxed on familiar roads. With this ecologic validity, the driver rehabilitation therapist can get an understanding of the traffic and roads that the stroke survivor normally encounters during driving and can get a picture of how well the driver plans his or her routes. If routes are dangerous, such as one that includes an unprotected left turn against heavy traffic, the driver rehabilitation therapist can counsel the driver about the danger of this maneuver and the high risk and accident potential of this situation and can assist in finding a safer route.

The therapist must be flexible during the road test, guiding the patient on and off the planned route as needed. For example, if a stroke survivor with poor insight and visual awareness starts to miss a stop sign or run through a yield sign without looking both ways or does not show any reaction to a lane ending sign, then this person should be taken off the planned route for instruction and practice to see whether improvement is possible. This driver should not be taken into more complex driving situations in which a hazard may be posed to other road users until the problem is corrected. A stroke survivor with expressive and receptive aphasia may be distracted from the driving scene while attempting to process the therapist's verbal directions during driving. In this case the patient may benefit from being taken around the familiar home environment and allowed to self-direct in driving from one destination to another such as the bank, drugstore, or doctor's office.

Common driving errors committed by elderly drivers may be related to vision, visual perception or cognitive dysfunction, or an overall decline (Box 21-7). The driver not only must see objects in the path of travel but also must understand their implications for safety to adjust

---

**Box 21-7**

**Common Driving Errors in Older Drivers**

Difficulty backing up and making turns
Not seeing traffic signs or other cars quickly enough
Difficulty in locating and retrieving information from dashboard displays and traffic signs
Delayed glare recovery when driving at night
Not checking rearview mirrors and blind spots
Bumping into curbs and objects
Not yielding to oncoming traffic or right-of-way vehicles
Irregular or slow vehicle speeds

---

driving accordingly. The most frequent citations for older drivers, noted by McKnight[22] in his report "Driver and Pedestrian Training," involved failure to heed stop signs, traffic lights, no left turn signs, and other signs and signals. Underwood[40] notes that "safe driving requires complex cognitive skills, including vigilance, rapid visual scanning with attention to environmental detail, rapid processing of multiple stimuli in several sensory modalities, adequate judgment, and rapid decision-making."

The therapist should have strong clinical experience and confidence in the ability to assess a stroke survivor's skill in each performance area of physical, visual, visual-perceptual, cognitive, and communication skills. Emotional and behavioral factors and characteristics also come into play many times. The therapist then must know the way the patient's performance level in each area may affect driving performance. Because of the importance of synergistic performance of many skills for safe driving, activity analysis is a valuable tool in which the occupational therapist is well trained. Breaking the driving task down to its simple performance components can assist greatly with relevant analysis of the clinical test results and in starting a patient in the car in a nonthreatening and stress-reducing fashion. Because driving requires certain abilities in each of the performance areas, the driver rehabilitation therapist should know the way to assess performance levels in each area in the evaluation vehicle and dynamic traffic situations (Box 21-8).

A well-planned road and traffic route for the on-the-road assessment has the following purposes:

- To assess the driver's ability to enter and exit the vehicle safely and store any mobility aids efficiently
- To assess the driver's understanding and operation of all vehicle primary and secondary controls
- To assess in the moving vehicle the driver's need for adaptive devices or techniques for driving safely (e.g., using two feet to operate the gas and brake pedals may be safer than using the right leg on both pedals if the patient has a leg brace, hip flexion weakness, or slow reaction time)
- To assess the driver's operational and strategic abilities in various traffic, speed, and road conditions

## Box 21-8

### Examples of Driving Behaviors to Be Observed During the In-Traffic Assessment

Visually searching traffic environment (20 to 30 seconds ahead)

Demonstrating safe physical control of the vehicle at all times

Maintaining safe speeds

Smooth braking

Demonstrating good lane selection

Maintaining a safe following distance

Backing the vehicle

Making turns

Navigating curves

Changing lanes and merging

Judging gaps at intersections

Making passing maneuvers

Performing parallel and angle parking

Interacting with traffic in a low-risk manner

Entering and exiting expressways

Using turn signals appropriately

Demonstrating proper use of all mirrors

Checking blind spots

Finding and using turn lanes properly

Observing and responding to road signs

---

- To assess the driver's memory for the roads and paths to various common locations
- To support the findings of the clinical assessment and be able to assess driving performance in the real dynamic driving environment

## ADAPTIVE EQUIPMENT MOBILITY PRESCRIPTION

After the stroke survivor has been through the predriving clinical screening, the vehicle and equipment assessment, and the on-the-road assessment, the driver rehabilitation therapist makes a decision regarding the stroke survivor's driving abilities. The occupational therapist's clinical reasoning and judgment skills are invaluable at this point to consider all observations, findings, and results from both the clinical assessment and the on-the-road assessment. Results from both phases, as well as conversations with family members and other team members, must be considered in drawing a final conclusion.

If the therapist determines that the stroke survivor can continue to drive, then the driver rehabilitation therapist should write an evaluation summary supporting licensure and specifying vehicle and equipment recommendations as needed. The 2000 edition of the American Heritage Dictionary of the English Language, Fourth Edition, defines *prescription* as "a formula directing the preparation of something." In the context of driving, the term *mobility prescription* is used to direct the patient, the equipment installer, and possibly a funding source to the specific equipment needs of the patient.[29]

The document should be easy to read and understand, written specifically for the stroke survivor and his or her vehicle. Sometimes the therapist may need to be more descriptive than just recommending a "left foot gas pedal." In other words, if the patient prefers a quick-release model so a spouse can drive the car without worrying about inadvertently stepping on the left gas pedal, then the therapist must include a specific brand. If the therapist finds that a right gas pedal block is necessary to prevent the patient from inadvertently stepping on the right gas pedal with the affected foot while using the left foot gas pedal, the therapist should describe a specific type. The prescription should be inclusive, considering every aspect of the vehicle, the driving task, and all related mobility factors such as the way the driver operates the steering column controls, loads or carries a manual wheelchair or quad cane, or opens the door or trunk of the vehicle.

The mobility prescription should not be guesswork or estimation but should be based on a thorough and objective assessment in stationary and dynamic modes after the stroke survivor was observed using each piece of equipment or device safely, efficiently, and easily. Finally, the prescription should not be written until the patient has had sufficient time in a moving assessment or training to demonstrate safe driving skills and safe use of the equipment. Many stroke survivors often need several driving sessions until they are deemed safe drivers. If the therapist writes the mobility prescription too soon, the patient may go to an installer and have the equipment put in the vehicle before he or she is ready to drive. The mobility prescription should indicate to all appropriate parties that the patient has completed a comprehensive driving assessment successfully, that the driver rehabilitation therapist has made an objective determination that the patient can drive safely, and finally that the equipment prescribed is necessary for the person to return to safe driving.[29]

Guiding the stroke survivor to a competent and qualified mobility equipment dealer or installer is important. The driver rehabilitation therapist should identify all of the appropriate dealers in the patient's community and communicate with the business by telephone or by sending the mobility prescription to them. The dealer should be factory trained or certified by the equipment manufacturer to install the specific devices prescribed. The dealer should respect the therapist's expertise and role so as not to overstep boundaries and install equipment without a prescription or substitute, delete, change, or add items on the document. Because the installer is the therapist's "pharmacist," the therapist must develop and maintain a solid working relationship with the installer.[29]

## FOLLOW-UP RECOMMENDATIONS

The final task for the driver rehabilitation therapist is to provide any necessary follow-up recommendations from the on-road assessment. These may include the following:

1. *Additional driver training:* This should be completed in the dual-controlled evaluation vehicle. If training is completed in the patient's vehicle, a rental training brake should be installed unless the patient is close to being finished with training and there is no need for the training brake.

2. A *final equipment inspection and fitting:* Inspection and fitting of equipment by the driver rehabilitation therapist should be done after the installation of the equipment and before the patient is released to drive the vehicle. The multiple purposes for the inspection and fitting by the therapist are as follows: (1) to verify that all mobility prescription items have been installed, (2) to verify that all equipment is installed and working properly, and (3) to observe the patient driving with the equipment to determine if any adjustments are needed so the therapist can supervise the adjustments. The dealer does not have the knowledge about the patient that the therapist has and may not know or understand the way to adjust equipment for a particular person's needs. Equipment may be installed properly and still not work optimally for the patient if it has not been adjusted for safe use. For example, the therapist may prescribe a spinner knob at the 5 o'clock position on the steering wheel. The dealer may ignore or forget the location specified and place the knob at 1 o'clock position. The stroke survivor has a weak right shoulder and fatigues quickly if the arm is held suspended against gravity for a long period. The lower position on the wheel allows the patient to maintain the arm in a resting position while steering straight and keeps the knob easily available for curves and turns. Another example is a patient, who wears a size 16 shoe, and the vendor does not account for this fact when determining the location of the left foot gas pedal in relation to the brake. The therapist must check the position of both pedals to make sure that the patient does not inadvertently hit both pedals simultaneously.

3. *Driver licensing or relicensing:* The driver rehabilitation therapist should inform the patient of the requirements of the department of driver licensing and provide assistance if necessary in obtaining a valid driver's license with the appropriate restrictions. The patient may need to be taken for a road test in the evaluation vehicle or may require the driver rehabilitation therapist's guidance and assistance to communicate with the medical review board of the department of driver licensing for having the driver's license reinstated after a suspension or lack of renewal.

4. *Communication with the rehabilitation team:* Written and/or verbal communication, particularly with the physician and the family regarding the outcome of the driving evaluation, is important so that all parties understand and support the final results and any follow-up services that may be necessary after the initial driving assessment. If the patient has a progressive condition such as the beginning of cataracts, macular degeneration, reflex sympathetic dystrophy or complex regional pain syndrome, Parkinson's disease, dementia, or Alzheimer's disease, the physician and medical review board should be notified of the need for periodic reevaluation of the patient's driving skills, the time frame for the reevaluation, and events that may indicate a need for reevaluation before the expected time.

5. *Patient and family counseling:* This is important at this point if the stroke survivor can no longer drive safely. This news requires the therapist gently to inform the patient directly with compassion, support, and understanding. The patient should not get the results by surprise in a letter or by telephone or by a written notice the following month from the medical advisory board that the license is being suspended. As hard as it is to complete this part of the job, this is an important aspect for the driver rehabilitation therapist to handle with respect of the person's dignity.

The loss of a driver's license changes a person's life dramatically. The person may no longer be able to live alone or remain in the house that has been home for decades. The person may become dependent on others for transportation and may have to cut out many social activities. The person may be forced to get to destinations important for purchasing services and goods for daily living by using a taxi, walking to a public bus stop, or calling on the cheaper but often unreliable local transportation services for the disabled that are available in many communities. The person should be informed that taxis are expensive means of transportation but are still cheaper than owning a car and paying for maintenance, gas, and insurance.

The occupational therapist can use his or her psychological background and holistic thinking to counsel the stroke survivor and the family on community mobility issues after driver cessation. The therapist needs to give the patient and family additional information and resources at this time and should discuss transportation needs and options. The following are suggestions to ease the psychological effects of learning about negative outcomes of a driving evaluation:

1. The therapist should give the person a frank and honest description of observable driving behaviors or problems areas that do not allow for safe driving. Discussion of the clinical results and the road test is helpful because time is needed for the information and

consequences to be processed. The therapist should give the person an opportunity to discuss the results and ask questions.

2. A significant other should be present with the stroke survivor at this point for psychological support, for help in deciding the best way of securing alternative transportation, and perhaps for a discussion of selling a vehicle and turning in a driver's license for a state identification card.

3. Available counseling through the doctor, psychologist, or other senior health counselor should be sought to assist the person psychologically. The patient likely will go through an expression of a variety of feelings and emotions such as denial, anger, resentment, and depression. Family members and friends should be available to check on the person in case depression becomes deep enough to require frequent and formal counseling.

4. Transportation problems must be resolved for the person who must give up driving. The therapist should recruit family members or friends for personal errands and appointments. Information about optional transportation for senior citizens and persons with disabilities should be given in detail and in writing. If necessary, the person should be taken on a city bus route to an appointment and instructed in the way to use the route and bus map guide. The therapist may discuss the option of keeping the personal car and hiring a neighbor or friend to drive it several days of the week for any necessary trips.

## LIABILITY CONSIDERATIONS

Because of the inherent nature of driving, all parties must address the degree of liability concerning the stroke survivor who drives, including the physician, the rehabilitation team, the clinical occupational therapist addressing driving as an IADL, the driver rehabilitation therapist, the patient, and the family. As American's passion for lawsuits continues to rise, the physician and other treating professionals of stroke survivors should be diligent in always recommending a formal driving assessment. Health care professionals working with stroke survivors must remember that protective privilege ends where public peril begins.[29] Every physician and rehabilitation staff member, if for no other reason than because of the liability, should consider the issue of driving after a stroke. If the facility does not have a driving program, a referral to a qualified program in the community should be made, and the referral should be documented in the chart. The driving network listserv of the AOTA or the Web site of ADED or Adaptive Mobility Services can help one locate a driver rehabilitation therapist or a certified driver rehabilitation specialist. A discussion of the concept of shared liability in each party follows.

### Patient's Liability

The driver has an ethical responsibility to avoid harming self or others. Each state department of motor vehicles grants a person the privilege of a driver's license based on criteria and regulations that vary from state to state. The driver must realize that the driving privilege can lead to potential disaster through injury to persons and destruction of property if residual functional deficits interfere with driving skills. Persons recovering from a CVA who cannot master the operational, tactical, and strategic skills necessary to operate a motor vehicle safely present a clear risk of injury to themselves, their passengers, pedestrians, and other operators of motor vehicles.[2]

The clinical occupational therapist carefully should address the liability issues for the family before discharge as an inpatient. The family should understand that following the rehabilitation team's recommendations for driving cessation until a driving assessment can be made will lessen their liability risk. Families are entrusted with ensuring compliance with the recommendations after discharge from the inpatient rehabilitation stay. They should be encouraged, if necessary, to take the stroke survivor's driver's license and/or vehicle keys and even relocate any vehicle to which the person may have access *before* the person is discharged from the rehabilitation facility. The entire rehabilitation team must reinforce this information so the family is informed properly, prepared, and willing to take their role and responsibility seriously and to follow through with the recommendations.

The rehabilitation team or family member should never hesitate to report the stroke survivor to the department of driver licensing if the person does not comply with the team's recommendations and is deemed unsafe to self or the public while driving. If the physician hesitates to address driving to a patient or thinks liability may be avoided by not addressing the issue, another team member should contact the department of driver licensing if allowable in that state. Each state differs in the requirements for reporting a person, so the occupational therapist should investigate the procedure for the patient's resident state. Obtaining a copy of the state's statute is important, as is talking to the department of driver licensing or medical review board. By performing a *Google* search using the letters "DMV," each state Division of Motor Vehicles website can be found.

The March 1993 AOTA physical disabilities special interest section newsletter discussed the legal considerations for driver rehabilitation programs in terms of the responsibility of the patient, physician, and occupational therapist.[29] To avoid any legal difficulties with the driver's insurance, the stroke survivor should notify his or her car insurance company about the stroke, the results of the driving evaluation, and the validation of the person's driving ability by the department of motor vehicles. Failure to notify the insurance company may result in a claim of fraud if the patient has an accident. As a result, the stroke survivor who is driving may be held completely or partially liable for costs rewarded in court judgments for property damage, bodily damage, pain, suffering, and loss of any parties involved in the accident because of contributory negligence.

## Physician's Liability

In the past 20 years, court precedent has established that physicians have responsibility for protecting the public health even if it conflicts with the patient's right to privacy and confidentiality. This duty to warn society for the greater good has been upheld by the courts. Consequently, the physician's liability to inform third parties has increased. Few, if any, exceptions to this rule exist, so any person who has had a brain trauma or damage should be assessed objectively for their safe driving skills. Failure to address these issues with the stroke survivor and concerned others may expose a health care provider to a charge of negligence.

Some states have mandatory reporting laws. A physician must report a new disability or diagnosis to the department of driver licensing. In states that lack this law, some physicians may overlook, ignore, or hesitate to report a patient for fear of losing a patient. The physician may feel a loyalty toward patients they have treated for many years. A patient may attempt to influence the physician's decision by indicating that he or she is the only driver in the family and driving is crucial to continued independent living. Although this may be true, the physician's first thought should be the safety and protection of the patient and the public. If the physician or others on the rehabilitation team are unsure the patient will comply with the recommendations as given regarding driving, the person should be reported to the department of driver licensing without hesitation.

The American Medical Association (AMA) now encourages physicians to make driver safety a routine part of geriatric medical services. The AMA in 2003 published the *Physician's Guide to Assessing and Counseling Older Drivers*. Information about this book and other resources is available through their website at www.ama-assn.org/go/olderdriver. The physician's decision to report a patient should be based on the amount of risk involved in allowing the person to continue driving. The physician should protect patients from further harm or injury to themselves or others. States that have a mandatory reporting law also protect individuals by a state statute who report medical conditions from being sued for slander or character defamation by divulging personal information to the department of driver licensing. For further protection, the name of the reporting person is not revealed to the licensee.

A review of past court opinions and judgments reveals rulings for and against physicians. Jacobs,[15] in a 1978 arti-

cle titled "Reporting the Handicapped Driver," cited several lawsuits against physicians. In a 1920 invasion of privacy lawsuit, *Simonsen v. Swenson*, the physician was vindicated of any wrongdoing by proving that the public welfare was being protected. In *Freese v. Lemmon*, 210 NW2d 576 (Iowa, 1973), a physician was found guilty of malpractice because he failed to warn and counsel a patient about the possible effects a medical condition might have on driving ability. In this case the patient had been diagnosed with epilepsy. The physician did not advise the person to stop driving. The person had a seizure while driving and struck a pedestrian. In a 1986 lawsuit *Tarasoff v. Regents of the University of California* (551 p. 2d 334, at 344 [1986]), a psychologist working in the student health department on campus was held liable because of his failure to alert and advise campus authorities properly when a student reported to him an intention to murder his girlfriend. The court ruled the psychologist had a duty to break confidentiality and warn the potential victim. The court's opinion concluded that the "protective privilege ends where the public peril begins." The court also stated the following[3]: "The physician treating a mentally ill patient, just as a doctor treating a physical illness, bears a duty to use reasonable care to give threatened persons such warnings as are essential to avert foreseeable danger arising from his patient's condition or treatment."

Antrim and Engum,[2] in an article titled "The Driving Dilemma and the Law: Patients Striving for Independence Versus Public Safety," describe other legal cases illustrating practitioner liability. In *Naidu v. Laird*, 539 A2d 1064 (Del. 1988), the court heard that Laird was killed in a car accident by a known psychotic person who had been involved in several similar accidents in which he drove his car deliberately into someone else's car. When taking his medication, the psychotic person was generally manageable, appropriate, and capable of living semiindependently. When not taking his medication, he had violent tendencies that presented a risk of harm to himself and others. Laird's widow sued the psychotic person and the treating physician, Dr. Naidu, for wrongful death. The court ruled in favor of the plaintiff. The court stated "a psychiatrist owes an affirmative duty to persons other than the patient to exercise reasonable care in the treatment and discharge of their patients." Antrim defines *reasonable care* as the degree of care, skill, and diligence that a reasonably prudent psychiatrist engaged in a similar practice and in similar conditions ordinarily would have exercised in like circumstances.

Antrim and Engum[2] further discuss the California case *Myers v. Quesenberry*, 144 Cal App 3d 888 (1983), which involved a car accident of a patient of Dr. Quesenberry's who was being treated for diabetes and receiving prenatal care. The doctor knew that his patient had been seriously affected during two previous pregnancies that resulted in one stillbirth. During the third pregnancy, the patient's diabetes could not be stabilized. During an office examination, the physician discovered the fetus had died. Dr. Quesenberry advised the patient to have a dilation and curettage procedure. He instructed her to drive immediately to a hospital. Emotionally distraught, the patient suffered a diabetic attack in route and lost control of her car, striking a pedestrian, Myers. The court noted that a fundamental principle of tort law held physicians liable for injuries caused by their failure to exercise reasonable care. A physician must warn a patient if the patient's condition or medications renders certain conduct such as operating a motor vehicle dangerous to others.

A physician must appreciate the complexity and dangers of driving and understand that certain conditions or deficits may impair driving performance. A physician should recognize limitations in having the tools and abilities to evaluate a person's driving skills fully in the office or hospital. A physician should be informed about the expertise and role of the occupational therapist and the driver rehabilitation therapist so as to refer patients for a medical-oriented and comprehensive driving evaluation.

## Occupational Therapist's Liability

The occupational therapist's responsibility can be as great and serious as the physician's is. The level of liability increases as the therapist's role and responsibility increase. In other words, the therapist seeing the patient in the acute care setting who is addressing only driving from a factual standpoint has little liability, if any. However, if the clinical occupational therapist chooses not to inform the patient or the family of their responsibility with this issue, then the therapist may be liable for an act of omission.

The driver rehabilitation therapist has the greatest degree of vulnerability to liability lawsuits compared with an occupational therapist in the clinic or hospital. The nature of the job, in which the therapist takes a patient in traffic, has inherent risks. A definitive legal case that eases the liability position of the driver rehabilitation therapist was *White v. Moss Rehab, et al.* (Philadelphia, 1995) when the court declined "to recognize a common-law third party cause of action for educational malpractice against a driving school." The driver rehabilitation program was found to not be liable for the driving mistake of a former patient that resulted in a motor vehicle accident that caused the death of a passenger in another vehicle.

The driver rehabilitation therapist should follow safe, accepted practices to lessen the liability risk (Box 21-9). The evaluation car must be viewed as an evaluation tool that must be adjusted to each patient's use and maintained in proper working order just as any machine in the occupational therapy clinic. Proper training by qualified professionals in the field and practice with in-car skills prepares the therapist for the work in the car. An

---

**Box 21-9**

### Reducing Liability Risk

The driver rehabilitation therapist can reduce liability risk by the following:

- Have a medical background with knowledge in driver education principles.
- Have specialized training in the field of driver rehabilitation.
- Have a working knowledge of each step of the comprehensive driving evaluation.
- Know and practice accepted standard of care in driver rehabilitation.
- Ensure that the evaluation vehicle is equipped properly with instructor's safety equipment.
- Set the vehicle up properly for each patient.
- Know how to control the vehicle from the right side, physically and verbally.
- Be a "see-all, know-all" passenger.
- Use sound judgment and good clinical reasoning.
- Use good observation and visual skills.
- Use good documentation and communication procedures.
- Carry personal professional liability insurance.

---

Adaptive Mobility Services, Inc. workshop titled *Take the Wheel: A Driver Education Workshop for the Therapist* provides this type of knowledge, instruction, and practice in a real evaluation vehicle with mock patients.

An occupational therapist must be credentialed adequately to enhance the value of his or her professional opinion. The therapist must have a strong working knowledge of each step of a comprehensive driving evaluation and must use the accepted practices in the industry conscientiously. The therapist must follow any industry guidelines, standards of practice, and code of ethics that exist for the therapy profession and the driver rehabilitation profession. Today the Association of Driver Rehabilitation Specialists has guidelines and a code of ethics that would be the measuring stick for any person desiring to work in the field of driver rehabilitation. In addition, an occupational therapist would follow any standards, guidelines, or code of ethics within the AOTA or state licensure laws. Wendy Kaplan-Stav,[17] in a 1999 AOTA physical disabilities special interest section quarterly newsletter article titled "The Occupation of Driving: Legal and Ethical Issues" stated that "Therapists should be aware of medical reporting requirements for impaired driving laws that exist in their state of practice. The AOTA Code of Ethics creates an obligation for administrative occupational therapists to be aware of the laws related the health care practitioners and driving as well as to disseminate that knowledge. It is the role of the manager to create departmental policies consistent with those laws and provide the administrative support necessary for observance of those policies." For legal protection, all therapists, and especially those in this specialty area, should have their own professional liability insurance in addition to coverage from the employer. If the therapist is ever drawn into a lawsuit, he or she must have representation by a personal attorney and not a third-party interest.

The driver rehabilitation therapist should possess all necessary clinical and vehicle tools, tests, and skills used to pass judgment fairly and accurately on a person's driving future. The therapist should evaluate a patient's driving ability fully, considering the safety of the patient and the public at large. The therapist should avoid zealousness as an advocate for the patient whose skills are in question. Rather, the therapist should respect the studied and influential analysis of disabilities on driving ability. The occupational therapist's perspective of looking at the whole person is key to making the best decision. While determining through a clinical assessment and in-traffic assessment whether the stroke survivor has the adequate level of skill performance in the occupation of driving, the therapist also must consider the strategic and tactical skill that the person uses. The community in which the person drives and the person's mobility in the community may have an effect on the therapist's overall opinion. If the patient will require a manual wheelchair permanently, then this may affect the opinions on the vehicle and equipment recommendations. If the person will be moving to a different location to be close to family and is unfamiliar with the area, then memory, learning skills, and directionality may be greater factors than when a person will be returning to a familiar environment in which he or she has resided for many years.

Antrim[2] is a practicing attorney and a member of the board of reviewers of the journal *Cognitive Rehabilitation*. He strongly suggests that current legal authority appears ready to impose liability on health care professionals for negligence in failing to address their patients' abilities to drive. Antrim recommends that health care professionals use a standard of care in making these recommendations and that their evaluation process should include guidelines for making those decisions reasonably and responsibly. No standardization is currently available for driving evaluation, so the driver rehabilitation therapist would develop or adopt a technique and process for his or her own program and patients based on what is considered the standard of practice for experienced driver rehabilitation therapists. To look at and model a program after others in the industry with experience and skill in the field would be prudent. The Association of Driver Rehabilitation Specialists offers recommended practices for driver rehabilitation services but the practices are written in general terms and do not identify the specific procedures or tests that must be used in the clinic or evaluator vehicle (Box 21-10). The therapist must rely on a

## Box 21-10

### The Recommended Practices for Driver Rehabilitation Services from the Association of Driver Rehabilitation Specialist

A driver rehabilitation program must have a qualified driver rehabilitation specialist and the appropriate vehicles and equipment to provide comprehensive services in the following areas:

1. Clinical evaluation: Applicable testing in the areas of physical functioning and visual/perceptual/cognitive screening; wheelchair and seating assessment
2. Driving evaluation: An on-the-road performance assessment of the patient in an actual driving environment using equipment similar to that being prescribed
3. Vehicle modification and prescription: Prescriptions based on the patient's demonstrated performance in an actual driving experience with equipment similar to that being prescribed, including appropriate descriptions and dimensions of the patient's vehicle and wheelchair
4. Driver education: Including sufficient practice and training to enable the patient to operate a motor vehicle with the prescribed equipment at a level that meets the patient's needs for a driver's license
5. Final fitting: A final fitting and operational assessment in the patient's modified vehicle

Courtesy Association of Driver Rehabilitation Specialists, Edgerton, Wis.

thorough literature search, available educational materials, other experienced driver rehabilitation therapists' opinions, and his or her own judgment regarding the driving performance skills to be tested for each person and the means for thoroughly and accurately testing them.

In a 1986 article, Steich[36] explained that the law holds professionals to a higher standard than it does the public because professionals consider themselves more highly skilled in their particular fields of expertise. For example, the driver rehabilitation therapist owes a greater duty of care to a patient and the public than does a parent teaching a child to drive. Steich goes on to explain that the occupational therapist must do something wrong or fail to do something that should have been done to be held liable. If the policies and procedures of a program define the steps that should be done to complete a comprehensive driver assessment but the therapist fails to use the tool or procedure defined, the therapist may be held liable for omitting that portion of the test. Legal counsel should review the wording of the driving program policies and procedures.

The therapist is responsible for ensuring that all evaluative or testing equipment is working when needed. For example, therapists can use several commercially available devices to test visual acuity and night vision. If the machine that measures night vision is not working when the therapist evaluates a patient with a diagnosis in which night vision could be a suspected problem (such as glaucoma), the therapist may be found negligent for not having the machine fully functioning when the patient was evaluated. The therapist may make a statement in the summary indicating that rendering an opinion on the issue was impossible; however, in making a final conclusion regarding the person's driving ability, night vision should be tested appropriately.

### Communication and Documentation

Communication and documentation are key to lessening everyone's liability throughout the entire process of addressing driving issues for the stroke survivor. The stroke survivor and the family need to be informed of the requirements of the state department of driver licensing. These requirements vary from state to state. In the rehabilitation phase the stroke survivor and family should sign a document that becomes a permanent part of the medical record that describes the information, recommendations, and follow-up plans given by the rehabilitation team regarding driving or transportation.

Documentation of a driving evaluation is crucial and necessary for several purposes. The evaluation and training report can be used to justify an adaptive equipment purchase for a third-party payer, inform the department of motor vehicles and a physician of the patient's driving performance, and help defend the therapist in a court of law or during a deposition in which professional judgment or expertise is deposed. The therapist should keep in mind that if something is not documented on paper, in the eyes of the court it was not done. This documentation is more vulnerable than usual because it is scrutinized far more than is the documentation of in-house therapy for ADL training. Because driving is an ADL that can kill,[27] the parties involved must maintain the highest degree of competence, thoroughness, and seriousness at all times. The documentation of a driving program is at greater risk to be subpoenaed by an attorney searching for liability for a lawsuit.

Occupational therapists should write their notes and summaries within 24 hours of assessment. Adherence to this recommendation ensures that memory of the information is fresh and subsequent documentation is more thorough and accurate. The detailed notes should document interactions with the stroke survivor, the way the patient performed in each step, and the clinical reasoning inherent in the decision making regarding the person's driving performance. Therapists should avoid statements such as "the patient has potential to be a safe driver." Rather, the therapist must have enough confidence with the patient's abilities and in his or her own professional judgment to document "the patient is a safe driver."

Another method of documentation is to say "today the patient drove safely in the following situations." The documentation should account for the time and days spent with a patient. The therapist should note positive and negative observations or scores. Brief, incomplete, illegible, and poorly written documentation is hard to defend in court if an expert witness is used to judge the driver rehabilitation therapist's work and decisions. As with the physician cases noted previously, an expert witness with similar practice to the therapist's may be called to testify regarding standard procedure in similar conditions. This witness may not be able to testify that the driver rehabilitation therapist acted with a reasonable care of duty if the documentation cannot support conclusions with evidence. The background, training, and experience of the driver rehabilitation therapist also often are compared with those of other driver rehabilitation therapists in the country. Attendance at driver-related workshops and professional conferences for the documentation of annual continuing education for updating the therapist's knowledge can validate the therapist's credentials.

After a complete driving evaluation, the therapist should explain final recommendations thoroughly to the stroke survivor and family members. The referring physician should receive written notification of the outcome of the evaluation. The therapist should document the results, recommendations, and follow-up services to be done in the patient's chart. The patient should sign the written recommendations to demonstrate legal proof of explanation of the findings. If the results of the evaluation are negative, a team member may inform the proper driver licensing authority in the patient's state of residency.

## SUMMARY

Driving must be included and addressed as an instrumental activity of daily living in the occupational therapy evaluation and treatment regimen for the stroke survivor. Driving after a stroke is possible for some persons, but a comprehensive driving evaluation with a qualified driver rehabilitation therapist is paramount to any decision regarding the person's ability to continue driving. The physician and other team members must educate stroke survivors and their families early in rehabilitation concerning the necessity and importance of the evaluation. The issues of liability and insurance arising from a stroke survivor driving without a valid license, without the doctor's approval, without necessary equipment, and/or without a documented formal driving evaluation should be explained carefully. Emphasis should be on the detrimental effects on the patient and family's finances, assets, and security if an accident occurs.

The occupational therapist is the logical team member to coordinate and be involved directly in driver evaluation procedures. Necessary specialized education and a period of practice and learning must take place to ensure the occupational therapist is confident and competent to make the important judgments regarding a stroke survivor's ability to drive. A stroke survivor presents unique problems that must be looked at individually. The final decision regarding the patient's driving future must be made on as much reliable, objective information as can be obtained.

## REVIEW QUESTIONS

1. Describe why the occupational therapist should include driving as an instrumental activity of daily living.
2. Describe at least five activities that illustrate the importance of community mobility to a patient who has had a cerebrovascular accident.
3. Describe the requirements for an occupational therapist to be a driver rehabilitation therapist.
4. What specific areas should be evaluated during a predriving clinical screening for a patient with left hemiplegia from a cerebrovascular accident?
5. Describe the liability issues involved for the patient, physician, therapist, and facility.
6. Identify four driving behaviors or errors that may be seen in a patient with left side neglect.
7. Identify specific performance skills (e.g., visual, perceptual, cognitive, and physical) used in the following steps of each driving task:
   Lane change to the right
   Rearview mirror check
   Right outside mirror check
   Right turn signal
   Right head check
   Gradual and small turn of wheel to right
   Cancel turn signal
   Accelerate as appropriate
8. List at least six factors influencing a successful driving evaluation process.
9. What is the purpose of the mobility prescription? List all its uses.
10. What adaptive driving equipment may be used for the following deficits?
    Use of one hand only for steering
    Nonuse of right lower extremity
    Nonuse of left upper extremity
    Lack of neck motion (particularly rotation)
11. List four purposes for the road test.
12. How can a therapist plan a driving route with ecological validity for the stroke survivor?
13. Describe why the occupational therapist is suited to perform the on-the-road assessment.

## REFERENCES

1. Committee for the Study on Improving Mobility and Safety for Older Persons: *Transportation in an aging society*, vol 1, Washington, DC, 1988, Transportation Research Board.
2. Antrim MJ, Engum ES: The driving dilemma and the law: patients striving for independence versus public safety, *Cognit Rehabil* pp. 16-19, March/April 1989.
3. Blum J: Keeping seniors on the move, *Columbus Monthly* 8:72, 1993.
4. Brooke MM, Questad KA, Patterson DR, et al: Driving evaluation after traumatic brain injury, *Am J Phys Med Rehabil* 71(3):177-182, 1992.
5. Carp FM: Significance of mobility for the well being of the elderly, *Transport Aging Soc* 2:2, 1988.
6. Diller L, Weinberg J: Evidence for accident-prone behavior in hemiplegic patients, *Arch Phys Med Rehabil* 51(6):358-363, 1970.
7. Engum ES: Criterion-related validity of the cognitive behavioral driver's inventory: brain-injured patients versus normal control, *Cognit Rehabil* 8:20, 1990.
8. Engum ES, Pendergras T, Cron L, et al: Cognitive behavioral driver's inventory, *Cognit Rehabil* pp 34-50, Sept/Oct 1988.
9. French D, Hanson C: Survey of driver rehabilitation programs, *Am J Occup Ther* 53:4, 1999.
10. Gianutsos R: Driving advisement with the elemental driving simulator (EDS): when less suffices, behavior research methods, *Instrum Comput* 26:183, 1997.
11. Gianutsos R: Personal communication, Sept 1996.
12. Gianutsos R, Suchoff IB: Visual fields after brain injury: management issues for the occupational therapist. In Scheiman M, editor: *Vision: screening and intervention techniques for occupational therapists*, Thorofare, NJ, 1996, Slack.
13. Gresham GE, Duncan P, Stason W, et al: *Post-stroke rehabilitation: clinical practice guideline*, No 16, AHCPR Pub No 95-0662, Rockville, Md, 1995, US Department of Health and Human Services, Public Health Service, Agency for Health Care Policy and Research.
14. Hibbard MR, Gordon WA, Stein DN, et al: Awareness of disability in patients following stroke, *Rehabil Psychol* 37:103, 1992.
15. Jacobs S: Reporting the handicapped driver, *Arch Phys Med Rehabil* 59(8):387-390, 1978.
16. Johansson C: Top 10 emerging practice areas to watch in the new millennium, 2000. Retrieved March 12, 2002, from http://www.aota.org/members/area7/index.asp.
17. Kaplan W: The occupation of driving: legal and ethical issues, *AOTA Phys Disabil Spec Interest Section Newsletter* 22:3, 1999.
18. Katz RT, Golden RS, Butter J, et al: Driving safety after brain damage: follow-up of 22 patients with matched controls, *Arch Phys Med Rehabil* 71:133, 1990.
19. Korner-Bitensky N, Sofer S, Kaizer F, et al: Assessing ability to drive following an acute neurological event: are we on the right road? *Can J Occup Ther* 61(3):141-148, 1994.
20. Launching a driver evaluation program, *AOTA OT Pract* 22:10, July 2002.
21. Legh-Smith J, Wade DT, Hewer RL: Driving after a stroke, *JR Soc Med* 79(4):200-203, 1986.
22. McKnight JA: *Driver and pedestrian training*, vol II, Washington, DC, 1988, Transportation Research Board.
23. Nouri FM, Tinson DJ, Lincoln NB: Cognitive ability and driving after stroke, *Int Disabil Stud* 9(3):110-115, 1987.
24. American Occupational Therapy Association: *Occupational therapy practice framework: domains and process*, Bethesda, Md, 2002, The Association.
25. On the road again, *AOTA OT Week* 5:16, Feb 1998.
26. Persson D: The elderly driver: deciding when to stop, *Gerontologist* 33(1):88-91, 1993.
27. Pierce S: A roadmap for driver rehabilitation, *AOTA OT Pract* 10(1):30-38, 1996.

28. Pierce S: Restoring competence in mobility. In Trombly C, Radomski M, editors: *Occupational therapy for physical dysfunction*, ed 5, Philadelphia, 2002, Lippincott Williams and Wilkins.

29. Pierce S, Blackburn C: *Building blocks for becoming a driver rehabilitation therapist*, Orlando, Fla, 2001, Adaptive Mobility Services.

30. Ramsey B: *Take the wheel: a driver education course for the therapist*, Course notes, Orlando, Fla, 1996, Adaptive Mobility Services Inc.

31. Rosenbloom S: The mobility needs of the elderly, *Transport Aging Soc* 2:26, 1988.

32. Scheiman M: *Understanding and managing visual deficits: theory screening procedures, intervention techniques*, Course notes, Atlanta, 1996, Vision Education Seminars.

33. Sivak M, Olson PL, Kewman DG, et al: Driving and perceptual/cognitive skills and behavioral consequences of brain damage, *Arch Phys Med Rehabil* 62(10):476-483, 1981.

34. Slavin S: Association of Driver Educators for the Disabled conference presentation, Keynote Speaker Address, Orlando, Fla, 1987.

35. Smith EE: Choice research time: an analysis of the major theoretical positions, *Psychol Bull* 69:77, 1968.

36. Steich T: Malpractice insurance important for occupational therapy personnel, *OT News* 40:7, 1986.

37. Stone SP, Wilson B, Wroot A, et al: The assessment of visuospatial neglect after acute stroke, *J Neurol Neurosurg Psychiatry* 54(4):345-350, 1991.

38. Stressel DL: American Occupational Therapy Association continuing education article: Driving issues of the older adult, *OT Practice* 5:CE1-CE8, 2000.

39. Toglia JP: Visual perception of objects: an approach to assessment and intervention, *Am J Occup Ther* 43:587, 1993.

40. Underwood M: The older driver: clinical assessment and injury prevention, *Arch Intern Med* 152:737, 1992.

41. Warren M: A hierarchical model for evaluation and treatment of visual perceptual dysfunction in adult acquired brain injury, part 2, *Am J Occup Ther* 47(1):55-66, 1993.

42. Weaver J: *Driver performance test*, Palm Harbor, Fla, 1989, Advanced Driving Skills Institute.

43. Wilson B, Cockburn J, Halligan P: Development of a behavioral test of visuospatial neglect, *Arch Phys Med Rehabil* 68(2):98-102, 1987.

44. Wilson T, Smith T: Driving after stroke, *Int Rehabil Med* 5(4): 170-177, 1983.

45. Van Zomeran AH, Brouwer WH, Minderhoud JM: Acquired brain damage and driving: a review, *Arch Phys Med Rehabil* 68(10): 697-705, 1987.

wendy avery-smith

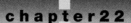

chapter22

# Dysphagia Management

**key terms**

alternative nutrition
aspiration
bedside evaluation
bolus
cervical auscultation

dysphagia
feeding trials
fiberoptic endoscopic evaluation
of swallowing

laryngeal penetration
modified barium swallow
silent aspiration

**chapter objectives**

After completing this chapter, the reader will be able to accomplish the following:

1. Describe the normal anatomy and physiology of the swallowing mechanism.
2. Discuss the effects of stroke on the swallowing mechanism.
3. Describe clinical and instrumental evaluation of dysphagia following stroke.
4. Describe various rehabilitative and compensatory techniques used to treat dysphagia after a stroke.
5. Discuss the efficacy of dysphagia intervention following stroke.

*Dysphagia* (dis-fa′-ji-a) comes from the Greek prefix *dys*, meaning *difficult*, and the Greek term *phagein*, meaning *to eat*. The occurrence of dysphagia, or difficulty swallowing, immediately after stroke is common, with a reported incidence as high as 51%.[55] In patients with brainstem stroke, the incidence may be as high as 81%.[40] Intervention for dysphagia is a part of occupational therapy care for patients with stroke in a variety of settings.

## NORMAL ANATOMY AND PHYSIOLOGY OF THE SWALLOWING MECHANISM

A prerequisite for successful management of patients with dysphagia is knowledge of the anatomy and physiology of the swallowing mechanism. Figure 22-1 represents a midsagittal view of the anatomic landmarks of the head and neck important in swallowing. Figure 22-2 represents

anatomic landmarks of the oral cavity. The act of swallowing may be divided into five separate stages: preoral, oral-preparatory, oral, pharyngeal, and esophageal. Figure 22-3 illustrates the anatomic division of the oral preparatory through esophageal stages.

### Preoral Stage

During the preoral stage, the patient engages in tray setup and preparation, visual and olfactory awareness of the food, and transportation of the food (feeding) to the mouth using a utensil, cup, or fingers.

### Oral-Preparatory Stage

During the oral-preparatory stage (Figure 22-4, *A*), the patient demonstrates adequate mouth opening, bolus reception, and containment in the oral cavity, oral sensation for the bolus, and appreciation of the flavor and

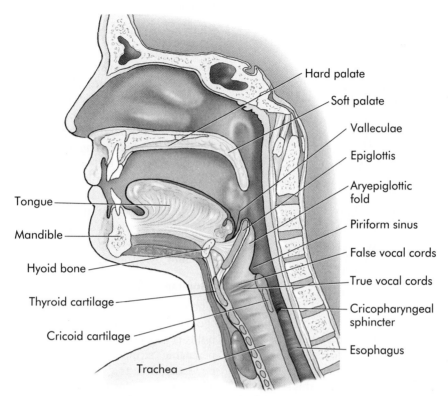

**Figure 22-1**   Midsagittal view of swallowing landmarks.

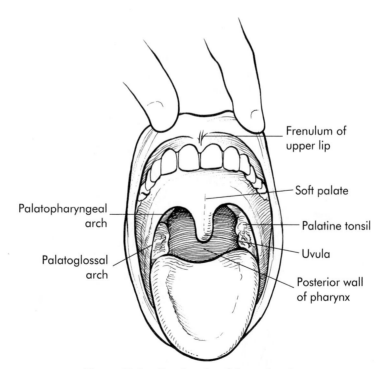

**Figure 22-2**   Landmarks of the oral cavity.

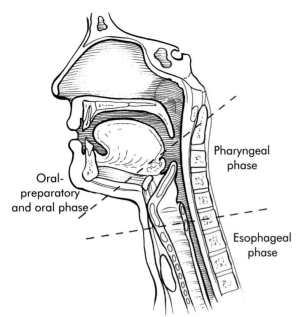

**Figure 22-3**    Stages of a normal swallow sagittal view.

texture of the bolus. The muscles of mastication prepare the food, if solid, into a bolus of suitable texture for swallowing by manipulating the bolus using the muscles of mastication, the jaw, and the cheek. During this stage, the soft palate rests on the back of the tongue to prevent food or fluid from trickling into the pharynx.

### Oral Stage

During the oral stage of the swallow, the prepared bolus is propelled through the oral cavity toward the pharynx (Figure 22-4, *B*). The lips and buccal muscles contract and transport the bolus posteriorly as the tongue sequentially pushes the bolus posteriorly against the hard palate,

propelling it through the oral cavity, to the base of the tongue.

### Pharyngeal Stage

During this stage of the swallow, the following events occur in rapid sequence, producing a swallow response. The soft palate elevates, closing off the nasopharynx. The vocal folds close, protecting the airway from aspiration and laryngeal penetration. The epiglottis folds over the opening to the larynx (the laryngeal vestibule) (Figure 22-4, *C*), also preventing airway penetration into the larynx and directing the bolus toward the piriform sinuses. The larynx rises and tilts anteriorly, and pharyngeal peristalsis squeezes the bolus downward through the pharnyx toward the cricopharyngeal sphincter (Figure 22-4, *D*). The cricopharyngeal sphincter, which is at the superior aspect of the esophagus, relaxes and allows the bolus to pass into the esophagus.

### Esophageal Stage

The esophageal stage begins as the bolus passes through the cricopharyngeal sphincter (Figure 22-4, *E*). The bolus is propelled through the esophagus by a sequential peristaltic "stripping wave." The lower esophageal sphincter, located at the base of the esophagus then relaxes, allowing the bolus to pass into the stomach.

### Neural Control of Swallowing

Cortical and subcortical centers control the voluntary aspects of the swallow, particularly during the preoral, oral-preparatory, and oral stages. The swallow response, which can be initiated voluntarily or involuntarily, is controlled by cranial nerves and their nuclei in the medulla, with input from cortical and subcortical centers. Six cranial nerves are involved in the swallow process[30] (Box 22-1).

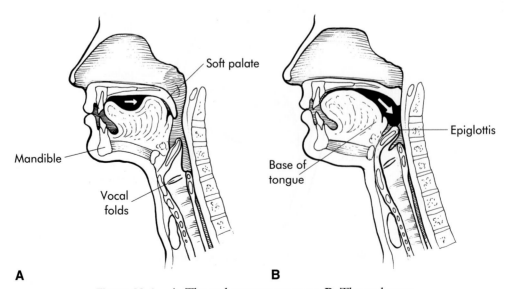

**Figure 22-4    A,** The oral-preparatory stage. **B,** The oral stage.

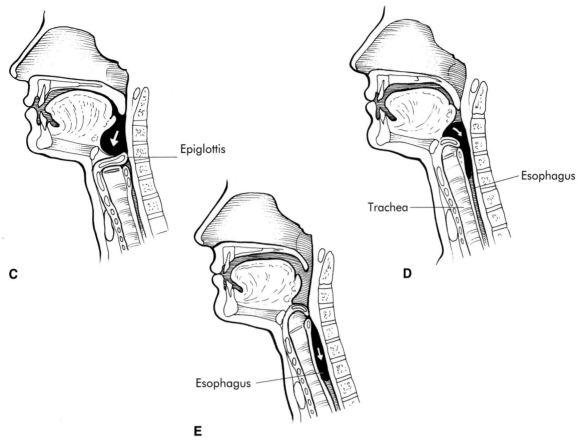

**Figure 22-4, cont'd**    C and D, The pharyngeal stage. E, The esophageal stage.

## Box 22-1

### Cranial Nerve Functions

**ORAL STAGE**

Cranial nerve V (trigeminal): tactile and proprioceptive sensation and motor
Cranial nerve VII (facial): taste and motor

**PHARYNGEAL STAGE**

Cranial nerve IX (glossopharyngeal): taste, pharyngeal peristalsis, salivation, and taste
Cranial nerve X (vagus): taste and motor, intrinsic laryngeal muscles, pharyngeal peristalsis, and swallow initiation
Cranial nerve XI (accessory): pharyngeal peristalsis and head and neck stability

**ORAL AND PHARYNGEAL STAGE**

Cranial nerve XII (hypoglossal): lingual movement and laryngeal and hyoid movement

## SIGNS OF DYSPHAGIA ASSOCIATED WITH STROKE

A variety of signs are observed directly or by videofluoroscopy during swallowing following stroke. Veis and Logemann[62] found that 75% of patients assessed by videofluoroscopy demonstrated more than one specific sign with their swallowing. Signs and symptoms vary with location and size of the lesion or lesions caused by stroke. Table 22-1 delineates specific impairments that one may observe. Figure 22-5 illustrates some of these impairments. Patients with dysphagia and stroke may have a tracheostomy and may require mechanical ventilation. Although this chapter does not cover these topics, the suggested reading will provide the reader with more information. Studies have observed the differences between dysphagia in stroke patients by lesion location.

### Hemispheric Stroke

Robbins et al[49] noted that persons with right hemispheric middle cerebral artery stroke tended to have greater incidence of laryngeal penetration and aspiration than those with left hemispheric middle cerebral artery stroke. This study also observed that persons with right hemispheric stroke took longer to initiate a swallow response than those with a left hemispheric stroke. Oral and pharyngeal bolus mobilization was slower in persons with right hemispheric stroke than in healthy individuals. Patients with left hemispheric stroke experienced slower bolus

**Table 22-1**

## Dysphagia Symptoms in Stroke Associated with the Stages of Swallowing*

| STAGE OF THE SWALLOW | BEDSIDE EVALUATION SYMPTOMS | MODIFIED BARIUM SWALLOW SIGNS | PHYSIOLOGIC SYMPTOMS |
|---|---|---|---|
| Preoral | Poor sitting posture | Suboptimal view | Reduced trunk control |
| | Reduced orientation to food | | Reduced cognition |
| | Inability to identify edibles from nonedibles or to recognize food | | Visual-perceptual or sensory deficits |
| | Inability to open packages or to prepare and cut food on plate | | Reduced upper extremity function, control, or coordination |
| | Inability to get bolus to mouth | | Apraxia/ataxia |
| Oral-preparatory | Reduced mouth closure | Loss of bolus onto lips, drooling | Reduced oral-motor strength, tone, range |
| | Reduced lip, tongue, and cheek control | Decreased ability to form bolus; incohesive bolus | Abnormal reflexes |
| | Perioral food residue (on lips and/or face); drooling | | Reduced perioral sensation |
| | Tongue thrust | Anterior tongue movements | Reflexive tongue movements |
| | Disorganized tongue movements | | Tongue tremors, weakness, reduced coordination |
| | Reduced mastication | Ineffective mastication, with unchewed bolus | Weakness, tone alterations |
| | Slow oral preparation time | | Weakness, poor sensory awareness |
| | Oral fatigue | Slow oral movements | Weakness, low muscle tone |
| | Lengthy mealtime | | Slow or poorly coordinated overall movements |
| Oral | Use of fingers to manipulate the bolus posteriorly | | Reduced awareness of or ability to propel the bolus posteriorly |
| | Holding of food in the mouth | | |
| | Pocketing of food in oral sulci (pooling) | Oral residue on tongue and sulci, lips, or palate | Reduced/absent muscle control to direct bolus |
| | Drooling | | Reduced or absent intraoral sensation |
| | Oral residue after attempts at swallowing | | Difficulty collecting or propelling the entire bolus |
| | Reduced tongue elevation to propel the bolus posteriorly | Tongue pumping | Apraxia, ataxia, tone alterations, discoordination |
| | Reduced anterior to posterior tongue movement/bolus propulsion; disorganized tongue movements | | |
| | Slow oral transit time | | Fatigue, poor coordination |
| Pharyngeal | Coughing/choking | Premature loss of bolus into hypopharynx | Cranial nerves X and IX: reduced/absent swallow, weakness of swallow response |
| | Wet/gurgly breath and vocal quality | Delayed or absent swallow response | |
| | Absent swallow response | | |
| | Difficulty initiating a swallow | | |
| | Weak cough | Repeated attempts at coughing/clearing | Reduced respiratory support/capacity |
| | | Ineffective cough; cannot clear aspirated or penetrated material | Bilateral or unilateral vocal fold paralysis |
| | | | Cranial nerves IX and X: reduced or absent sensation |

*This table is not an exhaustive list of signs and symptoms but is meant to suggest some causative factors for swallowing dysfunction.

**Table 22-1**

**Dysphagia Symptoms in Stroke Associated with the Stages of Swallowing\*—cont'd**

| STAGE OF THE SWALLOW | BEDSIDE EVALUATION SYMPTOMS | MODIFIED BARIUM SWALLOW SIGNS | PHYSIOLOGIC SYMPTOMS |
|---|---|---|---|
| | Complains of food sticking in throat<br>Increased throat clearing<br>Multiple swallows (more than two) | Pharyngeal wall residue<br>Valleculae<br>Piriform sinus pooling<br>Ineffective multiple swallows to clear residue | Cranial nerves IX and X:<br>Reduced pharyngeal peristalsis |
| | Nasal regurgitation | Penetration of bolus into nasopharynx<br>Penetration of bolus into trachea above level of vocal folds<br>Aspiration of bolus into trachea below level of vocal folds | Incompetence of palatal seal of nasopharynx<br>Reduced epiglottal movement; reduced laryngeal elevation<br>Reduced ability to prevent entry of food material into airway<br>Delayed swallow |
| Esophageal | Lengthy mealtime<br>Regurgitation, sour taste, heartburn, awaking with a wet pillow | Reflux: reduced upper esophageal sphincter opening caused by reduced pharyngeal/laryngeal movement; reflux | Esophageal or gastric reflux |

mobilization through the pharynx compared with healthy individuals. This same research demonstrated delayed oral time in those with left hemispheric stroke. Robbins et al[49] postulated that these oral and pharyngeal delays may be due in part to apraxia in those with left hemispheric stroke. A study by Irie and Lu[24] suggested that in general, patients with left hemispheric stroke tended to have primarily oral phase impairments and those with right strokes tended to have impairment of oral and pharyngeal phases. Robbins et al[49] corroborated that persons with left hemispheric stroke tended to require fewer dysphagia interventions and require alternative nutrition less than those with a right sided stroke. Pharyngeal and laryngeal sensory loss may play a role in reduced ability to respond to the presence of a bolus in some stroke patients.[4]

## Brainstem Stroke

Wallenberg's syndrome occurs with a lateral medullary infarction. Oral control may be near intact, but the ability to trigger a swallow is weak or absent. Reduced laryngeal elevation and unilateral pharyngeal weakness may be seen. Patients with pontine strokes may demonstrate high tone in the pharynx, resulting in a delayed or absent swallow response.[31] Veis and Logemann[62] noted that decreased laryngeal adduction causes aspiration during the swallow in persons with brainstem stroke.

## Lacunar Infarcts

Lacunar infarcts, often occurring in the periventricular areas, are not always associated with specific dysphagic signs.

## Multiple Strokes

Patients with multiple strokes may demonstrate slow oral movements and a delayed swallow response.[31] Often multiple deficits exist, resulting in a greater risk of aspiration. Patients with bilateral stroke are more likely to have sensory deficits in the pharynx and larynx.[4]

## Resolution of Dysphagia Following Stroke

Dysphagia clinicians and researchers have noted that difficulty with swallowing lessens in the 7 days following acute stroke, although in one study 27% of patients still were considered to be at risk by the physician. After 6 months, only 8% retained dysphagia, however 3% had developed new difficulty with swallowing.[55] Logemann[31] noted that 95% of patients with a single, uncomplicated stroke returned to full oral intake after 9 weeks, regardless of the location of the stroke. However, among that 95%, pharyneal function was not completely normal and possibly contributed to even more severe dysphagia with a subsequent stroke.

## MEDICAL COMPLICATIONS ASSOCIATED WITH DYSPHAGIA IN STROKE

Medical complications associated with dysphagia following stroke include aspiration pneumonia, dehydration, compromised nutrition, and death.

### Aspiration

*Aspiration* refers to the penetration of food or liquid into the airway, below the level of the vocal folds, before, during, or after the swallow. *Laryngeal penetration* refers to

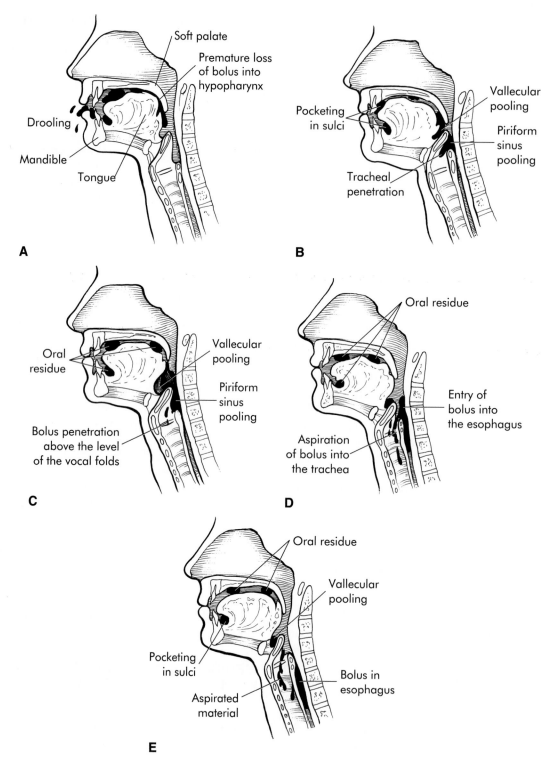

**Figure 22-5**    Pathophysiology of dysphagia after stroke.

the entrance of food or liquid into the larynx, above the level of the vocal folds.[31] *Silent aspiration* is defined as the entrance of saliva, food, or liquid below the level of the true vocal folds without a cough or any clinical signs of difficulty.[20] Aspiration and laryngeal penetration occur when the ability of the swallowing mechanism to prevent material from entering the airway is impaired.

Aspiration is common in the acute phase following stroke, with a greater incidence in severe strokes and in patients with pharyngeal sensory loss.[18] Approximately 40% of stroke patients with dysphagia who aspirate do not exhibit symptoms of aspiration during the bedside evaluation (silent aspiration).[20] Of stroke patients selected for a videofluoroscopic study, 48% to 55% were shown actually to aspirate.[13] Veis and Logemann[62] found that 32% of the subjects assessed by videofluoroscopy aspirated from pharyngeal stage problems, which the bedside evaluation cannot detect. Mann and Hankey[39] found that aspiration was correlated with delayed oral transit and incomplete oral clearance of the bolus. Sensory deficits in the larynx and pharynx may be associated with aspiration.[4] Patients with brainstem, subcortical, or bilateral stroke are at greater risk for aspiration.[13]

Tolerance for aspiration appears to be individual and may depend on the frequency, volume, and content of what is aspirated. Tolerance may also depend on the overall health of the individual patient. Information regarding who may tolerate aspiration and in what parameters is scarce. Therefore, counseling patients on the risks of continued oral intake despite aspiration is difficult because little data exists to support or negate its consequences.

### Aspiration Pneumonia

Aspiration can lead to aspiration pneumonia in patients with stroke,[37,44,51,56] which may lead to hospitalization or death.[51] Pneumonia is particularly common in stroke patients with multiple-location strokes, a history of airway disease, hypertension, diabetes, and aspiration during modified barium swallow.[13] Pneumonia may occur in 11% of those with brainstem stroke.[61] Saliva contains pathogens that may be causative factors for pneumonia when saliva is aspirated.[25,26]

### Dehydration and Compromised Nutrition

Dehydration is another possible consequence of dysphagia.[48] Schmidt et al[51] were unable to identify an increased risk of dehydration for patients with aspiration compared with those who did not aspirate. Dehydration may be caused by the use of dysphagia diets that provide only thickened liquids to avoid aspiration.[15,65] Dehydration also may be caused by the patient's inability to recognize thirst or to request a drink when thirsty. Nutritional status also may be compromised by stroke[56] for a variety of reasons, including dysphagia, loss of appetite, decreased mental status, depression and other psychosocial factors, and medication interactions.

## ASPIRATION AND SITE OF LESION

The correlation of stroke location with aspiration remains unclear[1,21,41]; this may be due to the fact that many parts of the brain contribute to safe swallowing. Teasell, Bach, and McRae[60] reported that aspiration occurred in at least 9.9% of all patients who had unilateral right hemispheric strokes, 12.1% of those who had unilateral left hemispheric strokes, 24% of those who had bilateral hemispheric strokes, and 39.5% of those who had brainstem strokes. Horner, Massey, and Brazer[21] reported that aspiration occurred twice as often in those with bilateral stroke compared with those with unilateral stroke. Aspiration after bilateral stroke may be caused primarily by incomplete laryngeal elevation and closure, which encourages aspiration during the swallow and reduces pharyngeal peristalsis after the swallow, causing aspiration of residue. Alberts et al[1] reported that patients with only small vessel infarcts had a decreased incidence of aspiration versus those with large and small vessel infarcts. All stroke patients should be screened and, if necessary, evaluated for dysphagia because aspiration cannot be predicted by lesion location.[1,49]

## ROLE OF THE SWALLOWING TEAM

The optimal swallow evaluation and management of dysphagia are performed by a multidisciplinary team. The team plays an important role in the identification, evaluation, diagnosis, treatment, and overall management of patients with dysphagia.

The multidisciplinary team should include the occupational therapist, speech-language pathologist, nurse, physician, respiratory therapist, and dietitian. The patient and caregivers also play an active role in decision making. For management of the dysphagic patient to be successful, *all* persons involved in the patient's care should understand the swallowing impairment and the management techniques used. Ongoing education and follow-up are often necessary.

## EVALUATION OF SWALLOWING

Dysphagia can be evaluated clinically and instrumentally. Clinical evaluation precedes instrumental evaluation because intervention may be initiated immediately thereafter. Clinical evaluation helps to determine whether instrumental evaluation is needed, and if so, which instrumental procedure is appropriate. In some settings, dysphagia screening identifies patients in need of a complete clinical evaluation. Several screenings are available in the literature, including the 3-oz water test[12] and the Burke Dysphagia Screening Test.[11]

## Clinical Evaluation and Assessment

Clinical evaluation is the process of gathering and interpreting information needed for intervention. Clinical dysphagia assessment uses specific assessment tools to gather evaluation data.[2]

When the physician suspects dysphagia, the physician orders a dysphagia evaluation. The physician, patient, nursing staff, and family also may identify the need for dysphagia evaluation. For patients who are NPO (not eating food by mouth), the physician must stipulate whether evaluation will include attempting trials of food by mouth with the patient. The evaluation examines factors that interfere with feeding and swallowing function, the patient's risk for aspiration, and factors that may contribute to a decrease in oral intake. The evaluation includes observational and direct examination components: chart review, patient and caregiver interview, functional status, oral motor examination, abnormal reflexes, pharyngeal examination, feeding trial, and a statement of impression and recommendations.

Specific assessment tools may be developed by facilities or a standardized assessment may be used. Appropriate dysphagia assessments for patients with stroke that are standardized include the Dysphagia Evaluation Protocol[3] and the Mann Assessment of Swallowing Ability.[38] The Mann Assessment of Swallowing Ability was standardized on a stroke population. Both of these assessments demonstrate a high degree of reliability.

### Chart Review

The therapist first must review the patient's chart carefully to ascertain pertinent facts from the medical and feeding history. Pertinent information includes the following:

- Age[33]
- Previous evaluations and tests indicating current status (positive infiltrate on chest x-ray examination; ear, nose, and throat evaluation)
- Primary diagnosis and date of onset
- History of present illness, secondary diagnoses, and medical history, including history of dysphagia
- History of aspiration pneumonia
- History of weight loss, appetite, and nutrition, especially with current inpatient admission
- Reduced oral intake and its possible relation to depression, pain, feeding dependence, and food preferences or dislikes
- Aspiration precautions
- Dietitian, chest physical therapy, and/or respiratory therapy evaluations
- Current method of nutritional intake
- Current type of diet ordered (dysphagia diet)
- Whether calorie counts are in place
- Length of time on current diet
- Dietary restrictions (diabetic: no concentrated sugars; cardiac: low sodium or low fat)

- Food allergies
- Current respiratory status

When reviewing the chart, the therapist must consider the patient's ability to participate in the evaluation, which contributes to the ability to feed and swallow safely. Factors to consider for mental status include primary language spoken, level of alertness, ability to follow directions, insight into swallowing difficulty, cognitive and perceptual status, and ability to communicate needs. Because eating requires a coordination of breathing and swallowing, respiratory problems may affect a person's ability to eat safely. The therapist should consider the following factors when evaluating the patient's ability to eat orally: excessive oral secretions, tracheostomy type, ventilator dependence and ability to wean, and frequency and route of suctioning.

### Patient/Caregiver Interview

Initial contact begins with medical nursing staff and in the patient's room, where the occupational therapist may ask questions of the patient, family, and caregivers regarding the patient's past and present eating function. This information may expand on that obtained during the chart review.

Observation begins as soon as the practitioner enters the patient's room. The therapist should observe the room for any types of food that may indicate the patient's recent diet. Details to observe include the presence of an untouched meal tray; residual food on the patient's face, clothing, bed, or tray; and wet or hoarse breath sounds and abnormal vocal quality. The patient's positioning in the bed or chair is also relevant.

### Functional Status

*Functional status* refers to the patient's ability to move in space and interact in the environment. Some functional interventions may be needed during evaluation to elicit optimal feeding and swallowing.

If a patient is unable to self-position to achieve an upright sitting position, this may interfere with feeding and swallowing. The occupational therapist should determine the amount of assistance required to position the patient in the bed or chair and whether the patient is able to maintain the position independently. Ideally the patient should sit upright in a chair with the pelvis in a slight anterior tilt, forearms weight bearing on the tabletop, and the head and neck at midline and upright. The therapist also evaluates upper extremity and hand function as they relate to feeding.

Adaptive equipment or environmental adaptations may enable patients to feed themselves if possible. Adaptations for positioning include supporting feet that do not reach the floor with a telephone book or foot rest, using wheelchair cushions and other devices to improve upright posture, and adjusting the table height as needed. Wheelchairs with removable or swing-away armrests allow the patient to eat at the table. Alternatively, a full lap tray can be used with a wheelchair (see Chapter 24).

The therapist should assess the patient's ability to initiate and complete oral hygiene. A clean mouth is necessary for sensory appreciation of food, and good oral hygiene has been shown to reduce rates of pneumonia in an elderly populations.[67] One-handed techniques and equipment create independence with oral care.

For feeding, helpful items include Dycem to prevent the plate from slipping, a rocker knife and plate guard for one-handed eating, a covered cup or straw for bringing beverages to the mouth without spilling, and built-up utensils for weak or poorly controlled grasp to encourage use of a hemiplegic dominant arm. Bent spoons for using a nondominant upper extremity to feed also may be helpful. Adapted cups with lids reduce spilling and provide handles for easy manipulation with a gross grasp; lids may have holes for straws, if that is appropriate. Specially angled dysphagia cups allow sipping without tilting the neck into extension.

Adaptations for reduced visual acuity, perception, and cognition may be useful at the table. The patient should wear eyeglasses if they usually are used at mealtime. A colorful piece of paper or "anchor" may be needed to draw the patient's attention or vision to the neglected side of the food array. A simplified presentation of one food item at a time can help to focus visual and general attention to the eating task. For stroke patients who are distractible, eating in a quiet, reduced-distraction setting promotes attention. Safety and pacing cues and supervision may be needed, especially for those with left hemiplegia. For right hemiplegic patients with aphasia and apraxia, minimal use of verbal directions and setup of the eating environment that makes the activity obvious are helpful (see Chapter 19).

## Oral Examination

The therapist must administer an oral motor examination of the lips, cheeks, tongue, jaw, and palate before presenting food to the patient. The occupational therapist determines whether range of motion, muscle tone, and sensation (intraorally and extraorally) are decreased, increased, or within normal limits. Strength of oral structures is observed but may not be appropriate to assess because of the presence of abnormal muscle tone, which invalidates strength testing.

## Abnormal Reflexes

If present, abnormal "primitive" reflexes can interfere with feeding. Primitive reflexes include the bite reflex, rooting reflex, and the jaw jerk. The gag reflex may be hypersensitive, and hypersensitivity of internal and external oral structures also may be present.

## Pharyngeal Examination

Although unseen, the therapist may assess aspects of pharyngeal function:

- *Dry swallow.* The ability to "dry" swallow (without food) provides information on the patient's ability to initiate a swallow response.
- *Vocal quality.* A wet, gurgly vocal quality can indicate pooling of secretions above the vocal cords, which normally are cleared by coughing or throat clearing. The patient may not perceive the presence of pooled secretions or may be unable to cough them up and clear the throat. Voice hoarseness or weakness may be due to unilateral or bilateral weakness of the vocal cords. Wet voice or a weak-hoarse voice suggests that weakness of the laryngeal structures may compromise the protection of the airway during swallow.
- *Volitional cough.* A volitional cough provides information about the strength of the vocal cords and breath support for coughing.
- *The gag reflex.* In normal individuals, the presence or absence of a gag reflex can vary. Horner and Massey[20] noted that a poor gag reflex proved to be a poor indicator of prognosis for safer swallowing. Triggering of the gag reflex with a tongue depressor is different from triggering the gag reflex by a misdirected bolus. Food does not (normally) trigger a gag, because it is not a foreign substance or a noxious stimulus. The presence or absence of a gag reflex in patients with neurologic impairments is not an accurate indicator of the patient's ability to swallow safely.[31] However, presence of a gag reflex does indicate some level of sensory and motor function of the tenth cranial nerve, which is responsible for innervating many structures that contribute to sensory and motor aspects of the swallow.

## Feeding Trial

Feeding trials are appropriate for patients who are alert, able to follow commands, and medically stable. Factors that may contraindicate feeding trials include absence of or significantly reduced laryngeal elevation during dry swallows, moderate to severe dysarthria, lethargy or severely impaired mental status, and severe pulmonary compromise.[3,46]

Therapists may observe patients in a formal evaluation setting or informally at mealtime. Informal mealtime observation provides an efficient indication of the patient's eating ability and allows the evaluator to assess the patient's ability to concentrate despite distractions and interruptions. An informal evaluation allows for observation of the rate of intake and the patient's reaction to the presentation of the meal.[46] If the evaluation takes place in a formal setting, or if this is the patient's first attempt at eating following a stroke, trials should begin with foods that are less likely to be aspirated, such as thick purees, which do not require much oral manipulation, since thin liquids are more difficult to control in the oral cavity and pharynx. The evaluation then progresses to include foods of more difficult consistencies, depending on the patient's tolerance and medical status. Box 22-2 shows the usual progression of consistencies (from easiest to most difficult).

The therapist may evaluate all the consistencies shown in Box 22-2 or begin at the consistency the patient currently is tolerating. During the feeding trial, the occupational therapist should pay close attention to the nature and quality of oral manipulation of food and to the following indicators of laryngeal function.

An automatic cough occurs under many conditions, including a dry throat, or when secretions have accumulated around the vocal cords even before eating begins. To some extent, coughing occurs with normal breathing and at times when swallowing. Although an automatic cough may be not heard during a meal or feeding trial, its presence may signal that the patient is making efforts to clear the airway of food or secretions and that there is difficulty with airway protection or aspiration of a particular texture or textures. In normal swallowing, laryngeal penetration occurs occasionally; material that is penetrated is cleared from the larynx with throat clearing and reswallowing and often does not result in a cough. However, laryngeal reaction to aspirated material below the true vocal folds is normally a cough, which ideally expels the aspirated material.[54] A strong cough is necessary to protect the airway well. Horner, Massey, and Brazer[21] reported that a weak cough is more likely to occur in aspirating patients than in nonaspirating patients. As with the gag reflex the presence of an automatic cough indicates that to some extent the structures of the larynx and pharynx innervated by cranial nerve X have sensory and motor function.

Full laryngeal elevation and depression indicates that a swallow has occurred. Perlman et al[46] concluded that reduced hyoid elevation impairs the pharyngeal stage of the swallow, thereby increasing the risk of vallecular residue and pharyngeal stasis. These factors may result in aspiration. Figure 22-6 demonstrates the proper positioning of the examiner's hand and digits on the patient's neck for palpation of the larynx to assess laryngeal elevation.

The therapist may assess breath and voice quality by the ear and by cervical auscultation with a stethoscope. Cervical auscultation is accomplished by placing the diaphragm of the stethoscope lateral to the trachea and inferior to the cricoid cartilage.[59] The therapist may adjust placement until hearing cervical breath sounds. The normal pharyngeal stage includes swallow initiation promptly after oral transit, an apneic period during the swallow, and exhalation immediately after the swallow, with clear breath sounds and vocal quality.[68] Breath and vocal quality differ in patients with dysphagia and often are characterized by gurgling sounds, increased throat clearing, and a "wet" vocal quality, which may indicate pooling. The therapist also may assess voice quality with the naked ear. Zenner, Losinski, and Mills[68] concluded that although cervical auscultation is an imprecise clinical method for the evaluation of aspiration, it has some correlation with aspiration found on a modified barium swallow (MBS).

Common dysphagia signs and symptoms in stroke are compiled in Table 22-1. The therapist should make observations relating to these signs and symptoms for the oral-preparatory, oral, and pharyngeal stages for each food and fluid consistency presented. Recommendations

---

**Box 22-2**

**Consistency Progression**

The usual progression of consistencies (easiest to most difficult)

**SOLIDS**

Puree
Soufflé/semisolid
Soft solid
Regular/chewable
Mixed textures (e.g., tablets with water)

**LIQUIDS**

Spoon-thick
Honey-thick
Nectar-thick
Thin

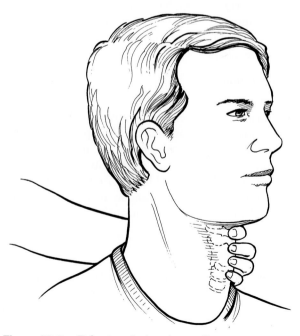

**Figure 22-6**  Palpation during the swallowing evaluation.

and intervention goals are based on these observations, medical history, prognosis, and instrumental assessment results.

## Evaluation Impressions and Recommendations

After gathering information from all aspects of the clinical assessment, the therapist must determine whether further instrumental evaluation of swallowing, discussed subsequently, is warranted. Often concerns about unseen pharyngeal function determine whether a referral for instrumental assessment is appropriate. Whether feeding should be oral or nonoral is a decision to be made by the team,[17] which should always include the patient. If, following a compete assessment, a patient clearly is aspirating, NPO is recommended. Langmore[29] lists the following factors relevant to the risk for aspiration:

- Activity level
- Level of consciousness
- Past aspiration with or without resultant pneumonia
- Prognosis of medical condition
- Prognosis for dysphagia to improve

The team should consider the impact of a decision for NPO on the patient and family.[27] The caregivers and patient provide information about the patient's quality of life and preferences regarding medical intervention. If oral feeding is initiated against medical advice, mealtime management guidelines should be provided to optimize safety and emphasize food consistencies least likely to be aspirated.

## Instrumental Evaluation of Dysphagia

*Instrumental evaluation* refers to diagnostic testing using instrumentation, the most important of which are modified barium swallow (sometimes referred to as *videofluoroscopy*) and fiberoptic endoscopic evaluation of swallowing (FEES) examinations.[6,28] These evaluations use diagnostic imaging techniques and provide information about the anatomy and physiology of the swallow. They also may be rehabilitative procedures to assess efficacy and progress of compensatory techniques. The MBS and FEES provide information regarding the oral stage and the unseen pharyngeal stage of the swallow and can provide information about the patient's ability to protect the airway during swallow, which clinical evaluation cannot. Other instrumental evaluations commonly used to assess dysphagic patients with stroke include ultrasound and electromyography.

### Modified Barium Swallow.
The MBS or videofluoroscopic evaluation of swallowing is the most widely used technique because it allows the clinician the opportunity to examine the oral-preparatory, oral, pharyngeal, and esophageal aspects of the swallow. The MBS also allows the clinician to observe aspiration before, during, and after the swallow.[34] The MBS ideally is performed by the radiologist and the occupational therapist. Food and liquid boluses are mixed with barium, which is radiopaque. Alternatively, some dysphagia clinicians prefer to present only barium, which is available in different thicknesses. The patient must be positioned in an upright position and preferably feeds himself or herself. The swallows are noted by a fluoroscopy unit and are recorded onto videotape. Thus, each stage of the swallow may be viewed during the assessment and reviewed later. The MBS not only allows the clinician to view swallow function and rule out aspiration but also provides useful information regarding compensatory swallowing strategies, discussed subsequently. Optimally, the MBS includes alteration in bolus volume, texture, and delivery and a determination of the amount, frequency, and quality of aspiration. The MBS also can assess the ability to clear aspirated material into the pharynx. The viewing of these modifications provides valuable information regarding dysphagia management and aspiration. The MBS does expose the patient to some levels of radiation, and the ability of the patient to cooperate and follow directions is important for the success of information gathering and to minimize radiation exposure. The MBS is difficult to achieve with patients who are in the intensive care unit, are difficult to position, and/or are difficult to transport to a radiology suite. Naturally, MBS presents function at a specific moment in time, and reliability with real-world swallowing function is not guaranteed; use of MBS results must take this into consideration. Additionally, interrater reliability of MBS performance assessment may vary.[58]

### Fiberoptic Endoscopic Evaluation of Swallowing.
Fiberoptic endoscopic evaluation of swallowing involves passing an endoscope with a light and camera through one of the patient's nares, down to the level of the valleculae. Before the assessment, lidocaine spray is used to numb the nares. Liquid and solid boluses are dyed with green food coloring for easy visualization. Images of the pharynx and larynx then are visualized and can be videotaped. This assessment is performed by an otolaryngologist, or trained occupational therapist or speech-language pathologist. The FEES allows the examiner to evaluate pharyngeal and laryngeal function and assess the amount of residue present on the vocal cords or pooled in the valleculae or pyriform sinuses after a swallow. Thus, one can assess aspiration and competence in protecting the airway. However, FEES cannot always explain the reason that aspiration is occurring, and the presence of the endoscopy tube inhibits a completely normal swallow. The FEES is minimally invasive, and the patient must be able to tolerate the procedure. This procedure is contraindicated for patients with cardiac arrhythmias, respiratory distress, bleeding disorders, anatomic deviations (narrow nasal passage), agitated or hostile patients, or patients with movement disorders.[57] The FEES is particularly useful

for patients who cannot undergo a modified barium swallow for the foregoing reasons or who require frequent reassessment. Clinical benefits of FEES include assessment of airway protection when vocal cord involvement or impaired adduction is suspected, assessment of laryngeal/pharyngeal sensation, and direct visualization of anatomy when it is believed to be a contributing factor in dysphagia.

*Ultrasound.* Ultrasound is the method of choice if only oral function is to be assessed. Ultrasound is a noninvasive, dynamic evaluation of swallowing that shows the anatomy. This procedure uses normal foods and liquids and is safe to use with patients who are unable to follow directions.[57] The disadvantage of ultrasound is that it can visualize only the oral preparatory and oral stages of the swallow.

*Electromyography.* Surface electromyography measures myoelectric impulses resulting from the firing of motor units. Surface electrodes are applied to the skin over specific muscles or muscle groups, producing a line tracing representing amplitude or strength of a contraction. Targeting of one muscle or the pharyngeal constrictor muscles is not possible. Placement of electrodes under the chin is used to detect motion of the suprahyoid muscles to assess whether a swallow has occurred.[22]

## ALTERNATIVE MEANS OF NUTRITION

Patients who are not candidates for oral feeding require alternative means of nutrition,[8] unless they or their designated surrogate have made a purposeful choice not be given artificial feedings. The medical team must determine the length of time the patient will be NPO and the optimal nutritional route. One study has suggested that stroke patients who are not tolerating spoon-fed thick fluids or purees by 14 days following their stroke will need an alternative nutritional route such as a percutaneous endoscopic gastrostomy, defined later.[66] Two primary feeding routes generally are used: enteral, which uses a gastrointestinal route, and parenteral, which uses an intravenous route. Table 22-2 summarizes the risks and benefits of alternative feeding routes.

### Enteral Feedings

*Noninvasive Tube Feedings.* Noninvasive tube feedings are most appropriate for short periods of time. A nasogastric tube is placed through the nose, pharynx, and esophagus into the stomach. Food in the form of an enteric feeding formula and water pass through the tube into the stomach (Figure 22-7). Feedings may be given intermittently via boluses with a large syringe or constantly using a pump.

*Invasive Feeding Methods.* Invasive feeding methods are best for prolonged, indefinite periods. With the patient under general anesthesia, a surgeon makes an incision in the abdomen and then places a gastrostomy tube directly into the stomach. Occasionally a tube is placed into the jejunum to reduce the reflux of stomach material into the esophagus, which gastrostomy tubes may cause. Food passes through the tube into the stomach.

Alternately, a percutaneous endoscopic gastrostomy is placed with the patient under local anesthesia. To place a percutaneous endoscopic gastrostomy, a surgeon inserts an endoscope through the mouth into the stomach, makes an incision in the stomach, and then threads a tube through the endoscope out through the abdominal wall. Special enteric formulae and water are administered as for tube feeding. A percutaneous endoscopic gastrostomy may be "advanced" into the jejunum, creating a percutaneous endoscopic jejunostomy, to help avoid reflux.

### Parenteral Feedings

Total parenteral nutrition administers a complete metabolic diet through a central vein, whereas peripheral parenteral nutrition administers the diet through a peripheral vein.

Table 22-2 outlines the risks and benefits associated with oral, enteral, and parenteral nutrition.

## DYSPHAGIA INTERVENTION IN STROKE

The goals of intervention include reduction of aspiration risk, improving the quality of the swallow, and improving independence in feedings skills and behaviors at mealtime. In the acute phase after a stroke, patients may require daily reevaluation and adjustment in the intervention plan because their status may change daily.

### Intervention Techniques

Interventions for dysphagia caused by stroke may be remedial or compensatory or a combination of both. Treatments for dysphagia include positioning, feeding techniques, facilitation of improved oral and pharyngeal responses, techniques to improve the quality of the swallow, therapeutic swallowing techniques, and diet modification.

*Positioning.* An upright seated position allows optimal function of the muscles of swallowing, maximizes alertness for the fatigued or somewhat lethargic patient, and minimizes reflux. An upright seated position can be achieved in a chair or wheelchair, at the edge of the bed if balance allows, or in bed if necessary. The section on functional status discusses specifics and adaptations for seating. Positioning should allow for proximity to the food for feeding (see Chapter 24).

*Feeding.* Feeding oneself allows the optimal coordination of upper extremity and oral motor responses and the

**Table 22-2**

**Risks and Benefits Associated with Oral, Enteral, and Parenteral Nutritional Support**

| TYPE OF NUTRITIONAL SUPPORT | RISKS AND DRAWBACKS | BENEFITS |
|---|---|---|
| Oral | Possible tracheal aspiration<br>Possible inability to ingest sufficient calories<br>Poor patient satisfaction (with limited dysphagia diet) | Psychologically pleasurable<br>Allows occupational performance of eating and feeding<br>Provides socialization experience<br>Promotes normal digestion |
| Nasogastric | Ulceration<br>Bleeding<br>Fistula<br>Gastroesophageal reflux; aspiration<br>Oropharyngeal discomfort<br>Poor patient satisfaction and compliance | Routine procedure<br>Affordable<br>Begins immediately<br>Easily reversible |
| Surgical gastrostomy | Requires general anesthesia<br>Bleeding<br>Gastroesophageal reflux; aspiration<br>Diarrhea<br>Stomal irritation | Common procedure<br>Good for long-term care if gastrointestinal tract is inaccessible<br>Easily replaceable<br>Removes tube from head/neck region<br>Nonsurgical placement available (PEG) |
| Jejunostomy | Peritonitis<br>Diarrhea<br>Difficult to replace | Minimizes gastroesophageal reflux<br>Can be used when stomach cannot tolerate diet<br>Nonsurgical placement available (PEJ) |
| TPN | Sepsis<br>Infection at site<br>Short-term alimentation<br>Pneumothorax<br>Expensive | Fewer complications in patients with dysphagia and malnutrition<br>For use in nonfunctioning gastrointestinal tract<br>Minimizes risk of aspirating stomach contents |

Adapted from Groher ME: Formulating feeding decisions for acute dysphagic patients, *Occup Ther Pract* 3:27,1992.
*PEG*, Percutaneous endoscopic gastrostomy; *PEJ*, percutaneous endoscopic jejunostomy; *TPN*, total parenteral nutrition.

best awareness of bolus approach. Awareness of the bolus, via visual and olfactory appreciation, provides oral readiness for the bolus.[32] The foregoing section on functional status discusses how to optimize self-feeding with stroke patients. Manual guiding for cerebrovascular accident patients with partial dominant upper extremity movement, particularly those with left cerebrovascular accident and apraxia, is a useful way to facilitate feeding in concert with upper extremity functional goals.

*Techniques to Improve Oral Responses.* Interventions begin with symmetrical body position and then are directed toward the affected side of the face to try to create symmetrical movement. When increased skeletal muscle activity is present, passive stretching of tight musculature such as a tight cheek with the back of a spoon or gloved finger is useful. When patients present with decreased motor control of the oral structures, the therapist encourages movement using functional speech and

eating tasks; for example, using oral exercises such as blowing or sucking tasks to elicit movement. The therapist can provide sensory stimulation for reduced sensation using a gloved hand inside and outside the mouth. Having the patient accomplish regular oral hygiene helps to establish sensory awareness and motor responses. For abnormally heightened sensation, graded sensory stimulation programs help the patient tolerate stimulation of the face and oral cavity so as to accept food and utensils. The therapist addresses abnormal reflexes with positioning and avoiding the stimuli that trigger the response.[10]

Weakness (as opposed to hypotonicity) of oral structures may be an issue with the debilitated stroke patient with reduced endurance. Some dysphagia therapists find that direct oral range of motion exercises are useful and often progress patients to gentle oral progressive resistive exercises. However, assuring good nutrition, maintenance of eating by mouth, oral hygiene programs, and use of oral and pharyngeal structures in conversation are also

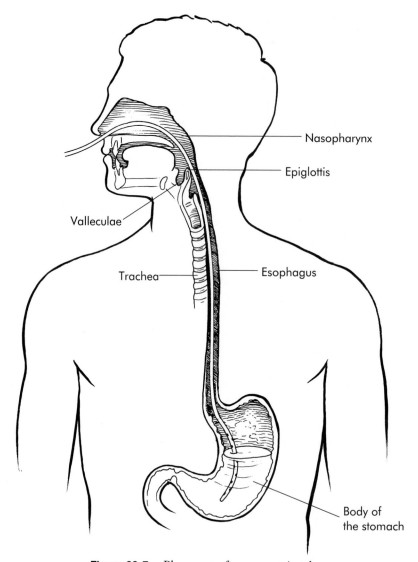

**Figure 22-7**    Placement of a nasogastric tube.

of utmost importance and may be just as useful as formal exercise programs.

While the patient eats, alteration in bolus qualities may help to trigger oral responses to food and thus improve the ensuing pharyngeal responses. Pushing down slightly with the spoon on the tongue as the bolus is introduced into the mouth can help with sensory awareness. Presentation of a cold bolus[7] or a sour bolus[36] can facilitate oral and also pharyngeal responses. Alternating food textures with each mouthful—for example, alternating fluids with solids—is a way of altering sensory input with each bite.[31]

***Facilitation of Pharyngeal and Laryngeal Movements.***
Exercises involving pulling the tongue back, yawning, and gargling with saliva serve to strengthen retraction of the base of the tongue,[63] which is necessary to execute a swallow. Shaker exercises strengthen laryngeal eleva-

tion.[53] To accomplish Shaker exercises the therapist has the patient perform repetitive tucking of the chin to the chest while supine. Shaker exercises have been shown to help patients with chronic dysphagia who are fed by tube to return to eating food by mouth.[52] Encouraging the patient to talk, cough, clear the throat intermittently provides functional exercise for motions of the pharynx and larynx.

***Facilitation of Swallowing.***    Different methods are available to facilitate a swallow when its initiation is weak or delayed:

- *Thermal-tactile stimulation* consists of stroking the faucial arches with a chilled laryngeal mirror before eating and has been shown to speed the onset of the swallow response and the total swallow time in stroke patients.[50]
- *Surface electromyography* has been used to retrain brainstem stroke patients with chronic dysphagia to eat

safely by mouth[9] and also has been demonstrated to be useful to provide biofeedback for relaxing high tone in laryngeal musculature, allowing an improved swallow response.[22]

- *Electrical stimulation.* A recent study describes the successful use of electrical stimulation using surface electrodes on the neck of stroke patients to stimulate a swallow response over a short duration.[16] The authors claim that electrical stimulation proved more successful than thermal-tactile stimulation.
- *Improving quality of the swallow.* Different techniques to improve the bolus direction during the swallow have been attempted with dysphagia patients. Patients with stroke often have residue in the affected cheek; using the tongue to clear the bolus or massaging the cheek with the hand are helpful to route the bolus back to the center of the tongue. Holding the affected lip closed with a finger to allow oral containment of the bolus may be necessary. Having the patient chew with the hemiparetic side of the jaw stimulates movement and function and helps the patient to practice transfer of the bolus between the two molar surfaces.

Using a chin tuck position during the swallow may be beneficial in decreasing aspiration in persons who experience a delayed pharyngeal swallow and reduced airway closure if the source of aspiration is material pooled in the valleculae.[54] The study by Shanahan et al[54] did not find a decrease in the risk of aspiration with pooling in the pyriform sinus with chin tuck. Chin tuck causes the structures of the pharynx to move posteriorly, reducing the size of the opening to the larynx.[64] Full rotation of the head causes the bolus to move away from the direction of rotation and can be used to direct the bolus down the more intact side of the pharynx.[35]

The "effortful swallow" is done by contracting the muscles of the throat hard during the swallow; this moves the base of the tongue posteriorly and helps to clear bolus from the valleculae.[47]

The Mendelson maneuver, accomplished by pushing the tongue into the hard palate while swallowing, has been demonstrated to open the cricopharyngeal sphincter better and for a longer period of time, allowing the bolus to pass.[5]

Throat clearing and reswallowing may be useful in clearing pooled residue and can be done with other swallowing techniques.

## Follow-Up Care

Follow-up dysphagia care is recommended to determine whether caregivers and patients understand and are complying with recommendations; a follow-up outpatient visit following inpatient care may be needed. Therapists should monitor patients to ensure that they are receiving the correct food and liquid consistencies for dysphagia.[19] Therapists can reassure caregivers and patients that

patients still can enjoy favorite foods and beverages, such as coffee, although with modification.

## Patient and Caregiver Education

The education process begins with initial contact with the patient and caregivers and continues with follow-up visits, informational pamphlets, and referrals to other health care professionals. Patients and caregivers must understand the concept of dysphagia, including the causes and consequences of aspiration, because they cannot follow recommended treatment without knowledge of the problem and its possible consequences. Anatomic pictures, handouts, and verbal explanations are useful educational tools. Precautionary signs placed by the bed also may be helpful in reinforcing the need to follow mealtime management guidelines.

## Efficacy of Intervention

Dysphagia intervention has been shown to improve aspects of oral and pharyngeal function,[42] as well as nutritional status, in patients with stroke.[14] Dysphagia intervention is associated with the ultimate ability to eat by mouth in those with neurologic diagnoses.[43] Intervention has been shown in one small study to enable those with chronic dysphagia requiring alternative nutrition sources to return to eating by mouth with the use of surface electromyography biofeedback.[23] Dysphagia intervention for patients with stroke has been shown to reduce the risk of aspiration pneumonia and thus is cost effective.[45]

### Case Study 1

#### SWALLOWING AFTER RIGHT HEMISPHERIC STROKE

Mrs. Jones was admitted to the hospital with a right middle cerebral artery stroke, resulting in a left hemiplegia with dysphagia. She had a nasogastric tube and was not referred for dysphagia evaluation until she was medically stable, a week after her admission. On evaluation, she demonstrated a left facial droop involving reduced muscle tone in the lip, cheek, and tongue. Drooling from the left side of her mouth was a problem because of reduced sensation. The gag reflex was reduced on the left side of the pharynx, although she could elicit a dry swallow with difficulty. Once her dentures were inserted and the nasogastric tube was removed, a feeding trial was done. During the feeding trial, Mrs. Jones demonstrated pocketing of food in her left cheek and in the sulcus between her lower jaw and cheek. She was able to swallow soft purees and honey-thick fluids, although thin fluids elicited a cough. A modified barium swallow further revealed pooling in the pyriform sinuses and occasional laryngeal

*Continued*

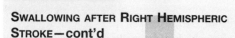

## Case Study 1

### SWALLOWING AFTER RIGHT HEMISPHERIC STROKE—cont'd

penetration with honey-thick fluids, which was alleviated with a chin tuck and by intermittent throat clearing. At this time she still had an intravenous line, so hydration was not a concern. She was able to feed herself with her dominant right hand once her tray was set up, with frequent cues to regard the left side of her plate because of left neglect. She also needed cues to swallow each mouthful and eat slowly because of reduced judgment and impulsivity. Mrs. Jones massaged her left cheek with tactile cues to move pocketed food back onto her tongue. Within a week Mrs. Jones was able to progress to soft solids and nectar-thick fluids, and her intravenous line was discontinued. The following week she progressed to thin fluids and ground solids and was able to prepare her tray independently. She still needed occasional safety cues to eat slowly, to take single sips, and to look at the left side of her plate.

## Case Study 2

### SWALLOWING AFTER LEFT HEMISPHERIC STROKE

Mr. Smith was admitted to the hospital with a left middle cerebral artery stroke and was referred for dysphagia evaluation the day after admission. His oral movements and ability to follow commands were difficult to assess formally because of aphasia. Active and fairly symmetrical motion of his lips, cheeks, and tongue were observed on attempts to speak. Mr. Smith's dentition was intact. His gag reflex was intact, although palatal movement was not observed because of inability to phonate on command; he was unable to produce an automatic cough. On the feeding trial, he initially demonstrated slow initiation of oral and hand-to-mouth movement characteristic of apraxia, but once he had eaten several bites, he was able to manipulate foods more efficiently during the preoral and oral-preparatory stages of the swallow. Mr. Smith was able to manage soufflé textures and soft chewable solids and to drink thin fluids using a dysphagia cup to prevent tipping his head back to swallow. He required some tactile guiding to self-feed with his dominant right upper extremity, which had exhibited isolated but weak movements. Within the week he was able to chew and swallow food with regular textures. Upper extremity function improved as well, and he was able to prepare his tray independently and cut solid foods using his right hand in dominant fashion.

## REVIEW QUESTIONS

1. Define aspiration.
2. Define laryngeal penetration.
3. Describe the five stages of swallowing. Indicate three signs or symptoms of dysphagia at each stage.
4. Name the cranial nerves and identify their functions in swallowing.
5. Name 10 items important for chart review.
6. Describe the elements of a dysphagia intervention program for a stroke patient.
7. Describe two advantages of fiberoptic endoscopic evaluation of swallowing.
8. Describe two advantages of a modified barium swallow.

## REFERENCES

1. Alberts MJ, Horner J, Gray L, et al: Aspiration after stroke: lesion analysis by brain MRI, *Dysphagia* 7(3):170-173, 1992.
2. American Occupational Therapy Association: Clarification of the use of the terms assessment and evaluation, *Am J Occup Ther* 49:1072, 1995.
3. Avery-Smith W, Rosen AB, Dellarosa DM: *Dysphagia evaluation protocol*, San Antonio, Tex, 1997, Therapy Skill Builders.
4. Aviv JE, Martin JH, Sacco RL, et al: Supraglottic and pharyngeal sensory abnormalities in stroke patients with dysphagia, *Ann Otol Rhinol Laryngol* 105(2):92-97, 1996.
5. Bartolome G, Neumann S: Swallowing therapy in clients with neurological disorders causing cricopharyngeal dysfunction, *Dysphagia* 8:146, 1993.
6. Bastian RW: The videoendoscopic swallowing study: an alternative and partner to the videofluoroscopic swallowing study, *Dysphagia* 8(4):359-367, 1993.
7. Bisch EM, Logemann JA, Rademaker AW, et al: Pharyngeal effects of bolus volume, viscosity, and temperature in clients with dysphagia resulting from neurologic impairment and in normal subjects, *J Speech Hear Res* 37:1041, 1994.
8. Ciocon JO: Indications for tube feedings in elderly patients, *Dysphagia* 5(1):1-5, 1990.
9. Crary MA: A direct intervention program for chronic neurogenic dysphagia secondary to brainstem stroke, *Dysphagia* 10(1):6-18, 1995.
10. Davies PM: *Starting again*, Berlin, 1994, Springer-Verlag.
11. DePippo KL, Hosas MA, Reding MJ: The Burke dysphagia screening test: validation of its use in patients with stroke, *Arch Phys Med Rehabil* 75(12):1284-1286, 1994.
12. DePippo KL, Hosas MA, Reding MJ: Validation of the 3-oz water swallow test for aspiration following stroke, *Arch Neurol* 49(12):1259-1261, 1992.
13. Ding R, Logemann JA: Pneumonia in stroke patients: a retrospective study, *Dysphagia* 15(2):51-57, 2000.
14. Elmstahl S, Bulow M, Ekberg O, et al: Treatment of dysphagia improves nutritional conditions in stroke patients, *Dysphagia* 14(2):61-66, 1999.
15. Finestone HM, Foley NC, Woodbury MG, et al: Quantifying fluid intake in dysphagia stroke patients: a preliminary comparison of oral and nonoral strategies, *Arch Phys Med Rehabil* 82(12):1744-1746, 2001.
16. Freed ML, Freed L, Chatburn RL, et al: Electrical stimulation for swallowing disorders caused by stroke, *Respir Care* 46(5):466-474, 2001.
17. Groher ME: Determination for the risks and benefits of oral feeding, *Dysphagia* 9(4):233-235, 1994.

18. Groher ME, Bukatman R: The prevalence of swallowing disorders in two teaching hospitals, *Dysphagia* 1:3, 1986.

19. Halper AS: Developing quality assurance monitors for dysphagia: continuous quality improvement, *Semin Speech Lang* 12:288, 1991.

20. Horner J, Massey EW: Silent aspiration following stroke, *Neurology* 38(2):317-319, 1988.

21. Horner J, Massey EW, Brazer SR: Aspiration in bilateral stroke patients, *Neurology* 40(11):1686-1688, 1990.

22. Huckabee ML: *Maximizing rehabilitative efforts for dysphagia recovery: SEMG biofeedback monitoring, 2001.* Retrieved April 11, 2002, from http://www.kayelemetrics.com/ProductInfo/ProductPages/SwallowWorkstation.

23. Huckabee ML, Cannito MP: Outcomes of swallowing rehabilitation in chronic brainstem dysphagia: a retrospective evaluation, *Dysphagia* 14(2):93-109, 1999.

24. Irie H, Lu CC: Dynamic evaluation of swallowing in patients with cerebrovascular accident, *Clin Imaging* 19(4):240-243, 1995.

25. Johnson ER, McKenzie SW, Sievers A: Aspiration pneumonia in stroke, *Arch Phys Med Rehabil* 74(9):973-976, 1993.

26. Kalra L, Yu G, Wilson K, et al: Medical complications during stroke rehabilitation, *Stroke* 26(6):990-994, 1995.

27. Kidd D, Lawson J, Nesbitt R, et al: The natural history and clinical consequences of aspiration in acute stroke, *Q J Med* 88(6):409-413, 1995.

28. Kidder TM, Langmore SE, Martin BJW: Indications and techniques of endoscopy in evaluation of cervical dysphagia: comparison with radiographic techniques, *Dysphagia* 9(4):256-261, 1994.

29. Langmore SE: Managing the complications of aspiration in dysphagic adults, *Semin Speech Lang* 12:199, 1991.

30. Linden-Castelli P: Treatment strategies for adult neurogenic dysphagia, *Semin Speech Lang* 12:255, 1991.

31. Logemann JA: *Evaluation and treatment of swallowing disorders,* Austin, Texas, 1997, Pro-Ed.

32. Logemann JA: Preswallow sensory input: its potential importance to dysphagic patients and normal individuals, *Dysphagia* 11(1):9-10, 1996.

33. Logemann JA: Effects of aging on the swallowing mechanism, *Otolaryngol Clin North Am* 23(6):1045-1056, 1990.

34. Logemann JA: Criteria for studies of the treatment for oral-pharyngeal dysphagia, *Dysphagia* 1:193, 1987.

35. Logemann JA, Kahrilas PJ, Kobara M, et al: The benefit of head rotation on pharyngoesophageal dysphagia, *Arch Phys Med Rehabil* 70(10):767-771, 1989.

36. Logemann JA, Pauloski BR, Colangelo L, et al.: Effects of a sour bolus on oropharyngeal swallowing measures in clients with neurogenic dysphagia, *J Speech Hear Res* 38(3):556-563, 1995.

37. Lorish TR, Sandin KJ, Roth EJ, et al: Stroke rehabilitation evaluation and management, *Arch Phys Med Rehabil* 75(5 Spec No):S47-S51, 1994.

38. Mann G: *MASA: The Mann assessment of swallowing ability,* Clifton Park, NY, 2000, Singular.

39. Mann G, Hankey GJ: Initial clinical and demographic predictors of swallowing impairment following acute stroke, *Dysphagia* 16(3):208-215, 2001.

40. Meng NH, Wang TG, Lien IN: Dysphagia in patients with brainstem stroke: incidence and outcome, *Am J Phys Med Rehabil* 79(2):170-175, 2000.

41. Miller AJ: The search for the central swallowing pathway: the quest for clarity, *Dysphagia* 8(3):185-194, 1993.

42. Neumann S: Swallowing therapy with neurologic patients: results of direct and indirect therapy methods in 66 patients suffering from neurologic disorders, *Dysphagia* 8(2):150-153, 1993.

43. Neumann S, Bartolome G, Buchholz D, et al: Swallowing therapy of neurologic patients: correlation of outcome with pretreatment variables and therapeutic methods, *Dysphagia* 10(1):1-5, 1995.

44. Noll SF, Roth EJ: Stroke rehabilitation. I. Epidemiologic aspects and acute management, *Arch Phys Med Rehabil* 75(5 Spec No):S38-S41, 1994.

45. Odderson IR, Keaton JC, McKenna BS: Swallow management in patients on an acute stroke pathway: quality is cost effective, *Arch Phys Med Rehabil* 76(12):1130-1133, 1995.

46. Perlman AL, Langmore SE, Milianti FJ, et al: Comprehensive clinical examination of oropharyngeal swallowing function: Veteran's Administration procedure, *Semin Speech Lang* 12(3):246, 1991.

47. Pouderoux P, Kahrilas PJ: Deglutitive tongue force modulation by volition, volume, and viscosity in humans, *Gastroenterology* 108:1418, 1995.

48. Robbins J, Levine RL: Swallowing after unilateral stroke of the cerebral cortex: preliminary experience, *Dysphagia* 3(1):11-17, 1988.

49. Robbins J, Levine RL, Maser A, et al: Swallowing after unilateral stroke of the cerebral cortex, *Arch Phys Med Rehabil* 74(12):1295-1300, 1993.

50. Rosenbek JC, Roecker EB, Wood JL, et al: Thermal application reduces the duration of stage transition in dysphagia after stroke, *Dysphagia* 11(4):225-233, 1996.

51. Schmidt J, Holas M, Halvorson K, et al: Videofluoroscopic evidence of aspiration predicts pneumonia and death but not dehydration following stroke, *Dysphagia* 9:7, 1994.

52. Shaker R, Easterling C, Kern M, et al: Rehabilitation of swallowing by exercise in tube-fed clients with pharyngeal dysphagia secondary to abnormal UES opening, *Gastroenterology* 122(5):1314-1321, 2002.

53. Shaker R, Kern M, Bardan E, et al: Augmentation of deglutitive upper esophageal sphincter opening in the elderly by exercise, *Am J Physiol* 272(6 pt 1):G1518-G1522, 1997.

54. Shanahan TK, Logemann JA, Rademaker AW, et al: Chin-down posture effect on aspiration in dysphagic patients, *Arch Phys Med Rehabil* 74(7):736-739, 1993.

55. Smithard DG, O'Neill PA, England RE, et al: The natural history of dysphagia following stroke, *Dysphagia* 12(4):188-193, 1997.

56. Smithard DG, O'Neill PA, Parks C, et al: Complications and outcome after acute stroke: does dysphagia matter? *Stroke* 27(7):1200-1204, 1996.

57. Sonies BC: Instrumental procedures for dysphagia diagnosis, *Semin Speech Lang* 12:186, 1991.

58. Stoeckli S, Huisman TA, Seifert B, et al: Interrater reliability of videofluoroscopic swallow evaluation, *Dysphagia* 18(1):53-57.

59. Takahashi K, Groher ME, Michi K: Methodology for detecting swallowing sounds, *Dysphagia* 9(1):54-62, 1994.

60. Teasell RW, Bach DB, McRae M: Prevalence and recovery of aspiration poststroke: a retrospective analysis, *Dysphagia* 9(1):35-39, 1994.

61. Teasell RW, Foley N, Doherty T, et al: Clinical characteristics of patients with brainstem stroke admitted to a rehabilitation unit, *Arch Phys Med Rehabil* 83(7):1013-1016, 2002.

62. Veis SL, Logemann JA: Swallowing disorders in persons with cerebrovascular accident, *Arch Phys Med Rehabil* 66(6):372-375, 1985.

63. Veis SL, Logemann JA, Colangelo L: Effects of three techniques on maximum posterior movement of the tongue base, *Dysphagia* 15(3):142-145, 2002.

64. Welch MV, Logemann JA, Rademaker AW, et al: Changes in pharyngeal dimensions effected by chin tuck, *Arch Phys Med Rehabil* 74(2):178-181, 1993.

65. Whelan K: Inadequate fluid intakes in dysphagic acute stroke, *Clin Nutr* 20(5):423-428, 2001.

66. Wilkinson TJ, Thomas K, MacGregor S, et al: Tolerance of early diet textures as indicators of recovery from dysphagia after stroke, *Dysphagia* 17(3):227-232, 2002.

67. Yoneyama T, Yoshida M, Ohrui T, et al: Oral care reduces pneumonia in older patients in nursing homes, *J Am Geriatr Soc* 50(3):430-433, 2002.

68. Zenner PM, Losinski DS, Mills RH: Using cervical auscultation in the clinical dysphagia examination in long-term care, *Dysphagia* 10(1):27-31, 1995.

## SUGGESTED READINGS

Agency for Healthcare Policy and Research: *Diagnosis and intervention of swallowing disorders (dysphagia) in acute-care stroke clients,* Evidence Report/Technology Assessment: No 8, 1999. Retrieved March 3, 2003, from http://hstat.nlm.nih.gov/hq/Hquest/screen/Direct/db/14.

Davies P: The neglected face. In *Steps to follow,* New York, 2000, Springer-Verlag.

Fornataro-Clerici L, Roop TA: *Clinical management of adults requiring tracheostomy tubes and ventilators,* Gaylord, Mich, 1997, Northern Speech Services.

Groher ME: *Dysphagia: diagnosis and management,* Boston, 1997, Butterworth-Heinemann.

Horner J, Buoyer FG, Alberts MJ, et al: Dysphagia following brainstem stroke: clinical correlates and outcome, *Arch Neurol* 48(11): 1170-1173, 1991.

jessica farman and
judith dicker friedman

**chapter 23**

# Sexual Function and Intimacy

## key terms

aging
disability
sexual dysfunction

sexual function
sexual rehabilitation

sexuality
sexuality counseling

## chapter objectives

After completing this chapter, the reader will be able to accomplish the following:

1. Identify and describe the normal human sexual response cycle and the changes that occur during the aging process.
2. Understand the effects of stroke on sexual function.
3. Identify the occupational therapist's role in sexuality intervention.
4. Understand and apply the levels of the PLISSIT model that are appropriate for occupational therapists.
5. Identify sexual impairments and how they affect function.
6. Plan treatment interventions for impairments affecting sexual function.

A discussion of sexuality includes not only specific sexual practices but also the attitudes, behaviors, thoughts, and feelings associated with sex and sexuality. These include an individual's perception of self as a sexual being, body image, self-esteem, participation and roles in relationships (sexual and other), sexual orientation (heterosexual, homosexual, or bisexual), and beliefs and attitudes toward a wide range of sexual behaviors, including masturbation, coitus, oral-genital sex, cuddling, and sensuality. Romano[55] defines sexuality expertly: "Sexuality is more than the art of sexual intercourse. It involves for most . . . the whole business of relating to another person; the tenderness, the desire to give as well as take, the compli-ments, casual caresses, reciprocal concerns, tolerance, the forms of communication that both include and go beyond words . . . sexuality includes a range of behavior from smiling through orgasm; it is not just what happens between two people in bed."

Everyone can enjoy sex. Health care professionals must be aware of their own attitudes toward sexuality. Our patients may be different from ourselves: they may be older, may be of a different sexual orientation, or may have permanent or temporary disabilities. And just as differences among human beings are inherent, therapists must consider and respect the variances in sexual behaviors, preferences, and beliefs among individuals.

# NORMAL HUMAN SEXUAL RESPONSE

One must have an understanding of the normal human sexual response cycle before one can explore the relationship between sexuality and disability. Masters and Johnson[38] divided the human sexual response cycle into four segments: (1) excitement, (2) plateau, (3) orgasm, and (4) resolution. In each phase, definite physical changes occur in both sexes. During the excitement phase, physiologic reactions occur as a result of somatosensory or psychogenic stimulation. In females, the nipples become erect, the vagina swells and becomes lubricated, the clitoris and the labia minora and majora swell, and the uterus and cervix retract. In males, the penis grows erect and the testes rise. In both sexes blood pressure and heart rate increase.

During the plateau phase, respiration increases and blood pressure and heart rate increase further. In females the areola surrounding the nipple swells, the orgasmic platform forms (vasocongestion of the outer two thirds of the vagina), and the color of the labia minora deepens from pink to red. In males, a full erection is achieved as the testes elevate further and the Cowper's gland secretes preejaculatory fluid.

Orgasms differ between the sexes; some women can achieve multiple orgasms. In both sexes, peak pulse rate, blood pressure, and respiration increase, as does muscle tone. Rhythmic contractions of the orgasmic platform and the uterus occur in women, and rhythmic contractions of the penis project semen forward in males.

Masters and Johnson[38] recorded cardiac response and found peak heart rates of 110 to 180 beats per minute during orgasm. However, the mean maximum heart rate during sexual activity was 117.4 beats per minute in a study of middle-aged men with postcoronary disease.[28] During sexual activity, systolic and diastolic pressure increase (from 30 to 80 and 20 to 40 mm Hg, respectively). Respiration rates of up to 40 breaths per minute have been recorded, depending on the level of intensity and duration of sexual activity.[38]

The resolution phase is characterized by the return to preexcitement status, including reductions in blood pressure, heart rate, and respiration. The genitals and breasts return to preexcitement size.

## Aging and the Human Sexual Response Cycle

In normal human development, changes occur during the aging process. Such changes affect sexuality[51] in males and females and already may affect patients who have sustained cerebrovascular accidents.

## Women

Generally between the ages of 40 and 50, women experience menopause, the cessation of menstruation caused by a lack of production of estrogen that occurs over a period of several months to a few years.[34] The major effects of menopause are as follows:

- Vasomotor syndrome (hot flashes)[34]
- Atrophic vaginitis (thinning of the vaginal walls)[34]
- Osteoporosis[34]
- A decrease in the rate, amount, and type of vaginal fluid, which can cause pain during intercourse and may lead to infection[61]
- Loss of contractility of vaginal muscles, which can cause shorter orgasms[61]
- Decreased size of the uterus and clitoris and atrophy of the clitoral hood[34]
- Loss of elasticity in breast tissue, causing sagging

According to Laflin,[34] regular muscle contractions help maintain the integrity of vaginal muscle tone, and "contact with the penis helps preserve the shape and size of the vaginal space." Therefore an active sex life can have a positive effect on genital function.

## Men

As men grow older the following changes occur:

- Erections are often less full, take longer to achieve, and may require direct stimulation.[61]
- Ejaculatory control increases, ejaculation may only occur every third sexual episode and is less forceful, and loss of erection after orgasm may occur faster.[34,61]
- The man may not be able to achieve another erection for 12 to 24 hours after orgasm.[31]
- Sperm volume decreases and the ejaculation may be less intense, which may affect the intensity of orgasm.[34,61]
- The size and firmness of the testes diminish.
- The testosterone level decreases.

Many elderly persons continue to enjoy sexual activity; however, a decline in sexual activity among elderly persons is not uncommon. Older persons do not necessarily lose their desire for sex, but circumstances can make it difficult for them to engage in active sexual relationships. Leading causes of altered sexual activity in the older adult include difficulty finding partners, illness, medication effects, widowhood, divorce, biases about masturbation, societal attitudes about sex and the elderly, and even their own biases and prejudices toward sexuality.[54] Elderly persons may view sex as something that only young, attractive persons do.

# SEXUALITY AND NEUROLOGIC FUNCTION

Sexual function is controlled by the brain, spinal cord, and peripheral nerves, whereas control of libido and sexual pleasure are mediated by several areas in the cortex, midbrain, and brainstem.[47] Men experience reflexogenic and psychogenic erections. Reflexogenic erections are caused by direct stimulation to the penis and may occur without conscious awareness, even in the absence of penile sensation. Psychogenic erections originate from mental activity such as sexual fantasies and stimulating visual input and do not require direct penile stimulation. Reflexogenic erections are controlled by the nervous system through the sacral roots, and psychogenic erections involve the sympathetic nerves between T11 and L2. Female sexual function is similar to that of males regarding nerve innervation.[64] The parasympathetic nerves S2 to S4 influence the clitoris and vaginal lubrication. "Contraction of the vaginal sphincter and pelvic floor occur with stimulation of the somatic aspect of the pudendal nerves (S2-S4)," according to Zasler.[64] Neurologic disability can cause organic impotence by altering the blood flow needed for penile erection and can cause problems with emission and ejaculation in males and with lubrication, clitoral engorgement, and orgasm in females. Some of the subcortical structures theorized to be involved in the neurology of sexuality are the reticular activating system and the hippocampus, amygadala, and hypothalamus. According to Zasler,[64] the thalamus and basal ganglia are hypothesized to be involved with the mediation of sexual function. Some of the cortical areas involved are the frontal lobes and the nondominant temporal lobe. "Lesions in the dominant hemisphere may produce aphasia or apraxia both of which could impede sexual activity. Nondominant hemisphere injury may result in . . . visuoperceptual deficits, denial and impulsiveness, all of which could impede expression of sexuality," according to Zasler.[64] Sexual stimulation is caused by stimulation of the brain or peripheral nerves, the former of which results from thoughts and psychological processes and the latter of which results from direct physical stimulation.[44,60]

## EFFECTS OF STROKE ON SEXUAL FUNCTION

The literature shows that common effects of stroke on sexual function are decreased libido, impaired erectile and ejaculatory function, decreased vaginal lubrication, impaired ego and self-esteem, and depression. The motor, sensory, cognitive, and physiologic effects of stroke have been shown to affect the desire and ability to engage in sexual activities in many ways. Some research has been focused on relating sexual dysfunction to the location of the lesion. Some of the scientific literature recommends counseling for patients following stroke but does not provide specific interventions.* As a result, therapists are left with insufficient information to treat sexual dysfunction adequately.

Studies by Korpelainen et al[32]; Korpelainen, Nieminen, and Myllyla[33]; and Monga, Lawson, and Inglis[43] found that among men and women who had sustained strokes, libido

was decreased, abilities to achieve erection and vaginal lubrication were impaired, and the frequency of intercourse was diminished. A small group (19 of 192 patients studied) indicated an increase in libido following stroke.[33] Isolated cases of hypersexuality and abnormal sexual behavior were found to occur in individuals with temporal lobe lesions and concurrent histories of poststroke seizure activity.[44]

In a study of 13 female stroke survivors, the most common complaint was found to be a decreased desire for sexual activity after the stroke; only 5% of the women reported actual impairment in the production of vaginal secretions after the stroke.[2] Most of the women reported no changes in their abilities to achieve orgasm or in their menstrual periods. In addition, although the stroke impaired sexual desire, physiologic function remained unimpaired. The authors concluded that nondominant hemispheric stroke is related to decreased desire; five of seven patients with decreased desire had right brain involvement.

The authors of several studies have attempted to determine cerebral hemisphere dominance on sexual function. Although some investigators found a greater decline in sexual function with left-sided cerebrovascular accident, others found little or no difference between right and left cerebral hemisphere strokes.[5,12,21,48] Garden[20] concludes, "There seems to be an overall consensus that stroke patients maintain prestroke sexual desire but commonly experience sexual dysfunction including erectile and libido problems. Changes in coital frequency and libido are also common. As a result there can be great potential for depression and loss of self esteem."

The individual's prestroke sexual activity is usually a better indicator of poststroke activity.[6,21,23,27] If the individual was leading an active sex life before a stroke, the likelihood of returning to sexual activities is good. Younger age is also a predictor of resumption of sexual activity, although less so.[27] Individuals who were without a partner before a stroke have less opportunity to develop new partnerships and resume sexual activity after a stroke. This decreased opportunity has to do with the effects of stroke itself and an individual's impaired social contact, possible placement in a nursing home or other long-term setting, depression, altered self-image, and the multitude of psychological effects caused by stroke. In a study of 192 stroke survivors and 94 spouses, the decline in sexual activity after stroke was associated largely with individuals' attitude toward sexuality, fears including erectile dysfunction, and the inability to discuss sexuality issues.[33]

Erectile dysfunction may occur as a direct result of stroke[27,32,57] and also may occur in men whose sexual partners have sustained strokes because of fear of causing another stroke or hurting the partner or averse feelings toward the disabled partner.[21,23,24] In women, vaginal

---

*References 5, 12, 19, 21, 23, 33, 56-58.

lubrication may be insufficient, causing painful intercourse.[2,20,21,32]

The presence of nocturnal erections indicates psychological versus organic reasons for erectile dysfunction. In a study by Korpelainen, Nieminen, and Myllyla,[33] all of the male subjects did experience nocturnal erections after stroke, although 55% had impaired nocturnal erections. Individuals with a history of taking cardiovascular medications and those who had diabetes mellitus exhibited a greater frequency of erectile dysfunction after stroke than those without. Similarly for women, impaired vaginal lubrication was more common in women who had taken cardiovascular medications prestroke.

Initiation of sexual activity after discharge from the hospital may be difficult. A couple may delay sexual activity because each partner waits for the other to initiate sex.[23,24] In a study by Goddess, Wagner, and Silverman,[23] one couple put off sexual activity for 15 months after the husband's stroke. The man was unsure whether his wife would find him attractive or a suitable partner, and the wife was concerned that sexual play for her husband may be unsafe.

Sensory impairment is common after stroke. Considering the significant role of touch in sexual expression, its dysfunction also may contribute to sexual dysfunction.[19,32] In subjective reports of 50 stroke survivors, 19% of the subjects reported sensory deficits as the reason for diminished sexual activity.[32] However, the research is inconclusive; a study by Aloni et al[1] of 15 male stroke patients showed that disturbed superficial and deep sensation were not correlated with decreased desire.

Motor impairment can affect sexual function. Decreased range of motion, strength, endurance, balance, abnormal skeletal muscle activity, impaired coordination, and oral motor dysfunction may interfere with intercourse or other sexual activities. However, some research suggests that the degree of hemiplegic impairment is not a major factor in sexual dysfunction.[19,21]

Cognitive deficits also may affect the stroke survivor's social and sexual function. Fundamental cognitive abilities such as attention and concentration are prerequisites for social and sexual activities; distractibility and overstimulation may cause anxiety and agitation, which prevent interaction. Decreased initiation, impulsivity, poor memory, decreased speed of processing, and impaired executive functions are possible effects of neurologic dysfunction and clearly can affect sexual relations.[59]

McCormick, Riffer, and Thompson[41] note that sexual activity is itself a form of human communication. When verbal or nonverbal communication is impaired, sexual activity may be affected.[64] One study found that sexual adjustment was easiest for physically intact individuals with aphasia with spared comprehension and nonverbal communication.[63] However, in one study involving 110 subjects, no correlation between aphasia and poststroke sexual activity was found.[58] Lemieux, Cohen-Schneider, and Holzapfel[35] report that individuals with moderate and severe aphasia are not included in most studies because they are difficult to interview, so little is known about their sexuality after stroke. In their small study of aphasia and sexuality in six couples, the researchers developed pictograms to facilitate communication with aphasic respondents. Although the effects of stroke on sexuality in this study were similar to those of previous studies, almost all the aphasic persons and their partners reported that aphasia had a negative effect on their sex lives.

The effect of stroke on psychological function is enormous. Korpelainen et al[32] found that the psychological impact of stroke was a greater factor in sexual function after stroke than associated neurologic deficits. The loss of function, including hemiparesis, sensory and balance disorders, pain, and cognitive, perceptual, and impaired communication skills may have an enormous negative effect on an individual's self-image. As Strauss[59] notes, the formulation of relationships, sexual or other, requires some level of self-esteem. An impaired image of one's body and appearance can affect the ability to make new relationships or maintain existing ones. Loss of confidence and decreased self-esteem may result from the following:

- Changes in appearance, including facial asymmetries and diminished facial expression
- Changes in clothing style (inability to don pantyhose or walk in high heels as a result of required ankle-foot orthosis
- Need for adaptive equipment or assistive devices such as a splint, wheelchair, or cane
- Dependence in activities of daily living (ADL), such as the need to have food cut and to have assistance with toileting

In addition to changes in self-perception, the stroke survivor suddenly may find a new role in relationships. For instance, a wife may discover that she is no longer able to carry out the functions related to her role as wife because of the effects of a stroke. The stroke survivor may depend more on other family members. Role changes could affect the quality of an existing relationship.[8,54] Such changes may be confusing and stressful for the patient and the partner, particularly if the stroke survivor requires assistance with self-care activities such as toileting or bathing. Dependence in ADL is a major predictor of decreased sexual activity level after a stroke. In a study by Kimura et al,[30] subjects who demonstrated ADL impairments also demonstrated a decline in sexual activity. Sjogren and Fugl-Meyer reported similar findings in their study in 1982.[58]

Impaired bladder function also may affect sexual activity. Strokes often occur in the elderly who may have underlying genitourinary dysfunction (prostatic hypertrophy, stress incontinence). Proper evaluation by a urologist is indicated.[37,52] Marinkovic and Badlani[37] recommend treatment of incontinence before addressing sexual dysfunction. Medications used to treat incontinence have side effects such as dry mouth, which can make kissing or other oral activities unpleasant. If the individual is taking additional medication for other reasons (for example, diuretic agents), urine output may be increased. For the individual with mobility impairments, quick and frequent access to the bathroom may be difficult, resulting in episodes of incontinence. Incontinence may affect self-esteem and may be a source of embarrassment.[29] Bowel incontinence is less common after cerebrovascular accident because stroke patients typically are constipated because of immobility and inactivity and poor food and fluid intake, which can cause bloating and discomfort.[62]

Hypertension is a major risk factor for stroke, and new research indicates that hypertension is associated with sexual dysfunction in men and women. Burchardt et al[7] report a higher incidence and greater severity of erectile dysfunction in men with hypertension compared with an age-matched population without hypertension. The study also suggested that the erectile dysfunction was linked to the hypertension and not to side effects of antihypertensive medications. Grimm et al[25] also found that "sexual dysfunction in hypertensive individuals may be related more to hypertension level than to drug treatment." Hypertensive women also report decreased lubrication, less frequent orgasm, and more frequent pain with sexual activity than women without hypertension; again, the effects were not related to the type of treatment.[16]

Individuals who have had strokes often have a history of other medical problems, including heart disease, which alone can cause functional impairments related to sexual activities. Often individuals with a history of myocardial infarction or bypass surgery fear the resumption of sexual activities.[25,36,46] Muller et al[46] studied 858 patients who were sexually active in the year preceding myocardial infarction and found that although the risk of myocardial infarction increases in the 2 hours following sexual activity, the risk is almost equivalent in patients with and without heart disease. The research indicated that the risk of myocardial infarction caused by sexual activity is 2 in 1 million for a person with heart disease and that individuals who experience periods of anger or heavy exertion have a greater increase in actual risk because these behaviors occur with more frequency than sexual activity. However, the overall risk of myocardial infarction is lower for patients who engage in regular exercise, which has been shown to decrease the amount of cardiac work required during sexual activity.

From a cardiac rehabilitation perspective, a patient is "safe" to resume sexual activity when the person can climb two flights of stairs or walk the length of a city block or its equivalent at a brisk pace with no discomfort.[28,36] This parameter may be difficult to assess in some stroke patients because of mobility deficits, and alternative activities may have to be explored (for example, propelling a wheelchair at a brisk pace with the use of unaffected arms and legs).

The effect of stroke on sexual function is difficult to assess without examining the types of medications patients are taking. Antihypertensive agents have been found to cause erectile dysfunction, impede ejaculation, and decrease libido.[11,19,21] Some β-blockers are known to affect erectile function and cause depression. One antihypertensive diuretic medication, spironolactone, is known to cause breast tenderness, galactorrhea (excessive secretion of the mammary glands), and gynecomastia (overdevelopment of the mammary glands), which is not always reversible in men.[11] In a study by Aloni, Schwartz, and Ring,[2] six of the seven women who reported decreased sexual desire were taking anticoagulant drugs, suggesting that the medications may affect sexual function. Medications other than those prescribed for stroke management or hypertension may have additional side effects such as rashes and feelings of fatigue that may affect a patient's desire to participate in sexual activities. Considering the potential side effects of various medications on sexual function and informing patients as necessary is the rehabilitation team's responsibility.

## SOCIETAL ATTITUDES

Attitudes on the part of the public or the patient's family members also may affect the patient emotionally or psychologically. Although the Americans with Disabilities Act has resulted in some improvement in public attitude, the fact remains that many persons still harshly judge individuals who appear "different" from the rest of society and regard disabled individuals with fear and shame. Stroke survivors and persons with other disabilities perceive these attitudes and as a result avoid social or public situations. The media seldom depict persons with disabilities as full partners in sexual relationships. The stroke patient and partner, family members, and others may share the view that persons with disabilities are sexless, "different," and undeserving of social and sexual fulfillment. These attitudes can affect patients' existing relationships and their willingness to pursue new relationships.

## ROLE OF OCCUPATIONAL THERAPY

When persons experience changes in sexual function, they may require professional intervention to cope with these changes in sexual function and sexuality. What is the role of occupational therapy in sexuality intervention for these patients, and what is required to fulfill this role?

Sexuality long has been considered an appropriate area for occupational therapy intervention. Andamo[3] states that "sexual function should be included in the occupational therapy evaluation as it relates to the identification of the patient's abilities and limitations in his daily living necessary for the resumption of his various roles." Neistadt[47] notes that as "holistic caregivers, dedicated to facilitating quality lives, occupational therapists should be prepared to address sexuality issues with their adolescent and adult patients." The American Occupational Therapy Association has confirmed the role of occupational therapy by including sexual activity as an activity of daily living within the areas of occupation in the Occupational Therapy Practice Framework.[50]

Occupational therapists are well prepared to address sexuality problems in stroke patients; the sensory, motor, cognitive, and psychosocial impairments that interfere with sexual function are the same ones that affect other performance areas addressed by occupational therapy, including other ADL and work and leisure activities. Occupational therapists' skills of activity analysis and adaptation, holistic orientation, and knowledge of biologic and behavioral sciences help them deal effectively with patients' sexual difficulties.[18] Research indicates that dependence in ADL is a major factor in decreased sexual activity after stroke,[30,58] further supporting the role of occupational therapists in sexual rehabilitation by restoring patients to the highest possible level of independence and role function.

Most occupational therapists receive some training in sexuality intervention. Even before the American Occupational Therapy Association listed sexual activity as an activity of daily living, the authors of a 1988 study reported that 88% of 50 occupational therapy programs included formal classroom training about sexual function, with an average of 3½ hours of class time devoted to this subject.[53]

## TEAM APPROACH

Although occupational therapists must be involved in sexual health care, effective sexual rehabilitation, like all rehabilitation, requires a team approach. The rehabilitation team must address all the individual's problems in a holistic way, and all team members should be knowledgeable about sexual issues and treatment options.[64] If each member of the treatment team is knowledgeable and skilled in this area, the patient can choose the team member with whom he or she is most comfortable to address sexual issues. In addition, each team member has different expertise from which the patient may benefit. The physician may best address problems related to erectile dysfunction, relationship changes may require social work intervention, and the speech and language pathologist may best address communication difficulties.

In reality, the health care team often ignores sexuality issues, especially for the stroke population. A support group of 37 wives of stroke patients at a Veterans Administration center reported that no one had spoken to them about poststroke sexuality.[41] In a 1988 study of sexuality counseling in an inpatient rehabilitation program, only 20% of non–spinal cord injured patients (55% of whom had a diagnosis of stroke) had received written materials on sex. Sexuality information was given voluntarily to 32%.[13] Rehabilitation professionals cite various reasons for not addressing sexuality with their patients, with the most common responses being that another team member is responsible for this intervention and that their knowledge is inadequate.[48] The physician, social worker, and psychologist most often are cited as responsible for sexuality intervention.

In yet another study on sexuality counseling following spinal cord injury, patients indicated a preference to speak with their occupational or physical therapist or nurse about their sexual concerns. Participants reported a positive response to therapists who used an open and direct style of communicating and otherwise were frustrated, embarrassed, or intimidated by therapists who did not. Although many of the subjects were not ready to discuss sexuality early in their rehabilitation, they concurred that knowing resources were available when they needed them was vital.[39]

Besides being neglected in the clinic, sexual rehabilitation has received little attention in research. However, a general positive correlation has been found between successful sexual rehabilitation and positive adjustment to disability. The literature shows that patients with disabilities are interested in the inclusion of sexuality in rehabilitation and give sexuality a high priority.[22] Recent studies confirm that stroke survivors and their partners are interested in information and/or counseling about sexuality after stroke.[17,33]

In clinical rehabilitation, "a job title does not always define competencies," and "no job title . . . excludes discussion of sexuality," according to Chipouras et al.[10] The qualities necessary in a competent sexuality counselor for persons with disabilities have been described variously. Chipouras et al[10] emphasize comfort with sexuality, including one's own; comfort with disability; empathy; nonprojection of one's own morals onto the patient; awareness of available resources; basic knowledge of human sexuality; and awareness of one's own competency and willingness to refer to others as necessary. The foundation of sexuality counseling consists of awareness and knowledge, which one can gain through reading, in-service education, coursework, and workshops. Therapists must develop skill in sexuality counseling through practice, as for all clinical skills. Discomfort in dealing with sexuality need be no different than discomfort with other difficult disability issues. Occupational therapists address many personal and sometimes painful issues with their patients. Increased competency, skill, and comfort comes with practice. Practice of sexuality interventions through role play with other staff members may be helpful in achieving greater comfort in conducting sexuality interventions.

## PLISSIT

The therapist may use various frameworks and models to address sexuality issues in health care. Among the earliest and most prevalent is the PLISSIT model, developed by psychologist Jack Annon.[4] *PLISSIT* is an acronym for four levels of intervention: *P*ermission, *L*imited *I*nformation, *S*pecific *S*uggestions, and *I*ntensive *T*herapy (Figure 23-1). Using this model, the practitioner can determine the type and extent of sexuality intervention needed, whether he or she has the skills to perform the intervention, and whether to refer to a more qualified counselor.

### Permission

Permission is the most basic and most frequently required intervention. Permission consists of reassuring patients that their actions and feelings are normal and acceptable. All occupational therapists should strive to perform permission-level sexuality interventions. Recognizing that sexual behavior varies widely and not

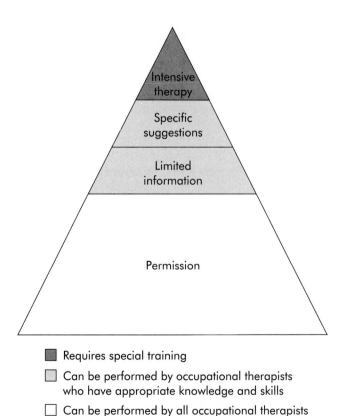

**Figure 23-1** The PLISSIT model. *PLISSIT*, Permission, Limited Information, Specific Suggestions, and Intensive Therapy.

projecting one's own values or morals onto the patient is most important.

The practitioner must be proactive to provide patients with permission. Waiting for the patient to bring up sexual issues is not enough; the therapist must let the patient know that expressing sexual concerns is acceptable. The simplest way to do this is to ask, "People who have had strokes sometimes have concerns or questions about how they will be affected sexually. Do you have any concerns or questions in this area?" This line of questioning serves to normalize the concerns and gives patients the opportunity to say "no" if they are not comfortable discussing sexuality with that person at that time. Asking also lets patients know that sexual concerns are considered legitimate and gives them permission to bring up sexual issues again if their needs change. The therapist should ask questions in a language appropriate for the patient's understanding, including the use of slang terms if necessary.

The best time to bring up sexuality is usually at the initial evaluation, when other ADL issues also are being addressed. If this is not feasible because of time constraints or because the evaluating therapist will not be treating the patient, sexuality should be brought up as soon as is comfortable. Sexual concerns should be explored before home visits and in the formulation of discharge plans because the patient's needs and concerns change throughout rehabilitation.

Opportunities to give patients permission to express themselves as sexual beings often occur spontaneously. On one rehabilitation unit, a 38-year-old Hispanic man with a diagnosis of right cerebrovascular accident was playing a getting-to-know-you game with the other patients, all of whom were older women. As part of the activity, each member of the group was asked to name something he or she liked. The women named things such as chocolate, flowers, and pets. The man said, "I like women." After a few seconds of silence, the occupational therapist running the group said, "Of course you do; what could be more natural?" The group members all nodded, and the activity continued.

### Limited Information

Sometimes simply reassuring patients about sexuality is not enough. If patients do have concerns or questions, they may require specific information related to their stated concerns. Most occupational therapists are qualified to provide patients with limited information. This level of intervention often is concerned with dispelling myths or misconceptions about sexuality. Limited information may be related to facts about the effect of disability on sexuality and sexual function. Handouts, pamphlets, and group education programs are good ways to provide limited information. The patients may read and absorb information on their own and ask the practitioner for clarification as needed. The important issue is to limit the information to the patient's specific concerns. The accuracy of the information is also paramount. If the therapist does not have the information, he or she should help the patient get it before making a referral to another practitioner. For example, a patient with a recent stroke and complex cardiac history asks whether it is safe to have sex. Although the patient's physician can provide the answer, it is not enough for the therapist to say, "Ask your physician." By bringing up the concern to the therapist, the patient has chosen that person as an advocate. The therapist might respond, "Your physician is best equipped to answer that question. Would you feel comfortable asking her yourself, or would you like me to contact her for you?"

## Specific Suggestions

If a patient is experiencing a sexual problem, limited information may not be enough to solve it. The next level of intervention is specific suggestions aimed at solving the specific problem. This type of intervention requires more knowledge, time, and skill from the therapist but is appropriate for some occupational therapists (Box 23-1). The therapist should meet with the patient (and partner, if appropriate) in a comfortable, private setting and obtain a sexual problem history. This history should include the following:

- The patient's assessment of the problem and its cause, onset, and course
- The patient's attempts to solve the problem
- The patient's goals

Just as the occupational therapist would not initiate treatment of other problems without a full evaluation, the therapist must understand the sexual problem fully before making specific suggestions. After obtaining the sexual problem history, the therapist should develop treatment goals in collaboration with the patient. These goals may address learning the effects of stroke on sexual function; adapting to changes in sensory, motor, or cognitive function; adapting to psychosocial and role changes; and improving sexual communication.

One male stroke patient reported sexual problems after a weekend visit home. A sexual problem history revealed that he had always preferred the male-superior position for intercourse. Since his cerebrovascular accident, increased leg extensor skeletal muscle activity and weakness had prevented adequate pelvic thrusting in this position. With his occupational therapist, the patient discussed various new positions to increase mobility: lying on the affected side with knees bent or sitting in a chair with his partner seated facing him.

## Intensive Therapy

If the patient's problems are beyond the scope of goal-oriented specific suggestions, he or she may require intensive therapy. This level of intervention is based on specialized treatment skills and is beyond the scope of most occupational therapists. Finding an appropriate referral for such patients, such as a psychologist, social worker, or sex therapist, is advisable. If the sexual problems predate or are not related to the onset of disability, the patient may require referral.

The PLISSIT model enables the health care professional to adapt a sexuality program to the needs of the setting and the population served. Although permission

---

**Box 23-1**

**Competencies for Sexuality Interventions at Each PLISSIT Level**

**PERMISSION**

To perform this level of sexuality intervention, the therapist should do the following:

- Acknowledge the sexuality of all persons.
- Be comfortable with his or her own sexuality.
- Believe that interest in sexuality is appropriate for everyone.
- Be comfortable speaking directly about sexual issues (or be willing to overcome discomfort).
- Refrain from projecting personal sexual morals and values onto others.

**LIMITED INFORMATION**

To provide this level of intervention, the therapist should fulfill the criteria listed for Permission and do the following:

- Have a basic understanding of human sexuality and its many variations.
- Understand the physiology of human sexual response.
- Be able to analyze the effects of physical disability on various sexual activities.
- Be willing to seek and provide accurate sexual information.
- Be aware of the limitations of his or her own knowledge base.

**SPECIFIC SUGGESTIONS**

To perform this level of intervention, the therapist should fulfill the criteria for Permission and Limited Information and do the following:

- Be familiar with various sexual activities.
- Be comfortable discussing specific sexual activities.
- Be able to conduct a sexual problem history.
- Be able to adapt various sexual activities to accommodate functional limitations.

**INTENSIVE THERAPY**

To perform this level of sexuality intervention, the therapist should fulfill the criteria for Permission, Limited Information, and Specific Suggestions and do the following:

- Have formal training in sex therapy, sexuality counseling, or psychotherapy.

to express sexual concern is universal, the need for limited information and specific suggestions varies. The best way to assess the need for sexuality intervention is to ask patients about their concerns. Occupational therapist Evelyn Andamo's treatment model[3] uses a written problem checklist in which the patient is asked to identify problems in whatever role he or she fills, including that of sexual partner. By addressing sexuality in a multiproblem context, this model helps normalize sexual concerns. The checklist includes two items related to sexual problems and concerns about sexual activity. Patients who check either item receive further intervention as needed, including problem clarification, sexual history taking, and the development of treatment goals and treatment planning. Therapists can adapt any evaluation to include verbal questions about sexual concerns and can repeat questions before home visits or as discharge approaches because patients' concerns change over time.

Underlying some health care workers' reluctance to address sexuality may be a fear of opening a Pandora's box of issues too difficult or intimate for them to handle. This is seldom the case. Most persons do not wish to disclose their sexual problems or to include strangers in their intimate relationships. They want and benefit from the least intervention possible to help them solve their sexual problems and deal with their concerns. Other therapists fear that providing permission to discuss sexual concerns will facilitate inappropriate patient sexual behavior. Recent literature indicates that many health care workers are exposed to inappropriate sexual behavior on the part of patients during their careers, and they often lack training in dealing with these behaviors. Less experienced therapists and students tend to ignore the behaviors even when they are severe, which may result in high stress and difficult working conditions.[40] Of course, any therapist who is exposed to sexual or other inappropriate behavior by anyone should address the problem immediately. Patient behaviors should be documented in the medical records; other staff members also may be affected. All new therapists and students should be encouraged to report harassment and seek help with difficult situations.

Providing permission to patients to address sexual issues directly actually decreases inappropriate behaviors. Flirting, sexual jokes, and innuendos are often a patient's way of indirectly expressing doubts and concerns about sexuality after disability. One stroke patient, M.G., overheard his occupational therapist inviting some co-workers to her home and asked, "When are you going to invite me over?" The therapist replied, "You know, M.G., that I am your therapist, and although you're a really nice person, it would be unethical for us to have a social relationship. But tell me, are you interested in developing new social relationships?" This question led to a lively discussion about M.G.'s returning interest in women and sex. The therapist was understanding and supportive.

The patient made no further advances to her. By refocusing attention on the patient, the therapist deflected the unwanted attention and responded to the patient's real need for permission to acknowledge his returning sexual feelings.

## DEVELOPING COMPETENCY

Competency in sexuality intervention comprises three elements (see Box 23-1): comfort, knowledge, and skill. These elements are interrelated; individuals are more comfortable with things they know well (knowledge) and do well (skill). Suggestions for improving these competencies follow.

### Comfort

- Reading (See resources and references at end of chapter.)
- Films (Be aware that many are related to spinal cord injuries.)
- Disability literature

### Knowledge

- Readings (See resources and references at end of chapter.)
- Lectures
- In-service education

### Skill

- Role playing with other staff members
- Acquiring skill through practice
- Seeking a mentor for private supervision who specializes in sexuality

## SPECIFIC SUGGESTIONS FOR TREATMENT

Many impairments that occur after cerebrovascular accident may affect sexual function and sexuality. These deficits include sensorimotor, cognitive, communication, and psychosocial changes. With sexuality, as with other ADL, determining the underlying causes of the performance problem can be challenging. The following section comprises a list of suggestions one may use during treatment.

### Hemiparesis/Sensory Loss

Patients with hemiparesis or sensory loss and their partners may try the following suggestions:
- Having the hemiplegic partner lie on the affected side frees the uninvolved side for touching; this position also provides support, permits active movement, and focuses attention on the intact side. Early treatment by the rehabilitation team (occupational and physical therapy) should include instructing the patient to lie comfortably on the affected side (Figure 23-2).

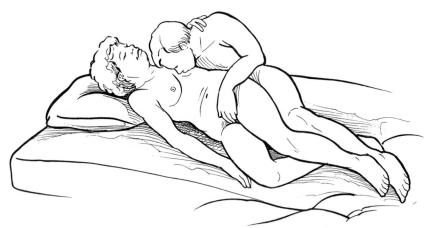

**Figure 23-2**    This position allows for genital fondling during rear entry vaginal or anal penetration and is appropriate for opposite or same-sex couples. Either partner can participate fully if lying on the hemiplegic side.

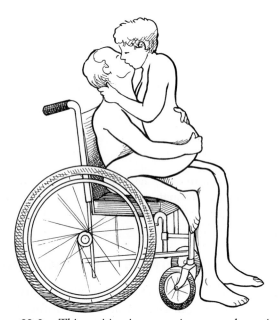

**Figure 23-3**    This position is appropriate as an alternative to lying on a bed or other surface; it is a nice alternative for wheelchair use and may break the barrier of the wheelchair being used only for transport.

- Impaired motor control (limb and trunk) may require a change in coital positioning because the hemiplegic partner may find it difficult to assume certain positions. Alternatively, the unaffected partner may assume the superior position in bed or on a chair or lying on his or her side (Figures 23-3 to 23-5).
- Positioning for comfort with the use of pillows can be incorporated into foreplay.
- Partners should discuss sensory loss beforehand; in hemiplegia there may be absent or diminished light touch, impaired proprioception, kinesthesia, or loss of stereognosis. Stimulation on areas of intact sensation

and incorporation of stimuli to intact senses (e.g., using scents, keeping lights on for visual stimulation, music, and stimulating language) may help improve sensory abilities.
- Individuals with severe sensory deficits must consider skin protection during sexual activity to prevent skin breakdown.
- In the case of impaired hand function, a vibrator can be attached with the use of Velcro to enable stimulation.
- Treatment of weakened muscles of facial expression to improve body image and facial expression and strengthening of oral-motor muscles may enhance oral sexual activities such as kissing and oral-genital sex.

### Cognitive/Perceptual/Neurobehavorial Impairments

Patients with cognitive/perceptual/neurobehavioral impairments and their partners may try the following suggestions:
- Simple positions are recommended (Figures 23-4 and 23-5). Achieving a routine of sexual activity may be helpful if the person has difficulty moving spontaneously. When the brain becomes used to a routine, it does not have to work as hard to plan movements and the patient does not have to concentrate on how he or she is moving.[48]
- Hemianopsia or unilateral neglect may cause a person to ignore parts of the partner's body or not respond when approached from the affected side. The unaffected partner must be sensitive to these deficits.
- Nonverbal communication such as touching and gesturing are encouraged with partners who may have speech or language disorders.[48]
- Distractions such as loud music should be kept to a minimum.[48]
- Individuals with memory impairment should keep a log of daily activities, including sexual activities, in an effort to remain oriented.[48]

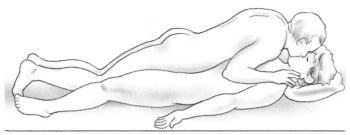

**Figure 23-4**  This position is recommended if the female partner sustained motor or cognitive impairment and requires less endurance for the partner on the bottom.

- Sexual role changes such as increased sexual initiation by the nondisabled partner can help minimize the effects of cognitive changes on sexual function.
- Partners may share fantasies or intimate thoughts in writing or by using augmentative communication devices before and after sexual activity.[48]
- A team approach may be helpful. Speech and language pathologists can help the patient improve or compensate for verbal and nonverbal communication deficits.

### Decreased Endurance

Patients with decreased endurance and their partners may try the following suggestions:
- Sexual activities should be planned. The patient should wait 3 hours after meals before engaging in activities and avoid sex when fatigued. Instead, this may be a good time for intimate cuddling, hugging, or participating in massage.
- Partners can deemphasize intercourse through exploration of other sexual activities such as mutual masturbation and oral-genital sex.
- Partners should consider sexual positions that use less energy (see Figures 23-4 and 23-5).
- Sexual activities may be easier to do in the morning, when energy may be greater, instead of the evening.

### Inadequate Vaginal Lubrication

Patients with inadequate vaginal lubrication and their partners may try the following suggestions:
- A water-based lubricant should be used.
- Foreplay should be extended to ensure adequate lubrication of the vagina before intercourse.
- Lubricated condoms may be helpful.
- Both partners should keep in mind that impaired vaginal lubrication also might be a normal age-related change.
- A consultation with a gynecologist may be warranted.

### Erectile Dysfunction

Patients with erectile dysfunction and their partners may try the following suggestions:

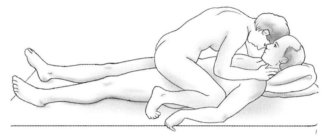

**Figure 23-5**  This position is recommended if the male partner sustained motor or cognitive impairment and requires less endurance for the partner on the bottom.

- Sildenafil citrate (Viagra), approved by the Food and Drug Administration in 1998, has revolutionized the treatment of erectile dysfunction.[9] The package insert warns that there is no "controlled clinical data on the safety or efficacy of sildenafil citrate in . . . patients who have suffered a myocardial infarction, stroke or life-threatening arrhythmia within the last 6 months."[45] However, sildenafil is safe and effective for patients with well-controlled hypertension receiving antihypertensive medications.[14,31] For any person with cardiovascular disease, a physician should assess the safety of sexual activity and use of sildenafil.[14] New oral medications for erectile dysfunction are currently in development by several manufacturers; the second generation of medications is expected to be more effective and less expensive and have fewer side effects.[15]
- Certain medications may have an effect on erection in addition to the stroke itself. The patient and physician should discuss this possibility.
- The patient and partner should consider alternatives to intercourse.
- If erectile dysfunction is related to depression or another psychological issue, the therapist should suggest that the patient discuss it with the appropriate team member, such as the psychologist or psychiatrist.
- A ring placed on the base of the penis may help maintain blood flow into the penis and help the patient maintain an erection.
- Other treatment options for erectile dysfunction require consultation with a urologist. These include vacuum constrictor devices, injection of vasoactive agents, and

penile prosthesis implantation.[26] Use of these therapies has not been studied in stroke survivors[42] and has decreased greatly since the advent of sildenafil.[15]

## Incontinence

Patients with incontinence and their partners may try the following suggestions:

- The patient should avoid fluids before engaging in sexual activity.[32]
- Men may wear a condom to prevent leakage onto the partner.
- Patients on a voiding schedule should be encouraged to adhere to the schedule to prevent accidents.
- Towels should be available in case of accidents, and the patient should discuss his or her situation before engaging in sexual activity to prevent embarrassment.
- The patient should empty his or her bladder before engaging in sexual activity.
- Pelvic muscle reeducation (with or without biofeedback) to improve strength and control of pelvic floor muscles may be indicated.[49]

## Contraception and Safer Sex

Most stroke patients are past the childbearing years; however, contraception remains an issue for those who are still fertile. Menses may be affected after a stroke, although studies are inconclusive.[38] However, the exploration of contraceptive methods may be necessary, depending on the patient's impairments. The functional abilities needed to use condoms, a diaphragm, or a cervical cap include fine motor abilities, motor praxis, and intact cognitive and perceptual function.[48] However, in some cases the nondisabled partner can assist with contraception and work it into the sexual repertoire. For example, if a woman had a stroke and her contraception of choice is the diaphragm but she cannot insert the device because of hemiplegia, her partner might do this for her. If the couple prefers, they can explore alternative methods of contraception. A review of other methods may be warranted, particularly if the patient previously used the pill or other contraceptive hormones, which have side effects, some of which affect circulation.[60]

Latex condoms are preferred for safer sexual practices against sexually transmitted diseases; however, an erect penis is required. If the male has difficulty maintaining or achieving an erection, it may not be possible for him to use condoms effectively. Female condoms or alternative sexual practices minimizing contact with body fluids may be explored, and individuals and couples should be educated on options such as mutual masturbation and oral sex with the use of a dental dam, which is a latex sheet placed over the vulva during cunnilingus. The therapist is responsible for staying updated on current guidelines related to safer sex practices if education on safer sex will be included in treatment.

## Case Study 1

### "WHEN WILL MY HUSBAND'S SEX DRIVE RETURN?"

P.R. is a 52-year-old married man who previously suffered a hemorrhagic left basal ganglia stroke. He was admitted to a subacute rehabilitation center with right hemiplegia and language and short-term memory deficits. His right upper and lower extremity sensation was absent for tactile stimulation. He demonstrated increased flexor activity and had no active arm movement. P.R. required maximal assistance with all transfers and activities of daily living, and his activity tolerance was poor. Before admission he had lived with his wife of 1½ years and ran a business requiring frequent travel. P.R.'s wife also worked full time and taught women's exercise classes in her free time.

By his 18-day team conference, P.R. had made substantial gains. He was independent in stand-pivot transfers and required minimal assistance in dressing. He demonstrated emerging sensation and motor control in his right arm and lower extremities. He was able to walk during physical therapy with a cane and assistance from a therapist. His language function had improved, with only some word-finding deficits remaining. He and his wife attended the team meeting. Her last question to the team was, "When will his sex drive return?" P.R. said, "Don't worry, Honey, it will come back like everything else." The staff recommended discussing this issue with the new neurologist, with whom the couple had an appointment the following day.

On return from his neurologist, P.R. reported to his speech therapist that he and his wife had "forgotten" to bring up sexuality. He reported achieving only partial erections. The therapist offered him a consultation with an occupational therapist on staff who was knowledgeable about sexuality and disability, and he agreed. The speech therapist had received no training or information about sexuality and had no experience in this area. P.R.'s treating occupational therapist, who was not present at the team meeting, was willing to use part of P.R.'s scheduled treatment time for the sexuality intervention.

The occupational therapist who specialized in sexuality issues introduced herself to P.R. and made an appointment to meet with him the next week in his private room. She asked whether he had any specific questions or concerns so she could prepare information for their meeting. He said the concerns were mostly his wife's and that he was confident his sex drive would "return just like use of my arm and leg are going to return." The occupational therapist suggested including P.R.'s wife in the meeting, but P.R. said she was unavailable during the daytime so the occupational therapist might as well speak to him alone.

A brief sexual history revealed that P.R. had been single for 11 years before this second marriage and that he had been sexually active with a variety of women during that time. He and his wife considered sex an extremely important part of their relationship. "People can be very sexy even though they don't look it," he explained. P.R. volunteered that he and his wife would not need help with sexual positioning for intercourse because they preferred the female-superior position. P.R. admitted to decreased sexual desire, which he attributed to fatigue, separation, and the nonconducive environment. He reported having erections that he estimated at "three quarters of normal hardness," which was an improvement. He reiterated that he was sure everything would come back.

The intervention included three levels of the PLISSIT model.

## PERMISSION

The therapist assured P.R. that concern about sexuality was common among stroke survivors and their sex partners and that, after a life-threatening event, sexual concerns are a sign of returning health. They discussed the myth that middle-aged persons are not attractive and society's insistence in portraying only young, thin, beautiful persons as "sexy." The therapist explained that although health care workers are sometimes reluctant to bring up sexuality, P.R. had the right to be assertive in getting any assistance he needed in this area.

## LIMITED INFORMATION

P.R. was provided a verbal summary of the research on stroke and sex. He was informed that some persons experience sexual dysfunction after stroke and that desire, libido, erection, ejaculation, and orgasm might be affected. The therapist emphasized the lack of correlation of sexual dysfunction to motor or sensory deficits and the high correlation between prestroke and poststroke sexual function. The therapist and P.R. discussed the effect of antihypertensive medications on sexual function. P.R. reported telling his physician that he would not take any medication that had side effects on sexual function. The physician prescribed a medication without sexual side effects.

## SPECIFIC SUGGESTIONS

Although P.R. reported no need for ideas to improve his sexual function, a level of denial was evident in his assurances that "everything would come back." The occupational therapist said, "Just as you're participating in therapy to improve your arm, leg, and speech, your sexual function will improve faster if you don't just sit around waiting for its return." P.R. agreed that he felt as if he had a new, different body and that he would find it helpful to explore and learn the responses of the new body. They discussed including his wife in the sexual explorations, but she was uncomfortable with the lack of privacy in the facility.

Because P.R. would be unlikely to have sexual relations with his wife before discharge, strategies were discussed for initiating sexual activity in a positive, nonthreatening way because early problems with erectile function are not necessarily predictive of continuing problems. Alternative sexual activities also are considered "real sex."

Because of their prestroke sexual function, motivation, interest, maturity, and willingness to communicate, P.R. and his wife were likely to make a good sexual adjustment to the effects of stroke. However, the therapist did offer information on treatment of erectile or other sexual dysfunction, for in the future, if problems arose, she would not be available to P.R. after discharge. She also reported the latest medical interventions for erectile dysfunction, which would be familiar to any urologist. Although he felt he would not need it, P.R. seemed glad to know that treatment was readily available.

At this facility, sexual concerns were not addressed by any rehabilitation discipline. While treating P.R., the therapist had provided written information on the sexual effects of cerebrovascular accident and the role of speech and language therapists in sexuality counseling to the speech therapist who referred him and summarized the results of the counseling session. Staff members became aware that other patients might have sexual concerns but lacked the comfort level or assertiveness to initiate the communication. The therapist was asked to provide an in-service on sexuality, which was well attended by members of the occupational therapy department and other interested staff.

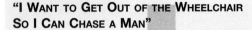

## Case Study 2

### "I WANT TO GET OUT OF THE WHEELCHAIR SO I CAN CHASE A MAN"

W.A. is a 62-year-old woman who previously suffered a right middle cerebral artery stroke with resulting left hemiparesis. After her initial and rehabilitation hospitalizations, she was discharged home for continued occupational and physical therapy. She lived in a senior housing development, which had a social room on the premises. W.A. had been widowed for more than 15 years and reported that her husband had been an alcoholic and a "terrible man." During W.A.'s initial evaluation at home, the occupational therapist asked what her goals for rehabilitation were. W.A. was quick to reply, "I want to be able to get out of the wheelchair so I can chase a man." Sexuality had not been addressed until this point in the evaluation. The therapist took the opportunity to ask W.A. whether she had a significant man in her life, to which W.A. replied "no." The therapist asked W.A. whether she had any concerns about resuming sexual activities after the stroke; again W.A. replied "no." She explained that she was not looking to marry again and simply wanted to be exposed to others so she could flirt. During this conservation the therapist realized that further exploration of sexual function was geared toward getting W.A. out into the community again. W.A. had been limited in this endeavor because of poor mobility and wheelchair dependency.

In this example, the therapist used the permission level of the PLISSIT model. The patient brought up the topic herself, and it was discovered through further questioning that W.A. was really referring to a need to socialize, not so much as to act on her sexual desires. In subsequent conversations, W.A.'s occupational therapist reassessed this situation, particularly as W.A. made progress with activities of daily living and functional mobility. After 6 months of treatment, W.A. was getting back out into the community, attending an adult day care center, and participating in bingo games in her building. She was taught how to transfer on and off the furniture in the social room to allow greater independence and a sense of normalcy. All areas of function, including sexuality, were reevaluated periodically during W.A.'s treatment program, and her goals remained unchanged from her initial evaluation.

In this example the issue of sexuality was related less directly to actual sexual activities than to socialization and flirting. Had the therapist neglected to pursue W.A.'s early statement about wanting to "chase a man," the patient's needs might never have been met.

## Case Study 3

### "WILL I EVER HAVE SEX AGAIN?"

L.E. was a 57-year-old woman with an unknown social history who was admitted to a rehabilitation hospital and who previously suffered a right cerebrovascular accident with left hemiplegia and perceptual deficits. At the initial evaluation the occupational therapist asked whether L.E. had any sexual concerns. "Yes, I want to know whether I'll ever have sex again," she said tearfully. The occupational therapist realized that such a question could not be answered and that the patient's concerns needed clarification. Was L.E. concerned about being able to find a partner? About "performing" sexually? The therapist helped L.E. clarify her question with some probing, "What are you concerned about specifically? What do you think might get in the way of your having sex again?" L.E. reported having a male friend with whom she had an active sex life. Her major concerns were whether she would regain enough function to return home and whether sexual activity would provoke further strokes. The occupational therapist reassured L.E. that most persons can resume sexual activity safely after a stroke and offered to help her consult her physician for medical clearance. The therapist provided the limited information L.E. was looking for through reassurance and by obtaining medical clearance through another team member (that is, the physician). The therapist was able to tie in all the rehabilitation goals with the patient's desire to return to her home and previous lifestyle, which strengthened the collaboration between L.E. and the rehabilitation staff.

## PROGRAM DEVELOPMENT

The therapist should have support, resources, and referrals available when addressing sexual issues. The therapist should inform supervisors and others on the rehabilitation staff of activities. Resources and referral services should be identified in other departments and outside the facility, if appropriate. The therapist should check the existing policies on sexuality (if any) at the facility and strive to be in compliance. The therapist should report experiences and provide education to others. If possible, an interdisciplinary committee should be formed to address sexual issues and develop appropriate programs.

## DOCUMENTATION AND BILLING

Sexuality interventions may be billed and documented in various ways, depending on the billing system and the issues discussed. Appropriate categories include activities of daily living training, patient and family education, discharge planning, and psychosocial training.

As in treatment, sexuality is best addressed in a multiproblem context. Patient privacy and confidentiality must be maintained. Examples of goals include the following:

1. Patient will identify proper bed positioning for sleep and sexual activity.
2. Patient's spouse will accurately assess patient's safety to engage in physical and sexual activities.

## SUMMARY

All persons are sexual, and sexual activity is important to most persons throughout their lives. Interest in or desire for sexual activity does not necessarily diminish as persons grow older. Stroke may interfere with sexual expression by affecting the survivor's desire, libido, erectile or lubrication response, orgasm or ejaculation, and sensorimotor, cognitive, psychosocial, activities of daily living, and role function. Stroke also may affect the partner's response or the patient's ability to find a sexual partner. Research has shown that sexual desire most often is affected; however, prestroke sexual activity is the strongest predictor of poststroke sexual activity. Occupational therapists can use a holistic approach and training in activity analysis and adaptation to assist persons who have had strokes to regain their desired sexual function. A team model is best for sexual rehabilitation, with each team member knowledgeable about sexuality and providing special expertise. The PLISSIT model helps the practitioner identify the type of sexuality intervention required. All occupational therapists should be able to provide patients with permission, limited information, and specific suggestions and should be able to make appropriate referrals for sexual concerns related to stroke. Therapists must be sensitive to the multiple components of sex.

## REVIEW QUESTIONS

1. What are the stages of the sexual response cycle and the associated physiologic changes in males and females?
2. What are some of the normal changes in sexual function in aging men and women?
3. Why does sexual activity decline among older persons?
4. What are the four levels of sexuality intervention in the PLISSIT model? Which may be performed by occupational therapists?
5. What skills are needed to provide sexuality counseling to patients who have had strokes?
6. What common effects of stroke interfere with sexual function and sexuality? What are the best predictors of poststroke sexual function?

## REFERENCES

1. Aloni R, Ring H, Rosenthal N, et al: Sexual function in male patients after stroke a follow up study, *Sex Disabil* 11:121, 1993.
2. Aloni R, Schwartz J, Ring J: Sexual function in post-stroke female patients, *Sex Disabil* 12:3, 1994.
3. Andamo EM: Treatment model: occupational therapy for sexual dysfunction, *Sex Disabil* 4:26, 1980.
4. Annon JS: The PLISSIT model: a proposed conceptual scheme for the behavioral treatment of sexual problems, *J Sex Educ Ther* 2:1, 1976.
5. Boldrini P, Basaglia N, Calanca MC: Sexual changes in hemiparetic patients, *Arch Phys Med Rehabil* 72(3):202-207, 1991.
6. Bray GP, DeFrank RS, Wolfe TL: Sexual functioning in stroke survivors, *Arch Phys Med Rehabil* 62(6):286-288, 1981.
7. Burchardt M, Burchardt T, Baer L, et al: Hypertension is associated with severe erectile dysfunction, *J Urol* 164(4):1188-1191, 2000.
8. Burgener S, Logan G: Sexuality concerns of the post-stroke patient, *Rehabil Nurs* 14(4):178-181, 1989.
9. Butler RN: The Viagra revolution, *Geriatrics* 53(10):8-9, 1998.
10. Chipouras S, Cornelius DA, Makas E, et al: *Who cares? A handbook on sex education and counseling services for disabled people*, ed 2, Baltimore, 1982, University Park Press.
11. Cole TM, Cole SS: Rehabilitation of problems of sexuality in physical disability. In Kottke FJ, Lehman JF, editors: *Krusen's handbook of physical medicine and rehabilitation*, ed 4, Philadelphia, 1990, WB Saunders.
12. Coslett HB, Heilman KM: Male sexual function: impairment after right hemisphere stroke, *Arch Neurol* 43(10):1036-1039, 1986.
13. Cushman LA: Sexual counseling in a rehabilitation program: a patient perspective, *J Rehabil* 54:2, 1988.
14. DeBusk R, Drory Y, Goldstein I, et al: Management of sexual dysfunction in patients with cardiovascular disease: recommendations of the Princeton Consensus Panel, *Am J Cardiol* 86(2):175-181, 2000.
15. Ducharme S: From the editor, *Sex Disabil* 20:105, 2002.
16. Duncan LE, Lewis C, Jenkins P, et al: Does hypertension and its pharmacotherapy affect the quality of sexual function in women? *Am J Hypertens* 13(6 pt 1):640-647, 2000.
17. Edmans J: An investigation of stroke patients resuming sexual activity, *Br J Occup Ther* 56:609, 2002.
18. Evans J: Sexual consequences of disability: activity analysis and performance adaptation, *Occup Ther Health Care* 4:1, 1987.
19. Fugl-Meyer AR, Jaasko L: Post-stroke hemiplegia and sexual intercourse, *Scand J Rehabil Med* 7:158-166, 1980.
20. Garden FH: Incidence of sexual dysfunction in neurologic disability, *Sex Disabil* 9:1, 1991.
21. Garden FH, Smith BS: Sexual function after cerebrovascular accident, *Curr Concepts Rehabil Med* 5:2, 1990.
22. Gatens C: Sexuality and disability. In Woods NF, editor: *Human sexuality in health and illness*, ed 3, St Louis, 1984, Mosby.
23. Goddess ED, Wagner NN, Silverman DR: Poststroke sexual activity of CVA patients, *Med Aspects Hum Sex* 13:16, 1979.
24. Goldberg RL: Sexual counseling for the stroke patient, *Med Aspects Hum Sex* June 1987.
25. Grimm RH, Grandits GA, Prineas RJ, et al: Long-term effects of sexual function of five antihypertensive drugs and nutritional hygienic treatment in hypertensive men and women, *Hypertension* 29(1 pt 1):8-14, 1997.
26. Hatzichristou DG, Bertero EB, Goldstein I: Decision making in the evaluation of impotence: the patient profile-oriented algorithm, *Sex Disabil* 12:29, 1994.
27. Hawton K: Sexual adjustment of men who have had strokes, *J Psychosom Res* 28(3):243-249, 1984.
28. Hellerstein HK, Friedman EH: Sexual activity and the postcoronary patient, *Arch Intern Med* 125(6):987-999, 1970.

29. Kaplan SA, Brown WC, Blaivas JG: When stroke patients suffer urologic dysfunction, *Contemp Urol* Jan 1990.
30. Kimura M, Murata Y, Shimoda K, et al: Sexual dysfunction following stroke, *Compr Psychiatry* 42(3):217-222, 2001.
31. Kloner RA, Brown M, Prisant LM, et al: Effect of sildenafil in patients with erectile dysfunction taking antihypertensive therapy, *Am J Hypertens* 14(1):70-73, 2001.
32. Korpelainen JT, Kauhanen ML, Kemola H, et al: Sexual dysfunction in stroke patients, *Acta Neurol Scand* 98(6):400-405, 1998.
33. Korpelainen JT, Nieminen P, Myllyla VV: Sexual functioning among stroke patients and their spouses, *Stroke* 30(4):715-719, 1999.
34. Laflin M: Sexuality and the elderly. In Lewis CB, editor: *Aging: the health care challenge—an interdisciplinary approach to assessment and rehabilitative management*, ed 2, Philadelphia, 1990, FA Davis.
35. Lemieux L, Cohen-Schneider R, Holzapfel S: Aphasia and sexuality, *Sex Disabil* 19:253, 2001.
36. Mackey FG: Sexuality in coronary artery disease, *Postgrad Med* 80(1):58-60, 1986.
37. Marinkovic SP, Badlani G: Voiding and sexual dysfunction after cerebral vascular accidents, *J Urol* 165:359, 2001.
38. Masters WH, Johnson VE: *Human sexual response*, Boston, 1966, Little, Brown.
39. McAlonan S: Improving sexual rehabilitation services: the patient's perspective, *Am J Occup Ther* 50(10):826-834, 1996.
40. McComas J, Hebert C, Giacomin C, et al: Experiences of student and practicing physical therapists with inappropriate patient sexual behavior, *Phys Ther* 73(11):762-769, 1993.
41. McCormick GP, Riffer DJ, Thompson MM: Coital positioning for stroke afflicted couples, *Rehabil Nurs* 11(2):17-19, 1986.
42. Monga TN, Kerrigan AJ: Cerebrovascular accidents. In Sipski ML, Alexander CJ, editors: *Sexual function in people with disability and chronic illness: a health professional's guide*, Gaitherburg, Md, 1997, Aspen.
43. Monga TN, Lawson JS, Inglis J: Sexual dysfunction in stroke patients, *Arch Phys Med Rehabil* 67(1):19-22, 1986.
44. Monga TN, Monga M, Raina MS, et al: Hypersexuality in stroke, *Arch Phys Med Rehabil* 67(6):415-417, 1986.
45. Mosby: *Mosby's Drug Consult 2003*, III-2858, St Louis, 2003, Mosby.
46. Muller FE, Mittleman MA, Maclure M, et al: Triggering myocardial infarction by sexual activity, *JAMA* 275(18):1405-1409, 1996.
47. Neistadt M: Human sexuality and counseling. In Hopkins HL, Smith HD, editors: *Willard and Spackman's occupational therapy*, ed 8, Philadelphia, 1993, Lippincott.
48. Neistadt ME, Frieda M: *Choices: a guide to sex counseling with physically disabled adults*, Malabar, Fla, 1987, Robert E Krieger.
49. Neuman B: Using behavioral treatment for urinary incontinence, *OT Pract* pp 10-16, Sept 30, 2002.
50. Occupational therapy practice framework: domain and process, *Am J Occup Ther* 56(6):609-639, 2002.
51. Parke F: Sexuality in later life, *Nurs Times* 87(50):40-42, 1991.
52. Patel M, Coshall C, Lawrence E, et al: Recovery from poststroke urinary incontinence: associated factors and impact on outcome, *J Am Geriatr Soc* 49(9):1229-1233, 2001.
53. Payne MS, Greer DL, Corbin DE: Sexual functioning as a topic in occupational therapy training, a survey of programs, *Am J Occup Ther* 42:227, 1988.
54. Purk JK, Richardson RA: Older adult stroke patients and their spousal caregivers, *J Contemp Hum Serv* 75:10, 1994.
55. Romano MD: Sexuality and the disabled female, *Accent Living*, winter 1973.
56. Sjogren K: Sexuality after stroke with hemiplegia. II. With special regard to partnership adjustment and to fulfillment, *Scand J Rehabil Med* 15(2):63-69, 1983.
57. Sjogren K, Damber JE, Liliequist B: Sexuality after stroke with hemiplegia. I. Aspects of sexual function, *Scand J Rehabil Med* 15(2):55-61, 1983.
58. Sjogren K, Fugl-Meyer AR: Adjustment to life after stroke with special reference to sexual intercourse and leisure, *J Psychosom Res* 26(4):409-417, 1982.
59. Strauss D: Biopsychosocial issues in sexuality with the neurologically impaired patient, *Sex Disabil* 9:1, 1991.
60. Szasz G, Miller S, Anderson L: Guide to birth control counseling of the physically handicapped, *Can Med Assoc J* 120:1353, 1979.
61. Thienhaus OJ: Practical overview of sexual function and advancing age, *Geriatrics* 43(8):63-67, 1988.
62. US Department of Health and Human Services: *Post-stroke rehabilitation*, Clinical practice guideline 16, AHCPR Pub No 95-0662, 1995, Rockville, Md, Public Health Service Agency for Health Care Policy and Research.
63. Wigg EH: Counseling the adult aphasic for sexual readjustment, *Rehab Couns Bull* Dec:110-119, 1973.
64. Zasler ND: Sexuality in neurologic disability: an overview, *Sex Disabil* 9:1, 1991.

## SUGGESTED READINGS

Finger WW: Prevention, assessment and treatment of sexual dysfunction following stroke, *Sex Disabil* 11:1, 1993.
Kroll K, Levy Klein E: *Enabling romance*, Bethesda, Md, 1995, Woodbine House.
Novak PP, Mitchell MM: Professional involvement in sexuality counseling for patients with spinal cord injuries, *Am J Occup Ther* 42(2):105-112, 1988.

## SEXUALITY RESOURCES

American Association of Sex Education Counselors and Therapists
435 North Michigan Ave., Suite 1717
Chicago, IL 60611
(312) 644-0828
www.aasect.org

American Congress of Rehabilitation Medicine
6801 Lake Plaza Drive, Suite B-205
Indianapolis, IN 46220
(317) 915-2250
www.acrm.org

American Stroke Association
National Center
7272 Greenville Ave.
Dallas, TX 52231
1-800-553-6321
www.strokeassociation.org

National Stroke Association
96 Inverness Drive East, Suite 1
Englewood, CO 80112-5112
1-800-STROKES
www.stroke.org

Planned Parenthood Federation of America (see local Yellow Pages for listing)
www.plannedparenthood.org

SEICUS (Sex Education and Information Council of the
    United States)
32 Washington Place
New York, NY 10003
(212) 673-3850
www.seicus.org

Sexuality and Disability Training Center
Boston University Medical Center
88 East Newton St.
Boston, MA 02118
(617) 638-7358

Stroke Clubs of America
805 Twelfth St.
Galveston, TX 77550
(409) 762-1022

The Task Force on Sexuality and Disability of the
    American Congress of Rehabilitation Medicine
5700 Old Orchard Road
Skokie, IL 60077
(708) 966-0095

**Specific Websites:**
Disability resources: www.menstuff.org
Sexuality in later life: www.nia.nih.gov/health/agepages/
    sexuality
Sexual Health Network: www.sexualhealth.com
Institute on Independent Living: www.independentliv-
    ing.org
Stroke Survivors without Partners: www.dateable.org

christine m. johann
and mary shea

chapter 24

# Seating and Wheeled Mobility Prescription

## key terms

| | | |
|---|---|---|
| patient education | mat evaluation | seating system |
| deformity prevention | pressure distribution | symmetrical postural alignment |
| functional mobility | product trial | team approach |
| functional positioning | seated posture | wheelchair |

## chapter objectives

After completing this chapter, the reader will be able to accomplish the following:

1. Understand the seating system and mobility base evaluation process.
2. Appreciate the difference between seating for rest and seating for activity performance.
3. Implement a treatment plan and identify the goals of the mobility device and seating and positioning system.
4. Appreciate the pros and cons of different mobility bases and seating system components.
5. Understand the influence of the seating system on carryover of treatment goals.
6. Appreciate the importance of the team process throughout the evaluation and fitting/delivery process.
7. Understand the importance of fitting and training with the recommended seating system and mobility device.

The statistics from the National Stroke Association indicate that stroke is the leading cause of adult disability in the United States.[8] Despite advances in rehabilitation and treatment approaches, many individuals have difficulty with mobility and performance of activities of daily living. An appropriate seating system and mobility base is essential to maximize each client's potential to achieve maximum independence and safety with activities of daily living. Consequently, it is important for a therapist to develop a working knowledge of assistive technology. *Assistive technology* is an umbrella term that includes seating and wheeled mobility, including manual and power wheelchairs, electronic aids to daily living (formerly known as environmental control units), computer access including workstation setup, and augmentative and alternative communication devices (see Chapter 26).

This chapter focuses on the basic principles of seating and positioning, the evaluation process, the fitting/delivery and training process, and the features of various seating system products and mobility devices. Although the emphasis is on the seating and wheeled mobility process specific to persons with a stroke, many of these principles are appropriate for use with all individuals with disabilities who have impaired functioning and disability.

The terms *client* and *individual with disability* are used interchangeably throughout the chapter for appropriate semantics. These terms consistently refer to the same person.

The wheelchair and seating system process is a collaborative process that begins with a client interview and ends with fitting and training of the recommended wheelchair and seating system. The complete process with a team approach is essential to ensure full achievement of safety and the client's goals. The ideal wheelchair and seating system team consists of the patient; health care practitioners such as a medical doctor, an occupational and/or physical therapist, and a speech pathologist (as needed); the caregiver and/or significant other; and an assistive technology supplier. The client is the central person in the wheelchair and seating system process, and the client's goals are given the highest priority.

If clients can communicate their needs and have the cognitive functioning to participate in decision making, then they are empowered, through education, to be more active in the decision-making process. If clients have had cognitive changes that limit their ability to function and be involved in the decision-making process, then they still are central; however, increased attention may be given to the caregiver's needs and goals.

In the past 30 years numerous changes have occurred in the health care industry. These changes were primarily at the environment level and include societal attitudes and expectations of persons with disabilities, rehabilitation service provision, manufacturer production of durable medical equipment, reimbursement policies, and system changes that include the development of authorities and organizations to organize, control, and monitor assistive technology services. As a result of these changes in the wheelchair industry, increased emphasis is on the client taking a more active role in medical care, increased expectations of returning to a previous level of activity and function, prevention of further deformities, actual evaluation of trial equipment, and the certification of a group of therapists and vendors with a comprehensive knowledge base of seating system and mobility device evaluation and provision.

## SOCIETAL ATTITUDES AND EXPECTATIONS OF PERSONS WITH DISABILITIES

For the past 30 years, individuals with disabilities have been lobbying for their needs and rights and have been relatively successful with the passage of several laws. The Americans with Disabilities Act has played a major role at the International Classification of Functioning, Disability and Health (ICF)[3] activities and participation level to increase access to transportation and public places. This increase in environmental accessibility has enabled many individuals with disabilities to pursue their education, employment, and leisure interests to become more active, productive members of society. These changes have fueled the wheelchair manufacturing industry to develop and provide appropriate equipment to meet these more active lifestyles.

## REHABILITATION SERVICES

The provision of rehabilitation services has changed drastically regarding length of stay on rehabilitation units and knowledge required to appreciate the variety of wheelchair and seating system options. Initially, patients had sufficient time in rehabilitation programs to adjust to the changes in their bodies and reach their full potential before they received a wheelchair and integrated into their discharge environment, preferably home. Today, because of the influence of managed care, patients are discharged from rehabilitation units once they are medically stable, have demonstrated restoration gains, and have a support system in place to enable them to be relatively safe with their basic activities of daily living. As a result, therapists are forced to look at a permanent seating system early to ensure that it will facilitate functional restoration and minimize the risk for increased deformity and secondary complications.

Years ago an overall one-size-fits-all philosophy prevailed, and a limited number of wheelchair and seating system options were available for individuals with disabilities. Because of changes in the manufacturing industry, a multitude of product options now are available to facilitate optimal positioning for individuals with a wide variety of needs. The knowledge base of therapists and the increased number of seating systems and accessories that are now available can help decrease the progression of deformities, pain, and other secondary problems. An individual who is seated appropriately can access more muscles, function with increased sense of security, and can lead a healthier, more enriching life. Specific product options are addressed later in this chapter.

## MANUFACTURER PRODUCTION OF DURABLE MEDICAL EQUIPMENT

The durable medical equipment industry has grown tremendously in the past 30 years to meet the increasing population of persons with disabilities and the increasing demand for more versatile, lighter-weight products. The increase in product options and advancement to lighter-weight materials such as aluminum and titanium has resulted in a vast selection of off-the-shelf products that have the potential to meet a wide array of needs. Manufacturers understand the need for persons with disabilities to try specific products to ensure they will meet their needs. Accordingly, they often provide evaluation equipment for patients to try.

## REIMBURSEMENT POLICIES

Insurance companies are the funding source for the majority of durable medical equipment provided for individuals with disabilities. As a result, the funding source often guides the decision-making process. This discussion focuses mainly on Medicare guidelines because many private insurance companies follow these guidelines and Medicare is the primary funding source for individuals who are older than 65 and have had a CVA. Medicare has specific codes and reimbursement guidelines for durable medical equipment. Medicare is concerned primarily about mobility within the home and considers payment for a device once a person has received it. As a result, vendors have to take the risk and supply equipment without receiving any guarantee of payment from Medicare. Consequently, differences exist between individual vendor policies and what wheelchair and seating system products vendors are willing to provide. As one can imagine, some vendors hesitate to provide more complex, expensive equipment for individuals with more involved needs. It is essential for the team to work together to ensure that each individual has access to the best product to meet his or her needs. If this is not possible under Medicare guidelines, the patient should notify the local congressional representative, and the team should consider other funding sources.

## SYSTEM AND POLICY CHANGES: DEVELOPMENT OF STANDARDS AND ORGANIZATIONS TO MONITOR ASSISTIVE TECHNOLOGY SERVICES

System changes have evolved over the past three decades and include the development of authorities and organizations to organize, control, and monitor assistive technology services. The Rehabilitation Engineers Society of North America (RESNA), the National Registry of Rehabilitation Technology Suppliers, the American Academy of Physical Medicine and Rehabilitation, and the Foundation for Physical Medicine and Rehabilitation have been created to develop or have been active in developing standards to ensure a higher standard of practice with wheelchair service provision. A monumental accomplishment was the (American National Standards Institute) ANSI/RESNA Wheelchair Standards. These standards provided the industry with increased consistency for wheelchair performance characteristics and measurements

that are widely used by manufacturers to categorize and test wheelchairs. Consequently, these standards provide the wheelchair team with the ability to compare similar products from different manufacturers easily.

Another major accomplishment has been the development of credentialing programs. The RESNA offers therapists and suppliers credentials for assistive technology practitioners and assistive technology suppliers. The National Registry of Rehabilitation Technology Suppliers awards a certified rehabilitation technology supplier credential. These credentials ensure that the professional members of the treatment team have a broad knowledge base of client's needs and assistive technology products.

Numerous outcome studies have been performed and are being performed at a multitude of levels to determine the efficacy of wheelchairs and wheelchair service provision. Specific topics studied include long-term wheelchair use, wheelchair design, repetitive stress injuries, propulsion methods, pressure relief techniques, and community integration. Many of these studies have focused on the spinal cord–injured population; however, the results are meaningful for all individuals who use wheelchairs as their primary means of mobility. The results from these studies have influenced manufacturing focuses and current practice with wheelchair prescription trends. This has translated into higher-quality products that decrease persons' risk of injury and increase their efficiency with mobility for increased integration into society. Continued involvement of health care practitioners in education, research, and product development is essential to ensure that all individuals with disabilities receive the best possible equipment to minimize their risk for secondary complications and maximize their ability to function indoors and outdoors.

## BASIC BIOMECHANICS OF SITTING

To appreciate and evaluate postural alignment, it is important to have a basic understanding of biomechanics. A therapist should understand basic anatomy of skeletal structures and their relationship to one another. The pelvis is the foundation for sitting; consequently, knowledge of the anatomy and biomechanical features of the pelvis and its relationship with the spine and lower extremities is essential to understand how changes in lower-extremity positioning influence the pelvis and subsequently the spine.

The pelvis moves anteriorly and posteriorly in the sagittal plane around a coronal axis, laterally tilting in a frontal plane around an anteroposterior axis and rotationally in a transverse plane around a vertical axis. A stable neutral position of the pelvis must be attained to provide the proper postural alignment of the spine (Figure 24-1). In a neutral pelvic position the anterior

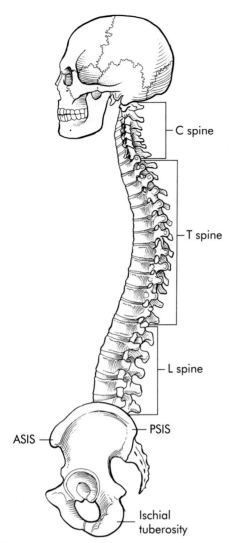

**Figure 24-1**  Lateral view of the spine and pelvis with appropriate alignment and spinal curvatures. *C*, Cervical; *T*, thoracic; *L*, lumbar; *ASIS*, anterior superior iliac spine; *PSIS*, posterior superior iliac spine.

superior iliac spine is level in a frontal plane and level with or slightly lower than the posterior superior iliac spine in the sagittal plane. A pelvis is also positioned in neutral when both ischial tuberosities are bearing weight equally (Figure 24-2). Palpating the anterior superior iliac spine (ASIS) and posterior superior iliac spine (PSIS) and then both right and left anterior superior iliac spine can help one determine the normal posture and/or alignment of the pelvis. Figure 24-3 shows optimal sitting posture with a stable neutral pelvic position and symmetrical positioning of the lower extremities and trunk.

## ASSYMMETRICAL PELVIC POSITIONS, CONCERNS, AND COMMON CAUSES

Figure 24-4, *A*, *B*, and *C*, shows changes in pelvic alignment. Part A demonstrates lateral tilting of the pelvis, in

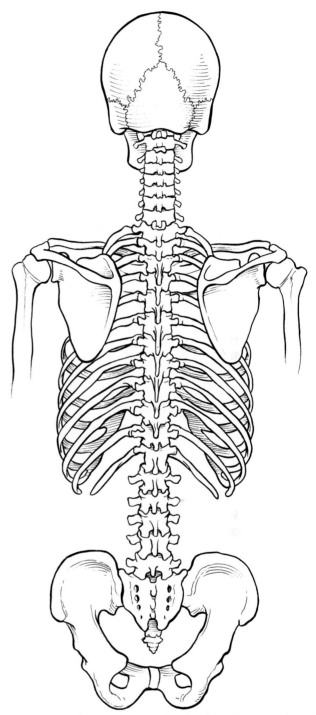

**Figure 24-2**  Appropriate spinal and pelvic alignment viewed posteriorly.

which one anterior superior iliac spine is higher than the other. This pelvic obliquity results in unequal weight distribution through the ischial tuberosities and a C- or an S-shaped spinal curve. This posture places an individual at a high risk for developing a pressure sore under the weight-bearing ischial tuberosity and secondary shoulder and neck problems. This problem is seen commonly in individuals with asymmetrical muscular strength,

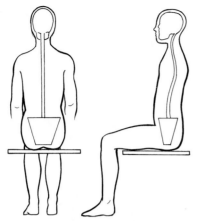

**Figure 24-3**  Appropriate alignment in seated posture. Note symmetrical pelvis and spinal alignment.

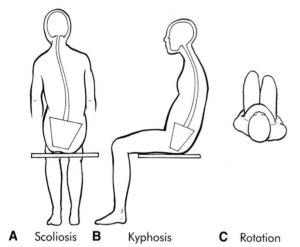

**A**  Scoliosis    **B**  Kyphosis    **C**  Rotation

**Figure 24-4**  Common posturing following a stroke. **A,** Lateral tilting of the pelvis in a client with right-sided weakness. **B,** Posterior pelvic tilt with kyphosis. **C,** Trunk and pelvic rotation (superior view).

asymmetrical muscle tone, limited hip joint mobility, lower extremity hip flexion or internal/external rotation range of motion limitations, asymmetrical lower extremity muscle strength, and midline orientation deficits.

Figure 24-4, *B,* demonstrates a posterior pelvic tilt. A posterior pelvic tilt occurs when the anterior superior iliac spine is higher than the posterior superior iliac spine. This abnormal pelvic position results in a kyphotic spinal posture. A posterior pelvis with lumbar and thoracic spinal kyphosis results in unequal weight distribution, with increased pressures on the sacrum and coccyx, and a compensatory cervical hyperextension. This posture can lead to pressure sores on the sacrum and coccyx, neck and back pain, limited neck range of motion, and a decreased visual field. Posterior pelvic tilt is commonly seen in individuals with trunk weakness, muscle imbalance, limited pelvic mobility, limited hip joint mobility, limited lower

extremity hip flexion, and/or limited hamstring muscle length.

With anterior pelvic tilt the anterior superior iliac spine is lower than the posterior superior iliac spine. This abnormal pelvic position can cause a lordotic curve in the spine. This posture is typically seen in individuals with decreased muscle recruitment and overall muscle weakness.

A pelvic rotation is present when one anterior superior iliac spine is farther forward than the other (Figure 24-4, *C*). The posture can present as unequal leg length posturing when an individual is seated. This abnormal pelvic rotation influences the spine to move into a rotated position and predisposes an individual to a scoliotic curvature of the spine. Pelvic rotation can create unequal weight distribution of the ischial tuberosities, which can lead to pressure sores. This posture is commonly seen in individuals with asymmetrical muscle strength, asymmetrical muscle tone, limited hip joint mobility, lower extremity abduction, or adduction limitations.

## WHEELCHAIR AND SEATING SYSTEM ASSESSMENT

### Basic Principles

Although accessibility and wheelchair technology have changed drastically over the past 30 years, Judai's study[4] is a reminder that the process still is evolving. Judai used the Psychosocial Impact of Assist Device Scale to assess the psychosocial impact of assistive devices on individuals 1 and 3 months following the stroke. His findings for individuals who used wheelchairs indicated that some individuals reported a negative effect on their self-esteem, competence, and adaptability. This is a reminder to be attentive to the social and attitudinal environment that includes the stigma associated with using a wheelchair. Approaching each treatment session with a positive tone and educating individuals about the benefits of increased comfort and the potential ability to function independently indoors and outdoors are important.[4] It is also helpful if the team has a working knowledge of community resources (i.e., support groups, transportation, and general accessibility) by which to educate the client about strategies for increased integration in the community.

Unfortunately, no specific formula exists to choosing the "right" seating system and mobility base. However, the set of guidelines discussed next can help the team achieve the best combination of mobility base and seating system with each client. The system involves an intricate balance of an individual's postural seated needs, personal preferences and goals, home and community environment, financial situation, and method of transportation. It is important to remember that the one-size-fits-all philosophy has no place in seating system and mobility device prescription.

The wheelchair and seating system assessment is specific to each individual's needs. After obtaining demographic data, the assessment process generally begins at the ICF activities and participation level and progresses to the body functions and structures level. Initially, an in-depth comprehensive interview with the wheelchair team takes place to develop an understanding of an individual's goals, environmental situation, funding sources, ability to participate in activities of daily living, and knowledge base of wheelchair and seating system needs. The assessment then continues to screen numerous body functions such as muscle strength, balance, and cognition and includes a mat evaluation, patient education regarding postural needs and seating and mobility base options, seating product and mobility product trial, fitting/delivery, and training on the use of the equipment selected. It is extremely important to take the time to perform a thorough assessment to avoid compromising to reach the end result and to minimize time spent fixing mistakes.[1]

## Step 1: Conduct a Comprehensive Interview

The therapist should lead the team and conduct a comprehensive interview that includes the patient's diagnosis; medical and surgical history; skin history; future medical and surgical considerations; allergies; precautions; pain; funding sources; social support network; use of splints or orthotics; previous and current level of functioning; likes and dislikes with current equipment; equipment fit in home environment, work environment, and community; transportation method(s) (car, van, taxi, or bus); and the patient's goals for the new or modified equipment. The interview should include psychosocial issues with respect to roles and lifestyle preferences; basic and instrumental activities of daily living performance, including indoor and outdoor mobility; and transfer status. A physical status screening should take place to ascertain passive and active range of motion, available movement patterns, muscle strength, sensation, endurance, balance, visual-perception, and cognition. If the client has moderate to severe oral-motor control issues, a speech pathologist is essential to ensure that the client's communication and/or augmentative communication needs are addressed thoroughly.

If this is a client's first wheelchair, a home evaluation form generally is provided and additional education is necessary to ensure that the patient and significant others understand environmental concerns.

## Step 2: Perform a Supine and Seated Mat Assessment

A mat assessment is an intimate evaluation that can be intimidating and confusing to the patient and significant others. The assessment involves therapeutic handling, palpation, and range of motion. The results of the mat assessment are essential to determine the amount of support an individual requires for upright sitting, the goals and overall setup of the seating system, and the mobility base options needed to accommodate the recommended seating system. The therapist must take the time to articulate the purpose and importance of the mat evaluation to ensure that everyone "understands what you are looking for, how you will be going about it, and why this information is important to reach a good end result."[1]

Before beginning a mat assessment, it is important for the therapist to understand some basic biomechanical and seating principles. One of the main concepts is the distinction between flexible, difficult to correct, and fixed postural deformities. These concepts clarify skeletal positions in the supine and seated mat assessment.

The initial focus with a mat evaluation is to determine whether neutral pelvic and trunk alignment can be achieved. If the pelvis is in an oblique position and lower extremity influence has been accommodated for or ruled out, the therapist should correct the pelvis manually.

If the pelvis stays in the corrected position, without handling, the deformity is considered flexible. If the pelvis goes back into the oblique position but is repositioned easily to neutral and requires gentle therapeutic handling to stay in neutral, the deformity is considered difficult to correct. If the pelvis cannot be repositioned manually into a neutral position, the deformity is considered fixed. A pelvic obliquity generally is measured by the height difference between each anterior superior iliac spine and is named for the side that is lower. A subsequent section discusses seating considerations for flexible, difficult to correct, and fixed body structures.

A thorough mat assessment can require two to four persons and consists of four major components:

1. Observation of the patient in the clinic with the present or loaned equipment; the therapist assesses postural positioning in the wheelchair and screens muscle tone and strength.
2. For a supine mat assessment the client is positioned on a mat. This is essential to determine the bony structure, muscle flexibility (including muscle tone), and range of motion of the client to achieve optimal spinal-pelvic alignment. The assessment provides the therapist with a "true" picture of each individual's potential to be seated with optimal spinal-pelvic alignment. The results from the supine assessment are essential to guide how an individual is positioned or supported for the seated mat evaluation.
3. A seated mat assessment is essential to determine the influence of gravity the individual's ability to sit upright. The therapist usually can perform the assessment with the client seated on the edge of the mat with therapeutic handling by the therapist and other members of the treatment team. At this time, muscle tone may be increased as the individual attempts to hold his or her body up against gravity. If a client has

moderate to significant postural needs, a simulator can be helpful to support the client in the upright position. A more detailed description follows.

4. Once an individual is positioned with maximum aligned posture on the mat or in the simulator, the time and location are ideal to take accurate measurements of the client's body. The five basic measurements for an active individual are seat width, seat depth, knee to heel (with shoe), elbow height, and distance from the seating surface to inferior angle of the scapula. All measurements can be documented in half-inch or inch increments (e.g., 17.5-inch seat width). Chest width, axilla, top of shoulder, and occiput measurements are important to obtain if an individual requires more aggressive support (Figure 24-5).

A simulator is a tool that permits the team to evaluate a sitting client more easily with various angles and amounts of support. The simulator permits therapists to evaluate the seated position with an individual, evaluate the level of function with different positions, educate the client on the potential to achieve the best possible resting posture, take more accurate measurements, visually document potential for increased alignment via pictures to funding sources, and save an enormous amount of time with evaluating different products. The simulator can help narrow the product options necessary for evaluation to provide optimal support.

### Step 3: Provide Client and Team Education

Education of the client about the mat evaluation findings and their effect on postural alignment in a seated position is important. At that time the therapist can review a client's goals and each team member should articulate their goals to ensure that all are headed in the same direction. Education is essential to enable an individual to participate actively in the wheelchair and seating system trial and decide what compromises he or she is willing to make to maximize the ability to function in a wheelchair. Although the client is the primary decision maker, the therapist and assistive technology supplier should freely discuss their professional opinions. Part of the educational process is to help a client prioritize what is most important, especially when future health, skin integrity, and secondary complications are a concern. No wheelchair and seating system is perfect for individuals with stroke; the solution is perfect only when a client makes informed decisions about what will work best for his or her lifestyle.

It is helpful to discuss wheelchair and seating system needs in a general way and then to select products so that a client can choose from two or three options. Using the mat evaluation results and understanding product features and benefits is essential and described in greater detail later in this chapter. The therapist and assistive technology supplier have the responsibility to articulate clearly the features, benefits, and pros and cons of various options to empower the clients to select products to best meet their needs. Providing this information empowers the client and significant others to be educated, reinforces their confidence in the decision of the team, and increases their satisfaction with the final product.

### Step 4: Equipment Trial

Actual trial of seating system and wheelchair options is the best case scenario; however, this is not always possible. If a manufacturer is unable to provide the team members with the equipment they are considering, simulating the type of seating design and components is important

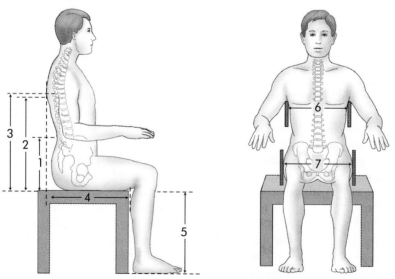

**Figure 24-5**   Measurements during the mat assessment. *1*, elbow height; *2*, seat to inferior angle of scapula; *3*, axilla; *4*, seat depth; *5*, knee to heel; *6*, chest width; *7*, hip width.

for the team to ensure that the product is accomplishing what they had hoped to achieve.

Actual trial of more complex, expensive equipment is highly recommended to minimize unseen compatibility and fit problems and ensure that the full system can meet the client's goals.

Once the ideal wheelchair and seating system is decided upon, the team gathers around the client in the "evaluation" wheelchair and seating system. At this point the team decides the measurements of the product, specifies wheelchair and seating system needs with order forms, and provides additional education about the pros and cons of specific features (such as pneumatic versus solid tires). In an ideal situation, this is truly a collaborative team process.

## Step 5: Documentation

At this point the therapist has gathered all the information needed to write a letter of medical necessity. This letter is a concise summary of the patient's functional level, mat evaluation findings, problems with existing equipment, wheelchair and seating needs, and medical and functional justification for the wheelchair, wheelchair features, and seating system recommendations. This is the letter that the medical doctor reviews and signs once the final additions are completed.

As the medical professionals are formulating the letter of medical necessity, the assistive technology supplier contacts each of the manufacturers for price quotes and creates a certificate of medical necessity. The doctor signs this insurance form and sends it with the letter of medical necessity and other insurance documents to the assistive technology supplier for funding approval.

## Step 6: Fitting and Delivery

After the team has recommended and documented the person's equipment needs, the job is only half over. It is not unusual for funding sources to question the team's recommendation. Responding as promptly as possible to these inquiries and clearly communicating the team's goals are important.

Once the assistive technology supplier is secure that the equipment will be funded and in some cases "approved" by the funding source, the equipment is ordered. All team members who were part of steps 1 to 5 will find it beneficial to be available for steps 6 and 7. During fitting and delivery, the wheelchair and seating system is set up and adjusted specifically to meet a patient's needs. At this time the therapist and assistive technology supplier educate the client and significant others regarding wheelchair and seating system parts management, care, and general maintenance about whom to contact if problems arise. For example, if a client needs replacement parts, he or she is advised to contact the assistive technology supplier; if a client experiences physical changes and is no longer comfort-

able, he or she is advised to contact the medical doctor and the therapist.

This fitting and delivery step is essential to ensure that the end product accomplishes the team's goals and minimizes an individual's risk for deformity and secondary problems. Another benefit to this step is that it significantly reduces the potential for product abandonment.

## Step 7: Functional Outcome Measurement and Follow-Up

The ideal situation would be for an individual to attend a follow-up treatment session 3 months after the fitting and delivery or at least to participate in a phone interview with the therapist to determine the success of the wheelchair and seating system intervention. This step is a true test to ensure achievement of the team's goals. Follow-up should focus on issues such as whether the equipment is holding up to the individual's specific needs and has made a difference on pain, quality of life, and independent functioning.

## MATCHING EQUIPMENT TO PATIENT FUNCTION: SEATING SYSTEM PRINCIPLES

### Translating the Mat Evaluation into the Seating System

Once the mat assessment is completed, the therapist must translate the measurements and ranges into the setup of the seating system and wheelchair. For example, if Mr. S. has only 80 degrees of hip flexion range, the seat-to-back angle must be set up to accommodate this 10-degree limitation. Most back canes have an 8-degree bend rearward and therefore a back support with some adjustability is provided with an additional 2 to 7 degrees of open seat-to-back angle. The extra 5 degrees is necessary to allow for some adjustment for comfort. It is important not to position an individual at the maximum range available. Likewise, if Mr. S. has hamstring tightness (–70 degrees of knee extension with his hip at 80 degrees of flexion), the therapist must be cautious about using an elevating leg rest, for it generally positions the lower extremity in –65 degrees of knee extension and overstretches the hamstrings. Because Mr. S.'s hamstring muscle cannot sufficiently elongate to tolerate this open knee angle, the body automatically compensates for this, which would result in Mr. S sitting with a posterior pelvic tilt. In this situation the team can order 70-degree standard footrest and use a longer heel loop for foot position rearward for a –70- to –75-degree knee angle, being mindful of castor (front wheel) clearance.

### Flexible, Difficult to Correct, and Fixed Deformities

Once therapists establish what type of deformity is present, they must figure out how to support the client to minimize his or her risk for increased deformity. If an individual has a flexible or difficult to correct deformity, the seating system should be set up to imitate the therapeutic handling and "correct" it. Client education regarding repositioning strategies is helpful at this point to ensure the client is aligned properly and to facilitate neuromuscular reeducation. Careful monitoring of a client's tolerance for correction and adjustment of the seating system accordingly are important. The process may require incremental steps to achieve increased alignment or may involve backing down from an aggressive start. If a deformity is fixed, as aggressive support as possible is important to support the client where his or her body is to decrease progression and minimize his or her risk for increased deformity.

With the more aggressive seating systems, a mobile person can be "locked" up by the aggressive supports used to achieve optimal spinal-pelvic alignment. Unfortunately, this often limits an individual's ability to function. With positioning for function, a compromise occurs to provide as much support as possible for the resting body position without affecting or limiting an individual's ability to function. Consequently, wheelchair seating is a continuum with safety and maximum postural support on one end and functional mobility on the other end. An ideal seating system should have some flexibility to provide optimal spinal-pelvic alignment and facilitate function. It is important to maximize the potential movement options of individuals who use wheelchairs as their primary means of mobility. Individuals with good motor control may choose to sit on a chair or stool for more active functioning. For individuals who do not have as many mobility options available, the wheelchair must have the ability to accommodate active and resting seated postures.

Although online resources for wheelchair and seating system products are an excellent source of information and education, online purchase of these products is not recommended because a client does not receive any of the benefits that an assistive technology supplier provides them with (i.e., assistance with setup and assembly, onsite adjustments, and personalized modifications).[6] In addition, an individual purchasing equipment online also may miss the opportunity for the team evaluation and product trial and may not be in-tune to mild physical changes that have occurred since last receiving a wheelchair and seating system.

## General Seating System Principles for Individuals with Stroke

Therapeutic intervention for individuals with brain damage caused by a stroke depends on the severity of the infarct and the amount of functional change that has occurred, including physical, visual-perceptual, and cognitive changes. Accordingly, wheelchair and seating system intervention also depends on the level of functional changes and confounding variables, including the environment in which the individual is functioning and the presence of other diagnoses such as diabetes, hypertension, and coronary artery disease. Seating systems for individuals with more involved needs may be more supportive because of decreased plasticity in the central nervous system and permanent brain damage.[2]

Individuals with hemiplegia resulting from stroke often have difficulty controlling posture, balance reactions, and smooth movement patterns that enable the performance of functional tasks. Davies[2] describes the typical patterns of adult hemiplegia (Table 24-1).

For individuals who use a wheelchair as their primary means of mobility, seating and mobility recommendations should address these typical patterns of adult hemiplegia. The following are typical seating system goals and seating principles specific to individuals with stroke.

### Goals of the Seating System

The primary goals of seating and positioning at the ICF body functions and structures level are as follows:
Provide adequate postural support
- to prevent deformity or minimize the risk of increased deformity
- to balance skeletal muscle activity
- to minimize compensatory postures
- to maximize pressure distribution and minimize the risk of pressure sores

**Table 24-1**

### Typical Patterns of Adult Hemiplegia

| BODY PART | COMMON POSTURE |
| --- | --- |
| Head | Flexion toward hemiplegic side, neck rotation toward unaffected side |
| Upper extremity (flexion pattern) | Scapula retraction, shoulder girdle depression, humeral adduction and internal rotation |
| | Elbow flexion, forearm primarily in pronation; occasionally supination dominates |
| | Wrist flexion and ulnar deviation |
| | Thumb and finger flexion and adduction |
| Trunk | Trunk rotation backward on hemiplegic side with lateral trunk flexion |
| Pelvis | Posterior tilt with obliquity (lower on unaffected side) |
| Lower extremity | Hip extension, adduction, and internal rotation |
| | Knee extension |
| | Foot plantar flexion and inversion |
| | Toe flexion and adduction |

- to enhance distal extremity control
- for adequate comfort to maximize sitting tolerance
- for autonomic nervous system functioning

The primary goals of seating and positioning at the ICF[3] activities and participation level are as follows: Provide adequate postural support

- to maximize ability to perform functional activities
- aesthetically to enhance dignity and self-esteem and quality of life
- to increase comfort for increased social interaction and participation in community activities

***Postural Stability and Control.*** Abnormal skeletal muscle activity and pathologic reflexes often influence the postural alignment of an individual with neurologic insult. A seating system should provide a stable foundation for maximum postural alignment to balance muscle activity, normalize muscle tone, and decrease compensatory posturing. Improved postural stability provides individuals with the freedom to interact, move their extremities, and hold their heads in the midline position.[1] Secondary benefits of improved stability and control are increased ability to attend to what is happening in the environment, increased interaction with the environment, improved ability to assist in or perform activities of daily living, and increased independence with mobility.

***Proximal Muscle Stability to Enhance Distal Muscular Control.*** A stable base of support for the pelvis provides individuals with the opportunity to develop control and balance of their trunk musculature. When the pelvis is stable, an individual's center of gravity passes through the base of support, which helps promote stability. This central stability allows for distal extremity control. The client is able to make better use of arm or leg movement, head control, or oral motor control to perform functional tasks (i.e., hand function for dressing, leg movement for wheelchair propulsion, midline head orientation for improved visual tracking of objects, and oral motor control for speech articulation or swallowing).

***Decrease Development of Muscle Contracture and Skeletal Deformity.*** Decreased pelvic control, muscle weakness, and muscle imbalance contribute to asymmetrical posturing. Asymmetrical postures can result in shortening or tightening of muscle groups, which can lead to a decreased range of motion in joints, increased tone, muscle contractures, and skeletal deformity. Asymmetrical posture must be corrected in a resting seated position to minimize an individual's risk for development of a fixed deformity. If soft tissue and skeletal flexibility is preserved, an individual can be encouraged successfully to sit with improved spinal-pelvic alignment through seating and seating system accessories. This positioning serves as a guide that eventually can promote

the development of more balanced muscle control in that desired position. If muscle control cannot be improved, good positioning provides adequate support.

***Enhance Comfort and Appearance.*** With optimal postural support in the seated position, individuals feel and look better. However, the process is not always a one-time event; seating system modifications can be introduced gradually to facilitate neuromuscular reeducation. Once an individual can tolerate increased postural alignment, the benefits are tenfold. Individuals who feel comfortable and feel good about themselves are much more productive and functional. This can lead to increased social interaction, communication, and an improved quality of life.

***Minimize Development of Pressure Sores.*** When impaired sensation, motor control, or judgment affect an individual's ability to shift body weight, the client is usually at risk for developing pressure sores. Essential aspects of seating are to focus on pressure-relieving cushions to maximize seating surface pressure distribution and to consider a method of pressure relief (power tilt or recline) that the client can operate independently or a tilt-in space or recliner wheelchair in which a caregiver can perform the pressure-relief technique.

***Improve Function of the Autonomic Nervous System.*** Abnormal posturing, muscle shortening, and the inability to shift weight can increase pressure on internal organs and other structures. When an individual is leaning forward or to the side because of poor pelvic or spinal muscle control, a strain on circulation, digestion, and cardiopulmonary function can result. Postural supports can facilitate optimal pelvic, spinal, and trunk alignment, which in turn can provide improved physiologic functioning of the autonomic nervous system. Sufficient head and neck support can decrease the potential for aspiration when swallowing problems exist.[1]

***Increase Sitting Tolerance and Energy Level.*** If an individual is well supported and can function from the wheelchair, sitting tolerance increases along with the ability to participate in therapy programs and functional activities. Individuals who receive adequate postural support experience less fatigue and pain than those who are fixing and stabilizing continually with a higher level of abnormal muscle activity and reflexes to support the body against gravity. The increased energy level associated with symmetrical postures increases sitting tolerance and an individual's ability to participate in functional activities within the home and the community.

***Functional Positioning: An Active Seating System.*** Although the primary focus for seating intervention thus far has been on symmetry and alignment, a therapist must remember that functional movement is asymmetrical and dynamic. As a result, consideration of seating systems that allow for function and activity performance and yet provide individuals with as much postural support as necessary to minimize their risk for increased deformity is essential. It is important to remember that "body control is interpreted and performed when the body understands its relationship to gravity, primarily through activation of the vestibular system."[5]

The pelvis is the foundation for seated posture. With this in mind, it is important to consider Kangas' perspective on pelvic stability. Kangas[5] states, "pelvic stability is not simply a musculoskeletal posture but rather is a movement of the body that includes an ongoing interaction of numerous systems, including the musculoskeletal, neuromuscular, circulatory, respiratory, gastrointestinal, and endocrinological systems." Pelvic stability is "not simply a musculoskeletal posture" and involves a position of actively holding still rather than being passively restricted. For individuals with a stroke, an active seating system generally provides as much seating surface as possible, a slightly anterior tilted seat, mild contour for upper leg positioning, and weight bearing of the feet on the floor to enable the individual to position them as he or she chooses. This base of support can provide the body with sufficient pelvic stability, and this position of active weight bearing allows an individual to assume an active task performance position for eating, writing a check, or working at a computer.[5]

An active seating system can be attained easily with minor adjustments to the wheelchair and seating system that is set up slightly higher on the continuum for increased safety and adequate support. This is beneficial for times when an individual is more active (i.e., meal preparation in the kitchen). A seat wedge can be placed under the cushion and the footrests and positioning straps removed to allow an individual to achieve a more active position. As with all intervention recommendations, the therapist and patient should evaluate this intervention together to ensure that it provides adequate stability for maximum safety with functioning. The art with mobility and seating system prescription is to achieve a balance between positioning for functional activity performance and symmetrical postural alignment for more sedentary activities (i.e., watching television) and to minimize an individual's risk for increased deformity.

## MATCHING EQUIPMENT TO CLIENT FUNCTION: SEATING SYSTEMS

Seating and positioning is a continuum that encompasses all of the foregoing goals and principles. It is important for clients to understand that the *wheelchair* is not uncomfortable; usually the *seating system* is. The seating system is the primary unit that influences body posture because it is the direct interface between the client and the wheelchair and provides the client with the foundation for adequate postural support to rest and function. The mobility base is a frame that has some seating components such as footrests and armrests; however, its primary focus is mobility indoors and outdoors. To have a seating system that provides sufficient postural support interfaced with a wheelchair frame set at the appropriate angles to facilitate optimal spinal-pelvic alignment is essential. Without appropriate postural support, an individual may be able to move about the environment; however, the risk for further deformity and pain is a major concern. A good rule of thumb for optimal positioning is to start with the pelvis and then proceed to the trunk and extremities. This approach follows the "support proximal to distal philosophy" inherent in numerous treatment approaches for individuals with neurologic dysfunction.

The importance of seating, goals, and assessment of biomechanics and posture were reviewed previously. This section describes the types of seating systems available and their various features. Three basic styles of seating exist: linear, contoured, and custom contoured. Each of these provides different levels of support to promote postural alignment and pressure distribution. The definition of each with their respective benefits and concerns follows.

### Linear Seating Systems

Linear seating systems (Table 24-2) are flat, noncontoured planes of support. Linear seat cushions or backs can be custom-made or ordered from the factory in various sizes, densities, and with different fabric covers.

Linear seating provides a firm, rigid seating base that can be beneficial for active individuals. Individuals with minimal musculoskeletal involvement typically benefit the most from linear seating. This seating is generally a lower cost option, and because of the flat surface, independent transfers are easy to achieve. Linear seating systems provide the least amount of postural support; however, because the human body is contoured, lack of support can result in higher peak pressures and pressure sores for individuals with prominent bony structures.

### Contoured Seating Options

Contoured seating system options (see Table 24-2) are designed to support the body ergonomically. They are generally available in predetermined shapes of varying contours in a wide range of sizes.

Contoured seating options provide a range of contours from mild to aggressive. This type of seating system provides an excellent surface area for support that can enhance postural alignment and pressure relief. Individuals with minimal neuromuscular or central nervous system insults can benefit from the gentle cues that

*Text continued on p.566*

**Table 24-2**

## Seating Systems

| SEATING COMPONENT | INDICATIONS FOR USE | POSTURAL AND FUNCTIONAL CONSIDERATIONS |
|---|---|---|
| Solid insert  | Insert can provide a level base of support on the sling wheelchair seat. Slide insert inside the cover, under the cushion and secure to cushion base with Velcro. The cushion cover usually has Velcro to attach the cushion securely to sling upholstery of the wheelchair. | A sling wheelchair seat encourages a posterior pelvic tilt with hip adduction and internal rotation. This sets an individual up for a "slumped" posture. A solid insert is essential to provide a firm and level base of support on the sling wheelchair seat. This facilitates more neutral pelvic positioning for upright posture and upper body movement for functional activities. |
| 1.5-inch seat wedge | Wedge slides inside the cushion cover, under the cushion. Wedge can provide an anterior or posterior seat tilt. | Wedge is a lightweight, easy to remove component to use for an anterior-sloped seat or a posterior-sloped seat. An anterior tilt would facilitate upright positioning for an individual who is working at a workstation or propelling with one arm and one foot. A posterior tilt can assist with decreasing extensor spasticity or creating a set, slight tilt for increased postural support in a standard wheelchair. Seat also encourages neutral pelvic alignment and lower extremity alignment. One concern is that it adds a significant amount of weight to the wheelchair. Unless necessary to achieve a low seat-to-floor height that cannot be achieved with a superlow wheelchair, the weight disadvantage outweighs the positioning advantages. |
| Solid seat | Remove wheelchair upholstery to install. To mount, solid seat hooks lock down on seat rails of wheelchair. The adjustable hooks on the solid seat can be positioned to provide an anterior or posterior tilt of solid seat and cushion on wheelchair frame. | Cushions can enhance sitting posture and pressure distribution, and increase comfort. |
| Foam cushion | Foam linear cushions provide a stable base of support for individuals with mild postural support needs. The foam comes in varying densities and can be layered in different densities to provide support, comfort, and some pressure relief. | The combination of stability and pressure relief is a major advantage to this cushion. The weight is a consideration; however, the advantage of a stable and pressure-relieving base of support minimizes the need for external supports. |
| Contoured foam cushion | Contoured foam cushion provides an increased surface area of support and pressure relief for individuals with mild to moderate support and pressure relief needs. A variety of foam densities are available. | These off-the-shelf cushions provide a superior level of pressure relief and good pelvic stability. This stability is important for improved balance and for adequate support. It can improve function at a wheelchair level and minimize compensatory posturing. |
| Pressure-relieving cushion (fluid medium) | A firm, contoured cushion base with pressure-relieving gel fluid pad on top provides stability and a high level of pressure relief appropriate for all individuals who need moderate to significant postural support and pressure relief. The gel bladder allows the pelvis to sink into it for full contact support for adequate pressure distribution to minimize the risk of pressure sores. | |

Continued

**Table 24-2**

## Seating Systems—cont'd

| SEATING COMPONENT | INDICATIONS FOR USE | POSTURAL AND FUNCTIONAL CONSIDERATIONS |
|---|---|---|
| Pressure-relieving cushion (air medium) 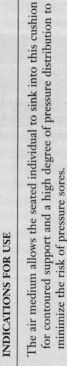 | The air medium allows the seated individual to sink into this cushion for contoured support and a high degree of pressure distribution to minimize the risk of pressure sores. | The pressure relief and lightweight qualities of this cushion are unsurpassed. However, this cushion does not provide any stability, and additional postural supports such as hip guides and adductors are essential for optimal alignment. These supports increase weight of the whole wheelchair system. Another concern is the ongoing maintenance required with this cushion. |
| Lumbar-sacral back support 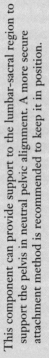 | This component can provide support to the lumbar-sacral region to support the pelvis in neutral pelvic alignment. A more secure attachment method is recommended to keep it in position. | This support is a low-cost method to provide minimal postural support for increased spinal-pelvic alignment. The support is easy to remove, which is an advantage for car transport but a disadvantage because the support is not stable and can shift out of place easily. |
| Solid back support | The solid back insert provides firm support to facilitate improved postural alignment for individuals with good pelvic and trunk control. The support is easy to remove for transportability of the wheelchair and usually is attached to the wheelchair back canes with Velcro straps. | This support is a low-cost method to provide minimal postural support for increased spinal-pelvic alignment. The support is easy to remove, which is an advantage for car transport but a disadvantage because the support is not stable and can shift out of place easily. |
| Pita back | This solid back insert provides a firm support to facilitate improved postural alignment for individuals with good pelvic and trunk control. The support is easy to remove for transportability of the wheelchair and slides into and out of a pocket in the back support upholstery. | This simple, low-cost back support can provide minimal postural support for increased spinal-pelvic alignment. The lack of foam makes the support easy to use; however, lack of sufficient padding is a concern for individuals using the wheelchair as a primary means of mobility. |
| Linear back support 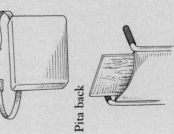 | This solid back insert provides a more durable back support for increased spinal-pelvic alignment, is beneficial for individuals with good postural control, is attached to the wheelchair frame with quick-release hardware, and usually is linear with a solid posterior base with foam in front. The support may be covered in vinyl or other materials. | This is a planar back support to enhance upright sitting. The adjustable mounting brackets makes it possible to open up seat-to-back angle to accommodate a hip range of motion limitation or for increased postural support and balance via gravity. This hardware is durable. One concern is the weight added to the wheelchair. |

*Continued*

**Adjustable-angle off-the-shelf back support**

This back support can be attached to the wheelchair with quick-release hardware. The support has generic, gentle contours that provide a guide for increased postural alignment for individuals with mild to moderate positioning needs and can be used in its original configuration or can accommodate a contoured foam in-place back support.

This back support provides mild contour to facilitate neutral trunk posturing and increased spinal-pelvic alignment. The angle can be adjusted to open up seat-to-back angle to accommodate a hip range of motion limitation or for increased postural support and balance via gravity. This support is a lightweight option that provides good support. One concern is that more durable hardware may be necessary for individuals with significant spasticity.

**Adjustable-angle custom back support**

This rigid back support can be attached to the wheelchair with quick-release or stationary hardware. The support often is positioned at an angle with a custom-contoured amount of support. The shell can be reused if the foam insert needs to be modified. This support benefits individuals with moderate to significant trunk weaknesses and/or flexible or fixed postural deformities.

This back support can provide moderate to significant support for individuals with flexible and fixed deformities. The hardware can open up the seat-to-back angle for the foregoing reasons. The contoured support provides maximum surface area contact to maximize alignment, accommodate deformities, and maximize pressure distribution to minimize the risk for increased deformities and pressure sores.

**Pelvic positioning belt**

Pelvic belts are designed to maintain optimal pelvic alignment and minimize an individual's risk for sliding out of the wheelchair. They are mounted to the seat frame via screws or straps and are available with various angles of pull and various buckles such as auto and airline style.

This support can be positioned at various angles depending on the individual's needs and functional level. A pelvic belt at the traditional 45 degrees can limit pelvic mobility for an anterior weight shift for forward reach and functioning at a table. Padded belts are available to minimize pressure concerns, and various buckles are available for maximum independence with opening/closing.

**Leg adductors**

The adductor can be attached to the wheelchair cushion base, under the seat, or on the footrest hanger and is designed to maximize lower extremity alignment and prevent the legs from rolling into abduction or external hip rotation.

Adductors can facilitate increased lower extremity alignment to minimize an individual's risk of increased deformity and pain. The size of the adductor can limit side-to-side transfers; a removable one can provide adequate support and increased safety with side transfers.

**Hip guides**

Hip guides provide support to maximize pelvic alignment, can be contoured or linear, and usually are made of different density foams with a solid back. Hip guides can be mounted onto the wheelchair armrests, seat pan, or back canes. The hardware can be fixed or removable.

Hip guides can provide a third point of control for individuals with fixed or flexible spinal curves or individuals who have a pelvic obliquity. Removable hardware is necessary for individuals who perform side-to-side transfers.

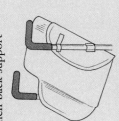

**Table 24-2**

## Seating Systems—cont'd

| SEATING COMPONENT | INDICATIONS FOR USE | POSTURAL AND FUNCTIONAL CONSIDERATIONS |
|---|---|---|
| Medial knee block (pommel) with flip-down hardware 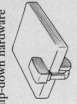 | Medial knee blocks or pommels can maximize lower extremity alignment. They prevent leg adduction and internal hip rotation. For optimal support the medial knee blocks are custom-made in a variety of shapes and sizes. This contour is essential for adequate contour and fit for increased pelvic and lower extremity alignment. The knee blocks and pommels typically are constructed of a variety of foams with a solid back and are attached to the wheelchair with various types of hardware. | Medial knee blocks are often necessary for individuals with severe spasticity. They are most successful when used with the other postural supports to maximize overall postural alignment. They can promote increased lower extremity alignment. Small pommels are helpful as a guide for more neutral lower extremity posturing. |
| Pelvic obliquity build-up  | This component usually is mounted under the gel pad or created with foams; it can be a gel or foam medium and can provide increased support under the weaker side to accommodate for muscle atrophy and level out the pelvis for improved pelvic alignment to provide a more level foundation from which the body can function. This component may be used with a hip guide to minimize lateral tilting of the pelvis for increased spinal-pelvic alignment. It also may be used under the higher side to support a fixed pelvic obliquity adequately and minimize the risk of increased deformity. | Foam or gel inserts are helpful for individuals with asymmetrical muscle strength. They can compensate for the decreased muscle bulk to facilitate a more level pelvic position. When used with hip guides, inserts can support optimal pelvic alignment in individuals who have a flexible pelvis. One concern is the amount of pressure the inserts place on the ipsilateral ischial tuberosity.[7] Monitoring of pressure with this treatment approach is important. |
| Lateral trunk supports, straight and curved 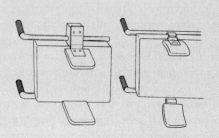 | These supports usually are mounted off the back support or back canes and are available in various sizes in planar or contoured levels of support. The hardware to mount to the wheelchair can be stationary or quick release, which is beneficial for individuals with trunk weakness or a tendency to lean to one side. Another point of control, usually via hip guides, is necessary for adequate trunk support to correct a flexible deformity or accommodate a fixed deformity. | Individuals who have decreased trunk support often hold themselves upright with their upper extremities. Lateral supports can provide increased trunk support to these individuals so that they can use their extremities for bilateral upper extremity tasks. Lateral supports also can provide the upper two points of control to correct or accommodate a lateral spinal curve for increased midline positioning in the wheelchair. The swing-away hardware is helpful with providing adequate support and shifting out of the way for transfers, dressing, and overall positioning in the wheelchair. Lateral support hardware that aggressively contours to the back support is necessary to get the hardware out of the way for adequate upper extremity mobility. Curved lateral support pads provide improved contour and support over planar lateral support pads. |

| | |
|---|---|
| Harness/anterior chest support | Anterior chest supports can be mounted to the wheelchair via the back support of back canes and seat rails. They are available in a variety of styles and are beneficial for individuals with severe trunk weakness. These supports often are used with a tilt or recline seating system to maximize postural support when more upright against gravity. | This component can provide anterior trunk support to allow an individual with poor trunk control to be more upright against gravity, which is helpful for more dynamic, engaging activities (i.e., working at a desk). Therapists should consider this component after evaluating a recline or tilt-in-space seating system for increased postural support in a more sedentary, posterior position. The component is helpful for maximum trunk support for increased safety and stability when negotiating varying terrain (i.e., ramps and door saddles). |
| Head/neck support | Head/neck supports can be mounted to the back support via quick-release hardware. They are essential to provide adequate head support for individuals with poor head or neck control. | This component is necessary for individuals with fair head control and for head and neck support when an individual tilts back for pressure relief or improved postural support. Additional pads and head bands are available for individuals with significant head positioning needs. This should be adjusted to support the head in neutral alignment for optimal functioning (i.e., respiration and feeding) and speech. |
| Wheel lock extension | Wheel lock extensions can be mounted over the existing wheel lock handle. They are available in various sizes. They provide a longer lever arm to make it possible to access and lock/unlock the wheel locks if an individual cannot negotiate the standard wheel lock. | Extensions are important for maximum independence and to stabilize the wheelchair for functioning and safety with transfers to and from the wheelchair. |
| Upper extremity support, full and half lap trays | Lap trays can be mounted over the armpad with "slide" hardware with an additional strap for stability, if necessary. They come in full or half tray models in various sizes. They can provide individuals with a support surface for their paretic upper extremity. | Adequate upper extremity support is essential to minimize an individual's risk for increased shoulder pain and deformity. A lap tray can provide a work surface for functional activities such as writing and feeding. The clear version can provide the individual with a clear view of the feet for maximum safety with wheelchair propulsion. Upper extremity edema is often present in individuals who are unable to move their upper extremity functionally. A lap tray can facilitate increased awareness of this extremity for edema management and positioning of the upper extremity to decrease the edema. |
| Arm trough | An arm trough can be mounted on the standard armrest in place of the armpad. The trough can provide more aggressive support for adequate upper extremity joint protection. | An arm trough provides optimal support for individuals with decreased upper extremity control, which is important to minimize the risk for pain, subluxation, and edema. An arm trough can provide an individual with a surface for upper extremity weight bearing for functional reaching activities or for repositioning the body in the wheelchair. |

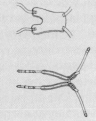

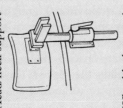

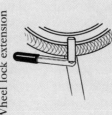

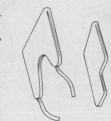

the slight contours of this seating system provide. Individuals can also achieve independent transfers with the less contoured options.

Individuals with moderate impairments benefit more from moderately contoured seating systems. These individuals are less likely to perform independent transfers, and the increased contours can meet their more involved postural support and pressure relief needs. An advantage to a contoured seating system is that it can be modified as an individual's needs change. It is important to remember that more aggressive contoured supports really hold and support an individual, which is great for postural alignment but can make transfers more difficult.

### Custom Seating Options

Custom seat cushions and backs provide customized support to meet an individual's specific needs.

Customized seating systems are essential to provide maximum support, accommodation, and comfort for individuals with moderate to severe deformities. The concerns with custom-molded seating systems is the lack of flexibility for changing postural support needs, the high cost, and the amount of labor to create a customized seating system. An experienced therapist and assistive technology supplier is essential to achieve a successful end product with this level of seating system.

In addition to the primary support surface contours, the angles and degree of postural support from gravity are major considerations. Two dynamic seating system options available are recline and tilt-in-space seating systems. Both of these systems can position a person posterior from the upright, 90-degree sitting for postural support from gravity. A recline seating system is one in which the back support can be shifted backward or forward for varying levels of support and upright posture (Figure 24-6). A tilt-in-space seating system is one in which the whole seating system (cushion and back support) tilts backward for increased postural support from gravity. Both of these systems can provide individuals with increased postural support and a method of pressure relief through movement of the seating system. A recliner

or a tilt-in-space wheelchair is often beneficial for individuals who need moderate to maximal support for upright sitting. These seating system options are available in manual and power wheelchairs. With a manual seating system, a caregiver is essential to perform the movement. A power-operated seating system can provide an individual in the wheelchair with the ability to shift position independently for pressure relief, increase postural support because of fatigue, decrease postural support for more upright seated functioning (i.e., feeding), or meet varying environmental demands (i.e., increased recline for improved support when descending a ramp).

The concept of reclining the back of the seating system or slightly tilting the seating system can be performed in 5- to 15-degree ranges in a standard wheelchair through add-on back supports and/or seat wedges. This is often necessary to accommodate hip range limitations or provide an individual with improved postural support and balance to function upright against gravity. One consideration is that this is a fixed, stationary position in a standard wheelchair. The stability of a recliner or tilt-in-space wheelchair specifically designed for tilt or recline is essential for this position to be a dynamic seating function.

Table 24-2 describes a variety of seating system products and secondary support products for seating systems and depicts the seating component, its indications for use, considerations for use, and the functional benefit.

## FITTING THE PERSON BASED ON FUNCTIONAL STATUS

The following list describes body structures and the seating components that can be used for individuals with hemiplegia and flexible deformities. The list encompasses individuals who have a wide range of functional abilities. One concept that is ever present throughout seating and positioning is always to provide proximal support first and then support distally. An example of this concept with an upper extremity support is first to provide sufficient trunk support before supporting the upper extremity on a half-lap tray. This is essential to minimize the risk of injury to the shoulder girdle.

■ Pelvic positioning: Wheelchair upholstery stretches over time; consequently, the sling facilitates poor postural alignment with a posterior pelvic tilt, a pelvic obliquity, and lower extremity adduction and internal rotation. A cushion with a solid base of support (such as a wood insert) is highly recommended to provide a firm and level base of support for the pelvis on the sling wheelchair seat. This is essential for all individuals at various stages of the rehabilitation process. Initially, the support can facilitate carryover of rehabilitation restoration goals and later can provide a good seating surface for upright functioning at a wheelchair level.

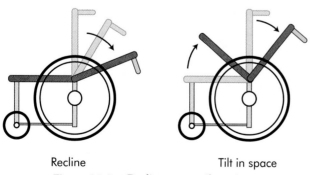

Recline                    Tilt in space

**Figure 24-6**    Recline versus tilt options.

- Lower extremity positioning: The affected side typically is postured in a position of hip adduction and internal rotation.[2] This posture can be decreased significantly with a mild contoured cushion and a solid insert. For individuals with more significant positioning needs, postural support via gravity, a padded pelvic belt, hip guides, and medial knee support should be considered. Medial knee blocks are beneficial for individuals with severe adduction and internal rotation concerns to minimize the risk for hip dislocation.
- Trunk: The affected hemiplegic side typically postures with lateral trunk flexion.[2] The lateral trunk flexion is often a consequence of decreased pelvic alignment. Optimal pelvic positioning with a good cushion and sacral support with a mild contoured back support can significantly decrease or fully correct the lateral trunk flexion. For individuals with severe weakness, hip guides and a build-up in the cushion can compensate for asymmetrical muscle loss and provide optimal pelvic alignment. In addition, lateral trunk supports can be added as needed to support the body in alignment. Three points of control are essential for optimal trunk support. Figure 24-7 shows placement of these supports. It is important to remember that a fixed deformity is supported to minimize the risk of increased deformity. A flexible deformity can be corrected; however, the therapist should monitor an individual's tolerance of this correction.
- Upper extremity: The affected upper extremity requires adequate scapula and glenohumeral support and stability from a lap tray or arm trough to minimize the risk for increased pain and subluxation. Appropriate positioning is essential to facilitate optimal upper extremity alignment and to maximize function. For a paretic upper extremity, optimal upper extremity alignment is with the shoulder in 5 degrees of abduction and flexion with neutral rotation, the elbow in 90 degrees of flexion and positioned slightly forward of the shoulder joint, the forearm in a neutral or pronated position, and the hand in a functional resting position. Functional hand splints often are integrated into the seating system for optimal wrist and hand support with the forearm supported on a lap tray. More aggressive supports are used for individuals with more severe spasticity.
- Head/neck: Typically, if an individual is seated with a stable base of support at the pelvis and lower extremities and has adequate trunk control or support, the asymmetrical neck posture decreases or disappears. For individuals with moderate to severe involvement who require more support, a head or neck rest can be placed on the chair to ensure proper support of the cervical spine and head. This is important to address, especially if the client has a reflex activity, visual field neglect, or visual-perceptual difficulties.
- Feet: Foot support typically is determined by the person's functional level. Most individuals with hemiplegia who propel their wheelchairs prefer to propel with the unaffected arm and leg. Consequently, the top of the cushion to floor (seat-to-floor height) is a crucial measurement. The seat-to-floor height must allow the person's heel to access the ground for a successful heel strike to propel the wheelchair effectively. It is also important to consider the depth of the seat cushion. This should be slightly shorter than a client's seat depth or have an undercut/beveled base of the cushion for adequate freedom of movement. A leg rest or footrest should support the affected lower extremity. In general, individuals with stroke do no benefit from elevating leg rests. Elevating leg rests tend to cause overstretching of hamstring muscles and facilitate posturing with a posterior pelvic tilt when muscle imbalance or spasticity is present.

## MOBILITY BASE CONSIDERATIONS

The primary goals of the mobility base at the ICF[3] body functions and structures level are to increase safety and independence with mobility and to provide an efficient method of mobility. The primary goal of the mobility base at the ICF activities and participation level is to maximize an individual's ability to interact with the environment (indoors and outdoors).

### Manual Wheelchair Frame Styles

Two basic types of manual wheelchair frame styles are available: rigid and folding. Rigid wheelchairs tend to be

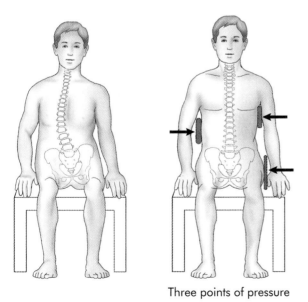

Three points of pressure

**Figure 24-7**  Three points of support for a lateral spinal curve.

lighter weight and more maneuverable than their folding counterparts. This is because of fewer moving parts and a shorter base length resulting from the integrated footrest design. Folding wheelchairs are designed with a cross brace that allows the chair to be folded in half for transport and storage. The wheelchair style commonly recommended for individuals with stroke is the folding style, primarily because the style is traditional and most familiar to medical professionals, fits into certain reimbursement codes, and is recognized easily by the general public.

An individual's medical condition, functional status, seating system needs, home environment, method of community mobility, and funding source are important variables that determine the style of wheelchair frame that is recommended. Wheelchair frames are made of different materials to meet various chair weight requirements. The weight of the wheelchair is important if the person's strength, endurance, and propulsion abilities are in question. A basic wheelchair is constructed of aluminum, is relatively heavy, and is appropriate for persons who are not active and do not use a wheelchair as their primary means of mobility. These wheelchairs are durable enough for everyday use and are reasonably priced. Ultralightweight wheelchair frames typically are constructed with aircraft aluminum or titanium. These chairs are durable but more costly than standard wheelchairs. In general, these wheelchairs are not recommended for individuals with stroke primarily because of the principal funding source, Medicare, and the documentation necessary for this level of wheelchair.

Because of the increased incidence of repetitive stress injuries in individuals who use wheelchairs as their primary method of mobility, a strong case can be made for justification of an ultralightweight wheelchair for individuals who have sustained a stroke. The trunk weakness and use of one upper extremity for all mobility, transfers, and activity of daily living performance is of great concern. Lighter-weight wheelchairs typically have an adjustable axle that can be adjusted for increased balance and an optimal hand-to-wheel relationship. This adjustment can decrease the mechanical forces required for wheelchair propulsion and is essential for energy conservation and adequate joint protection of the upper extremity. For the same reasons, power mobility can be considered as a viable option to preserve upper extremity function and maximize overall functioning and community mobility for individuals who have sustained a stroke.

Figure 24-8 shows the basic wheelchair frame style. Consideration of frame style, wheelchair accessories, and the seating system is crucial to ensure adequate postural support and maximum function at a wheelchair level.

The following are wheelchair and wheelchair frame features that are important to consider when recommending a folding manual wheelchair.

### Wheelchair Frame Seat-to-Floor Height
Three common seat-to-floor heights are these (Figure 24-9):
- Standard: 19.5 inches from seat to floor
- Hemiheight: 17.5 inches from seat to floor
- Superlow: 14.5 inches from seat to floor

The seat-to-floor height is the height from the floor to the sling seat of the wheelchair. It is important to remember that the height of the cushion chosen also influences the seat-to-floor height. The wheelchair frame height decision is based on the individual's lower extremity knee-to-heel measurement and what type of wheelchair propulsion the client uses.

If an individual is pushing the wheelchair with both arms or not independently propelling the wheelchair, the footrest clearance is a major concern. After the patient is

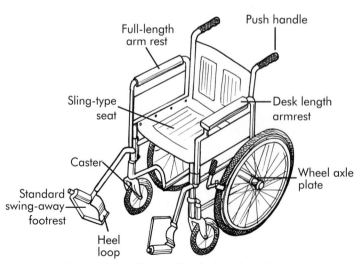

**Figure 24-8**  Basic style of wheelchair frame.

positioned with good femoral support on the wheelchair cushion, approximately 3 inches of clearance should be between the footplate and the ground. This is essential so that the patient can negotiate ramps and uneven surfaces without scraping the footplates on the ground. This seat-to-floor height is often compromised to 2 inches of clearance to allow for improved table and desk access.

If an individual is a negotiating the wheelchair with one arm and one foot, then the seat-to-floor height is crucial for comfort of the hemiparetic lower extremity on the foot rest and adequate heel access for propulsion of the wheelchair with one or both lower extremities. The individual's knee-to-heel measurement (taken with shoe on) is generally the exact measurement from the top of the wheelchair cushion to the floor. The wheelchair should not be too high because the client will slide into a posterior pelvic tilt to obtain improved heel contact for efficient mobility.

***Wheel Style.*** Several styles of inner wheel support structure are available. For the purpose of this chapter, discussion is limited to mag wheels and spoke wheels. Wheel style is chosen based on an individual's ability to care for and maintain the wheelchair.

The team should consider the following:

- The advantage of mag wheels is that they do not require maintenance. However, they do not have as much shock absorption as spoke wheels and can be slightly heavier.
- Spoke wheels are lighter than mag wheels; however, they require periodic tightening of the individual spokes. A local bicycle shop can perform this adjustment.

***Rear Wheel Size.*** Wheelchair wheels are measured from the ground to the top of the wheel. They are available in 12-, 20-, 22-, 24-, 25-, and 26-inch diameters. For individuals with stroke, the seat-to-floor height needs of the individual primarily determines the size of the rear wheel.

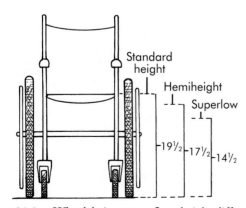

**Figure 24-9**  Wheelchair seat-to-floor height differences.

The team should consider the following:

- The standard wheel size is 24 inches.
- If an individual requires a superlow wheelchair height to fit a petite frame and/or for foot propulsion, the size of the rear wheel can be 20 inches.

***Tire Style.*** Numerous tire options are available; however, for simplicity this section focuses on the types of tires available for standard, folding wheelchairs: pneumatic, pneumatic with flat-free inserts, and polyurethane.

The team should consider the following options:

- Pneumatic tires provide a smoother ride because of good shock absorption ability. The traction of the tires provides good wheelchair stabilization for safety with transfers, and the tires handle varying terrain better than the other two options. The disadvantages are maintenance of air pressure and the risk of a flat tire.
- Pneumatic tires with flat-free inserts are pneumatic tires with an insert to replace the air. This eliminates the need for air pressure maintenance and the possibility of flats. The benefit of this combination is the traction of the tire that results in increased stability of the wheelchair for safe transfers. Unfortunately, the flat-free inserts decrease the shock absorption potential and add weight to the tire.
- Polyurethane tires are the least expensive and are durable; however, they are heavier than pneumatic tires, provide no shock absorption, and handle varying terrain poorly. In addition, the smoothness of the tire does not provide any traction of the wheelchair wheel on smooth flooring. Often these tires are the reason wheelchairs slide when persons are transferring to and from them.

***Wheel Handrims and One-Arm Drive Wheelchairs.*** Handrims are the circumferential rim on the outside of the tire to allow stroking and propulsion of the wheel. Hand rims are available in aluminum, plastic-coated, or projection styles. One-arm drive wheelchairs have two hand rims on one wheel only (Figure 24-10).

The team should consider the following options:

- Aluminum or composite hand rims are standard on most wheelchairs. Aluminum hand rims can become slippery or cold in different weather conditions. As a result, most active wheelchair users wear specific gloves to compensate for this.
- Plastic-coated hand rims are beneficial for individuals with decreased grasp. The plastic coating provides traction against an individual's hand or a Dycem glove. The one disadvantage is that individuals cannot let the rim run through their hands as they descend hills and ramps because the friction will burn the skin on their hands.
- Projection handrims are occasionally used for individuals with decreased grasp. The disadvantages are that

they can increase the overall width of the wheelchair if they are not vertical and the propulsion method is more labor intensive because one has to look continually at the handrim to hit the projection.

One-arm drive wheelchairs have right- and left-hand rims on the same side. This wheelchair was designed for individuals with only one functional upper extremity (see Figure 24-10). The double hand rim allows one upper extremity to control the wheelchair in all directions. Use of these wheelchairs takes much strength and a high degree of coordination to move straight. In addition, this propulsion method has a longer learning curve because the concept is difficult to master. Asking an individual to use his or her one functional upper extremity for wheelchair propulsion is an excessive request if one considers that the client also uses this one extremity for all other activities of daily living. I feel that a power wheelchair should be strongly considered for independent mobility along with adequate upper extremity joint protection and energy conservation.

***Wheel Axle Positioning.*** Standard wheelchairs allow minimal or no axle adjustment. If a standard wheelchair allows for this adjustment, it only allows the wheel to go up and down to create a hemi- or standard-height wheelchair. Several lightweight wheelchairs provide a middle level of axle adjustment. On ultralightweight wheelchairs, an adjustable wheel axle plate allows for wheel positioning up and down and back and forth.

An adjustable axle position allows the chair to be fine-tuned by adjustment of the wheel to the best position for propulsion. This is essential for optimal wheel setup for an energy-efficient propulsion stroke and to minimize an individual's risk for upper extremity repetitive stain injuries. As the wheel is shifted slightly into a forward position, wheel access is improved and propulsion is easier for an individual. This adjustment should be performed with caution as it affects the balance of the wheelchair. One concern is for individuals who have had

a lower extremity amputation (because of a compounding diagnosis such as diabetes); the axle is better placed in a rear position to stabilize the wheelchair adequately.

***Casters.*** Casters are the front wheels of the wheelchair (see Figure 24-8). They are available in several diameters (3, 4, 5, 6 and 8 inches) and two thicknesses (1 and 1.5 inches).

The team should consider the following:

- Large casters handle uneven terrain and door saddles well; however, they increase the turning radius of the wheelchair and provide higher rolling resistance to the user.
- Small casters are typical in superlow and ultralightweight, rigid wheelchairs. They provide the client with a lower front seat-to-floor height and improved maneuverability in small areas. The disadvantage of small casters is that they get stuck in cracks and bumps on sidewalks and streets.
- Narrow-width casters handle smooth surfaces well but can get stuck easily in uneven terrain.
- The 1.5-inch width is available on the 5- and 6-inch diameter casters. This option balances maneuverability and performance over uneven surfaces; the smaller diameter provides improved maneuverability in tight areas and the increased width facilitates transitioning over different surfaces such as door saddles and prevents the casters from getting stuck in sidewalk cracks.

***Elevating Leg Rests and Footrests.*** Elevating leg rests can raise or lower the lower extremities if an individual requires this because of a medical condition (Figure 24-11). Footrests have a fixed knee angle and support the lower extremity in sitting.

The team should consider the following:

- Elevating leg rests typically are recommended for individuals with limited knee angles (because of arthritis or other orthopedic diagnosis), poor circulation in the lower extremities, or edema. These leg rests typically

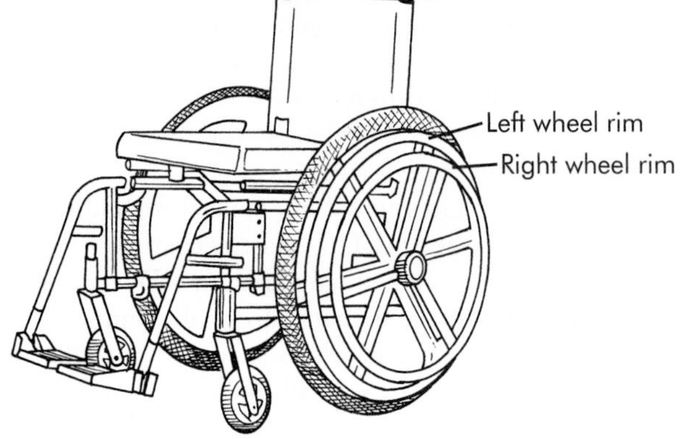

**Figure 24-10**   One-arm drive wheelchairs have two hand rims on one wheel only.

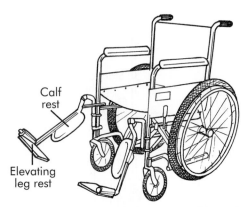

**Figure 24-11**   Elevating leg rests raise or lower the lower extremities.

are overprescribed and should be considered carefully. An elevating leg rest usually protrudes out farther than a footrest. This increases the overall length of the wheelchair and compromises maneuverability. If an individual does not have adequate hamstring muscle elongation to tolerate this large knee angle change, he or she will sit with a posterior pelvic tilt to compensate for the lack of muscle flexibility (Figure 24-12).[9]

- The circulation benefits of these leg rests are questionable, since they do not raise the lower extremity above the heart in a standard wheelchair.
- A major disadvantage to elevating leg rests is the significant amount of weight they add to the wheelchair.
- Footrests are available in different knee angles, typically 60, 70, and 75 degrees. The angle recommended should be based on the individual's knee range and hamstring range from the mat evaluation. Proper adjustment of the footrest length is important to ensure lower extremity stability and support in sitting. Swing-away removable footrests enable the footrests to be shifted out of the way for increased safety with transfers and improved table accessibility.
- A 70-degree angle is usually a standard option and provides a shorter turning radius than a wheelchair with the 60-degree angle footrest.

***Footplates.*** Footplates are available in different materials such as composite and aluminum and are available in different sizes with different angle options: angle adjustable or standard.

The team should consider the following:

- The aluminum option is heavier and more durable than a composite footplate.

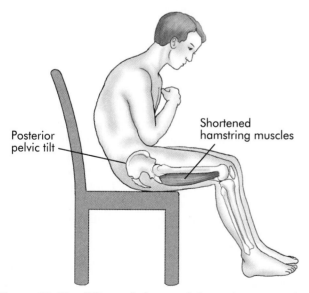

**Figure 24-12** Effect of shortened hamstrings on pelvic positioning.

Posterior pelvic tilt

Shortened hamstring muscles

- An angle-adjustable footplate is essential to accommodate ankle range of motion limitations and can be helpful in accommodating hamstring muscle limitations.

***Armrests.*** Depending on the level of wheelchair, armrests (see Figure 24-8) are available in different styles: (1) fixed or removable with different height options: fixed and adjustable height, and (2) with two different length options: full and desk length.

The team should consider the following:

- Fixed armrests are welded to the frame and set at a standard height; they cannot be adjusted. This is good for an individual who stands from the wheelchair; however, this design does not work for an individual who needs to transfer sideways to and from the wheelchair.
- Removable armrests can be positioned out of the way to allow an individual to transfer sideways into and out of the wheelchair. The armrests also can be removed from the wheelchair frame for more compact storage locations such as the trunk of a car.
- Adjustable-height armrests allow for height adjustment to provide sufficient glenohumeral support. This is important for individuals with hemiparesis and shoulder subluxation.
- Full-length arms provide full arm support at rest and upper extremity support during sit to stand and stand-pivot transfers.
- Desk-length armrests are shorter. This can provide an individual with the ability to maneuver close to desks and tables for functional activities such as feeding or writing.

### Power Mobility Products

Power mobility products frequently are recommended for individuals who do not have the strength, endurance, or coordination to negotiate a wheelchair manually. Power mobility can provide individuals with increased independent and safe mobility within the home and the community. This mobility is essential to provide individuals with increased ability to perform activities of daily living and to perform their life roles. It is important for clients to present with a basic level of visual-perceptual and cognitive functioning and be available for power wheelchair mobility skills training for this to be a safe method of mobility. The wheelchair industry has exploded in the past 15 years; consequently, a wide array of products now exists to meet specific client needs. This section gives an overview of power wheelchair products with a general list of advantages and disadvantages of each option.

***Power Scooters.*** Scooters provide individuals who have good upper extremity control with a means of power mobility. They are available in a three- or four-wheel bases (Figure 24-13). Scooters have a long and narrow

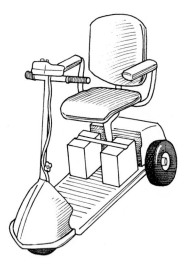

**Figure 24-13** Clients are appropriate for power scooters if they have good functional control of their upper extremities and appropriate visual, perceptual, and cognitive skills.

base, and as a result they are great for open areas and general outdoor community mobility. They can be disassembled for car transport; however, this is an awkward task to perform, and some components are heavy.

The team should consider the following:

■ Scooters generally have mildly contoured seating systems. These are similar to car seats, with a limited number of options. As a result, they cannot provide sufficient postural support for individuals who need a moderate level of trunk support.

■ In general, scooters are long and narrow, and as a result they have a large turning radius and often do not fit in small rooms.

■ Four-wheeled scooters handle outdoor terrain better but are less maneuverable in smaller areas. In addition, they are heavier and therefore are more difficult to break down for car transport.

### Power Wheelchairs

Power wheelchairs are available with a folding frame or a power-base frame with the drive wheel in the front, middle, or rear position. For ease of discussion, power wheelchairs are divided into the front-, center-, and rear-wheel drive bases with the understanding that each of these models can be classified further into a basic-level wheelchair and a power-base wheelchair.

After the therapist determines that an individual has the range of motion to sit in most wheelchair styles and the sufficient visual-perceptual and cognitive level abilities to move safely, the next important consideration is fit of the wheelchair into and within an individual's home environment. This fit is critical and often influences the type of drive-wheel base selected.

***Front-Wheel Drive Wheelchairs.*** A front-wheel drive wheelchair is a base with the large drive wheel in the

front. This style of wheelchair is the most stable base and is beneficial for individuals with significant hamstring muscle limitations. This is the only base that can accommodate positioning the feet as far back as possible without compromising on the seat height and interfering with casters or motors. Accommodation of hamstring tightness in a rear-wheel drive base compromises driving, and an individual often has to be positioned high up to keep the feet above the castor wheels.

The team should consider the following:

■ A front-wheel drive wheelchair is an excellent option for individuals who have environmental limitations. This style of wheelchair is excellent for tight turns into doorways at the end of a hall and maneuvering at a desk or table.

■ A portable ramp is necessary for individuals to negotiate curbs or one-step entrances more than 3 inches high.

■ Because of the design of this base, turning occurs in the rear, outside of the driver's visual field. Consequently, an individual requires excellent proprioception to know where the wheelchair is for safe mobility. This wheelchair base generally is not recommended if an individual has visual or cognitive limitations.

***Mid-wheel Drive Wheelchairs.*** For the purpose of this chapter, the term *mid-wheel drive wheelchair* includes center-wheel drive wheelchairs. A mid-wheel drive wheelchair is a wheelchair base that has the drive wheel in the center of the wheelchair with smaller wheels in the front and the rear. This base requires wheels in the front and the back for maximum stability of the wheelchair base. Because the drive wheel is in the middle, this wheelchair usually has the smallest turning radius and is the most maneuverable in tight areas.

The team should consider the following:

■ A portable ramp is necessary for individuals to negotiate curbs or one-step entrances more than 3 inches high.

■ Because of the design of this base, turning occurs at the center, which is the same axis on which the body turns. As a result, some individuals feel that this is an easier drive method to learn; however, one concern is that some of the turning occurs in the rear, outside of the driver's visual field. Consequently, an individual requires good proprioception to know where the wheelchair is for safe mobility. This wheelchair base generally is not recommended if an individual has more involved visual or cognitive limitations.

***Rear-Wheel Drive Wheelchairs.*** A rear-wheel drive wheelchair is the traditional power wheelchair with which most persons are familiar. Because the drive wheel is in the rear position, most of the weight of the wheelchair is in the rear. As a result, this style of wheelchair has little "anti-tipper" wheels in the back for maximum safety ascending inclines.

The team should consider the following:

- This wheelchair base is easier to control at higher speeds than the comparable front-wheel drive and mid-wheel drive models.
- This wheelchair base can be assisted up higher steps and curbs, if necessary. When a wheelchair is tipped back onto the tippers, the amount of caster clearance determines the actual height one can negotiate with assistance of another person. This is important for one-step entrances and curbs that are 6 to 8 inches in height. This feature is not a luxury but a necessity for individuals to access their favorite restaurants and stores without a ramp.
- This wheelchair base operates similar to a car, and consequently, many individuals find it easy to operate.
- Because of the design of this wheelchair base, the turning wheels are in front of the driver. As a result, all turns happen within the driver's visual field. This is the optimal situation for individuals with sensory (auditory), visual, or cognitive limitations because this base provides the driver with the maximum amount of visual input about the environment they are negotiating.
- Because of the design of this wheelchair base, the footrests have to be positioned in front to allow the casters to turn. This increases the overall length of the wheelchair and results in a larger turning radius. Consequently, a rear-wheel drive base is not as maneuverable in tight areas as a mid-wheel drive base.

*Basic Power Wheelchair.* A basic power wheelchair is fairly durable and can handle relatively level terrain. Most basic power wheelchairs operate by joystick. The joystick controls the speed and direction of the wheelchair. Some basic power wheelchairs can even be folded for car transport.

The team should consider the following:

- Basic power wheelchairs have basic electronics with little programmability. Consequently, if an individual requires a higher degree of electronics adjustments because of tremors, spasticity, or ataxia, a power base with more flexible electronics may be indicated.
- If an individual requires a moderate or aggressive level of postural support, including a tilt or recline seating system, this wheelchair base would not meet that person's needs.
- Power folding frames are practical in theory but deceiving in reality. Although the frame can be folded by pulling out the batteries and battery tray, the unit is still heavy. Two strong adults can lift the folded power frame in and out of a van or car; however, everyday use with one person assisting the individual with a stroke is difficult and unrealistic. Because of its folding crossbar and flexible frame, a power folding frame does not handle terrain as well as a power base. However,

for basic power mobility, the model is an efficient and reasonably priced alternative.

*Power Wheelchair Bases.* Power wheelchair bases are much more durable than basic power wheelchair frames. The frame style is more rigid, which translates into increased durability, increased ability to handle uneven terrain, and a smoother ride. In addition, this higher-level base is often available with the option for more flexible, higher-level electronics, and the option for a more supportive seating system such as a tilt or recline seating system.

The team must consider that power bases cannot be disassembled for car transport. Transportation availability by bus, ambulette, or accessible van is essential for individuals to be able to travel with this wheelchair base.

*Power Wheelchair Options.* For most power wheelchairs, a wide array of joystick handle and joystick mounting options are available to position the joystick in the best location for an individual with a stroke. These include larger ball joystick handles, built-up cylindrical-type joystick handles, swing-away joystick mounts, and midline joystick mounting brackets.

On power wheelchairs with more advanced electronics, alternative drive methods such as a single-switch scanner, a head array, or a pneumatic controller can be easily set up. This is essential for individuals who do not have the upper extremity control to operate a joystick or modified joystick to maneuver the wheelchair safely and independently.

## REVIEW QUESTIONS

1. What are the most important considerations when recommending a wheelchair and seating system?
2. Why is a mat evaluation an important first step before considering a wheelchair and seating system?
3. What is the difference, in treatment approaches, for a fixed and a flexible deformity?
4. What is a wheelchair contributing factor to sitting with a posterior pelvic tilt?
5. What are the basic differences between a rigid and a folding wheelchair?
6. In addition to the mat evaluation, what are important areas to screen when considering power mobility?
7. What are the differences between a front-wheel drive, mid-wheel drive, and rear-wheel drive power wheelchair?

## REFERENCES

1. Bergen A: Assessment for seating and wheeled mobility systems, *Team Rehab Rep* p 16, April 1998.
2. Davies PM: *Steps to follow: a guide to the treatment of adult hemiplegia,* Heidelberg, Germany, 1985, Springer-Verlag.

3. *International classification of functioning, disability and health: ICF short version*, Geneva, 2001, World Health Organization.
4. Judai JW: Psychosocial impact of assistive devices in stroke. Proceedings of the twenty-sixth International RESNA Conference on Technology and Disability: Research, Design, Practice, and Policy, Atlanta, June 2003.
5. Kangas KM: The task performance position: providing seating for accurate access to assistive technology, *Physical Disabilities Special Interest Section Quarterly* 23(3), 2000.
6. Lipka DD: BuyerBeware.com, *Physical Disabilities Special Interest Section Quarterly* 23(3), 2000.
7. Shea M: A wheelchair cushion insert and its effect on pelvic pressure distribution. Proceedings of the twenty-third International RESNA Conference: Technology for the New Millennium, Orlando, Fla, June 2000.
8. www.stroke.org: Main stroke page. International Center for Disability Resources on the Internet, 2002, retrieved 3/8/03.
9. Zollars JA: *Special seating: an illustrated guide*, Minneapolis, 1996, Otto Back Orthopedic Industry.

## SUGGESTED READINGS

Angelo J: *Assistive technology for rehabilitation therapists*, Philadelphia, 1997, FA Davis.
Axleton P, Chesney D, Minkel J, et al: *The manual wheelchair training guide*, Santa Cruz, Calif, 1998, Pax Press.
Axleton P, Minkel J, Chesney D: *A guide to wheelchair selection: how to use the ANSI/RESNA wheelchair standards to buy a wheelchair*, Washington, DC, 1994, Paralyzed Veterans of America.
Bergen AF: *Positioning for function*, Valhalla, NY, 1990, Valhalla Rehabilitation.
Carr EK: Positioning of the stroke person: a review of the literature, *Int J Nurs Stud* 29(4):355, 1992.
Ferido T: Spasticity in head trauma and CVA persons: etiology and management, *J Neurosci Nurs* 20(1):17, 1988.
Lange ML: Tilt in space versus recline: new trends in an old debate, *Tech Spec Interest Section Q* 10(2):1-3, 2000.
Lange ML: Positioning the upper extremities, *OT Practice* May 1999.
Lange ML: Power wheelchair access methods, *OT Practice* July/Aug 1999.
Minkel JL: *Sitting solutions: principles of wheelchair positioning and mobility devices*, New Windsor, NY, 1996, Minkel Consulting.
Pedersen JP: Providing a stable, yet unrestricted posture, May 2000. Article archives of rehabcentral.com.
Ramsey C: Power mobility access methods, *Tech Spec Interest Section Q* 9(3):1-3, 1999.
Sparacio J: The effects of seating on upper-extremity function, *Tech Spec Interest Section Q* 9(2):1-2, 1999.
Sweet-Michaels B: Alternative methods for power wheelchair control: then and now, *Tech Spec Interest Section Q* 9(3):1-4, 1999.
Taylor SJ: The head control dilemma, *Tech Spec Interest Section Q* 9(2):1-3, 1999.
Trefler E: Then and now: simulators have evolved from simple positioning chairs into devices with multiple uses and benefits. Is it time your facility purchased one? *Team Rehab Rep* p 32, Feb 1999.
US Department of Health and Human Services: *Pressure ulcers in adults: prediction and prevention*, AHCPR Pub No 92-0050, Rockville, Md, 1992, US Department of Health and Human Services.
Vogel B: Maintaining your chair, *New Mobility* p 25, June 2003.

## RESOURCES

### Clinician Websites
www.rehabcentral.com
www.resna.com

### Manufacturer Websites
www.bodypoint.com
www.invacare.com
www.pridemobility.com
www.sunrisemedical.com
www.supracor.com
www.whitbio.com

### Consumer Websites
www.pva.org
www.rolli-moden.com
www.spinlife.com
www.sportaid.com
www.stroke.org
www.wheelchairjunkie.com
www.wheelchairnet.org

### Accessibility Websites
www.access-board.gov
www.dot.gov

catherine a. duffy

chapter 25

# Home Evaluation and Modifications

**key terms**

accessibility

adaptations

architectural barriers

durable medical equipment

home environment

mobility

safety

## chapter objectives

After completing this chapter, the reader will be able to accomplish the following:

1. Apply methods of assessing the home environment for barriers.
2. Understand architectural guidelines as established by the American National Standards Institute.
3. Implement methods for modifying the home environment and increase safety and mobility independence for patients recovering from cerebrovascular accident.

A barrier-free environment in the home and community is essential to successful independent living for individuals who are elderly or physically disabled and particularly for individuals who have suffered stroke.[2] Throughout the rehabilitation process, therapists work with patients toward the goal of achieving independence in mobility and self-care. However, this process usually occurs in an institutionalized setting that is relatively free of architectural barriers. *Architectural barriers* are defined as architectural features (e.g., stairs and doors) in the home and community that make negotiating at will difficult or impossible for an individual.[3]

Most individuals with disabilities wish to return to their own homes. For many, some type of durable medical equipment and home modifications are necessary to achieve easy access.[4]

Understanding the patient's home environment is an integral part of treatment and discharge planning. A home visit with the patient should occur well before the discharge date to provide recommendations to facilitate safety and independence. The therapist uses information gained from this home visit to modify the existing treatment plan and establish appropriate therapy goals. This chapter focuses on architectural barriers commonly found in the home, ways to eliminate them, basic wheelchair information, and a general overview of methods for assessment appropriate for patients who have had a cerebrovascular accident. This chapter—with its bulleted, quick-reference format—is intended to be used as a resource for practical suggestions that will assist the occupational therapist's clinical reasoning process when evaluating the homes of stroke survivors.

## BASIC GUIDELINES AND WHEELCHAIR INFORMATION

The wheelchairs shown in Figures 25-1 to 25-6 are based on a standard adult-size chair. Dimensions vary with the size of the patient using the chair. See Chapter 24 for information regarding specific wheelchair adaptations. The therapist must know the specific size and type of wheelchair being prescribed for the patient before making recommendations for home modifications.

## EVALUATING THE HOME

Evaluation for architectural barriers usually is organized by room.[5] In this approach, the therapist considers the following information during a home evaluation:

### Exterior

Suggestions include the following:
- Assess type of residence: Note whether dwelling is a house or apartment building; determine whether dwelling has elevator or staircase access; examine steps (their number, height, width, and depth); note walkway railings and width; and assess distance and grade between the dwelling entrance and the curb or driveway.
- Note protection from the weather: Examine the condition of surfaces over which the wheelchair must travel (e.g., grass that becomes mud, concrete with cracks, shaded bricks covered with moss, and asphalt that softens in the hot summer sun).
- Examine driveway: Note size and ability to accommodate a wheelchair van; assess composition (solid or boulevard style with a strip of dirt in the middle); and determine whether surface is paved or gravel.
- Survey surrounding area: Look for trees that drop nuts, branches, leaves, and pine cones; note location of mailbox.

### Entrances

Suggestions include the following:
- Consider all entrances to evaluate accessibility; note any entrances inaccessible to the patient.
- Measure steps and landings and note the presence and height of railings.

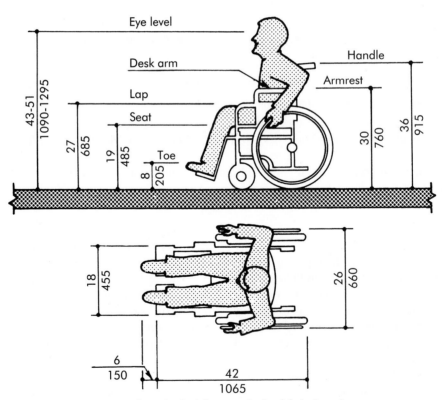

**Figure 25-1**  Dimensions of standard adult manual wheelchair (metric measurements are in millimeters). Width: 24 to 26 inches from rim to rim. Length: 42 to 43 inches. Height to push handles from floor: 36 inches. Height to seat from floor: 19 to 19½ inches (excluding cushion). Height to armrest from floor: 29 to 30 inches. NOTE: Footrests may extend farther for very large persons. (From American National Standards Institute: *Accessible and usable buildings and facilities,* New York, 1992, The Institute.)

- Measure all doorway widths and heights, including interior doors to closets and between rooms.
- Note the direction of each door swing, the presence and height of any sills, and the height of any installed locks; determine whether screen doors open outward

and solid doors open inward and assess the weight of the doors and whether they can be moved from a wheelchair.
- If the patient lives in a building with an elevator, note whether the chair can be maneuvered into the elevator; assess whether the elevator stops flush with the landing; and consider whether the patient can reach the buttons.

### Interior

Suggestions include the following:
- Assess the number of levels and whether the bedrooms are located upstairs or downstairs; consider relocating a bedroom downstairs for improved mobility.
- Count and measure all steps (their height, width, and landing), and note whether handrails exist on both sides.
- Measure the dimensions of the staircase; note the stair height, width, and depth.

### Living Room and Hallways

Suggestions include the following:
- Consider phone accessibility; height of light switches, thermostats, and electrical sockets; furniture arrangement; floor covering; and doorway width and thresholds. Note the width of the hallway and number of turns.
- Determine whether the patient will be able to open and close windows; note whether the windows slide up and down or swing outward; and measure the height of the latches.

### Bedroom

Suggestions include the following:
- Measure doorway width, threshold height, and mattress height.

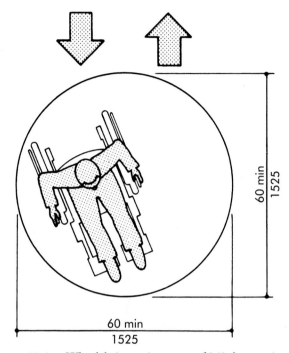

**Figure 25-2** Wheelchair turning space of 360 degrees (metric measurements are in millimeters). A 360-degree turn requires a clear space of 60 by 60 inches. This space enables the individual to turn without scraping the feet or maneuvering multiple times to accomplish a full turn. *min,* Minimum. (From American National Standards Institute: *Accessible and usable buildings and facilities,* New York, 1992, The Institute.)

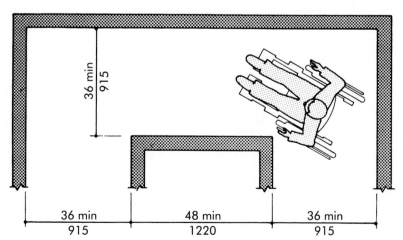

**Figure 25-3** Wheelchair turning space of 90 degrees (metric measurements are in millimeters). A 90-degree turn requires a minimum of 36 inches for the wheelchair user to have clear space for the feet and prevent scraping the hands on the wall. *min,* Minimum. (From American National Standards Institute: *Accessible and usable buildings and facilities,* New York, 1992, The Institute.)

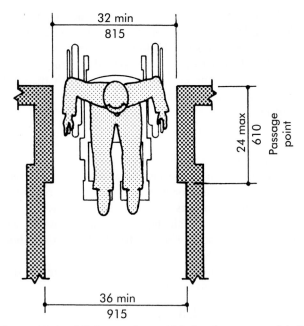

**Figure 25-4** Minimum clear width for doorways and halls (metric measurements are in millimeters). A minimum of 32 inches of doorway width is required; the ideal is 36 inches. Hallways should be a minimum of 36 inches wide to provide sufficient clearance for wheelchair passage and allow the user to propel the chair without scraping the hands. *max*, Maximum; *min*, minimum. (From American National Standards Institute: *Accessible and usable buildings and facilities*, New York, 1992, The Institute.)

- Consider space for hospital bed and bedside commode; note floor space and covering (i.e., carpet, wood, tile, or linoleum) because these may have an effect on walking and wheelchair mobility.
- Note whether the bed is stable for transfer.
- Assess the accessibility of dressers and closets.
- If a mechanical lift is being prescribed, ensure enough room is available to maneuver it around the bed.

**Bathroom**

Suggestions include the following:
- Measure the door width and threshold height, and note the direction of the door swing (inward or outward).
- Measure the entry width and note the type of entry of the shower or bathtub; determine the inside and outside sill height and sill width; measure the length, width (inside top and bottom), and height of the faucet; and note the type of shower head.
- Note whether the wall is plasterboard, tile, or fiberglass; the type of wall affects the installation of grab bars.
- Measure the height of the toilet, the available space on the left and right, and the space in front of it; check whether the toilet paper roll is within easy reach; and

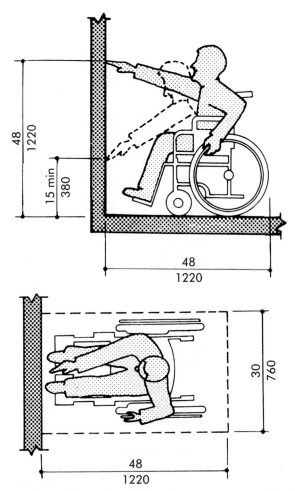

**Figure 25-5** Forward reach (metric measurements are in millimeters). The maximal height an individual can reach from a seated position is 48 inches. Height should be at least 15 inches to prevent the wheelchair from tipping forward. *min*, Minimum. (From American National Standards Institute: *Accessible and usable buildings and facilities*, New York, 1992, The Institute.)

consider the sink height and counter distances to the left and right.
- Determine the presence of any nonslip treatment in the tub; note whether the patient has a shower curtain or a glass door.

**Kitchen**

Suggestions include the following:
- Measure the height and depth of the basin of the sink, the distance to the faucet knobs, cabinet and counter heights, and refrigerator door heights.
- Consider table height in relation to wheelchair fit.
- Note outlet height and location, type of controls and location on the stove and microwave, and height and accessibility of light switches.

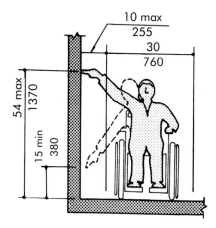

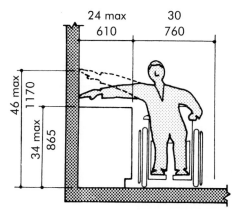

**Figure 25-6** Side reach (metric measurements are in millimeters). The maximal height for reaching from the side position without an obstruction is 54 inches. If an obstruction such as a countertop or shelf is present, the maximal height for side reach is 46 inches. *max,* Maximum; *min,* minimum. (From American National Standards Institute: *Accessible and usable buildings and facilities,* New York, 1992, The Institute.)

## Laundry

Suggestions include the following:
- Note the location and measurements of the washer and dryer if relevant.
- Determine whether the washer and dryer are front loading or top loading.
- Assess whether the washer and dryer are installed permanently or must be moved into place and set up each time for use.

## Basement

The therapist should examine the staircase, railings, windows, furnace controls, fuse box, and lighting.

Sketches of each room with notations of problematic areas are useful for the therapist attempting home simulation during treatment sessions. The therapist should provide a brief summary of findings with recommendations for modifications and safety to the family.

## HOME EVALUATION FORMS

Evaluation formats range from simple to complex, depending on the therapist's and patient's needs. Figures 25-7 to 25-10 show samples of home assessments.

## MODIFICATIONS

The therapist's recommendations should meet the patient's need to function with the greatest level of independence and safety. The therapist must consider the patient's budget and the extent of the structural changes necessary to attain the patient's goals. The therapist should consult building contractors and obtain bids for extensive reconstruction needs and to assist with determining the feasibility of structural modifications. Generally, modifications should be made in accordance with the guidelines established by the American National Standards Institute.[1]

The American National Standards Institute publishes the document *American National Standards for Buildings and Facilities,* which provides specifications to make buildings and other facilities accessible and usable for individuals with physical disabilities. The examples provided are reprinted to increase occupational therapists' understanding of specifications needed for patients who are recovering from a cerebrovascular accident and who rely on wheelchairs for independent mobility.

### Exterior

A parking space with a 4-foot aisle adjacent to it allows an individual to maneuver a wheelchair alongside the car. Pathways and walkways should be a minimum of 48 inches wide and have smooth surfaces to prevent tipping and difficult wheelchair mobility. Motion-sensitive or automatically timed lighting along walkways provides safety. At least one entrance to the home should have easy access. If all entrances are reached by stairs, the number of steps influences the solution to creating a no-step entrance. Options include ramps, stair gliders, or porch lifts.[6]

#### General Comments on Ramps
The therapist should consider the following:
- Ramps should be a minimum of 36 inches wide and have nonskid surfaces.
- The ideal ratio of slope to rise is 1:12—every inch of vertical rise requires 12 inches of ramp (Figure 25-11).
- Ramps should have level landings at the top and bottom of each run; the landing should be at least as wide as the ramp; and to allow for unobstructed ability to open the door, a 24-inch area is needed.

# OCCUPATIONAL THERAPY
## HOME ASSESSMENT WORKSHEET

Address visited _____

Date of assessment _____

**Exterior:**

Type of residence:                                    Type of terrain:

☐ House        ☐ Own        ☐ Rent        ☐ Incline        ☐ Concrete/asphalt
☐ Apartment                                 ☐ Smooth         ☐ Rough
☐ Care home

Distance from parked car to home: _____        Walkway width: _____ inches wide

Distance from home to curb: _____

Ramping space:   1 foot of ramp to 1 inch of elevation

Maximum length: 30 ft

Level platform:   5 square ft

Platform at door: 5 square ft

Railings

| AREA | IDEAL | ACTUAL | COMMENTS/DIAGRAM |
|---|---|---|---|
| **Entrance:** | | | |
| Most accessible entry: | | | |
| Front   Rear   Side | | Front   Rear   Side | |
| Steps (ground to porch) | 7 inches high with nonskid stripes | Number<br>Height _____<br>Width _____<br>Depth _____<br><br>Carpet<br>  Nonskid strip<br>  Artificial turf _____ | |
| Landing | | Number _____<br>Width _____<br>Depth _____ | |
| Railings (ascending steps) | 32 inches high—extends 1½ ft beyond top and bottom step | Left _____   Right _____<br><br>Height _____ | |
| Porch size | 4 or 5 square ft | Width _____<br>Depth _____ | |
| Height of step from porch to house level | 7 inches high | | |
| Doorway width | 36 inches wide | | |
| Swing of door | | In _____ Out _____ | |
| Screen door swing | | In _____ Out _____ | |
| Threshold | Level with floor | | |

Staff _____          Date _____          Time _____

**Figure 25-7**   Occupational Therapy Home Assessment Worksheet. (Courtesy K. Hatae, V. Tully, N. Wade; Honolulu, Hawaii.)

| AREA | IDEAL | ACTUAL | COMMENTS/DIAGRAM |
|---|---|---|---|
| **Interior:** | | | |
| Number of levels within the house | | | |
| Number of steps | | | |
| Steps | 7 inches high | Number _____ Height _____ Width _____ Depth _____ Left _____ Right _____ | |
| Railings (ascending steps) | | Left _____ Right _____ | |
| Landing | | Height _____ Number _____ Width _____ Depth _____ | |
| **Living room:** | | | |
| Threshold | Level with floor | | |
| Doorway width | 36 inches wide | | |
| Floor covering | Wood/tile | | |
| Furniture arrangement | 5 square feet turning space | | |
| Favorite chair | Wheelchair height | Height _____ | |
| Density | Firm | | |
| Armrest | Both sides | | |
| Phone accessibility | No long wire Cordless | | |
| Television accessibility | Remote control | | |
| Outlets | 18 inches from floor | | |
| Light switches | 36 inches from floor | | |
| **Hallways:** | | | |
| Width | 36-48 inches wide | Turns _____ Straight | |
| Turns | Straight | | |
| Floor covering | Wood/tile | | |
| **Bedroom:** | | | |
| Doorway width | 36 inches wide | | |
| Door swing | | In _____ Out _____ | |
| Threshold height | Level with floor | | |
| Floor covering | Wood/tile | | |
| Telephone accessibility | Next to bed | | |
| Bed size | Single, double, queen, king | | |
| Mattress height | Wheelchair height | | |
| Mattress density | Firm | | |
| Space for hospital bed | 36 inches × 88 inches | | |
| Space for bedside commode | 24 inches × 24 inches | | |
| Night light | Next to bed | | |

Staff _____    Date _____    Time _____

**Figure 25-7, cont'd**

*Continued*

| AREA | IDEAL | ACTUAL | COMMENTS/DIAGRAM |
|---|---|---|---|
| Bell | Next to bed | | |
| Outlets | 18 inches from floor | | |
| Light switches | 36 inches from floor | | |
| Wheelchair turning space | 5 square ft × 5 square ft | | |
| Dresser accessibility | Toe space below | | |
| **Closets:** | | | |
| Accessibility | Bifold, curtain | | |
|    Rod height | No higher than 48 inches | | |
| **Bathroom:** | | | |
| Threshold | Level with floor | | |
| Door width | | | |
| Door width (with door) | 36 inches wide | | |
| Door swing | | In _____ Out _____ | |
| Shower/tub: | | Entry width _____ | |
|    Entry width | | | |
|    Type of entry | Curtain | Curtain, glass door | |
|    Sill height (outside) | | | |
|    Sill height (inside) | | | |
|    Sill width | | | |
|    Sill width—wall | | | |
|    Width (inside top) | | | |
|    Width (inside bottom) | | | |
|    Length (inside top) | | | |
|    Length (inside bottom) | | | |
|    Faucet height | | | |
|    Shower head (type) | Removable for hose | | |
| Wall type (e.g., tile, fiberglass) | | Tile, fiberglass | |
| Toilet | | | |
|    Height | | | |
|    Distance on left (sitting on toilet) | 3-9 inches minimum | | |
|    Distance on right | 3-9 inches minimum | | |
|    Distance in front | 30 inches | | |
| Lavatory | | | |
|    Height | 26-30 inches | | |
|    Distance on left | | | |
|    Distance on right | | | |
|    Distance in front | | | |
|    Accessibility below | | | |

Staff _____    Date _____    Time _____

**Figure 25-7, cont'd**

| AREA | IDEAL | ACTUAL | COMMENTS/DIAGRAM |
|---|---|---|---|
| Electric outlets | Open for knee space | Yes _____ No _____ | |
| Wall surface | Wood | | |
| Floor covering | No scatter rugs Tile/linoleum | | |
| Wheelchair turning space | 5 square ft | | |
| **Kitchen:** | | | |
| Door width | | | |
| Sink | | | |
|   Height | | | |
|   Knee space | | | |
|   Basin depth | 6½ inches deep | | |
|   Type | | Double/single | |
|   Faucet control | | Double/single | |
|   Distance to faucet | | | |
| Cabinets | | | |
| Stove | | Gas/electric | |
|   Height | | | |
|   Controls | Front | Front/back/top | |
|   Oven-handle height | | | |
|     Type | | Wall/integral | |
| Refrigerator | | | |
|   Door height | | | |
|   Door hinge | | Left/right | |
| Freezer | | | |
|   Door height | | | |
|   Door hinge | | Left/right/side | |
| Outlets | | | |
| Light switches | 36 inches from floor | | |
| Table height | | | |
| Chair height | | | |
| Counter height | 30 inches high | | |
| Telephone accessibility | | | |
| **Appliances:** | | | |

Staff       Date       Time

**Figure 25-7, cont'd**

*Continued*

| AREA | IDEAL | ACTUAL | COMMENTS/DIAGRAM |
|---|---|---|---|
| **Laundry:** | | | |
| Location | | | |
| Doorway width | 36 inches | | |
| Number of steps | | Number _____ | |
| | | Height _____ | |
| | | Width _____ | |
| | | Depth _____ | |
| Railings (ascending steps) | | Left _____ Right _____ | |
| | | Height | |
| Washer door | Front opening | | |
|   Controls | Front panel | Front/back | |
| Dryer door | Front opening | | |
|   Controls | Front panel | Front/back | |
| Clothes line location | | Height _____ | |
| **Patio:** | | | |
| Doorway width | 36 inches | | |
| Type of door | | Sliding/hinged | |
| Threshold | Level with floor | | |
| Steps | | Number _____ | |
| | | Height _____ | |
| | | Width _____ | |
| | | Depth _____ | |
| Railings (ascending steps) | | Left _____ Right _____ | |
| | | Height _____ | |

_____

Staff                Date          Time

**Figure 25-7, cont'd**

## HOME VISIT EVALUATION

Name of patient: _____ M/F    Age: _____

Address: _____ Phone number: _____

Diagnosis and disability: _____

_____

_____

**Status of patient on discharge:**

*Ambulatory Status*

Is patient ambulating independently?    Yes _____ No _____

Does patient use assistive device? If yes, what type? _____

Wheelchair?    If yes:  Standard _____ Motorized _____

*Cognitive Status*

Is patient alert and oriented?    Yes _____ No _____

Does patient have memory deficits?    Yes _____ No _____

Judgement and safety awareness:    Intact _____ Impaired _____

_____

Vision: _____

Hearing: _____

Who will be home to assist patient?

   Family member _____ Home attendant _____ hours per day

In what capacity?

   Self-care _____ Domestic _____ Total _____

For whom will patient be responsible?

   Self _____ Spouse _____ Children (number) _____

For which activities of home management was patient formerly responsible?

   Cooking _____ Laundry _____ Cleaning _____

   Shopping _____ Child care _____

For which activities of home management will patient now be responsible?

   Cooking _____ Laundry _____ Cleaning _____

   Shopping _____ Child care _____

**Actual home visit**

Type of residence patient lives in:

   House _____ Apartment _____

                        What floor? _____

                        Is there an elevator?    Yes _____ No _____

                        Width of elevator (for w/c) _____

Are there stairs to enter house/apartment?    Yes _____ No _____

   How many? _____

Are structural alterations allowed in residence?    Yes _____ No _____

How many rooms in house/apartment? _____

Can patient get to all rooms?

   Bedroom _____ Kitchen _____ Bathroom _____ Living room _____

   (If patient is in a w/c, width of doorway must be at least 30 inches.)

If private house:

   Can patient sleep on ground floor?    Yes _____ No _____

   Are there bathrooms on every floor?    Yes _____ No _____

**Figure 25-8**   Home Visit Evaluation. (Courtesy K. Hatae, V. Tully, N. Wade; Honolulu, Hawaii.)

*Continued*

*Bedroom*

Width of doorway: _____

Height of bed: _____

Is there room for bedside commode?    Yes _____  No _____

*Kitchen*

Width of doorway: _____

Height of:    Sink _____  Stove _____  Cabinets _____  Table _____  Chair _____

Where are meals eaten?    Kitchen _____  Dining room _____

How far is table from cooking area? _____  From refrigerator? _____

*Living room*

Width of doorway: _____

Height of:    Sofa _____  Chair _____

Do chairs have armrests?    Yes _____  No _____

*Bathroom*

Width of doorway: _____

*Toilet*

Height: _____

Width of space to nearest surface (e.g., wall, sink):    Right _____  Left _____

Are walls sturdy enough for grab bars?    Yes _____  No _____

Is there a shower stall? _____  Bathtub? _____  Bathtub with shower? _____

Does patient shower? _____  Bathe? _____  Shower in tub? _____

*Shower stall*

Glass doors _____  Shower curtain _____

Is there a step up or down? _____  Height _____

Are there grab bars?    Yes _____  No _____

Height of faucets: _____

Width of shower stall: _____

Length of shower stall: _____

*Bathtub*

Glass doors _____  Shower curtain _____

Facing tub—where are faucets?    Right _____  Left _____  Straight ahead _____

Height of faucets: _____

Height of bathtub: _____

Width of bathtub: _____

Length of bathtub: _____

*Miscellaneous*

Carpeting? _____  Area rugs? _____

How many telephones does patient have? _____  Wall phones _____  Desk phones _____

Does patient currently own any adaptive equipment? What type? _____

_____

**Figure 25-8, cont'd**

**Equipment recommendations**




**Home adaptation recommendations**




**Follow-up**

Equipment ordered from _____, _____
                                                       (Vendor)                      (Phone number)

on _____.
                (Date)

Equipment to be delivered to _____ on _____.
                                                                (Date)

Date of home visit: _____

Did patient go? _____

_____    _____
         (Name of occupational therapist)                   (Phone number)

**Figure 25-8, cont'd**

To:_____

Address:_____

From:_____

Date:_____

Purpose:

## RECOMMENDATIONS FOR PREVENTING FALLS AND/OR INCREASING ACCESSIBILITY WITHIN THE HOME

### Exterior

☐ Entrance:   Use ☐ Front ☐ Back ☐ Side ☐ Other ☐ Entrance

☐ Stairs:    ☐ Use nonskid stripes on step edges.
            ☐ Reinforce stairs.    ☐ Remove: _____

☐ Handrails:  ☐ Install: Right/left   ☐ Secure handrails.

☐ Walkway:   ☐ Cover with nonslip material.   ☐ Remove: _____
            ☐ Repair broken walkway.

☐ Door:     ☐ Assist with door.
            ☐ Install door-closing mechanism.
            ☐ Add hook to door and _____

Notes:

### Living Room

☐ Entrance:  ☐ Locate lamp close to entry of room.

☐ Floor:    ☐ Remove throw rugs.   ☐ Tape or tack down carpet.
            ☐ Clear walking path of electrical/phone cords.

☐ Space:    ☐ Clear room of furniture and other obstacles.

☐ Furniture: ☐ Ensure that tables and chairs can provide support if leaned on.
            ☐ Remove furniture with wheels or unsteady bases.
            ☐ Remove low-lying objects (e.g., coffee tables).

Notes:

### Hallway/Stairwell

☐ Lighting:  ☐ Install light.   ☐ Change light bulb.

☐ Handrails: ☐ Install: Right/left   ☐ Secure for sturdiness.

☐ Other:    ☐ Remove obstacles: _____

Notes:

### Bedroom

☐ Lighting:  ☐ Install nightlight and/or bedside lamp.

☐ Path from bed
   to bathroom: ☐ Remove obstacles: _____

☐ Bed:     ☐ Rearrange: _____
           ☐ Lower/elevate bed: _____

☐ Clothes:  ☐ Arrange closet: _____

☐ Other:   ☐ Install bell/intercom.

Notes:

**Figure 25-9**  Recommendations for Preventing Falls and/or Increasing Accessibility Within the Home. (Courtesy K. Hatae, V. Tully, N. Wade; Honolulu, Hawaii.)

| AREA OF CONCERN | PROBLEM | RECOMMENDATIONS | RESPONSIBLE PERSON |
|---|---|---|---|

**OCCUPATIONAL THERAPY**
RECOMMENDATIONS FOR HOME MODIFICATIONS
FOR SAFETY AND ACCESSIBILITY

Patient name:_____

**Bathroom entrance**
- ☐ Doorway is too narrow.
- ☐ Tub/shower entrance is too narrow: _____ inches wide.
- ☐ Towel rack is unsteady as support.
- ☐ Throw rugs pose a trip hazard.

Recommendations:
- ☐ Remove/widen door.
- ☐ Remove tub/shower door and replace with curtain.
- ☐ Remove and replace with grab bars.
- ☐ Remove rugs.

**Bathing**
- ☐ Balance is unsteady.
- ☐ Rinsing is difficult.
- ☐ Tub/shower floor is slippery when wet.

Recommendations:
- ☐ Sit to bathe.
- ☐ Use a bath bench.
- ☐ Use grab bars.
- ☐ Use a flexible shower hose.
- ☐ Use a nonskid bath mat.

**Dressing**
- ☐ Balance is unsteady.
- ☐ Dress on _____.

**Using toilet**
- ☐ Difficulty getting on/off toilet is difficult.
- ☐ Toilet is too low.

Recommendations:
- ☐ Keep toilet seat raised.
- ☐ Use right/left toilet guard rails.
- ☐ Use grab bars on _____.

**Kitchen**

**Laundry**

**Comments**

Occupational Therapist          Date

**Figure 25-10** Occupational Therapy Recommendations for Home Modifications for Safety and Accessibility. (Courtesy K. Hatae, V. Tully, N. Wade; Honolulu, Hawaii.)

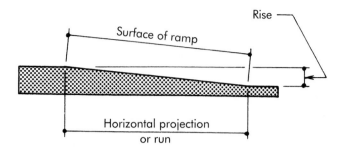

| | Maximum rise | | Maximum horizontal projection | |
|---|---|---|---|---|
| Slope | in | mm | ft | m |
| 1:12 to 1:15 | 30 | 760 | 30 | 9 |
| 1:16 to 1:19 | 30 | 760 | 40 | 12 |
| 1:20 | 30 | 760 | 50 | 15 |

**Figure 25-11**  Slope and rise of ramps. This diagram provides the components of a single ramp run and a sample of ramp dimensions. The slope ratio is an important consideration when designing a ramp; slope creates hazardous wheelchair propulsion conditions if it is too steep. (From American National Standards Institute: *Accessible and usable buildings and facilities,* New York, 1992, The Institute.)

- Handrails should be waist high for individuals who can walk (a minimum of 34 to 38 inches) and should extend a minimum of 12 inches beyond the top and bottom runs.
- Ramps require railings or curbs at least 4 inches high to prevent individuals from slipping off the ramp

### General Comments on Stairs
The therapist should consider the following:
- According to American National Standards Institute, all steps on a flight of stairs should have uniform riser heights (a maximum of 7 inches) and tread depth (a minimum of 11 inches)
- All stairs should have handrails; the handrail grasping surface should be ½ inch to 2 inches in diameter and have a nonslip surface; and handrails should be mounted approximately 1½ inches away from the wall to allow for adequate grasping space.

### General Comments about Doors and Landings.
Standard door width should be a minimum of 32 inches. Several solutions to narrow door problems do not require replacing the entire frame and door with a wider doorway. Existing hinges may be replaced with swing-clear hinges. Thus the clear opening of the door may be enlarged by 1½ to 2 inches. Doorstops may be removed, adding an additional ¾ inch to the clear opening width of the doorway. Removal of existing doors can provide an additional 1½ to 2 inches. Removing doors and

doorstops can increase door width a total of 2¼ to 2¾ inches.[5]

Small landings on either side of the door present problems for a wheelchair or walker user because pulling a swinging door open is difficult if the assistive device already is occupying the landing area over which the door must swing.[6] A minimum of 18 inches for walkers and 26 inches for wheelchairs is needed outside the door swing area (Figure 25-12). Rather than enlarging a landing by removing walls and partitions, three options are available. The door can be removed, an automatic door opener can be installed, or a door pull loop with Velcro-type attachments can be devised. The latter can assist individuals with closing a swing-in door. The loop can be constructed from 2-inch wide webbing material and should be at least 30 inches in length. A loop sewn at one end assists patients with weak grasps. The other end can be fastened to the door lever or knob using 1-inch wide Velcro-type loops and hooks.

If doors are to be replaced, several options are available. If space is a limiting factor, sliding doors are useful (Figure 25-13). However, their weight and lateral movement can make maneuvering difficult. Moreover, some sliding doors require floor tracks, which are obstacles for wheelchairs and persons who have difficulty walking. Pocket doors are effective if only occasional privacy is necessary (Figure 25-14). Folding doors require lateral movement but are lighter in weight (Figure 25-15). Door thresholds higher than ¼ inch should be removed or beveled to prevent tripping hazards and to remove barriers for wheelchair users.

***Hardware.***  Lever door handles or doorknob adapters are preferable to round twist doorknobs. Slide bolts, which can be reached from a seated position, may replace dead bolt locks. Kick plates can be installed on doors to prevent gouging and scratches from wheelchairs and walking aids. They should be as thin as possible to allow clear door width opening. They should extend from the bottom of the door to a height of 10 to 16 inches.

### Interior

***Hallways, Living Room, and Dining Area.***  Hallways should be a minimum of 36 to 48 inches wide. They should be free of protruding objects such as low tables, coat racks, and planters. Thresholds should be eliminated. Nonslip and low-friction surfaces are recommended. Scatter rugs should be removed. Carpeting should be removed or tacked or taped down to eliminate trip hazards. Furniture should be rearranged to accommodate a wheelchair turning area of 5 square feet. Coffee tables, ottomans, and other trip hazards should be eliminated for patients who walk with assistive devices. A favorite chair can be increased in seat height by adding medium-density foam cushions. Telephone and appliance

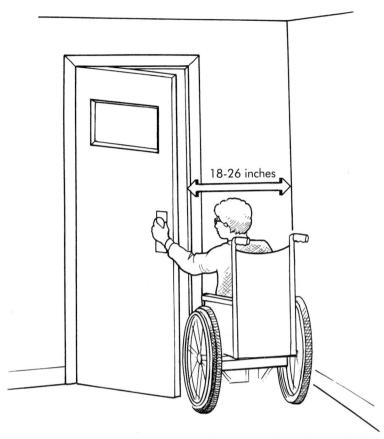

**Figure 25-12** Door swing area. A minimum of 18 inches for walkers and 26 inches for wheelchairs is needed outside the swing area.

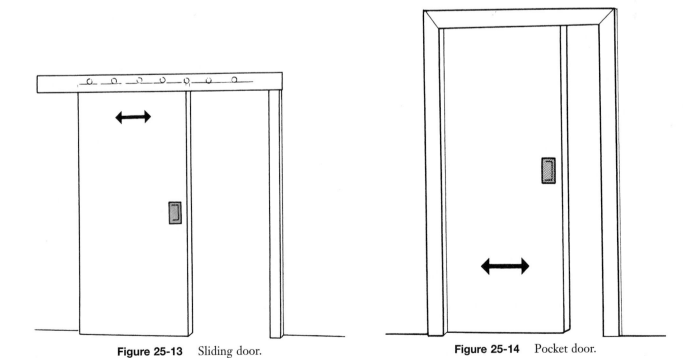

**Figure 25-13** Sliding door.

**Figure 25-14** Pocket door.

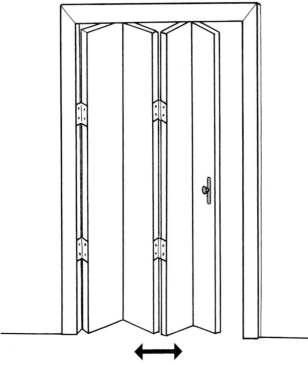

**Figure 25-15**    Folding door.

wires should be taped or tacked down. Easy access to light fixtures and outlets is recommended. Appropriate height for wall switches is 36 to 48 inches. Outlets should be a minimum of 18 inches above the floorboard. Rocker switches and dimmer switches can reduce the fine manipulation required for operating light switches, or automatic timer lights can be installed. Inexpensive environmental control units can aid in independent operation of television sets, radios, and other appliances (see Chapter 26).

**Bedroom.** The bedroom should be free of clutter and scatter rugs. A minimum of 3 feet should be available on the side of the bed to allow for wheelchair transfers.[3] The height of the bed should be equal to the height of the wheelchair for safe transfers. If the bed is too low, it may be elevated on blocks or a platform. Raising the bed also increases ease for sit-to-stand transitions if the patient is ambulatory. A firm mattress is recommended to improve bed mobility. A trapeze can assist with mobility in bed if necessary. Side rails provide safety from falls and also can be used as assistive devices for rolling in bed. Dressers should have toe space underneath and easy-glide drawers. Stackable baskets may be a substitute for clothing storage. Closet doors should be removed or replaced with folding doors or a curtain. The height of the clothing rod should be a maximum of 48 inches.

**Bathroom.** Doorway width may preclude bathroom access for the wheelchair user. Removing the door,

installing a pocket or sliding door, or using a narrow rolling commode chair are options for entry to the bathroom for nonambulatory individuals. The optimal toilet seat height should be 17 to 19 inches, which allows for level transfers from a wheelchair and decreases the amount of bending required to get up and down for those who can stand. Options for raising the height of the toilet include a raised toilet seat, an over-toilet commode, or a drop-arm commode. For individuals who have greater weakness in their lower extremities than in their upper extremities, a toilet safety frame may assist with sit-to-stand transitions. Grab bars should be installed throughout the bathroom because surfaces become slippery and falls are more likely. The height of horizontal bars should range from 33 to 36 inches above the floor. The width of the bar should be 1¼ to 1½ inches to accommodate grasp efficiently. When bars are mounted adjacent to the wall, the distance between the wall and the bar should be 1½ inches so that the patient's fingers can reach around the bar but the arm cannot slip through. Walls around the tub or shower stall should be reinforced. Bars should be mounted securely into the wall studs. Towel racks should be removed if they are likely to be used for support.

Glass doors on tub and shower stalls should be removed and replaced with a curtain. Glass doors can detach from tracks and fall on the person. This renovation increases accessibility for transfers and improves safety conditions. The recommended height for tub rims is 17 to 19 inches. Shower stall thresholds should be ½ inch high. A roll-in shower may be recommended for nonambulatory individuals and should be a minimum of 30 by 60 inches. Some tubs have rounded bottoms. This can present stability problems if a stationary leg of a tub bench is supposed to be positioned inside. A clamp-on tub bench is more suitable for such tubs. Regardless of the type of tub, the therapist should evaluate the individual's balance and transfer method and architectural constraints carefully to determine the most appropriate and safest type of seat. A flexible shower spray unit assists with rinsing; the hose should be a minimum of 60 inches long. The handle can be adapted for individuals with limited hand dexterity. Nonskid tub strips or a rubber bath mat should be applied to the floor of the tub or shower stall and outside the tub to prevent falls. Figure 25-16 gives samples of shower stall and shower seat dimensions.

**Sink and Lavatories.** The height of the sink should be a maximum of 34 inches above the floor. Wheelchair users need a minimum of 29 inches of height underneath the sink to enable them to have close access to the faucets and basin. Access problems may be eliminated by removing cabinets or doors. The mirror above the sink should be angled ¼ to ½ inch for individuals who are seated. Water pipes should be insulated to prevent contact burns. Hot

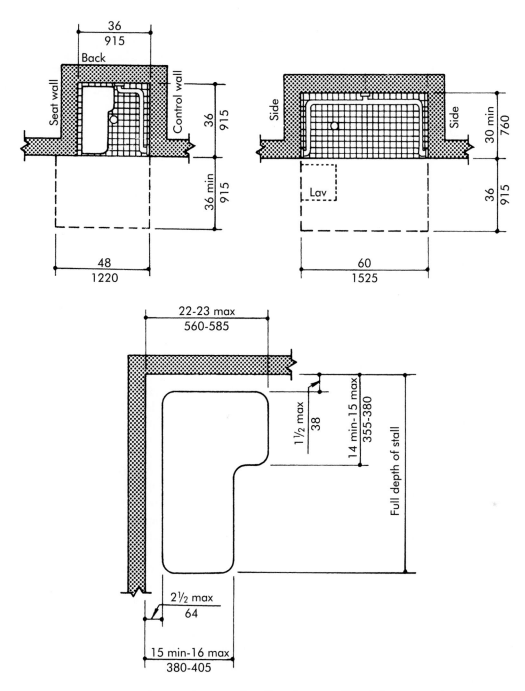

**Figure 25-16**  Transfer-type shower stall, roll-in shower stall, and shower seat design (metric measurements are in millimeters). *Lav*, Lavatory; *max*, maximum, *min*, minimum. (From American National Standards Institute: *Accessible and usable buildings and facilities*, New York, 1992, The Institute.)

and cold water should mix and empty through a single faucet to mix water of variable temperatures. Water temperature controls should be set no higher than 115° F. Ordinances in some cities mandate a fixed maximum temperature for hot water for safety. Single-lever faucet controls are recommended because they provide visual indication of water temperature and do not require fine motor dexterity to operate.

*Kitchens.* The three most common kitchen layouts are L-shaped, aisle, and U-shaped. The L- or U-shaped configuration can improve efficiency (Figure 25-17).[5] Work surfaces should be free of clutter, and small appliances that are used frequently should be placed within reach.

Countertops are generally 36 inches high, making accessibility difficult for wheelchair users. Alternate counter or work surfaces can be adapted by adding pullout

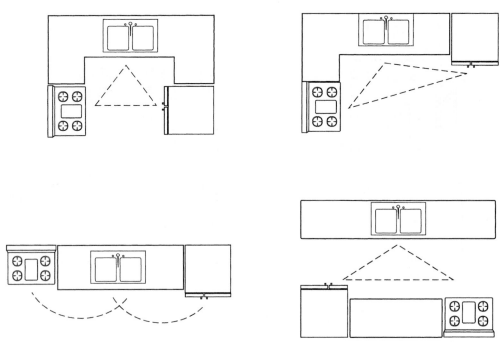

**Figure 25-17**    Common kitchen layouts.

cutting boards or placing a cutting board on top of a drawer that has been opened partially. Height-adjustable countertops and cabinets provide easy access for individuals with limited reach; however, this option is expensive. The countertop should have a maximum depth of 24 inches. The corners and edges should be rounded. Base cabinets should have enough toe space at the bottom to accommodate wheelchair footplates. Retractable doors and lazy Susans increase accessibility to stored items. Adapted knobs or D-loop handles assist individuals with decreased coordination and grasp strength. Easy-glide drawers and pullout shelves may decrease energy expenditure.

The therapist also must take appliances into account. A side-by-side refrigerator is recommended for increased access to the refrigerator and freezer. Shelves should be adjustable; lazy Susans may provide easier access to stored food items. A wall-mounted oven and range top with staggered burners are recommended for wheelchair users. A mirror placed above the stove allows seated individuals to see the cooking process. Transparent pots are another alternative. Range controls should be located at the front or side to eliminate the need to reach over hot elements. Controls can be adapted for individuals with limited hand dexterity. Tactile or audible cues can assist individuals with limited vision. For wall-mounted ovens, the controls should be no higher than 40 inches above the floor for wheelchair user access.[5] Microwave and toaster ovens may be convenient and safe alternatives for cooking.

Sink basins should be a maximum of 6½ inches deep. A plastic or wooden rack can be used to raise the work-ing level. A retractable hose can increase the ease of rinsing dishes. Single-lever faucet controls are recommended and should be positioned no farther than 21 inches from the edge of the counter.

***Moving Around the Obstacles.*** General mobility and transfers will be difficult for the individual who has severe motor deficits. After a discussion of prognosis for motor return, it may be appropriate to recommend a safe mechanical transfer system for the primary caregiver to use within the home.

From a historical perspective, standard lift systems were difficult to use because they generally required more than one person to operate and were difficult to maneuver in limited spaces. Modern advances in technology have resulted in effective, safe, and more affordable equipment available to mobilize the more physically involved individual.

An example of one system is the Barrier Free Lift. With this system, tracks usually are custom installed on the ceilings in patients' homes. They allow the caregiver or home attendant to stay close to the patient during the transfer process but do not require physical exertion from the caregiver. Several benefits to using a Barrier Free track system include prevention of caregiver injuries and ensuring that furniture, carpets, and other equipment do not get in the way of the lift (Figure 25-18).

## FALL PREVENTION

The checklist in Figure 25-19 is an adaptation from the fall prevention checklist used at the Rehabilitation

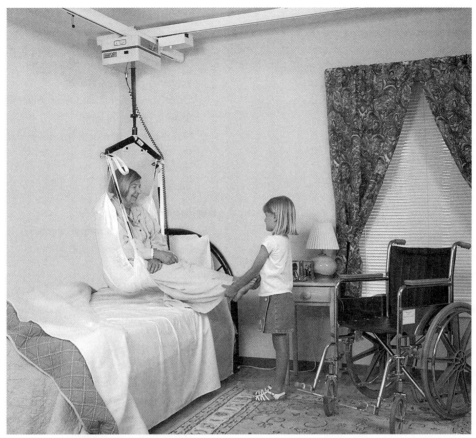

**Figure 25-18** Using a Barrier Free Lift, caregivers can now come in all sizes. (Courtesy Ted Hensley, Barrier Free Lifts Inc.)

Hospital of the Pacific located in Honolulu, Hawaii. This checklist originally was used as a tool to provide education to family members and caregivers after the home evaluation process. The adjustments incorporate options for durable medical equipment.

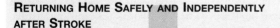

## Case Study

### RETURNING HOME SAFELY AND INDEPENDENTLY AFTER STROKE

J.J. is a 72-year-old woman who was admitted to the hospital with a diagnosis of right cerebrovascular accident. Her hospital course was uncomplicated, and she was transferred to the rehabilitation unit 4 days later.

An occupational therapy evaluation was performed and clinical findings were reported. Passive range of motion was within functional limits throughout all joints in the upper extremities bilaterally. Strength was good in the right upper extremity. Minimal active movement was present in the left shoulder, and one-finger subluxation was noted. Sensation was intact for light touch, pain, and temperature. Functional abilities were impaired moderately because of decreased ability to bear weight on the left upper and lower extremities. Sitting balance was fair. Standing balance was poor. J.J. required moderate assistance for bed mobility. Sit-to-stand required maximal assistance of one person, and transfers required moderate to maximal assistance depending on the surface. She was unable to walk at the time of evaluation, and wheelchair mobility skills required moderate assist. In self-care, a left neglect was noted during all activities. J.J. required setup assistance for eating and grooming. Dressing and bathing required moderate to maximal assistance.

J.J. was treated in occupational and physical therapy for 6 weeks. During her fourth week of treatment, a home evaluation was scheduled. The therapy team felt that having the patient present during the visit would be useful because she lived alone and still required the use of a wheelchair. She lived in a two-bedroom rental

## Exterior

___ Walkways have a smooth surface and are clear of objects.

___ Outdoor lighting is sufficient for safe ambulation and wheelchair maneuvering at night.

___ Step surfaces are nonslip and edges are clearly marked to prevent tripping.

___ Steps are sturdy and handrails are secure.

## Living Room

___ Entryway and room are free of clutter to allow safe walking or wheelchair mobility.

___ Stepstools, ottomans, coffee tables, and other low-lying objects are out of the way to prevent trip hazards.

___ Chairs have armrests and are sturdy.

___ Telephone and lighting are accessible; cords are tucked down.

___ Environmental controls are accessible.

## Hallway

___ Doors that open into halls are removed.

___ Floor is clear of objects.

___ Carpet borders and runners are secured.

## Bathroom

___ Door width is wide enough to permit wheelchair access.

___ No thresholds are trip hazards.

___ Scatter rugs are removed.

___ Grab bars are installed near toilet, tub, and entryway.

___ Toilet is proper height.

___ Nonskid bath mat or strips are installed on floor of tub or shower.

___ Tub or shower seat is available for bathing.

## Bedroom

___ Doorway entry is proper width.

___ Bed is proper height and firmness.

___ Night lights are present.

___ Hospital bed is available.

— Side rails are installed.

___ Bedside commode is available.

## Kitchen

___ Table is sturdy.

___ Frequently used items are located at waist level.

___ Use of range top is avoided.

___ Microwave or toaster oven is available.

___ Throw rugs are removed.

___ Electrical cords are tied up or taped down.

**Figure 25-19**    Fall prevention checklist.

---

### Case Study

#### RETURNING HOME SAFELY AND INDEPENDENTLY AFTER STROKE—cont'd

apartment in a building with a no-step entry and elevator. The apartment had large rooms, but wheelchair accessibility was limited because of excessive furniture and thick carpeting. The hallway was narrow. Her bedroom and bathroom were located off to the right of the hallway, and the second bedroom was located at the end of the hallway. She was unable to negotiate the turn into her bedroom with the wheelchair because of the hall and door width. The therapist suggested that she switch bedrooms and use the second bedroom as her own. The bed was low with a soft mattress and the closet was not accessible because of narrow paths and excessive furnishings. The bathroom was spacious and easily could accommodate a wheelchair; however, the door was only 19 inches wide, preventing wheelchair access. The bathroom had a combination tub and shower with sliding glass doors. The toilet was located behind the door. The sink had round fixtures that were difficult to turn. The kitchen was wheelchair accessible. The refrigerator door opened to the right, and the stove had controls at the back of the range top. The cabinets were high and not accessible from a seated position. The following recommendations were made:

#### Living Room

1. Remove one couch and coffee table.
2. Remove the area carpet and scatter rugs.
3. Relocate the lamps for easier access.

#### Bedroom

1. Elevate the bed 4 inches on cinder blocks to equal the height of the wheelchair.
2. Place a plywood board beneath the mattress to increase firmness.

## Case Study

### RETURNING HOME SAFELY AND INDEPENDENTLY AFTER STROKE—cont'd

3. Remove the closet door and one dresser.
4. Lower the height of the closet rod to 40 inches above the floor.
5. Place a drop-arm commode chair next to the bed.
6. Place a night-light in the wall socket.

#### Bathroom

1. Remove the sliding glass doors and replace with a shower curtain.
2. Use a tub transfer bench and flexible shower hose for bathing.
3. Place a 24-inch grab bar on the wall of the tub 33 inches from the floor.
4. Park the wheelchair in front of the bathroom door and walk with assistance.
5. Place a chair in the bathroom in front of the sink to perform grooming and dressing tasks.
6. Tilt the mirror ½ inch.

#### Kitchen

1. Reverse the door swing on the refrigerator.
2. Relocate frequently used items to the counter.
3. Relocate the toaster oven to the kitchen table.

#### Communication

1. Purchase a portable cordless phone.
2. Consider registration with an emergency call service.

J.J. agreed with the foregoing recommendations and requested permission from the landlord to install the grab bar. During the rest of her inpatient rehabilitation stay, the focus of treatment was placed on achieving independence in bed-to-commode transfers, short-distance walking, light meal preparation, and kitchen tasks from wheelchair level in a home-simulating environment. At the time of discharge, J.J. was independent in all self-care, transfers, and meal preparation. She required contact guard for short distance ambulation with a hemiwalker and was independent with wheelchair mobility. She was recommended for home care services for follow-up therapy and assistance from a home health aide.

## SUMMARY

In 1991, Cooper, Cohen, and Hasselkus[2] published an article in the *American Journal of Occupational Therapy* titled "Barrier-Free Design: A Review and Critique of the Occupational Therapy Perspective." In their review of occupational therapy literature regarding barrier-free design, they identified insufficient research on this topic and a lack of a common conceptual base with which to guide the development and use of environmental assessments.

Two themes emerged from the literature: an increased awareness among occupational therapists regarding accessibility standards as developed by the American National Standards Institute and a consistent reference to accessibility and mobility concepts. The review makes clear that occupational therapy has declared an interest in barrier-free design.

The educational curriculum of occupational therapy includes the teaching methods used to conduct home evaluations and modifications for functional and architectural features. Despite the emphasis placed by the profession on the importance of barrier-free design, a computer search of the major international occupational therapy journals revealed that few articles of relevance on the topic have been published during the past 20 years.

Among the articles reviewed from 1971 to 1991, the earliest article, a position paper of the American Occupational Therapy Association, presented a historical perspective on architectural barriers in relation to persons with physical disabilities. In 1984, another historical overview focused on the needs of the geriatric population. In that overview, four survey studies resulting from occupational therapy class projects were described. A funded study described in the overview addressed public building access. This study revealed that none of a variety of public buildings was completely compliant with American National Standards Institute standards. A grocery and convenience store accessibility study yielded descriptive results indicating little difference in the compliance with American National Standards Institute standards between urban and rural centers. A subsequent follow-up indicated that 25% of the stores had complied with accessibility standards and recommendations. The authors described the role of occupational therapists as advocates for community accessibility as being key to the resultant changes.

The present review appears to indicate that research on barrier-free design is in an early stage of development. The home-based checklist found in occupational therapy educational programs is evident in the literature but lacks a common conceptual framework. Because the demand for accessible environments is increasing, occupational therapy consultation and input also can be expected to increase. To provide optimal care and improve quality of life for stroke survivors, this area of intervention must continue to be challenged and researched.

## REVIEW QUESTIONS

1. What options can an occupational therapist consider if existing doorways are too narrow for a wheelchair?

2. What issues does an occupational therapist need to address for a wheelchair-dependent patient recovering from stroke who is returning home?
3. What modifications should be considered to make bathrooms safe and accessible?
4. What are architectural barriers?

## REFERENCES

1. American National Standards Institute: *Accessible and usable buildings and facilities*, New York, 1992, The Institute.
2. Cooper AB, Cohen U, Hasselkus B: Barrier-free design: a review and critique of the occupational therapy perspective, *Am J Occup Ther* 45(4):344-350, 1991.
3. Datona R, Tesster B: Architectural barriers for the handicapped, *Rehabil Lit* Feb 1967.
4. Law M, Stewart D, Strong S: Achieving access to home, community, and in workplace. In Trombly CA, editor: *Occupational therapy for physical dysfunction*, ed 4, Baltimore, 1995, Williams & Wilkins.
5. Salmen JPS: *AARP: the do-able renewable home*, Washington, DC, 1991, American Association of Retired Persons.
6. Shamberg S, Shamberg A: Blueprints for independence, *Occup Ther Pract* 1:22, 1996.

beverly k. bain

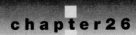

**chapter 26**

# Assistive Technology

## key terms

assistive technology

assistive technology devices

assistive technology services

augmentative alternative
communication

control site

electronic aids for daily living

monitoring systems

powered mobility

powered scooters

Rehabilitation Engineering and
Assistive Technology Society of
North America

## chapter objectives

After completing this chapter, the reader will be able to accomplish the following:

1. Integrate assistive technology interventions into treatment plans focused on increasing the independence of the stroke survivor.
2. Identify commonly used assistive technology for the following performance deficits: communication dysfunction, mobility dysfunction, and decreased ability to access the environment.
3. Understand the use of electronic aids for daily living (formerly known as environmental control units), augmentative communication, powered mobility, and computer access in the stroke population.

George is aphasic and has minimal use of his right upper and lower extremities because of a stroke he sustained 2 days ago. When he wants to turn on the hospital television, he can use a portable augmentative alternative communication (AAC) device to call for assistance or use his left hand to press the large buttons on a remote electronic aid for daily living (EADL) that has been attached within easy reach with the use of Velcro.

Marie has been discharged from the hospital to her daughter's home and will undergo outpatient rehabilitation. She will be alone several hours a day. Rather than hurry to answer the telephone, she can use an answering machine or a small cellular telephone she carries in her pocket. She can prepare a cup of coffee by using a remote EADL to turn on the coffeemaker and other electronic appliances.

Harry can move about his apartment with a cane, but when he wants to go shopping or to visit friends, he uses a one-arm drive wheelchair or add-on power pack attached to a standard wheelchair or a powered scooter. Rather than travel to the post office, he can use his computer to send e-mail to his granddaughter working in another state or to pay bills or check his bank statement.

These examples are a few ways in which assistive technology can improve the quality of life for persons who have had strokes. A reflective therapist can be creative in evaluating patients in this age of technology. Persons of all ages and abilities can use assistive technology to increase their function, compensate for loss of bilateral function, conserve energy, ensure safety, develop self-reliance, and enhance independence.

Historically, occupational therapists have used adaptive equipment to enhance the functional abilities of the patients they treat. Assistive technology devices (ATDs) are an extension and expansion of adaptive equipment and are wondrous tools in the total rehabilitation process of persons who have had strokes. Assistive technology services are the therapeutic processes that therapists use to evaluate, select, train, and reevaluate the assistive technology user, tasks, environments, and devices that are most appropriate. According to the American Occupational Therapy Association Technology Competencies,[20] "low-technology" devices are inexpensive, readily available, and easy to adapt, and "high-technology" devices may be expensive, be available only from select rehabilitation vendors, require special training for the professional and the assistive technology user, and require modifications or fabrication by a rehabilitation engineer. A computer is considered a high-technology assistive device for written communication, and a communication board is considered a low-technology assistive device; however, a creative therapist might use a low-technology universal cuff to help a patient use a computer.

Occupational therapists are vital members of the assistive technology rehabilitation team. They are educated to evaluate a patient holistically, to analyze tasks, and to consider all environments in which the individual must perform these tasks to become independent. In addition, occupational therapists usually work with interdisciplinary teams—an attribute in the area of rehabilitation technology—which requires collaboration with physical therapists, therapeutic recreation specialists, nurses, physicians, speech pathologists, social workers, and most important, the patient and caregiver.

## DEFINITIONS

The 1988 Technology-Related Assistance for Individuals with Disabilities Act—referred to as the Tech Act—defined an ATD as "any item, piece of equipment, or product system, whether acquired commercially off the shelf, modified, or customized, that is used to increase, maintain, or improve functional capabilities of individuals with disabilities."[34] Examples range from a $15 device purchased from an electronics store or through a catalog that may be screwed into a lamp for touch activation to a $3000 voice-activated computer purchased from an assistive technology vendor. The Tech Act defines an assistive technology service as any service that directly assists an individual with a disability in the selection, acquisition, or use of an assistive device.[34] This act also provided grant

appropriations for the development of projects to provide states with information and technical assistance. In 1994, after a year of congressional hearings and deliberations, the second Tech Act was passed. This act requires states to conduct activities leading to the development of systems change and to encourage advocacy services.

## ASSISTIVE TECHNOLOGY MODEL

When an occupational therapist determines that a patient might benefit from adaptive equipment, an effective and efficient treatment model has four elements the therapist must consider: (1) the patient/user, (2) the tasks the user must perform and wants to perform, (3) all the environments in which the tasks will be performed, and (4) the devices required to accomplish the tasks. The four parts are interdependent and must be considered if a device is to be used to its fullest potential by a contented person who wants to enhance functional abilities at home or in the community. In the past 10 years, the development of technology devices to enhance quality of life has exploded. The prudent therapist must have a model to follow when selecting assistive technology devices and rendering assistive technology services as part of the total rehabilitation process (Figure 26-1).

In this interdependent model the patient's physical, cognitive, and psychological needs are considered along with those of the family and caregivers. Not every new device is appropriate for every person. The tasks most persons must accomplish are (1) hand manipulations (e.g., to turn on appliances or write), (2) communicating with others verbally with the use of gestures or writing, and (3) mobility (transverse, up and down, for short or long distances). Most tasks are performed in various environments (e.g., home, school, workplace, community, and clinic). The therapist must consider all present and future environments so the patient does not underuse or abandon the device.[11,30] The ATDs most commonly used

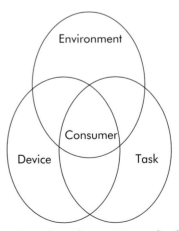

**Figure 26-1**   Interdependent assistive technology model.

by persons who have had strokes are powered scooters, adapted vehicles, verbal communication aids, EADLs, and computers.

## THERAPEUTIC FOUNDATION

The therapeutic foundation for the use of assistive technology as a tool in occupational therapy rehabilitation is based on three frames of reference: (1) biomechanical—specifically energy conservation and work-simplification principles, (2) acquisitional—learning theories, and (3) rehabilitational—adaptation of devices and the environment.

The use of a powered scooter to travel long distances, use of a remote control to activate appliances, and use of a computer are in the biomechanical frame of reference. By reducing the energy expended for these activities, patients can increase their endurance for other activities of daily living and leisure activities. When patients use assistive technology to increase function, they also conserve the energy of the caregiver.

The acquisitional frame of reference is associated with a person learning new ways of performing desired tasks,[28] perhaps with the use of a computer or AAC device. The appropriate application of ATDs can enhance a person's ability to interact in the environment and accomplish purposeful activities. For example, a person who could write before a stroke (but not after) could learn to use a computer and again correspond with family and friends. By learning to use an augmentative communication device, the patient conveys needs and holds meaningful two-way conversations.

Compensation and adaptation of equipment and the environment are the elements in the rehabilitational frame of reference that form the theoretical bases for using ATDs.[22] Devices such as "stove minders" that signal a person when a pot is boiling or automatically turn off the burner at a preset time may be considered adaptive or low-technology equipment. Such devices also compensate for memory loss as a result of a stroke. Environmental modifications have been enhanced by tool redesign, such as electric door openers, adapted one-hand computer keyboards, special computer wrist supports, and electric lifts for powered scooters and wheelchairs. In addition, the use of EADLs can reduce the number of needed modifications of home, school, and work environments while increasing the patient's quality of life.[21]

## ASSESSMENT

No standard assistive technology assessment instrument exists. Table 26-1 summarizes a systematic nine-step problem-solving approach to evaluating each component of the model.[10] The occupational therapist is familiar with sensorimotor, cognitive, and psychosocial standard and nonstandard evaluations of patients. All ATD assessments should include the input, throughput, output, and feedback characteristics and the safety and reliability of all devices. Other references for assistive technology assessment are the American Occupational Therapy Association technology special interest newsletters.[7] Samples of assistive technology assessment instruments are available.[8,9,32,33,37] The key factor in all assessments is the collaboration of the patient with the assistive technology rehabilitation team members.

## GUIDELINES FOR USING ASSISTIVE TECHNOLOGY EQUIPMENT

Because most ATDs contain electronic components, professionals, users, and caregivers must be aware of and should check routinely the following parts when using assistive technology equipment:

- All appliances, wall outlets, lamps, electrical cords, and extension cords should be checked carefully.
- All electrical cords should be kept out of pathways.
- Electrical cords never should be wrapped around appliances or bound tightly because the extra stress can damage the wires.
- Batteries should be recharged or replaced routinely (especially in powered scooters, AAC devices, and infrared or radio frequency EADLs).
- Batteries have memory and require a full charge the first time they are used. (Read and study the manufacturer's label.)
- Cellular telephone batteries must be recharged.
- Telephone answering machine tapes should be checked for readiness.
- Computers always should be connected to surge protectors (especially in old buildings).
- Any ATD selection starts with readily available devices that can be purchased from reliable electronics stores or catalogs.
- A conventional backup for electronic high-technology devices (especially AAC devices) should always be available. Some manufacturers have devices they will loan for patients to use while equipment is being repaired.
- Written instructions, catalogs, diagrams, telephone numbers, and pictures of ATDs should be given to the user, caregiver, or both.
- The warranty of any equipment should be checked. (The warranty is not valid if modifications are made.)
- All environments should be barrier free. (Small scatter rugs should be removed, hallways and stairs illuminated, and door widths checked.)
- Many persons who have had strokes are older and may have decreased vision, hearing, sensation, and cognitive abilities. They should be observed daily for changes.

**Table 26-1**

**Problem-Solving Approach to the Assessment of Patients for Assistive Technology Devices**

| STEP | PART OF SYSTEM | PROBLEM | ACTION |
|---|---|---|---|
| 1 | Task | Tasks the patient must accomplish with the assistive technology device:<br>■ Communication<br>■ Mobility<br>■ Electronic aids for daily living<br>■ Computer adaptation<br>■ Switch interface | Review records; interview patient, caretakers, and family; and observe. |
| 2 | Patient/user | Patient's abilities in the lying, sitting, and standing positions | Conduct formal testing: motor, manual muscle testing, reflexes, range of motion, coordination, endurance, sensory, psychosocial, cognitive, and social; interview; and observe. |
| 3 | Assistive technology device | Based on information from steps 1 and 2, determine possible devices patient can use. | Characteristics to consider include input, processing, output, and display; commercial availability; safety and reliability; practicality; and affordability. |
| 4 | Environment | Present and future:<br>■ Bed/chair<br>■ Home<br>■ School/work<br>■ Community | Interview, observe, and conduct on-site visits. |
| 5 | All | Trial period | Try various devices in a variety of environments. |
| 6 | Assistive technology device | Selection | Order, adapt, or fabricate. |
| 7 | Patient/user | Application | Train in use and maintenance. |
| 8 | All | Documentation | Record in all intradepartmental and interdepartmental files. |
| 9 | All | Reevaluation | Periodically reevaluate patient, assistive technology device, environment, and tasks. |

■ Many older persons are not as familiar with computers and high technology and may be reluctant to try ATDs. Devices should be kept simple to increase the user's function; too many gadgets may overburden or infringe on their independence.

■ The therapist should keep a network list of long-time ATD users, professional consultants, reliable manufacturers, and dependable vendors.

■ As a patient's physical, cognitive, and psychosocial abilities change, environmental changes occur, or tasks and needs change, ATD requirements also may change; therefore, reevaluation is an ongoing process. If a patient cannot return to the occupational therapy department, a telephone call or a mailed checklist can substitute.

## MOBILITY

Most individuals who have had a stroke use standard wheelchairs that they learn to propel with the nonaf-

fected arm and leg during the early phase of rehabilitation. Some persons progress to using only a cane, a leg brace, or both; a few need powered mobility in the home or immediate work environment. However, many mobility technology devices have been developed for the comfort of older patients that may enhance the function of persons who have had strokes: powered scooters; add-on powered systems for standard wheelchairs; electronic lifts; porch lifts; and portable, lightweight ramps. See Chapters 14, 15, 24, and 25.

### Powered Scooters

In the past 5 years, major advances have been made in powered scooter design: bucket seats, adjustable telescopic handle or tillers, front- or rear-wheel drive option, and ease in disassembly or folding for transport in cars or vans. (Several electronic trunk lifts are also available.) The new scooter seats provide additional comfort and stability, with armrests that may be flipped up for ease in transfer. Some seats swivel and may be fitted with special seat cushions or custom molded seats, depending on the person's sitting balance (see Chapter 24).

One should note that front-wheel drive scooters have small wheels that maneuver well in tight spaces and on hard surfaces but not on thick carpet, grass, or uneven surfaces. Rear-wheel drive scooters have greater traction to maneuver over grass, dirt, gravel, and hills (10-degree incline or less). All scooters require a battery charger. Most have built-in battery chargers permanently mounted in the base, meaning the entire scooter must be taken in for service; others have external chargers that must be transported separately if the user plans a trip or the scooter needs an unexpected charge. Careful evaluation of the user's visual ability and all environments is highly recommended, as is an interdisciplinary team making a decision after the user has practiced with different models. Scooters have many advantages for patients in need of mobility technology because they are lighter, easy to disassemble for transport in a car, easy to maneuver, and cost less than powered wheelchairs. Many stores and most shopping malls have scooters available for use by their patrons.

### Add-On Power Units

Another ATD that may increase function for persons who sometimes need power mobility are known as "power pack" or portable power conversion or add-on power units that fit most manual wheelchairs. Some of their advantages are ease of assembly and portability in the overhead storage compartments of airplanes. However, the large rear wheels of a manual wheelchair (which uses friction drive) may wear down when one uses a pack for a prolonged time, they are expensive if used infrequently, and their availability is limited. As with any ATD, the therapist must discuss with the user a careful evaluation of the advantages and disadvantages of the ATD.

## VERTICAL MOBILITY

Mobility in some environments may require vertical mobility, which can be accomplished with a chair lift; chair glide; or small, wall-mounted elevator. All can be expensive. When the assistive technology user needs to use stairs only to reach a bedroom, the environment may be modified with a downstairs room (e.g., dining room, study, or den if bathroom facilities are available on the same level) as the bedroom. Many homes, buildings, and workplaces have one flight of stairs outside that may be fitted with a porch lift for a wheelchair; portable ramps also may be used for inside or outside accessibility.

Other ATDs to conserve energy and increase the mobility of users are electrical, hydraulic, and battery-operated lifts. An Abledata[1] search is an excellent way to find information on the various available lifts. All caregivers should know all lift operations, and the manufacturer should supply the user with warranties, instructions, and catalogs.

### Powered Wheelchairs

If a severely affected person does need a powered wheelchair, the therapist should take the following steps:
- Proper positioning is essential (see Chapter 24).
- The therapist should evaluate the user for an appropriate control site and switch mounting.
- The therapist should determine whether the patient will use an AAC device or EADL.
- Add-on equipment should be mounted securely.
- An interdisciplinary team should select all the equipment with collaboration from the user and caregiver.[35]

### Public Transportation

With the passage of the Americans with Disabilities Act,[4] accessible public transportation for persons with disabilities has increased. Buses, trains, airplanes, and ship companies have made an effort to improve this accessibility. Persons who have had strokes must plan each trip carefully and consider the following:
- Getting to and from the station or bus stop
- Getting up and down stairs
- Locations of elevators or escalators
- Getting through turnstiles
- Getting through doors
- Walking distances in the station
- Availability of accessible bathroom facilities
- Available assistance
- Availability of lifts into and out of mode of transportation

Persons always should use seat belts in automobiles, and any wheelchair or scooter should be securely tied down and the wheels locked. Therapists should note that many states require a person who has had a stroke to be evaluated and then to pass a practical driving test before returning to driving a car. In addition, if necessary, most cars and vans can be adapted for one hand and one leg driving by a competent company.

## ELECTRONIC AIDS FOR DAILY LIVING

An EADL is "a means to purposefully manipulate and interact with the environment by alternately accessing one or more electrical devices via switches, voice activation, remote control, computer interface, and other technologic adaptations. The purpose of an EADL is to maximize functional ability and independence in the home, school, and leisure environment."[10]

Commercially readily available EADLs are the devices of choice for patients who need to turn lights and appliances off and on, use portable telephones and telephone answering machines, and in some cases use devices to summon assistance. Electronic aids for daily living can be practical for use in the hospital or long-term care facility, at home, in bed, in chairs, or any situation in which a person needs to increase the function of manipulative skills.

## Assessment

In assessing an individual for an EADL (or any assistive technology or adaptive device), the therapist should consider first proper positioning of the patient in bed and when mobile. Next, the therapist should evaluate the patient's abilities in the following areas:

- Physical/motor: Range of motion, reflex coordination, and endurance. Usually, the unaffected extremity can be used to activate the device, but an assessment of the person as a whole is important, especially for bilateral activities.
- Sensory, visual, and auditory ability: Assessments of these areas are important to determine the best means of access and feedback.
- Cognitive ability to follow instructions: For example, can the patient remember which device is activated by which button and in what sequence?
- Psychosocial factors: Patient and caregiver expectations and motivation to use an EADL should be determined.

After evaluating the patient's abilities, the therapist should discuss the goals, needs, and all tasks that could be accomplished with an EADL now and in the future. One suggestion is a written list of needs that the therapist discusses with the family and all caregivers (Figure 26-2).

The therapist then should evaluate the characteristics of the EADL with an emphasis on (1) input method and required distance of the throughput or transmission (e.g., one room, several rooms in a small apartment, and inside and outside a house), (2) the output (the number of lights and appliances that must be controlled), (3) portability (because most EADLs are used in bed, in a wheelchair, or in various rooms in a home or office), (4) safety, reliability, and durability, (5) ease of assembly, operation, and maintenance, and (6) current and future affordability.

## Electronic Aids for Daily Living Remote Transmission

The major means of EADL transmission are infrared; radio frequency; sound, ultrasound, or voice; and alternating (house) current. Most EADL are controlled remotely with no physical attachment between the input (switch,

---

Name _____ Date _____ Age _____ Sex _____

Date of Onset _____ Diagnosis _____

Reason for Referral _____

Major Functional Problem Areas: Communication _____ Manipulation _____ Motor _____ Other _____

### I. DEVICES TO BE CONTROLLED

| Devices | Quantity | Comments<br>Location (bed, wheelchair, school, workplace, other); Remote transmission: IR, ultrasound, RF |
|---|---|---|
| Call Bell | | |
| Emergency Call System | | |
| Telephone | | |
| Intercom | | |
| Lights:<br>    Lamps | | |
|     Overhead | | |
| Bed Control | | |
| Television | | |
| VCR | | |
| Stereo | | |
| Radio | | |
| Tape Recorder | | |
| Fan | | |
| Temperature | | |
| Computer | | |
| Page Turner | | |
| Door Opener | | |
| Door Lock | | |
| OTHER | | |

**Figure 26-2** Environmental control systems needs assessment form. (Courtesy American Occupational Therapy Institute; Bain B, DiSalsi M, Gold J, et al, 1991; revised 1995.)

## II. POSSIBLE ACCESS METHODS

Direct Selection _____ Scanning _____ Encoding _____ Voice Activation _____

Switch(s) _____ Mounting Hardware _____

Comments:

## III. FEEDBACK

Offered by ECU:   Auditory _____   Visual _____

Offered by USER: Auditory _____   Visual _____

## IV. INTEGRATION WITH OTHER EQUIPMENT (check all that apply)

| Equipment | Manufacturer/Model |
|---|---|
| Wheelchair | |
| Computer | |
| Communication Aid | |
| OTHER: | |
| Comments: | |

## V. EXPENDABILITY FOR FUTURE USE

A. What are the user's goals?

Vocationally:

Avocationally:

Educationally:

B. Medical Status (Prognosis/Potential for Improvement)

## VI. FUNDING

Additional Comments:

**Figure 26-2, cont'd**

button), throughput (transmission), battery or power source, and output (lights, appliances) (Figure 26-3).

### Guidelines for Electronic Aids for Daily Living Transmission Selection

The therapist, caregiver, and patient should consider the following qualities of EADLs:

- Infrared transmission travels only in line-of-sight, but the distance can be extended with the use of extending devices such as Powermids or Leap Frogs. An infrared controller can teach a television controller or an X-10 infrared receiver to accept signals (Figure 26-4).
- Sound waves, voice and ultrasound, travel in only one room. Ultrasound waves can bounce off walls, and voice-activated EADL may require a microphone or close proximity to the controller. Use of ultrasound devices is easy to learn because it involves color-coding of modules and buttons. Ultrasound devices have several methods of input (e.g., large buttons, large pads, or joysticks).
- Radio frequency transmission travels from room to room. The signal is sent from a portable input device to a radio frequency receiver (plugged into a house outlet) that sends the signal through an X-10 module and house current to an appliance or light.

- Using house current, EADLs can transmit inside and outside a house or building. This method uses a controller to send signals to designated modules that have plugged in lights or appliances. Each controller has a "house code," and each module must have the same house code and a "unit code" for each light or appliance. The controller and module must be connected to the same house circuit. However, different controllers can be used in the same house if different house codes are designated. For example, if two patients were sharing the same hospital room, one patient's house code would be set on A and the other patient's code would be set on C. The patients would be able to control their own nurse call button, television, radio, lights, or fan. The patient with house code A could use unit code 1 for the lamp, 2 for the television, and 3 for the nurse call button; the patient with house code C could use unit code 1 for the nurse call button, 2 for the fan, and 3 for the television (Figure 26-5). Many EADLs incorporate the X-10 system into their units; therefore the occupational therapist must understand the basis of this means of transmission. A variety of input controllers are commercially available, so the therapist must evaluate the number of devices that need to be controlled carefully. A point to remember about an

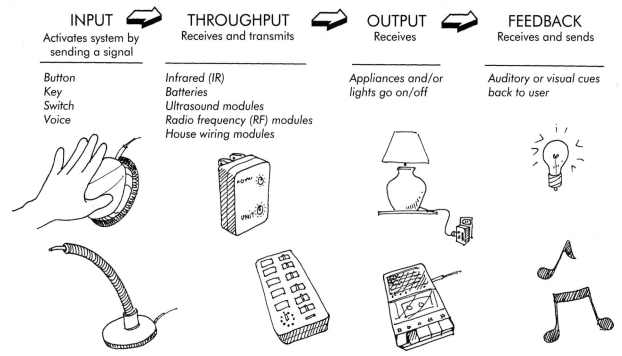

**Figure 26-3**    Electronic aids of daily living control sequence.

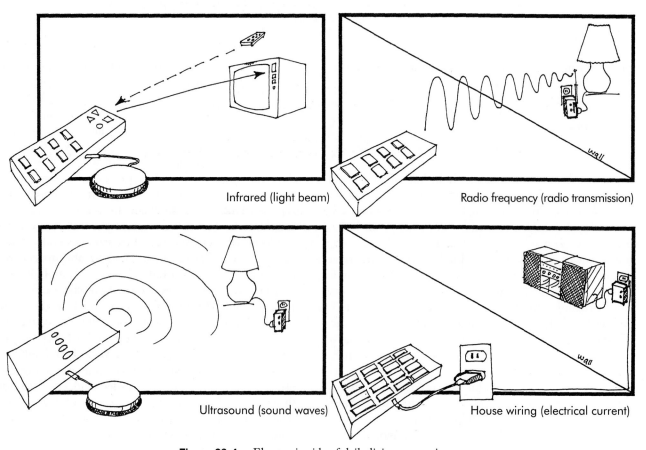

**Figure 26-4**    Electronic aids of daily living transmitters.

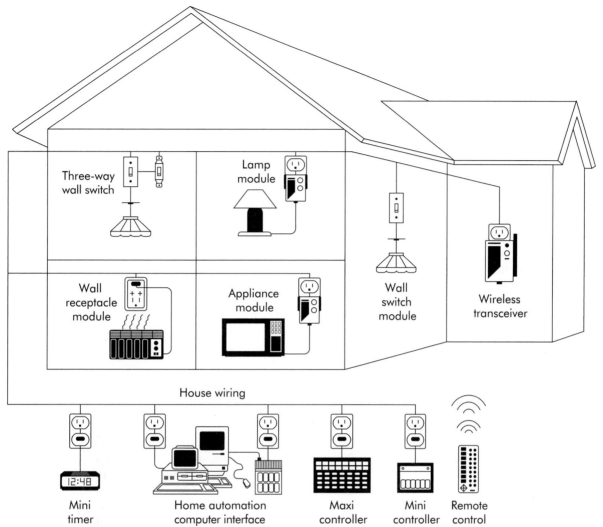

**Figure 26-5**   Control of lights and appliances throughout the house with an electronic aid of daily living. (Courtesy X-10 Inc [USA], Closter, NJ.)

EADL using house current is that it can receive stray signals from airplanes, radio-operated garage door openers, and electrical storms. Additional information on EADLs is available.*

- Recently, with the development of pocket or handheld computers, appliances can be programmed and then remotely controlled without the need to be tethered to a desktop computer.

## TELEPHONES

Telephones are important for safety, convenience, and socialization for persons with disabilities. Many technologic telephone advances benefit persons with hearing, speech, visual, and motor impairments. For visual impair-

ments, telephones are available that have enlarged number pads or enlarged stick-on numbers that may be applied to any telephone. For the person who can function with one hand, speaker phones, shoulder holders, gooseneck holders, and telephone clips are available. For severely impaired persons who need assistance dialing an operator, an overlay may be placed over the buttons that requires only a gross motion to push down the 0 button. Telephones also may be controlled by desktop computers, pocket or handheld personal computers, AAC devices, and EADLs. Today cellular phones have become readily available because they are small, portable, and convenient for use. They can be attached to a wheelchair arm with Velcro or carried in a pocket. Other modifications include the following:

- Portable, lightweight headset telephones
- Telephones with a four-button emergency attachment
- Memory storage of frequently called numbers

*References 9, 10, 13, 14, 16, 24, 27.

- Battery backup
- Redial capacities

For persons with poor voice quality, electronic artificial larynxes are available; for those with poor voice volume, telephones are available that amplify the voice. Several voice-activated telephones have been developed and refined in recent years. The great advances in technology have increased the telephone capabilities of older persons with hearing impairments and those who are deaf. Individuals with hearing impairments may attach small amplifiers to any handset or purchase a handset with adjustable amplification built in. With the passage of the Americans with Disabilities Act, many more public telephones also have amplification capabilities. Special telephone modifications can be purchased at local telephone stores and electronics stores and through office supply catalogs. Fax machines and e-mail are also convenient means of communicating for persons with speech or hearing impairments.

The occupational therapist must assess the patient's telephone needs, collaborate on the selection, train the user and the caregiver, be sure the installation is satisfactory, and conduct routine follow-ups. In a study of aging by the Rehabilitation Engineering Research Center, the State University at Buffalo found that when older subjects were satisfied with their telephone systems, they actually increased their use by almost 50%. Another important result of this study was the finding that the cost for telephone solutions equipment averages $70.45, not including labor charges.[26]

Persons who have had strokes rely on the telephone to communicate daily, call for assistance if they fall, report a fire, or call police in an emergency. The assistive technology rehabilitation team must consider telephones as necessities.

## MONITORING SYSTEMS

Personal-response systems are technologic devices worn or carried by persons who live alone. These devices are activated with minimal pressure; some have voice activation. The switch sends a signal to a monitoring center that puts the user in touch with a relative, friend, neighbor, or emergency services. Most users with cardiac problems are linked directly to hospital monitoring centers. This device can be cost-effective in reducing nursing home or hospital stays while granting safe independence to the user and comfort to relatives who cannot offer constant care.[23] Several systems exist throughout the United States and in many European countries. Most require a monthly monitoring fee, and some equipment is rented or must be purchased. The 24-hour monitoring centers have all the patient's vital information. The patient, therapist, and family must evaluate each system according to the user's and family's needs.

A low-technology solution for monitoring persons in the same house is an inexpensive (i.e., less than $50) portable baby monitor, which is sensitive enough to hear breathing anywhere in the house. These monitors are available in department stores and electronics stores.

## COMPUTERS

Computers have become part of daily life and can be used to compensate for deficits in written communication, conserve energy, socialize on the Internet or by e-mail, and build self-esteem by helping the patient accomplish "tech age" tasks and play games such as bingo, chess, mah-jongg, or bridge. Occupational therapists with basic computer skills can use computers as an effective tool for those with visual, cognitive, or physical impairments.

### Assessment

The assessment of the patient (which should begin with proper positioning) includes the following:

- Cognition—especially attention span, short-term memory, following directions, and decision making
- Visual ability—with emphasis on lateral neglect, figure-ground, visual attention, and acuity
- Motor control—noting whether the person can use the affected hand to assist in simultaneous striking or only the unaffected hand is being used and whether the person has sufficient range of motion to reach all the keys on the keyboard

An interview or discussion with the patient is necessary to determine which tasks he or she wants to accomplish with the computer because many persons have "computer phobia." (Another patient who can demonstrate the ease of word processing to write a letter or show a computer-prepared flyer to a computer novice often is helpful.) A grandparent's task might be to increase social interaction skills; playing computer games with grandchildren could help the individual meet this goal if the occupational therapist evaluates the cognitive and visual skill requirements of several games.[29]

The therapist also should assess all present and future environments in which the computer will be used. Considerations are physical factors (e.g., accessibility of the room, computer table height, and light in the room) and psychosocial factors (e.g., determining who will be sharing the computer and who will set up the computer).

After evaluating the characteristics of the computer, the therapist should consider the following factors:

- Input methods—single- or two-handed, scanning or direct-selection, mouse, keyboard, voice
- Throughput or processing—by batteries or alternating current, model type (e.g., desktop, notebook, or handheld PC)
- Output—print size, color, contrast of letters on the background

- Feedback—size and color on the monitor, auditory sounds of printer and central processing unit

An excellent computer assessment resource is Deterding and Dustman's *Computer Access Checklist*,[15] which contains two parts: an evaluation of the patient's performance components (motor, sensory, cognitive) and contextual issues related to the patient's computer use. Another beneficial resource is the article by Anson[6] that has flow charts to describe physical access and sensory and performance enhancements. The therapist can modify an illustrated checklist designed for health and education professionals to identify computer access for individuals with cerebral palsy.[19]

## Computer Adaptations

Computer adaptations might be required to help an individual to compensate for deficits in cognitive, visual, and motor skills (Table 26-2). Low-technology solutions should be attempted first, followed by software and hardware solutions.

Most major computer companies have accessibility and disability group information one can access through the company website.

Additional considerations when assessing a computer include the following:

- Hardware should be adapted so that the top of the monitor is lined up with the top of the user's head.

- The keyboard and central processing unit should be separate from the monitor to allow positioning flexibility.
- Desk height and width should be adjustable to accommodate a wheelchair.
- Proper seating position should never be compromised.
- Users with hearing loss or who work in a noisy environment may require visual prompts.
- Synthesized speech computers can be useful as communication devices or training aids for users with aphasia.

## Computer Activities

In the rehabilitation process, computer applications are used to compensate for deficits, conserve energy, and enhance psychosocial skills. The therapeutic applications for persons who have had strokes are numerous. Besides the previously mentioned activities, other examples are word processing a favorite recipe book, preparing and keeping schedules of important names and dates, corresponding through electronic mail, shopping from catalogs by faxing and using databases to research information on specific equipment, learning safety and wellness measures, and socializing on Internet support groups. The current trend in computer use is the handheld or pocket PC. These devices are useful for organizing schedules, preparing shopping

**Table 26-2**

### Computer Problems and Solutions

| PROBLEM AREA (PATIENT'S DEFICITS) | POSSIBLE SOLUTIONS (LOW TECHNOLOGY, SOFTWARE, HARDWARE) |
|---|---|
| Visual<br>- Acuity<br>- Figure-ground<br>- Light sensitivity<br>- Eye control<br>- Lateral neglect | - Large, color stick-on tabs<br>- Enlarged text size<br>- Large monitor<br>- Magnifier on monitor<br>- Enlarged screen commands<br>- Screen reader<br>- Antiglare screen |
| Motor<br>- Simultaneous key striking (holding one key, pressing one or more keys at the same time)<br><br>- Mouse use<br>- Energy conservation | - Key latches/locks<br>- Key guard locking adapters<br>- Holding typing stick in affected hand<br>- Track ball<br>- Mouse-key program<br>- Mini keyboard<br>- Word prediction programs<br>- Macros<br>- One-handed keyboard |
| Cognitive (mainly software retraining programs)<br>- Attention span<br>- Short-term memory<br>- Following directions<br>- Decision-making | - Help key<br>- Abbreviation expansion<br>- Work prediction<br>- Macros<br>- Synthesized speech<br>- Gradation from one step to multiple steps |

or "to do" lists, and keeping track of expenses. In addition, users can use handheld PCs with telephones, faxes, digital cameras, and remote EADLs. Only the occupational therapist's experience and the user's motivation limit the possibilities.

Additional information about computers is available.[9,13,14,17,25]

## AUGMENTATIVE ALTERNATIVE COMMUNICATION

The basic areas of communication are verbal, conversational, written, and gestural. Usually the occupational therapist screens, evaluates, and trains persons in the area of written communication. Use of computers as writing aids and speech synthesizers is increasing.

The term *augmentative communication* is defined as any form of communication that does not require speech. An aphasic person may communicate through gestures, facial expressions, body or sign language, picture-letter-word boards, communication boards, AAC aids, or a combination of these. An effective speech system includes standard nonelectronic and electronic aids.

*Communication aids* are defined by the American Speech-Language-Hearing Association as "physical objects or devices used to transmit or receive messages (e.g., a communication book, board, chart, mechanical or electrical device or computer)."[3] Augmentative alternative communication systems "attempt to compensate (either temporarily or permanently) for the impairment and disability pattern of individuals with severe expressive communication disorders."[2]

For AAC aids, the therapist must consider the speed at which the user can locate and select a key, the number of required selections before the aid offers an output, and the quality of the output, as well as the user's sex, age, and dialect. The most frequently used nonelectronic communication system requires the user or communication partner to point to choices to convey messages. The patient may point using the unaffected hand.

An electronic AAC system uses a form of electronic technology, usually with batteries as throughput. The input must be mounted properly and be readily accessible to the user. Output can be conducted by spelling; abbreviation; pictographic; coding of words, phrases, and sentences by synthesized speech; visual display; printed copy; or a combination of these outputs.

### Assessment

A communication evaluation should begin with the identification of all the tasks, needs, and goals of the patient and his or her communication partners. The therapist should assess the cognitive, motor, and hearing abilities of the patient because communication is a sender-receiver feedback system. The therapist should assess all the environments in which the aid will be used, including factors such as mounting of the aid (e.g., in bed, for walking, or in a wheelchair), sound level, and light. (Some AAC aids use light-emitting diodes that decrease in visibility in bright sunlight.)

The key characteristics of any communication system are the following:

- Speed at which a message can be conveyed
- Portability of the aid
- Accessibility of the aid to the user in various positions
- Dependability of manual and electronic power sources
- Quality of the output
- Durability of the aid
- Independence of the user
- Vocabulary flexibility (programmable or fixed)
- Time required for repairs and maintenance of the aid[9,13,14,18,27]

### Role of the Occupational Therapist

Team cooperation is required to deliver the appropriate augmentative communication services to a patient and to integrate the AAC aid with other ATDs. In the service delivery of electronic communication, the four substantial contributions of the occupational therapist are (1) a holistic evaluation of the patient that includes an evaluation of physical abilities (e.g., seating and positioning, range of motion, and coordination), cognitive skills (e.g., following directions, memory, and sequencing), and sensory abilities (visual and auditory); (2) evaluating and recommending the most effective control interface and selection technique; (3) training the person to use the aid (especially if switches are used); and (4) collaborating with other team members.[5,13,14,27]

The speech therapist usually determines the individual's communication needs, assesses the language ability, collaborates in the selection of the aid, and trains the patient and his or her major communication partners. Other professional members of the team may include a physician, who is required to sign orders for equipment; a social worker, who may counsel the patient and family members; a rehabilitation engineer, who may modify the control interface and mounting system; and the vendor or manufacturer, who designs and produces the electronic aid. To be effective, this professional team must work closely with nonverbal patients and their communication partners.

In addition, the occupational therapist should be aware of various aids that are available—from simple, small, battery-operated aids that can be used at the bedside for nonverbal persons, to complex, programmable, wheelchair-mounted systems that integrate with computers and EADLs. Communication is required all day in many different situations; therefore, any AAC device should not interfere with other activities and should use an appropriate power source.

For additional information, speech pathologists, manufacturers, and vendors are available for in-service training, workshops, and training institutes. Three valuable comprehensive resources are the American Speech-Language-Hearing Association booklet *Augmentative Communication*[2]; the International Society for Augmentative and Alternative Communication journal, which includes proceedings of its biennial conference; and the *Trace Resource Book*.[12] The occupational therapist must know what equipment is available and the most appropriate control interface. The speech pathologist is responsible for evaluating the patient's language communication abilities and training the patient in communication.

## SUMMARY

Recently, occupational therapists have learned to use assistive technology to extend the abilities of patients of all ages and with varying degrees of function. The occupational therapist should seek more information, knowledge, skills, and competency by attending conferences and workshops, enrolling in technology courses, visiting electronics stores, reading catalogs, and talking with other professional groups and users. For additional information on general aspects of assistive technology, see references 9, 14, 20 to 22, and 36.

In 1991 the American Occupational Therapy Association formed a special-interest group in technology; additional information can be obtained from the American Occupational Therapy Association Division on Practice. Another informative interdisciplinary professional group is Rehabilitation Engineering and Assistive Technology Society of North America, which publishes a journal, newsletter, proceedings of conferences, special topic booklets, and other excellent resources in their *Assistive Technology Sourcebook*.[17] The society holds regional, national, and international meetings each year; in addition, some states have local groups that meet bimonthly.

As with any specialty area, assistive technology builds on the body of professional knowledge. The occupational therapist first must learn low-technology solutions and then progress to the areas for which the occupational therapy department or clinical site is responsible: positioning, mobility, EADLs, AAC aids, and computers. Staying informed about the rapid advances in technology often seems impossible, but discussion with occupational therapists, other professionals, and patients is beneficial. Assistive technology is one of many tools of the occupational therapy profession. As Mary Pat Radabough said, "For most people, technology makes things easier. For people with disabilities, however, technology makes things possible."[30]

### Case Study

#### ASSISTIVE TECHNOLOGY SOLUTIONS FOR MARIE

Marie, a 64-year-old widow, had a stroke 6 months ago. She lives alone on the second floor of her married daughter's house.

Marie independently carries out all personal hygiene tasks except bathing. The day Marie had her stroke, her daughter found her on the bathroom floor, unable to speak or to move her right hand and leg. Now, she can lightly clean her one-bedroom apartment, prepare meals, and do laundry by hand. She needs assistance shopping for food. Marie attends outpatient therapy once a week, plays cards with friends once a week, and attends church when someone drives her.

Marie was referred to the assistive technology rehabilitation team so that she could increase her mobility on stairs and over long distances and learn to use safety devices in cases of emergency so she can continue to live independently.

While in the hospital, Marie used a simple augmentative alternative communication device until her speech became clear. She also used an on/off electronic aid to daily living to control her television, radio, and lights. After discharge, she was transferred to her daughter's home, where she used her grandson's bedroom on the first floor. She attended outpatient rehabilitation 3 times a week. Marie's occupational therapist taught her work-simplification and safety skills such as using a microwave oven placed at table height to prepare meals and an automatic electrical teapot that turns off after boiling; using bathroom bars installed near the toilet and bathtub; using an answering machine for telephone messages; and carrying a simple electronic aid to daily living in her pocket to control her lights, fan, television, and radio. Marie's physical therapist continued to work on her gait and stair-climbing ability. She no longer needs speech therapy.

The assistive technology rehabilitation team recommended that (1) Marie and her daughter investigate a "life emergency system" to summon assistance (preferably a pendant that Marie would wear at all times to summon her daughter and then the hospital), (2) the daughter contact a rehabilitation technology supplier to determine whether a porch or stair lift or a one-floor elevator might be installed to allow her mother to continue to live on the second floor (to avoid disrupting her daughter's family life and to increase Marie's independence and quality of life), (3) the occupational therapist supply Marie with literature about the emergency system and suppliers, and (4) the social worker discuss funding of the assistive technology equipment with Marie and her family.

## REVIEW QUESTIONS

1. When considering whether a person should use an assistive technology device, which factors must be evaluated according to the technology model presented in this chapter?
2. What are the three frames of reference that form the theoretical basis for using assistive technology with stroke patients? Give an example of each.
3. Which powered mobility devices would you recommend for a stroke patient to use while shopping in a mall? State your rationale.
4. What are the four major transmission methods for electronic aids for daily living? Give examples of each.
5. What would be the most cost-effective and safe electronic aid for daily living for a patient whose tasks include turning lights and appliances off and on and who also needs a telephone system?
6. Give two possible solutions for a problem in each of the three problem areas that might limit a stroke patient using a computer (visual, motor, cognitive).
7. What are the major occupational therapy contributions of the assistive technology team in the area of augmentative alternative communication?
8. Briefly discuss the value of the Rehabilitation Engineers Society of North America for the occupational therapist working in the area of assistive technology.
9. Give two examples of assistive technology devices that could enhance the function of stroke patients in (1) mobility, (2) manipulation, and (3) communication tasks. State your rationale.
10. List five ways an occupational therapist can increase knowledge about and skills in assistive technology.

## REFERENCES

1. Abledata, National Rehabilitation Information Center, Silver Spring, Md.
2. American Speech-Language-Hearing Association: Report: augmentative and alternative communication, *ASHA* 33(suppl 5):9-12, 1991.
3. American Speech-Language-Hearing Association: Report: Competencies for speech-language pathologists providing services in augmentative communication, *ASHA* 31:107, 1989.
4. Americans with Disabilities Act, Public Law 100-366, 42, USC 12101, 1988.
5. Angelo J, Smith RO: The critical role of occupational therapy in augmentative communication services. In *American Occupational Therapy Association technology review '89: perspectives on occupational therapy practice*, Rockville, Md, 1989, American Occupational Therapy Association.
6. Anson D: Finding your way in the maze of computer access technology, *Am J Occup Ther* 48(2):121-129, 1994.
7. Bain BK: Assessment of assistive technology, *AJOT Technology Special Interest Section Newsletter* 5(2):1-3, 1995.
8. Bain BK: Assessment of clients for technological assistive devices. In *American Occupational Therapy Association technology review '89: perspectives on occupational therapy practice*, Rockville, Md, 1989, American Occupational Therapy Association.
9. Bain BK, Leger D: *Assistive technology: an interdisciplinary approach*, New York, 1997, Churchill Livingstone.
10. Bain BK, Okoye R: Technology. In Hopkins H, Smith H, editors: *Willard and Spackman's occupational therapy*, ed 8, Philadelphia, 1993, Lippincott.
11. Batavia AI, Hammer GS: Toward the development of consumer-based criteria for the evaluation of consumer-based criteria for the evaluation of assistive devices, *J Rehabil Res Dev* 27(4):425-436, 1990.
12. Borden P, Lubich J, Vanderheiden G: *Trace resource book: 1996-97 edition*, Madison, Wis, 1996, Trace Research and Development Center.
13. Church C, Glennen S: *The handbook of assistive technology*, San Diego, 1992, Singular Publishing Group.
14. Cook A, Hussey S: *Assistive technologies: principles and practice*, St Louis, 1995, Mosby.
15. Deterding C: Computer access options. In Hammel J, editor: *Technology and occupational therapy: a link to function*, Rockville, Md, 1996, American Occupational Therapy Association.
16. Dickey R, Loeser A, Specht E: Environmental control for persons with disabilities. In Bedford J, Basmajian J, Trautman P, editors: *Orthotics: clinical practice and rehabilitation technology*, New York, 1995, Churchill Livingstone.
17. Enders A, Hall M: *Assistive technology sourcebook*, Washington, DC, 1990, RESNA Press.
18. Fishman I: *Electronic communication aids*, Boston, 1987, College-Hill Press.
19. Fraser BA, Bryen O, Morano CK: Development of a physical characteristic assessment (PCA): a checklist for determining appropriate computer access for individuals with cerebral palsy, *Assist Technol* 7:26-33, 1995.
20. Hammel J: *Technology and occupational therapy: a link to function*, Rockville, Md, 1996, American Occupational Therapy Association.
21. Hammel J, Angelo J: Technology competencies for occupational therapy practitioners, *Assist Technol* 8(1):34-42, 1996.
22. Hopkins HL, Smith HD, editors: *Willard and Spackman's occupational therapy*, ed 6, Philadelphia, 1983, Lippincott.
23. Joe BE: International symposium focuses on emergency response devices, *Occup Ther Week* 4:4, 1990.
24. Lange M: Selecting environmental controls, *Team-Rehabil* 6:43, 1995.
25. Lee K, Thomas D: *Control of computer-based technology for people with physical disabilities*, Toronto, 1990, Toronto Press.
26. Mann WC, Hurren D, Charvat B, et al: The use of phones by elders with disabilities: problems, interventions, costs, *Assist Technol* 8(1):23-33, 1996.
27. Mann WC, Lane JP: *Assistive technology for persons with disabilities*, Bethesda, Md, 1995, American Occupational Therapy Association.
28. Mosey AC: *Psychosocial components of occupational therapy*, New York, 1986, Raven.
29. Nunnally MR: Technology as a therapeutic modality for older adults: a continuum of tasks for improved function, safety, and quality of life. In Hammel J, editor: *Technology and occupational therapy: a link to function*, Rockville, Md, 1996, American Occupational Therapy Association.
30. Phillips B: Technology abandonment from the consumer point of view, *NARIC Q* 3:2, 1992.
31. Radabough MP: Keynote address. RESNA Conference, Washington, DC, June 1990.
32. Scherer MJ: Assistive technology device predisposition assessment. In *The Scherer MPT model: matching people with technologies*, Rochester, NY, 1991, Scherer Associates.
33. Smith R: *Administration and scoring manual: OT fact*, Rockville, Md, 1990, American Occupational Therapy Association.

34. Technology-Related Assistance for Individuals with Disabilities Act, 29 USC 2202 (2) and (3), 1988, 1994.

35. Warren CG: Powered mobility and its implications. In Todd SP, editor: *Choosing a wheelchair system*, Washington, DC, 1990, Veterans Health Services and Research Administration.

36. Webster JG, Cook AM, Tompkins WJ, et al: *Electronic devices for rehabilitation*, New York, 1985, John Wiley & Sons.

37. Williams BW, Stemach G, Wolfe S, Stanger C: *Lifespace access profile: assistive technology planning for individuals with severe or multiple disabilities*, Sebastopol, Calif, 1993, Lifespace Access.

patricia a. ryan
and jennie w. sullivan

**chapter27**

# Activities of Daily Living Adaptations: Managing the Environment with One-Handed Techniques

**key terms**

adaptive devices

adaptive techniques

basic activities of daily living

energy conservation

environmental modifications

instrumental activities of daily living

work simplification

**chapter objectives**

After completing this chapter, the reader will be able to accomplish the following:

1. Explore a variety of adaptive techniques and assistive devices to allow for completion of activities of daily living.
2. Enhance performance of activities of daily living using principles of energy conservation and work simplification.
3. Explore environmental modifications to enhance safety and ease of mobility in the performance of activities of daily living.

Occupational therapy intervention for stroke survivors is geared toward ameliorating deficits resulting from stroke and varies tremendously from one patient to another. For certain individuals, limited return of functional use of the involved extremity makes performance of self-care and instrumental activities of daily living (IADL) uniquely challenging. According to the study described in "Compensation in Recovery of Upper Extremity Function After Stroke,"[2] the emphasis of intervention during rehabilitation for patients with extensive upper extremity paralysis should be on teaching one-handed compensatory techniques. The occupational therapist is called to use creative problem-solving abilities to enhance independence in a wide range of activities, helping the patient achieve meaningful, realistic goals. (See Chapter 20 for a comprehensive overview of IADL.)

## BASIC ENVIRONMENTAL CONSIDERATIONS

Before initiating basic activities of daily living (BADL) training, the therapist should address the variety of environments in which the patient is required to perform. While surveying the patient's environment, the therapist should consider the following criteria:
1. Safety factors
2. Ease of mobility and performance of activities of daily living (ADL)

### Safety

Helping patients negotiate the bedroom environment safely is a priority because this is an area in which many self-care activities are performed. The height of the bed should allow the patient to sit comfortably with both feet flat on the floor so as to provide a good base of support. If the bed is too high or too low, the therapist can consider the following adaptations. Several inches can be sawed off or added to the bedposts of a wooden bed to adjust the bed height. Leg extensions are commercially available from a variety of rehabilitation catalogs. Another alternative is to remove the bed frame entirely and use only the box spring and mattress. Ideally, a double mattress should be used to improve ease of mobility and provide an increased sense of security. The mattress should be firm to allow for increased postural stability and improved balance. The bed should be placed within the room to allow access from both sides. Use of a transfer handle positioned on the patient's noninvolved side improves safety and ease of mobility in and out of the bed (Figure 27-1).

Bedroom furniture should be rearranged to eliminate obstacles hindering the patient from negotiating a path to the bathroom or room exit. If possible, changes in the floor surface should be avoided. Bare floor surface changing to raised carpeting, for example, may increase the risk of falls.

The sensory environment is another component to consider. Factors such as sufficient lighting and a comfortable room temperature must be ensured. If inadequate, both conditions present safety obstacles. For example, if the room temperature is too cold, the patient may experience an increase in muscle activity, possibly decreasing postural stability and the ability to perform self-care tasks successfully. (See Chapter 25 for a detailed review of home modifications.)

### Ease of Mobility and Performance of Activities of Daily Living

In addition to the safety of the environment, the therapist also must consider arrangement of the bedroom to increase ease of mobility and performance of ADL. The therapist may use energy conservation and work simplification techniques to teach the patient ways to prioritize,

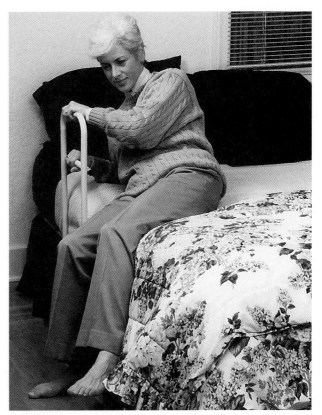

**Figure 27-1** Transfer handle. (Courtesy North Coast Medical, San Jose, Calif.)

organize, and limit work to save time and energy and to enhance the successful outcome of task performance. The following techniques should be considered:
1. Eliminate excess space. Enough space must be available for ease of mobility without excess. Excess space forces a patient to travel greater distances, draining personal energy resources. For example, the bathroom ideally should be directly off the bedroom rather than down the hall. If this arrangement is not possible, a bedside commode and sitting table with a mirror that can be set up to allow for performance of toileting and grooming are useful modifications. A living room can be used to replace an out-of-the-way bedroom.
2. Arrange the room so that sequential tasks can be performed with minimal travel time in between.
3. Place appliances and controls where they can be accessed easily. Lamps, alarm clocks, and telephones should be placed where they are needed most often and are most convenient for the patient. The use of environmental control units should be considered (see Chapter 26).
4. Eliminate clutter. Thorough cleaning and organization is essential to allow for easy retrieval of commonly needed items.
5. Arrange for easy access of clothing and toileting supplies by eliminating excess reaching and bending.

Shelves are easier to access than drawers. If drawers are used, they are easier to open with a central knob rather than handles. Also, closet rods can be lowered to eliminate excess reaching. An alternative solution includes use of a reacher.

Therapists must be aware of the neurobehavioral deficits that affect BADL and IADL. These deficits influence equipment choices and training techniques (see Chapters 17 and 18).

## BASIC ACTIVITIES OF DAILY LIVING

The U.S. Department of Health and Human Services has published poststroke rehabilitation guidelines that describe several BADL instruments, including the Barthel index and the Functional Independence Measure. Each assessment is psychometrically strong and is recommended for this population. The therapist can gather information regarding validity, reliability, sensitivity, and strengths and weaknesses of each instrument by reviewing the guidelines in depth. Guidelines can be obtained by contacting the U.S. Department of Health and Human Services.[3]

### Grooming and Hygiene

When performing hygiene and grooming, assistive devices and alternative methods often provide increased independence and safety and decreased energy expenditure.

*Toileting.* A toilet tissue dispenser should be mounted within easy reach of the unaffected side and allow for easy, one-handed retrieval of tissue sheets. Two possibilities include a tissue box dispenser mounted on the bathroom wall or an easy-load toilet paper holder, which eliminates excessive paper roll waste. This alternative gives a more aesthetic appearance, possibly improving acceptance by the patient (Figure 27-2). Moist towelettes can be used in place of toilet paper and are a viable alternative for patients with urgency or impaired sphincter control.

Two devices that are available and recommended to increase independence in bladder care for women who have survived a stroke include the Asta-Cath and the Feminal. Both products are available from A+ Products. The Asta-Cath female catheter guide is a simple device that assists women in locating their urinary meatus. As the Asta-Cath is inserted into the vagina, it spreads the labia and one hole aligns with the urinary meatus. The patient then can pass a No. 14 French or smaller catheter into the bladder for emptying. The three alignment holes allow for most anatomic differences (Figure 27-3). The Feminal is designed so that a woman can urinate in a reclined, seated, or standing position. When gently pressed against the body, the unique shape creates a leak-proof seal (Figure 27-4).

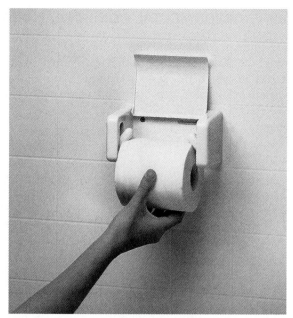

**Figure 27-2** Easy-Load toilet paper holder. (Courtesy Sammons Preston, Inc, a BISSELL Company.)

*Showering and Bathing.* Transferring from a slippery tub, controlling water temperature, and washing adequately in a slippery tub are safety factors to consider during bathing. No-slip mats should be placed inside and outside the tub. All toiletries should be placed where they can be reached easily. Articles should be moved close together if the individual is sitting on a tub bench to ensure safe reaching. To ensure safety of water temperature and ease of bathing, a handheld shower hose with control of water flow may be used to prevent scalding. This device can be purchased through a variety of catalogs.

Long-handled scrub sponges and bath brushes are excellent assistive devices for washing. A flex sponge is able to bend in any direction to wash all of the body, including the nonaffected arm, axilla, and shoulder, which may be difficult to reach (Figure 27-5). Soap on a rope or a suction soap holder may be used to prevent soap from slipping about or getting lost in the water. The soap on the rope is hung around the neck or hung within easy reach. Another alternative is to use liquid soap in a pump container. A soaper sponge also may be used to wash without having to hold a slippery bar of soap. If grasp is limited, the patient can use a terry cloth wash mitt with a pocket to hold the bar of soap. The aforementioned devices may be purchased through a variety of rehabilitation catalogs. For those who must rely on another to bathe them, a mechanical lift positions the person in a body sling. This lifting device has a swing arm to allow a person to be suspended in a shower or over a tub.

*Shampooing.* Shampoo in a pump spray bottle helps avoid waste and reaches a broader area of the scalp. A full-spray handheld shower is convenient for rinsing.

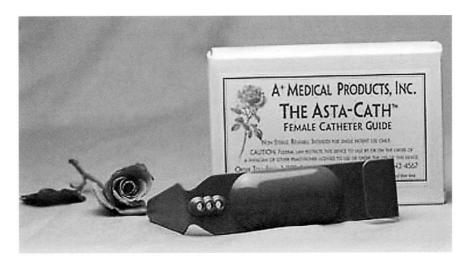

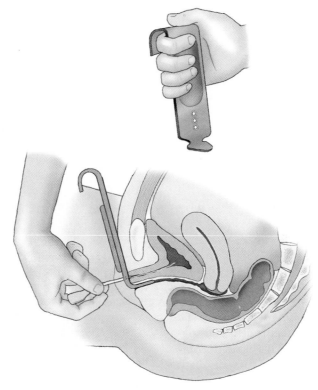

**Figure 27-3** The Asta-Cath (Available from A⁺ Products, www.aplusproducts.biz, [888] 843-3334.)

***Drying.*** To decrease energy expenditure while drying, an extra large towel or terry wraparound robe can be worn to absorb most of the water. The back and nonaffected arm are the most difficult areas to dry. The following procedure can be incorporated:

1. Place the towel over one shoulder.
2. Reach behind and grasp the other end, pulling the towel down across the back.
3. Repeat the same procedure over the opposite shoulder.

An alternative method is to toss the towel over the top of a doorway and shut the door as much as possible to hold the towel in place. The patient then can pull the towel across the back and shoulder with the nonaffected extremity.

***Washing at the Sink.*** Some individuals may have difficulty showering or bathing for a variety of reasons. An alternative method is to have body washes at the sink. The easiest position in which to wash the affected arm is to place the arm and axilla in the sink basin. To wash the unaffected arm, the individual steadies the soapy washcloth over the edge of the sink and rubs the arm and hand

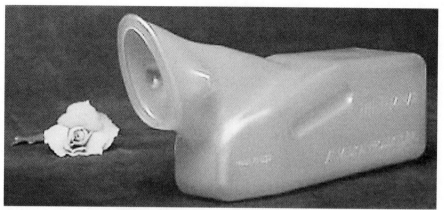

**Figure 27-4**    The Feminal (Available from A+ Products, www.aplusproducts.biz, [888] 843-3334.)

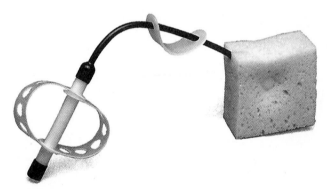

**Figure 27-5**    Flex sponge. (Courtesy Sammons Preston, Inc, a BISSELL Company.)

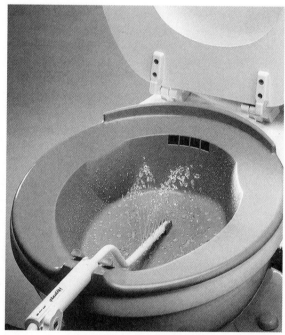

**Figure 27-6**    Hygenique Plus Bidet/Sitz Bath System. (Courtesy North Coast Medical, San Jose, Calif.)

over it. The patient then washes the rest of the body with one hand. Again, a flex sponge is useful to wash all of the body, including the nonaffected extremity. A supplement to washing at the sink is the use of a bidet. The Hygenique Plus Bidet/Sitz Bath System is designed specially for personal hygiene needs. This system combines a spray wand for bidet cleansing and a sitz bath (Figure 27-6).

For individuals with low endurance who are unable to shower or bathe at the sink, a total-body, pH-balanced cleanser may be used for shampooing, bathing, and incontinence care. This product is available through a variety of rehabilitation catalogs. Drying techniques are the same as previously described.

***Performing Oral Hygiene.*** Oral hygiene care can be done easily with one hand. A toothpaste dispenser can dispense the correct amount of toothpaste on the brush for individuals with limited hand function (Figure 27-7). The method of brushing (electrical or manual) is a personal choice. The use of an electrical toothbrush may decrease energy expenditure because the brush vibrates up and down, and the patient holds the arm in one posi-

tion. A Waterpik attachment is excellent for massaging the gums and rinsing between the teeth. Suction toothbrushes may be attached to a suction unit to prevent dysphagia-related aspiration in individuals who cannot tolerate thin liquids.

The simplest method for denture care is to soak the dentures overnight in a commercial denture cleanser. If additional cleansing of dentures is needed, the patient can use a suction denture brush.

Flossing teeth with one hand can be performed easily and effectively with a dental floss holder (Figure 27-8).

***Applying Deodorant.*** Aerosol sprays are easier to apply to the unaffected arm unless the individual has sufficient

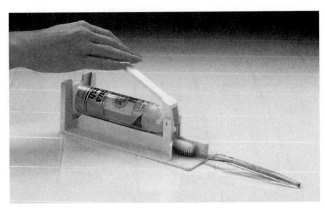

**Figure 27-7** Toothpaste dispenser. (Courtesy Sammons Preston, Inc, a BISSELL Company.)

function to reach the axilla with a roll-on or stick applicator. The affected axilla must be placed passively away from the body to apply deodorant. This can be accomplished by bending forward at the hips and allowing gravity to assist the arm away from the body.

***Caring for Fingernails.*** Nail care of the affected hand can be done easily with the noninvolved hand. Cleaning, cutting, and filing the nails of the unaffected hand are more difficult.

The following strategies may be used to ease nail management:
1. To clean the unaffected hand, a nailbrush with suction cups for cleaning fingernails can be used.
2. To cut the nails of the unaffected hand, the patient may use a one-hand fingernail clipper. When the patient presses down on the board, the jaws of the clipper close (Figure 27-9).
3. Filing the nails of the unaffected hand can be done in a variety of ways. A suction emery board is useful. Other individuals may choose to use a homemade device such as an emery board or sandpaper glued to a piece of wood, a nail file secured to a table with masking tape, or a file wedged in a drawer.
4. Applying nail polish to the unaffected hand can be done by mounting a clothespin on a piece of wood with a C-clamp to hold the polish brush. The polish is applied when the person moves the nail in relation to the brush.

***Caring for Toenails.*** Cleansing toes can be accomplished with the use of a footbrush or Footmate System (Figure 27-10). Clipping toenails is easier if the feet are soaked in warm water first. A pistol-grip remote toenail clipper is one of several devices designed for one-handed use to clip toenails; it allows one to reach the foot with less bending (Figure 27-11).

***Hairstyling.*** Simple, short hairstyles are the easiest to manage with one hand. Combing or styling long hair

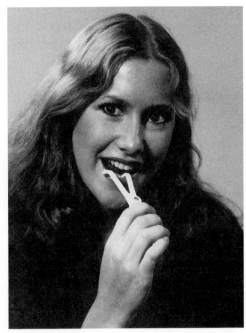

**Figure 27-8** Floss Aid dental floss holder. (Courtesy Maddak, Pequannock, NJ.)

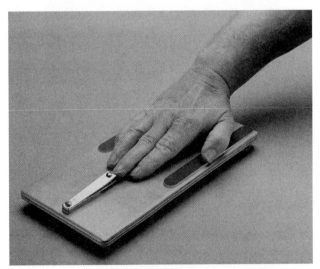

**Figure 27-9** One-hand fingernail clipper. (Courtesy Maddak, Pequannock, NJ.)

may be easier using adjustable, long-handled grooming accessories, available through various rehabilitation catalogs. Lightweight splinting material also may be used to extend the handles of an individual's favorite grooming tools.

Blow-drying hair can be made easier by using a commercial product called the Hands-Free Hair Dryer Holder, which allows the unaffected hand free operation to style hair (Figure 27-12). An alternative method is a home-devised product such as a position-adjustable hair

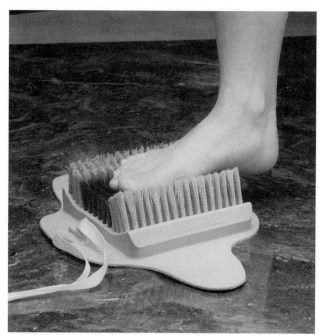

**Figure 27-10**    Footmate System. (Courtesy North Coast Medical, San Jose, Calif.)

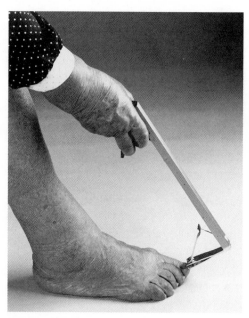

**Figure 27-11**    Pistol-grip remote toenail clipper. (Courtesy Maddack, Pequannock, NJ.)

dryer. A lightweight blow-dryer, a desk lamp with spring-balanced arms, a tension control knob at each joint, and a mounting bracket are the only materials needed to fabricate the device. The position-adjustable hair dryer requires limited body movement because the dryer can be positioned in any plane desired.[1]

Brush attachments to the hair dryer also can be used for blow-drying styles. A hot brush curling system can be used for setting hair in simple hairstyles.

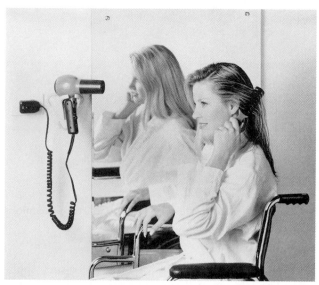

**Figure 27-12**    Hands-free hair dryer holder. (Courtesy Sammons Preston, Inc, a BISSELL Company.)

***Shaving.*** Shaving can be done one-handed with any type of razor. If a patient is unsteady with the motor skills, a Silk Effects razor reduces the risks of nicking the skin. An electric razor is easy to manage with one hand and is recommended for safety to prevent nicks.

***Applying Makeup.*** The patient may apply makeup one-handed with practice. Grip and bottle makeup holders are useful to stabilize supplies; suction cups and rubber mats also help stabilize grooming items.

### Feeding Techniques

***Positioning at the Table.*** The affected extremity should be supported in a good weight-bearing position on the table. This position promotes appropriate upper extremity alignment, visual awareness of the extremity, and trunk symmetry.

***Use of Adaptive Devices.*** To avoid embarrassment while dining with others and to reach full independence with feeding, the patient often uses compensatory strategies and adaptive equipment. The following equipment is recommended:
- Nonskid mats should be used to prevent slippage of plates and bowls and to hold them steady during meals.
- Plate guards and scoop dishes are recommended to eliminate food getting pushed off the plate while scooping or when buttering bread.
- A rocker knife or knife with serrated and curved edges is easy to use with one hand if safety awareness is intact.
- Combined implements such as knife and fork or knife, fork, and spoon are available for purchase. Safety in

using these combined instruments is a concern if loss of sensation or weakness in oral-motor structures is present. Utensils with built-up handles also may be used to assist a weak grasp.

## Dressing

Retraining an individual with hemiplegia who is limited to the use of one hand to dress presents challenges to the patient and the therapist. Specific deficits that the therapist must address include the following:

1. Impaired postural stability and balance
2. Decreased dexterity and work speed
3. Impaired ability to stabilize clothing articles and body parts
4. Decreased endurance accompanied by increased energy demands on the body
5. Impaired sensory capabilities
6. Possible cognitive and perceptual limitations

When retraining the patient in dressing techniques, the therapist should incorporate adequate time and allowances for rest breaks into the session. The patient should be able to achieve success without undue effort. Loose-fitting clothes should be selected. Roomy clothes with limited fasteners allow for increased ease of movement and easier donning and doffing.

Dressing and undressing invariably involve awkward movement patterns and a certain amount of sitting down and standing up. Care must be taken to ensure that the danger of falling is minimized. Management of clothes is always difficult at first; the occupational therapist should reinforce to the individual that independence and efficiency are achieved through practice.

### Fasteners

Many individuals with hemiplegia can learn to manage fasteners if the following requirements are met:

■ Garments fit loosely.
■ Buttons and hooks are of a larger size.
■ Fasteners are positioned in front of or on the nonaffected side of the garment and are within sight.

*Buttons.* If the patient is unable to manage fasteners, the therapist can use the following adaptation:

1. Remove the buttons from the garment and then sew them back on over the buttonholes.
2. Using Velcro squares, sew the loop side of the Velcro over the original button side of the garment.
3. Sew the hook side of the Velcro under the buttonholes.

The patient then simply uses hand pressure to close the garment. A standard collar extender also can be used. With this item, collars and cuffs are increased by ½ inch, increasing ease of management.

*Zippers.* Zippers may be easier to manage if a ring or loop is added to the zipper tab. Patients should avoid open-ended zips. Patients can leave the zip fastened at the bottom and don the garment by pulling it on over the head. A large safety pin left fastened can prevent the zipper from sliding all the way down and detaching during overhead donning.

*Adaptive Dressing Techniques.* Before initiating dressing training, the therapist should ensure the patient is seated on a stable, supportive surface, preferably a sturdy armchair. Both of the patient's feet should be securely positioned on the floor to establish a solid base of support and increase postural stability. Clothing should be placed within easy reach and in the order in which each item is required. This helps maximize energy preservation.

A wide variety of dressing techniques are described in the literature, depending on the particular treatment theory incorporated by the therapist. Some general principles that facilitate ease of one-handed dressing are described in the following sections.

### Upper Extremity Dressing

*Donning Garments with Front Fasteners.* The patient should follow these instructions for donning garments with front fasteners (Figure 27-13):

1. Pull the shirtsleeve onto the affected arm.
2. Pull the shirtsleeve over the affected shoulder.
3. Swing the garment around until the other sleeve hangs down the back or pull the sleeve over the head and around the neck. The patient may even anchor it by biting the sleeve.
4. Reach to the back with the nonaffected arm and place it into the opening of the remaining sleeve.
5. Using a shrugging motion with the nonaffected arm, straighten the sleeve into place.

Shirtsleeves may need to be expanded or loose fitting to be pulled over the noninvolved hand. This can be achieved by sewing a piece of elastic into the sleeve cuff to allow for easy passage over the hand[3] and to eliminate the difficulty of managing a cuff button.

The top button of a shirt collar is often difficult to fasten. The button is usually small, and the collar fits snugly around the neck. The problem can be eliminated by replacing the button with a Velcro fastener.[3]

*Donning Ties.* Ties are difficult to manipulate single-handedly. The simplest solution is to use a conventional, already-tied tie. A piece of elastic may be inserted into the back of the tie to replace a small part of the fabric. This allows for easy passage of the tie over the head. Clip-on ties also are convenient to use.

### Donning Pullover Shirts

The patient should follow these instructions for donning pullover shirts:

1. Use shirt tags or labels to identify the front and back sides of the garment.

2. Pull the correct sleeve onto the affected arm, and pull the garment onto the affected shoulder.
3. Bend the head forward through the neck opening.
4. Put the unaffected arm into the other sleeve.
5. Straighten the sleeve by rubbing the arm against the leg.
6. Pull the garment over the torso.

***Donning Brassieres.*** Front-fastening bras are easier to manage than bras that fasten in back. The bra should be donned by putting the affected arm in first. Another method is to fasten the bra first and then put the bra on by donning it over the head. Larger hooks can be substituted for smaller hooks, or a Velcro strap and D ring may be sewn in as substitutions for the fastener. A bra extender can be purchased and interchanged between bras; increasing the girth accommodation can ease donning.

Patients may manage back-closure bras in the following way[3]:

1. Align the bra around the waist so that the cups face backward. The strap can be held in place by hugging it with the affected arm, by tucking it into the elasticized panty waist, or by using a clothespin to hold it onto the pants.
2. Fasten the hooks in front.
3. Swivel the bra around so that the cups are in front.
4. Pull the strap over the affected shoulder.
5. Using the thumb of the unaffected hand, pull the strap over the unaffected shoulder.

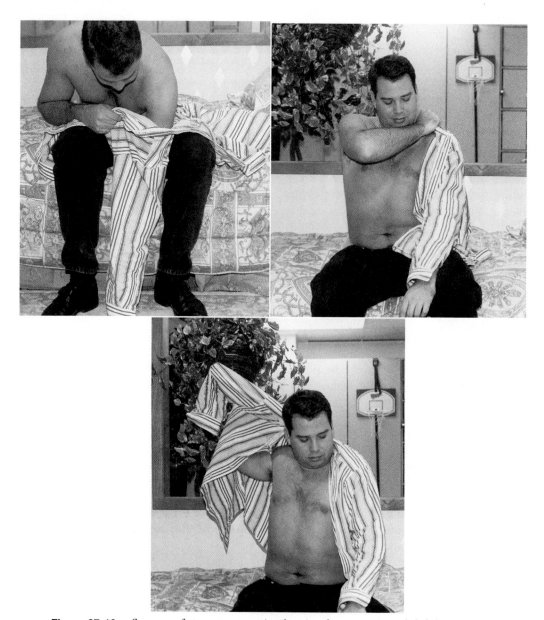

**Figure 27-13**    Sequence for upper extremity dressing for a patient with left hemiplegia.

The easiest solution, although not necessarily the most aesthetic, is a fully elasticized bra such as a sports bra, which can be slipped on over the head. A hook-and-eye bra can be adapted by sewing the back fasteners together.

## Lower Extremity Dressing

### Donning Pants and Underwear While Lying in Bed

The patient should follow this procedure for donning underwear and pants in bed:

1. Bend the affected leg until the foot is within reach. The patient may use the unaffected leg to assist with this.
2. Place the pants over the affected foot and allow the leg to straighten into the pant leg.
3. Put the unaffected leg into the pants and pull the pants up as far as possible.
4. Using the unaffected leg, or if possible both legs, lift the pelvis off the bed. Wriggle the pants up to the waist.
5. Fasten the pants. (Velcro may be used in place of buttons.)

### Donning Pants and Underwear While Sitting Up

The patient should follow this procedure for donning underwear and pants while sitting up (Figure 27-14):

1. While sitting (preferably on a firm surface), cross the affected leg over the unaffected leg. Use clasped hands to lift the leg.
2. Put the correct pant leg over the affected foot and pull it onto the leg.
3. Dress the unaffected leg.
4. Pull the pants up as far as possible while sitting; shift weight over each buttock.

5. Stand up to pull the pants up around the waist. If balance is impaired, lean against a wall or sturdy piece of furniture to provide support and minimize the risk of falling. The patient also can use a pant clip. The pant clip attaches to the pants and an upper body garment, the clip holds the pants up while the patient transitions to standing, thereby improving safety and function.

### Donning Skirts

The patient should follow this procedure for donning skirts:

1. Put the skirt over the head and then pull it down.
2. Make sure to maneuver the fasteners to the front or the unaffected side for increased ease of fastening.
3. Twist the skirt around to the correct position.

A skirt with an elasticized waist that expands to pass over the head may be simpler.

### Donning Socks

The patient should follow this procedure for donning socks (Figure 27-15):

1. Cross the affected leg over the other leg, using clasped hands to lift the leg.
2. With the leg in place, open the sock using the thumb and index finger of the unaffected hand. Roll the sock down to the heel before slipping it on for greater ease in donning.
3. Bend forward at the hips to assist in reaching the foot. Pull the sock over the foot.
4. Don the sock on the unaffected foot in the same fashion.

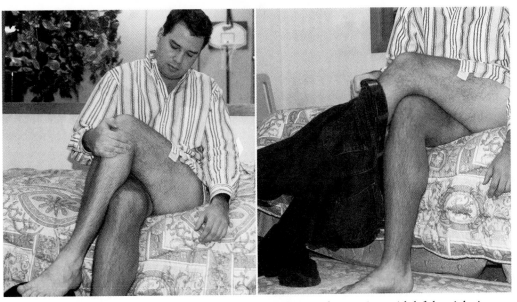

**Figure 27-14** Sequence for donning pants and underwear for a patient with left hemiplegia.

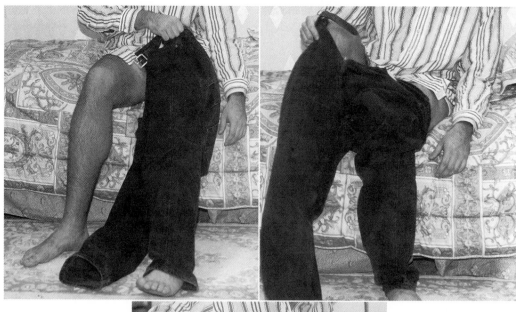

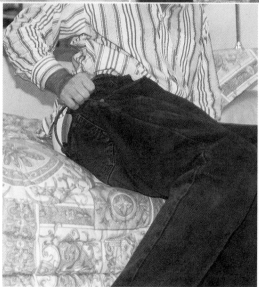

**Figure 27-14, cont'd**

### Donning Shoes

The patient should follow this procedure for donning shoes (Figure 27-16):

1. Choose shoes that provide good support. A broad heel can provide better stability if balance is poor. Men's standard dress shoes have a toe spring built into the front. For a patient recovering from stroke, the toe spring may assist with toe clearance during the swing phase of gait.

2. Bring the affected foot closer to the body by crossing it over the unaffected leg or by using a small footstool.

3. With the leg in place, open the shoe as much as possible before attempting to put it on.

4. Bend forward at the hips to reach the foot. Place the shoe over the ball of the foot and pull it on. A helpful technique to aid with getting the shoe over the foot is to mold a small piece of splinting material onto the shoe heel and allow it to harden. This helps to keep the heel rigid, preventing it from buckling under as the foot slides in.

5. Shoes with Velcro closures are easy to manage with one hand. Shoelaces can be substituted with elastic laces or coilers that do not require tying.

### Donning Lower Extremity Orthotics.

Lower extremity orthotics can be difficult for patients to manage one-handed, and patients may require assistance. In general, the donning of orthotics is easier if placed into the shoe first. An adaptation to the pant leg that may be helpful in donning the orthotic is to open the inseam of the pant

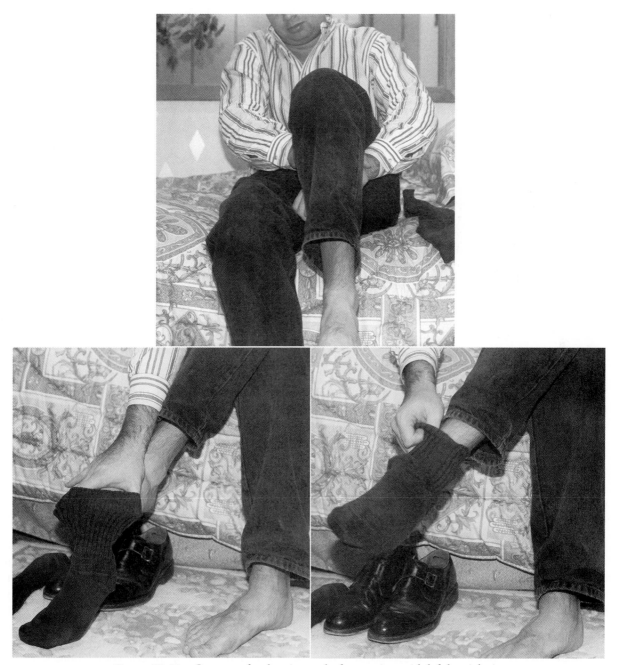

**Figure 27-15**   Sequence for donning socks for a patient with left hemiplegia.

cuff to the desired length. Stitch the loop side of a Velcro strip underneath the top of the seam and the hook side to the front of the seam. The pant leg then can be opened up, allowing for easier manipulation of the orthotic over the calf.

**Adaptive Devices**

The therapist should introduce adaptive dressing devices only if the patient cannot otherwise perform dressing safely or efficiently. Dressing devices to consider might include the following:

- A reacher, particularly if a patient has poor trunk control
- A dressing stick, which can be useful to extend reach if trunk balance is impaired and to push garments off the affected side
- A long-handled shoehorn, which may assist the patient in slipping on shoes

All of the aforementioned devices are available from a variety of rehabilitation catalogs.

Walker, Drummond, and Lincoln[4] completed a randomized crossover study. One group (*n* = 15) received

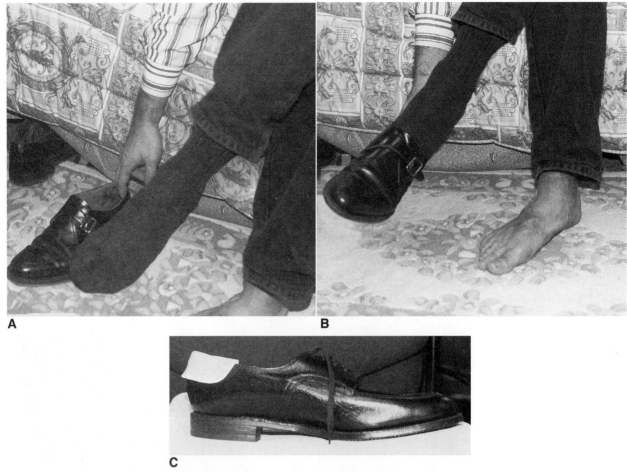

**Figure 27-16**    **A** and **B**, Sequence for donning shoes for a patient with left hemiplegia. **C**, Heel support fabricated from low-temperature plastic.

3 months of no intervention followed by 3 months of treatment; the other group (*n* = 15) received 3 months of treatment followed by 3 months of no treatment. Treatment was provided by an occupational therapist and focused on dressing training for the subjects and their families. The subjects were assessed by an independent evaluator using the Nottingham Stroke Dressing Assessment; the Rivermead ADL Assessment, self-care section; and the Nottingham Health Profile. Both groups showed statistically improved performance during the treatment phase, neither group showed a change during the nontreatment phase, and subjects who received treatment in the first 3 months maintained their improvement.

## INSTRUMENTAL ACTIVITIES OF DAILY LIVING

### Kitchen Activities

An individual with hemiplegia can accomplish kitchen tasks safely with adequate activity pacing; properly placed, secured equipment; and provision of adaptive devices.

***Energy Conservation and Work Simplification.*** A consequence of weakness and impaired upper extremity function is that the individual with hemiplegia tires more quickly and thus needs to work at a slower pace. The following energy conservation guidelines should be included in treatment plans focusing on increasing IADL:

- Allow increased time for task completion.
- Take frequent, short rest breaks.
- Sit when working, when possible.
- Avoid complicated procedures.
- Use ready-prepared foods when possible.
- Use labor-saving equipment. (Electrical equipment such as microwaves and food processors with easy-to-control on-off switches and self-cleaning ovens and self-defrosting freezers reduce manual labor requirements.) A variety of cookbooks are available for use with microwave ovens. Recipes tend to be simpler and require less preparation as well as shorter cooking times.
- Arrange work surfaces at a height that allows for maximal efficiency.

- Avoid excessive reaching and bending.
- Reduce clutter.

To allow for easy access to supplies, items needed most often should be kept on convenient shelves at the front of the most accessible cupboards and drawers or at the back of the work surface.

### Storage

A variety of storage devices can be purchased that enhance easy equipment access:

- Plastic-covered racks slide under or clip to the underside of shelves, increasing visible storage space. They can be purchased at hardware stores.
- Peg-Boards can be hung on the wall and used to hang small pots, strainers, kitchen tongs, and spatulas.
- Magnetic knife racks can be placed over a counter top and can be used to store knives, peelers, and kitchen scissors.
- Lazy Susans, which can be placed in easy-to-reach cupboards or at the back of a counter, are useful for persons who have trouble bending or reaching beyond the front of the cabinet; they allow for convenient storage of jars, cans, and bottles.

**Transport.** Moving supplies safely about the kitchen is another significant challenge for the person with hemiplegia. To avoid lifting and carrying, the patient can use a rolling cart for transporting items from one side of the kitchen to the other. Ideally, the cart should have a handle at one end to provide support while walking. Dycem can be used to help secure items on the cart shelves. A clip secured to the side of the cart with glue can be used to hold a cane or walking device while the person pushes the cart with the noninvolved hand.

**Stabilization.** Patients can accomplish cooking activities successfully single-handedly with adequate stabilization of items. Tasks such as opening packages and containers, peeling, slicing, making sandwiches, stirring, and mixing create problems that usually can be solved by a variety of self-help devices. The following paragraphs describe commonly used and readily accessible items for self-help.

The Zim jar opener is mounted easily to the wall or underside of a cabinet and allows for one-handed screw cap removal of lids measuring from ½ to 3½ inches in diameter (Figure 27-17).

A Sure Shot jar opener combined with a Belliclamp allows for easy opening of jar lids for individuals with weak grasps or use of only one hand. The Belliclamp holds jars and bottles securely during use of the jar opener. The Spill Not Jar and Bottle Opener has a plastic nonskid base with three rubber-lined openings to accommodate jars from 1 to 3 inches in diameter. A rubber lid opener provides a firm grip for easy opening of jar tops. Lightweight electrical or cordless can openers are

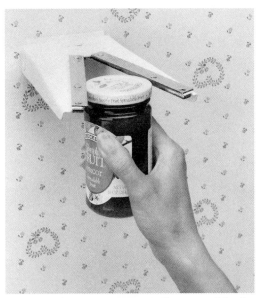

**Figure 27-17** Zim jar opener. (Courtesy North Coast Medical, San Jose, Calif.)

easy to use with one hand and are available from a variety of product catalogs and appliance stores. An example is the E-Z Squeeze One Handed Can Opener (Sammons-Preston).

Patients can open cardboard boxes containing cereals, rice, and instant potatoes one-handed by stabilizing them firmly in a kitchen drawer and then carefully using scissors or the point of a knife to slit the boxtop open. Box toppers are inexpensive devices that easily slide open box tops and are ideal for one-handed use (Figure 27-18).

Pan holders keep pots and pans stabilized on a range top while the individual stirs or sautés one-handed and are important to prevent spillage of hot food (Figure 27-19).

A common device for stabilizing equipment and food items during food preparation is Dycem. The product is made from gelatinous material, is nonslip on both sides, and is an easy, inexpensive alternative to help secure items such as pans and mixing bowls in place during cooking. The Stay Put Suction Disc provides another means of securing bowls and plates to any smooth surface using vacuum pressure (Figure 27-20). Mixing bowls with suction bases are available from a variety of product catalogs and allow for more vigorous one-handed stirring without sliding or tipping. Similarly, the Little Octopus Suction Holders are inexpensive and provide double acting grip to anchor glasses, dishes, bowls, and other common objects during meal preparation. Other items such as suction bottom nail brushes can useful during meal preparation to clean fruits and vegetables.

Cutting boards designed for one-handed use and designed from wood, formica, or plastic come equipped with rubber suction feet to secure the board in place.

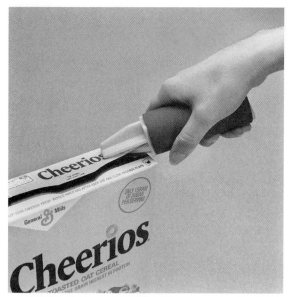

**Figure 27-18**    Boxtopper. (Courtesy North Coast Medical, San Jose, Calif.)

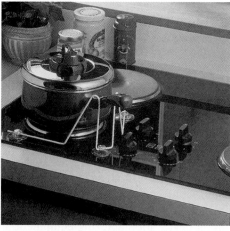

**Figure 27-19**    Pan holder. (Courtesy Sammons Preston, Inc, a BISSELL Company.)

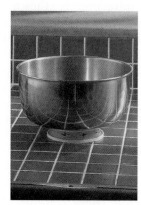

**Figure 27-20**    Stay Put Suction Disc. (Courtesy Sammons Preston, Inc, a BISSELL Company.)

Stainless steel nails hold food in place for cutting and chopping. Food guards keep food from sliding while the individual spreads butter or sandwich spreads. Cutting boards can be fabricated easily using 2-inch thick wood and nails.

*Food Storage.* Rigid plastic containers with overlapping lids usually are easy to open and seal with one hand.[3] Plastic containers with screw-top lids are ideal for storing rice, sugar, flour, and other items that pour. Aluminum foil molds easily with one hand and is useful for covering containers and wrapping food that requires refrigeration.

*Dish Washing.* Nonstick cooking utensils are easy to clean and make the cleanup process go quicker. Oven-to-table cookware cuts down on the number of supplies used. Pots and pans can be stabilized for scrubbing by positioning them on a wet dishcloth positioned in the corner of the sink. For washing cups and glasses, the patient can use a brush suctioned to the inside of the sink, such as a suction bottle brush (Figure 27-21).

## Home Maintenance

Work simplification methods should be applied in the performance of household tasks. Housework requires a great deal of mobility and necessitates getting into awkward positions. Housework can be made easier by removing clutter from the house. Time spent dusting is cut in half without added clutter. To conserve personal energy and ensure ease of performance, adaptive devices such as

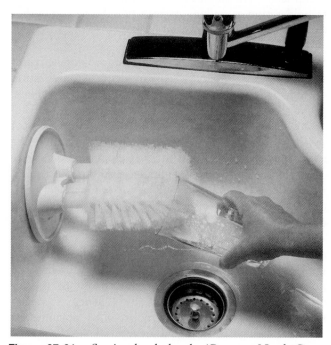

**Figure 27-21**    Suction bottle brush. (Courtesy North Coast Medical, San Jose, Calif.)

lightweight, long-handled, and electronic tools may serve as useful supplements.

***Caring for the Floor.*** Long-handled, freestanding dust-pans; self-wringing sponge mops; electrical floor scrubbers; light upright vacuum cleaners with helping hand attachments; and no-wax floors can ease the maintenance of floor care. While mopping the floor, the individual should use a rectangular bucket. This allows the sponge mop to be soaked fully with water in a half-filled bucket as opposed to partial soaking in a round bucket. The bucket should be filled and emptied on the floor with a plastic jug to avoid heavy lifting.

***Cleaning the Bathroom.*** The patient should use a long-handled reach sponge mop to clean the bathroom. This product is available through a variety of rehabilitation catalogs. The risk of falling is great, and kneeling or sitting should be considered in the performance of this household task.

Extra cleaning materials should be kept upstairs and downstairs to avoid unnecessary journeys. Items can be transported in an apron with large pockets, a shoulder bag, or a wheeled cart.

***Bed Making.*** Bed making can be difficult with only one hand. Beds should be positioned so that access to both sides is easy. To conserve energy, the patient can make the bed by completing each corner of one side from the undersheet to bedspread before moving to the other side to repeat the operation.

***Changing Sheets.*** Patients can manage sheets easily if they are folded or unfolded in position on the bed. Pillows should be kept on the bed during changing of the pillowcases so that the bed takes the weight of the pillow.

## Laundry

***Machine Washing Clothes.*** The patient should select fabric and garment designs that are completely machine washable and dryable and should use automatic machines.

***Hand Washing Clothes.*** Soaking articles overnight in soap or detergent can minimize the effort to remove dirt with one hand. A washboard can be useful for scrubbing out dirt and stubborn stains.

***Wringing Clothes.*** Small articles can be rolled in a towel and squeezed to remove excess water. Clothes can be wrung out with one hand. Drip-dry clothes should be placed on a hanger before they are removed from the sink.

## Ironing

The patient should use a lightweight iron. Steam irons are efficient at removing creases from many materials.

Most ironing boards are height adjustable so that the individual can sit or stand when using them. Ironing boards can be difficult and heavy to manage with one hand. The board may be left permanently standing if space permits. Ironing also can be done on the kitchen table or a counter covered with a folded towel or sheet.

## Sewing

***Threading Needles.*** A patient can thread a needle easily with one hand if the needle is held in a pincushion, padded armchair, or bar of soap. Self-threading needles and automatic needle threaders also are available at most major department stores.

***Cutting.*** A patient can cut material if it is stabilized by weight to prevent slipping. Although most scissors are for right-handed use, scissors and shears for left-handed use are available.

***Hand Sewing.*** The patient can perform hemming and sewing seams easily by placing material over a curved object such as an armchair and holding it down with weights.

***Machine Sewing.*** A patient can use a sewing machines with one hand with practice according to safety guidelines.

## Communication

***Writing.*** Individuals whose strokes have affected their dominant sides need to consider dominance retraining to learn to write with the noninvolved hand. An important goal for such individuals is to be able to sign their names legibly.

Writing practice begins with exercises consisting of continuous circles and connected up and down strokes. Patients practice large strokes first and progress to smaller ones. With increasing proficiency, patients practice alphabet letters. At the initiation of training, patients should use a larger-size pencil, crayon, or rubber pencil grip attached to a standard pencil. The paper may be stabilized with Dycem or a clamp or by weighting the paper down.

Except for meeting the requirement of a functional signature, individuals may prefer to use another method of written communication. Individuals with hemiplegia can access equipment such as personal computers, tape recorders, and word processors easily.

***Using the Telephone.*** Providing for easy access to the telephone is not a significant problem. Use of a speakerphone can facilitate telephone use. Another product, the commercially available phone holder, frees the noninvolved hand for dialing or taking messages. This device consists of a flexible arm clamped to a table, which holds the telephone receiver in a stationary position; the device is available through product catalogs (see Chapter 26).

## COMMUNITY-BASED ACTIVITIES

### Marketing and Grocery Shopping

Energy conservation should be applied in marketing and grocery shopping. The individual should make a list of necessary items and anticipate weekly expenses to minimize trips to the cash machine. The patient should categorize items according to aisles, thus limiting excess walking around the store. The patient can use a lightweight pushcart to carry items around the store and home if a car is not available. An alternative solution is phone and mail shopping. Individuals using wheelchairs require assistance with shopping trips. The patient should place money in an easily accessible pocket or purse to ensure easy retrieval at the checkout line. An alternative is mail, phone, or online shopping.

### Banking

Banking has become easier during the past decade. Individuals can go the bank, access money through automatic teller machines, and bank by phone or online. If the patient's signature has been altered because of loss of function in the dominant hand, the bank must be notified. Banks have varying policies regarding this situation. For the most part, the new signature can be placed on file easily. Some banks, however, require a written and notarized letter from a physician before a new signature can be authorized.

### Case Study

#### ONE-HANDED TRAINING AFTER STROKE

E.B. is a 74-year-old male recovering from a left stroke with right hemiplegia and a medical history of significant hypertension. E.B. was employed as an engineer for 50 years but has been retired for the past 2 years. He currently is married, and his wife is employed full time. E.B. resides in a ground-floor apartment with three steps up to enter the building.

E.B. was referred for home care services on discharge from the hospital. Initial occupational therapy evaluation revealed the following: He was alert and oriented to person, place, situation, and time. His cognitive perceptual status was intact. Before his stroke, E.B. was right-hand dominant. On evaluation, his right upper extremity was flaccid. His left upper extremity had functional range of motion and strength. Sensation was intact throughout. Static and dynamic sitting balance was good. When standing, however, he was unsteady while performing challenging tasks. His endurance for light activity was poor. E.B. required assistance with the following activities of daily living tasks: bathing, grooming, feeding, dressing, simple meal preparation, writing, and community-based activities.

The therapist established a number of treatment goals with the patient:

#### Long-Term Goals

1. E.B. will be independent in managing basic activities of daily living using adaptive techniques and assistive devices as required.
2. E.B. will be independent with simple meal preparation.
3. E.B. will participate in instrumental activities of daily living, such as shopping and banking.

#### Short-Term Goals

1. E.B. will independently bathe himself using assistive devices.
2. E.B. will independently clean and floss his teeth with use of assistive devices.
3. E.B. will be able to cut and butter food independently with a rocker knife.
4. E.B. will independently dress himself using adaptive techniques and devices.
5. E.B. will independently prepare himself lunch.
6. E.B. will independently perform home-based financial responsibilities.
7. E.B. will participate weekly in food shopping outings.

## ADAPTATIONS

Before initiating basic activities of daily living training, the therapist surveyed the environment to ensure safety and ease of mobility. The following changes were recommended and implemented:

1. Excess clutter was removed from the bedroom, bathroom, kitchen shelves, and drawers to ensure easier access of needed supplies. Closet rods were lowered to allow for easier access of clothing.
2. The bathroom floor rug was replaced with no-slip mats inside and outside the tub. A tub transfer bench with handheld shower attachment was provided.
3. A board was placed under the mattress to increase firmness, and a bedrail was placed on E.B.'s uninvolved side to increase safe transfers in and out of bed.

4. A lamp was placed on a bedside table next to E.B. to ensure sufficient lighting.

Activities of daily living training was initiated with implementation of several adaptations:

## Bathing

1. Soap on a rope was used to stabilize the soap.
2. A flex sponge enabled E.B. to reach all body parts successfully.
3. A pump spray shampoo bottle was used to avoid excess waste and keep shampoo from getting into eyes.
4. E.B. reviewed one-handed drying techniques.

## Oral Hygiene

1. A toothpaste dispenser allowed for easy one-handed access.
2. The Floss Aid dental floss holder allowed E.B. to floss his teeth.

## Nail Management

1. A one-handed home device was fabricated from a nail clipper secured to a piece of plywood with suction feet attached.
2. A pistol-grip toenail clipper enabled E.B. to cut his toenails with less bending.

## Dressing

1. Energy conservation techniques were reviewed because of E.B.'s poor endurance.
2. E.B. was able to don and doff shirts but unable to manipulate fasteners. Velcro was substituted for buttons.
3. E.B. was able to don his pants successfully with the support of a sturdy dresser placed next to the bed, which he leaned against to pull up his pants safely while standing.
4. E.B. was able to don his shoes after a piece of splinting material was molded into the shoe heel. Elastic laces allowed for easy fastening.

## Feeding and Simple Meal Preparation

A rocker knife, nonskid mat, and plate guard allowed E.B. to cut and butter his food successfully and without spillage.

E.B. also was required to make lunch for himself while his wife was at work. His favorite lunch was a ham and cheese sandwich with lettuce and tomato and a glass of apple juice.

The following kitchen adaptations were made:
1. E.B. used a rolling cart to gather necessary supplies at one time and maneuver them to the kitchen table, where he could sit to complete the task.
2. A cutting board was fabricated using 2-inch thick wood, nails, and a plastic food guard glued to the side of the board. Using the board, E.B. was able to cut tomato slices successfully, stabilize lettuce, and spread mayonnaise on a slice of bread while stabilizing it against the food guard.
3. Presliced ham and cheese were stored in a plastic zipper bag that E.B. could access easily and seal using the zipper bag sealer.
4. Using a Zim jar opener, E.B. was able to open the apple juice bottle top.

## Dominance Retraining and Financial Management

E.B. was initially right-hand dominant. An important goal for him was to be able to sign his name legibly on legal documents. He was put on a program of writing practice exercises. After obtaining a legible signature, E.B. contacted the bank and was required to submit a copy of his new signature to be placed on file.

## Marketing and Grocery Shopping

As E.B.'s endurance improved, shopping outings with his wife were encouraged. The following energy conservation guidelines were incorporated:
1. E.B. made a list of necessary items and grouped them according to aisles to limit excess walking.
2. A lightweight pushcart was purchased to carry items around the store and into the home.
3. Before leaving home, E.B. would place his money in an easily accessible pocket from which he could retrieve it quickly at the checkout line.

## SUMMARY

This chapter describes equipment recommendations and practical and creative solutions that the occupational therapist can incorporate to assist patients in becoming more independent in performing basic activities of daily living and instrumental activities of daily living. For individuals with limited functional return of the involved upper extremity, compensatory techniques are crucial during the rehabilitation process and maximize the potential for reaching meaningful goals. As always, the therapist should concentrate on activities the patient finds most meaningful and curtail activities the individual does not want to perform. For individuals with extensive paralysis resulting from stroke, family members or hired outside help may be required to assist with ADL.

## REVIEW QUESTIONS

1. When is use of compensatory strategies most advantageous as part of the rehabilitation process?
2. What environmental considerations need to be taken into account before the initiation of activities of daily living training?
3. Where can specific information regarding the reliability and validity of basic activities of daily living evaluation instruments be obtained?
4. What are some compensatory techniques and adaptive devices an individual may use during grooming and hygiene to compensate for loss of one upper extremity?
5. Which specific deficits need to be considered before the initiation of dressing training?
6. What energy conservation and work simplification techniques should be considered during instrumental activities of daily living training?
7. Which compensatory techniques and adaptive devices should be considered to compensate during kitchen-based activities for loss of one upper extremity?
8. What types of adaptive devices should be considered for easier performance of home-maintenance activities?
9. If a signature has been altered as a result of loss of function in the dominant hand, what issues need to be addressed before the patient resumes financial responsibilities?

## REFERENCES

1. Feldmeier DM, Poole JL: The position-adjustable hair dryer, *Am J Occup Ther* 41(4):246-247, 1987.
2. Nakayama H, Jorgensen HS, Raaschou HO, et al: Compensation in recovery of upper extremity function after stroke: the Copenhagen stroke study, *Arch Phys Med Rehabil* 75(8):852-857, 1994.
3. US Department of Health and Human Services: *Clinical practice guideline #16: post stroke rehabilitation*, Rockville, Md, 1995.
4. Walker MF, Drummond AER, Lincoln NB: Evaluation of dressing practice for stroke patients after discharge from hospital: a crossover design study, *Clin Rehabil* 10:23, 1996.

## SUGGESTED READINGS

Berger PE, Mensh S, Whitaker J: *How to conquer the world with one hand . . . and an attitude*, ed 2, Merrifield, Va, 2002, Positive Power Publishing.
Mayer TK: *One-handed in a two-handed world*, ed 2, Boston, 2000, Prince-Gallison Press.

glen gillen,
nancy c. whyte,
and denise a. supon

**chapter 28**

# Leisure Participation
# after Stroke

## key terms

| | | |
|---|---|---|
| adaptive equipment | leisure | leisure satisfaction |
| extrinsic barriers | leisure attitudes | models of leisure |
| intrinsic barriers | leisure roles | types of leisure |

## chapter objectives

After completing this chapter, the reader will be able to accomplish the following:

1. Define leisure, types of leisure, and functions of leisure activities.
2. Discuss the changes in an individual's ability to engage in leisure tasks after a cerebrovascular accident.
3. Describe problems that may interfere with a patient's participation in leisure tasks.
4. Present possible solutions to these problems.
5. Discuss research addressing leisure participation and occupational therapy interventions after stroke.
6. Outline ways occupational therapists can adapt leisure tasks to allow partial or full participation by someone with a disability caused by a stroke.

Occupational therapy includes the consideration of leisure. Although insurance companies may be reluctant to cover this area of intervention, occupational therapists are obligated professionally to address changes in patients' leisure roles and to use patients' leisure interests to plan treatment sessions. This area of functioning is critical in the assessment of patients' motivation, quality of life, and self-esteem. Effective approaches to improving leisure skills and participation may require a team approach (e.g., therapeutic recreation and occupational therapy) to meet the complex needs of stroke survivors. This chapter was written from an occupational therapy perspective.

This chapter provides a conceptual framework to help therapists evaluate the leisure skills and improve the leisure participation of patients who have survived a stroke. Its focus is to increase the ability of occupational therapists to improve the leisure skills and the quality of life of this population. Readers are encouraged to review Chapter 3 with this chapter.

## LEISURE, STROKE, AND OCCUPATIONAL THERAPY

In their review of the literature regarding the role of occupational therapy and leisure after stroke, Parker, Gladman, and Drummond[34] summarize the following:

- Stroke survivors often fail to resume full lives, regardless of whether they make a good physical recovery.
- Participation restrictions such as a decline in social and leisure pursuits are prevalent.
- Customary goals of rehabilitation are focused on mobility and independence in self-care, but recovery in a broader sense may not be maximized if health professionals concentrate exclusively on these goals.
- Leisure has been shown to be associated closely with life satisfaction and is a worthwhile goal of rehabilitation.
- Elderly persons show a decline in leisure activity that has been well studied. This information may provide a useful model for the more rapid decline seen in stroke patients.
- Further research is needed to confirm the finding that specialized occupational therapy can be effective in raising leisure activity and to show whether this translates into improved psychological well-being.

Widen-Holmqvist et al[46] studied a community-based sample of 20 patients living at home 1 to 3 years after hospitalization for stroke and who perceived that they were in need of rehabilitation services. Their results included the following:

- Most of the subjects reported a change in activity and interest patterns after stroke.
- Subjects had high motivation for current activities.
- Cognitive functions were within normal limits for all tested subjects.
- Motor abilities and verbal performances frequently were affected and varied considerably.
- Social and leisure activities outside the home were identified as the most promising goals for community-based rehabilitation programs and that by focusing on such activities, potential improvement in quality of life for this population possibly could be achieved by individually planned rehabilitation programs.

## DEFINITION OF LEISURE

Many definitions of leisure appear in the literature.[37-39,42,44,47] *Leisure* can be defined according to various theories, including cognitive, sociologic, psychological, and cultural perspectives. A combination of these theories is necessary to ensure a complete understanding of the complex phenomenon of leisure.

The Practice Framework[1] of the American Occupational Therapy Association includes leisure under the heading Performance in Areas of Occupation. Leisure is described as being nonobligatory behavior, intrinsically motivated, and engaged in during discretionary time. The Practice Framework includes the following two subcategories:

1. Leisure exploration: identifying interests, skills, opportunities, and appropriate leisure activities
2. Leisure participation: planning and participating in appropriate leisure activities, maintaining a balance of leisure activities with other areas of occupation, and obtaining, using, and maintaining equipment and supplies as appropriate

Leisure definitions can be divided into four categories: temporal, activity-based, work-related, and psychological.

Several authors have defined leisure in temporal terms. *Leisure* may be defined as planned time off from scheduled, necessary activities such as self-care, sleep, home management, work, and school. Patients who have had strokes may require excessive time to complete their basic self-care routines. Self-care methods may require adaptation to allow time for leisure pursuits. This definition is limited because it addresses only the time spent performing the activity, not the content of the leisure activity. Experiences at work may be similar in quality and fulfill the same purpose as the leisure activity experience.[36]

*Leisure* also can be defined as an activity, free time, or a state of mind or being.[6] *Leisure* refers not only to a quantity of time but also to a sense of freedom, a decrease in obligations, the chance to gain knowledge, an opportunity for socialization, a symbol of social status, and a physiologic or emotional necessity.[3] Common definitions of leisure are as follows:

- An attitude or feeling of freedom
- A kind of social activity
- A specific time period

*Leisure* also has been defined according to activities. Activity-based definitions of leisure are the least common.[29] *Leisure* can be defined as any activity undertaken by choice. Examples include a specialized group task or lesson, a day trip, and a favorite craft activity. These activities have various functions, including rest, relaxation, stress relief, enjoyment, social networking, and skill development.

Some definitions define *leisure* according to an individual's work and leisure roles. These definitions focus on the balance of work and play, the perceived needs that are met, and the roles that are performed. A person may develop a professional career based on a leisure interest. For example, someone who enjoys sailing may become a sailing instructor. In this example, work and leisure roles are similar, as opposed to those of a surgeon who also enjoys sailing. The way individuals incorporate leisure into their workday is also relevant. An example of this is eating lunch in an alternate environment, such as a garden. These work-leisure definitions are difficult to apply to children, persons who do not work because of medical problems, and persons who are retired.

Psychological definitions focus on the human experience of leisure. Concepts such as state of mind, perceived freedom, and intrinsic motivation are used commonly. These definitions emphasize the person's subjective view of the leisure experience, including the amount of perceived freedom, level of leisure satisfaction, and motivation for the leisure activities. Responses to the same activity vary among individuals. For example, the sailing instructor may experience a low degree of freedom while sailing because it is the primary source of income. The hospital worker, however, may experience a high degree of freedom while sailing because performance or participation does not affect income.

Many writers have outlined various models of leisure.[14,15,18,19,36] These models draw from various categories in an attempt to explain leisure fully. Box 28-1 summarizes three models of leisure based on the work of Krauss, Murphy, and Neulinger (see Neulinger[32]).

The classic view of leisure is best represented by Aristotle, who defined *leisure* as "a state of being in which activity is performed for its own sake."[32] According to Primeau,[36] "the state of mind definition provides us with the qualities that distinguish leisure from non-leisure activities. Some qualities include freedom of choice, intrinsic motivation, enjoyment, low work-relation, low role constraint, aesthetic appreciation, relaxation, novelty, self-expression, companionship, intimacy, and lack of evaluation."

According to James F. Murphy, the five views of leisure are categorized according to the classical or traditional view, the discretionary-time concept, the idea of leisure as a social instrument, the antiutilitarian view, and the holistic model.[32]

### Box 28-1

### Models of Leisure

**RICHARD KRAUS**

Classic view (state of mind)
Symbol of social class (social status)
Form of activity (nonwork task)
Unobligated time (free time)

**JAMES F. MURPHY**

Classic view (state of mind)
Discretionary time (free time)
Social instruments (social interactions and networking)
Antiutilitarian (leisure as an end in itself)
Holistic view (person considered as a whole)

**JOHN NEULINGER**

Subjective view (meaning of leisure experience to individual)
Objective view (free time)

Kelly determined that individuals participate in leisure tasks for a variety of reasons. Kelly classified four types of leisure performance: unconditional leisure, compensatory and recuperative leisure, relational leisure, and role-determined leisure.[23] Usually a leisure task is chosen based on the individual's needs.

The type of leisure activity chosen for personal pleasure or enjoyment is known as *unconditional leisure*. The individual is free from social influences or limitations.[23] Examples include reading the newspaper and painting.

Rest and relaxation are the purpose of compensatory or recuperative leisure activities.[23] For example, someone may require rest and relaxation to cope with job-related stress. These leisure activities promote relaxation. Examples include knitting, going to a movie theater, and watching television. All individuals have unique stress-reduction strategies; consequently, each individual responds differently to a given activity.

Building and maintaining personal relationships are the goals of relational leisure activities.[23] Examples of this type of leisure include dining with friends, playing with children, and going on outings with a significant other or family. This type of leisure task enables an individual to build supportive social systems, develop social skills, and maintain relationships.

Obtaining the approval of others is the purpose of role-determined leisure activities. The expectations of family members, friends, and co-workers affect the individual's choice of activity and perceived performance or skill level.[23] These leisure activities are an inherent part of the individual's identity. Participation in this type of leisure task varies according to cultural role expectations (Box 28-2).

Many factors affect an individual's participation in leisure tasks. The next section reviews and discusses these factors and the role of occupational therapists in evaluating and enhancing the leisure skills of patients who have sustained a cerebrovascular accident.

## FACTORS AFFECTING LEISURE PERFORMANCE

Many factors affect leisure participation, including the following:

- Skills, physical and intellectual
- Types of leisure tasks available

### Box 28-2

### Types of Leisure

Unconditional leisure
Compensatory or recuperative leisure
Relational leisure
Role-determined leisure

- Stage of life
- Social and cultural environments
- Leisure attitudes, roles, and satisfaction
- Use of time
- Barriers to leisure participation

A strong, well-coordinated person may prefer physical leisure activities such as baseball, soccer, and basketball. Persons with less developed physical skills may be interested in more intellectual leisure tasks such as reading, playing chess, and working puzzles. They also may be interested in creative leisure pursuits such as painting, photography, and quilting.

Geographic location also may affect participation in leisure activities. If a person lives in a rural environment, leisure activities may include hiking, horseback riding, swimming, and fishing. Someone in an urban environment may go shopping or to theaters, lectures, and museums.

Leisure assumes various forms throughout life. The amount and type of leisure activities depend on the person's developmental stage.[20] Brightbill[3] makes the following observation: "Sustaining leisure interests during middle age and later adulthood is important for constructive use of time, happiness, and quality of life." During adulthood, leisure pursuits are important for establishing and maintaining social networks. A balance between work and play is important. Factors that influence participation in active leisure activities include financial constraints, decreases in functional skills, and decreases in social supports. Many elderly individuals replace active leisure tasks with more passive ones after experiencing decreases in physical and cognitive abilities.

The family structure often reveals the influence of social and cultural factors. Leisure attitudes, roles, and satisfaction are shaped by the family system, which provides the child with a forum to explore play activities and learn appropriate behaviors. Parents value leisure activities to varying degrees. The occupational therapist must appreciate the significance of the family and the culture on activity participation. Godbey and Parker[16] describe the importance of culture as follows: "Many people in Western societies view solitary activities as a poor use of time and as nonproductive. On the contrary, many Eastern societies place emphasis on time spent engaging in solitary, reflective activities."

*Leisure attitude* is defined as the expressed amount of affect toward a given leisure-related object. According to Feibel and Springer,[11] "this attitude is a multiplicative function of a person's beliefs that an object has certain characteristics and a personal evaluation of these characteristics." Many factors affect an individual's leisure attitudes. These factors include social influences, personality, past experiences, and motivation. Leisure attitudes play an important role in the choice and pursuit of leisure activities. A positive experience during an activity usually results in the person continuing to engage in this pursuit.

A *leisure role* is defined as a perceived identity associated with a leisure task. Changes in a person's roles throughout life are accompanied by shifts in leisure participation. Role changes resulting from disability may cause role strain and role conflict: "*Role strain* refers to the difficulty an individual experiences when attempting to meet role obligations. Role conflict occurs when the occupant of a position perceives that he or she is unable to meet role expectations."[22]

Use of time is an important factor in leisure participation. If a person spends most of the day at work and returns home with additional work, participation in leisure may be limited. Although the person may derive satisfaction from this schedule, participation in leisure is low. The therapist should analyze the person's schedule to determine whether intervention is necessary. Assistance with time-management skills or strategies to combat stress may be necessary. An individual's leisure participation also is influenced by internal, environmental, and communication-related barriers[24] (Box 28-3).

## LEISURE ACTIVITIES DURING OCCUPATIONAL THERAPY

Occupational therapists working with patients who have had a stroke are concerned with the way these individuals spend their time. Often leisure and play interventions are considered secondary during the rehabilitation process as therapists focus on self-care and instrumental activities of daily living. However, leisure activities can be equally meaningful to patients as they redefine their life roles.[41] Occupational therapists can integrate leisure activities into the rehabilitation process in two ways: "occupation-as-end" and "occupation-as-means."[43]

Occupation-as-end[43] refers to activities and/or tasks that comprise a role. The patient chooses the occupation as a meaningful activity he or she wants to perform, needs to perform, or has to perform. Therapists may become aware of these activities (e.g., bowling, crossword puzzles, and making jewelry) via an interview process or a semistructured interview such as the Canadian Occupational Performance Measure (COPM). When a (leisure) activity is defined by the patient, the therapist collaborates with the

---

**Box 28-3**

**Factors That Affect Leisure Performance**

Skills
Types of leisure tasks
Stage of life cycle
Social and cultural environments
Leisure attitudes, roles, and satisfaction
Use of time
Barriers to leisure participation

patient to accomplish the goal through a variety of interventions including adaptation (e.g., enlarged print on books), education (e.g., providing information regarding transportation methods to and from a local pool), using remaining abilities, and/or remediation. Trombly[43] points out that when a therapist uses occupation-as-ends, the therapist is *not* focused on using leisure activities to make a change at the impairment level (e.g., improve scanning ability), although this may occur as a secondary gain. Trombly suggests that the therapist use the following principles to implement occupation-as-end:

- Organize the subtasks to be learned so that the patient will succeed.
- Give clear instructions.
- Use feedback to promote success (see Chapter 5).
- Structure the practice to ensure learning (see Chapter 5).
- Make adaptations when needed (see Chapter 27).

Occupation-as-means[43] may be described as using (leisure) occupations as a treatment to improve body system and body structure impairments. In other words, the (leisure) activity is the change agent. The therapist may use leisure activities to remediate impairments such as weakness, postural dyscontrol, and neglect. Valued leisure activities may be incorporated into the treatment plan to improve other functional areas. For example, the patient may be achieving postural and motor goals in a standing position while engaging in a game of air hockey. See Chapter 10 for examples of using occupation-as-means to remediate upper extremity motor control dysfunction and Chapter 19 for examples to improve cognitive-perceptual dysfunction (Box 28-4). A note of caution for therapists who rely too much on using occupation-as-means during treatment sessions: Patients should be given a clear explanation related to why the activity was chosen. For example, when a patient has mild inattention, the therapist might say "As we've both discovered, you are forgetting to look for items on your left, such as not finding your tooth brush on the left side of the sink or the juice in the left side of the refrigerator. We are going to try to get you to look left more often. We are going to play dominoes, and I will put all of your dominoes on the left side. Try to look left as often as possible, and

I will remind you as needed." After the activity, processing should occur related to whether the patient met the goals of the session (see Chapter 19). If patients are not given this information, they will not be able to make the connection between the activity and their functional goals.

## Evaluation of Leisure Skills

When evaluating the leisure roles of patients, therapists must consider seven factors that can affect leisure performance:

1. Evaluation findings related to impairments and performance in areas of occupation
2. Types of leisure activities that interest the patient
3. Patient's stage in the life cycle
4. Physical, social, and cultural environments
5. Patient's previous leisure attitudes, roles, and satisfaction
6. Patient's past and present use of time
7. Premorbid barriers

These factors can guide therapists in identifying leisure activities that must be modified and in assisting patients with leisure exploration. A checklist (Figure 28-1) can assist therapists in determining the type of leisure tasks patients enjoyed before their stroke.[17,30]

Other usual and customary assessments can assist therapists in making decisions regarding leisure interventions. For example, information regarding range of motion, skeletal muscle activity, strength, endurance, postural control and alignment, motor control, praxis, fine motor coordination, and visual-motor integration is critical. The complete cognitive and perceptual assessment provides necessary information regarding the level of arousal, orientation, recognition, attention span, initiation and termination of activities, memory, sequencing, categorization, concept formation, spatial operations, problem solving, learning, and generalization.

The type of leisure activities the patient performed before the cerebrovascular accident is important to review. For instance, someone who participated in unconditional leisure tasks most of the time may have been content with little social contact. If the person enjoyed relational leisure tasks, social interactions may assume a greater importance.

The therapist must consider the patient's stage in the life cycle because participation in leisure changes during the aging process. During adulthood, an individual's participation in leisure activities decreases because of demands such as work, household maintenance, and childcare. The importance and meaning of leisure also change as a person matures.

The physical, social, and cultural environments are critical in the development of leisure practices and the pursuit of leisure activities during adulthood. Information on the patient's social and cultural networks helps the therapist focus the treatment plan.

### Box 28-4

#### Role of the Occupational Therapist

Evaluate patient's physical, cognitive, and perceptual skills and environmental factors (social and cultural) that affect leisure participation.

Provide treatment to improve patient's limitations.

Provide adaptive equipment and adapt techniques to improve leisure participation.

Provide education about various community resources and alternative transportation methods to increase participation.

Date _____

Occupation _____

Name _____

Marital status _____

Age _____

Onset of stroke _____

Cultural background _____

Children's ages _____

Favorite leisure task _____

Male _____ Female _____

Please answer the following questions to enable your therapist to assist you in resuming/pursuing your leisure interests:

1. When do you perform leisure activities?

____ Morning     ____ Afternoon     ____ Evening     ____ Weekdays

____ Weekends     ____ Holidays     ____ Vacations

2. What type of leisure activities do you enjoy?

____ Physical     ____ Intellectual     ____ Arts     ____ Social

____ Solitary     ____ Structured     ____ Unstructured

3. Place a check mark next to the persons who are involved in your leisure activities.

____ Significant other     ____ Spouse     ____ Children     ____ Parent

____ Sibling     ____ Friend     ____ Co-worker     ____ Pets

____ Relatives     ____ Grandparents     ____ Grandchildren

4. Do you want to resume your past leisure activities?

____ Yes     ____ No     ____ Do not know

5. If you do not want to resume past leisure activities, please place a check mark next to the reasons.

____ Loss of skills     ____ No time     ____ Depressed     ____ Resources not available

____ Afraid     ____ No transportation     ____ Decreased leisure performance

____ Decreased communciation skills     ____ No interest

____ Other—Please state the reason. _____

_____

6. Are you satisfied with your present leisure activities?

____ Yes     ____ No—why? _____     ____ Do not know

**Figure 28-1**     Leisure interest checklist.

The patient's leisure attitudes, roles, and satisfaction before the stroke are important factors to consider after the stroke. The therapist should identify the importance of the selected leisure tasks and the patient's level of satisfaction with them. Identifying the specific aspects of the activity the patient finds enjoyable is helpful. The therapist also should document the patient's leisure roles by discussing topics such as family expectations.

The therapist can address past and present use of time by asking patients to describe the way they spent their time before the stroke, whether they achieved a balance between work and play, and whether they now require additional time for nonleisure activities.

The therapist must address premorbid barriers to leisure participation. These are obstacles that kept patients from participating in the full scope of leisure activities before their stroke. These barriers include intrinsic, environmental, and communication barriers (Box 28-5).

Many ways are available to assess an individual's leisure interests, such as a leisure interest checklist (Figure 28-1), a structured interview form, and a time log (Figure 28-2) that requires the patient to record previous and current use of time. Therapists should strive to use assessments that are standardized.

Examples of assessments the therapist can use to assess leisure skills and participation in stroke survivors include the following:

- Nottingham Leisure Questionnaire[10]: This assessment was developed to measure the leisure activity of stroke patients. The results of the interrater reliability study

Please check the types of leisure activities you enjoy:

**Music**

____ Attending concerts
____ Singing
____ Playing instruments
____ Conducting
____ Watching concerts on television
____ Listening to the radio

**Dance**

____ Tap
____ Ballet
____ Folk
____ Jazz
____ Ballroom
____ Modern
____ Other

**Arts and Crafts**

____ Carpentry
____ Sewing
____ Knitting
____ Needlepoint
____ Painting
____ Quilting
____ Ceramics
____ Model making
____ Drawing
____ Sculpture
____ Photography
____ Other

**Community**

____ Volunteering
____ Travel
____ Church
____ Temple
____ Other

**Sports**

____ Skiing
____ Softball
____ Baseball
____ Football
____ Running
____ Jogging
____ Biking
____ Hockey
____ Basketball
____ Skating
____ Sailing
____ Other

**Table Games**

____ Table tennis
____ Cards
____ Scrabble
____ Dominoes
____ Puzzles
____ Chinese checkers
____ Checkers
____ Othello
____ Chess
____ Monopoly
____ Backgammon
____ Trivial Pursuit
____ Other

**Relaxation**

____ Meditation
____ Yoga
____ T'ai chi
____ Horticulture
____ Pet care

**Figure 28-1, cont'd**

were "excellent," and "excellent" or "good" for the test-retest reliability study. More recently the Nottingham Leisure Questionnaire has been shortened (from 37 to 30 items) and the response categories have been collapsed (from five to three categories) to make it suitable for mail use.[8] Higher Nottingham Leisure Questionnaire scores were associated with higher subscores on the Nottingham Extended Activities of Daily Living Scale, and lower Nottingham Leisure Questionnaire scores were associated with living alone and worse emotional health.

**Box 28-5**

**Factors Affecting Leisure Performance after Stroke**

**TYPE OF LEISURE TASKS**

- Unconditional
- Compensatory or recuperative
- Relational
- Role-determined

**STAGE IN THE LIFE CYCLE**

- Childhood
- Young adult
- Middle age
- Later life

**SOCIAL AND CULTURAL ENVIRONMENTS**

- Support system (i.e., family and friends)
- Nationality
- Religion

**LEISURE ATTITUDES, ROLES, AND SATISFACTION**

- Attitudes
- Roles
- Satisfaction

**USE OF TIME**

- Present
- Past

**BARRIERS TO LEISURE PARTICIPATION**

- Internal barriers
- Lack of knowledge
- Decreased skills
- Decreased opportunities
- Environmental barriers
- Attitudes
- Architectural
- Transportation
- Rules and regulations
- Barriers of omission
- Economic
- Communication barriers
- Social skills
- Ability to speak
- Ability to listen

- Activity Card Sort: The card sort is used to measure an individual's participation or lack of participation in instrumental, leisure, and social activities. See Chapter 3 for a full description.
- Canadian Occupational Performance Measure: This semistructured interview covers three areas: leisure, self-care, and productivity. The patient identifies and ranks areas of occupational performance that are meaningful and rates the level of performance and satisfaction. See Chapter 20 for further information.

- Leisure Competence Measure[25]: This measure provides information about leisure functioning and measures change in leisure function over time. The tool includes nine areas: social contact, community participation, leisure awareness, leisure attitude, social behaviors, cultural behaviors, leisure skills, interpersonal skills, and community integration skills. Items are rated on the 7-point Likert scale.
- Leisure Diagnostic Battery[4]: The original version includes 95 items, whereas the newer, shorter version includes 25 items. Items are rated on 3-point scale. Assessment areas include playfulness, competence, barriers, and knowledge.
- Frenchay Activities Index[45]: This tool is used for assessing general (i.e., other than personal care) activities of stroke survivors. The tool comprises 15 individual activities summed to give an overall score from 0 (low) to 45 (high).

**Interventions to Improve Leisure Skills**

The intervention process begins with obtaining the patient's leisure history. The therapist then reviews the results of the evaluation and determines the patient's strengths and limitations in relation to the performance components. Leisure tasks may be used to achieve the goals of occupational therapy treatment. Leisure activities may be used during treatment sessions to remediate component skills, enhance the skill itself, or adapt the leisure activity itself. Therapists must identify the skills necessary to perform the tasks and modify them according to each patient's ability. The occupational therapist may provide treatment for neuromuscular and cognitive deficits that will enable the patient to engage in the leisure activity.

The National Therapeutic Recreation Society proposes a continuum model of leisure service delivery. According to one description, "the 'Leisure Ability Model' serves as a guide for community recreation professionals to facilitate the movement of individuals with disabilities from more intrusive, specialized recreation services into integrated leisure environments."[40] This model consists of a continuum with four levels:

1. Noninvolvement
2. Segregated
3. Integrated
4. Accessible

At the first level—noninvolvement—the person who has the disability does not participate in any leisure tasks. At the second level—segregated—the patient participates in structured activities developed for group members with the same disability group. Examples include community activities through local stroke organizations, stroke support groups, and specialized sports programs (aquatics).

The third level—integrated—"provides persons with disabilities the opportunity to be mainstreamed into regular community recreation programs and to participate

| Time | Activity | Environment | Physical assistance | Cognitive skills required | Feelings |
|------|----------|-------------|---------------------|---------------------------|----------|
| 6:30 AM | | | | | |
| 7:00 | | | | | |
| 7:30 | | | | | |
| 8:00 | | | | | |
| 8:30 | | | | | |
| 9:00 | | | | | |
| 9:30 | | | | | |
| 10:00 | | | | | |
| 10:30 | | | | | |
| 11:00 | | | | | |
| 11:30 | | | | | |
| 12:00 PM | | | | | |
| 12:30 | | | | | |
| 1:00 | | | | | |
| 1:30 | | | | | |
| 2:00 | | | | | |
| 2:30 | | | | | |
| 3:00 | | | | | |
| 3:30 | | | | | |
| 4:00 | | | | | |
| 4:30 | | | | | |
| 5:00 | | | | | |
| 5:30 | | | | | |
| 6:00 | | | | | |
| 6:30 | | | | | |
| 7:00 | | | | | |
| 7:30 | | | | | |
| 8:00 | | | | | |
| 8:30 | | | | | |
| 9:00 | | | | | |
| 9:30 | | | | | |
| 10:00 | | | | | |
| 10:30 | | | | | |
| 11:00 | | | | | |

**Figure 28-2** Patients can use a time log to record their previous and current use of time.

alongside nondisabled participants. It appears that this approach goes a long way toward helping to change the negative attitudes, stereotypes, stigma and myths associated with persons with disabilities and the systems that serve them."[40] The occupational therapist can instruct patients in the use of adaptive equipment and methods to pursue leisure activities successfully in the community.

The fourth level—accessible—occurs when the individual with a disability "is able to select and access preferred recreation programs with no more effort than his or her counterpart who is non disabled. . . . The participant is able to realize his or her ultimate goal of achieving a satisfying leisure lifestyle, free of any significant individual and external constraints."[40]

The therapist can use these levels to improve an individual's level of involvement gradually. For instance, if a patient enjoys bowling and wants to return to this activity, the therapist may locate or form a specialized bowling program. When the patients develop skills, they may join an integrated bowling program and eventually an accessible bowling program.

This model can serve as a guide for occupational therapists when introducing resources for leisure services. Occupational therapists can assist patients in exploring alternative types of leisure tasks that fulfill their needs. This may include expanding their leisure activity repertoires to improve the quality of their lives. Occupational therapists educate patients on available services.

Treatment also can focus on helping patients and family members overcome barriers to leisure participation. Common barriers are intrinsic, environmental, and communication-related.

Intrinsic barriers are the results of the disability. These barriers may include lack of knowledge about leisure activities and programs, decreased educational activities, health problems related to the disability, psychological and physical dependence, and decreased skills.[24]

Occupational therapists can address intrinsic barriers in a variety of ways. Remaining informed about current community resources, support groups in the area, and professional leisure organizations designed to serve individuals who have a physical disability is essential.[5] These organizations include stroke support groups, wheelchair sport leagues, and the American Heart Association.

Environmental barriers include attitudes, architectural and ecologic obstacles, transportation, rules and regulations, and barriers of omission.[24]

The attitudes of others are a serious problem for persons who have disabilities. Attitudinal barriers result in negative behaviors, stigmas, and decreased acceptance and participation in leisure tasks. Occupational therapists can suggest strategies that patients can use to address social prejudices.

Architectural barriers prevent individuals who have physical disabilities from participating in leisure activities. The main problem is accessibility. Many buildings and sport facilities are not wheelchair accessible. Occupational therapists can consult with architects, builders, and contractors to determine necessary modifications, such as installing a lift for a swimming pool.

Transportation barriers are another issue. Many persons who have disabilities cannot drive or take public transportation independently. Public transportation is not always wheelchair accessible. When public transportation is accessible, it does not always foster independence because it may require a driver to operate the lift to enter or a brake-locking mechanism, for example. The Americans with Disabilities Act is correcting this problem gradually by requiring wheelchair-accessible transportation. Occupational therapists can educate patients about the Americans with Disabilities Act and alternate methods of transportation.

Economic barriers also play a role in preventing individuals with disabilities from performing leisure activities. For example, gym memberships are too costly even for many able-bodied persons. Disabled individuals often live on a fixed income and have many medical and living expenses. Occupational therapists can educate their patients about available resources and community groups and encourage participation.

Barriers of omission occur when leisure programs are developed without consideration of all members of society.[24] For instance, a barrier of omission exists when a new leisure program is being developed and the site is in a building inaccessible to persons in wheelchairs. Occupational therapists should instruct their patients to become advocates for themselves and make the public aware of their needs.

The final barrier involves communication. Disabilities that affect the ability to speak, listen, or respond lead to poor social interaction during the leisure task. By training patients in the use of assistive technology to improve communication skills, occupational therapists can play an active role in correcting this environmental barrier (see Chapter 26).

## LEISURE INTERVENTIONS FOR STROKE SURVIVORS: EVIDENCE-BASED PRACTICE

A number of research studies address the issue of leisure activities after stroke. This literature can provide occupational therapists with valuable information about assessment and adaptation of leisure skills for stroke patients.[7,26,28,33]

Research has demonstrated that many individuals who sustained a stroke do not resume many of their favorite social and leisure activities.[21,31] Factors that affect leisure participation after stroke include the following:

- Time
- Meaningfulness of activities
- Personal standards
- Internal/external control
- Range of interests
- Performance
- Transportation
- Social relations

Other studies have found the following:

- Individuals who sustained strokes do not resume leisure tasks because they do not have time. Their days usually are filled with exercises and self-care tasks. In addition, subjects reported that time passed slowly and they were bored.[21,31]
- Disabilities resulting from stroke can lead to changes in family roles and social relationships, which may result in role strain or role conflict.[22]
- Depression after stroke is related strongly to a decrease in social activities.[11]
- Stroke survivors do not resume normal social activities after stroke. Factors include social and environmental issues, emotional difficulties, and organic brain dysfunction. Activities outside the home appear more difficult to resume than activities in the home.[27]
- Factors that affect life satisfaction after stroke include depression, poor activities of daily living performance, and decreased social activity outside the home.[2]

Of paramount importance is for occupational therapists to document what types of intervention are most successful related to improving engagement in leisure activities after a stroke. At this point, clinical trials focused on this issue are conflicting.

Parker et al[35] evaluated the effects of leisure therapy and conventional occupational therapy via a randomized controlled trial (multicenter) using the outcomes of mood, leisure participation, and independence in activities of daily living. Subjects included stroke survivors 6 and 12 months after hospital discharge. In total, the study included 466 patients from five centers in the United Kingdom. The standardized assessments used in the trial included the General Health Questionnaire (12 items), the Nottingham Extended ADL Scale, and the Nottingham Leisure Questionnaire, assessed by mail, with telephone follow-up for clarification. Eighty-five percent of survivors and 78% of survivors responded at 6- and 12-month follow-up, respectively. At 6 months and compared with the control group, those allocated to leisure therapy did not have significantly better General Health Questionnaire scores, leisure scores, and extended activities of daily living scores. The group assigned to activities of daily living did not have significantly better General Health Questionnaire scores and extended activities of daily living scores and did not have significantly worse leisure scores. The results at 12 months were similar. The authors concluded that in contrast to the findings of previous smaller trials, neither of the additional occupational therapy treatments showed a clear beneficial effect on mood, leisure activity, or independence in activities of daily living measured at 6 or 12 months.

Gilbertson and Langhorne[12] evaluated a short postdischarge home-based occupational therapy service for stroke patients, including an assessment of the patients' satisfaction with occupational performance and service provision using a single-site, blind, randomized, controlled trial. One hundred thirty-eight patients were assigned randomly to a conventional outpatient follow-up or conventional services plus 6 weeks of home-based occupational therapy. The data were collected before discharge and at 7 weeks and 6 months after discharge using the COPM, the Dartmouth COOP Charts, the London Handicap Scale, and a patient satisfaction questionnaire. At 7 weeks the intervention group reported significantly greater changes in performance and satisfaction on the COPM, better emotional scores (Dartmouth COOP Charts), and improved work and leisure activity scores (London Handicap Scale). The authors concluded that a 6-week postdischarge home-based occupational therapy service could improve patients' perceptions of their occupational performance and satisfaction with services but may not have a long-term effect on subjective health outcomes.

Drummond and Walker[9] carried out a randomized, controlled trial to evaluate the effectiveness of a leisure rehabilitation program on functional performance and mood. Subjects were allocated randomly to three groups: a leisure rehabilitation group, a conventional occupational therapy group, and a control group. The subjects assigned to the leisure and conventional occupational therapy group received individual treatment at home after discharge from hospital. Baseline assessments were carried out on admission to the study and at 3 and 6 months after discharge from hospital by an evaluator blind to the trial.

The results showed an increase in the leisure scores for the leisure rehabilitation group only despite an age imbalance in the study. The authors also concluded that subjects receiving leisure rehabilitation performed significantly better in mobility and psychological well-being than the subjects in the other two groups.

Gladman and Lincoln[13] reported findings of the DOMINO study that compared home-based and hospital-based rehabilitation services for stroke patients via a randomized, controlled trial. A total of 327 subjects were enrolled after discharge from the hospital. No difference between the services had been found at 6 months, but home therapy was better than outpatient therapy related to improving household ability and leisure activity in the subjects who originally were discharged from a stroke unit.

Jongbloed and Morgan[21] designed a study to determine the efficacy of occupational therapy intervention related to the leisure activities of stroke survivors. The study included 40 discharged stroke patients who were assigned randomly to an experimental group, which received occupational therapy intervention related to leisure activities, or to a control group. An independent evaluator assessed the patients' involvement in activities and satisfaction with that involvement on three separate occasions. The authors found no statistically significant differences between the experimental and control groups in activity involvement or satisfaction with that involvement. The authors point out that the lack of significant differences may be due to the intervention being limited in scope (five therapist's visits) and the observation that many environmental factors strongly influence activity participation and satisfaction.

## ADAPTING THE LEISURE TASK

Reintroducing leisure activities to patients who have sustained a stroke is important. If the patient does not regain the skills needed to perform these leisure tasks, many adaptive devices are on the market to enable full participation in these tasks. To select the most effective adaptive aid, the occupational therapist analyzes the skill components necessary to perform the chosen activity. After identifying the components that limit performance, the therapist selects and introduces an appropriate adaptive device. Occupational therapists provide patients with information about various organizations, adaptive methods, and adaptive equipment that enhance and promote participation in leisure activities. Use of these resources enables patients to lead meaningful and productive lives.

Many types of adaptive equipment enable patients who have use of one hand to participate in leisure tasks (e.g., card holders, knitting-needle holders, fishing-pole holders, and needlepoint holders). These products are available from the Internet, catalogs, occupational therapists, and specialized organizations and stores.

## SUMMARY

Leisure is a complex phenomenon. A review of the literature reveals that leisure may be defined in various ways. Many factors influence an individual's participation in leisure activities, such as roles, attitudes, satisfaction, stage in the life cycle, and intrinsic and extrinsic barriers. The role of the occupational therapist is multifaceted, including assessment, intervention through techniques and adaptive equipment, and patient and family education, with an emphasis on community resources. Leisure activities may be used to improve a patient's motivation, quality of life, and self-esteem.

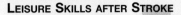

## Case Study

### LEISURE SKILLS AFTER STROKE

R.S. is a 74-year-old woman who sustained a right-sided cerebrovascular accident 4 months ago. After completion of the central nervous system assessment, interest checklist, time log, and activity analysis form, the occupational therapist established goals with R.S.

Briefly, the results of the central nervous system assessment were as follows: Right upper extremity function was within normal limits. Left upper extremity function revealed poor motor control with synergistic patterns present and impaired sensation throughout. Ability to shift weight anteriorly and laterally while in a seated position was fair. Sustained attention skills were limited. She had a minimal left-sided inattention to self and environment and minimal impairments with spatial relations.

R.S. has been widowed for 5 years and reported feeling lonely, depressed, and fearful of falling. Her three adult children live out of state, and her social network consists of supportive neighbors, church members, and her dog.

Currently a home health aide assists R.S. with self-care and home management tasks. R.S. requires activity setup for grooming and upper body hygiene, minimal assistance with upper body dressing and bathing, moderate assistance with lower body dressing and bathing, moderate assistance for stand-pivot transfers, minimal assistance for bed mobility, and moderate assistance with meal preparation from a seated level. She is not performing her favorite leisure task of knitting. How can an occupational therapist assist R.S.?

## REVIEW QUESTIONS

1. Describe leisure according to the temporal definition.
2. List and define the types and purposes of leisure tasks.
3. What are the seven factors the therapist must address when evaluating an individual's leisure participation and performance after sustaining a cerebrovascular accident? Describe how these factors affect leisure participation and performance.
4. What are leisure attitudes, roles, and satisfaction?
5. List and describe the environmental barriers that affect leisure participation.
6. What is the role of the occupational therapist in assessing and improving a patient's leisure participation after a cerebrovascular accident?
7. How would the occupational therapist assist a patient and family members in resuming leisure activities in their community?

# REFERENCES

1. American Occupational Therapy Association: Occupational therapy practice framework: domain and process, *Am J Occup Ther* 56(6):609-639, 2002.

2. Astrom M, Asplund K, Astrom T: Psychosocial function and life satisfaction after stroke, *Stroke* 23(4):527-531, 1992.

3. Brightbill C: *Man and leisure: a philosophy of recreation*, Englewood Cliffs, NJ, 1961, Prentice Hall.

4. Chang Y, Card JA: The reliability of the leisure diagnostic battery short form version B in assessing healthy, older individuals: a preliminary study, *Ther Recreation J* 28:163, 1994.

5. Dattilo J: *Inclusive leisure services: responding to the rights of people with disabilities*, State College, Pa, 1994, Venture Publishing.

6. DeGrazia S: *Of time, work and leisure*, New York, 1962, Twentieth Century Fund.

7. Drummond AE: Leisure after stroke, *Int Disabil Stud* 12(4):157-160, 1990.

8. Drummond AE, Parker CJ, Gladman JR, et al: Development and validation of the Nottingham leisure questionnaire (NLQ), *Clin Rehabil* 15(6):647-656, 2001.

9. Drummond AE, Walker MF: A randomized controlled trial of leisure rehabilitation after stroke, *Clin Rehabil* 9(4):283, 1995.

10. Drummond AE, Walker M: The Nottingham leisure questionnaire for stroke patients, *Br J Occup Ther* 57:11, 1994.

11. Feibel JH, Springer CJ: Depression and failure to resume social activities after stroke, *Arch Phys Med Rehabil* 63(6):276-277, 1982.

12. Gilbertson L, Langhorne P: Home-based occupational therapy: stroke patients' satisfaction with occupational performance and service provision, *Br J Occup Ther* 63(10):464, 2000.

13. Gladman JR, Lincoln NB: Follow-up of a controlled trial of domiciliary stroke rehabilitation (DOMINO Study), *Age Ageing* 23(1):9-13, 1994.

14. Godbey G: *Leisure in your life: an exploration*, State College, Pa, 1994, Venture Publishing.

15. Godbey G, Goodale T: *The evolution of leisure*, State College, Pa, 1988, Venture Publishing.

16. Godbey G, Parker S: *Leisure studies and services: an overview*, Philadelphia, 1976, Saunders.

17. Holbrook M, Skilbeck CE: An activities index for use with stroke patients, *Age Ageing* 12(2):166-170, 1983.

18. Iso-Ahola S: *Social psychological perspectives on leisure and recreation*, Springfield, Ill, 1980, Charles C Thomas.

19. Iso-Ahola S: *The social psychology of leisure and recreation*, Springfield, Ill, 1980, Charles C Thomas.

20. Iso-Ahola S, Jackson E, Dunn E: Starting, ceasing and replacing leisure activities over the life span, *J Leisure Res* 26:3, 1994.

21. Jongbloed L, Morgan D: An investigation of involvement in leisure activities after a stroke, *Am J Occup Ther* 45(5):420-427, 1991.

22. Jongbloed L, Stanton S, Fousek B: Family adaptation to altered roles following a stroke, *Can J Occup Ther* 60:70, 1993.

23. Kelly J: Leisure styles and choices in three environments, *Pac Sociol Rev* 21:187, 1978.

24. Kennedy D, Austin D, Smith R: *Special recreation opportunities for persons with disabilities*, Dubuque, Iowa, 1987, WC Brown.

25. Kloseck M, Crilly RG: *Leisure competence measure: adult version I*, London, Ontario, 1997, Data System.

26. Krefting L, Krefting D: Leisure activities after a stroke: an ethnographic approach, *Am J Occup Ther* 45(5):429-436, 1991.

27. Labi ML, Philips TF, Gresham GE: Psychosocial disability in physically restored long-term stroke survivors, *Arch Phys Med Rehabil* 61(12):561-565, 1980.

28. Lawrence L, Christie D: Quality of life after stroke: a three year follow-up, *Age Ageing* 8(3):167-172, 1979.

29. Loesch L, Wheeler P: *Principles of leisure counseling*, Minneapolis, 1982, Educational Media.

30. Matsutsuyu J: The interest check list, *Am J Occup Ther* 23(4):323-328, 1969.

31. Morgan D, Jongbloed L: Factors influencing leisure activities following a stroke: an exploratory study, *Can J Occup Ther* 57:223, 1990.

32. Neulinger J: *To leisure: an introduction*, Boston, 1981, Allyn & Bacon.

33. Niemi M, Laaksonen R, Kotila M, et al: Quality of life 4 years after stroke, *Stroke* 19(9):1101-1107, 1988.

34. Parker CJ, Gladman JR, Drummond AE: The role of leisure in stroke rehabilitation, *Disabil Rehabil* 19(1):1-5, 1997.

35. Parker CJ, Gladman JR, Drummond AE, et al: A multicentre randomized controlled trial of leisure therapy and conventional occupational therapy after stroke, TOTAL Study Group, trial of occupational therapy and leisure, *Clin Rehabil* 15(1):42-52, 2001.

36. Primeau LA: Work and leisure: transcending the dichotomy, *Am J Occup Ther* 50(7):569-577, 1996.

37. Roberts K: *Leisure*, New York, 1970, Longman Group.

38. Rojek C: *Leisure for leisure*, New York, 1989, Routledge Chapman & Hall.

39. Rosenfeld M: *Wellness and lifestyle renewal*, Rockville, Md, 1993, American Occupational Therapy Association.

40. Schlelen S, Ray M: *Community recreation and persons with disabilities: strategies for integration*, Baltimore, 1988, Paul B Brookes.

41. Soderback I, Ekholm J, Caneman G: Impairment/function and disability/activity 3 years after cerebrovascular incident or brain trauma: a rehabilitation and occupational therapy view, *Int Disabil Stud* 13(3):67-73, 1991.

42. Torkilkdsen G: *Leisure and recreation management*, London, 1992, Thompson Science.

43. Trombly CA: Occupation. In Trombly CA, Radomski MV, editors: *Occupational therapy for physical dysfunction*, ed 5, New York, 2002, Lippincott Williams & Wilkins.

44. Veblen T: *The theory of the leisure class*, New York, 1899, Economic Classics.

45. Wade DT, Legh-Smith J, Langton Hewer R: Social activities after stroke: measurement and natural history using Frenchay activities index, *Int Rehabil Med* 7(4):176-181, 1985.

46. Widen-Holmqvist L, de Pedro-Cuesta J, Holm M, et al: Stroke rehabilitation in Stockholm: basis for late intervention in patients living at home, *Scand J Rehabil Med* 25(4):173-181, 1993.

47. Yukic T: *Fundamentals of recreation*, New York, 1970, Harper & Row

salvatore dimauro*

chapter 29

# A Survivor's Perspective

## THE EVENT

It happened during breakfast, on a bright December morning, unannounced, almost gently, and absolutely painlessly. I was wearing a thick terry cloth robe, which buffered my slumping to the floor and gave it (at least in my visual memory) a slow-motion appearance.

I ended up on my left side on the parquet floor, rejecting my father-in-law's offers of help, thrashing my right leg, holding onto the seat of my chair with my right hand, a little embarrassed and miffed that I did not seem able to stand up. I also remember distinctly my irritation at my mother-in-law's plaintive demands that her husband remove a piece of bread I was chewing on when the stroke hit. She, a keen observer with an artist's eye for detail, had noticed that chewing motions had ceased on the left side of my mouth and food was stuck under the cheek.

Because I was recuperating from open heart surgery—a mitral valve repair that had been performed 2 weeks earlier—little diagnostic acumen, especially for a neurologist, was required to conclude that I had suffered a stroke. Lying on my dining room floor waiting for the ambulance, I ruminated about the inappropriateness of the word *stroke* to describe what had happened to me, which had been more like the gentle snuffing of a candle than a violent hit. Nevertheless, the term *stroke* (from the Latin *ictus*, which is still widely used in medical jargon) is universally accepted and has equivalent words in most Western languages. I concluded one of two things: either stroke referred to the suddenness of the event rather than to its outward manifestations or I had had an unusual stroke. Now I know both things are probably true.

The fact that I was musing about words minutes after my stroke illustrates the most important "lucky" feature of this unfortunate event: it had spared mentation and speech. Although at times I suspect that my friends and relatives may have welcomed a little aphasia on my part, talking, reading, and, soon enough, working have been a vital part of my recovery, and I am certainly grateful for whatever forces, natural or supernatural, pushed the blood clot into the right rather than into the left carotid artery.

Finding myself totally incapacitated in a hospital bed was not as traumatic an experience as it would be now, maybe because it occurred so shortly after a similar postoperative intensive care experience. Or else, unbeknown to me, I was in a slightly stuporous state that blessedly quenched the emotional reactions to what was happening. Although I seemed to remember every detail of those first days after the stroke, later I discovered some curious gaps. For example, I have no memory of having received a Doppler scan. Months later, when a repeat scan was performed and I was shown the results of the first examination, I had to admit to myself that I must have been in that same laboratory, which I did not remember, subjected to the same procedure, which seemed new to me, by the same technician, who greeted me cordially but whom I did not recognize.

The question most often asked, especially by other neurologists, is "What does it feel like to be hemiplegic?" I had asked myself the same question when seeing patients who had lost various degrees of motor control. The answer, again, at least in my case, is disappointingly simple: it really felt like nothing, like I had never been able to use my left limbs; no exasperating feeling of formulating a mental command and getting no action occurred. Nor do I think that this was because of loss or diminution of left-body awareness (asomatoagnosia) or sensation, because I had neither to any detectable extent.

---

*This chapter is dedicated to Maria Laura, Beppe, Giorgio, and Alessandra. My recovery would have been a lot slower without their loving assistance and support.

Peculiarly, the frustration and anger with the sluggish and clumsy left limbs, especially in the hand, came later as I was gradually regaining function and continue to this day. I do not remember how many times I have cursed and actually punched my left hand for not performing adequately, knocking things over, being in the way, or simply being ridiculously (and embarrassingly) tremulous in reaching for objects.

However, at the time of admission to neurology, my only frustration was related to being totally dependent on others for everything, from turning in bed to performing bodily functions. As an intensely (maybe a bit neurotically) private person as I had been all of my life, the loss of privacy that comes with major illness was initially a big problem for me. The "silver lining" has been, in fact, the acceptance of my physical frailty as a matter of fact.

How does a neurologist live with a neurologic disease? I cannot answer this question appropriately because I lived my stroke as a patient, not as a neuroscientist. I asked few neurologic questions and never wanted to see my magnetic resonance imaging films. As I had done at the time of my heart operation, I had full trust in the skill of my physicians and colleagues first and my physical and occupational therapists later and took a passive though cooperative attitude throughout the healing process. I think this consciously ignorant and trusting position may have done me more good than a critical, controlling approach.

Of course, seeing my own left toe go up in a classical Babinski's sign, witnessing my own excessive knee jerk, feeling odd paresthesias in the left side of my body and "pins and needles" in my left hand were strangely interesting experiences. Some peculiar phenomena may have escaped an untrained observer; for example, I noticed at some point (perhaps 2 months after the stroke) that a spontaneous Babinski's sign occurred whenever I initiated urination. This happened without exception and consisted of two or three jerky dorsiflexions of the left toe that promptly subsided as the stream of urine became steady. This "urinary Babinski" persisted throughout the first year after the stroke and continues to occur sporadically to this day. My colleagues in the stroke unit swear they have never heard of a similar phenomenon, but physicians and therapists may find inquiring about this systematically with patients recovering from stroke a worthwhile task. Who knows, perhaps the "urinary Babinski" (DiMauro's sign?) will be added to the spontaneous Babinski's sign observed by H. Houston Merritt on removing a patient's slippers.

As every patient does, I worried about the extent of recovery I could expect. I was encouraged by the fact that I could bend my leg from the very beginning. I would show this proudly to visitors and colleagues with the expectation of rosy prognostic pronouncements. I was concerned by the total lack of movement in my left arm, but I learned later from a good friend, a pediatric neurol-ogist, that he had felt optimistic about my future recovery because from the first day I could flex my fingers. Wisely, however, he kept his own council about his positive prognosis until much later, when my arm had in fact regained a good deal of function.

Another weird aspect of my stroke (and as it turned out a positive one) has been the complete lack of spasticity, which has greatly facilitated the rehabilitation process. The only hint of spasticity appeared during automatic reactions such as stretching and yawning, when both left limbs would spontaneously and uncontrollably go into extreme flexion.

## THERAPY

When one of the editors of this book, who had been my occupational therapist, asked me to write about my experiences as a patient recovering from stroke and suggested the title "Notes of a Survivor," I asked him whether he meant survivor of the stroke or survivor of physical and occupational therapy. Lest my later comments sound too enthusiastic or be considered self-serving on the part of the editor, let me start with a few negatives.

Both physical and occupational therapy are boring, consisting as they must of highly repetitive exercises and activities: the patient soon learns to count "reps," longing to reach the magic number (usually 10—do therapists have a functional rationale for this quota?) requested by the therapist. And no cheating is tolerated; therapists have mastered a secret way of keeping track of reps automatically and privately even as they keep up a conversation with you, and they will not be defrauded of even a few reps.

Another thing—therapists have a bit of a sadistic trait that may be innate and predisposing to the job or else part of their professional training. As soon as you feel comfortable doing the required number of reps for any given exercise, the number of reps usually goes up by five. The idea, I think, is to keep you challenged, and you are. Furthermore, consider pain; did you know that therapists distinguish between "good" pain and "bad" pain? Good pain is the muscle soreness that comes from those five cycles of ten reps, a guarantee for the therapist that you are doing your exercises and using the proper muscles. Bad pain is classified in imaginative ways; my occupational therapist, a man, used a scale of severity that ranged from "paper cut pain" to "labor pain," at which point the secretary on the occupational therapy floor, a woman, invariably reminded us that we men did not know what we were talking about.

One other piece of good news and bad news—exercise works, but only as long as you keep exercising. The moment you stop, you start losing ground, so that you are in fact condemned to exercising for life, which to a Mediterranean soul such as I is a pretty harsh sentence.

My way of surviving this torture is to make exercise part of a highly routinized wake-up ritual, something I do almost automatically, like brushing my teeth. This way I feel slightly guilty when I skip the routine and, conversely, when I do exercise, I enjoy that little heady virtuous feeling I remember from my jogging days.

So much for the negatives. The positive side of the ledger is much larger. As a neurologist and a student of neuromuscular diseases, I am ashamed to confess that I had virtually ignored physical therapy and occupational therapy—a never-never land where patients usually ended up after the physicians concluded their brilliant diagnostic workups—and I had a vague notion of physical and occupational therapists as robotlike technicians. A few sessions of occupational therapy and physical therapy sufficed to change my views drastically. The first thing that impressed me was their knowledge of muscle anatomy and physiology; I thought I knew muscles! Throughout the rehabilitation process, I was amazed at their understanding of movement and lack thereof, muscle coordination, and compensatory mechanisms. Thus, I had at all times the comforting notion that all exercises and activities were rationally planned on the basis of my specific deficits and needs and were not part of a "canned" program. Another encouraging sign was the therapists' obvious satisfaction at every sign of improvement; far from being automata, these people clearly loved their profession and took pleasure in a job well done. In fact, I came to admire both the dedication and the professionalism of my therapists so much that I developed the conviction—which I expressed to the chairman of our Department of Neurology—that all neurology residents ought to spend at least a few weeks observing occupational and physical therapists at work. All too often we neurologists are content with our diagnostic workup of stroke patients and our intervention in the acute phase, only to lose sight of patients' progress.

I developed a pain syndrome in my left shoulder that not only gave me sleepless nights (partly because of pain, partly because of an exaggerated fear of dislocating my arm by sleeping on the left side) but also resulted in a "frozen shoulder," a very painful condition that interfered with my occupational therapy. Again, I was impressed by the variety of approaches used by my therapists not just to alleviate the pain but also to resolve the problem, including slinging, supporting my arm on an over-the-shoulder bag, and taping my shoulder in conjunction with passive mobilization and massage. On that occasion, I found myself in another situation I usually experience from the other side; I volunteered to be the subject of a teaching conference for occupational therapy trainees. Although I derived some satisfaction from being materially useful to the medical profession (something akin to but fortunately short of donating your body to the Department of Anatomy) at our clinical conferences, I am now much more aware of the discomfort caused to the patient by being an object of study.

## GOING HOME

Falling is, of course, the big fear. I had fallen once in my hospital room, and I fell once again a few days after my return home. Finding myself on both occasions next to a wall, I went through the steps my therapists had so carefully rehearsed with me in the hospital gym, and on both occasions I got up on my own. However, after my relatives left, I had nightmares about falling in the middle of a room and not being able to get up and reach the phone or the intercom. The problem was solved by the acquisition of a portable phone, which I slipped into my pocket every night as soon as I entered my house. I never had to use it, but it served its purpose as a "security blanket."

Showering and getting dressed in the morning also took some adjusting, but I soon learned that what had appeared in the hospital as slightly ridiculous procedures (left sleeve and pants leg first; hook the sock on your big toe first, then slip in the other toes) were in fact precious clues to a highly routinized and reasonably rapid process. I took several months to remaster the tie knot, but I remember with joy the pride of my occupational therapist when I appeared at a clinic appointment wearing shirt and tie instead of the usual turtleneck.

Lest all this appear an exceedingly smooth return to normal life, let me dwell for a moment on the frustrations to which I alluded in my opening paragraphs. Even a mild residual hemiparesis is an endless source of frustration in just about every aspect of daily life. I find dropping objects especially irritating and often remember with new empathy my son's frequent outbursts as a clumsy adolescent—"I hate gravity!" Buttoning shirts, especially cuffs, can be a trying experience, and I have more than a few shirts with ripped-off buttons to prove it. Frustration at times turns to rage, and I have occasionally punched my sluggish left hand with my agile right one; even worse, I have punched a table, with the only result of having still a sluggish left hand and a painful right one. One less disruptive way to deal with frustrating experiences is to curse; I have invented a peculiar English/Italian hybrid curse (unprintable in either language) that I use as a mantra many times a day. Naturally, the level of frustration and the threshold for the "tantrums" vary considerably from day to day and are influenced by mood; on some "bad days," I notice that I am almost looking for a frustrating experience so I have an excuse to explode, thus using the stroke as a scapegoat for my bad mood.

Although I have never been a sportsman (library mouse would be a more fitting definition), as my rehabilitation progressed I have repeatedly had vivid dreams in which I ran, I just ran for the sake of running, and it felt both exhilarating and as easy as it had been before the stroke. I actually tried the motions of running while holding onto a shopping cart in the hallway of my apartment building, but somehow the exhilaration of the dream wasn't there.

## CONCLUDING REMARKS

Although I cannot run, I can walk without a cane, I am independent in my daily activities, I have been able to resume my (fortunately sedentary) job, and I travel around the world. To be sure, this is not the typical outcome of stroke. Every patient is different, and I have been unusually lucky in that I was spared speech impediments and spasticity. This in turn has made my rehabilitation easier and more effective.

However, my left side was totally paralyzed only 2½ years ago (at age 54), and I am now enjoying a nearly normal life. Much of my progress has been because of the patient, steady, intelligent, and compassionate work of my physical and occupational therapists. The punchline of these "Notes of a Survivor" has to be that not only can one survive a stroke, but brain plasticity does exist, and good physical and occupational therapy does improve the condition of every patient recovering from stroke to a remarkable degree. Some improvement continues to occur (if you exercise, that is!) for a long time, although at a reduced pace. So,

who knows, maybe I will be able to run again before I turn 60.

■ ■ ■

P.S. Just as Alexandre Dumas père felt obliged to write "Twenty Years Later," a follow-up to "The Three Musketeers," so 10 years after my stroke I also feel obliged to offer a follow-up. The good news is that I still walk independently, work full time, and travel extensively. The bad news is that I never ran again—although running remains a recurrent subject of my dreams—and I still have paresthesia in the left side of my body, mostly in the hand. Additional problems are due to two situations, one of which is totally outside my will, while for the other I have to take full responsibility. The first has to do with aging and related troubles (still preferable to the alternative, to quote Woody Allen). Thus, generalized arthritis has necessitated a total left hip replacement, adding insult to the injury of the stroke and accentuating my limp. The second has to do with my physical laziness and my weakness for the Mediterranean diet (which is the opposite of the Atkins diet): lack of exercise and excessive weight are not what my physical therapist recommended. And I hear about it about every day because my physical therapist and I have developed a wonderful personal relationship. You can call this development a positive side effect of the stroke for me, and an occupational hazard for her. But it is a happy ending for both, and who does not like a happy ending?

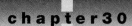

# A Survivor's Perspective II: Stroke

Somehow, I thought it would never happen; cancer, yes, but not this. My right arm lay lifeless at my side, and my right leg was too weak to lift from the sheet. For the second time in a week I was in a hospital bed. My left arm was hooked up to a plastic bottle suspended from an IV [intravenous] pole, and a slender tube was relaying medication via my veins to the rest of my system. At least my body was someone else's problem now, and I did not have to pretend any longer that everything was all right. But rather than feeling relaxed, my mind was racing, replaying the events of the past 6 days.

"I've had a TIA." On Monday morning I finally had to admit this to myself. It was the third day of gradually increasing weakness of my entire right side, and I knew I had a transient ischemic attack, which temporarily interrupts the flow of blood to the brain but then generally resolves itself within 24 hours. It is often the first warning of a stroke.

I was strangely calm—nonfeeling—but then, the topic of stroke was no stranger to me; for over 40 years I had been an occupational therapist and was familiar with neurological problems. It was ironic—too ironic even for my ability to find humor in the darker side of life. I had worked with men and women who themselves were the survivors of strokes and other serious illnesses, and I had found great satisfaction as I showed them how to manage daily life during their recovery. I had listened to the stories men and women told me of their strokes, recalling exactly where they were and what they were doing when they were struck. Most stories included a dramatic part of losing consciousness and falling. These stories and many like them formed the content of the teaching that was the natural progression of my career from practice to education. Until retiring 2 years ago, I had been a professor at Columbia University, and patient vignettes that helped to illustrate a particular point punctuated many of my classes.

It took getting used to the new experience as a patient. It differed from other patient stories in many ways. I never lost consciousness, nor did I suddenly collapse. I watched for 3 days and went about my business while my right side got weaker. It was a busy time for me, since I was anticipating a vacation trip to Europe with my brother and sister-in-law, and we exchanged frequent phone calls to discuss plans. I felt I had no time to pay attention to the annoying weakness that hardly interfered with my ability. On Sunday night a friend came to dinner. The symptoms were still not fully in my consciousness, and I was able to prepare the meal by compensating with my left side. On the return from walking my friend to the bus, I felt a strange urgency to get home to do the dishes before I got weaker. When I finally got to bed, I fell into a fitful, uneasy sleep. The next morning I couldn't ignore that I had had what the textbook refers to as a transient ischemic attack.

I had to repeat the hated phrase, "I think I've had a TIA," two more times; first, to the doctor's receptionist to get an appointment, then to my brother in New Jersey, asking him to take me to the doctor, since I knew I couldn't maneuver the car.

I tried to keep myself busy until my brother's arrival. Although I was still trying to deny the reality, I packed an overnight bag just in case I had to stay in the hospital. An added unpleasantness was the slurring of my speech that I couldn't control.

Much to my satisfaction, once we had arrived in his office, the doctor confirmed my diagnosis and made an appointment for me right away to see a neurologist who specializes in stroke. This was truly weird; just 2 months before, in my role as a retired adjunct professor, I had been coordinating a course for student occupational and physical therapists covering neurological problems, and this doctor had been our guest lecturer on the topic of stroke. I had liked his calm, confident manner and the clarity with which he sketched out to the students the various areas of the brain that might be affected. I had even remarked to a colleague that he was definitely someone I would consult if I ever needed a neurologist. All of this played back to me now as I sat in his waiting room, anxiously anticipating my turn.

Luckily, I was in familiar territory. The neurologist's office was only three stories below where my own office had been. I felt a slight twinge of embarrassment as he came out to greet me.

"I'm wearing a different hat today," I slurred and forced a weak smile. His smile was warm and reassuring. His neurological examination further established that I had had a stroke, and he confirmed the need to be hospitalized for further tests.

While the doctor made the necessary phone calls to admit me, my brother and sister-in-law took me to the fifth floor of the adjoining hospital building where a single room overlooking the Hudson was waiting for me. When my family was satisfied that I was in capable hands, I urged them to leave. I needed some time to myself and yet, when the door closed behind them, I felt like a little girl on the first day at camp after the parents have gone home.

It was difficult for me to grasp the seriousness of my condition, although a slow dread began to hover in the back of my mind. I had no pain and did not feel really sick, so the idea of getting into an ill-fitting hospital gown in the middle of the afternoon seemed ridiculous. What was this going to do to my plans for the trip? Before I had much time for reflection, a very young resident stood at my bedside, poised to take blood from my arm; her deft handling of the needle belied her youthful appearance. She was the first of a long line of men and women who entered my room at all hours of the day and night to perform some service which was much more useful to them than it was for me. The idea of using the hours around midnight for sleeping was not part of their thinking.

Sometime during the next several hours I was roused from a restless sleep by something metallic banging into my bed. It was a stretcher on wheels.

"Your doctor ordered a CT scan," the orderly said with false cheeriness.

"Now?" It was hard to believe that my neurologist would suddenly awaken with one thought in his mind— to order a CT [computed tomography] scan to be carried out during the next hour. Obediently I slid from my mattress to the stretcher that was parked alongside the bed. The orderly covered me with a blanket and without another word, whisked me rapidly down numerous corridors and elevators to another section of the hospital. We were now clearly in the basement approaching the double doors of the CT scan suite where two technicians were waiting for me. Without interrupting the flow of their

conversation, each of them grabbed one end of the sheet on which I was lying, and similar to the motion used to move sacks of meal to a waiting truck, transferred me onto the cold, hard surface of a narrow table. With two swift movements the technician wrapped the sheet around me in mummy fashion.

"Let me have your glasses." His outstretched hand was close to my face, and I surrendered my last link with a world I could see. "First, you'll hear the motor start, and then the scan will start to turn. Don't move until I tell you." With that he and his companion left the room.

I tried to dredge up all the things I had read about CT scans, but all I could focus on was the cold and my temporary blindness. The machine had started to whir at a considerable volume. A lighted circle above my head began to rotate and then gathered speed as the entire halo moved slowly back and forth. I shivered with cold and felt terribly vulnerable and alone. If I called for help, no one would hear me above the din of the machine.

After what seemed like an interminable time, the motor slowed down and stopped. The door was flung open, and the technician returned. It was only after the noise had stopped that I became aware of its unnerving effect. An unparalleled fatigue took over my body.

"Here are your glasses. I've called for a pickup," were the last words the technician spoke before he vanished again, this time for good. The silence in the room now became as frightening as the noise had been before. I closed my eyes and must have dozed off. When the orderly arrived, he seized the stretcher silently and retraced the circuitous route until I was back in my room.

Although my body felt exhausted, I could not get comfortable in the bed. Each time I awoke from what seemed hours of sleep, the large clock on the wall indicated that only a single hour had passed since I last checked. Now I had ample time to study the view from the large window by my bed. I looked out on the majestic Hudson, a coal-black ribbon bordered by the blinking lights of the Jersey edge. Finally, the first hues of the morning began to lighten the sky, and the hospital came to life. Someone entered my room and switched on the bright overhead lights.

"I've come to take your blood pressure." The speaker in white slacks and a pink T-shirt could have been anyone. Through my years as a therapist I was familiar with the subtle signs of hospital dress and behavior code; a stethoscope loosely slung around the neck meant that you were a nurse.

"Can you wash yourself?"

"I think so."

"Someone will bring you the basin in a few minutes."

"Can I go to the bathroom first?"

"When the aide comes to wash you, she'll give you a bed pan. We don't have time to take you to the bathroom now. All the patients have to be washed before the shift ends at seven." With that she left the room. It was the first example of hospital rules, made for the convenience of the staff, without consideration of patients' needs. A feeling of utter powerlessness swept over me, and I knew that, like thousands of others before me, I had now entered the world of the patient, aptly named for the quality that is the keystone for survival in the hospital setting.

The day was punctuated by more tests and the visit of a hierarchy of doctors who represented all the developmental steps in a physician's career. Each of them questioned and probed. All of them wanted to feel my extremities, to see the amount of movement I could demonstrate, and to ask about my medical history. For all of them, I was the cheerful, cooperative patient, an approach that came to haunt me in the days that followed.

Evaluations by the physical therapist, occupational therapist, and speech and hearing therapists were part of the day's schedule. The physical therapist that I recognized from sight as a sweet, gentle young woman went over most of the leg motions I had performed for the various doctors, but then she asked me to move back and forth in the bed and to sit on the edge. It was clear that my right side hardly took part in carrying out all the requested movements, but the years of keeping fit were paying off; I could support myself on my left side and even hobbled around the room, firmly hanging on to Kathy, the physical therapist.

I had never met the speech pathologist before. Her manner was cheerful and matter-of-fact. Her role was not only to listen to the formation of sounds and words but also to test my comprehension and memory. I was appalled when I listened to myself; no matter how much I tried to enunciate clearly, certain words came out slurred. I fared better with the comprehension and memory tests. Thank goodness, that part of me seemed to be intact.

When I returned from more tests in another part of the hospital, the occupational therapist entered the room. I was very familiar with most of the occupational therapists in the rehabilitation department; 12 of them had been research subjects in a study I had conducted and published last year, and I was currently gathering information from their patients for a study that I was conducting with one of them. Fortunately, I was not acquainted with the two who worked with the patients on the stroke service but knew that a former student was doing her internship there. My patient role was still too new for me, and I was not ready for the exchange that would inevitably result from seeing a colleague-in-becoming.

As soon as I saw the occupational therapist, I knew I was in good hands. She was in her mid-20s, short, with Asian features. She spoke with a slight accent, but I could not identify her country of origin. She moved and talked with an air of competence. Directly behind her was the student.

"I'm Romana, the occupational therapist, and I've brought a friend of yours to do the evaluation with me."

I hoped that my discomfort at seeing Yaffa was not too obvious; I remembered her well from my class 2 years ago. I was certain that she felt an equal degree of unease. Romana checked me over carefully, noting on her clipboard all the areas of function that I could or could not do. Occasionally, she asked a question of the student. She left me some therapy putty and a piece of theraband, both familiar parts of the beginning exercise program for the hand and arm.

"You know what to do with these," she laughed somewhat apologetically; I returned the laugh.

"You want me to squeeze the putty?" She nodded and then watched my efforts to close my fingers around the apple-green mass. Although I squeezed as hard as I could, I had not even dented the putty and felt utterly defeated. Our eyes met briefly and Romana said the thing that I had offered lamely a hundred times when I had overestimated a patient's ability, "Try using the putty every day; you'll see that it will get easier each time you try."

After Romana and Yaffa had left, I had little time to take stock of my situation before a new round of people stood in my doorway. This time it was Dr. Mitchell, the neurologist, with seven residents in tow. I recognized some of them from the interviews and blood tests of the day before. Dr. Mitchell greeted me with a question, "May we come in and talk to you for a few minutes?" I appreciated his consideration and was eager to cooperate. Between asking me to move my right side, he addressed the young doctors, asking them questions and sharing information about my condition. Then he turned to me. "The CT scan shows a very small lesion deep in the brain. The weakness should resolve itself in a few days, and you can go for outpatient therapy. You may call your brother now to take you home. I'll sign the necessary discharge papers." With a cheery wave he and his entourage walked out. I was left with a million unanswered questions.

Although I should have been ecstatic about the verdict, the news left me stunned. Nothing had changed in my condition since I had arrived yesterday. The fingers on my right hand could hardly move, my leg could barely support me, and I had to hold on to furniture to move around the room. I had expected more improvement than this before being allowed to go home. But hadn't the doctor said that I would get my strength back? The most important thing now was to share the good news with my brother and sister-in-law before the staff members changed their minds.

My family's delight made me feel a tinge of guilt at my own lack of enthusiasm. They offered to take me to their spacious house for a few days, a prospect I always enjoyed. Why wasn't I glad to be going home? Aside from a loss of appetite, I did not feel ill, but I could not shake a vague uneasiness that dampened my spirits. But as I waited, once again, for their arrival, I passed the time getting into my clothes as best I could. I recalled the hours of sitting with a patient, giving him or her advice on how to put a paralyzed arm into a sleeve, putting on slacks while supported by the bed. Fastenings like shoelaces I left for my sister-in-law to do; we were on such good terms that I did not hesitate to broach this subject with her.

The genuine pleasure at seeing my family pushed aside the uncomfortable feeling that was gnawing at the back of my mind. I was grateful for the wheelchair that was required by the hospital to take me to the front door. Was it really only 24 hours since I had entered? Aside from the numerous black-and-blue marks left from the blood tests on both forearms I was certainly no worse, but was I better? Again, I reminded myself that I needed more time to get stronger.

Once we were in the car, Jeff and Helen told me that they had made numerous phone calls in the morning to cancel our European trip.

"But why shouldn't *you* go? I'll surely be able to take care of myself by next Sunday," I protested. "You were so much looking forward to seeing our cousins and your friend. Why should you give it all up on my account?"

"We wouldn't go without you." Their reply was almost in unison. "Anyway, we can go next year." For the first time in 24 hours I was near to tears, perhaps because it was the first moment when I had dared to think about my feelings. All I could mutter was a bland, "Thank you; I know I've spoiled the trip for all of us, and I'm truly sorry." Helen reached over from the driver's seat and squeezed my hand.

As we headed toward their home in New Jersey, I knew I would be well cared for, and I began to feel better. Our conversation turned to everyday matters and to the things we might do together now that the pressure of the trip was off. Having an unexpected guest presented no problems to Helen and Jeff. As the parents of five children and grandparents to four, life was a never-ending chain of filled and empty beds and the feeding that were a part of this. I knew I was welcome in every family activity, but in spite of our intimate relationship, each of us had maintained separate lives with a different set of friends and daily responsibilities.

"Do you know, this is the first time I will be staying overnight at a time other than Christmas," I volunteered as we approached their house. I had always loved the canopy of old trees that joined branches over the street; they were an important part of keeping the summer heat from their large old house. It sat at the top of a hill with a steep driveway that had been the bane of my existence on many winter nights after a family gathering.

"Oh, yes!" Helen was genuinely excited by the prospect of being together for several days.

The walk from the car was supported by Jeff; it seemed doable. When I got into the house, I found refuge in the first available chair and stayed there for most of the evening. Not until it was time to go to bed did I realize that the stairs would create a real obstacle, especially since the banister was only on the right side and my right hand was too weak to hold on to pull my body from stair to stair. The only sensible, but thoroughly undignified, way was to go up on all fours, getting little help from the right side. I saw myself as a lame wolf I had recently seen in a nature film; my heart had gone out to the wolf that kept collapsing onto his weak side and was no longer able to keep up with the pack.

By the time I got into a bed where I had slept many times before, I was totally exhausted. I had not realized that every move involved a carefully strategized plan that required the mental layout of the room and each piece of furniture in relation to and its distance from its nearest neighbor. As long as I did not have to traverse any wide-open spaces, I would be all right. With that thought in mind, I fell asleep.

For the next 2 days, we spent the hours with all the routines that kept us close to the house. Knowing that I was safe, Helen and Jeff went for their usual swim in their large backyard pool while I stayed at the kitchen table or in a comfortable chair, reading. The canceled trip was still preying heavily on my mind, and it was hard to keep my attention focused on a printed page. My usual non-flagging energy had not returned, and I was most content to stay in one place. In the afternoon Helen suggested that the two of us might drive to the two stores from which we had purchased gifts for the cousins in Germany and Switzerland. Now we were taking the gifts back to the stores where we had spent such a pleasant afternoon choosing items that were suited to the temperaments of our friends and relatives.

I was grateful to Helen for suggesting this outing, since she and I always enjoyed doing things together. I knew that she would understand when I declined the chance to go into the stores with her; I just did not have the energy to walk from the car. While I waited for Helen to return to the car, I tried to move my fingers and my leg and had to admit that I could not voluntarily move them any better than the day before. Why was it taking so long to get my strength back? Actually, in my 11 years of practice, I had never worked with anyone who had only a temporary stroke; by the time patients were referred to therapy, they were recovering from much more serious conditions, but I could not shake the knowledge that I was not getting better.

That evening, we decided that since it would be easier for me to manage in my apartment, Jeff and Helen would take me home and stay with me there for a few days.

After all, the cancellation of the trip had left us with lots of free time. An overnight visit by Jeff and Helen was a real novelty; the thought of it buoyed up my spirits immediately. They could sleep in my room, while I would be comfortable on the couch in my study. What I failed to remember at the time of making these plans was that a major repair of the outside of my apartment building was underway, and all tenants had been asked to move all terrace furniture and plants inside. Since I thought that I would be away for several weeks anyway, I had piled most of the planters on the floor in the study, with just enough room to move to the desk and the bed.

We retired at a reasonable hour, and I was glad not to have to climb stairs tonight. Sometime in the night I got up to go the bathroom. Apparently, my right leg had become even weaker and when I tried to stand next to the couch I lost my balance and fell backwards into one of the planters. I was conscious of a cracking sound, fortunately not of a bone but the branch of a flowering geranium plant that had cushioned my fall and now held me captive. The ridiculousness of the situation made me laugh in spite of myself, and for a moment I simply enjoyed the humor without having to figure out a way to return to my bed. Then I saw that I could not rely on my body only to get me out of this predicament. I reached for a solid piece of furniture, pulled myself up with my left arm and stood firmly on my left leg. Thank goodness, it supported me well.

Once back on the couch, I could not get to sleep. My mind was racing almost as fast as my heart. I knew that I wasn't getting better, and somehow I was not prepared for this. Would I just keep getting weaker and weaker? So far, my sensation was intact; I could feel everything that touched my right side, but was it only a matter of time before that too disappeared?

My bodily needs became all too clear for me. I again had to leave the couch to go to the bathroom. In almost a Xerox copy of my previous escapade into the flowerpot, I fell again into one of the plants. This time I did not laugh, but again, unhurt, I was able to extricate myself quickly. At this rate, I would not have any flowers left. I was becoming a hazard to myself as well as to the environment.

When I had returned from the bathroom a second time by holding onto all the pieces of furniture along the way, I tried in vain to find some rest. I stared at the ceiling, contemplating what lay ahead. I dared not face up to the reality of what my body had imposed on me. Like a worn-down music box that is ready to stop, the same tune played over and over again, "You know you're getting worse and worse. Why did you leave the hospital?" Finally the first pink stripes along the visible sky told me that another hot day had started. I couldn't bear lying there any longer, and I got up to take a shower; the warmth of the water had often cleared my head after sleepless nights and always made me feel better.

Although there was nothing to hold on to around the tub, at least it wasn't dark. Probably that was why I had fallen during the night. The water felt soothing to my skin, and for a moment I felt cleansed of the demons that had become a part of my thinking. I turned off the water and approached the edge of the tub to get out. I would have to sit down on the edge and then lift my legs out one by one. Somehow I lost my footing and came crashing down. When I finally came to rest on the floor of the empty tub I noticed with relief that my head was about three inches from the wall while I was lying on my back. Once again I was unhurt but, like a beetle that had been turned on its back, I felt utterly helpless for fight or flight. If I called loudly enough Helen or Jeff would no doubt hear me. Considering that option for a moment, I decided I was not ready to capitulate to that extent; the thought of being pulled out of the bathtub stark naked by my brother did not appeal to me even in my helpless state. "Calm down!" I firmly told myself. "You're supposed to be a problem-solver." I was able to call on the dormant forces that are part of our emergency system, and they did not desert me. I turned over and with my left arm and leg, got myself first to a kneeling position with the left side holding all my weight and then to sitting on the edge of the tub. Holding onto the sink, I pulled myself to standing next to the tub. I found that I was shaking, totally exhausted by the ordeal. Somehow I got myself dressed and returned to the study where I had spent the night.

By now Helen was up and came to look for me.

"I've got to go back to the hospital," were my words of greeting. I then relayed the details of the three falls to her.

"I'm so glad you've decided to go back; we were thinking the same thing as we watched you last night." She seemed as relieved as I was that the decision had been made.

When I called Dr. Mitchell, his secretary told me he was on rounds but would call me as soon as he got back to his office. If he was at all surprised by my call, his voice certainly did not reflect this when he called back. Instead, he said calmly we should come right over.

Our departure from the house this time did not go unnoticed by my fellow tenants who were just leaving for work. It was not so easy to flash a cheery "Hi!" to neighbors from the compromised position of being held up by Jeff and Helen while we made our way through the lobby out to the car. This time we drove right up to the busy front door of the hospital.

"There are always wheelchairs there," I told Jeff, grateful that I could give in to my inability to walk the long corridors to Dr. Mitchell's office. As an automatic gesture on approaching the hospital doors, I slipped the chain with my ID over my head; "This will give us much faster entree to the different buildings," I told Jeff and

Helen. What I did not tell them was that the simple act of wearing the ID firmly established my role as faculty member rather than having to yield completely to the patient role.

For the second time in 4 days Dr. Mitchell confirmed my diagnosis following the neurological examination. "I thought I was supposed to be getting stronger, not weaker." My voice did not hide the indignation I felt.

"You're experiencing a progressive stroke, which can go on over several days." In my long experience I had not heard of this, and I questioned him further about the length of time it would continue. "Usually it is finished by the fifth day." Silently I counted back to the day I had felt the first signs of weakness; that was 6 days ago. By the time I figured it out, Dr. Mitchell had left the room to ask his assistant to make the necessary calls to get me readmitted to the hospital.

When Dr. Mitchell returned, he stayed just long enough to tell me to go to the admitting office where they would tell us when the room was ready. "I'll stop in to see you later on," was all he said as a sign that the session was over.

I was very grateful for the wheelchair that Jeff now pushed through the many corridors that took us back to the hospital. At the admitting office, they already had papers for me that I now had to sign. I had not expected that I would be totally unable to sign my name. After several futile attempts at guiding the pen, I had to admit that this was impossible for me.

"Just do the best you can; you can even put an X if you want."

The humiliation was almost more than I could stand; I choked back the tears as best I could. We were told to wait until the bed was ready, and we sat in the waiting room along with other patients. At first it was rather interesting to watch and listen to the different snatches of life stories unfolding around us. I was comfortable in the wheelchair with two good friends at my side; I had made all needed decisions for the moment and was ready to relinquish my body to the wonders of the healing sciences.

It was hard to sustain my interest in the fate of other people when my own had a much higher priority. Repeated inquiries of the clerk at the desk about the readiness of my bed resulted in the same answer: "They should be calling from the floor any minute now." It was the first of a chain of broken promises that I came to recognize as one of the hallmarks of patient treatment. No one wants to give a straight answer when they know how unpleasant the truth may be to the patient; it is far easier to promise a fulfillment of the patient's request than to be in the role of the bad guy. And so the minutes turned into hours. Finally, 3 hours after we had entered the waiting area, we were told that the bed was indeed ready, and I could report to the fifth floor of the hospital. My room—

with only one bed—was again on the river side. After another wait to get the necessary hospital paraphernalia, I was able to convince Jeff and Helen that I was in good hands, and they left for home. It was then that I became aware of the enormous fatigue in my body, but even more so, the seriousness of my condition now faced me squarely. I had to admit to myself I had lost the exhausting battle with denial, and I gave full expression to the overriding despair that gripped me. My body shook with sobs that I did not try to control.

After a few moments of this, when I had begun to collect myself, the door burst open and the first of the ever-present residents came in, sporting the now familiar blood-taking kit.

"We'll be checking your blood every few hours." Her manner was friendly but business-like. Hardly had she left when a nurse entered, carrying the floppy plastic bag filled with clear fluid; this meant that I was to have an infusion. Without a word she hung the sack of liquid on an arm of the pole that she wheeled from the corner of the room to my bedside. With a minimum of wasted motion, she inserted the needle in my left forearm and held it in place by a strip of adhesive tape. She fitted the slender tube that extended from the bag of liquid into the needle, turned the valve, and the liquid began to drip slowly into my veins. In response to my inquiry, she told me that I was to receive an infusion of heparin, which I recognized as a so-called blood thinner. I let out a long sigh of relief; at last someone was doing something that seemed vaguely helpful, and for a moment I relaxed. Then I realized that I was not only tethered to the IV pole, but that this virtually made my left arm as useless as my right. Before I allowed myself to go into a full-blown panic, I tested the slack in the tube, how far I could reach with my arm before a tweak reminded me that I had reached the limit of my arm motion. I had to admit that this wasn't too bad; after all, I could reach as far as the top of my head, and if I sat up, I could reach my knees. These were the limits of my world for now; I let out a sigh of resignation and fell into an exhausted sleep.

After what seemed to be only moments later, I woke up to the cheery sound of a man's deep bass voice humming a tune as he entered my room.

"Hi, I'm Malcolm, your night nurse," he smiled broadly, and his rich Caribbean accent was undeniable. "I've come to check your pulse and blood pressure."

"Could you also call someone to help me to the bathroom? I need help with walking. Besides, I don't know how I can manage with the IV pole."

"Sure. I can take you."

This was not exactly what I had bargained for. The idea of a man taking me into the bathroom was not very appealing, but since I could not think of a graceful way of getting around this, I moved myself to the edge of the bed in anticipation of getting up.

Malcolm turned out to be a great help. He held me up effortlessly with his right arm while wheeling the pole with the other hand. In spite of my sorry condition, I smiled inwardly. We were indeed an odd couple as we headed toward the bathroom door. Once inside the bathroom I had to face another hurdle. Could I balance my body by standing solely on my left leg, and use my left hand to pull down my pants? I decided to risk it, rather than ask Malcolm to perform this task for me. There was a limit how much I was willing to ask for assistance, and I needed to prove to myself that I was not totally helpless.

"I'll be all right now, Malcolm. Thanks a lot for your help," I managed a smile.

"Just pull this cord when you're finished." Malcolm handed me a slender cord that was attached to the switch for the bell. A fleeting thought crossed my mind; whatever needs my body or soul now had had to be carried out with the help of other people or exclusively by my less skilled left hand. This, like everything else that was happening to my independent lifestyle, would take some adjustment on my part.

The 3 days that followed were filled with the dull hospital routine, frequent visits by doctors in all stages of their development, always physically probing and asking for more information, and the change in nursing shifts and the actions performed by each, depending where they found themselves on the hierarchy of professionals and helpers. Some were extremely cheerful and encouraging; some showed the strain of severe staff shortages.

There were also the small annoyances like a stuck window that took 5 days to get fixed. Of greater consequence to me were the details of my care that suddenly loomed larger than reality and reminded me at every moment just how helpless I really was. Perhaps in an effort to be kind, perhaps in a moment of absentmindedness, someone had shut my door at night, thereby leaving me at the mercy of my left hand to call the nurse. The first time the beeper announced that the heparin bag was empty, I rang the bell, and the remote voice at the end of the intercom told me that a nurse would come right away. The beeper screeched unceasingly, without the appearance of the promised nurse. I began to feel my heart pounding fiercely, certain that I would have another stroke because my blood was not getting the required dose of heparin. I tried feebly to call for help, but I had to admit that my voice barely reached to the door. At last the nurse arrived with the new bag, totally unmoved by my near-panic state.

"A short interruption like this doesn't make any difference." Her matter-of-fact response to my concern made me realize that I was losing my cool and had become just like all the frightened patients whom I had tried to reassure during my professional life.

I had struggled to view the whole experience with an objective clinical gaze, but I found myself forced into the role of docile sufferer, lacking the necessary willpower to do otherwise. Nothing seemed to be happening that was changing my condition; I began to feel very sorry for myself.

I was aroused from this "blue funk" by the arrival of an exquisitely blooming exotic plant sent by my colleagues at the University. How had they learned of my whereabouts? According to the calendar I was supposed to be on my way to Europe! I thought that since no one was expecting me back for 3 weeks, my secret was safe. But there were enough people in the hospital that knew me, and the news soon leaked out. From then on, during the weeks of my stay in the hospital, the wide windowsill of my room was always filled with fresh flowers or potted plants, thanks to the dozens of people whose good wishes were expressed in this touching way. I felt ashamed of the feelings of self-pity that I had allowed to take over.

Soon after the flowers, the first of a steady flow of visitors from the University arrived. They managed to squeeze in friendly calls before, during, and after their work hours in the University. Now I had to face my deficits head-on, and I experienced a sense of shame, especially at my slurred speech. It was also exhausting to answer "How did it happen?" again and again. Still, the visitors were bright spots in the monotony of the hospital days. The ones I anticipated with the greatest pleasure were Helen and Jeff, my sister-in-law and brother. They always brought fresh news of their family and also delivered my mail. I could count on them for all the support and understanding I needed. Jeff had taken over the management of my finances; Helen took the bag of dirty clothes from the floor of my closet, and when I started to object, she silenced me. I surrendered a further aspect of my independence, this part more willingly.

Another break in the routine was the daily visits of the therapists. I was concerned that nothing was being done for my arm. I had seen too many tight, painful shoulders and permanently weak wrists to risk similar complications, frequently the result of lengthy disuse. When I voiced this to Romana, she brought me two wrist splints to try. I also began to exercise my arm with my other hand. It was the first action toward resuming charge of my life, and it felt good.

Now the next hurdle to be overcome was the decision by the doctors and therapists if and when I could be moved to the rehabilitation floor. Of course, I was still receiving the heparin infusion; the needle would have to be removed before I could begin a strenuous rehabilitation program. Finally, 6 days after my second admission, the order came from the doctors; my blood had been thinned to the required level, and I was to be moved to the eighth floor.

As promised, the two needles were removed from my arm, and I was liberated from my tether. In spite of my relief at the prospect of starting the rehabilitation program,

I felt the slightest twinge of sadness, much as I felt in grade school when I advanced to the next grade. I had begun to think of the familiar routine of the fifth floor as more or less safe, and I had become used to the staff. I knew that on the rehabilitation floor patients were in double rooms; there were also much higher expectations for helping oneself placed on the patients; would I be able to measure up? As always, there was a long wait ahead until finally, an attendant with a stretcher announced that he was moving me. But why the stretcher?

"Oh that," he explained, "That's not for you. That's for all your plants and stuff. I'll come back for you in a little while with a wheelchair." Then he left me sitting in bed, once again feeling abandoned. There was nothing to do but wait; to amuse myself I looked out at the river, which was changing to its evening glow in preparation for the sunset. Most of my life I had lived within sight of a river; first, during my early childhood, it was the Danube with its rushing brown current in spring, and during many of my adult years, it was the Hudson. Now the steady flow had become a source of comfort and assurance of the continuity of life. The lights on the side of the river were already starting to blink when the door was flung open by the returning orderly, this time pushing a wheelchair. He lifted me nimbly into the chair and whisked me toward the elevator to the eighth floor. Halfway down the hall he pushed me into a large double room with a similar picture window facing the Hudson. My new roommate approached me, pushing a walker.

"Hi, I'm Virginia," she extended her hand in a confident way, and I shook it with my left. Virginia was a tall, black woman with a matter-of-fact manner and a smile that hovered just behind her eyes. I liked her immediately.

"Why are you here? Did you have a stroke?" I knew that I bore all the signs of patients with whom I shared this diagnosis, but Virginia's direct query caught me off guard. For the first time in days, I burst into tears.

"No sense feeling sorry for yourself." Virginia was right, and her words became my special mantra during the weeks that followed. But for now I was content to let Virginia talk; it was obvious that she knew the routine of the floor. When we said good night, I felt relieved that there was a person on the other side of the curtain that was drawn during sleeping hours.

I woke frequently during the night; each time I awoke, the big clock on the wall showed that only an hour and a half had passed. Now that I was free to move in the bed, I realized that I couldn't change my position much more than I had when my left arm was held in place by the tubes. Besides, my right side kept getting in my way and I needed to move both the arm and the leg with the other side. I was once again grateful that at least I knew the technique, but that didn't make the situation more palatable nor me more comfortable. I watched the sky for the first signs of summer dawn that arrived at the same time as the noise in the corridor that announced that the rehabilitation floor was coming to life. Shortly thereafter, a hand reached for the light switch that changed night into day.

"Time to get up," the raspy voice of the nurse called loudly; I noticed that the clock confirmed that it was only 5:30.

"Do you want to bathe yourself in bed, or sit by the sink in the bathroom?" I had noticed with satisfaction that each of us had a private bath.

"The sink," I responded, eager to have the chance to fend for myself.

"Do you have slacks and a shirt to wear? Here we expect people to wear their own clothes." To be able to shed the hospital gown after a week! Suddenly I realized how much I wanted to be restored to my former self and to leave the patient role behind.

The nurse brought a wheelchair into our large room and parked it next to my bed.

"Can you transfer into this?" Her voice sounded friendlier than before, and although I hadn't attempted to move from the bed to the wheelchair by myself, I had worked with dozens of patients to teach them this skill. I sat on the edge of my bed, slid down to stand on my left leg, pivoted around and grasped the left armrest before letting myself down in the chair. I had to gather each garment I wanted to wear from the drawers of the nightstand and the closet and wheel myself the bathroom door. Moving the wheelchair with only my left foot and arm took a lot more skill than I remembered, but after several attempts to stop myself from merely going in a circle, I got the knack. The nurse moved an armchair into the bathroom to the small space between the wall and the sink. "Once you're in the bathroom, I'll help you transfer to the chair and then take the wheelchair out. Otherwise, you won't be able to close the door." I welcomed the privacy that this would give me; how I would get back the wheelchair when I had finished was too far in the future to consider.

Now began the long, arduous process of washing and dressing myself, but the idea of doing all of this by myself behind a closed door seemed like the best thing that had happened to me in a week! For the next 50 minutes I was fully occupied in breaking down each task into tiny steps and then, mostly by trial and error, carrying out each step with my left arm and leg, as well as my teeth and any working part of my body that I could involve in completing a given task. I had never thought of myself as even remotely ambidextrous, and my left hand had only complemented my right for any task that naturally called for bilateral skill. Now I not only had to resort to being one-handed but also confining all hand use to the left.

One of the first challenges was putting toothpaste on the toothbrush before I brushed my teeth. Like all of the activities of daily living, I had worked with patients on this, so there was no mystery connected to it, but the frustration I experienced before I even had toothpaste on the brush was enormous. Flipping up the top of the tube presented no problem, although it meant grasping the tube without my thumb, since I needed the thumb free to push open the top. Obviously, I was out of practice; otherwise, I would have remembered that the toothbrush has to be laid flat and braced against an object to keep it from moving while the toothpaste was squeezed onto the bristles. Now I had to put the toothpaste down; why wasn't there at least a ledge on the edge of the sink on which to place the toothbrush? When I put down the toothpaste to pick up the brush, the heavy tube fell into the sink where I left it momentarily; at least it couldn't fall on the floor. Once I had wedged the toothbrush against the left faucet in hopes that it would stay there, I was ready to retrieve the toothpaste and squeeze it onto the waiting toothbrush. Then, finding a place for the toothpaste, I picked up the toothbrush with my left hand. However, before it reached my teeth, the toothpaste had fallen off the brush and was clinging in a soggy mess to the edge of the sink. The second time I repeated the whole routine I was successful and began to brush my teeth rather clumsily with my left hand. When I had at last advanced to my socks, I was already so tired that the thought of the struggle was almost more than I could face. Then the "achiever half" of me chided the "flagging half"; I picked up the first of two socks that were the only remaining garments on the arm of the chair in which I was sitting. Surely I could do this last step. Happily, I had not lost the agility that has always allowed me to squeeze through narrow spaces and bring my knees close to my chest! At least I could bring my left foot up to rest it on my right knee. I decided to tackle the left sock first and found that my left foot cooperated nicely in the task by extending the big toe so I could hook the sock over it. Then it was just a question of pulling the sock first over the rest of the toes and the heel.

It was a different story with the right sock. I lifted the right foot up to the left knee but without the muscle power to hold it, it slid down to the floor. I remembered that I could expect no help from my right side. I leaned over and brought my body closer to the foot, but I was afraid that if I leaned over too far I would tip over. I sat back as far as I could in the chair and leaned forward again but when I was ready to hook the sock over the toe, the foot stayed flat on the floor. No sooner was the sock on the toe than I would pull it off accidentally in attempting to move the sock over the foot. After several more tries, I succeeded in getting the sock over the toe and gradually working it over the static foot. In my delight at seeing socks on both feet, I was glad to overlook that the right sock was completely stretched out and hung limply at the ankle.

"Oh, well," I sighed to myself with resignation. I realized that I would have to lower my standards for achieving anything. I would have to settle for just doing a task without looking for quality. And I had to muster all the patience I had slowly learned in the socialization process of becoming a therapist; only now it was not a question of sitting on my hands in order not to give in to my desire to help a struggling patient. I had to serve as my own cheerleader, goading myself on and applauding when I was done.

When the nurse came back to check on my progress, I reported triumphantly that I needed help only with fastening my bra and putting on the sneakers that were still in the closet. It was then I felt my exhaustion; I had used up every ounce of energy of my body before the day had even officially started.

Virginia was already seated in her chair fully dressed, her walker at her side.

"I'm supposed to graduate to a cane today," she announced, "I'll be going home when I can walk by myself." How I envied her! She seemed so competent with everything. A funny thought crossed my mind; I had often told my students how patients compared their own progress to that of other patients even when they had quite different diagnoses, "You should have seen me two weeks ago; I couldn't do anything." Invariably, the second patient would gather hope from seeing that progress. Now I had reached that stage of using Virginia as a role model, even though she had undergone thigh surgery only and her arms and hands were totally intact. In spite of everything, this type of black humor never ceased to amuse me!

Three hours after our untimely reveille, breakfast arrived. I realized that I was also weak from hunger and fell on the food for the first time since leaving home. Just as we finished, one of the physical therapists came to introduce herself as the person who would be working with me. I recognized her immediately as a graduate of the physical therapy program whose students shared many science classes with our occupational therapy students. She had been working several years and had fortunately lost some of the tentativeness of novice therapists. After we had talked for a few minutes and she had given me a quick once-over, she promised to return later with my total therapy schedule; the rest of the day I could relax! I was terribly disappointed and had to keep myself from crying again. For this I had gotten out of bed at 5:30!

Thank goodness, the day's visitors and several phone calls took my mind off the letdown. Virginia returned from therapy sporting her new cane and mighty proud of herself. Would I ever get to use a cane? It was hard to think beyond today, and I was not ready to create a new image of myself as anything other than my former self. In the effort to get used to so many new things, time had ceased to exist for me. I lived from moment to moment, and the outlandishness of my current existence enveloped me totally. Once again, I was grateful that all responsibilities had been taken from me, and no one was expecting anything more from me than being a good patient for my caretakers, a role that I had described at great length to my students. Although never expressed, the message was, "Be compliant, don't complain, don't ask too many questions, get well, and go home!" Here I was, very quickly behaving just like every good patient in the hospital.

Now that I was on the rehabilitation floor, life had a peculiar déjà vu feel; just a week before I became ill, I was interviewing patients in many of the rooms on this floor for a research project I was conducting with the occupational therapy department. Before I had time to dwell on this, Dr. Mitchell appeared, as always cheerful and energetic and seemingly very interested in my condition.

"I'd like to get an MRI on you. You're not claustrophobic, are you?" The question was almost rhetorical, but it hit me hard. For years I had heard reports of this procedure and had seen videotapes of patients' heads encased by the confining cagelike structure; I had often remarked that I would die of fright—how easily we speak of death when it is not imminent—if I ever had to have an MRI [magnetic resonance imaging].

"Yes, I'm terribly claustrophobic," I said and remembered the time I thought I was suffocating when I woke in the upper bunk at camp with the ceiling ostensibly only inches from my face. "Do I *have* to have an MRI?" I felt ashamed of my childish, almost petulant question.

"I think you'd better, so we can tell the exact place of the lesion. I'm conducting a research project on brain function during hand movement at various points of recovery after stroke, and I'll be there with you." The dual possibility of contributing to research in an area that had always fascinated me and having Dr. Mitchell close by quickly convinced me, and I gave my consent. Besides, it was to be scheduled for next week and that seemed far in the future.

Meanwhile, I had to face the weekend without having started any therapy. My disappointment was mixed with the fear that I would begin to see in myself many of the complications that were the result of disuse. At night, during several sleepless hours, I suddenly discovered that I could slide my arm and leg across the sheet. That meant that a small amount of strength was returning to my limbs! I was so excited that I had to fight my urge to wake Virginia, who was sleeping soundly. After that, each time I awoke after a period of sleep, I had to move first my leg and then my arm to make sure that it had not been a dream. As I knew, the slight movement did not have any functional value, but the feeling that resulted from it gave me a boost that got me through the rest of the weekend. I had hoped that perhaps we would be allowed to sleep longer on Saturday and Sunday, but the routine was unchanged, since the only purpose of the early rising was the schedule of the night nurses; their duty ended at 7 AM, by which time all the patients had to be washed and dressed. "Patient-centered care," one of the buzzwords of the 1990s, this was not. Like much of hospital practice, it served the staff and the administration long before the wishes of the patients were taken into consideration.

Finally, it was Monday, and today therapy was to begin for me. As promised, Ilsa, the physical therapist, stopped in our room before she started working and had attached my therapy schedule to the back of my wheelchair in order to let the staff know where I was to be at any time during the day. Until I became familiar with the routine, Ilsa had told me, the therapists would come for me at the appointed hour. I was to start with physical therapy at 9:30, then on to occupational therapy at 10:10, followed by speech therapy until 11:30. Luckily for me, Romana was to remain as my occupational therapist, although she usually worked with the acute patients only. I felt that it was better to have someone who was new to me, rather than any of the 12 occupational therapists who had served as subjects for a study I had conducted last year and which meanwhile had been published in a professional journal. As a patient I had been stripped of all the professional trappings that one is bound to accumulate, but after 15 years of serving as director of a university program, I was afraid that my history would serve to intimidate the young therapists. It was quite different with the physical therapists, most of whom I did not know and from whom I could expect ordinary patient treatment. When it came time to meet the speech therapist, we recognized each other immediately as colleagues who had shared the same monthly administrative department meetings for many years. Anne-Marie was nearer my own age than some of the others, and I felt we understood each other right away. And yet I felt the stigma of being a disabled patient more acutely in speech than I did in either of the other two therapies.

As expected, the first morning in therapy was taken up by a detailed assessment by each of the therapists. I was glad to show off the movement in my arm and leg and was pleased that these were not the only things that were recognized as strengths. Rather than experiencing the depression that was common when patients realized how much they couldn't do, I felt a surge of the need to excel that had driven me from my earliest years. As a child I had responded to the desire to please a very critical father whom I adored; now I wanted to be the "best" rehabilitation patient.

From frequent visits to the rehabilitation floor, I knew that both occupational therapy and physical therapy were extremely lively places. The large, airy physical therapy gym had mats in several places where patients with diverse problems were working with their therapists on strengthening exercises or resting between the different parts of their program. While I sat in my wheelchair waiting for Ilsa to finish with her first patient of the morning, I had a chance to survey the other patients with whom I would be sharing rehabilitation. I knew that in coming to this floor I had become part of a distinct society who were bound together only by the fact that each of them had incurred a temporary and not-so-temporary loss of function, of self-image, of role. I knew nothing of my new associates except that they were patients; they, in turn, knew nothing of me. Once again, I was reminded of one of the topics I had chosen for lectures: "People in the Patient Role." Was it part of a self-fulfilling prophesy? I decided that here I had an opportunity to fashion a totally new personality, but the thought seemed entirely too fatiguing. True to my old self, curiosity took over; I made up my mind to experience the new role as a fully participating member rather than an inquisitive spectator. Besides, I thought ruefully, I actually had little choice. The realization of this made me feel teary. I turned my attention to the bustling environment; I did not want to start my first physical therapy session as an emotional disaster.

Approximately eight other patients were engaged in some type of exercise or walking practice with their own therapist. Laughter and jokes resounded everywhere; it was obvious that therapists and patients enjoyed working together. One woman with a newly fitted artificial leg was practicing walking in the parallel bars; she was perspiring with the effort of lifting the heavy prosthesis in preparation for each step, but she wanted us all to know that she was there. A man, who seemed younger than the rest of us, was learning to step up and down simulated curbs using a cane. A very old and frail-looking lady was objecting strenuously that she couldn't stand on her operated side; the therapist firmly but gently insisted that she try in spite of the pain, and in a few minutes the patient was on her feet, tightly clenching the walker in front of her. Then it was my turn to begin.

Ilsa approached me with a broad smile and told me to wheel myself to one of the mats that was raised about 18 inches from the floor. I was told to transfer from the wheelchair to the mat pivoting on my left leg. It was an activity I had performed countless times with patients of all sizes and in need of varying degrees of help; I remembered how I was filled with dread at the sight of patients who were taller and heavier than myself and needing a great deal of assistance. Thank goodness, I was well schooled in this task and needed no help to get to the mat. Ilsa then checked every muscle for active and passive motion and pain. I was glad to be able to show the slight motion I had in both arm and leg; Ilsa told me that was a very good sign. Before the session ended, she let me try one of the walkers in the gym, but since I couldn't hold on with my right hand, this was still too difficult for me to attempt. It became a goal for a future session, some-thing that seemed a distinct possibility. I had concluded my first session in physical therapy; Romana now pushed my wheelchair to occupational therapy.

This place was extremely familiar to me; first, from my years as a clinician in similar departments, and more recently, as the place where I had been coming to gather information on the patients who were the subjects in my current study. Conducting research in occupational therapy was one of the retirement projects I had promised myself, and since this department had accepted my offer with enthusiasm, I had been a weekly visitor on this floor, interviewing patients about their perceptions of occupational therapy. I had chosen the supervisor of occupational therapy as a research partner; Glen and I had known each other for many years and knew that we could work well together. He was also a favorite clinical instructor of our students. Glen and one of his colleagues were editing a book on stroke rehabilitation, and several months before, much to my surprise, had asked me to write the foreword. I had told Glen that I was no longer as well versed with the topic as I had been when I was teaching clinical courses, but when he asked a second time, I agreed. The book was to appear on the market in several weeks. I thought of this when Romana and I entered the occupational therapy clinic and I spotted Glen working with a young man.

This was the place where I felt at home. In one of the momentary flashbacks that catch one unaware, I recalled the reason for my becoming an occupational therapist over 40 years ago. I was still in high school searching for a career in medicine without blood when I heard about occupational therapy. It allowed for direct work with people using my hands and a great deal of creativity of a special sort; assisting patients with the kinds of day-to-day physical, cognitive, and emotional problems that were preventing them from living ordinary lives. All of the patients here, like myself, were learning to live with what they had left after injury or disease had robbed them of a part of their function. In occupational therapy, they found a place and people who allowed them to mourn their losses and then to move ahead to learning new ways of accomplishing tasks. The aspect of my clinical work that I found most satisfying was literally to get into patients' heads, to discover which tasks had the most meaning for them, and then to elicit each patient's readiness to work on those tasks together until a satisfactory solution had been found. This had allowed me to glimpse deeply into other people's lives and to discover what kinds of activities were most important to people at different points in their lives. It had also given me a chance to be a partner in the roller coaster experience of recovery with men and women from all walks of life. Now I was acutely aware that a long process of moving through all the emotions from despair to exhilaration that probably lay ahead for me as well.

The occupational therapy clinic was a room with two distinct parts. There were also two large raised mats where people were practicing all sorts of movements in preparation for carrying out some functional activity. The other part was the "Easy Street" unit that had arrived only several months before. "Easy Street" had received much publicity in professional journals several years ago, and one of its features was that, depending on the needs of the particular rehabilitation center, it could include one or more daily life units such as a model apartment, a supermarket, a street with curbs and a traffic light, a factory setup, a golf driving range, or a stationary car. I remembered the discussions we had as a faculty, wondering whether this highly touted and equally highly priced equipment would really be worth the price and the large amount of space that was needed to house the various components. But even before I arrived as a patient, I had my answer. The majority of subjects in my recent study had all remembered some aspect of their occupational therapy that they practiced with their therapist in "Easy Street." I had never dreamed that I would be a candidate for validation of the equipment.

But clearly there was much I had to do before I got to that point. Romana first asked me to demonstrate all the motion I had and also checked strength and coordination in both arms. Then she asked me to describe a typical day, making sure that I mentioned not only major tasks and responsibilities, but also what I did for pleasure, where, and with whom. At the end I felt she had quite a complete picture of who I was and the types of skills, manual as well as cognitive and social, I needed to approach my previous lifestyle. We ended the session with setting long-range and more immediate short-term goals. If the whole procedure would not have been so familiar and right to me, I suppose I would have been more bewildered and overwhelmed than I was; I knew what I had to do to get where I was going, but would I find the strength to do the work that would get me there?

Across the hall from occupational therapy was Anne-Marie's office, where I was to go for speech therapy. We talked about old times, especially the monthly meeting both of us had attended; Anne-Marie filled me in on details of the current politics in the department, and I responded to her news. This gave her the opportunity to listen to my thick, slurred speech and also to assess the extent of the breathlessness that had plagued me since the stroke. The deficient speech was of far greater concern to me than the paralyzed arm and leg, perhaps because speech and intellect are so closely linked on the social measurement scale. It was good that Anne-Marie and I could laugh together when I bungled sounds; otherwise, the situation would have been even harder to face.

At 11:30, when I was totally exhausted, I was told that during the hour before lunch each patient was assigned to a group for further physical activity, depending on one's needs. I was sent to the strengthening group, which on that day consisted of about 10 other people. Seated in a circle in our wheelchairs, we were an odd cross-section of New York City demographics: black, white, and Hispanic men and women, dressed in sweat suits or shorts, shirts, and sneakers, we vaguely resembled a crowd at Yankee Stadium on a Saturday afternoon, although the average age was certainly above 50. Most of us were recovering from strokes, with varying degrees of disability on either the right or the left side. Some people were obviously seasoned members and knew the routine, which was not difficult to understand. Far more difficult for all of us was to carry out the commands issued by one of the therapists in charge. The purpose of the group was to encourage use of our limbs in sport or recreational activities that were simplified to make it possible for all of us to participate in games like beanbag toss with a laundry basket as the target or modified soccer with the goal of kicking a big but light ball to each other. A very important aspect of the group was clearly socialization, and most of us got into that component effortlessly. It was amazing to see the inventiveness and enthusiasm of our leaders; I was quickly caught up in the laughter and the chance to be utterly ridiculous. During moments of waiting for my turn, I was reminded once again of my own incapacity; the newly regained motion in my arm and leg was of little help to me, and I had to confront the reality that I was one of thousands of people who were hemiplegic— "hemis," as we affectionately used to call them as therapists. I recalled the group traits that characterized the "hemis," depending on the side of the brain where the lesion was located; thank goodness, I thought once again, I'm a right hemi whose dominant side was affected but who was not expected to have problems in thinking or behavior. My experience as a therapist had borne out much of the textbook information, and I had always enjoyed working with right hemis, many of whom had aphasia, a language problem, or, like myself, dysarthria, which is a problem involving the clarity but not the content of speech. I had liked the challenge of developing a partnership with a patient with aphasia and together discovering a new mode of communication, something like a secret language between us at first. But I was awakened from this reverie by a large balloon being tossed my way and struggling to catch it with my left hand before it hit me squarely in the face. "Go, Barbara, go!" the therapist encouraged; no one seemed to mind that I dropped the ball. So ended my first morning in therapy. I was too drained by the morning's activity to acknowledge the fact that in an hour and a half the therapy routine would begin again.

In the middle of the week, my roommate Virginia went home, feeling satisfied that the recovery from the surgery had progressed to the extent that she could carry on alone at home. For one night I had the room all to myself, and I welcomed the solitude between the steady pace of visitors—professional and friends and family—that was continuing. I longed for a chance to be left alone, at least long enough to appraise where I was, not fully 2 weeks since the onset of the stroke. I also wished for an opportunity to take off the cheerful mask that I was wearing, but the anticipated depression still had not come. I was just glad to be alive, and aside from the obvious paralysis of my right limbs and the breathless exhaustion, I felt perfectly well. This came as a total surprise to me. In all the conversations I had with patients who were recovering from a stroke, it always seemed they had pain or other discomfort. The movement in my arm and leg was definitely returning; I could not yet move even against gravity. I still wore the splint on my right wrist to keep that joint from tightening up in a contracted position.

Before I got too used to the luxury of having the large sunny room all to myself, my new roommate arrived. My first impression of her was quite favorable; in a few sentences, Mrs. Gold told me not only her medical history, but also enough details about her life that I knew she lived near me, "in a very good section" of the neighborhood as she emphasized, that she liked good quality and always bought the best, and that she had a daughter in California whose marriage to a penniless college professor—at least 20 years ago—she still did not approve. Her daughter had come East to transfer her mother from another hospital, "a regular hellhole" she noted, where she had been taken after being hit by a van while crossing the street. Now her only remaining injury was a small tear in her bladder. She also needed to practice walking, since she was off her feet a number of weeks. She was greatly relieved when, in response to one of her first questions, I told her that yes, I was Jewish, too. She then asked for my marital status and many other details about my personal life that I had not expected to divulge within the first half-hour of our meeting.

When Mrs. Gold had been put to bed for the night, she began to rummage in her pocketbook for her checkbook, declaring it stolen after a few moments. I urged her to look again, then suggested that it might be in her night table. Sure enough, there it was! She began to flip through the check register and announced that her daughter, who now had power of attorney over Mrs. Gold's finances, was squandering her money on God knows what.

"Why, here is a check for one hundred dollars to Channel Thirteen! I never told her to do that."

For the rest of the evening she repeated the action of getting the checkbook from the drawer and narrative of the check. I tried to reassure her by saying that she could ask her daughter about the money the next day. This resulted in a new cascade of accusations against her daughter. Finally, after both of us were exhausted, Mrs. Gold fell asleep. For the next 3½ weeks Mrs. Gold and I

shared the room, and she became both the much-needed scapegoat on whom to vent my anger and the equally needed comic relief. How much of her confusion was her normal state and how much could be attributed to the accident I never found out, but although she had moments of complete clarity, she also was beset by feelings of persecutions and paranoia that made ordinary conversation almost impossible. Luckily, we spent many hours attending our respective therapies, and thus I did not encounter Mrs. Gold for most of every day.

When Dr. Mitchell next came to see me, he told me that the MRI had been scheduled for the following day. While he spoke very reassuring words, I could feel the familiar cold dread spreading over me that was part of a childhood fear of suffocating. To my knowledge, the closest I had ever come to that state was in third grade when we were rehearsing for a play. As a prank, one of the boys in my class decided to wrap me in the dark red velvet curtains that hung open at the edge of the stage. Before I could object, I felt myself being spun around as the heavy material enveloped me. I can still smell the thick dust that saturated the curtain; I felt trapped and unable to breathe. I let out a piercing shriek, and the boy released the curtain. While I sobbed hysterically, the curtain fell away from me and I stood free, feeling utterly humiliated in front of my laughing classmates. That image stayed with me all these years and became particularly vivid while Dr. Mitchell spoke further about the procedure.

"I'll be with you in the room; you'll be able to see me through a mirror, and I'll tell you exactly what to do, first with your left hand and then with your right." Since I had already told him about my anxiety, I decided that my telling him again would change nothing. If the procedure were really life threatening, I decided, I would have read about the consequences by now. "I'll meet you down there tomorrow," with a breezy wave of his hand, Dr. Mitchell was gone, and I was left alone with my irrational fear.

At least I would have a respite for an hour tomorrow from the twice-daily therapy that consumed 6 hours of every day. With that small bit of comfort, I fell asleep. The next morning, an orderly arrived with the now-familiar stretcher that took patients to special services in other parts of the huge hospital. We arrived in one of the basement corridors clearly marked with a large sign that announced that we were approaching the MRI suite. "Caution—Electromagnetic Equipment—No Unauthorized Personnel beyond this point!" a second sign heralded ominously. In response to a special bell pressed by the orderly, the double doors swung open and closed behind us as soon as we were inside.

Contrary to the CT scan room where I had been alone with the machine, this room was a lively place, mostly occupied by outpatients and a variety of technicians.

After a long wait where no one seemed aware of my presence, a man in shirtsleeves greeted me.

"You're Doctor Mitchell's patient, aren't you? I'm Doctor Timoshenko, his assistant, and will prepare you for the actual procedure. Please remove everything metallic you are wearing, like your watch and your rings."

A nurse holding a little plastic box was standing next to me, her hand outstretched in anticipation.

"I can only remove the ring on my left hand," I volunteered, "my other hand is paralyzed." Didn't she realize that herself? Without a word she slipped the ring from my right finger, removed my watch, and proceeded to tackle my earrings. I wanted to scream! I was systematically being stripped of my identity, and felt the last vestige of myself disappearing into the little white box.

"I need to take your glasses, too." Reluctantly, I relinquished my remaining hold on reality. Anything could happen to me now, and I couldn't even see my aggressors!

Dr. Timoshenko wheeled me into another room where I could dimly see several people in lab coats seated before computers. Beyond this outer room was the actual chamber with the large white machine into which I would be placed during the test. Now Dr. Timoshenko and another man seized the sheet on which I was lying on both sides and at the familiar count of three hoisted my body onto the platform of the machine. I felt the hard, cold surface against my spine and hoped that I would not have to remain in this position very long. With deft hands, the two men strapped me down to the table, first making sure that I was covered by a flannel sheet. Then a strip of adhesive tape across my forehead tethered my head to the platform and gave the finishing touch to my immobilized, mummylike state.

"Here are earplugs to block out the noise made by the machine." What else was part of the preparation? I was beginning to feel utterly dehumanized, and this was only the preparation! With their work apparently completed, the two men left me alone. A dull, whirring sound came from somewhere in the machine; I could vaguely hear voices on the other side of the window that looked into the next room. Just then the door was flung open, and Dr. Mitchell entered with a technician. His usual cordial greeting sounded oddly remote through the rubber earplugs that a moment later, when the machine was turned on, did little to drown out the penetrating noise like a jackhammer all around my head. Before I was fully aware what was happening, the entire platform on which I was lying slid soundlessly into the machine that now encased my head. I could only make out that the top of the enclosure was just inches from my face. This was the moment I had been dreading, and I sensed raw panic flooding over me. I could feel my breath coming in short gasps, and in spite of the chilly air that had bothered me moments before, I felt that I was burning up and had to get out of this place. But before I could act on this impulse, I told myself that I was not the third grader wrapped in a curtain and that there was plenty of air inside the box enclosing my head so that I would not suffocate. I closed my eyes, took several deep breaths and slowly felt my equilibrium returning. I then surrendered myself to the state of imprisonment and waited for whatever was ahead.

After what seemed to be hours, I saw Dr. Mitchell's striped shirt through the small overhead mirror.

"How are you doing?" I could hardly distinguish his voice over the clanging knock of the jackhammer. "Are you ready to begin? First, with your left hand and then with your right, open and close your fist as quickly as you can for thirty seconds. Wait until I say 'go.'" He glanced at his watch, then signaled with his hand and voice that I was to begin. The left hand was easy, but when the procedure was repeated with the right hand, I could not make the fingers move, no matter how hard I tried. The sheer effort of racing against the clock with nothing to show for it, was overwhelming, but I remembered my discussion of this with Dr. Mitchell before the test.

"I'm only looking for brain activity while you attempt the movement." His response had been reassuring, at least for the moment. This got me through the second half of the test, touching each of my fingers to the thumb with equal lack of success on the right side.

At the end of this trial, Dr. Mitchell patted my hand approvingly.

"You did very well." He gave me a broad smile. "In about ten minutes you'll be finished." He left the test chamber, and I was once again by myself. The clanging abated slightly. At least, I could expect an end to the ordeal.

I wondered why, after Dr. Mitchell had completed his experiment, I had to remain in the machine, but all signs of human staffing of the machine had vanished on the other side of the window, and I was once again all alone. Time seemed at a standstill; I recalled a story from the *New Yorker* that my father had told me when I was a little girl. An elderly lady lived alone with her servants in a brownstone house with an elevator. On a Friday night, after the butler and cook had gone off for the weekend, the woman got stuck in the elevator. She knew she could not expect anyone to find her until the servants returned on Sunday night, and in order to maintain both her mental and physical health until that time, she fashioned a totally rational plan for spending the next 48 hours in the elevator. When her servants found her on Sunday night, she was not only quite composed, but aside from feeling parched and empty, in good condition. Although I had long since forgotten the details of the woman's ordeal, her resourcefulness and self-control remained as a metaphor for survival under adverse conditions. I now invented a plan for an eventual escape if no one came back to liberate me within a reasonable time. But what was reasonable? I asked myself, and how would I know how much time had elapsed? Before I could ponder these questions, one of the technicians entered, removed the adhesive tape and the other fetters, and placed me back on the mattress of the stretcher that was a welcome relief from the granitelike surface of the machine platform.

The nurse with the little white box was no longer in the outside room. Who would return my belongings to me? An attendant with a Herculean build approached my stretcher.

"Do you know where my glasses and other belongings are?"

"Yes, I have them." He handed me my glasses and one by one brought out my rings, earrings, and watch.

"I need help with putting on everything except my glasses and one ring. I don't suppose you've ever put a pair of earrings on a woman?" I teased him, secretly hoping that he would become flustered at my question.

"Oh, sure, I have a wife and two daughters." Undaunted, with deft fingers, he replaced my earrings. Once again, as he leaned over me with his big hulk, I felt my private space invaded, but he sensed nothing of this and after completing his task wheeled me outside the MRI suite to a "holding station," where other patients on stretchers and in wheelchairs were also waiting to be returned to their floors. We were not a happy group; on the stretcher next to me a tiny, shriveled old woman was weeping quietly to herself, while a heavyset middle-aged man on the other side moaned loudly in pain. In the far corner of the room, a seemingly disoriented figure in a hospital gown swore loudly and effusively at no one in particular. Yet no one at the desk paid the slightest attention to any of us. The laughter and teasing of the orderlies and nurses at the desk continued. I recalled an illustration of the powerlessness of the individual patient I had frequently used in my teaching: a ladderlike hierarchy of the hospital staff with a small, nondescript patient on the bottom rung. I was struck again by the feeling of powerlessness not only in terms of myself, but more importantly, any of the other patients to whom the hospital was a strange, bewildering place where no one was willing to listen, much less understand their fear, pain, or loneliness. And I, a supposed helper, was just as vulnerable as they were. I was relieved when a female attendant, without a word, took hold of my stretcher and wheeled me back to the eighth floor.

By the end of the first week in therapy, I was standing upright with a walker and with one of the therapists at my side, taking the first halting steps. From the sheer social acceptance of devices, the wheelchair had always seemed preferable to a walker, but I was glad to be able to move forward from a standing position. At first, my grip was still so weak that I needed an auxiliary upright grab bar for my right hand, but at least I was putting my right side to some good use. Ilsa had built up the handle with ace

bandages to make the grasping surface thicker, but unless I concentrated on my hand, it would slip off inadvertently and needed to be replaced in the required position. Within days I was walking all over the rehabilitation floor and felt elated when I was able to see my visitors to the elevator.

With Romana, occupational therapy was also taking on a more functional note, albeit with simulated tasks. My least favorite activity—I groaned at the mere sight of the plastic milk crate that held plastic bottles and containers of various sizes and weights—was picking up these items one by one and placing them on the raised mat on which I was sitting. As I remembered from my clinical practice days, grasping an object was far easier than letting it go, unless the item was so heavy that I would drop it before I had a decent grip on it. This activity was clearly the most tiring I attempted, and there was a noticeable point of no return, when all of Romana's encouraging remarks could not restore the required strength to pick up another object, no matter how small or light. After the first few times of hating myself for being a quitter, I was glad that Romana recognized my readiness to work on something else until my strength had returned.

Romana had provided me with elastic shoelaces that stayed laced up and knotted in place and did not require tying. Now there were just two dressing items with which I needed help: my bra and the strap of my watch. I remembered trying to teach a one-handed bra technique to patients and usually decided with the patient that it was not worth the enormous strain nor the equally great frustration that this entailed. I had not been part of the bra-burning generation, and therefore never understood the symbolism of going without a bra. Getting into the bra was high on my priority list, and I was willing to spend the time it took to learn this elusive skill. The idea was to fasten the bra first, then slip the involved arm and the head into the opening as if putting on a tee shirt, and finally pushing the healthy arm into the other armhole. Theoretically, this works, but the reality was, at least with me, that I was left with the bra hanging on my right shoulder and around the neck. It was the closest I had come to screaming, but before I uttered a sound, I began to see the ridiculousness of the situation, and I laughed instead. I decided to put on the bra without fastening it and dressing the rest of my body; sooner or later some female would appear in the room, and I could ask her to fasten my bra.

I enjoyed speech therapy simply because Anne-Marie and I were definitely on a compatible wavelength, but I saw little progress in the clarity of my speaking. We spent much time working on silly word exercises, and I even practiced these in my room, but certain consonants like "d" and "p" were slurred and ugly sounding. When any of my colleagues or former students came to see me, I felt very self-conscious about my speech, but no one ever mentioned it, although my family often commented on the low volume of my voice during our conversations.

Although I was very grateful for the good wishes and cheerful conversation they brought, the many visitors from the University were becoming a real burden, mainly for their unpredictability. I had always found that the ID card that allowed university employees carte blanche access to the hospital to be a great help when we needed some clinical information or even for using one of the corridors as a short cut. Now the privilege of going into the hospital at any time came back to haunt me; at any hour of the day, I could expect visitors in my room, and I felt I had to be "on stage." When I told Anne-Marie that these visits were even more fatiguing than 5 to 6 hours of therapy, she suggested that I tell my drop-in guests that I had to rest my voice during mealtimes, a measure I accepted and applied gratefully.

Far better were the announced or mutually arranged visits that I anticipated with pleasure. Such a visit was from Marie, a colleague and friend who telephoned one Saturday and announced that she was bringing dinner. Marie, of Italian descent and a marvelous cook, was certain that I wasn't eating enough and needed some home cooking. She came bearing not only a delicately prepared dinner but also a bright tablecloth, real silver, cloth napkins, and pottery plates! At one of the round tables, Marie spread out her wealth, and we proceeded to have a gourmet meal while the other patients ate the usual hospital fare nearby, casting envious glances in my direction. For a moment I almost forgot that I still couldn't cut meat and had to eat everything except finger food with an awkward left hand.

After my first days on the rehabilitation floor, I decided that eating a meal alone or with a roommate in the same room that served as a bedroom was not conducive to stimulating my still lagging appetite, and so I chose to take my meals in the day room, a large open space that served as a recreation or meeting room for both patients and staff. A folding wall could be closed off to divide the space in half, thereby allowing it to be used for several purposes simultaneously. The last activity of the morning—the "upright" group—was held on one side of the wall at the same time as members of the staff met on the other to discuss the progress and eventual discharge of patients. At mealtimes, the large round tables were pulled into the center of the room and patients who wished could take their meals there. Some of us chose this setting, while others preferred the privacy of their own rooms. Since most of the staff were in the day room with the majority of the patients, it was easier there to get assistance with any aspect of a meal. Perhaps if I had not been used to watching people with chewing and swallowing difficulty eat, I too would have preferred to stay in my room during mealtimes, but after working with both chil-

dren and adults who experienced these problems, I knew the atmosphere would not be as unpleasant for me as it appeared to be for patients who did not return to the day room after their first meal there. Besides, I knew that my own eating was not up to the aesthetic standards I had been taught as a child. For a strongly right-handed person like me it was awkward to eat with the left hand, and I often ended with much of the meal in my lap.

Although the quality and the quantity of most meals were quite adequate, and those of us who had no dietary restrictions could ask for as many dishes as we wished, the plastic wrapping of the utensils and much of the food was a daily source of frustration to those of us who did not have use of two hands. Certain wrappings could be removed only by helping with the teeth or developing other questionable methods for tearing the plastic. When one of us had devised a technique that seemed particularly effective, we quickly shared it with the others. To me, this teaching aspect was particularly important; it was the first small sign that I was reclaiming a part of my former self.

Mealtimes were also useful for seeing the similarities and differences among patients in response to their disability. I marveled at the way that premorbid personality surfaced and either aided or impeded progress in different patients. A tiny, very old lady whose strong accent I recognized as Viennese complained and demanded things in a penetrating voice throughout each meal. She was quite deaf and could not hear when one of the nurses told her she would come right away and so continued calling for help. I soon found out that the only way to calm her down was to sit next to her and engage her in conversation close to her ear. She then cheered up instantly and listened to my shouted explanations that help was on its way. Mrs. Siegel told me repeatedly about many aspects of her life, particularly her age—she was 93—and the fact that she was now cut off from her sister in California because she could not hear her on the telephone. At home she had a special phone; in fact, since she had no family here, she had to rely on a friend who was not really a friend. Her repertoire of conversation topics remained constant from meal to meal, and I soon became familiar with her litany of complaints. She frequently whimpered that the physical therapists made her work too hard by forcing her to stand with her walker and take steps. Looking at the tiny, frail, and unhappy woman, I almost agreed with her, but I was pleasantly surprised when several days after our first encounter, I saw her slowly taking steps pushing the walker, still complaining about working too hard.

Seating arrangements for meals in the day room were up to us—one of the few choices we had. I usually sat with the same crowd who was by nature, and as a circumstance of their diagnoses, most communicative. Mrs. Gold, who at first could not find her way anywhere on the rehabilitation floor, was my steady companion as we dragged our walkers along the hall to the dayroom for meals. Once there, we would sit together because that seemed to be the simplest way to deal with her. According to Mrs. Gold, she never got the dishes she had ordered, but when I looked at the menu on her tray that she herself had completed the day before, she usually had not circled the missing items on her order, and I had to listen to her complaints during the whole meal. When I could not seem to satisfy her demands, she called whatever staff person whom she could see in the day room, addressing them with a loud, "Mi-iss!" no matter who they were. The residents often visited their patients at meals, when the doctors knew that the patients were not in one of the therapies. They were frequently the only staff in sight, but Mrs. Gold did not discriminate in the persons selected to carry out her demands; generally, the young doctors chuckled at these requests for help and good-naturedly said they would call one of the aides. Mrs. Gold and I then agreed that it would be more reasonable if I helped her fill out the menu for the following day to assure that she would get the dishes she had selected. Filling out the menu then became part of our daily ritual; I would read aloud the choices to Mrs. Gold who said that she could not see enough to read the menu. When she had made her selection, I held the pencil and circled the items with my very awkward left hand much as I did when I completed my own menu. I marveled that the helpers in the kitchen could decipher which dishes I had actually circled since my scribbles on the page hardly resembled circles. But I knew that handwriting difficulties were a rather commonplace deficit among most of the patients on the rehabilitation floor.

Almost every one of us was eager to take advantage of the therapies. Although we each had at least two 30-minute sessions of individual treatment of each type of therapy daily, there were always other people around who were simultaneously working with their therapists. Only speech therapy was private, a fact that made it much easier for me. As a result of spending so much time with the rehabilitation patients, I became very familiar with the rate or degree of progress of other people and they with mine. Pretty much everything we did in therapy was public knowledge, and for me, this served as a strong motivation to try to succeed at everything I was asked to do. Both Ilsa and Romana expected more of us each day, and in spite of being naturally fearful and in a constant state of fatigue, I tried to rise to the challenges of their demands. When I was successful, my flickering battery of self-esteem felt recharged. But at the end of each day of therapy, in spite of steady progress, I was so drained of energy that I dragged myself back to my room just to sit and relax a few moments before it was time to walk back to the dayroom for dinner. Usually there were already visitors waiting for me, and I was forced to muster a new round of power for conversation and answers to the well-meaning inquiries about my progress.

After 3 weeks in rehabilitation my life had settled into a routine that served as a stable background for the changes in my body and, I suppose, my soul. I became aware that I was living only in the present; I did not dwell much on the past because that could be painful, but I also did not think ahead about my future. As long as I was in rehab, I must still be moving ahead, and so I really did not think of myself as a fixed being, but rather as a work in progress. Since I was still sleeping fitfully, I often found myself at night in a state of semiconsciousness, when I envisioned the same image of myself. I was a paper doll folded at the waist because the upper half of my body was not strong enough to allow me to stand upright. By morning this had faded back into my subconscious, but every night it returned. During the day, there were many opportunities to prove to myself that I could indeed do more than stand upright. My activities with both Ilsa and Romana had taken on a more practical tone; in occupational therapy, we practiced getting in and out of the bathtub, and I actually went to the grocery store of Easy Street to do some "shopping." There was a small shopping cart in the store, the kind found in New York City neighborhood grocery stores. My task was to pick up various items from the shelf, place them in the shopping cart, and walk to the cash register. Each of the plastic fruits and vegetables and the empty boxes of cereal or containers of detergent were filled with a substance that calibrated its approximate real weight. I was expected to use my right hand for all one-handed tasks and could use my left hand only to assist with normally bilateral activities. After picking up a simulated tomato, a cucumber, and a banana out of the vegetable bin, my arm was totally worn out. Letting go of the objects was almost harder than picking them up; my right hand hovered over the basket until I was able to release whatever I held in my hand. Although I had done similar tasks with patients for many years, I had never imagined that fatigue was the constant companion of even the simplest tasks.

Although I still tired quickly with any type of physical activity, I experienced the massive fatigue more totally when using my right hand. When I reached the end of my muscle power, I felt literally like a windup toy that had run down and needed a new boost, one that was not immediately available to me. I was surprised how long it took before I felt ready to use the hand or arm again for a task requiring lifting of any but the lightest items. This was one of the few areas where I felt that the therapists did not fully understand that when a patient states unequivocally, as I did on several occasions, "I can't do it again; I'm exhausted!" that a 2-minute rest period won't restore the expended energy. I began to wonder whether, as a practicing therapist, I had been as sensitive to each patient's fatigue as I should; I sent a silent apology to the many patients I had treated years ago.

I had never experienced the kind of massive exhaustion that now held my body in its grip. It was probably apparent to others in the breathlessness I experienced many times during the day, especially when I was walking and talking at the same time. This brought to mind the old dare we tried on one another as children: "Try rubbing your stomach and patting the top of the head at the same time!" I did not succeed even as a child, and the memory of that made me smile somewhat ruefully each time I had another breathless episode. When I mentioned these to Anne-Marie, she suggested I try to slow down my speech in normal conversation and continue to practice in my room the breathing exercise I did with her twice every day—blowing as hard as I could into a thick tube that was connected to a plastic bottle with a calibrated gauge that registered the volume of my lung capacity. The gauge was useful in measuring my progress, but I never advanced beyond a certain point, in spite of Anne-Marie's motivating cheers. For the rest of my body, there did not seem to be an immediate remedy. I always knew I had reached the end of my energy supply when I began to experience actual nausea and a strong desire to lie down and shut off the world. I never acted on the impulse, however; instead, I simply sat down on whatever surface was available and waited for my equilibrium to be restored. Generally, that did not take longer than 5 minutes, and no one ever questioned my "time out."

My days took on another dimension when a patient called Ben became more visible on the rehabilitation floor and took his meals with the rest of us. He was younger than I by about 10 years, but like me, he had survived a stroke that affected his right arm and leg; he also had considerable slurring in his speech and, because the paralysis affected his chewing and swallowing muscles, he was on a special pureed diet. As a result, his tray always included many small dishes of unappetizing-looking pureed food of varying colors and several soft desserts. At first, he preferred to eat alone in his room or at a table by himself in a corner of the large day room, but one day I asked him to move to our table, mainly because I sensed he would be a better communicator than some of the other people.

I recognized him from the various therapies, especially the movement group where his attempts at kickball or ring toss were as unsuccessful as mine most of the time. He caught my immediate attention by his unfailing sense of humor that resounded readily with me. I had decided that among other sequelae of the stroke, the slow, awkward way of carrying out most every day activities would appear utterly ridiculous if compared to my past life; I could tolerate my present lack of speed only if I looked upon my performance as being a caricature of myself. Many of the quips that Ben tossed out to the group in general indicated to me that he operated on an equal wavelength with me. When we were not sitting at the table with the others, we sat in other parts of the day-room, from where he and I could joke or make sarcastic comments about the food, the routine, and the other patients without being heard. Our favorite topic was, of course, Mrs. Gold, who gave us ample material for a new script each day. She felt that most therapy was a waste of time and was quite vocal about this, especially in the "upright group," individually adapted to meet the needs of every member of the group. A staff person carefully monitored each of us, since most were unsteady at best in an upright position. During one of our particularly lively games that must have looked grotesque to the uninitiated, Mrs. Gold announced in a loud voice, "I think this is a big waste of time!" Thereafter, from our corner Ben and I invented situations where we would tell Mrs. Gold that the doctors and therapists had selected her as captain of all team sports or other similar crazy ideas. Ben grew so enamored with his ideas that at times I felt I had to restrain him from carrying out the pranks. Although this was surely not my proudest hour, it helped to diminish the reality of our condition that confronted us every waking moment of each day. With Ben I could count on being amused, and our shared laughter had a beneficial effect on both of us. Every afternoon just before dinner Ben's wife Charlotte appeared and stayed with him until visiting hours had ended. From what I learned, they had married less than 10 years ago, and she appeared to be a housewife, free to spend many hours of each day at the hospital. The couple readily accepted me in their hospital dinners, and I was grateful to have one meal daily away from the complainers.

I knew that I was progressing well, but I was still walking with a walker and using my right hand only to assist my left. The walker was light to move about, but it was wider than I was and required enough space to get into the places that were part of my present environment. As a result I missed most of my phone calls, because the phone was on the nightstand on the right side of my bed and meant walking around the bed to answer it. Maneuvering the walker and myself into the narrow space between the window and the bed took me much longer than most callers were willing to wait. No matter how quickly I tried to move—and my quickest pace still resembled that of a sloth—I never reached the phone before the caller had hung up. Much as I tried to tell my callers that they should let the phone ring at least a dozen times, anyone who called for the first time did not reach me. At first, this was a source of frustration and disappointment, but after a while I realized that I was not in control of this, and I accepted the missed calls as a matter of course.

I had now reached the third week in rehab. One of the most dramatic physical challenges was climbing the set of four or five practice steps in the gym. Even with the aid of the banister on the left, going up was bad enough, but when I arrived at the platform on the top and faced forward, the sight of the steps below me was a daunting prospect that made my heart beat madly. How would I get down? I was suddenly transported back to my childhood to the Sunday hikes in the German evergreen forest that frequently ended with a climb of the deserted observation tower for hunters and forest rangers. My father deemed that this activity would be a healthy challenge to my brother and me. Although Jeff was quite unathletic and much preferred reading to sports, he did have the advantage of being older by a year and a half and thereby having longer legs. Outwardly, at least, he showed no fear. Scaling the ladder meant going up the rickety rungs that were much too far apart for my short legs, but I was expected to follow my brother. Under loud protestations I actually reached the top. My immediate expression of victory was clouded by the dreaded moment when I would have to descend. As the simultaneously ambitious and compliant child that I was, I never thought of refusing the climb up, especially when my older brother accomplished this without difficulty, but when I saw how far I had come and realized that the tiny man below with the smiling upturned face was really my father, I froze and sobbed that I couldn't come down. Eventually, my father's encouraging words and explicit directions on placement of each foot guided me down, but it spoiled the hike for me for that day and many days to come when I realized the performance had to be repeated. Now I could feel the same terror, but Ilsa was less than 6 feet below; the sight of her brought me back to the present, and to the entirely achievable task of descending the steps, again holding on to the banister on the left side.

When I saw how difficult it was to accommodate to the early bedtime routine of the hospital—if I went to sleep at 9 o'clock, as many of the patients did, I woke at 2 AM and lay awake waiting for dawn and the 5:30 reveille without ever falling asleep again—after a week of this, I decided to go into the deserted day room and read. No one objected to my being there, since by now all the nurses knew that I did not need help getting myself ready for bed. I soon discovered that this was the hour and place for the aides' dinner, but they tolerated my presence on the other side of the room with cheerful indifference. Instead of reading—I still found it difficult to concentrate for an extended period of time—I watched whatever "drama" the aides had selected as their dinner accompaniment on the large-screen television and listened to their high-spirited banter in the Caribbean patois I had come to love after many visits to the islands. The performances on the screen fascinated me by their sheer novelty; in my white, middle-class culture I had never tuned in to an all black channel. Now I watched the screenplays and commercials in which all black stars were featured, accompanied by the comments of the aides. A favorite topic of conversation was the Caribbean food that some of them brought from their homes. Although I was extremely interested to see what they were eating, I did not want to spoil my coveted role of silent participant-observer in their mealtimes. At the end of an hour, with a collective sigh as someone glanced at her watch, the dinner break ended, and they quickly cleaned up the remains of their meal before returning to their posts. One of them always passed close to my chair to hand me the remote control. Now I was truly on my own, sitting in the semidark with only the huge screen of the television coming between me and the drowsiness that overcame me shortly after I was left alone. I don't think I ever saw the end of a program that I had selected. With my last bit of energy I pushed my walker through the silent corridor to my room, where I soon joined Mrs. Gold in sleep.

Whether it was part of the denial that carried me through the first few days following the onset of the stroke or another part of my psyche, I found myself on several occasions using the "magical thinking" that many of my patients employed to escape a painful reality. More than once, when I arrived in my room after a particularly exhausting day, I found myself wishing for a miracle. A soundless voice from a part of myself that I rarely used would say to me, "For just five minutes, I would like to feel normal again so I could move with ease!" I never considered what would happen when those 5 minutes were up; that was part of the magical thinking, of course. Once I had uttered that wish and cried for a moment with the certainty of knowing I was asking for the impossible, I somehow felt empowered again to carry on.

I was really so much better than I had been; I no longer wore the splint during the day and began to use my right hand more spontaneously. At night, as a precaution, I put the splint on for several additional days, and then developed the habit of putting my hand under the pillow so that the weight of my head would keep the fingers from curling up and the wrist supported. In occupational therapy, Romana and I were working on my handwriting; at this point we were still unsure whether I should switch to using the left hand. As children we had all practiced writing with the left hand, as many of my classmates did, but I never perfected this skill and now found it awkward and fatiguing. With the right hand, at first, the pen or pencil often fell from my grasp. Romana had a large selection of adapted pens, all of which I tried with limited success. Whenever I practiced writing, I was reminded of a visit by one of the rehabilitation physicians who, after reading my chart, quipped in an almost jovial way:

"You should do very well, but you'll never get your handwriting back." With that, he left the room. I was furious and hurt. How could he predict my recovery merely from reading my medical chart? Since I never saw him again, I did not even have the satisfaction of asking him to explain the basis of his prognosis. Nevertheless, Romana and I continued in our efforts to find a writing utensil that was really useful for me. I was given sheets of writing exercises (large script on wide lines not unlike the ones that I remembered from elementary school when learning to write for the first time). I traced over the sample letters and then completed the sheet on my own with varying results. Like with everything else, I tired rapidly; I also found this activity to be terribly boring, and I had to force myself to do it in the rare moments without prescribed activity or visitors.

At the end of the fourth week, the entire rehab team discussed my case as reported to me by Dr. Stuart, who had been my attending physician and in charge of all the patients on our floor. She and I related easily to one another, first, because we had attended the same department meetings for several years, and second, because as women, we had a similar perspective on many aspects of life. Now she reported that the team had agreed that I should be ready for discharge in 7 days, exactly 5 weeks from the date of my second admission. This would give me time to work on additional tasks that were important for my particular lifestyle—living alone in an apartment on the northern fringes of New York City. My initial reaction was neither surprise nor alarm. I was familiar with the regulations that medical insurance dictated the maximum length of stay by diagnosis, not status. I knew that by the date that Dr. Stuart mentioned, I would have received the maximum number of days of inpatient treatment covered for a stroke.

Until that moment I had not allowed myself to think a great deal about discharge; now I had to face the outside world with the residual changes wrought by the stroke. The first thing that came to mind was that I really was ashamed to be seen in my community with a walker that to me signified a far greater degree of dependency than I was willing to accept. It also would place me in a large group of elderly people who, for one reason or another, used walkers to get around our community, usually accompanied by another person. I hated the thought of joining that group at this point in my life, and again I realized the importance for me to get on the cane as quickly as possible. The cane had become a metaphor for an older but independent person.

My three therapists, Romana, Ilsa, and Anne-Marie, all talked to me about the discharge date and the goals I wanted to attain before leaving the hospital. Clearly, I had to be able to prepare meals for myself, and increase my endurance, not only for speaking without getting out of breath but also for tackling the five-block walk to the grocery store. Before we could put into practice any of these plans, I was faced by another weekend without therapy, and this time I really resented the forced idleness imposed by the 5-day treatment schedule. On Saturdays

the two recreation therapists were in charge of keeping our minds and bodies stimulated, and since I had seen for 3 weeks that attendance at the morning current events group and the afternoon cooking group was sparse, I decided to join the groups once more in a show of collegial solidarity. I felt much closer to the other patients during therapy and meals where our disabilities formed a common bond. It was much harder to feel the same connection when we had a somewhat artificial conversation about sports or the latest scandal from the *Daily News*. Still, I gave the two young therapists a great deal of credit for their enthusiasm and inventiveness week after week.

On Monday, my rehabilitation took on a new note of immediacy; there were only 4 days of therapy before leaving the hospital! Both Ilsa and Romana had prepared a list of very practical activities they wanted me to perform before Friday, which included preparing my habitual lunch from a shopping list prepared by myself, as well as walking outside and taking a ride on a city bus with Ilsa along in the event that I needed assistance. Ilsa and Romana had also planned a home visit with me to see if any changes were needed in the setup of my apartment. It seemed to be an awful lot for me to accomplish in the short time, but the therapists assured me that we could get everything done. After this afternoon's walk outside on the street, Ilsa would be able to judge if I could exchange the walker for a cane.

Wisely, Ilsa had decided that I needed to save my energy for the actual walk in the street; I could therefore use the wheelchair until we were outside. Our first stop on this venture was the elevator that would take us down to the lobby. I realized that there were many hurdles along the way that 6 weeks before would have been just routine parts of dealing mindlessly with the interaction of human beings and technology. Suppose I could not wheel myself through the open doors of the elevators before they closed again automatically? Was I strong enough to manage the various doors that led to the busy hospital lobby? Thank goodness, Ilsa was there to ward off any real danger. I could feel the fierce beating of my heart as the elevator stopped on our floor. I rolled over the threshold into the narrow space left by the other passengers before the doors closed behind us and then rolled out again at the lobby level. One hurdle had been conquered. I exhaled gratefully and approached the entrance to the lobby feeling somewhat less anxious.

As we left the hospital building I realized that this was the first fresh air I had breathed in 5 weeks. I had missed most of July and within the air-conditioned rooms of the hospital had forgotten how oppressive the August heat could be in New York. Now it hit me as I stood up and took hold of the walker. Before I took the first steps on the sidewalk Ilsa bent toward me: "There's a good chance that you'll meet up with some of the people you know around here; do you think that will that bother you?"

I was touched by her sensitivity. In the same way that I had felt when the first colleague had approached my bed when the news of my stroke reached the university, I decided that only the first encounter would be difficult. Before I had a chance to ponder this, I saw a colleague crossing the street and approaching me.

"Hi, how are you? It's good to see you again!" He treated me quite normally, and I knew I would have little difficulty relating to other colleagues in the same way. Not until I left the hospital environment would I have to deal with the questions I expected from my neighbors. At this moment, I was much more concerned with managing the uneven pavement and the hazards of crossing the street that Ilsa had included in the itinerary.

For the last 25 years of my professional life, this had been one of the most familiar corners; it was the intersection where the university and the hospital met. How many times in all seasons had I crossed here, running to and from classes, going to my office and the administration building? It was a bustling, unruly place, teeming with students, medical personnel, and ambulatory patients, some patiently waiting for the light and others, perennially rushed, darting between the traffic to make it quickly to the other side. Gypsy cabs, unmindful of either traffic lights or the people, were everywhere, adding to the noise and confusion by blasting their horns at the slightest provocation. Did Ilsa really expect me to get into the midst of this?

"I don't think I can make it across before the light changes." I hoped that she would agree with me, and we could call the whole thing off.

"Of course you can! Just don't stop walking. Besides, I'll be right next to you."

I knew that I could trust Ilsa not to set a challenge beyond my ability to meet it, and so, when the light turned the next time, I stepped off the curb and met the onrushing pedestrian traffic. Again I could hardly breathe for the wild beating of my heart. Was this going to be my partner in every new situation facing me? This time I felt almost overwhelmed; Ilsa's presence served both as a protective and an empowering mantle whenever a menacing task was ahead, and now, too, I made it safely to the other side. But I was not yet free to gloat over my victory.

"Now let's go back. Cars will stop when they see the walker," Ilsa was as confident as ever, and I could not disappoint her. I held my breath and dragged myself back across the street. The waiting wheelchair was a welcome haven, and I sank back into it, too exhausted to speak. Would every outing require that much courage as well as energy? Where would I find an endless supply of both? Once again I was reminded how much the stroke had taken from me. Could I really reclaim the missing parts of my former self?

Ilsa's cheerful voice roused me.

"You made it, you see! You also showed me that tomorrow we can start with the cane." I immediately cheered up and could hardly wait to tell my family about my accomplishments.

Helen then told me of her decision to stay with me at my apartment for at least a week, thereby eliminating the need for home care from a stranger. This piece of news cheered me enormously, since the thought of having a stranger stay with me was thoroughly unappealing and had caused me a great deal of concern. After my outing with the walker, there were only four days of hospitalization left. As promised, Ilsa had a cane waiting for me in physical therapy the next morning. I took my first steps rather unsteadily, with Ilsa holding the back of my slacks for support. It was difficult to think of all the parts of walking simultaneously and sequentially. Compared to the walker, the cane had a much narrower base of support. I was grateful that I was not totally on my own as I walked along the long corridor. In order to give me additional practice, a young male therapy aide was given the job of walking with me twice each day around the extended quadrangle that covered the entire eighth floor.

I had done my homework for Romana for the next day: making a list of all the items I would need for the salad I was to prepare in the occupational therapy kitchen. It had taken me almost half an hour to print out the names of six vegetables! And they were barely legible. At least I had found a built-up pencil that I could grasp, and Romana had given it to me to take home. However, for today I was to remove and replace the sheets on the bed in the Easy Street apartment. This was a task I remembered well from my days of being a clinician: one-handed bed making is a slow, arduous procedure; the help that my right hand could offer at this point reduced neither the effort nor the length of time that elapsed until the bedspread was safely back on the bed. Changing the pillowcase was especially hard; all the two-handed steps that turn this into an efficient, easily done task now became mostly unilateral. Since I was still too unsteady with the cane, I had to use the walker. I circled the bed a dozen times to tuck in sheets and the blanket, but I proved to Romana and myself that I was capable of performing this task by myself; once I got home, only I would need to know how much time and energy it cost!

I had progressed sufficiently to be eating most of each meal with my right hand in an awkward manner. At first, my hand often overshot its mark, and the food dropped back on the plate or in my lap. I was plagued more by the lack of coordination now than by the weakness. Also, I had discovered another annoying aspect of hand function over which I had no control; whenever I coughed or was surprised by an unexpected noise, my hand shot up and I dropped whatever I was holding. Worst of all, if I was startled while I held a cup of juice or coffee, I would spill the liquid all over the table. The first time this happened was during lunch at our large round table. I was holding a roll in my right hand and was ready to take a bite when an uncontrollable cough shook my body. My hand shot up and flung the roll across the room in what must have looked like very crazy behavior. I looked around quickly to see if anyone had noticed, but luckily, everyone was too absorbed with his or her own meals. Though I was initially amused at my action, it was a painful reminder of the extent of neurological damage I had incurred. How many years I had explained to my students that "a brain injury can actually 'undo' the learning that has occurred in the neurological system in the course of normal development of an infant. All of us are born with a 'startle' reflex that makes an infant raise its arms in response to a loud noise or sudden striking of the surface on which the baby lies. This reflex is suppressed as part of normal development. A stroke will undo the suppression, and the reflex operates as in early infancy." Now as I lay awake in the early hours of the following day, I recognized that this had actually happened to me as part of the larger picture of irreversible neurological loss. All of my recovery thus far was probably due to the fact that the brain is such a versatile organ with spare neurological pathways that can take over lost functions. This was powerful stuff, and while I accepted it as theoretical information, I was not ready to accept it as inevitable fact. When I next saw Dr. Mitchell, I asked him whether I would ever lose the startle reflex. His answer was terse but friendly, "Probably not."

As planned, Ilsa and Romana met me at 10 AM the next morning to do the home visit at my apartment. At the front door of the hospital, one of them hailed a cab. Since neither of them knew the way to my house, I felt totally in charge of this outing. I gave the driver instructions of the route that had brought me home every day—not seated in the back of a taxi, to be sure—but relishing the short, pleasant drive along the Hudson in back of the wheel of my own car. Now as I watched the trees and the sky flash by, I wondered whether I would ever be capable of enjoying the degree of independence that both night and day driving of my car had allowed. Thank goodness, that was not one of my immediate concerns.

I was surprised at the amount of anticipation that I now felt as the taxi turned the last corner and swung into the driveway of the apartment building. Except for one brief visit by Helen to fetch me more shirts and slacks, no one had entered the apartment since I had left it almost 5 weeks ago. A quick composite of Sleeping Beauty and Rip van Winkle flashed across my mind; would the rooms be covered by cobwebs?

The doorman rushed from the building when the cab pulled up; his face lit up with a huge smile as he opened the door.

"Welcome back! How are you?" He extended his arm and helped me out of the car, flanked by the two therapists. Before we could enter the building, however, I had to mount the single step that led up to the front door. In more than 10 years of living in this place, I had never noticed that there was no railing and was genuinely surprised to see that oversight now.

"Yipes!" was the only word I could utter. In her usual calm manner, Ilsa called out.

"Just use the technique you used on the practice curbs in the gym." I was very glad that she was standing next to me as I mounted the step.

Everything looked pleasantly familiar as I crossed the lobby and went up the three steps to the elevator, this time firmly holding on to the banister. Even taking stairs with the cane presented few problems now that I could carry the cane in my right hand while the left grasped the railing.

I felt as if I were welcoming new friends to my home as I unlocked the door. My absence from the familiar rooms suddenly seemed much longer than the actual 5 weeks. I could recall coming home from college after a semester away from home; there was always a comfortable recognition of the furnishings, but I was no longer the same person who had left. This time I was returning from a journey to unexplored terrain, and my physical relationship to the objects was changed as well.

Romana's voice brought me back to reality.

"Is it OK if we just look around?" I knew the considerations of a routine home visit, and I pointed out to Romana all the features of accessibility and safety they would be looking for: no scatter rugs to trip on, the placement of kitchen utensils and dishes that I had to use every day, the location of the telephone, and the layout of the bathroom.

"You'll need a bench for the shower, and we'll order that in the hospital today. Otherwise, the apartment looks good and you should be able to manage everything."

"Did you really think that an occupational therapist's apartment would be full of hazards?" I couldn't resist the chance to tease the therapists.

Leaving the apartment after such a brief visit was less difficult than I had thought it would be. There were several things I needed to practice while I was still in rehabilitation, such as the cooking experience and the ride on the city bus. Besides, Mrs. Gold was going home today, and I actually looked forward to the next 2 days alone.

That evening for the first time I allowed myself to think about what it would be like at home. I realized how much I had employed denial as a useful method of dealing with an unpleasant or unacceptable reality. I could make the problem disappear temporarily by just not thinking about it; when it next confronted me, as it inevitably did, I was more ready to face it and work on a solution. Although I would not recommend this style of problem solving to anyone else, it had certainly worked for me until now. Therefore, I was finally ready to concentrate on life at home, fully aware that there were hazards and hurdles that would have to be surmounted, and

I would somehow manage them as I had all the previous ones during my rehabilitation. Thank goodness, I had learned long ago to hide my fears quite well and thereby keep face. I recognized once again how unacceptable it was to me to lose face. With these thoughts I finally drifted off to sleep.

Practicing the various curbs while using the cane was my assignment in physical therapy next morning. At one point, Ilsa made a seemingly innocent comment about doing this alone once I was home. Suddenly, all the emotions that I had kept to myself for 5 weeks broke the thin shell that held them in check; I was caught completely off guard and burst into uncontrollable tears. Ilsa, seeing my state, quickly ushered me into an empty back room, where I spent the next 20 minutes sobbing noisily in a way that was completely foreign to me. Try as I might, I could not stop crying. Ilsa tactfully left me alone and even brought me moist paper towels for my red eyes when the torrent seemed to be abating. The enormity of what had happened had finally dawned on me. I was totally overcome by the thought of leaving the safe haven of the rehabilitation floor where we all had problems and had been completely sheltered from the outside world. No explanation about one's condition was necessary, and if anyone needed medical or psychological help, it was always available. Now I would have to cut through all the red tape that stood between the health care system and me. And then the dreaded "S" word flashed through my mind; suppose I would have a second stroke! I knew that the threat of a second stroke was much greater than that for the first time; the only preventable factor in my own case was keeping the blood pressure under control. The twice-daily reading of blood pressure had made me painfully aware that it fluctuated considerably from day to day. Before this episode I had never been concerned about my blood pressure, which, as I was repeatedly told by my doctor at my annual checkup, was within normal limits for my age. In the hospital I was on the verge of panic when it seemed particularly high one day. I asked to see Dr. Mitchell since I was sure I was having a second stroke. He reassured me that this was not the case and to be prepared for the frequent ups and downs. After his visit I felt ashamed about my hysterical reaction, but it was a fear that did not leave me. Who would respond to my cries for help from home? As always, I calmed myself by calling on my reasoning system.

At last I felt that my equilibrium was at least partially restored. Although I was drained by the experience, it was a necessary part of the healing process.

I realized how long I had been in the back room when I saw Romana searching for me; she was ready to take me through the salad-making experience that would give her a chance to observe my performance in the kitchen. I hoped that my red eyes were not too obvious as I followed her into the occupational therapy kitchen where a bag with the salad ingredients on my shopping list was waiting for me.

"I know I don't have to show you any of the equipment or the techniques," she laughed, "You probably know them better than I do. I'll just observe you from here. I'd like to try out a new test on you; it includes such aspects of your performance as safety, sequencing, and time. Please use your right or both hands whenever you can, especially for removing dishes from the cabinets."

Romana was right; I had been through countless cooking experiences with patients. In fact, cooking and baking had been among the most successful therapy sessions I had with many types of patients who needed not only to reacquire the physical skill but also to restore their self-concept and self-confidence. While I was washing lettuce and peeling the cucumber, I felt vaguely like the schoolmaster Mr. Chips, who in his dreams recalled dozens of his former pupils marching in front of him.

Romana watched me wordlessly from a corner of the large table at which I worked, sometimes standing, sometimes sitting, while the salad slowly took shape. The sequential steps were in and of themselves not difficult for me to do, mostly one-handed. I was appalled to realize how long the simple process of washing, peeling, and cutting six vegetables took—45 minutes—and all my remaining energy went into the process. Walking from sink or counter to the table meant holding the cane in my left hand. This left the weak right hand to carry objects. After the first attempt I found that this was still too difficult for me. Romana had pointed out the teacart on which I placed all the objects that ordinarily I would have carried in both hands. This, too, was familiar, but nevertheless it struck me as totally wrong that now I was the patient rather than the teacher who showed patients how to carry objects on the cart that also served as a support while walking. My reward for completing the activity was the finished salad that Romana carried to the dining room for me. Although I knew, theoretically, that walking and carrying objects would be a problem at home, the cooking experience reminded me that I still had a lot of work to do at home.

I found it difficult to believe that this had been my last full session in occupational therapy, since the afternoon's therapy would be cut short as a result of the planned bus trip to Fort Tryon Park, and, after getting off the bus and crossing the street, taking the bus back to the hospital. This was an outing I did not anticipate with pleasure. Even with Ilsa's guidance I could not see myself being able to hold the rail with my left hand while mounting the bus step in the time New York bus drivers usually allow before starting up the bus again.

The ride on the elevator and walk to the front of the hospital was almost routine for me. I was glad that I did not need many repetitions of a procedure to overcome my greatest fears. However, when the bus approached our corner, I would gladly have told Ilsa that I was not ready for this challenge. This was my last chance to practice this skill with supervision, and once more, reason took charge. I noticed that there were several other men and women of my vintage with canes waiting for the bus. I would let some of them precede me and try to watch the technique they employed. But then it was my turn. With Ilsa following close behind I moved the cane to my right hand, grasped the handrail with my left hand and pulled myself up. Ilsa managed the tokens for us while I walked to one of the seats in front that had been vacated by a younger rider when he saw me coming. Gratefully, I fell into one of the places designated "For elderly and disabled," a seat that only 5 weeks before I would gladly have left for the people who fit one of these groups. Now, involuntarily, I had joined their ranks. I was so totally preoccupied with these thoughts that I paid no attention to the passing scene or my fellow passengers, which would have been unthinkable for me before the stroke. Ilsa stood in front of me and reminded me that the next corner was the last stop, and once the bus had come to a stop, we would be getting out. Again, I feared that I would not be able to get out in time and slid to the edge of my seat to be ready as soon as the bus came to a halt. Ilsa preceded me on the way out so she could supervise my getting down the bus steps. In my eagerness to descend the steps I stumbled and would have landed on the sidewalk had Ilsa not caught me. By now I was trembling all over.

"The bus drivers will always wait until you are well outside." Ilsa's voice was reassuring, but I could tell she was not pleased by my performance. "Let's cross the street since the bus is coming." I was still completely rattled when I remounted the bus steps, but both the ascent and descent were accomplished without further incident. Still, I did not think I could ever find the courage again to ride a city bus.

I was too excited to sleep more than a few hours that night, anticipating all the good things connected to life in my own apartment. One of the most annoying things of sleeping in the hospital bed had been the rubber covering of the mattress that was stiff, hot, and noisy each time I changed my position. The thing I hated most, though, were the light blue hospital gowns, most of them too big for me, so that they resulted in a rakish, off-the shoulder look that gave me at the same time a waiflike appearance not helpful to my sagging self-confidence. Worst of all, in spite of daily washings in the hospital laundry, was the acrid smell of having been worn by too many bodies, each with its personal odor. Tomorrow I could return to my own bed and wear my own nightgown!

When dawn finally came, I relished the sight of the Hudson whose steady, relentless flow had had such a calming influence on me during the past 5 weeks. It had been a source of silent, steady support that spoke of the continuity of life even in the face of changing seasons and circumstances. It was comforting to know that it would always be there, whether I regarded it or not. The view of the river had served me well, and I wished that the sight of it would be equally calming to future inhabitants of this bed.

Even the early reveille and the sponge bath at the sink were easier to bear today, knowing that a few hours hence I would be able to put hospital life behind me. But every small part of the morning routine was tinged with a bit of sadness, nevertheless. Would I ever have that much guidance and support again from the people around me?

The head nurse breezed into my room.

"I've come to give you the prescriptions for all the medications Doctor Mitchell wants you to take. Get these filled as soon as you get home." She handed me several prescriptions in an envelope. Her visit started a procession of various staff members, each with his or her written orders for my new life. Dr. Stuart, who had checked on me almost daily, left me a prescription for another rehabilitation center where I was to take a driving evaluation when I felt ready. At this point that seemed like a distant goal, but I was pleased that she considered me a future candidate for resuming driving. Even the social worker that I had hardly ever seen told me that a visiting nurse would evaluate my need for a home health aide. For the moment, Helen would be my helper, and I was relieved that I would not need other assistance.

I had been told that I would not have therapy this morning, but my three therapists were available for final questions and instructions. It was hard to say good-bye to all three: Anne-Marie and I had laughed together over the small successes and rough going as the slurring slowly left my speech; Romana, kindness personified, yet nevertheless very businesslike when it came to all of the activities of living; and Ilsa, to whom I had formed a deep relationship based on her understanding and unfailing confidence in my ability; all three had guided my progress in a way that far exceeded my expectations. I knew I would be back for occasional visits, since I still had the unfinished research project that I was hoping to complete, and this made it easier to leave them behind. I felt I owed the therapists so much; I could never adequately express my feelings to them without breaking down.

When I returned to my room, Helen was already waiting, and I was eager to go. The obligatory wheelchair was brought by an orderly who took me down to the front door, where I happily exchanged the wheelchair for my cane and the front seat of Helen's car. At last I was free and could put life in the hospital behind me!

I felt the same kind of euphoria that always signaled the end of an examination in college. Suddenly I could understand patients with whom I had worked who relied on magical thinking that "everything will be all right once I get home." It was a way of avoiding unpleasant challenges in the hospital or confronting realities that seemed too awful to face. In my case, it was somewhat different; I was tired of practicing in simulated situations and wanted to try what is was really like to have to solve a particular problem.

On the drive home, Helen and I talked about the way we would spend the days together; her goal was to make sure I could manage taking care of myself and preparing meals with minimal help from a home care worker, whose salary for a few hours each day was covered by my insurance. We would practice walking as much as I could to build up my endurance. It seemed like a practical plan, and I was eager to get started.

My arrival at home was similar to my visit, except for one important difference; since it was later in the day, many of my neighbors were passing through the lobby on their way in or out, and I was warmly greeted by several people.

"We heard about your illness from Carlos." Leave it to the doorman to inform the entire building population! I was touched by so much concern and offers of all kinds of help by tenants I hardly knew.

When we reached my apartment, I was overcome by exhaustion and sank into an easy chair where I stayed for several hours, grateful that no one was expecting me to be anywhere or do anything. Helen plied me with food and drink, after which I felt a new surge of energy. I was surprised that the visiting nurse that was scheduled to look in on me called to announce her house call in an hour. When the doorbell rang, I picked up my cane and walked to the door to let in the visitor.

"Hello, I'm Donna Vasquez. Are you the patient?" When I nodded my head, she continued, "I expected you to be in bed! I've never had a patient greet me at the door before, you made my day!" With that she began her interview and evaluation, reviewed my medications and said she would call me the next day, but since I was already so independent and had Helen for the present, she felt that her services were not required. Besides, the home therapists were to evaluate me the next day to determine what type of physical therapy and occupational therapy were to be ordered.

Her assessment increased my confidence to the extent that, almost giddily, I suggested to Helen that we celebrate by going out to dinner, since we had no food in the house.

"Are you sure you're up to it?" Her query was prompted by genuine concern, but when I answered in the affirmative, she was ready to take me up on the suggestion. I thought it would be a good idea to face the public while I was feeling so high.

People did not even look up from their dinners when we entered. I became aware of the number of diners using canes, crutches, and wheelchairs who passed our table; I felt I was in good company. It was the last time I ever worried about the cane in public. Far more worrisome was my tortoiselike gait; everyone on the sidewalk easily passed me. In the hospital this was the normal speed with which patients progressed. Now obviously I had to compete primarily with able-bodied individuals, and the match was not a good one. Nevertheless, Helen and I enjoyed our first outing; I was beginning to shed my patient skin.

It was heavenly to sleep in my own bed again, and I slept soundly. Next morning I stepped into the tub gingerly, holding on to the sink for support and was glad to sit on the shower bench that Romana had ordered for me. The fall in the shower 5 weeks before was still fresh in my memory, and I did not want to repeat it. On the other hand, a nurse had given me a shower only twice during more than a month in the hospital, and I was ready for the experience of feeling really clean and refreshed.

As expected, the physical therapist came to assess my strength and gait. She was very young but appeared competent in checking my status. When she was finished, she gave me some exercises to do on my own but said I was too advanced for the home therapy to which I was entitled. Shortly after she had left, the occupational therapist arrived, and like Romana on the home visit, she wanted to inspect the apartment for safety hazards, after she had determined my functional status. She was older than the physical therapist and experience had seasoned her to be more thorough. We enjoyed talking shoptalk for a few minutes before she rose to leave.

"You're really doing very well, and I don't believe you need any home therapy. Just do the exercises on the staircase that I'll show you." With that she took me to the apartment house staircase where she demonstrated a number of exercises for strengthening my ankle. Then she, too, took the elevator down, leaving me in the questionable position of having lost all eligibility for further therapy because I was too well! Instead of feeling elated that all three health professionals independently of each other had pronounced me in such good condition, I felt rather abandoned and let down. Helen considered the therapists' verdict as good news, and so I agreed with her.

Now we were really on our own, rejoicing in the fact that we could schedule the time together in any way that suited our fancy. It was delightful to be free of the rigid hospital schedule!

We filled the next days with short walks and frequent rests to build up my endurance. During a trip to the supermarket by car, I found that I could use the grocery cart almost like a walker, and so could look forward to shopping by myself. I was aware that the store made deliveries, and I decided to investigate the possibility at a future time.

With every day we added another block to my destination, and although I was completely exhausted each time I reached my house, I saw that an increased distance was well within the realm of possibility. Helen allowed me to try everything in the kitchen; she knew that I would not risk doing the impossible. Finally, 7 days after I came home, I was able to walk to the supermarket and back—the goal I had set for myself. Helen and I agreed that I could carry on by myself.

As she packed her bag, we talked about the fact that my illness had brought us even closer together. Difficult though it was to say good-bye, I was eager to try to fend for myself as the new person I had become during the last 6 weeks. Seven weeks ago, the chance of my having a stroke at this time was not even in my realm of possibilities. I was anticipating many years of the good health that I enjoyed and that I considered my responsibility. Six weeks ago, when I first took my place among the seriously ill men and women in the hospital, I did not remotely envision that exactly 42 days later I would be well enough to resume my former life with only a few adjustments. But would I ever get back my prior self? Perhaps not, but as I had learned, I had been blessed with a rich dose of the resilience that allows both body and spirit to seize the second chance.

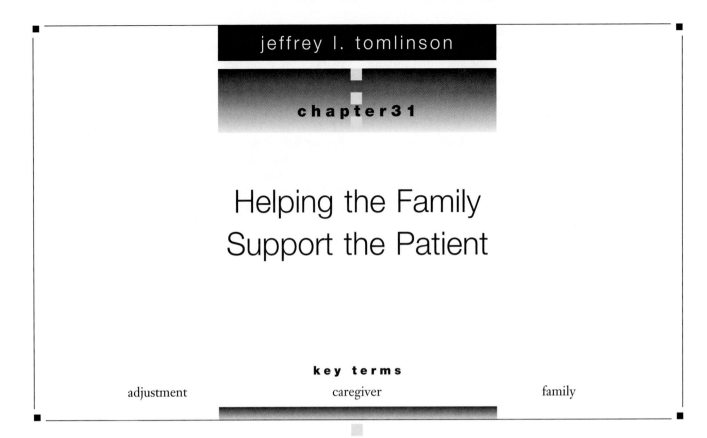

jeffrey l. tomlinson

chapter 31

# Helping the Family
# Support the Patient

**key terms**

adjustment                    caregiver                    family

**chapter objectives**

After completing this chapter, the reader will be able to accomplish the following:

1. Develop treatment plans that integrate families and caregivers.
2. Recognize the family's influence on the recovery of the stroke survivor.
3. Develop strategies to deal with difficult families.

## FAMILY'S ROLE

The patient who sustains a stroke is thrown quickly into crisis, physically and emotionally. Survival and recovery take all the patient's resources. The patient's family is one of the most important resources. The stroke patient may need extensive support in many facets of life: emotional support, financial aid, physical assistance, and long-term care. As Caplan[4] states, "During the frustration and confusion of struggling with an at-present insurmountable problem, most individuals feel weak and impotent and tend to forget their continuing strengths. At such times, their family reminds them of their past achievements and validates their pre-crisis self-image of competence and ability to stand firm."

The family serves many functions in our society. One of the first, most important, and most natural roles is caring for those in need of physical and cognitive assistance in the family. Initially, a family usually focuses on the care and nurturing of children. However, in later years the same function often applies to the care of an individual who is ill. The family provides assistance and resources such as food, shelter, money, clothing, and transportation. Families also interpret the meaning of events in the outside world and their meaning to the affected family member. This function may affect how the patient responds to health care providers and their services. The family functions as a source of ideology, values, and codes of behavior that guide its members in how to respond to the events of life. This effect on the family member of course also affects how the patient responds to the stroke and the subsequent care by health professionals.[4]

Because the family's influence on recovery from a stroke is not completely clear,[19] several investigators have attempted to determine the contributing factors involved. In one study of 60 families of stroke patients, the patients and families were assessed 5 months after the patient's discharge from the hospital. The authors examined the relationship between family functions and adherence to treatment. Family function was assessed with the

McMaster Family Assessment Device, a 60-item evaluation of seven family dimensions. The authors found a strong correlation between compliance with treatment regimens and families that had effective involvement, functional communication, and problem-solving skills.[11] Evans et al[12] state, "If rehabilitation services can affect family behavior early in the course of recovery, there is often a positive influence on other outcomes." For example, education of the family about the stroke has been shown to improve communications between the family and the patient.[12] Another investigator noted that patients with positive, constructive attitudes toward the challenge of a stroke were more likely eventually to achieve their fullest potential.[2] Finally, a study of 43 first-stroke patients that assessed functional status and the extent of family support concluded that the quantity of social support had a significant relationship to functional outcomes. In this study, the Family Support Scale was developed by the investigators and included subscales regarding compliance with therapeutic instructions, instrumental support such as direct care, and emotional support.[24]

The family's role as an important resource for fostering these positive attitudes may be one of its most important contributions to recovery. The shared positive outlook of the family and the patient provides a sense of support and hope and focuses collective energies toward recovery. Finally, as a patient begins to recover, families who have taken over some of the roles and tasks of the patient must once again have the flexibility to allow and even encourage the patient to resume some productive occupational role in the family. Dysfunctional families may have great difficulty shifting roles in the home. Such role changes also can be difficult for family members who have benefited from their present roles.

Patients who do not recover fully from a stroke may depend on others for extensive assistance and care. This care often is provided, at least partially, by the family. Of the home care recipients in the United States, 80% receive part of their care from a relative.[19] Of those relatives providing care, 72% are women. Adult daughters represent 29%, and wives represent 23%. The demands on family most likely will continue to grow as the population ages. Those older than 65 years represented 31.2 million in the 1990 census. By 2020 this part of the population will have grown to approximately 52 million. Population projections suggest that the number of potential family caregivers will keep pace with this aging population because the caregivers will be composed of the baby boomer generation. However, the availability of these relatives will depend on many other factors, including the continued increase in the number of women in the workforce and divorce rates.[13]

In addition to the aging population, the growing emphasis in the economy on control of health care costs—including long-term care—will put greater pressures on families to provide even more care for their aging and disabled members. Efforts to control costs may include abbreviated rehabilitation contacts and increasing use of family members to perform rehabilitation activities.

In consideration of the natural caregiver role, the resources of the family, and the socioeconomic trends in communities, one must conclude that the rehabilitation of a stroke patient must include the active involvement of the family as a team member.

## FAMILY RESPONSE TO ILLNESS AND DISABILITY

In collaboration with a family, one must consider the possible responses of the family. Often therapists and other health care providers feel burdened or exasperated when families act angry, demanding, controlling, or unrealistic. Such behavior may affect the therapist's ability to work with the family, the rehabilitation outcome, and finally the success of the discharge plan.

The initial onset of a stroke is generally sudden and not anticipated. The family may experience a sense of loss of control or helplessness. Seemingly little can be done by the family initially to speed recovery. The family may have a deep sense of loss and disruption, especially when the patient and the family had expected a vital, productive future for the patient. Disruption of the family may be especially severe when the patient's disability affects the other family members' activities and hopes for the future.

Retired couples often speak of the plans they once had to travel or pursue other interests that they had delayed until retirement. Adult children of stroke victims who become caregivers may complain of loss of freedom to leave the home, the problem of social isolation, or the loss of time for personal interests. Families also may be fearful for the patient's safety.[14] Concerns about avoiding any stimulus that might cause another stroke is not uncommon. Family members understand the embolic or hemorrhagic process of stroke at a rudimentary level and generally perceive the patient's condition as delicate. Information from physicians indicating that future strokes may occur often adds weight to this concern. The family may be fearful of physically moving the patient because they worry it may affect vascular stability. The family may avoid exciting or upsetting the patient because they are concerned it will increase the patient's blood pressure and cause another stroke. These concerns lead families to change their behavior around the patient and transmit a message of fear to the patient that may be detrimental.

The response of the family to the stroke changes over time. An interesting note is that during recovery, the patients and their health care providers—who have known the patients only since the stroke—generally compare gains in function with the patient's disabled state after the stroke, whereas the family is much more likely to compare recovery gains with the patient's previous level of function.[2] The authors of one study examined families 7 to 9 months after a member had a stroke and found a substantially higher prevalence of depressive symptoms among the primary caregivers and the patient.[22] The responsibilities of caring for a family member who has sustained a stroke may lead to greater social isolation for the patient and the caregiver. Aphasia can cause even greater changes in social function, often resulting in social withdrawal by the patient and the family.[16] The caregivers of patients with aphasia are more likely to identify their relationship as worse than before the stroke.[2] The family's complaints may include changes in the patient's behavior, mood lability, confusion, constant demands, and changes in sleep patterns.

The need to appreciate the responses of families to the sustained, long-term care of a family member is a growing concern in health care; indeed, some consider family caregivers unidentified patients. Families that functioned well before the onset of illness generally have the capability to adapt to the challenges posed by the illness. Families that have been disrupted naturally strive for a new balance. Roles and responsibilities in the family gradually are reapportioned in an unconscious adjustment process that protects the function of the family.[1] For example, a husband, who previously paid the bills and handled insurance forms, is hospitalized with a stroke. His tasks are considered the father's role of family financial manager. The wife lacks confidence in assuming the responsibility for this task and part of her husband's role. Indeed, a time of such great stress is a difficult time to assume any new responsibility. These responsibilities may be transferred to an adult child, a man if possible. Likewise, when a wife becomes disabled, her husband may have difficulty assuming many of the traditional roles that the wife had assumed.

When a person with a disability from a stroke plans to return home, the assignment and assumption of caregiver roles may be stressful for the family. Assisting with activities of daily living, home management, and cooking can be time-consuming and physically demanding. Many activities of daily living tasks such as bathing, grooming, and toileting are intimate, and some family members may be uncomfortable assisting the patient with them at first. Although home care services are available in many regions, the extent of care may be limited. In addition, increased effort by the health care industry to control the costs of health care (e.g., managed care and utilization review) decrease the availability and increase the cost of home care supports for the family.

The assumption of new roles in the family, especially the caregiver role, may lead to the abandonment of previous roles. This shifting of roles may affect more than one household and may affect others indirectly. Other roles family members may assume include source of emotional support, energy source, spiritual guide, organizer, comedian, cleaner, and initiator of events. In one study of 10 wives whose spouses had become disabled by a stroke, the Buxbaum Marital Role Questionnaire was applied during hospitalization and 2 weeks after discharge. The study results confirmed that the wives' responsibilities had increased to include "nontraditional responsibilities." In addition the study found that the degree of the wives' happiness with the marriage had decreased.[10]

Dysfunctional families and families that were in conflict before the stroke have greater difficulty adjusting to the challenges imposed on them. Marital relationships that were strained before the stroke may be strained further by this crisis.[7] Families with maladaptive patterns of function provide less constructive support and at times may hinder rehabilitation efforts.[11] Families with idiosyncratic, paranoid, or negative ways of interpreting events in the outside world may have a negative effect on the patient. In a study of family functioning after a stroke, 60 stroke patients, 46 spouses, and 25 other family members were evaluated using the McMaster Family Assessment Device and the competence scale of the Australian ADL Index. The study supported earlier studies that suggested a high degree of family dysfunction before a stroke. Family functioning deteriorated even further after the stroke, most notably in problem solving, communication, and role definition.[6]

Families characterized as centripetal in their function are focused inward: family activities, emotional investments, values, interests, and expectations are directed toward the family. The members of such a family have been socialized to fulfill their needs with only family assistance and have difficulty using outside resources.[26] Therapists working with this type of family may sense that they are not openly and completely accepted and that the suggestions made about management of the illness and adaptations of the home are met with skepticism or hesitation. To enhance a more collaborative relationship with a centripetal family and increase the chances that the family follows through with the treatment and management plans suggested, the therapists may have to make a greater effort to gain trust and acceptance. Without such an effort, other therapy interventions offered to the patient may be rendered ineffective by an unsupportive family.

Therapists who must work with angry, demanding families may try to reduce the extent of their contact with them. Contact may make therapists uncomfortable and defensive. Such a reaction diminishes the opportunity for effective communication of the information necessary for continued treatment. Therapists must consider families' emotional responses to a stroke objectively. Families often become anxious or angry because they are frightened by the trauma and loss created by the illness. Families often vent or focus their anger on individuals unrelated to the events that have caused the anger. Indeed, experiences in hospitals often do little to comfort families and sometimes add to their distress. When responding to a family's anger or complaints, the therapist's must remain calm and be an empathetic listener. The therapist should address the family's complaints and concerns. Attention to complaints is not only a basic responsibility of a therapist as a member of the health care team but also an initial opportunity to demonstrate respect for and responsiveness to the family, which in turn helps the family feel more in control at a time when they feel out of control. The therapist should validate the family's emotional reaction to the traumatic event. Validation is not indiscriminate agreement with everything the family says, it is empathetically listening to the family's reactions, helping them clarify their thoughts and feelings, and sharing similar experiences of other families and individuals. Consider the following scenario, and note the therapist's responses.

Deborah, a 76-year-old, was returning home from the hospital after 5 weeks of rehabilitation. The occupational therapist from the home care agency immediately received complaints from Deborah's family about the hospital care. The therapist focused on Deborah's physical needs, ordering durable medical equipment and initiating treatment. However, the family then complained about the equipment. The home care agency addressed these complaints quickly by providing satisfactory replacements. Rather than becoming defensive, the therapist listened to the husband's multiple complaints. At the beginning of the third session, the husband, feeling more comfortable and becoming more trusting, started to express his concerns about his wife's condition. He was worried about how frail his wife had become, that she could have died as a result of the stroke, and that she was still at risk for another stroke. The therapist recognized these concerns as the core issues driving the husband's anxiety. The therapist listened carefully and validated the husband's concerns. This allowed the husband to disclose his fear that he would lose his wife and be alone. The therapist was able to offer some reassurance that Deborah was in stable condition. The therapist then shared this information with the social worker, who was able to counsel the husband and help him come to terms with Deborah's stroke and her health status.

Therapists must also have the support of the administrators of their facilities to intervene with families who may display extreme dissatisfaction. Administrators must understand the family's reactions and be willing to empower their staff to handle family complaints.

## COLLABORATING WITH THE FAMILY

Because the family has such an influence on the patient's ability to respond to health care services and may actively deliver some of the care and services during later phases of rehabilitation, engaging of the family in the functions of the treatment team is essential. The initial stages should include an assessment of the family's understanding of the patient's status and the intent of the services being offered. Family members, especially spouses, feel they are given little information about the stroke and treatment. Communication problems related to educating the family may include the use of medical jargon by health professionals.[5] The therapist simply should listen to the type of questions asked by the patient and pose a few evaluative questions in return. The health care team then should educate the family about the illness so that members may use the information effectively to respond appropriately to the patient and health care providers. Each member of the treatment team collaborates with the family in a different context. The physician most likely will educate the family about the cause and anatomy of a stroke, as well as the course of medical treatment during onset and throughout the course of illness. The social worker may be the person who will make initial and continuing formal contact with the family, first to assess the family and home environment, and then to help the family develop a long-term care plan and discuss financial needs. The nurse may educate the family about daily management and the new needs of the patient: how to handle and position the patient safely, comfortably, and therapeutically to prevent the development of a decubitus ulcer and how to administer medications and other treatments.

The occupational therapist must educate the family about many aspects of managing the care of a stroke patient.[13] The family must learn about paralysis, ineffective movement, and protection of the impaired extremity: how to manage and adapt to perceptual deficits, hemianopsias and unilateral neglect; how to apply positioning devices and orthotics, keep schedules of orthotic wear, care for the skin, and clean the orthosis; and how to position the patient in bed. Learning safe transfers of the patient to a variety of surfaces may require many practice sessions with the family. The therapist may think every transfer situation has been taught to the family until an accident occurs, such as the patient injuring an ankle falling off a street curb while entering the family car. Transfer training should include transfers to automobiles, beds, toilets, regular chairs, and bathtubs. Education about the handling and care of wheelchairs and the proper use of adaptive equipment helps ensure proper use and increased patient safety. Sharing a supplier's durable medical equipment catalog with the family may help give the family a better idea of available products and generate some questions or ideas about other home adaptations that may be needed. Home visits by the occupational therapist before the patient's discharge may help the family predict adaptations that will be needed in the home and reduce the number of obstacles encountered and frustrations experienced in the first few days at home. The therapist's suggestions for changing the home environment should be tempered by sensitivity to personal property and financial limits (see Chapter 25).

The occupational therapist should share detailed information with the family about the patient's ability to perform various activities of daily livings because the family may overestimate or underestimate the patient's abilities. Instructions on setting up tasks and providing proper assistance helps the family members feel they are contributing to the patient's recovery and may relieve the family's worry that all tasks will have to be done for the patient. At the same time, the therapist must be sensitive to the family's need for activities of daily living to be completed in a reasonable time to maintain a home routine. (Allowing 15 minutes for the patient to don a shirt may seem reasonable in a hospital, but it may not be practical in a busy home.) The therapist should instruct the family or primary caregiver on helping the patient perform safe, passive range of motion and active exercises and perhaps practice these exercises with the family. When designing an exercise or therapeutic program for the family to perform with the patient, the therapist must consider the availability and needs of the family and caregiver. Tasks that are time-consuming, that are detailed, or that cause discomfort or pain for the patient may discourage the family from following through with the program. Tasks that fit into the family's routine and perhaps incorporate activities the family enjoys may meet with greater compliance.[3]

The therapist should encourage the family members to maintain their previous relationship with the patient as much as possible and not assume the role of therapist or home health aide. This can be a naturally occurring problem when family members are used as service extenders to provide exercises or therapeutic activities for the patient. Although assuming this role may seem to be a constructive way for family members to respond to the negative effects the stroke, it alters the existing patient-family relationship and may be considered an additional problem for the patient. In a qualitative study conducted in the Netherlands, 20 stroke patients in rehabilitation wards of nursing homes were interviewed. The study concluded that overprotection and paternalism by family members had a negative influence on the patient's sense of autonomy and self-determination.[20]

The patient and family should be involved in the goal-setting process. Evaluations such as the Canadian Occupational Performance Measure are helpful in this process. If the family is to support the patient and the rehabilitation effort, they must understand and be invested in the goals. This involvement begins with the therapist asking the patient about goals for rehabilitation and then making the patient aware of what is realistic and which goals are priorities. The therapist then asks the family what they consider to be important goals and then gives this information to the patient. This process can be cumbersome, especially when the family and patient disagree or have set unrealistic goals. However cumbersome, the goal-setting process is an opportunity to clarify perceptions about the patient's status; the prognosis and course of the illness; the expected efficacy of the rehabilitation; the restorative and compensatory approaches; and short-term, step-by-step incremental goal setting.

The treatment planning process is an opportunity to make certain that expectations and demands on all parties are reasonable and consensual. When the family, patient, and therapist have different goals, the therapist should help them compromise. Usually the therapist can identify similarities in goals and help all reach a common goal. When a compromise cannot be reached, the therapist should help the patient and the family prioritize or sequence goals. The patient's wishes should be given some extra consideration. If the patient and the family have been involved actively in treatment planning and the measure of outcomes, they will understand better and accept the eventual end of rehabilitation services. The patient and family members more likely will agree with the therapist's observation that the patient has reached the optimal level of recovery for the present setting and is therefore ready to move to a different level of care or to be discharged from treatment.

A common assumption of families is that the more therapy the patient receives, the better the patient's recovery. The therapist must explain how much therapy is appropriate and why and should teach families that rest, socialization, and recreation are essential aspects of recovery (see Chapter 28). Too many hours of intensive therapy may be overwhelming to someone trying to recover.

The therapist and other health care providers can educate the family more subtly by modeling appropriate behaviors. The therapist's comfortable and positive interactions with the patient can help put the family at ease and encourage more natural interactions. Humor can play an important role in this process. The therapist's comfort with touching, holding, and handling the patient, especially the paralyzed extremities, may help the family begin to do the same. An illness and subsequent physical disability may cause the patient or the patient's partner to avoid intimacy and sex (see Chapter 23). In addition, many hospitals and residential health care facilities deter physical intimacy. The authors of one study found that only 17% of couples continued sexual contact.[8] Touching and embracing may be the first way a couple begins to become intimate again. Physical intimacy can be comforting and affirming for the patient. Accepting and discreetly handling situations in which the patent is incontinent also can set a good example for the family. If the therapist is to help the family address these issues, therapy sessions occasionally should be open for family members to observe or participate. This may seem an additional burden on the therapist and meet with some objections by administrators; however, the benefits of engaging the family in this way can be immeasurable, especially because treatment periods are becoming shorter and greater reliance is being placed on families to become caregivers and extend therapy.

Some hospitals and outpatient clinics have developed structured educational series for families. Indeed some hospitals have developed structured educational programs for the patient and the family and have received positive responses from the participants.[9] Hinckley, Packard, and Bardach[17] describe a successful family education program focused on patients with aphasia and their families. The topics of the program included communication, intimacy and sexuality, vocations, driving, and volunteering. This type of program can be labor intensive, which should be considered when developing similar programs. The authors were unable to identify outcomes related to more effective management of the patient by family members; however, attendance by families and positive results on satisfaction surveys suggested that the families benefited from this program.

## HELPING THE FAMILY ADJUST

Professional assistance in helping the family adjust to the stroke and its effects can have positive long-term results by strengthening the natural family support system for the patient. The educational approach discussed previously is one step toward that adjustment. Professionals can help the family in several other ways. The therapist should acknowledge the efforts the family is making to be with, assist, and care for the affected family member.[22] Often families and caregivers who devote significant effort to caring for their family member feel their devotion is not being reciprocated. Reciprocity is a natural element of social relations. When an object or service is offered to one individual, that individual usually reciprocates in some manner.[23] In a relationship in which someone is ill and dependent, reciprocation is altered. For health care providers, reciprocation can be indirect—remuneration by a third party, an altruistic sense of social reward, or a focus on the further development of professional skills. Some patients and families with limited socioeconomic resources whose services are paid for by government or other programs may feel an absence of social reciprocation and try to reciprocate with a gift or friendly gesture. For family caregivers the absence of reciprocation from the affected family member may leave them feeling angry, empty, or unrewarded. However, the findings of one study suggest that many caregivers experience reciprocity in a dependent relationship. In one

study, mothers who received care from their daughters were able to reciprocate through expressions of love. Of the daughters in a caregiving relationship, 87% were able to identify some form of reciprocation that they valued, such as sharing information and advice.[25]

The professional can support family members by acknowledging their efforts and appealing to the family's sense of altruism. Professionals can also help family caregivers identify small, everyday forms of reciprocation. Often this reciprocation occurs in the context of an activity: a smile of appreciation after assistance with care or the reintroduction of music, old recipes, or a craft from a previous era or culture of origin. The identification, spoken or unspoken, of these rewards may help the caregiver sustain their efforts and care for the family member with an increased sense of the value of their assistance.

As noted previously, one aspect of family dysfunction can be a deterioration in problem-solving abilities. One approach recommended for this issue is "social problem-solving therapy," provided by telephone contacts. The problem-solving therapy involved a four-step systematic approach to problem identification, prioritization, and solving by caregivers.[16]

Professionals also may support family caregivers by monitoring their health promotion activities. Asking caregivers periodically about their own health and feelings can remind them that their health and stress levels are important also and allow them an opportunity to share their experiences and feelings. The therapist should observe caregivers for signs of fatigue or excessive stress and encourage them to schedule and pursue social and leisure interests. The occupational therapist can help caregivers identify these interests and determine how they fit into the routine of caring for the affected family member. The family and the caregivers should be encouraged to use respite periods for travel or leisure.[18]

Respite can be achieved in several ways, including temporarily placing the patient in a residential program, hiring a 24-hour attendant, or relying on other family members to provide temporary care. The therapist should not be discouraged if the family and the caregivers do not respond immediately to these suggestions. The therapist should encourage the family to increase use of home care and day care programs to help reduce stress. Health care providers should help the family identify when the extent of care needed by the patient exceeds the family's resources, capabilities, and home care supports. Consideration of long-term residential care may be necessary. The family and the patient may have some emotional difficulty discussing this issue. Professional support, clear information about nursing homes, and assistance in finding the best home for the patient can help make this transition smoother and more successful.

## DYSFUNCTIONAL CARE

The demands of caring for a family member who has sustained a stroke not only may exceed the family's resources but also may exacerbate dysfunctional aspects of the family or the individual caregiver. Previously strained relationships may be placed under greater stress and can lead to a breakdown of the family.

Estimates indicate that 3.2% of older Americans are victims of abuse or neglect[21]; chronic disability is believed to be one of the risk factors.[15] It is also estimated that only one out of six cases of elder abuse is brought to the attention of authorities.[15] Therapists working with patients disabled by a stroke should be sensitive to the signs of abuse and neglect and should be prepared to contact authorities. Often more disagreement occurs among professionals about what constitutes neglect than what constitutes inadequate care. Fulmer and O'Malley[15] suggest that defining neglect and abuse cases as situations of inadequate care helps reduce resistance when attempting to deal constructively with the issue—the welfare of the patient.

## DOCUMENTING FAMILY CONTACTS

Many therapists who traditionally have focused on physical rehabilitation express concerns about documenting their work with the family. Often therapists believe they must document only the physical and functional restoration for reimbursement purposes. This leads therapists to avoid intervening in family-related problems or to avoid reporting these interventions to others. This decision is unfortunate because it eventually harms the patient and the family and does not promote the idea that family interventions need to be provided and reimbursed.

Many interventions with family members can be tied directly to improving the patient's level of function or increased safety in the home. Interventions can help the family to assist the patient safely and effectively with transfers, dressing, and bathing. Other goals the therapist may be document include the following:

- The family will encourage the patient to perform the self-exercise program daily.
- The family will demonstrate a more accurate understanding of the patient's safety needs by maintaining a hazard-free home environment.
- The family will engage the patient in an active leisure pursuit at least twice a week.

## REVIEW QUESTIONS

1. Which natural functions does the family provide for its members?
2. How should a therapist respond to an angry, complaining family?
3. What are some of the family attributes that may lead to difficulty helping a member who has sustained a stroke?
4. How should the therapist educate the family?
5. What can a therapist do for family caregivers to improve compliance with treatment?
6. How should the family and the patient be engaged in treatment planning?
7. How can the therapist help the family adjust to the stroke and chronic disability?

## REFERENCES

1. Ackerman NW: *The psychodynamics of family life*, New York, 1958, Basic Books.
2. Anderson R: *The aftermath of stroke: the experience of patients and their families*, New York, 1992, Cambridge University.
3. Anderson J, Hinijosa J: Parents and therapists in a professional partnership, *Am J Occup Ther* 38(7):452-461, 1984.
4. Caplan G: The family as a support system. In Caplan G, Killilea M, editors: *Support systems and mutual help: multidisciplinary explorations*, New York, 1976, Grune & Stratton.
5. Clark MS: Patient and spouse perceptions of stroke and its rehabilitation, *Int J Rehabil Res* 23(1):19-29, 2000.
6. Clark MS, Smith DS: Changes in family functioning for stroke rehabilitation patients and their families, *Int J Rehabil Res* 22(3):171-179, 1999.
7. Diller L: Hemiplegia. In Garrett J, Levin E, editors: *Rehabilitation practice with the physically disabled*, New York, 1973, Columbia University.
8. Drummond AE: Stroke: the impact on the family, *Br J Occup Ther* 51:193, 1988.
9. Easton KL, Zemen DM, Kwiatkowski S: Developing and implementing a stroke education series for patients and families, *Rehabil Nurs* 19(6):348-351, 1994.
10. Enterlante TM, Kern JM: Wives' reported role changes following a husband's stroke: a pilot study, *Rehabil Nurs* 20(3):155-160, 1995.
11. Evans RL, Bishop DS, Matlock AL, et al: Family interaction and treatment adherence after stroke, *Arch Phys Med Rehabil* 68(8):513-517, 1987.
12. Evans RL, Connis RT, Bishop DS, et al: Stroke: a family dilemma, *Disabil Rehabil* 16(3):110-118, 1994.
13. Evans RL, Held S: Evaluation of family stroke education, *Int J Rehabil Res* 7(1):47-51, 1984.
14. Figley CR: Catastrophes: an overview of family reactions. In Figley CR, McCubbin HI, editors: *Stress and the family*, vol 2, *Coping with catastrophe*, New York, 1983, Brunner-Mazel.
15. Fulmer TT, O'Malley TA: *Inadequate care of the elderly: a health care perspective on abuse and neglect*, New York, 1987, Springer.
16. Herrmann M, Britz A, Bartels C, et al: The impact of aphasia on the patient and family in the first year poststroke, *Top Stroke Rehabil* 2:5, 1995.
17. Hinckley JJ, Packard MEW, Bardach LG: Alternative family education programming for adults with chronic aphasia, *Top Stroke Rehabil* 2:53, 1995.
18. Kahana E: *Family caregiving across the lifespan*, Thousand Oaks, Calif, 1994, Sage.
19. Norris VK, Stephens MAP, Kinney JM: The impact of family interactions on recovery from stroke: help or hindrance? *Gerontologist* 30(4):535-542, 1990.
20. Pillemer K, Finkelhor D: Causes of elder abuse: caregiver stress versus problem relatives, *Am J Orthopsychiatry* 59(2):179-187, 1989.
21. Proot IM, Crebolder HF, Abu-Saad HH, et al: Stroke patients' needs and experiences regarding autonomy at discharge from nursing home, *Patient Educ Couns* 41(3):275-283, 2000.

22. Schulz R, Tompkins CA, Rau MT: A longitudinal study of the psychosocial impact of stroke on primary support persons, *Psychol Aging* 3(2):131-141, 1988.
23. Silliman RA, Fletchner RH, Earp JL, et al: Families of elderly stroke patients: effects of homecare, *J Am Geriatr Soc* 34:643, 1986.
24. Tsouna-Hadjis E, Vemmos KN, Zakopoulos N, et al: First-stroke recovery process: the role of family social support, *Arch Phys Med Rehabil* 81(7):881-887, 2000.
25. Walker AJ, Pratt CC, Oppy NC: Perceived reciprocity in family caregiving, *Fam Relat* 41:82, 1992.
26. Walsh F: *Normal family processes*, New York, 1993, Guilford.

## SUGGESTED READING FOR CHILDREN

de Paola T: *Now one foot, now the other*, New York, 1980, GP Putnam's Sons.

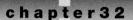

# ann burkhardt

## chapter 32

# Total Quality Management of the Adult Stroke Population

### key terms

process improvement

quality assurance

quality improvement

risk management

total quality management

### chapter objectives

After completing this chapter, the reader will be able to accomplish the following:

1. Understand the concept of total quality management.
2. Articulate the difference between quality improvement and the process of improvement.
3. Conceptualize how incident reporting relates to risk management.
4. Describe several clinical monitors for the care of individuals surviving stroke.
5. Share tools available in a clinical setting that address the concerns of case management of individuals surviving stroke.

One of the criticisms often made concerning the cost-effectiveness of rehabilitation services is the general lack of sufficient outcomes research. This assertion in particular has been used as a basis by some health maintenance organizations and managed care organizations as a reason to deny coverage of occupational therapy services. The occupational therapy profession needs to focus on how to measure its benefits so that others can appreciate its value. One of the ways to generate clinical research is through preliminary investigation by clinically based continual quality improvement (CQI) monitors.

Total quality management (TQM) comprises two levels: CQI and risk management.[10] The aim of each CQI monitor is to define an aspect of care that is the essence or crux of professional interventions. One quantifies the goals of intervention in measurable terms, which allows gathering of data that will predict a reproducible and ver-

ifiable outcome. Through the provision of a reporting structure, the TQM process assists the therapist with formulating outcome measures and setting the standards for provision of patient care according to the process of performance improvement standards (benchmarking).

Continual quality improvement monitors direct outcomes of prevention of disease complications or success in treatment. These data should be readily retrievable from charts or through surveys of patients and health care workers (e.g., nurses). Follow-through of the monitors with the recommendations of occupational therapy affects the success of the treatment intervention. The process now called *process improvement* once was called "quality assurance." The terminology and underlying management philosophy changed, resulting in a model that is progressive and less based on monitoring the status quo. The term *improvement* clearly suggests that quality

*684*

patient care or treatment must increase continually and also implies that change is an inherent aspect of the monitoring process.

In contrast, risk management defines morbidity, or aspects of patient care that could put the individual or a caregiver at risk for personal injury. Occupational therapists may work with individuals who have survived a stroke in an inpatient hospital, clinic, home, or work setting. One of the more common risk management issues concerns the risk of falling because of changes in balance and equilibrium.[2] Therapists often are consulted to recommend the parameters for safely participating in activities. Physical or chemical restraints may be needed for patients with cognitive changes impairing judgment, attention, or short-term memory to reduce the risk of injury. Federal law limits the conditions under which one may use restraints. Therapy staff and other members of the interdisciplinary team must be aware of the law and adhere to compliance measures yet continue to act in the best interest of the patient. Misuse of exercise equipment may result in injury. For example, if a person who has had a stroke and has glenohumeral joint malalignment uses an upper body exerciser, such use could lead to tendonitis and development of a pain syndrome. When limbs have decreased sensation, particularly when the patient's protective sensation is impaired, participation in activities places the patient at risk for a cut or burn. Certain physical agent modalities also carry a risk when protective sensation is impaired because patients could get burned (e.g., by superficial or deep heat modalities) or shocked (by electrical modalities) if health care professionals do not follow precautions and consistently check equipment for safe operation (Figure 32-1). Speculation also exists that as more occupational therapists use complementary and alternative medical techniques in treatment, liability may increase. Therefore, in settings in which one uses complementary and alternative medicine, an additional risk management concern is overuse of nonallopathic treatment techniques that may or may not affect outcome of overall case management for a person who has had a stroke.

Total quality management is an essential part of any occupational therapy setting today. Not only do credentialing agencies such as the Joint Commission on the Accreditation of Healthcare Organizations or the Commission on Accreditation of Rehabilitation Facilities require TQM activities, but so do individual contracts for private practices with managed care companies. The managed care industry promotes the idea that cost-effectiveness does not imply reduced quality. All practitioners must see practice from this perspective if they are to continue practicing within the changing health care system. Probably the most current trend within TQM models is the concept of best practice.

Best clinical practice initiatives focus on asking critical questions about care delivery; choosing what is believed to be best, given current research and practice knowledge; and standardizing and measuring outcome of care. Some questions a therapist might ask in developing best practice models of care are as follows:

- What evidence am I using to help make clinical decisions or formulate local standards and criteria for good practice?
- How can I involve patients in making choices about their care?
- How do I update my knowledge and practice?
- What strategies do I use for implementing changes in practice?
- How am I evaluating the care that I provide?

Best clinical practice models often embrace the concept of evidence-based practice. For example, Burkhardt[1] documented a clinical example of evidence-based practice. The article discusses how an occupational therapy rehabilitation unit in a hospital setting used evidence-based practice through journal review and meta-analysis to reassess the clinical reasoning to determine whether one should or should not use a sling or a splint for management of the hemiparetic upper extremity.

In her 2003 American Occupational Therapy Association presidential address,[9] Barbara L. Kornblau, JD, OT/L, FAOTA, DAAPM, ABDA, spoke about evidence as existing more naturalistically, including in anecdotal reports and patient statements when patients state they felt positive change or stated that a technique or approach helped them during the care they received. Best practice initiatives form the basis for care that is driven by providing the best specialty care through centers of excellence in many health care facilities in the United States at present. The concept behind this initiative is marketing, but marketing that depends on providing the best care possible. Occupational therapists are being challenged to think and to provide care in support of these approaches to care. For example, in tertiary care settings, care may be based

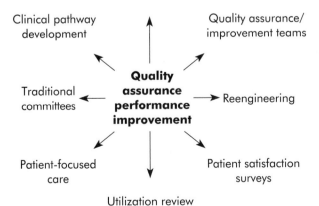

**Figure 32-1**  The relationship of quality assurance performance improvement to hospital-based care.

on advanced technology: organ and tissue transplants, robotic cardiac surgery, artificial heart pumps (e.g., ventricular assistive devices). The knowledge and skills that all supporting services provide is beyond the scope of general practitioners in each of their fields. Best practice supports acquisition of knowledge of technology advances and how they are applied to practice under the circumstances.

Another way in which implementation of treatment and rapid discharge are combined is through the use of critical pathway models.[14] Critical pathways are standardized, multidisciplinary care plans through which care is introduced on a timed continuum. Critical pathways efficiently coordinate inpatient care so that the patient receives intervention from all critical care services and is discharged to the community as rapidly as feasible. The rapid discharge reduces the inpatient length of stay (LOS) and is financially desirable for the system providing primary care. Occupational therapists must seek opportunities to participate in the critical pathway planning committees that coordinate the design and implementation of the pathway. Therapists must define the parameters of their staff members' involvement, an optimal treatment time frame, and the content of evaluation and treatment to ensure the patient has the skills needed to survive at home following discharge. The level of anticipated function at the time of the discharge should be defined as well. Discharge planning is still the method for recommending the appropriate level of home care or outpatient service for each case.

Most of the resources concerning TQM arise out of the medical and nursing literature. Early articles on the topic describe the necessity for defining functional outcome in reference to quality of life.[3] When physicians generate studies, the outcomes tend to be measured in terms of the development of medical complications following inpatient discharge or an inpatient LOS.[12] These factors are related to issues of delaying discharge from the hospital or readmitting a patient to an inpatient setting because of a medical complication. These issues are related directly to reimbursement for care[15] and funding to the provider calculated using the diagnosis-related groups. The facility receives a flat rate to treat the patient for the primary medical diagnosis, regardless of complications. The rate is controlled regionally and is derived by averaging the actual length of hospital stay for persons with a particular diagnosis. The system promotes treating the disease quickly and discharging the patient early. Theoretically, this lessens the possibility of complications such as nosocomial infections.[5,16] The problem with the system is that it fails to account for the differences in the recovery times of the healing organ systems and the effect delayed healing has on the ability to participate in basic and instrumental activities of daily living.

For example, joint replacements following fracture usually heal more rapidly than brain tissue damaged because of a stroke. The predicted complications associated with bone healing are more readily quantifiable by nature than those of the central nervous system. For example, learning to dress the lower extremities is less cumbersome if the two upper extremities are functionally intact and visual perception is intact. This concept is simple but may not necessarily be accounted for in physician- or nursing-generated morbidity reviews. An inherent dichotomy exists in nursing-generated CQI because a physician's ability to control a patient's medical status is not necessarily correlated positively with the patient's functional recovery or ability to participate in the activities that define the patient's life goals.[11] Conflict for therapists working within these models occurs when a philosophical difference in opinion results from team members using professional terms inconsistently because understanding those terms in different ways impedes discharge planning.

Other models attempt to evaluate the severity of effect of disease sequelae on LOS. Thomas and Longo[13] described several measurement methods in 1990. Individual case review is a method by which charts are peer reviewed retrospectively in an attempt to determine factors that may be prolonging care (and thus increasing cost) beyond the point at which functional ability improves. Difficulties arise when the person reviewing the charts is a member of another profession or not a specialist. A reviewer who is a member of the profession but not a specialist may not understand the nuances or standards of the subspecialty area of practice. Despite these concerns, less than 5% discrepancy exists between accurate charts and the peer reviewers' findings.[11]

Thomas and Longo[13] also describe measuring the effect of disease sequelae on function using several scales including the Acute Physiological Assessment and Chronic Health Evaluation II (APACHE II). Although generally used to measure functional impairment severity in intensive care units compared with general acute care, factors used in this scale include the effects of acute illness, age, and chronic disease. The shortcoming of the scale from an occupational therapist's perspective is that it fails to consider that occupational therapy can restore functional control of the human and nonhuman environments with or without the use of adapted technology and regardless of the severity of disease.

In comparison, scales have been developed in an attempt to measure categories of function in relation to physical demand. One such scale is the Sickness Impact Profile.[10] The profile has 12 categories, including ambulation, mobility, body care, and movement. Another similar scale used widely is the Functional Independence Measure.[7] Although these scales are quantifiable, they fail to account for individual idiosyncrasies or foibles that can enhance or impede functional recovery. In addition, little if any consideration is given to the functional influence of cognition on an individual's ability to participate successfully in and achieve practical or actual desired outcomes in daily life. To an occupational therapist, this fact is incredulous because learning is based on cognition and the ability to use problem solving to plan and complete tasks successfully.

One could argue that the relationship of cognition to survival from stroke varies so much that using treatment methods that disregard the influence of this relationship may be the only means of achieving any function at all with any degree of consistency.[6] If the goal of treatment for a person with impaired cognition is subcortical execution of daily tasks with habits used before the stroke, then perhaps measurement scales originating from occupational therapy sources are best to consider; the Árnadóttir OT-ADL Neurobehavioral Evaluation (A-ONE) (see Chapter 18) and the Assessment of Motor and Process Skills (see Chapter 20) are two such scales. The A-ONE is used to demonstrate the influence cognitive impairment has on an individual's ability to complete basic activities of daily living, and the Assessment of Motor and Process Skills is used as a valid indicator of instrumental activities of daily living activity. A similar index, the Activities Index, was used to determine whether the speed of intervention initiation following stroke had an influence on recovery. This possible relationship has implications for occupational therapists working in inpatient settings with interdisciplinary team case management plans. Abbreviated scales with universal application have great value in inpatient and subacute settings in which an interdisciplinary approach is used.

Gross mobility is also an important risk management factor, especially in patients with demonstrated motor or sensory impairments, because they are at greater risk for falls.[2,4] Falls increase the risk of developing comorbidities such as fractures and soft-tissue injuries. The therapist should consider a person with a known central nervous system disorder diagnosis at risk and must educate the patient and caregivers about the implications of community mobility. Therapists must teach patients the least harmful way to fall and the way to get up from the ground if they do fall. If patients get up from a fall alone, a system must be in place for them to gain assistance. Supervision is one solution but may be intrusive to an adult patient who is otherwise cognitively intact and able to live alone. For higher-functioning individuals a medical alert system, such as a beeper-activated device worn around the neck, may allow independence in the home environment. A fracture superimposed on a neurologically weakened limb will have decreased circulation and delayed healing time. The presence of a fracture necessitates rehospitalization and a second course of rehabilitation intervention. This clearly is a measurable CQI indicator in the inpatient setting and on community questionnaire follow-up activities.

## CRITICAL PATHWAYS

Because managed care has become more prominent in health care systems, provider groups have formed multidisciplinary teams to address cost containment.[8] Two heavily weighted factors affecting cost containment in inpatient settings are LOS and the development of comorbidities. Therefore, strategies are being developed to decrease the LOS and provide essential services more quickly and efficiently.

Critical pathways are interdisciplinary team case management plans.[14] The team decides on the ideal inpatient LOS and then tailors an in-depth care map, or treatment plan, that describes the timing and extent of multidisciplinary services. The underlying issues for any health care provider are (1) determining whether participation in the planning committee is beneficial for a critical pathway, (2) streamlining intervention plans without sacrificing what managed care organizations deem quality or cost-effectiveness, resulting in realistic staffing that will support a positive outcome, (3) providing the best quality care at the least cost to aid the competitiveness of the institution in the managed care marketplace, (4) being proactive in support of the marketability of services, and (5) continuing to guide practice using ethics.

During the planning process for a critical pathway, often an aura of open bidding exists for the time or opportunity to intervene with the patient. Understanding the timing of making referrals for services and the mechanism used to make referrals is important. If a physician will have to write a prescription for a therapist to initiate an intervention plan, one benefit is for the pathway to indicate that the referral is to be written the day before the planned intervention. One way to simplify this process is to use a general checkoff referral form. The physician checks off or initials the request for therapy services; the request indicates the usual time frame for initiation of services (e.g., the first day after a stroke). If blanket referrals are not acceptable, the process of making and receiving referrals increases the multidisciplinary team's labor and decreases available time. For example, reliance on utilization reviewers increases to locate the documentation of the physician referral, and the process of relaying the referral to the ancillary services takes the caregiver more time to locate the referral in the written chart.

Once the team has established that each service will deliver care according to the care map, the team must establish a mechanism to monitor whether the plan is carried out. A care map can be put into the main frame system of the hospital computer. As caregivers intervene, they can initial the computer care map grid. A note usually also is needed to specify the details and outcome of the caregiver sessions (e.g., whether the patient was willing to participate and the patient's tolerance for activity).

The acute inpatient LOS for a stroke patient is currently 4 days. At the end of 4 days, the patient returns home with or without home care (depending on the recovery and resources available for treatment), goes to an inpatient rehabilitation setting for a short LOS (e.g., 2 to 4 weeks), or goes to a long-term care facility for rehabilitation followed by maintenance care. Many long-term care facilities now accept acute care patients and are being reclassified as subacute care facilities. This trend has changed the common perception of a nursing home stay—that it is a terminal care facility and a last resort—because more and more individuals are being discharged to their homes and the community after a short-term nursing home stay.

The role of acute care therapists has become more consultative. Therapists are now members of the primary care team in many acute hospital settings. Because of knowledge of function and safety, they often lead the team when determining discharge planning projections.

As consultants, primary care therapists rapidly evaluate sequelae of stroke and recommend proper positioning and needed equipment for immediate intervention. Because of the limited LOS and therefore of time, therapists must emphasize patient-centered caregiver education and training.

Handling and alignment during activity participation are duties that home care or subacute care therapists often assume. Handling and alignment always must be a part of functional tasks because outcome is measured by function alone. Therapists can no longer use hands-on treatment methods for months or years on the same patient. Although neurodevelopmental treatment techniques commonly are used with the stroke population, professional survival in the current economic environment ultimately is defined by functional success of patients. Function is the only reimbursable commodity according to third-party payers. Documentation of treatment intervention efficacy is necessary to continue to provide occupational and physical therapy care in the future.

## CONTINUOUS QUALITY IMPROVEMENT

The development of CQI monitors should be tied to the context and content of treatment provided to a given population. Therefore the CQI monitors of a stroke population should track the outcome of the care according to the underlying clinical intervention philosophy. For example, if clinical evaluations are used to measure function, one CQI monitor should focus on the outcome of treatment as measured by functional improvement

according to the particular measurement tool. Two of the tools used in rehabilitation units are the A-ONE and the Assessment of Motor and Process Skills. The A-ONE measures basic self-care functioning in relation to cognitive impairment and recovery after a stroke. The therapist observes and documents baseline functioning. The therapist reevaluates the patient weekly and on discharge. The test is in the form of prefabricated progress note formats and discharge evaluations. Use of prefabricated notes helps therapists adhere to documentation parameters while reporting functional improvements applicable to the deficits identified at the initiation of therapy. Improvement of function continues to be documented throughout the LOS. Although a patient's neurologic status can improve without therapy, many cases reveal clinical trends. If CQI monitoring demonstrates an inability to reach projected benchmarks, the therapist could demonstrate need to change the focus of therapy.

Another CQI monitor that one could use on a stroke service is tracking the development of secondary conditions, such as painful shoulder. Therapists using shoulder protection or positioning programs for their patients, the clinical standards for positioning the shoulder, training the caregivers, and providing education to the patients and caregivers could be monitored routinely. Patient compliance also could be documented. The outcome (i.e., percentage of patients who develop shoulder pain) could be compared with current data on the national norms. The effectiveness of the program could be demonstrated if the outcome is above the national average.

Interdisciplinary CQI monitors are intrinsically valuable to credentialing agencies such as the Joint Commission on the Accreditation of Healthcare Organizations or the Commission on Accreditation of Rehabilitation Facilities. An area of stroke patient care that naturally lends itself to interdisciplinary monitoring is dysphagia assessment and treatment outcome. Individuals who develop dysphagia are at greater risk for increased in-hospital LOSs or repeatedly being admitted to the hospital because of resulting aspiration pneumonia. The interdisciplinary team treating dysphagia often consists of representatives from occupational therapy, speech pathology, nutrition, radiology, nursing, and otolaryngology. Information could be collected about whether a swallowing assessment was done, the incidence of aspiration pneumonia, the appropriateness of the alternative methods recommended to the patients, and findings when the patient is reassessed.

Another emerging issue is the use of conscious (physical or chemical) restraints. The Omnibus Budget Reconciliation Act of 1981 mandates that restraints of any kind cannot be used without proper justification and/or agreement from the patient or the appointed proxy. This decision must be documented in the medical chart and communicated to the interdisciplinary team. Many facilities have formed restraint committees to set facility standards that comply with federal and state laws.

Patient satisfaction may be difficult to assess in the stroke population because of the potential sequelae of stroke and patients' overall dissatisfaction with quality of life, issues over which the therapist has no control. These are inherent problems associated with studying CQI potential in this specific population. Satisfaction must be defined specifically in quantifiable terms and directly relate to functional improvements in basic self-care activities and instrumental activities of daily living.[17,18]

Safety is a key area of concern in the stroke population. Continual quality improvement monitors could track risk management issues such as reducing the incidence of falls in the inpatient or the home setting. Compliance with therapists' recommendations for removing potential safety hazards (e.g., throw rugs) could be monitored. Documenting safety education is often a good way to contain risk management liability.

Theoretically, a CQI monitor could be a pilot for a clinically based outcomes research project. The data could be saved over extended periods of time and retrospectively studied. If therapists could not carry out this degree of analysis independently, graduate students or academic peers could assist with analyzing and documenting the outcomes. Pairing clinical practice with academic preparation for practice may help future generations of therapists develop the skills to collect and analyze their practices routinely, which could improve the efficacy of professional involvement in health care.

## RISK MANAGEMENT

Liability—one of the key underlying concepts of risk management—is always a concern when an industry provides a service to the public. Responsibility for injury must be contained to protect the public and the industry providing the services. In a patient care setting, numerous risk factors exist, the most common of which are (1) a physical environment that is unsafe, (2) management of injury under conditions that are not ideal, (3) mishandling by a trained care provider or professional resulting in injury or harm, (4) mishandling by nonprofessional personnel resulting in injury or harm, and (5) equipment malfunctions.

A key to risk management is documentation of incidents. When anyone is involved in an incident, whether it initially appears to have resulted in injury, the incident should be documented within the time frame required by the credentialing agency or institutional policy. In many settings, this window of time is 24 to 48 hours. The forms usually require a description of the incident, a list of witnesses, the location of the incident, findings of a medical review, and a plan for action to change the contributing factors and decrease the chance of an incidence recurring. Institutional policy may require that these incidents be reported to the state and become part of the morbidity and mortality review standards by which the institution is judged.

## DOCUMENTATION OF THE TOTAL QUALITY MANAGEMENT PROGRAM

The TQM (CQI and risk management) policies and procedures should be kept in the departmental policy and procedure manual. If the practitioner is in sole practice or private practice, the practice also should have a policy and procedure manual. In addition to having general policies and procedures, the practice should have a mission statement that agrees with the TQM documents. The staff should participate in risk management and quality improvement initiative training that is documented on a yearly basis. If CQI monitors indicate a need to revise the departmental policies and procedures, the plans for the revision can be documented in the CQI plan. For consistency and context validity, changes should be monitored for efficacy to ensure that they result in improved care and management.

## REVIEW QUESTIONS

1. What types of administrative activities should be included in any occupational therapy department's program to ensure quality? (That is TQM = RM + PI/QA, where *TQM* is total quality management, *RM* is risk management, *PI* is performance improvement, and *QA* is quality assurance.)
2. Describe a method to measure and monitor risk in any practice setting.
3. Name three clinically based performance improvement initiatives that could be developed for a setting in which persons who have survived a stroke are treated.
4. What benefit is there for therapists to use the A-ONE, Canadian Occupational Performance Measure, and Assessment of Motor and Process Skills scales to measure function in comparison with other researched and popular tests or scales?
5. From a rehabilitative manager's perspective, what benefits or hindrances are inherent in the use of critical pathways?

## REFERENCES

1. Burkhardt A: Evidence-based practice in occupational therapy: implications for hospital-based practice, *AOTA Admin Manage SIS Q* 17(4):1-3, 2001.
2. DeVincenzo DK, Watkins S: Accidental falls in a rehabilitation setting, *Rehabil Nurs* 12(5):248-252, 1987.
3. Deyo RA, Inui TS: Toward clinical applications of health status measures: sensitivity of scales to clinically important changes, *Health Serv Res* 19(3):275-289, 1984.

4. Hamrin E: Early activation in stroke: does it make a difference? *Scand J Rehabil Med* 14:101, 1989.

5. Holloway JJ, Thomas JW: Factors influencing readmission risk: implications for quality monitoring, *Health Care Financ Rev* 1(2): 19-32, 1989.

6. Kalra L: The influence of stroke unit rehabilitation on functional recovery from stroke, *Stroke* 25(4):821-825, 1994.

7. Kalra L, Dale P, Crome P: Improving stroke rehabilitation: a controlled study, *Stroke* 24:1462, 1994.

8. Kalra L, Fowle AJ: An integrated system for multidisciplinary assessments in stroke rehabilitation, *Stroke* 25(11):2210-2214, 1994.

9. Kornblau BL: Presidential address: a vision for our future, as viewed on 12/21/2003 at http://www.aota.org/nonmembers/area2/links/link15.asp.

10. Nelson E, Conger B, Douglass R, et al: Functional health status of primary care patients, *JAMA* 249(24):3331-3338, 1983.

11. Stewart AL, Greenfield S, Hays RD, et al: Functional status and well-being of patients with chronic conditions: results from the medical outcomes study, *JAMA* 262(7):907-913, 1989.

12. Tarlov AR, Ware JE Jr, Greenfield S, et al: The medical outcomes study: an application of the methods for monitoring the results of medical care, *JAMA* 262(7):925-930, 1989.

13. Thomas JW, Longo DR: Application of severity measurement systems for hospital quality management, *Hosp Health Serv Admin* 35(2):221-243, 1990.

14. Underwood R: Developing critical pathways: management strategies, *AOTA Admin Manage SIS Newsletter* 12(2):1, 1996.

15. Ware JE, Brook RH, Rogers WH, et al: Comparison of health outcomes at a health maintenance organization with those of fee-for-service care, *Lancet* 1(8488):1017-1022, 1986.

16. Weinberg J: Which rate is right? *New Engl J Med* 314:317, 1986.

17. Wells KB, Burnam MA, Leake B, et al: Agreement between face-to-face and telephone-administered versions of the depression section of the NIMH diagnostic interview schedule, *J Psychiatr Res* 22(3):207-220, 1988.

18. Wells KB, Stewart A, Hays RD, et al: The functioning and well-being of depressed patients: results from the medical outcomes study, *JAMA* 262(7):914-919, 1989.

## RESOURCES

American Occupational Therapy Association
- Administration and Management Special Interest Section (membership benefit)
- Quarterly newsletter, subscriber's listserv, electronic bulleting board, continuing education at annual conferences

www.aota.org

Institute for Health Improvement
http://www.ihi.org/

Institute for Healthcare Improvement
375 Longwood Ave., Fourth Floor
Boston, MA 02215
Telephone: (617) 754-4800
Fax: (617) 754-4848
E-mail: info@ihi.org

# Glossary

**acalculia**  An acquired inability to solve basic mathematic problems

**accessible environment**  An environment that is usable by an individual, including those with mobility impairments

**accommodation**  The adjustment of the eye to variations in distance

**activities of daily living (ADL)**  The activities usually performed in the course of a normal day, such as eating, toileting, dressing, washing, and grooming

**activity analysis**  A process by which properties inherent in an activity or task are gauged for their ability to elicit individual motivation and fulfill patient needs in occupational performance and performance components

**acuity**  The clarity or sharpness of perception (e.g., visual acuity)

**adaptation**  Coping with the changing characteristics of a task, the environment, or the method of carrying out a task so that an activity can be completed

**adhesive capsulitis**  Thickening and contracture of a joint capsule (specifically the glenohumeral joint) in which the capsule adheres to the humeral head; also known as a *frozen shoulder*

**adjustment to disability**  The point at which an individual with a disability demonstrates self-acceptance and capability of adjustment to disability by using productive strategies for dealing with the handicapping effects of the disability

**Affolter approach**  A treatment approach that emphasizes habit formation and relies heavily on the use of nonverbal stimuli (specifically tactile-kinesthetic input) to guide movement during functional activities

**aging**  The process of becoming older during which cells replace themselves more slowly and are lost through infections and disease

**agoraphobia**  An anxiety syndrome manifested by an abnormal fear of being in open or public places

**agraphia**  An acquired writing disturbance

**alexia**  An acquired inability to read or comprehend written language as a result of brain damage

**alignment**  The placement or maintenance of body structures in their proper anatomic positions

**anatomy of the eye**  The structure of the eye, which is a spheric body contained in a bony orbit and is composed of the iris and pupil, lens, retina, vitreous humor, and eyelids

**angioplasty**  The surgical repair of a narrowed blood vessel (e.g., unclogging a vessel by inserting a balloon-tipped catheter and blocking a weakened area of the vessel wall [aneurysm] or by replacing or remodeling a part of the vessel)

**ankle strategy**  An automatic postural response that occurs when movement is centered about the ankles to maintain the center of mass over the base of support; used to control small, slow, upright sway

**anomia**  Loss of the ability to name objects or remember names of people

**anosognosia**  Denial of ownership of a paretic extremity accompanied by a lack of insight about the paralysis

**anteroposterior splint**  An orthotic device that has points of contact on both the front (anterior or volar) and back (posterior or dorsal) surfaces of a limb or the trunk

**antihypertensives**  Drugs used to lower blood pressure in individuals with abnormally high blood pressure

**anxiety**  A disorder characterized by a sense that something bad will occur; tension, fear, or worry out of proportion to the situation, racing thoughts, physiologic symptoms (such as a dry mouth, heart palpitations, cold hands and feet, stomach and bowel upset, and bladder frequency or incontinence)

**aphasia**  The loss of the ability to speak or understand spoken or written language

**apraxia**  The inability to plan or execute a movement to function or participate in activity

**aprosody**  Difficulty expressing or recognizing emotions; often associated with nondominant parietal lobe lesions

**architectural barriers**  Obstacles inherent in the structure or design of buildings that hinder individuals with impaired mobility

**arousal**  The general state of readiness in which an individual is prepared to process sensory information and organize a response

**aspiration**  Penetration of food or liquids into the airway below the level of the vocal folds before, during, or after swallowing

**assistive devices**  Tools that allow an impaired individual to function

**assistive technology device**  Any item, piece of equipment, or product system that is used to increase, maintain, or improve functional capabilities of individuals with disabilities

**astereognosis**  Failure to recognize objects, sizes, and shapes of objects by touch alone; also called *tactile agnosia*

**attention**  The ability to focus on an interaction or activity long enough to grasp its meaning and prepare an appropriate response

**auscultation**  Listening for sounds in the body for evaluation purposes either directly or with a stethoscope; used during dysphagia evaluations to detect signs of swallowing dysfunction

**balance** The ability to control the center of mass over the base of support within the limits of stability, resulting in the maintenance of stability and equilibrium

**benchmarking** Setting goals for process improvement; formerly known as "threshold"

**biofeedback** A process that provides a person with visual or auditory information about physiologic aspects of the body (such as muscle tension)

**biomechanical approach** An approach that is applicable to the ability and capacity levels of physical function; deals with increasing strength, range of motion, endurance, and alignment in patients with physical dysfunction

**bivalve cast** A cast that has contact with both surfaces of the limb it surrounds and has been cut in half lengthwise to allow it to be removed and replaced

**blocked practice** Practice that consists of drills and requires many repetitions of the same task in the same way

**bottom-up assessment** An evaluation that focuses on the deficits or components of function (e.g., strength, range of motion) that are believed to be prerequisites to function

**Broca's aphasia** Expressive aphasia characterized by a loss of speech ability

**caring** Compassion for others and concern for their well-being

**carotid plaque** A hardened, abnormal deposit on the wall of an artery believed to be related to elevated serum cholesterol blood levels

**casting** Use of casting tape and plaster or fiberglass (which forms a solid when placed in water) to immobilize a limb in a position of function; when used with neurologically impaired individuals, is usually applied to provide slow, prolonged stretch to a limb with excessive skeletal muscle tightening and/or shortening

**cataracts** An abnormal progressive condition of the lens of the eye characterized by loss of transparency and a gray-white opacity that can be seen in the lens behind the pupil

**center of mass** The midpoint or center of body weight

**cerebellar strokes** Strokes or cerebrovascular accidents involving the cerebellar lobes or blood vessels of the cerebellum of the brain

**cerebrovascular accident (CVA)** A stroke; can be caused by numerous factors including cardiac factors, hemorrhagic factors, abnormally increased platelet levels, carotid plaques, infection, and neoplasm

**circumduction** The circular motion of a limb or the eye

**client-centered practice** An approach to providing occupational therapy services that embraces a philosophy of respect and partnership with the persons receiving services

**closed tasks** Activities that take place in a stable and predictable environment; consistent methods of performance over time

**cognition** The thought process combining sensory function, learning, and the ability to choose an effective response; knowing, thinking, learning, and judging

**coital frequency** The incidence of periods of coitus; may diminish with aging or disability

**color agnosia** A deficit in ability to recognize colors as a result of a brain lesion; characterized by an inability to name or recognize colors

**concrete thinking** Interpreting thought strictly, without processing implied meaning; inflexible thinking

**cone** A photoreceptor cell in the retina of the eye that enables a person to visualize colors

**confabulation** An unconscious fabrication of stories or excuses to fill in memory gaps

**confrontation** Movement of an object through the visual field toward the observer

**context** Circumstances associated with a particular environment or setting

**contextual interference** Factors in the learning environment that increase the difficulty of initial learning

**contracture** An abnormal and usually permanent condition of a joint; characterized by flexion and fixation and caused by atrophy and shortening of muscle fibers or by loss of the normal elasticity of the skin

**convergence** Coordinated turning of the eyes inward to focus on a certain point

**coping** Psychologically adjusting to change

**cortical blindness** Blindness that results from a lesion in the visual center of the cerebral cortex of the brain

**cranioaxial tomography (CT) scan** A serial radiograph that can create an image using multiple attenuation readings

**deconditioning** Decreased body tolerance to fluctuations in vital function (e.g., blood pressure, heart rate, respiratory rate) in response to exercise or activity

**decubitus** Skin breakdown (usually adjacent to a bony prominence or weight-bearing surface) that is observed in individuals who continuously remain in a static position; caused by a loss of oxygen in the skin surface that causes tissue necrosis (death), resulting in an ulceration

**deep venous thrombosis (DVT)** A blood clot positioned statically in a deep vein of a limb

**degrees of freedom** Elements or variables that are free to vary; a term used to classify the number of planes in which joint segments move or the number of primary axes they possess (e.g., joints that move in one plane such as the elbow joint—1 degree of freedom)

**denial** Lack of acceptance or disavowal that a circumstance or condition exists

**depression** A state of being characterized by sadness, feelings of helplessness and hopelessness, low self-esteem, sleep and appetite disturbances, and psychomotor agitation or retardation; in stroke survivors, may be reactive or organic in origin

**diabetes** A disease resulting from decreased functioning of the islets of Langerhans (which produce insulin to utilize sugars in the blood stream) in the pancreas resulting in organ damage caused by the free circulating sugars; also causes small blood vessel disease, which contributes to the organ tissue death (including target organs such as the heart, kidneys, peripheral nerves, retina of the eyes, and blood vessels)

**diabetic retinopathy** A disorder of retinal blood vessels characterized by capillary microaneurysms, hemorrhage, exudates, and the formation of new vessels and connective tissue; most often occurs in patients with longstanding, poorly controlled diabetes

**disability** The inability to perform daily life tasks

**disorientation** The inability to give personal information regarding self, disability, hospital stay, and time without language disturbance

**dissociation** The separation of body parts during movement patterns (e.g., dissociation of the scapula from the thorax while reaching)

**distractibility** Diversion of attention

**divergence** A separation or movement of objects away from each other (e.g., a simultaneous turning of the eyes outward)

**drop-out cast** An immobilization cast that has a portion cut out in the direction of desired movement so that the person can volitionally move the limb after initial muscle relaxation is gained (or gravity can assist stretch)

**dual obliquity** Refers to the anatomy of the hand and has two anatomic ramifications: (1) the progressive decrease of length of the metacarpals from the radial to the ulnar aspect of the hand and (2) the immobility of the second and third metacarpals in relation to the first, fourth, and fifth metacarpals

**durable medical equipment**   Devices primarily manufactured to assist persons with impaired mobility; includes wheelchairs, bathtub equipment, bedside commodes, and ambulatory devices

**dynamic splinting**   Employing traction devices in a splint to alter the range of passive motion of a joint

**dysarthria**   Weakness or altered neuronal control of the muscles responsible for speech production or defective sensory feedback regarding their movement

**dysphagia**   Impairment of the ability to swallow

**ejaculatory dysfunction**   An interruption in the ability to ejaculate or reach sexual plateau; may be caused by a lack of available seminal fluid for the ejaculate and premature loss of the ejaculate

**embolism**   A blood clot that is moving; may travel to an organ and enter a vessel smaller than itself, blocking circulation and contributing to organ dysfunction; can be life threatening

**empathy**   The ability of a person to have compassion for others who are dealing with issues and feelings the person has never experienced

**endarterectomy**   Surgical removal of the lamina of an artery to eliminate plaque and restore blood flow

**enteral feeding**   Provision of nutrients through the intestinal tract

**environment**   The external and internal surroundings that influence a person's development (including the person's own psyche)

**environmental control unit**   A device such as a switch, voice activator, remote control, computer interface, or other technologic adaptation used to purposefully manipulate and interact with the environment

**epiglottis**   The cartilaginous structure that hangs over the larynx like a lid and prevents food from entering the airway

**erectile dysfunction**   Difficulty achieving or maintaining an erection during sexual relations until plateau is reached; inability to ejaculate and resolve an erection

**executive functions**   The skills used in problem solving, recognition, goal formulation, planning and organization, initiation, and self-regulation and monitoring

**extracranial-intracranial bypass**   A surgery originating outside the cranium in which the cranium is entered, and circulation is rerouted around an obstruction

**far transfer**   Introduction of an activity that is conceptually the same but physically different from the initial task initially performed

**feedback**   Information about a person's environment and the person's relationship to it; can provide knowledge of performance as well as knowledge of results

**fiberglass casting tape**   Soft, rolled synthetic tape that is combined with water and hardens as it cools; used to immobilize a limb

**fiberoptic endoscopic evaluation of swallowing (FEES)**   A functional, diagnostic test of deglutition in which a contrast dye, a flexible endoscopic catheter (inserted nasogastrically), a light source, and an air source (which is used to test sensation of the cricopharyngeal region) connected to a videocamera to test and document the oropharyngeal phase of a swallow reflex

**figure-ground discrimination**   Discrimination of the foreground from the background (e.g., locating a particular object in a cluttered drawer)

**fixation patterns**   A natural strategy used to maintain select body parts in certain positions when in posturally threatening situations

**force control strategy**   A movement strategy characterized by frequent stops and steplike movements requiring more effort or force for progression

**fovea**   The center of the retina in which cone cells (color receptors) are concentrated and rod cells (low-light adapting cells) are absent

**functional optometry**   Analyzes active ocular ability and perception

**gait analysis**   Observation and qualification of rhythm, pattern, cadence, and speed while walking

**gait training patterns**   Combinations of intact aspects of gait (rhythm, cadence, and speed) that are used to train persons in an attempt to restore functional ambulation

**glaucoma**   An abnormal, usually progressive condition in which elevated eye pressure caused by obstruction of the outflow of aqueous humor results in decreased visual acuity and vividness of perception and generally involves the entire visual field; progression controlled by treatments such as use of medicated eye drops

**handicap**   Social dysfunction resulting from outward signs of disease or impairment; a limitation in social role performance

**handling**   The manner in which therapists use their hands to provide input to a patient to enhance the quality of motor output and prevent abnormal movement; is associated with NDT/Bobath

**hemianopsia**   Defective vision or blindness often in half of the visual field; may involve a portion of the field of each eye and tends to follow predictable patterns associated with the decussation (crossing over) of ocular nerve fibers

**hemiplegic gaits**   Ambulation patterns used as a response to unilateral weakness involving a lower extremity

**hemorrhage**   External or internal loss of a large amount of blood in a short time

**heterotopic ossification**   A benign overgrowth or deposition of bone in soft tissues that is usually associated with an increase in the blood level of alkaline phosphatase; may be increased by forced, resisted movement of the affected body part; active (rather than active assistive or passive) movement emphasized in rehabilitation

**hip strategy**   An automatic postural response involving movement about the hips that maintains or restores equilibrium

**hydrocephalus**   A pathologic condition characterized by an abnormal accumulation of cerebrospinal fluid that is usually under increased pressure in the cranial vault

**hyperopia**   Farsightedness; a condition resulting from an error of refraction in which rays of light entering the eye are brought into focus behind the retina

**hypertension**   A common disorder characterized by elevated blood pressure persistently exceeding 140/90 mm Hg; may be caused by a number of factors including failure of the organs regulating homeostasis such as the cardiovascular and renal systems; tends to be a strong hereditary component; can usually be well controlled by a variety of oral medications including diuretics and beta-blockers, but poor control can increase risk of stroke, renal failure, and cardiopulmonary disease

**hypertonia**   Abnormally increased muscle tone or strength

**ideational apraxia**   A breakdown in the ability to perform a task because of a loss of neuronal model or mental representation of the procedure required for performance

**impaired initiative**   The inability to initiate performance of an activity when the need to perform is present

**impairment**   Organ dysfunction; the motor and cognitive residuals of pathology

**impingement**   Restriction of movement of a body part, usually involving soft tissues, because of anatomic limitation; tends to increase as the degrees of freedom of a given joint increase because tendons, muscles, and ligaments act as pulley systems or ceilings to a joint, which structurally protects the joint but causes pain and motion limitation when structures overlap abnormally (e.g., fluctuations in tension of soft tissue during repetitive motion or abnormal posturing)

**inhibitory casting**  A casting technique used to decrease spasticity and increase functional movement through slow, prolonged stretch of an involved limb

**insight**  The ability to foresee and comprehend implications of actions on circumstances

**instrumental activities of daily living (IADL)**  Complex activities of daily living performed to maintain independence in the home or community

**integrated functional approach**  An approach in which functional activities are used to directly treat sequelae of a stroke

**intermediate transfer**  Changing a moderate number of task parameters while keeping some similarities to the initial task performed

**ipsilateral pushing**  A syndrome associated with stroke in which the individual physically pushes the body toward one side because of a misperception of the actual center of gravity

**ischemia**  A decreased supply of oxygenated blood to a body or organ part

**jargon aphasia**  A language disorder characterized by speech that cannot be understood by others

**knowledge of performance**  Information about the processes used during task performance

**knowledge of results**  Terminal feedback about the outcome of an action in terms of accomplishing a goal

**larynx**  The voice organ; a part of the air passage connecting the pharynx with the trachea that is protected at its proximal end by the vocal folds (cords)

**learned nonuse**  Lack of use of a body part in normal daily activities or spontaneous movement resulting from weakness, diminished perception, or neglect of the impaired body part that leads to a change in its normal, functional use

**learning**  The acquisition of information or skills that is personalized through experience

**lens**  The anatomic crystal of the eye that functions by refracting (i.e., directing the path of) light onto the retina

**limbic system**  A group of structures in the rhinencephalon of the brain that is associated with various emotions and feelings such as anger, fear, sexual arousal, pleasure, and sadness

**limits of stability**  The boundaries of an area of space in which the body can maintain its position without changing the base of support

**long-term memory**  Consolidated and retained information that has passed through the short-term memory

**low-load prolonged stretch**  A stretch obtained by holding a tissue in a moderately lengthened position for a significant amount of time

**macular degeneration**  Progressive degeneration of the macula (a central spot) of the retina and choroid of the eye that leads to central visual blindness; is commonly managed by ultraviolet-blocking lenses (because sun exposure is considered a contributing factor) or high doses of niacin (vitamin B)

**mania (stroke related)**  A state of being characterized by euphoria, pressured speech, unfocused and prolific thoughts, grandiose thoughts and delusions, insomnia, hallucinations, poor judgment, paranoia, or hypersexuality

**memory**  The mental faculty or power that enables a person to retain and recall (through unconscious associative processes) previously experienced sensations, impressions, ideas, concepts, and information that has been consciously learned

**mental imagery**  A concept or sensation produced in the mind through memory or imagination

**metacognition**  The knowledge and regulation of one's own cognitive processes and capacities

**modeling**  The use of drawings, photographs, videotapes, therapists, or patients as models to enhance motor performance

**motor adaptation**  The ability to adapt postural responses to changing tasks and environmental demands

**motor apraxia**  Loss of access to kinesthetic memory patterns that leads to an inability to perform purposeful movement because of defective planning and sequencing of movements (even though the idea and the purpose of the task is understood)

**motor control**  Control of movement and posture

**motor learning**  The study of the acquisition and/or modification of movement; a set of processes associated with practice or experience leading to relatively permanent changes in the ability to produce skilled movement

**mourning**  A reaction to loss of function, a change in appearance, and a loss of potential or existing life roles; commonly associated with hostility and anger

**multicontextual approach**  An approach in which a combination of remedial and functional learning is used to regain functional participation of persons recovering from stroke

**myopia**  Nearsightedness caused by the elongation of the eyeball or an error in refraction causing parallel rays to be focused in front of the retina

**near transfer**  Performance of an alternate form of the initial task performed

**negative symptoms**  A disturbance in normal behavior or a performance deficit

**neoplasm**  An abnormal growth of new tissue (benign or malignant); also called a *tumor*

**neurobehavior**  Any behavioral response resulting from central nervous system processing that forms the basis for task performance in activities of daily living

**neurobehavioral deficit**  A functional impairment characterized by defective skill performance resulting from neurologic processing dysfunction that affects performance components

**neurophysiologic approach**  A theoretic framework in which external stimuli are used to influence the functional systems of the body

**NPO**  Abbreviation for "nothing by mouth"

**occupation**  The engagement in daily life activities that are meaningful and purposeful, including self-care, instrumental, vocational, educational, play and leisure, and rest and relaxation activities of daily living

**occupation as end**  Teaching an activity or task by using participation in the particular activity or task

**occupation as means**  Using occupation as the therapeutic change agent to remediate impaired abilities or capacities

**occupational functioning**  The ability to perform the tasks that have a role in their natural context

**occupational performance**  The ability to accomplish the tasks required by a certain role

**open tasks**  Tasks requiring adaptation to unpredictable events because objects in the environment are in random motion during task performance

**optical flow**  Movement of an image on the retina

**organization**  The ability to organize thoughts so that a task can be performed in an organized way with properly sequenced and timed steps

**orthokinetics**  A therapy for spasticity in which an orthotic device is used to enable contraction of one muscle while inhibiting its antagonist

**orthotic device** An external appliance that supports a paralyzed muscle, promotes a certain motion, or corrects a deformity

**parenteral** Through a route other than the digestive system

**pathology** The direct anatomic and physiologic effects (e.g., of a stroke)

**penetration** Entrance of food or liquid into the larynx above the level of the vocal folds

**perception** The ability to meaningfully interpret sensory information

**performance areas** Broad categories of human activity that are typically part of daily life

**performance components** Fundamental human abilities that are required for successful engagement in performance areas

**performance contexts** Situations or factors that influence engagement in desired and required performance areas

**peripheral vision** A capacity to see objects that reflect light waves falling on areas of the retina distant from the macula

**perseveration** Repeated movements or acts during functional performance resulting from difficulty in shifting from one pattern of response to another; refers to initiation and termination of performance and inertia

**pharynx** The throat; serves as a passage for the respiratory and digestive tracts

**plaster** A composition of liquid and powder that becomes chemically active on contact with water and hardens when it dries; used to shape a cast

**PLISSIT model of sexual counseling** Permission, limited information, specific suggestions, and intensive therapy

**positive symptoms** Spontaneous, exaggerated disturbances of normal function; symptoms that are reactive to specific external stimuli

**postural adjustment** Automatic, anticipatory, and ongoing muscle activation to maintain balance against gravity; maintain alignment; and orient the head, trunk, and limbs to the environment

**postural control** The ability to control the body's position in space for stability and orientation

**postural stability** The ability to maintain the position of the body in space

**praxis** Ideation; the programming and planning necessary for the execution of skilled, purposeful movement

**problem solving** The ability to manipulate a fund of knowledge and apply it to new or unfamiliar situations

**procedural memory** Recall and/or motor implementation of the steps of a task; situational use of learned sequential behaviors

**process improvement** Use of an assessment tool or mechanism to monitor problem resolution in a care delivery system; part of quality assurance

**prosopagnosia** The inability to recognize previously familiar faces

**quality assurance** Any evaluation that compares services provided and results achieved with accepted standards

**quality of life** The ability to carry out activities of daily living in patterns and configurations that are acceptable to the individual, have personal meaning, and fit into the context of life

**random practice** Practice of tasks that vary in the same session

**recurvatum** Backward thrust of the knee by weakness or a joint disorder that results in hyperextension of the joint

**reflexes** The involuntary functioning or movement of any organ or part of the body in response to a particular stimulus

**refraction** The deflection of light from a straight path through the eye by various ocular tissues, including the lens and its muscles

**refractory** Resistant to treatment

**remedial approach** Using splinter skills to transfer skills to functional applications

**reticular activating system (RAS)** A functional system in the brain essential for wakefulness, attention, concentration, and introspection; closely related to the limbic system

**risk management** An administrative function directed toward identification, evaluation, and correction of potential risks that could lead to injury and legal liability

**rod** One of the eye structures that is perpendicular to the retina and detects low-intensity light

**saccadic eye movements** Fast, voluntary, coordinated movements of the eye that allow the eyes to fix accurately on a still object in the visual field as the person moves or the head turns

**selective attention** The ability to select or focus on one type of information and exclude others

**sequencing** Efficiently ordering and timing events

**serial casting** The process of applying casts of increasingly greater degrees of joint motion to stretch a limb away from a contracted position

**sexual dysfunction** A change in sexual function that is viewed as unsatisfactory, unrewarding, or inadequate

**sexuality** The quality of being sexual; the sum of a person's sexual attributes, attractiveness, and sexual impulses

**sexual phases** Excitement, plateau, orgasm, and resolution

**short-term memory** Information that is consciously retained and manipulated for brief periods; the registration and temporary storing of information received by the different sensory memory modalities; refers to working memory

**shoulder-hand syndrome** Classified under the general term *reflex sympathetic dystrophy*; characterized by severe pain, stiffness, swelling, and marked reduction in function of the upper extremity

**silent aspiration** Penetration of saliva, food, or liquid below the level of the true vocal folds without a cough or outward sign of difficulty

**somatoagnosia** A body scheme disorder; diminished awareness of body structure and the failure to recognize own body parts and their relationship to each other

**somesthetic** Pertaining to tactile and proprioceptive sensation

**spasticity** One type of hypertonus that increases with the velocity of joint movement; attributed to hyperactive stretch reflexes mediated by muscle spindle stretch receptors

**spatial relations dysfunction** Difficulty in relating objects to each other or self

**static splinting** Splinting that does not allow movement of the body parts; used to provide support, alignment, stretch, and immobilization

**stepping strategy** A postural strategy used to widen the base of support in which a step is taken when the base of support is expanded in the direction of the center of mass movement

**stereopsis** The quality of visual fusion

**strabismus** An abnormal condition in which the eyes are unable to have their axes cross because of an imbalance of the extrinsic eye muscles, resulting in an inability to accurately focus an object in the visual field that is usually accompanied by impaired saccades

**tonic arousal** A change in muscle tone and response that occurs as a person wakens from sleep

**top-down assessment** An assessment that focuses on the evaluation of performance areas

**topographic disorientation** Difficulty finding way in space as a result of amnesic or agnostic problems

**Trendelenberg's sign** Occurs when a person stands on the affected limb and the opposite gluteal fold falls rather than rises

**unilateral body neglect**  Failure to report, respond, or orient to a stimulus presented to the body contralateral to the cerebral lesion; refers to personal space

**unilateral spatial neglect**  Inattention to or neglect of stimuli presented in the extrapersonal space contralateral to the cerebral lesion

**urinary tract dysfunction**  Dysfunction of the organs and ducts involved in the secretion and elimination of urine from the body

**vergence**  Movements of the two eyes in opposite directions

**videofluoroscopy**  A technique in radiology for visually examining a part of the body or function of an organ using a fluoroscope; used for dynamic evaluation of swallowing

**visual pathways**  Anatomic, physical conduits through which visual information is transmitted from the retina to the brain

**visual perception**  The receipt and interpretation of visual sensation that provides information about the environment

**Wallenberg's sign**  Horner's syndrome; cerebellar ataxia and contralateral loss of pain and temperature

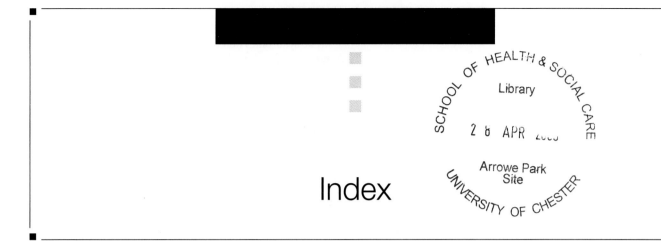

# Index

Page numbers followed by "f" denote figures, "t" tables, and "b" boxes.